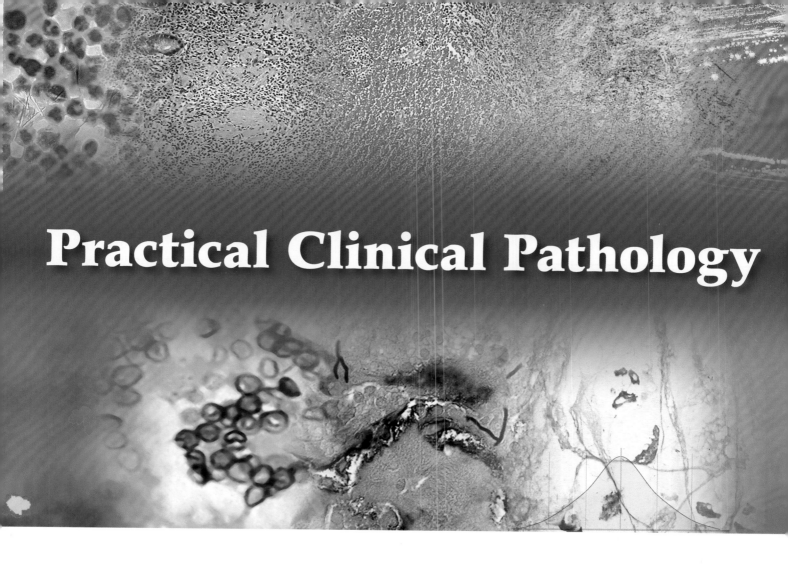

Practical Clinical Pathology

Daniel D Mais, MD

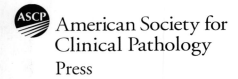
American Society for
Clinical Pathology
Press

Publishing Team
Aimee Algas (reference editing)
Beena Rao (proofreading)
Erik Tanck (production)
Joshua Weikersheimer (publishing direction)

Notice
Trade names for equipment and supplies described herein are
included as suggestions only. In no way does their inclusion
constitute an endorsement or preference by the American
Society for Clinical Pathology. The ASCP did not test the
equipment, supplies, or procedures and therefore urges all
readers to read and follow all manufacturers' instructions
and package insert warnings concerning the proper and safe
use of products.

Printed in Hong Kong

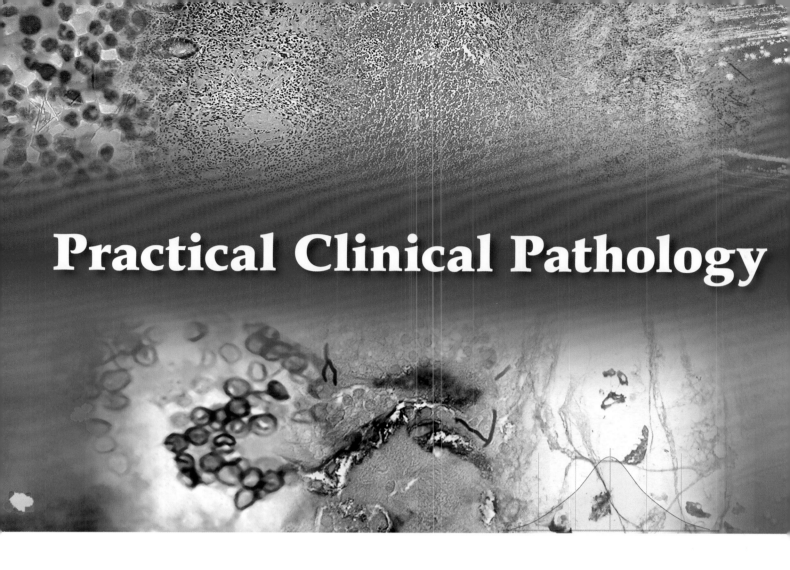

Practical Clinical Pathology

Daniel D Mais, MD
Chief of Pathology
Baptist Medical Center
San Antonio, Texas

American Society for
Clinical Pathology
Press

Dedication

To Sarah, Diana, the Davids & Emily

Contributors

John A Branda, MD
Associate Director, Clinical Microbiology Laboratories
Massachusetts General Hospital
Assistant Professor of Pathology
Harvard Medical School
Boston, Massachusetts

Anand S Dighe, MD, PhD
Director, Core Laboratory
Massachusetts General Hospital
Associate Professor of Pathology
Harvard Medical School
Boston, Massachusetts

Dina N Greene, PhD, DABCC
Scientific Director, Chemistry
Northern California Kaiser Permanente Regional
Laboratories
Berkeley, California

Daniel T Holmes, MD, FRCPC
Division Head, Clinical Chemistry
St Paul's Hospital
Clinical Associate Professor of Pathology & Laboratory
Medicine
University of British Columbia
Vancouver, Canada

George T Leonard, MD, PhD
LTC, MC, USA
Chief, Department of Pathology
Madigan Army Medical Center
Tacoma, Washington
Assistant Professor of Pathology
Uniformed Services University of Health Sciences
Bethesda, Maryland

Mary M Mayo, PhD, DABCC, MT(ASCP)
Director of Clinical Chemistry, Special Chemistry, POCT
Associate Professor of Pathology, Pathology Residency
Training Program
St Louis University School of Medicine
St Louis, Missouri

Bobbi S Pritt, MD, MSc, (D)TMH
Director, Clinical Parasitology
Division of Clinical Microbiology
Mayo Clinic
Rochester, Minnesota

Kimberly W Sanford, MD, MASCP
Medical Director, Transfusion Medicine
Medical Director, Stony Point Laboratory
Department of Pathology
Virginia Commonwealth University
Richmond, Virginia

Patricia J Simner, PhD
Clinical Microbiology Fellow
Department of Laboratory Medicine & Pathology
Mayo School of Graduate Medical Education
Rochester, Minnesota

Additional contributions by

Imad Bakri, MS, CG(ASCP)
Laboratory Supervisor
CorePath Laboratories
San Antonio, Texas

Wes Schreiber, MD
Professor, Clinical Chemistry, University of British Columbia
Consultant Pathologist, Vancouver Coastal Health
Vancouver, British Columbia, Canada

f7.12, f7.13, f7.35 & f7.39 are courtesy of the ASCP Asset Warehouse

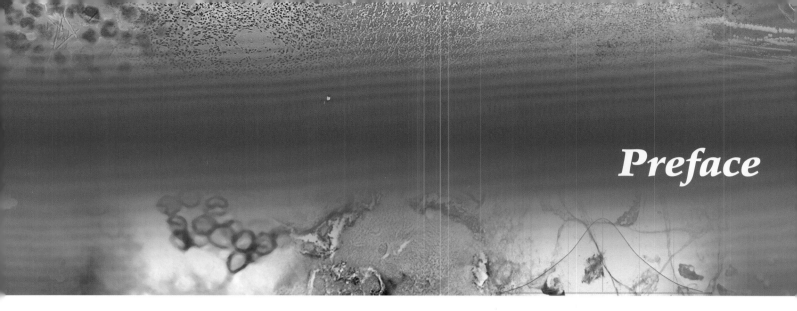

Preface

For most of us, the perfect day might well be one spent hugging a microscope in quiet contemplation. Inevitably, however, this does not describe a typical day. Instead, such moments must be stolen between the myriad clinical laboratory difficulties that crop up every day. Even to those of us with keen interest in it, the clinical laboratory is a mystery. The truth is that many of us spend our days in the realm of anatomic pathology, where through immersion we are able to keep most important facts at the forefront of our brain. But when heaved into clinical pathology, we often must relearn things, comb through patient charts, ask questions, and synthesize it all into a plan of action. When the problem is first posed, we don't always have a good answer; in this instant, we sympathize, promise to investigate, and promise to follow up.

This state of affairs comes as a surprise to most young pathologists. It is in fact normal and is no reflection upon one's training or dedication. A willingness to engage with and assist clinicians in such moments is in large measure the value of the local pathologist. The help we offer in these situations is a large part of what defines us as a specialty. Furthermore, small improvements in the clinical pathology laboratory are quickly leveraged to impact a large number of patients in ways that anatomic pathology can rarely achieve. Last, it is our duty; in that humming and whirring place toil the too-often nameless face shield-wearing people who are the long arm of our own medical licenses.

The original *Quick Compendium* began as a publication of my personal notes, begun when I was a resident, because I thought that somebody might like to use them. Unexpectedly, many came to depend upon them not only for board preparation but also, alarmingly, for the practice of clinical pathology. That certainly was outside the intended scope of use!

Practical Clinical Pathology hopes to provide a comprehensive and up-to-date working review of clinical pathology; the making of it required help from experts in a variety of disciplines. So please pay attention to the Contributors' page that faces this Preface. With their help, we mean to bring a text that encompasses what, to date, is of greatest practical necessity for general pathologists and others wanting more than can ever be included in a *Quick Compendium*.

Daniel Mais

Acknowledgements

The existence of *Practical Clinical Pathology* is credited to Joshua Weikersheimer, who saw the value of expanding from the *Quick Compendium* idea to create a book better suited to the everyday needs of general pathologists. My mentor, Dr James Kelley, exemplified the real value one could bring as a general pathologist: by being always available to assist or consult, always forthright in explanations and corrections, and fearless in taking on new problems and in correcting entrenched old ones. I hope that this is the sort of book that he might have made good use of.

Last, I acknowledge those close to me who put up with me (and without me) for so long while I was absorbed in doing this book.

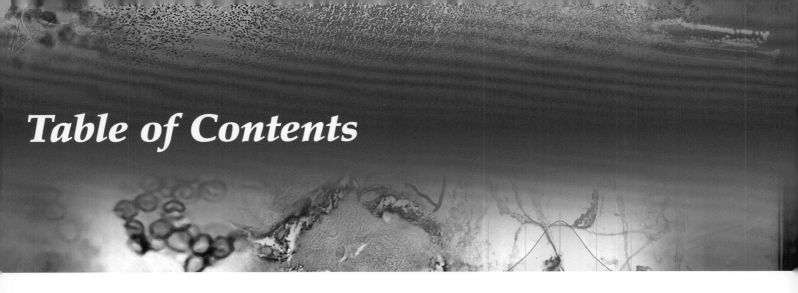

Table of Contents

Chapter 1: *Chemistry*

Anand Dighe, Dina Greene, Daniel Holmes & Daniel Mais

ISBN 978-089189-5985

Chapter 2: *Blood Banking/ Transfusion Medicine*

Kimberly Sanford & Daniel Mais

ISBN 978-089189-5985

Chapter 3: *Microbiology*

John Branda, Bobbi Pritt, Patricia Simner & Daniel Mais

Chapter 4: *Hematopathology*

Daniel Mais

ISBN 978-089189-5985

Chapter 5: *Coagulation*
Daniel Mais

Chapter 6: *Immunology*
Kimberly Sanford & Daniel Mais

Chapter 7: *Molecular Pathology*

George Leonard & Daniel Mais

ISBN 978-089189-5985

Chapter 8: *Medical Directorship*
Mary Mayo & Daniel Mais

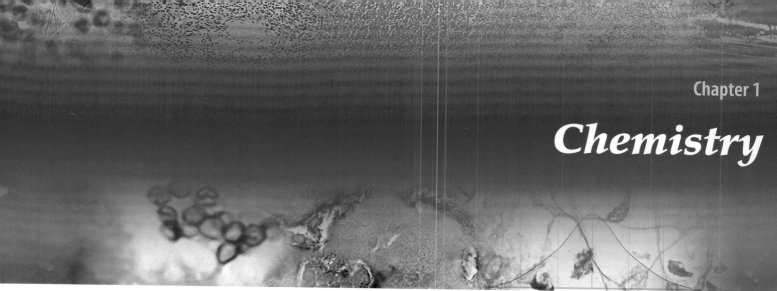

Chapter 1

Chemistry

The liver
Liver function tests
Aspartate aminotransferase (AST) & alanine aminotransferase (ALT)

Together, AST and ALT are referred to as the "liver transaminases" or "aminotransferases." Formerly, AST was known as SGOT (serum glutamic oxaloacetic transaminase), and ALT was SGPT (serum glutamic pyruvic transaminase). Neither is entirely liver specific. AST is present in cardiac muscle, liver, skeletal muscle, kidney, brain, lung, and pancreas (in decreasing order of concentration). ALT distribution is more restricted, confined primarily to liver and kidney.

Generally speaking, the higher the level of transaminase elevation, the more likely it is of hepatic origin. Low level transaminase elevation (from 1-2× the upper limit of normal) is highly nonspecific. Both AST and ALT may be elevated in heparin therapy to 2-3× the upper limit of normal. Strenuous exercise raises the AST, as does hemolysis.

Nonetheless, significant elevations in both ALT and AST (>3× the upper limit of normal) are rarely observed in nonhepatic disease, the exception being rhabdomyolysis. Both AST and ALT activities are higher in adult males compared to adult females, and both are slightly higher in African Americans. Intra-individual variation is more significant for ALT than AST, with marked diurnal variation (highest in the afternoon) and day to day variation of up to 30%. The half life of AST is ~16-18 hours and the half life for ALT is ~40-48 hours.

The AST:ALT ratio is called the DeRitis ratio. In healthy adults and in most forms of liver injury, the ALT exceeds the AST (the AST:ALT ratio is <1). This is attributed to the fact that AST is found primarily within mitochondria (~80% of it), while ALT is located entirely within the cytoplasm. In alcohol abuse and cirrhosis there may be reversal of the DeRitis ratio. Alcohol has been shown to result in the release of mitochondrial AST into the blood, accounting for the increased AST:ALT ratio.

The asymptomatic patient with mild transaminase elevation (<3× upper limit of normal) is a common clinical problem. As with other unexpectedly abnormal laboratory results, the first step is to repeat the test. Patients who subsequently test normal probably do not need further evaluation; however, chronic hepatitis C is notorious for fluctuating transaminase levels, so this must be considered.

Those with persistent transaminase elevation should undergo further evaluation, keeping in mind the nonspecificity of the transaminases, at levels below 3× the upper limit of normal, for liver disease. A careful history and physical may point towards a specific explanation and the following tests may be useful if clinically indicated: hepatic related tests (alkaline phosphatase and bilirubin, see below), serum creatine kinase (CK) (to exclude muscle disorders), hepatitis serologies (anti-HCV, HBsAg, HBcAb, anti-HBs, anti-HAV total and IgM), serum protein electrophoresis, autoimmune serologies (anti-mitochondrial antibody, anti-smooth muscle antibody, antinuclear antibody), iron studies (hemochromatosis), and ceruloplasmin (especially in patients <40).

Lactate dehydrogenase (LD)

LD is widely distributed and is separable into 5 isoenzymes by electrophoresis. The fastest moving isoenzymes, LD1 and LD2, are found in greatest abundance in heart, red blood cells, and kidney, with a significantly greater proportion of LD1 than LD2. The slowest isoenzymes, LD4 and LD5, are found in liver and skeletal muscle. LD3 is found in lung, spleen, lymphocytes, and pancreas. The comparative concentrations found in normal serum are LD2>LD1>LD3>LD4>LD5.

When LD1 is elevated, particularly when there is a "flipped LD ratio" such that LD1>LD2, the 3 most likely explanations are acute myocardial infarction, hemolysis, or renal infarction. Elevated LD4 & LD5 suggests liver damage, but other possibilities include skeletal muscle insults. An additional LD, LD6, is sometimes seen migrating cathodal to LD5. Its presence is thought to be a dire finding, and may be noted in the sera of severely ill patients.

LD isoenzymes currently are infrequently measured with the development of improved assays (eg, cardiac troponins) for the diagnosis of myocardial infarction. Total LD activity remains a commonly performed test. LD activity is elevated in numerous disease states including hemolysis, megaloblastic anemias, and disorders of muscle, liver, kidney and lung. LD may also be highly elevated in neoplastic states including leukemia, lymphoma, and a wide variety of carcinomas.

Alkaline phosphatase

There are 2 types of phosphatases: alkaline (pH optimum of 9) and acid (pH optimum of 5). Acid phosphatases (ACP) are found in greatest concentrations in prostate, red blood cells, and bone. Traditionally, red cell acid phosphatase was distinguished from other ACPs by its susceptibility to inhibition by 2% formaldehyde and resistance to inhibition by tartrate. Red cell ACP, also known as tartrate-resistant acid phosphatase (TRAP), may be found in the leukemic cells of patients with hairy cell leukemia. Further, a type of non-TRAP acid phosphatase (prostatic acid phosphatase) has been investigated as a serum marker for prostatic adenocarcinoma.

Alkaline phosphatase activity is present in most tissues of the body and is especially concentrated in the bone, liver, intestine, and placenta. Clinically, elevated alkaline phosphatase commonly originates from the liver or bone. Discovering the tissue source of elevated alkaline phosphatase traditionally required a labor intensive laboratory investigation t1.1. By electrophoresis, alkaline phosphatase can be resolved into 4 isoenzymes, each of which displays characteristic degrees of inactivation with heating, urea incubation, and L-phenylalanine. Heating produces significant (90%) inactivation of bone alkaline phosphatase ("bone burns"), 50% inactivation of biliary alkaline phosphatase, and 0% inactivation of placental alkaline phosphatase. Sensitivity to urea incubation parallels heating.

t1.1 Characteristics of alkaline phosphatase isoenzyme

Source	Heat/urea inhibition	L-phe inhibition	Anodal mobility
Biliary	+	−	1
Bone	+++	−	2
Placenta	−	+++	3
Intestinal	+	+++	4

A form of alkaline phosphatase, known as the Regan isoenzyme, is observed in a small proportion of individuals with malignant disease. It appears to be identical to placental alkaline phosphatase and seems to occur due to derepression of the placental alkaline phosphatase gene in tumor cells.

Electrophoretic methods and other means of assessment of alkaline phosphatase isoenzymes have largely been supplanted by the use of adjunctive tests (see below), including GGT and 5' nucleotidase. If these analytes are within the normal range, then the excess alkaline phosphatase is most likely of bone origin.

Alkaline phosphatase is affected by a wide range of nonpathologic conditions. Both normal growth (in childhood) and pregnancy are causes of significant elevation in alkaline phosphatase; separate reference intervals are required for children. Intestinal alkaline phosphatase can be the cause of factitious elevations in nonfasting individuals, particularly in Lewis positive group B or O secretors. Ingesting a meal can elevate the alkaline phosphatase by 30% for 2-12 hours in such individuals. A repeat fasting alkaline phosphatase may be useful in such settings. Numerous medications including oral contraceptives may elevate alkaline phosphatase levels. Alkaline phosphatase is typically slightly higher in men than women. In women, values increase in the perimenopausal period to levels similar to those found in men.

A minor elevation in alkaline phosphatase is a common clinical problem. Many advocate a threshold of 1.5× the upper limit of normal as an indication for further investigation, particularly if this threshold is breached on 2 separate occasions >6 months apart. Common clinical situations associated with a mildly elevated alkaline phosphatase include liver disease (especially cholestatic or infiltrative, such as metastasis), unrecognized pregnancy, bone disease (Paget, osteomalacia, rickets, metastasis), congestive heart failure, hyperthyroidism, and exposure to certain drugs (ibuprofen, acetaminophen). Alkaline phosphatase is a sensitive marker of hepatic metastases. In the appropriate clinical setting, imaging studies are indicated to evaluate for mass lesions and to assess the status of the hepatobiliary tree. In women approaching middle age, investigation of an elevated alkaline phosphatase may include assay for anti-mitochondrial antibodies, as primary biliary cirrhosis may be in the differential diagnosis. Note that bone alkaline phosphatase is produced by osteoblasts and reflects bone forming activity. While it is reasonable to exclude osteomalacia and hyperparathyroidism, one of the most common causes of a raised bone alkaline phosphatase in older people is Paget disease.

A major elevation in alkaline phosphatase (>3× upper limit of normal) points to a more limited differential diagnosis. Causes of major elevations of alkaline phosphatase include extrahepatic biliary obstruction, primary biliary cirrhosis, severe drug induced hepatocellular cholestasis, and Paget disease of bone.

Decreased alkaline phosphatase is found in hypophosphatasia (an inborn deficiency) and malnutrition. Hemolysis may falsely lower alkaline phosphatase. Low levels have also been reported in Wilson disease, theophylline therapy, and estrogen therapy in post-menopausal women.

γ-glutamyl transferase (GGT)

GGT measurement may be used to confirm that an elevated alkaline phosphatase is from the biliary tree. GGT is produced in biliary epithelial cells, particularly those lining the small interlobular bile ducts and bile ductules, and is a highly sensitive indicator of biliary injury. The specificity is not as high as the sensitivity, and GGT is elevated in many other types of liver disease.

GGT is present within the smooth endoplasmic reticulum of hepatocytes, and may be induced in the presence of an excess toxin. Thus, GGT is increased in patients exposed to warfarin, barbiturates, dilantin, valproate, methotrexate, and alcohol. GGT may be elevated ~2-3× the upper limit of normal in heavy drinkers. Upon abstinence the GGT level returns to normal in ~3 weeks, and can then be followed as a marker of alcohol consumption.

GGT is not exclusive to the liver, being found in renal tubules and pancreatic ducts; therefore, it may be elevated in renal failure and pancreatic disease. GGT may also be elevated in diabetes, hyperthyroidism, rheumatoid arthritis, acute myocardial infarction, and chronic obstructive pulmonary disease. GGT is considerably lower in women than men, and considerably higher in African Americans.

5′ nucleotidase

Biliary epithelium is the main source of 5′ nucleotidase, and levels are highest in cholestatic conditions. Due to this specificity, the 5′ nucleotidase can be used to confirm that an elevated alkaline phosphatase is due to hepatobiliary disease. Its relatively low sensitivity has kept its utility below that of GGT.

Ammonia

The main sources of ammonia in the body are skeletal muscle (urea cycle) and the gut; in the gut, ammonia is derived from enteric bacteria that break down protein and release ammonia. The normally functioning liver removes this ammonia from the portal circulation and discards it in the form of urea, which is excreted in the urine. In a patient with liver failure, when there is significant hepatocyte dysfunction, too much collateral circulation, or excess protein in the gut (for example, excess hemoglobin from a variceal bleed), blood ammonia may be elevated and ammonia is highly neurotoxic.

In adults, hyperammonemia is nearly always the result of liver failure or the result of preanalytic error (see below). In children, hyperammonemia should raise suspicion for an inborn error of metabolism, especially urea cycle enzyme deficiencies. Additional causes of hyperammonemia are listed in t1.2

t1.2 Causes of hyperammonemia

Liver failure
Inborn errors of metabolism affecting urea cycle (eg, ornithine transcarbamoylase (OTC) deficiency), fatty acid oxidation (eg, carnitine deficiency), organic acidemias (eg, carboxylase deficiency)
Total parenteral nutrition
Atonic bladder with superimposed urinary tract infection with urease producing bacteria (eg, *Proteus*)
Ureterosigmoidostomy
Valproic acid therapy
Cigarette smoking

Ammonia measurement requires a specimen that has been placed on ice during transport and has undergone no hemolysis. The ammonia level in a blood sample increases over time, ~20% in the first hour, so immediate measurement is important. Further, a patient who smokes should abstain for several hours preceding the blood draw, as smoking may raise the ammonia level.

Bilirubin

Unconjugated (indirect) bilirubin is a water-insoluble compound produced in the breakdown of heme. In the bloodstream, unconjugated bilirubin is bound to albumin. It is removed from blood as it passes through the liver. There, bilirubin undergoes glucuronidation to produce the water-soluble conjugated (direct) bilirubin. Conjugated bilirubin is then excreted in the bile, and intestinal bacteria convert a portion of it to urobilinogen. While much of the urobilinogen ends up in the feces, some is reabsorbed and excreted in the urine. Furthermore, some urobilinogen is converted by colonic bacteria into brown pigments (complete biliary obstruction results in white-yellow acholic stool—so-called silver stool of Thomas). Note that unconjugated bilirubin, even when quite elevated, does not appear in urine; thus, bilirubinuria indicates conjugated hyperbilirubinemia.

If conjugated hyperbilirubinemia is prolonged, conjugated bilirubin can become covalently linked to serum albumin, resulting in a moiety known as δ-bilirubin. Both the liver and kidney are incapable of excreting δ-bilirubin; thus, even after resolution of the underlying cause, conjugated hyperbilirubinemia (in the form of δ-bilirubin) may persist for some time.

Understanding the methods used to measure bilirubin is essential to proper interpretation of results. The *diazo-colorimetric methods* rely on the formation of a colored dye through the reaction of bilirubin with a diazo compound. Without the addition of an accelerator (such as an alcohol), mainly conjugated bilirubin is measured (direct reaction). Addition of accelerators permits unconjugated bilirubin to react as well, providing a measurement of total bilirubin. The difference between total and direct bilirubin is an estimate of the unconjugated (indirect) bilirubin. *Direct spectrophotometry* can determine the bilirubin concentration by measuring absorbance at 455 nm; potential interference by hemoglobin is corrected for by subtracting the absorbance at 575 nm (hemoglobin's other absorbance peak). This method is only capable of measuring total bilirubin. The urine foam test is a crude way of assessing for bilirubinuria—shaking urine creates foam that is typically white; yellow foam indicates bilirubinuria. Dipstick methods are discussed later in this chapter.

Hyperbilirubinemia can be classified according to the type of bilirubin that is elevated t1.3, t1.4. Conjugated hyperbilirubinemia (said to be present when >30% of serum bilirubin is conjugated) is caused by an excretory defect of already-conjugated bilirubin. Unconjugated hyperbilirubinemia is caused by increased production (hemolysis) or a hepatic defect that prevents uptake or conjugation.

t1.3 Pathophysiologic differential diagnosis of hyperbilirubinemia

Step of bilirubin metabolism	Pathologic processes	Type of hyperbilirubinemia
Excess conversion of heme to unconjugated bilirubin (hemolysis)	Hemolysis (extravascular) Ineffective hematopoiesis (intramedullary hemolysis) Large hematoma (resorbed heme)	Unconjugated hyperbilirubinemia
Excess delivery of unconjugated bilirubin to liver	Blood shunting (cirrhosis) Right heart failure	Unconjugated hyperbilirubinemia
Poor uptake of unconjugated bilirubin into hepatocyte	Gilbert syndrome Drugs, especially rifampin & probenecid	Unconjugated hyperbilirubinemia
Impaired conjugation of bilirubin in hepatocyte	Crigler-Najjar syndrome Hypothyroidism	Unconjugated hyperbilirubinemia
Impaired transmembrane secretion of conjugated bilirubin into canaliculus (hepatocellular jaundice) t1.4	Hepatitis/hepatic injury Endotoxin (sepsis) Pregnancy (estrogen) Drugs: estrogen, cyclosporine Dubin-Johnson syndrome Rotor syndrome	Conjugated hyperbilirubinemia
Impaired flow of conjugated bilirubin through canaliculi & bile ducts (cholestatic jaundice) t1.4	Intrahepatic: primary biliary cirrhosis, medication, alcohol, pregnancy, sepsis Extrahepatic: primary sclerosing cholangitis, tumor, stricture, stone, AIDS choledochopathy	Conjugated hyperbilirubinemia

t1.4 Differential diagnosis of conjugated hyperbilirubinemia

	Hepatocellular jaundice	Cholestatic jaundice
Alkaline phosphatase	<3× upper limit of normal	>3× upper limit of normal
Transaminases	>3× upper limit of normal	<3× upper limit of normal
Serum cholesterol	Normal	Increased
Pruritus	Absent	Present

Unconjugated hyperbilirubinemia, when caused by hemolysis, is rarely severe unless there is underlying liver disease. The total bilirubin in the setting of hemolysis and a normal liver is usually in the 2.5-3.0 mg/dL range. A blood film should be examined in such cases, looking for morphologic findings that suggest hemolysis or suggest a specific cause (eg, dyspoietic findings, spherocytosis). Laboratory findings consistent with hemolysis include reticulocytosis, elevated LD, reduced haptoglobin, and urine hemosiderin (microscopic finding of hemosiderin within urinary nucleated cells). Intramedullary hemolysis, caused by ineffective erythropoiesis, may be more subtle. Measurements of serum folate and B_{12}, serum iron studies, and serum lead levels should be considered, as appropriate. If these are excluded, then medication related hemolysis should be considered.

Gilbert syndrome is a common autosomal dominant cause of unconjugated hyperbilirubinemia that affects ~5% of the Caucasian population. Although provocative measures may be used (nicotinic acid administration or fasting) to stimulate an abnormal increase in unconjugated bilirubin, generally Gilbert syndrome is a diagnosis of exclusion. The patient presents typically in adolescence or young adulthood with episodic unconjugated hyperbilirubinemia that is provoked by fasting, infection, or other stress. To establish the diagnosis, the alkaline phosphatase and transaminases should be normal, and hemolysis should be excluded.

Crigler-Najjar syndrome is an autosomal recessive cause of unconjugated hyperbilirubinemia that comes in 2 varieties—type 1 and type 2. Type 1 is severe disease caused by complete absence of UDP-glucuronidase and presents in infancy. In type 2 there is diminished UDP glucuronidase activity that presents clinically in childhood or infancy.

The causes of conjugated hyperbilirubinemia include hepatocellular and cholestatic disorders, the latter including intrahepatic and extrahepatic disorders. In most cases, there are abnormalities in other liver function tests. The distinction between hepatocellular and cholestatic disorders may be difficult but generally depends upon history, physical examination, and imaging studies. From the laboratory standpoint, a comparison of the magnitude of alkaline phosphatase and liver transaminase elevation may provide some guidance t1.4.

The most common hepatocellular causes of jaundice include alcoholic steatohepatitis, autoimmune hepatitis, viral hepatitis, drug toxicity, α_1 antitrypsin deficiency, and hemochromatosis. History and the relevant laboratory assays can usually identify the specific problem. Cholestatic disorders are initially evaluated with imaging. Anatomic abnormalities in the biliary tree suggest extrahepatic causes. If the biliary tree is normal, then an intrahepatic cause of cholestasis is suspected.

In the case of a patient with conjugated hyperbilirubinemia when all other liver function tests are normal, one should consider the unlikely possibility of Rotor or Dubin-Johnson syndrome. Both are rare but benign diseases that are inherited in autosomal recessive fashion. The main distinction between them is the presence of diffuse hepatic hyperpigmentation in Dubin-Johnson syndrome and absence of this feature in Rotor syndrome.

Prothrombin time (PT)

Most coagulation factors are synthesized in hepatocytes and have short half lives, particularly factor VII with a T½ of 12 hours. The PT can therefore be used as a marker of impaired hepatic synthetic function. Extensive hepatic injury must be present for the PT to be prolonged, so its sensitivity is limited. Most patients with chronic liver disease have a normal PT; however, in acute fulminant hepatic injury, the PT serves as a useful marker of hepatic synthetic function.

The short half life of the coagulation factors makes the PT a better marker of acute injury than albumin, whose half life is 3 weeks. It is important to note that impaired bile secretion can lead to vitamin K deficiency, since bile salts are required for vitamin K absorption. A prolonged PT due to cholestasis or other causes of impaired vitamin K absorption can be distinguished from a prolonged PT due to hepatocyte injury by administering parenteral vitamin K. In absorptive defects, the prothrombin time will shorten by 30% within 24 hours of parenteral vitamin K administration.

γ globulins

The brisk infiltrate of lymphocytes and plasma cells that histologically characterizes autoimmune hepatitis is reflected in serum hypergammaglobulinemia. In autoimmune hepatitis, there is a marked polyclonal increase in IgG, and in primary biliary cirrhosis, there is a polyclonal increase in IgM. Furthermore, the combination of impaired hepatic synthesis and enhanced immunoglobulin synthesis results in a decreased albumin:globulin (A/G) ratio; an A/G of <1.0 is usually the result of liver disease.

Albumin

Albumin, which is discussed in further detail below, is synthesized in the liver and is therefore a marker of hepatic synthetic function. The causes of a decreased serum albumin are many, however, limiting its specificity. The sensitivity of albumin for liver disease is also limited, with normal values found in over half of patients with cirrhosis.

Neonatal jaundice t1.5

Most cases of neonatal jaundice are benign—so-called physiologic jaundice—and result from hepatic enzymes that are not yet at full capacity, leading to a build-up of unconjugated bilirubin. Physiologic jaundice has the following characteristics:

1. it is usually noted between days 2-3 of neonatal life

2. it rarely rises at a rate >5 mg/dL/day

3. it usually peaks by day 4-5

4. it rarely exceeds 20 mg/dL

t1.5 Causes of neonatal hyperbilirubinemia

Unconjugated	Conjugated
Physiologic jaundice	Biliary obstruction (extrahepatic biliary atresia)
Breast milk jaundice	Sepsis or TORCH infection
Polycythemia	Neonatal hepatitis (idiopathic, Wilson disease, α_1-antitrypsin deficiency)
Hemolysis (HDFN, hemoglobinopathies, inherited membrane or enzyme defects)	Metabolic disorders (galactosemia, hereditary fructose intolerance, glycogen storage disease)
Increased enterohepatic circulation (Hirschsprung disease, cystic fibrosis, ileal atresia)	Inherited disorders of bilirubin transport (Dubin-Johnson syndrome, Rotor syndrome)
Inherited disorders of bilirubin metabolism (Gilbert syndrome, Crigler-Najjar syndrome)	Parenteral alimentation

The most common causes of severe hyperbilirubinemia in neonates are hemolytic disease of the fetus and newborn (HDFN) and sepsis. The poorly developed blood-brain barrier permits unconjugated bilirubin to cause damage to the central nervous system (kernicterus). The pathologic correlates of kernicterus include yellow staining of the subthalamic nucleus, hippocampus, thalamus, globus pallidus, putamen, cerebellar nuclei, and cranial nerve nuclei.

The problem facing the clinician is when to worry about neonatal jaundice. Features suggesting that hyperbilirubinemia is not due to benign physiologic jaundice include:

1. the appearance of jaundice within the first 24 hours of life

2. a rising bilirubin beyond 1 week of age

3. persistence of jaundice past 10 days

4. total bilirubin that exceeds 12 mg/dL

5. a single-day increase of >5 mg/dL

6. conjugated (direct-reacting) bilirubin >2 mg/dL

In the healthy term infant, phototherapy should be considered when bilirubin is >10 mg/dL before 12 hours of age, >12 mg/dL before 18 hours of age, and >14 mg/dL before 24 hours of age. Exchange transfusions are considered when the bilirubin is >20 mg/dL. Phototherapy converts unconjugated bilirubin into a molecule that can be excreted without conjugation; phototherapy is not useful for conjugated hyperbilirubinemia.

The differential diagnosis for neonatal hyperbilirubinemia depends upon the predominant type of bilirubin—conjugated or unconjugated—and the time of onset. Jaundice appearing in the 1st 24 hours suggests erythroblastosis fetalis, concealed hemorrhage, sepsis, or TORCH infection. Jaundice appearing between the 3rd and 7th day suggests bacterial sepsis, particularly of urinary tract origin. Jaundice arising after the 1st week suggests breast milk jaundice, sepsis, extrahepatic biliary atresia, cystic fibrosis, congenital paucity of bile ducts (Alagille syndrome), neonatal hepatitis, galactosemia, or inherited forms of hemolytic anemia (eg, PK deficiency, hereditary spherocytosis, G6PD deficiency).

Transcutaneous bilirubin has become an important technology in an era wherein it has become common to discharge newborns after 24 hours in hospital. A transcutaneous bilirubin measurement can be used to screen otherwise healthy term infants to determine which may benefit from a serum bilirubin assay, thus sparing the great majority of infants a venipuncture. Transcutaneous bilirubin measurements can detect hyperbilirubinemia before jaundice is visible, and transcutaneous measurement has been shown to correlate reasonably well with serum bilirubin measurement. Several caveats are worth noting. There is a small impact of skin color, with the effect being least pronounced in measurements taken from the trunk, more pronounced with forehead measurements. The effect of maturity and postnatal age is unclear. Lastly, correlation appears to be best in the low range of bilirubin concentrations, with negative bias (underestimation) observed in many systems in the higher range.

Acute hepatic injury

Acute hepatic injury may present in several ways, including with jaundice, elevated transaminases, or constitutional symptoms. It may be caused by acute viral hepatitis, autoimmune hepatitis, toxins, drugs, ischemia, or Wilson disease. Hepatitis serologies, ANA, ceruloplasmin, and clinical history often point to the specific etiology. With regard to drug history, most hepatic injury occurs within the first 4 months of drug administration. The pattern of changes in liver function tests—particularly transaminases, bilirubin, and the prothrombin time—may be useful to suggest an etiology and to estimate the degree of hepatic injury.

Acute viral hepatitis due to HAV or HBV most often leads to complete recovery; however, acute HCV hepatitis leads to the development of chronic hepatitis C in >80% of cases. Serologic testing for HAV and HBV (IgM anti-HAV, IgM anti-HBc, HBsAg) are in general reliable for diagnosing acute infection. However, the anti-HCV antibody test has only ~60% sensitivity in acute infection. HCV RNA testing has ~90-95% sensitivity.

Transaminases may follow typical patterns. Acute hepatic injury due to ischemic or toxic insults produce the most profound elevations in transaminases—often >100× the upper limit of normal (ULN). Such elevations are rare in acute viral hepatitis. When the AST is >3,000 U/L, the etiology is a toxin in >90% of cases. AST is >10× the upper limit of normal (ULN) in >50% of patients with acute viral hepatitis; however, it reaches this level only rarely in alcoholic hepatitis. The AST:ALT ratio is >2 in 80% of patients with toxic, ischemic, and alcoholic hepatitis. It is usually <1 in viral hepatitis. Unlike the PT and bilirubin, the degree of transaminase elevation poorly reflects the extent of hepatic injury.

Bilirubin also may take on predictable patterns. Jaundice occurs in 70% of patients with alcoholic hepatitis and acute hepatitis A. Jaundice is present in only ~20-30% of patients with acute hepatitis B and acute hepatitis C. Jaundice is rare in children with acute viral hepatitis, and it is rare in toxic or ischemic hepatic injury. The distribution of bilirubin (direct vs total) in acute hepatic injury and obstructive jaundice is similar: usually >50% direct. The aminotransferases begin to fall before the bilirubin peaks in all forms of acute hepatic injury. Bilirubin >15 mg/dL is indicative of severe liver injury and an unfavorable prognosis.

The prothrombin time (PT) is probably the best indicator of prognosis in acute hepatic injury. PT prolongation of >4.0 seconds indicates severe liver injury and an unfavorable prognosis.

The pancreas
Pancreatic enzymes
Amylase

Serum amylase consists primarily of salivary (S-type) and pancreatic (P-type) isoenzymes. Typically, when serum amylase is subjected to electrophoresis, 6 bands result. The first 3 are salivary, while the slowest 3 are pancreatic. Immunoassays based on monoclonal antibodies directed against specific isoenzymes can now accurately quantitate P-type and S-type amylase; however, these assays are rarely clinically indicated.

In a patient with uncomplicated acute pancreatitis, serum amylase rises within 2-24 hours of onset and returns to normal in 2-3 days. Higher levels do not correlate with greater severity of injury, but higher levels are more specific for the diagnosis of acute pancreatitis. The persistence of elevated serum amylase beyond 5 days suggests a complication such as a pseudocyst.

The sensitivity of amylase for acute pancreatitis is limited. Up to 10% of cases of acute pancreatitis are associated with normal levels of amylase. This occurs most often in relapsing and chronic pancreatitis. The sensitivity of amylase is also lower in alcoholic pancreatitis.

The specificity of amylase for acute pancreatitis is even more limited. Up to 30% of amylase elevations are caused by nonpancreatic disorders. The nonpancreatic causes of hyperamylasemia include diabetic ketoacidosis, peptic ulcer disease, acute cholecystitis, ectopic pregnancy, salpingitis, bowel ischemia, intestinal obstruction, macroamylasemia, and renal insufficiency. Amylase may also be raised somewhat by the administration of opioid analgesics, presumably due to contracture of the sphincter of Oddi. In all of these instances, the degree of elevation tends to be lower than that seen in acute pancreatitis, but with substantial overlap. Amylase is primarily cleared by glomerular filtration; thus renal insufficiency spuriously elevates the serum amylase.

Macroamylasemia has a prevalence in the general population of ~1% and is thought to account for up to 5% of elevated amylase levels. It is an acquired condition in which apparently healthy individuals have an elevated serum amylase (with an accompanying low urine amylase) due to immunoglobulin-amylase complexes.

Lipase

Unlike amylase, lipase is highly specific for the pancreas. Its rise parallels that of amylase, but it remains elevated for up to 14 days. It is less dependant on renal clearance than amylase, requiring greater renal impairment to falsely elevate lipase. For these reasons, it is often considered superior to amylase in the diagnosis of acute pancreatitis.

Laboratory evaluation of acute pancreatitis
Confirming acute pancreatitis

Amylase has limited sensitivity and specificity, for the reasons described above. In addition to acute pancreatitis, there are numerous causes of an elevated serum amylase, including other intraabdominal inflammatory conditions (eg, bowel infarction, salpingitis), salivary gland pathology, renal insufficiency, and macroamylasemia. At the often-applied cutoff of 3× the upper limit of normal, the specificity is 95%, and the sensitivity is 60-80%.

Lipase remains elevated for longer than amylase (up to 14 days), giving greater sensitivity in patients with a delayed presentation. Like amylase, lipase may be elevated in other intraabdominal diseases and in renal insufficiency. At a cutoff of 3× ULN lipase specificity and sensitivity for the diagnosis of acute pancreatitis approaches 90%. Both serum lipase and serum amylase are less sensitive for acute exacerbations of chronic pancreatitis, likely the result of less acinar tissue available to spill enzymes into the blood.

Prognosis

Acute pancreatitis is fatal in ~10% of cases. Aggressive management—ICU admission, parenteral feeding, and systemic antibiotics—is undertaken in those patients felt to be at risk for fulminant pancreatitis and death. To help identify patients at risk for this outcome, several indices have been developed. For example, the Ranson criteria t1.6 provide a specificity of 90%; however, these criteria predict severe disease in only 50% of those who subsequently develop it. Furthermore, a Ranson score cannot be assigned until 48 hours after admission. Serum amylase and lipase levels are poor predictors of severity.

t1.6 Ranson criteria

Criterion	Value	At
Age	>55 years	Admission
WBC Count	$>16 \times 10^9/L$	Admission
Glucose	>200 mg/dL	Admission
AST	>250 U/L	Admission
LD	>350 U/L	Admission
BUN	>5 mg/dL increase	48 hours
Calcium	<8 mg/dL	48 hours
PaO$_2$	<60 mm Hg	48 hours
Base deficit	>4 mEq/L	48 hours
Fluid sequestration	>6 L	48 hours
Hematocrit	>10% decrease	48 hours

Etiology

Detecting stone disease as the cause of acute pancreatitis is clinically important, since endoscopic retrograde cholangiopancreatography (ERCP) can significantly improve outcome. Tests for additional causes of acute pancreatitis include triglycerides, calcium, and viral serology titers (mumps, coxsackievirus, cytomegalovirus, varicella zoster virus, herpes simplex virus, hepatitis B viruses, and HIV).

Inherited diseases may underlie a small but significant minority of cases, particularly when there is a history of recurrent episodes of pancreatitis beginning in childhood. Mutations in cationic trypsinogen (PRSS-1), pancreatic secretory trypsin inhibitor (PSTI), and cystic fibrosis transmembrane conductance regulator (CFTR) have been identified in some patients with familial recurrent acute pancreatitis.

Finally, serum IgG4 levels may be of assistance in patients with suspected autoimmune pancreatitis, which may present mildly without episodes of acute pancreatitis.

Tests of pancreatic exocrine function

Secretin-CCK test

The secretin-cholecystokinin (CCK) test may be used to evaluate for pancreatic exocrine insufficiency, an indicator of chronic pancreatitis. An endoscope is introduced, and after discarding the initial secretions, CCK is administered intravenously. The duodenal concentrations of pancreatic exocrine products (bicarbonate, amylase, lipase, trypsin) are measured for 80 minutes, generally submitted as 4 20-minute aliquots.

Noninvasive tests

Noninvasive tests include fecal fat, fecal chymotrypsin, and fecal elastase-1. The traditional test, still the gold standard for detection of steatorrhea, is the 72-hour fecal fat quantitation. The test is performed by ingesting a high-fat diet for 6 days (3 days before collection and 3 days during collection). Under these circumstances, >7 g of fat/day in the stool is abnormal. In chronic pancreatitis, fecal fat often exceeds 20 g/day. This test has certain limitations. First, the reliability of outpatient 72-hour fecal collection is poor. Control of diet in outpatients is likewise poor. Admission for 72 hour stool collection is not cost-effective. Lastly, steatorrhea has other causes, including malabsorption. Therefore, other testing is often pursued.

The "spot" fecal fat, assessed by Sudan black staining of a random stool sample, is considered positive when there are >6 droplets of fat/high power field. The test is relatively insensitive, however. Fecal fat is detected by this method only when >25 g/day, and sensitivity for steatorrhea is only 70% overall.

Both stool elastase-1 and stool chymotrypsin are decreased in pancreatic exocrine insufficiency. Neither test is as sensitive as the 24-hour fecal fat. Both tests have a sensitivity of 60-80% for advanced chronic pancreatitis, but both are relatively insensitive to early exocrine insufficiency. Note that the D-xylose test is a measure of small bowel mucosal absorptive capacity and not a test of pancreatic exocrine function.

Laboratory evaluation of pancreatic cyst fluid

Pancreatic cyst aspirates are submitted for laboratory analysis. The combination of clinical features, chemical analysis, and cytologic evaluation allows proper characterization of such lesions t1.7 in most instances.

t1.7 Pancreatic cyst evaluation

Cyst type	Clinical findings	Cyst aspirate	Chemistry
Pseudocyst	Associated with pancreatitis, ovoid unilocular lesion with thick wall adjacent to pancreas	Amorphous material, inflammatory cells; no epithelium	↑ Amylase; Nl CEA; ↑CA 19-9
Serous cystadenoma	Elderly female, microcystic lesion within pancreas	Bland cuboidal epithelial cells	↓Amylase; ↓CEA; ↓CA 19-9
Mucinous cystadenoma (mucinous cystic neoplasm)	Middle-aged female, macrocystic lesion within pancreas	Bland mucinous epithelial cells	Nl Amylase; ↑ CEA; ↑ CA 19-9
Intraductal papillary mucinous tumor	Elderly male or female, variable appearance, dilated duct	Bland to atypical mucinous epithelial cells	↑ Amylase; ↑ CEA; Nl-↑CA 19-9
Solid-cystic (solid-pseudopapillary tumor)	Adult female, solid & cystic lesion	Bland, neuroendocrine-like cells, myxoid stroma	↓Amylase; ↓CEA; ↓CA 19-9

The heart

Myocardial markers

Creatine kinase (CK)

CK has 3 isoenzymes distinguishable by electrophoresis: CK-MM, CK-MB, CK-BB. The fastest migrating is BB (CK1), followed by MB (CK2), then MM (CK3) f1.1. CK-BB (CK1) is found primarily in the brain, with lesser amounts in bladder, stomach, and prostate. Of the 3, CK-BB is the most widely distributed, with nearly all tissues in the body having some percentage of their CK composed of BB; nevertheless, virtually no CK-BB is found in normal serum. CK-MM (CK3) is found in skeletal and cardiac muscle. Skeletal muscle is made up of ~99% MM, and cardiac muscle has ~70% MM. In healthy individuals MM makes up ~100% of serum CK, mostly from skeletal muscle. CK-MB (CK2) is found in cardiac and skeletal muscle. Cardiac muscle is ~30% MB, and skeletal muscle has ~1% MB. Skeletal muscle is the source of nearly all MB circulating in the serum of normal individuals.

Although electrophoresis is the traditional means to detect CK-MB, immunoassays (CK-MB "mass assay") are now widely used for this purpose. Immunoassays provide much faster results and better accuracy, particularly in the low (clinical decision making) range. Total CK is usually measured by an enzymatic assay. Measuring and calculating the ratio of CK-MB to total CK (the "relative index") improves the specificity of CK-MB for myocardial infarction. A relative index of >5% is suggestive of a cardiac source.

There are 2 additional types of CK that are found only in isolated circumstances. *Macro-CK* (Macro-CK type 1) is a CK-immunoglobulin complex. On electrophoresis, it migrates between MM and MB. Macro-CK is generally found in healthy elderly women, but it may be a manifestation of autoimmune conditions. *Mitochondrial CK* (Macro-CK type 2) migrates very close to MM, usually slightly slower than MM. It is seen in patients with advanced malignancy and is associated with a poor prognosis.

CK isoforms are metabolic breakdown products of CK. In serum, CK released from damaged myocardial cells undergoes enzymatic cleavage. It takes several (>4) hours for cleavage to begin. With the advent of high-resolution electrophoresis, it was found that CK-MB actually resolves into 2 bands, and CK-MM resolves into 3 bands. The forms initially released from myocardium are CK-MB2 (CK-MB1 being the cleaved type) and CK-MM3 (CK-MM1 and 2 being cleavage products).

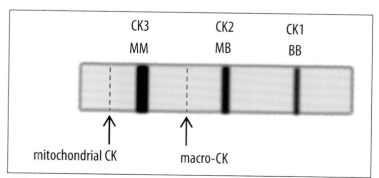

f1.1 Creatine phosphokinase electrophoresis

ISBN 978-089189-5985

Thus, persons with an elevated ratio of CK-MB2/CK-MB1 or CK-MM3/CK-MM1 are likely to have had a recent enzyme leak. These CK/CK isoform ratios provide ~90-100% sensitivity for acute myocardial infarction (AMI) when tested within 4-6 hours after onset. They perform comparably with CK-MB. Assays for CK isoforms are not widely available, and published reports do not appear to display significant advantages over CK-MB.

Troponin

Troponin is a group of proteins consisting of troponin T (TnT), troponin I (TnI) and troponin C (TnC) that are involved in mediating the actin-myosin interactions that result in muscle contraction. While the same gene encodes cardiac and skeletal muscle TnC, separate genes encode TnI and TnT in cardiac and skeletal muscle. Immunoassays can distinguish cardiac troponin (cTnI and cTnT) from skeletal muscle troponin.

While a small proportion of cardiac muscle troponin is free in the cytoplasm, the vast majority is bound to actin and myosin. Thus, there is both an immediate release of cytoplasmic troponin by infarcted cardiac muscle (within 4-8 hours) and a sustained release of bound troponin over the next 10-14 days.

TnI and TnT are similar in many respects, including their kinetics following myocardial infarction. Studies have consistently demonstrated the exceptional cardiospecificity of cTnI and cTnT. Unlike CK-MB and myoglobin, cTnI and cTnT are not usually elevated in skeletal muscle injury or in vigorous exercise. However, both may be elevated in nonischemic forms of cardiac injury—cardiac contusion, myocarditis—albeit at lower levels.

For most laboratory tests, the reference interval ("normal range") is selected to encompass the central 2 standard deviations (2SD) of a normal population. For troponin I (TnI), the definition of normal has evolved. Initially, when troponin assays were relatively imprecise at the low end, it was suggested that the cutoff should be set at the lowest point that a particular assay could achieve a 10% coefficient of variation (CV). With the advent of assays that can achieve precision at very low levels of troponin ("high-sensitivity" troponin assays), the definition of abnormal was changed, such that current international guidelines suggest that the reference interval include all values *up to the 99th percentile of healthy adults*. Thus, an "abnormal" TnI would be any above the 99th percentile.

Myocardial ischemia cannot be excluded with a single normal troponin. But the evidence is abundant that an admission and 3-hour TnI together may facilitate early exclusion of AMI. In fact, recent studies utilizing high-sensitivity TnI assays indicate that after the 3-hour TnI measurement, one can exclude MI with nearly 100% sensitivity, and that the subsequent 6- and 12-hour measurements are minimally informative. On the other hand, *a significant change in the TnI level from admission to 3 hours may help establish an MI diagnosis*, even in patients with very low TnI.

Utilizing current assays, an abnormal troponin (above the 99th percentile) usually indicates myocardial ischemia. But sometimes it does not. There is a large body of literature on the subject of patients with elevated troponin and no other evidence of myocardial ischemia; ie, "false positive" troponin. In a variety of single-institution retrospective reviews, the rate of these "false positives" ranges from 0.2-4.8%. These "false positives" fall into 3 categories. First, some are related to nonischemic pathology such as acute pulmonary embolism, myocarditis, pericarditis, heart failure, intracranial insults, rhabdomyolysis, sepsis, shock, and renal insufficiency. Second, some reflect the 1% of healthy adults whose TnI is normally above the 99th percentile. Third, there are analytical false positives. Widely reported in cardiology and emergency medicine literature, analytical false positive troponin is a phenomenon that is an inherent weakness of the available assays, which are predominantly immunoassays and thereby susceptible to a multitude of interferences such as heterophile antibodies. Importantly, whereas, nonischemic causes of TnI elevation (eg, renal insufficiency, congestive heart failure [CHF], toxin) are generally associated with low level elevations, *most analytic false positives are actually quite high.*

The newest issue is the normal but detectable troponin. It used to be that any measurable troponin was abnormal, because early assays were insensitive to very low levels of troponin. But troponin assays have evolved. A decade ago, no assay on the market could measure troponin at the 99th percentile with reasonable precision. Now, commercially available troponin assays can reliably measure troponin as low as 0.01 ng/mL, and some in development as low as 0.001 ng/mL. It is still unclear what is to be done with the patient with detectable TnI at a concentration beneath the 99th percentile. It seems that patients with detectable TnI have higher 1-year mortality than matched patients with undetectable TnI. The published studies have findings similar to those of high-sensitivity C-reactive protein.

The rate of false positives for any test is inextricably affected by the prevalence of disease in the tested population. Without changing anything about the test itself, *the rate of false positives is higher if the prevalence of disease is lower*. So, if you test every patient in the ER who has pain above the waist, then you must be prepared to deal with a lot of false positive troponins.

Myoglobin

Myoglobin is a highly sensitive cardiac marker and is an early marker of acute myocardial infarction, being elevated within 1-2 hours after symptom onset. However, it is present in both cardiac and skeletal muscle, and may be elevated with any type of injury to skeletal muscle, reducing its utility in AMI diagnosis.

B-type natriuretic peptide (BNP)

The natriuretic peptides, including atrial natriuretic peptide and brain-type natriuretic peptide, are involved in the regulation of fluid balance and blood pressure. Their actions tend to antagonize those of the renin-angiotensin system; that is, the natriuretic peptides cause vasodilation, natriuresis (sodium excretion in urine), and lowered blood pressure.

Brain-type natriuretic peptide (BNP), now called B-type natriuretic peptide, was so-named because it was first discovered in the brains of pigs; nevertheless, its main source in humans is ventricular myocytes. Synthesis of BNP correlates directly with ventricular wall tension. It is rapidly degraded following its production and has a half life of 20 minutes. The N-terminal peptide fragment (NT-proBNP), which is cleaved from pro-BNP to make the active hormone BNP, is more stable (half life of 1-2 hours).

BNP and NT-proBNP are elevated in patients with heart failure. Both are useful in distinguishing cardiac from non-cardiac causes of dyspnea. Both prove useful in stratification, prognostication, and differential diagnosis in patients with congestive heart failure and acute coronary syndromes. Once a patient is diagnosed with heart failure, the BNP level can be used to monitor treatment efficacy.

Acute coronary syndrome (ACS)

ACS is a term that is meant to encompass several clinical situations having myocardial ischemia in common: stable angina, unstable angina, acute myocardial infarction (AMI), and sudden cardiac death (SCD). While laboratory assays are very good at diagnosing acute myocardial infarction, they are quite poor, overall, in the diagnosis of other acute coronary syndromes.

Nonacute myocardial infarction acute coronary syndromes (non-AMI ACS) include angina, unstable angina, ventricular arrhythmia, and other manifestations of transient ischemia without infarction. To date, there has been little progress in finding biochemical markers of transient myocardial ischemia. The usual markers of myocardial necrosis, such as CK-MB, myoglobin, and troponin, are overall poor markers of non-AMI ACS. Elevated troponins in non-AMI ACS somewhat blur the boundary with AMI but may serve to indicate which patients with non-AMI ACS are at risk for increased morbidity and mortality. In some studies, up to a third of those diagnosed with unstable angina have elevation in troponin, and mortality in these patients approaches that of traditionally defined AMI.

Studies suggest that the likelihood of progression to clear-cut AMI and the mortality in these patients (those with non-AMI ACS having elevated troponin) can, like AMI, be reduced with aggressive intervention. CK-MB and myoglobin have little or no demonstrated role in the diagnosis of non-AMI ACS. Elevated BNP in non-AMI ACS is predictive of both recurrence and a higher likelihood of sudden cardiac death. C-reactive protein (CRP) and high-sensitivity CRP (hsCRP) appear to be independent predictors for the development of ACS in healthy individuals, and predict short term prognosis following non-AMI ACS. Elevated hsCRP values within 6-24 hours after symptom onset indicates an increased risk for recurrent cardiac events within 30 days to 1 year. Further, in patients with unstable angina, elevated hsCRP values may predict a higher rate of myocardial infarction or mortality.

Acute myocardial infarction (MI)

The current universal definitions of MI, promulgated by the European Society of Cardiology (ESC), American College of Cardiology (ACC), American Heart Association (AHA), and World Heart Federation (WHF) are in their third iteration. The definition most applicable to patients presenting to the emergency department is as follows:

1. an alteration in troponin (rise and/or fall in cTn with at least one value above the 99th percentile upper reference limit)

2. one of the following:

- symptoms of ischemia

- new significant ST–T changes or new left bundle branch block

- development of pathological Q waves

- imaging showing new loss of viable myocardium or new regional wall motion abnormality

- identification of an intracoronary thrombus by angiography or autopsy

The preferred biomarker is cTn. The authors of the third universal definition recognize no diagnostic role for myoglobin or CK or CK-MB. Blood samples for cTn should be drawn initially and repeated 3 and 6 h later. Later samples are required only if further ischemic episodes occur or when the timing of the initial symptoms is unclear.

In patients whose initial cTnI value is abnormal (initial cTnI >99th percentile), there is increased risk for AMI. In these patients, >20% change in cTnI values at 3 or 6 hours indicates myocardial necrosis. This combination plus clinical evidence of ischemia indicate MI.

In patients with normal initial cTnI value (initial cTnI <99th percentile), serial monitoring is indicated. In these patients, >50% change in cTnI values at 3 or 6 hours indicates myocardial necrosis. This combination plus clinical evidence of ischemia indicate MI.

Note that the demonstration of a *rising and/or falling pattern is needed to distinguish acute from chronic* elevations in cTn concentrations that are associated with structural heart disease. Troponin elevations related to conditions such as chronic renal failure or congestive heart failure may be marked but do not change acutely. However, a rising or falling pattern is not absolutely necessary to make the diagnosis of MI if a patient with a high pretest risk of MI presents late after symptom onset.

Cardiac reperfusion

An indication of successful reperfusion following thrombolysis is the so-called washout phenomenon. In successful reperfusion, all of the cardiac markers peak earlier than normal, although their sequence of peaks parallels that of normal MI. In addition, their peak concentrations may be higher than they would have been with unreperfused MI.

Myocarditis

An endomyocardial biopsy is required to fulfill the conventional Dallas criteria for myocarditis, which requires an inflammatory myocardial infiltrate. Some have advocated the application of immunohistochemistry (eg, CD3, CD20) and molecular testing for viruses to improve sensitivity.

Most cases of myocarditis are attributed to virus, especially Coxsackie B, adenovirus, HIV, and parvovirus B19; however, other possibilities to consider include *Trypanosoma cruzi* (Chagas disease) and *Borrelia burgdorferi* (Lyme disease). Medications and sarcoidosis must be considered in the appropriate clinical contexts. Lastly, giant cell myocarditis should be considered in patients with systemic autoimmune diseases and/or thymoma.

Most patients present with acute dilated (congestive) cardiomyopathy. There may be an antecedent viral syndrome within the past 2 weeks. Other well defined clinical presentations include an acute MI-like presentation with normal coronary arteries and sudden cardiac death.

Laboratory findings in myocarditis include elevated CK-MB and troponin, but the sensitivity of these assays is low. The diagnosis primarily relies on other clinical tests, including echocardiography, MRI, and ECG. Laboratory studies do aid in the identification of etiologies, with the endomyocardial biopsy and viral serologies important in this regard.

Chemotherapy induced cardiac toxicity

Anthracycline (eg, doxorubicin, daunorubicin), alkylating agents (cisplatin, ifosfamide), and trastuzumab (anti-EGFR monoclonal antibody) are currently the most common agents implicated in chemotherapy induced cardiac toxicity. The presentation may be acute or chronic, manifesting as congestive heart failure or conduction disturbances.

The left ventricular ejection fraction is the most common means of assessing for cardiac toxicity, with baseline and serial measurements forming the basis for the diagnosis. Recently, there has been investigation of serum cardiac markers, including troponin and BNP in this context, although it is not clear that serial monitoring of patients for troponin and/or BNP improves outcomes.

Proteins
Major serum proteins t1.8
Albumin

Albumin is the most abundant serum protein, constituting ~2/3 of it, and is synthesized primarily in the liver. Albumin has many functions, chief among them the maintenance of serum osmotic pressure and provision of serum transport for numerous substances. α-fetoprotein is the albumin equivalent in fetal blood. Interestingly, congenital absence of albumin (analbuminemia) is not a serious problem, only resulting in mild edema and hyperlipidemia. There are several alleles for albumin, the most common of which is albumin A. When a variant albumin is present, it may electrophorese at a slightly different rate than albumin A, leading to bisalbuminemia, a benign condition in which 2 peaks are seen in the albumin band.

Albumin's clinical utility resides in the assessment of hepatic synthetic function, nutritional status, and diabetic control. In assessing nutritional status, it is important to remember that the half life of albumin is 17 days. In addition, hepatic synthetic function is somewhat poorly reflected in the albumin level, since only in end-stage liver disease is serum albumin noticeably decreased. The greatest decrements in serum albumin are seen in protein losing conditions such as protein losing enteropathy and nephrotic syndrome. Albumin is a negative acute phase reactant; that is, in inflammatory conditions, albumin decreases t1.9.

Glucose becomes nonenzymatically linked to a variety of serum proteins, resulting in the natural formation of glycoproteins such as glycated albumin and glycated hemoglobin. Concentrations of glycoproteins increase in relation to the concentration of serum glucose and can be used as indicators of glycemic control in diabetic patients. The short half life of albumin (~2 weeks) makes glycated albumin an indicator of short term glycemic control; in contrast, the half life of hemoglobin (120 days in patients without hemolysis) makes glycated hemoglobin an indicator of long term glycemic control.

t1.8 Serum proteins

Electrophoretic band	Major constituent(s)	Notes
Prealbumin	Prealbumin	Indicator of nutritional status Binds thyroid hormones, binds retinol binding protein Negative acute phase reactant
Albumin	Albumin	Maintains serum oncotic pressure Binds numerous substances Negative acute phase reactant
Alb-α_1 interface	α_1-lipoprotein	HDL
α_1	α_1-antitrypsin	Positive acute phase reactant α_1 antitrypsin deficiency detectable with serum protein electrophoresis (SPEP)
α_1-α_2 interface	Gc globulin	Binds vitamin D
	α_1-antichymotrypsin	Positive acute phase reactant
	α_1-acid glycoprotein	Positive acute phase reactant
α_2	α_2-macroglobulin	Elevated in nephrotic syndrome
	Haptoglobin	Positive acute phase reactant
	Ceruloplasmin	Binds copper Low ceruloplasmin not detectable with SPEP Positive acute phase reactant
α_2-β interface	Usually empty	Hemoglobin, usually absent from serum, may be present here when there is hemolysis—a possible pseudo-M-spike
β_1	Transferrin	Transferrin may be high in iron deficiency—a possible pseudo-M-spike
β_1-β_2 interface	β-lipoprotein	LDL
β_2	IgA	Fibrinogen, usually absent from serum, may be present in the β-γ interface when there is incomplete clotting—a possible pseudo-M-spike
	C3	Positive acute phase reactant, C3 breakdown products—a possible pseudo-M-spike
γ_1	γ globulins	Positive acute phase reactants
γ_2	CRP	Positive acute phase reactant

t1.9 Acute phase reactants (APR)

	Protein	Acute inflammation	Chronic inflammation
	Prealbumin	↓	↓
	Albumin	↓	↓
α_1	α_1-antitrypsin	↑	↑
	α_1-antichymotrypsin	↑	↑
	α_1-acid glycoprotein	↑	↑
α_2	Haptoglobin	↑	↑
	Ceruloplasmin	↑	↑
β	Complement (C$_3$)	↑	↑
	Transferrin	↓	↑
	Fibrinogen	↑	↑
	Ig (IgA, IgM)	→↓	↑
γ	Ig (IgG, IgA, IgM)	→↓	↑
	CRP	↑	↑

Prealbumin

Prealbumin is the fastest migrating protein on serum protein electrophoresis (SPEP). Due to its low concentration, however, it is not normally seen on traditional SPEP and seen only faintly on high-resolution SPEP. It has 2 main functions: it binds ~10% of circulating thyroxine (it is also called transthyretin [TTR] and thyroxine binding prealbumin [TBPA]), and it binds and carries the retinol binding protein:vitamin A complex.

There is a rare prealbumin variant whose very high affinity for thyroxine leads to elevated total T4 in a euthyroid individual. In addition, normal sequence transthyretin is the amyloid precursor protein in senile cardiac amyloidosis, and mutant versions of transthyretin are responsible for certain familial forms of amyloidosis (eg, familial amyloid polyneuropathy).

Prealbumin's clinical utility resides mainly in the assessment of nutritional status. In this regard, its short half life of 48 hours makes it particularly useful. Elevations in prealbumin are seen in corticosteroid therapy and with decreased renal function. Like albumin, prealbumin is a negative acute phase reactant.

Prealbumin crosses the blood-brain barrier and is actively secreted into the cerebrospinal fluid (CSF) by the choroid plexus. Thus, it is a relatively prominent component of CSF protein, and a sharp prealbumin band is a hallmark of CSF protein electrophoresis.

α₁-antitrypsin (AAT)

AAT is the major component of the α_1 band. Its main function is to inactivate various proteases such as trypsin and neutrophil elastase. The AAT gene (*SERPINA1*) is highly polymorphic, with >100 genetic variants described. The most common allele is PiM, and the most common genotype is PiMM.

Inheritance of homozygous Z allele ("PiZZ") leas to deficiency of AAT, a condition in which affected individuals are at high risk for development of neonatal hepatitis, emphysema, cirrhosis, and hepatocellular carcinoma.

The SPEP can detect AAT deficiency (homozygotes for PiZZ), in which the serum will display a markedly diminished α_1 band. In addition, AAT produced from the Z allele migrates slower (more cathodal) than the normal M allele. Depending upon the gel system used, electrophoresis may detect some heterozygotes (PiMZ).

α₁-acid glycoprotein

α_1-acid glycoprotein (orosomucoid) is also a positive acute phase reactant. It is a minor component of the α_1 band normally, but it is a major component of the increased α_1 band in acute inflammatory states.

α₂-macroglobulin

α_2-macroglobulin is a protease inhibitor whose serum concentration is elevated in liver and renal disease. In particular, its large size prevents its loss in nephrotic syndrome, leading to a relative 10-fold rise in concentration.

Ceruloplasmin

Ceruloplasmin functions in copper transport. Although a decreased serum ceruloplasmin is an important marker for Wilson disease, the differential diagnosis of a decreased serum ceruloplasmin also includes hepatic failure, malnutrition, and Menkes syndrome. A falsely normal or elevated ceruloplasmin may be seen in inflammatory states, because ceruloplasmin is an acute phase reactant, and in pregnancy.

Haptoglobin

Haptoglobin is the third major component of the α_2 band. It is a protein that binds free hemoglobin; hence, it is rapidly depleted in acute intravascular hemolysis. Since only tiny amounts of free hemoglobin are necessary to deplete the serum of haptoglobin, it is a very sensitive marker of hemolysis. Haptoglobin does not bind myoglobin, such that serum haptoglobin may be useful in the workup of a urine dipstick that is positive for hemoglobin. Haptoglobin is an acute phase reactant, so that acute inflammation may mask the decrease in haptoglobin produced by hemolysis.

There are 2 common haptoglobin alleles: Hp1 and Hp2. Based upon these alleles, 3 haptoglobin genotypes are possible: Hp1-1, Hp1-2, and Hp2-2. The Hp2-2 genotype appears to be an independent risk factor for cardiovascular disease in diabetics.

Transferrin

Transferrin is the major β globulin. Its function is to transport ferric (Fe^{3+}) iron, with which it is normally ~30% saturated. There is a marked increase in serum transferrin in iron deficiency. The total iron binding capacity of the serum may be assayed and is a reflection of the amount of transferrin present. Transferrin is also increased in pregnancy and estrogen therapy. Transferrin decreases in the early stages of an acute phase response, but later increases if the inflammatory state persists.

The blood-brain barrier transports transferrin into the CSF, but not before modifying a percentage of it to create asialated transferrin (so-called tau protein), while the rest is unmodified. Thus, a hallmark of CSF protein electrophoresis is a double transferrin peak.

A form of transferrin in serum—carbohydrate-deficient transferrin—may be superior to GGT as a marker for alcohol use.

Fibrinogen

Fibrinogen is also considered a β globulin with a couple of caveats. Firstly, in the normal course of events there is no fibrinogen in serum, most of it having been consumed in the clot. However, if the specimen clots incompletely (eg, a heparinized patient), then fibrinogen may be seen. Secondly, fibrinogen can straddle the β-γ interface. All of these features may combine to form a pseudo-paraprotein on SPEP.

C-reactive protein (CRP)

The name "C-reactive protein" derives from its reaction with streptococcal capsular (C) polysaccharide. CRP is produced in the liver. In protein electrophoresis, it is found in the γ region, with the immunoglobulins, where it can on occasion produce a small apparent band.

Formerly, assays for CRP had an analytical sensitivity of ~5 mg/L. This was appropriate, as the CRP test was used to support such diagnoses as bacterial endocarditis, appendicitis, active collagen vascular disease, and the like, in which CRP values tended to be well >10 mg/L. However, attention has recently been turned to the predictive value of low level CRP elevations (>2-3 mg/L) for cardiac events, and as a result high-sensitivity CRP (hsCRP) assays have become available which have analytical sensitivity of <0.5 mg/L.

An exact cutoff for CRP, in the context of cardiovascular risk, is difficult to determine. About half the population has CRP >2 mg/L, and about a third has CRP >3 mg/L. Interestingly, a population distribution of CRP levels is not an evenly-distributed Gaussian curve; instead, it is significantly skewed, with a dense cluster in the very lowest CRP levels and a long tail extending into the >10 range.

Thus, there are 3 categories based upon CRP concentration. Normal CRP concentration is <3 mg/L. High level CRP elevations are those >10 mg/L, usually indicative of active inflammation. Low level CRP elevations are those between 3 and 10, indicative of cellular stress. Low level CRP elevation may indicate a wide array of minor disease states, genetic factors, demographic variables, and behavioral patterns. There are seasonal variations in CRP, varying up to 0.5 mg/L over the course of the year, with highest levels in winter and lowest levels in summer. An individual's set point appears to be inherited. Low level CRP elevation is known to predict poor outcome following cardiovascular events, but have also been shown to correlate with mortality in noncardiac diseases as well as in apparently healthy individuals. Several reports indicate that elevated CRP is a risk factor for subsequent coronary and cerebrovascular events. For example, in the Physician's Health Study, men with CRP >2.11 mg/L had 3× the risk of suffering an acute myocardial infarction as compared with men having CRP <0.55 mg/L.

Patterns in serum protein electrophoresis

Normal serum f1.2

Normal serum is characterized by a nearly invisible prealbumin band and a very large albumin band. This is followed by a small peaked α_1 band, a somewhat broader α_2 band, a bimodal β, and broad γ.

Bisalbuminemia

Bisalbuminemia is seen in heterozygotes for albumin alleles. The SPEP shows double albumin spike. This is of no clinical consequence.

α_1-antitrypsin (AAT) deficiency f1.3

AAT deficiency can be detected with SPEP (though it is not the most sensitive or specific assay), since AAT is the major component of the α_1 band. Genotypic PiZZ individuals have a visibly and quantitatively decreased band.

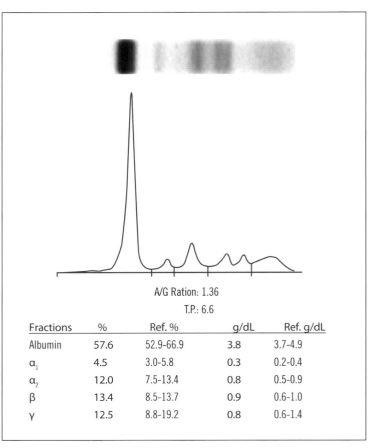

Fractions	%	Ref. %	g/dL	Ref. g/dL
Albumin	57.6	52.9-66.9	3.8	3.7-4.9
α_1	4.5	3.0-5.8	0.3	0.2-0.4
α_2	12.0	7.5-13.4	0.8	0.5-0.9
β	13.4	8.5-13.7	0.9	0.6-1.0
γ	12.5	8.8-19.2	0.8	0.6-1.4

A/G Ration: 1.36
T.P.: 6.6

f1.2 Normal high-resolution serum protein electrophoresis; the most anodal band is albumin, followed by α_1, α_2, β_1, β_2, and the broad, faint γ region

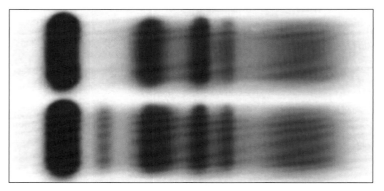

f1.3 SPEP showing patient with α_1 antitrypsin deficiency (top) & normal SPEP for comparison (bottom)

Nephrotic syndrome

Nephrotic syndrome results in massive loss of small serum proteins, particularly albumin. In minimal change disease, there is a selective loss of albumin (selective proteinuria). In other forms of nephrotic syndrome, nearly all proteins are lost, including γ globulins. In all types of nephrotic syndrome, very large protein molecules are retained. The result is a decrease of all the electrophoretic bands, most prominently the albumin band, with the conspicuous exception of the α_2 band that contains the very large protein α_2-macroglobulin.

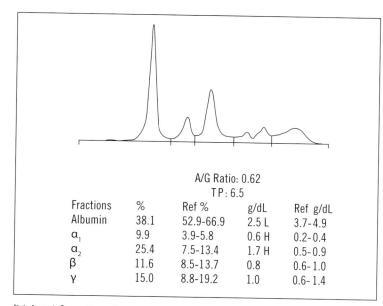

Fractions	%	Ref %	g/dL	Ref g/dL
Albumin	38.1	52.9-66.9	2.5 L	3.7-4.9
α_1	9.9	3.9-5.8	0.6 H	0.2-0.4
α_2	25.4	7.5-13.4	1.7 H	0.5-0.9
β	11.6	8.5-13.7	0.8	0.6-1.0
γ	15.0	8.8-19.2	1.0	0.6-1.4

A/G Ratio: 0.62
T P: 6.5

f1.4 Acute inflammation pattern

Acute inflammation f1.4

Inflammatory states are characterized by increased acute phase reactants, accounting for an increase in the α_1 and α_2 bands. Albumin is slightly decreased. Initially, the γ globulins are unchanged, but with prolonged inflammation, these are polyclonally increased.

β-γ bridging

This is the hallmark of cirrhosis. Additional features include hypoalbuminemia and blunted α_1 and α_2 bands. β-γ bridging is primarily due to the increased serum IgA typically found in cirrhotic individuals.

Monoclonal gammopathy f1.5-f1.8

A monoclonal gammopathy (paraproteinemia) is a condition in which there is an immunochemically homogeneous immunoglobulin (M protein) in the serum. The SPEP shows a prominent, discrete, dark band (M-spike) usually within the γ region but sometimes in β or α_2. An M protein is usually an intact immunoglobulin, composed of 2 heavy and 2 light chains. Sometimes it is composed of a light chain only and (rarely) a heavy chain only. Biclonal gammopathy (2 M-proteins) occurs in 3-4% of cases. When what appears to be a biclonal gammopathy turns out to be composed of IgA spikes having a single light chain, this is most likely due to the appearance of both monomers and dimers in the SPEP and should be considered monoclonal rather than biclonal.

~10% of patients with myeloma have an SPEP showing only hypogammaglobulinemia. Hypogammaglobulinemia, when not due to myeloma, may be the result of a diverse group of conditions including congenital hypogammaglobulinemia, lymphoma, nephrotic syndrome, and corticosteroid treatment. Patients with myeloma whose SPEP shows only hypogammaglobulinemia are likely to have free light chains in their serum and urine (Bence Jones protein).

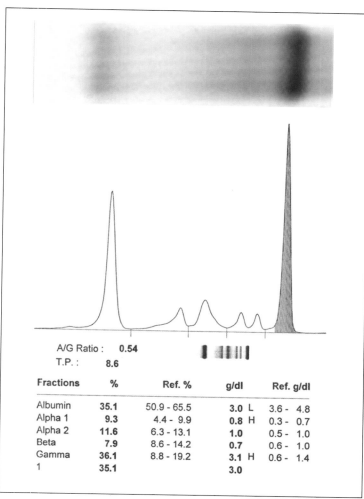

Fractions	%	Ref. %	g/dl	Ref. g/dl
Albumin	35.1	50.9 - 65.5	3.0 L	3.6 - 4.8
Alpha 1	9.3	4.4 - 9.9	0.8 H	0.3 - 0.7
Alpha 2	11.6	6.3 - 13.1	1.0	0.5 - 1.0
Beta	7.9	8.6 - 14.2	0.7	0.6 - 1.0
Gamma	36.1	8.8 - 19.2	3.1 H	0.6 - 1.4
1	35.1		3.0	

A/G Ratio : 0.54
T.P. : 8.6

f1.5 SPEP showing typical M spike; most IgG paraproteins are found in the γ region on the gel (above) & densitometry tracing (below)

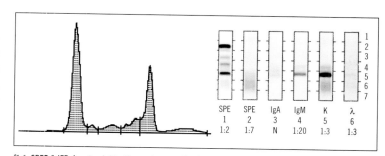

SPE 1 1:2 | SPE 2 1:7 | IgA 3 N | IgM 4 1:20 | K 5 1:3 | λ 6 1:3

f1.6 SPEP & IFE showing IgM κ M protein; note that IgM paraproteins tend to migrate near the β-γ interface

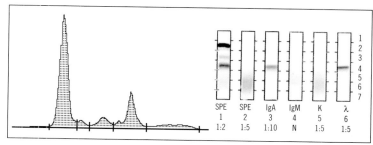

SPE 1 1:2 | SPE 2 1:5 | IgA 3 1:10 | IgM 4 N | K 5 1:5 | λ 6 1:5

f1.7 SPEP & IFE showing IgA λ M protein; note that IgA paraproteins tend to migrate into the β region)

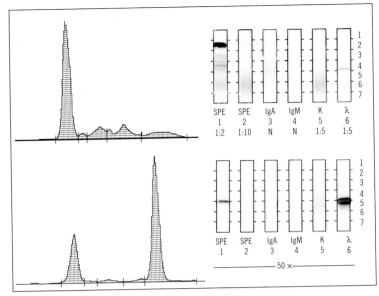

f1.8 SPEP (upper left), serum IFE (upper right), UPEP (lower left), urine IFE (lower right) showing λ light chain only M protein

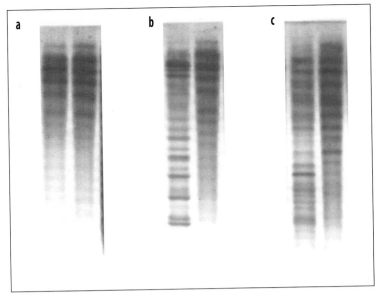

f1.9 CSF protein electrophoresis
a CSF (left) & serum (right) from the same patient, neither demonstrating oligoclonal bands
b CSF (left) & serum (right) from the same patient, in which oligoclonal bands are present in the CSF but not in the serum, a result supportive of the diagnosis of MS
c CSF (left) & serum (right), both with oligoclonal bands, in which case the CSF bands would be discounted

Immunofixation or immunosubtraction is indicated to characterize the M-protein. Even when an M-spike is not evident on SPEP, an immunofixation may be indicated if (a) there is a strong clinical suspicion of myeloma, (b) there is systemic AL amyloidosis, or (c) there is hypogammaglobulinemia. In patients with negative serum screens in whom the clinical suspicion is high, the urine should be screened for the presence of monoclonal free light chains by electrophoresis and immunofixation and serum free light chain levels should be evaluated.

An M-spike is most commonly the result of a plasma cell neoplasm, Waldenström macroglobulinemia (lymphoplasmacytic lymphoma), or chronic lymphocytic leukemia/small lymphocytic lymphoma.

Pseudo-M-spikes, abnormal distinct bands resembling M-spikes but with negative confirmation (immunofixation, immunoelectrophoresis, serum free light chains), have numerous causes. Most commonly, pseudo-M-spikes result from normal constituents: fibrinogen (incompletely clotted sample), hemoglobin (hemolyzed sample), elevated C-reactive protein, or elevated transferrin. Certain antibiotics and some radiocontrast agents absorb light at the wavelengths used to quantify proteins in capillary electrophoresis and can be excluded by repeating the assay using conventional electrophoresis with dye binding techniques. Very high levels of serum tumor markers, such as CA 19-9, may also produce pseudo-M-spikes.

After making the diagnosis, serum protein electrophoresis is used to follow disease progression and the efficacy of treatment. 3 quantitative immunochemical results are important in disease monitoring. The M-protein quantity, routinely carried out by nephelometry (or turbidimetry), is important to classify and to follow the disease. Secondly, it is important to quantify the other major immunoglobulin classes—IgG, IgA, and IgM—to determine the degree to which they are suppressed.

The quantity of serum free light chains is important both diagnostically and in the monitoring of disease status. Using sensitive serum free light chain assays >95% of patients with myeloma will have an elevation in either the free light chains themselves and/or an abnormal κ:λ ratio. The utility of the serum free light chain assays extends to patients previously classified as having nonsecretory myeloma; with the use of serum free light chain assays the majority of these patients will have elevation in either the free light chains themselves and/or an abnormal κ:λ ratio. The free light chain assay is extremely sensitive to myeloma recurrence after treatment.

Serum viscosity is typically calculated as relative viscosity (ratio of serum viscosity to water) and is normally in the range of 1.5-1.8. The symptoms of hyperviscosity syndrome occur when the serum viscosity is in the range of 6-7 but may develop at lower levels. Hyperviscosity syndrome may present with nasal bleeding, blurred vision, retinal vein dilation (with flame shaped retinal hemorrhages) and/or neurologic symptoms (headache, vertigo, nystagmus, tinnitus, hearing loss, ataxia, and diplopia). Serum viscosity should be measured when an IgM M-protein exceeds 4 g/dL or an IgA or IgG exceeds 6 g/dL as these patients are at risk for hyperviscosity syndrome.

CSF protein electrophoresis

Electrophoresis of normal CSF appears distinctly different from serum. The CSF normally contains essentially all the proteins present in serum, although in smaller quantities. The most characteristic features of the normal CSF electrophoresis are: a prominent prealbumin band and a double β (transferrin) band; additional subtler features are a faint albumin and α_2 band. The main purpose of CSF electrophoresis is to support a diagnosis of multiple sclerosis by finding oligoclonal bands—several distinct bands in the γ region reflective of several clonal immunoglobulins f1.9. These bands should be absent from the patient's serum, run concurrently, to be specific.

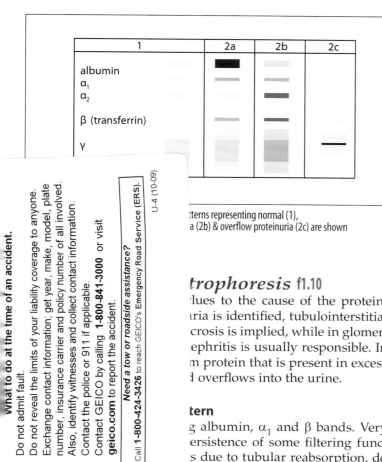

	1	2a	2b	2c
albumin				
α₁				
α₂				
β (transferrin)				
γ				

...terns representing normal (1),
...a (2b) & overflow proteinuria (2c) are shown

...trophoresis f1.10

...lues to the cause of the protein-
...ria is identified, tubulointerstitial
...crosis is implied, while in glomer-
...ephritis is usually responsible. In
...m protein that is present in excess
...d overflows into the urine.

...tern

...g albumin, α₁ and β bands. Very
...ersistence of some filtering func-
...s due to tubular reabsorption, do
... urine. This leaves the proteins in
... albumin, AAT, and transferrin.

Tubular proteinuria pattern

The urine contains a weak albumin band, and strong α_1 and β bands. This pattern results from the impaired tubular reabsorption of low molecular weight proteins normally freely filtered by the glomerulus such as α_2-macroglobulin, β_2-microglobulin, and polyclonal light chains.

Overflow proteinuria pattern

Most commonly this is a monoclonal light chain (Bence Jones proteinuria). Other possibilities include myoglobin and hemoglobin.

Cryoglobulinemia

Cryoglobulins

Cryoglobulins are immunoglobulins that precipitate reversibly at low temperatures. To detect cryoglobulins, blood is drawn and kept at 37°C until clotted, then centrifuged at 37°C. The serum is then placed at 4°C for ≥3 days, then centrifuged at 4°C. Any precipitate that forms is a cryoprecipitate. The cryoprecipitate can then be washed and subjected to electrophoresis and immunofixation for characterization.

3 types of cryoglobulins are recognized: type I and the mixed types, II & III. Type I cryoglobulins are monoclonal immunoglobulins that are found in association with multiple myeloma or Waldenström macroglobulinemia. Type II cryoglobulins are a mixture of a monoclonal IgM and polyclonal IgG. The IgM has rheumatoid factor activity (anti-IgG). This is the most common type of cryoglobulin. Type III cryoglobulins are a mixture of 2 polyclonal immunoglobulins, typically IgG and IgM. The polyclonal IgM in type III cryoglobulins also has rheumatoid factor activity.

Mixed cryoglobulinemia (types II & III)

Mixed cryoglobulins can be found in the serum of individuals with a variety of clinical conditions, including lymphoproliferative disorders, chronic infections, chronic liver diseases, and autoimmune diseases (especially SLE). Historically, about half of cases were associated with no identifiable underlying disorder and were termed *"essential mixed cryoglobulinemia."* It is now known that most such cases are the result of chronic hepatitis C virus infection. Currently, HCV is the most common cause of mixed cryoglobulinemia.

Cryoglobulinemia is a systemic immune complex disease characterized by a distinctive clinical syndrome of palpable purpura (leukocytoclastic vasculitis), arthralgias, hepatosplenomegaly, lymphadenopathy, anemia, sensorineural deficits, and glomerulonephritis. Purpura is a constant feature, usually distributed over the lower extremities. Most patients are variably hypocomplementemic, reflecting the immune complex nature of the disease.

Renal involvement, which may appear only several years after initial presentation, manifests as either nephrotic or nephritic syndrome, and is associated with severe hypocomplementemia. In renal biopsies, the most common finding is membranoproliferative glomerulonephritis (MPGN) type II. In some cases, usually when acute, the deposits produce the appearance of thrombotic microangiopathy. In all tissues, as in the kidney, the basic pathologic lesion is vasculitis. Electron microscopy demonstrates large subendothelial immune complex deposits with a fibrillary or tubular structure in a fingerprint like pattern.

Laboratory methods

Protein electrophoresis

Protein electrophoresis is the movement of proteins due to an electrical potential. In this technique, a charge is applied across a medium that is composed of a solid support and a fluid buffer. This charge creates an electromotive force. The solid support has a slight negative charge and is drawn towards the positive pole (anode), but, being a solid support, it cannot move. There is instead a flow of the positively charged fluid buffer towards the negative pole (cathode). This buffer flow is called endosmosis and has the capacity to carry with it substances suspended within the medium.

Thus, if proteins are added to the medium and the charge is applied, 2 forces act on each protein: electromotive and endosmotic. Since most proteins bear a net negative charge at pH 8.6, electromotive force tends to pull them towards the anode (positive pole), whereas endosmosis pulls them towards the cathode. In the case of γ globulins, which have a weak net negative to positive charge, the endosmotic force displaces the proteins towards the cathode. In the case of most other proteins, the electromotive force exceeds the endosmotic force, and they move to variable extents towards the anode.

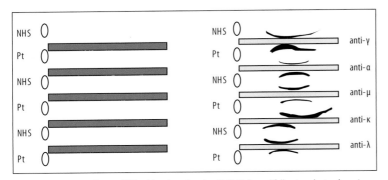

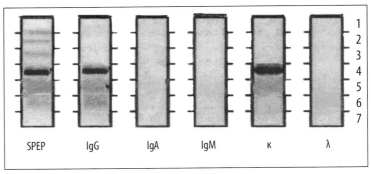

f1.11 Immunoelectrophoresis (IEP) with uninoculated wells (left) & a gel following electrophoresis, diffusion, fixation & staining (right) demonstrating an IgG κ monoclonal protein

f1.12 Immunofixation electrophoresis (IFE) demonstrating an IgG κ monoclonal protein

When electrophoresis is carried out on serum at pH 8.6 on an agarose gel, fixed, and stained, 5 distinct bands can be seen. The fastest moving band is albumin, followed by the 2 α bands (α_1 and α_2), the β band, and finally the γ band. The γ band consists of proteins that move very slowly or actually move towards the cathode. Individual bands can be measured by densitometry.

Capillary zone electrophoresis is similar in many respects to gel electrophoresis. Instead of occurring in a gel that contains buffer, however, capillary electrophoresis occurs in a narrow-bore capillary tube that contains buffer. A small volume of sample is aspirated into the capillary tube, the interior of which has a strong negative charge. In these conditions, the effect of endosmosis is greater than it is in gel, resulting in strong flow towards the cathode. Rather than staining as in gels, absorbance measurements note the elution time and quantity of the different protein fractions. The tracings produced, however, are similar to those seen with high-resolution gel electrophoresis.

Immunofixation & immunotyping

Immunofixation electrophoresis (IFE), immunotyping, and immunoelectrophoresis (IEP) are methods for characterizing a suspected monoclonal band observed on SPEP or UPEP.

IEP f1.11 is no longer commonly used. The procedure is performed by first placing patient serum in every other of a series of wells that are arranged alongside troughs in an agarose gel. In the remaining wells is placed an aliquot of normal serum. The gel is then subjected to electrophoresis. After electrophoresis, antiserum is added to each trough. After a period of time, precipitation arcs form between the antisera in the troughs and the electrophoresed proteins in the gel. Interpretation depends on visual comparison of the arcs formed with patient serum and the arcs formed with normal serum. If there is no M protein in the patient's serum, then the arcs should be symmetrical and in the same location (mirror images).

IFE f1.12 is much simpler to interpret than IEP. The procedure involves placing patient serum into each of 6 wells in an agarose gel. The gel is then subjected to electrophoresis. Finally, 5 different antisera are applied to the gel: anti-IgG, IgA, IgM, κ, and λ. The entire gel is then stained. Interpretation is relatively straightforward.

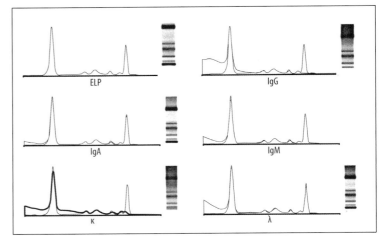

f1.13 Immunotyping (IT) or immunosubtraction demonstrating an IgG κ monoclonal protein

Immunotyping (IT, immunosubtraction) f1.13 is often used in conjunction with capillary electrophoresis to identify the M protein. The serum sample is incubated with different solid-phase sepharose beads attached to antibodies against γ, α, μ, κ, or λ. After incubation, the supernatants are subjected to electrophoresis to determine which of the reagents resulted in the removal of the abnormal spike.

Acid-base & electrolytes
Sodium

Hyponatremia

Hyponatremia is defined as serum sodium below the reference interval, which is typically 135 mmol/L in non-pregnant adults. It is considered severe when <125 mmol/L. Hyponatremia is a fairly common abnormality among the elderly and among hospitalized patients. It is perhaps the most common electrolyte abnormality in hospitalized patients, occurring in up 30%. Hyponatremia can cause marked morbidity and mortality, especially if severe or if corrected with excessive rapidity.

The differential diagnosis begins with excluding spurious hyponatremia, pseudohyponatremia, and hyperglycemia. Spurious hyponatremia is an anomaly of the preanalytic phase, in which blood is drawn proximal to an intravenous infusion or from a central venous line.

Pseudohyponatremia is a true anomaly of the analytic phase, affecting any instrument that utilizes "indirect" method of measurement, in which the sample is prediluted before analysis. Such analyzers measure sodium by ion-selective electrode and then calculate the plasma/serum sodium on the assumption that the water content of the plasma is 93%. In the presence of hypertriglyceridemia, hypercholesterolemia, and hyperproteinemia, this assumption is incorrect, as the water content in the original sample is lower. 2 approaches to investigating this possibility have been suggested. First, serum osmolarity can be determined; it is normal (>280 mOsm/kg) in pseudohyponatremia, and there would be a wide discrepancy between the osmolality calculated from the measured sodium and the measured osmolarity. Second, direct potentiometry, as performed on blood gas analyzers, is not affected by pseudohyponatremia. Again, a significant difference in the direct and indirect measurement suggests pseudohyponatremia.

In hyperglycemia, there is a true physiologic shift in sodium ions. Excess glucose draws water into the extracellular space, producing hyponatremia that is real but unrelated to any intrinsic defect in sodium homeostasis. The degree of change in sodium concentration attributable to glucose can be calculated by following formula (glucose expressed in mg/dL):

$$\frac{1.6 \times (\text{serum glucose} - 100)}{100}$$

If this accounts for the change in sodium, then there is no additional anomaly in sodium homeostasis. For example, if the measured glucose is 600 mg/dL and the measured sodium is 128 mEq/L, then the formula gives an expected change in sodium of $1.6 \times (600-100)/100$ or 8 mEq/L. 8 mEq/L, added to 128 mEq/L, gives 136 mEq/L; thus the altered sodium can be attributed to hyperglycemia. Hypertonic (>295 mOsm/kg) hyponatremia suggests marked hyperglycemia, but may also be seen in patients given mannitol in order to reduce their intracranial pressure.

True hypotonic hyponatremia (<280 mOsm/kg) is further classified according to the patient's volume status through clinical parameters (eg, edema, skin turgor).

In patients who are hypovolemic, the major consideration is sodium loss through renal or extrarenal routes. Renal losses are suggested by elevated urine sodium (U_{Na}>30 mmol/L); this may be caused by diuretics, renal medullary disease, primary adrenal insufficiency (Addison disease), renal tubular acidosis type I (RTA type I), and cerebral salt-wasting syndrome (see discussion below, in conjunction with SIADH). Extrarenal sodium losses may occur in the gastrointestinal tract (vomiting, diarrhea) or result from third spacing (eg, peritonitis or pleuritis). Extrarenal sites of sodium loss are suggested by low urine sodium (U_{Na}<30).

In patients who are euvolemic, the syndrome of inappropriate antidiuretic hormone secretion (SIADH) is suggested. SIADH itself has numerous causes; traditionally, it was thought that the hyponatremia and increased ADH found in some patients who had suffered cerebral insults, such as neurosurgical intervention, was a secondary form of SIADH. However, such cases are now largely classified as cerebral salt-wasting syndrome (CSWS), differentiated from SIADH by the presence of a hypovolemic state, a differing pathophysiology, and, importantly, different treatment (CSWS is responsive to infusion of normal saline and generally corrects itself over time).

After SIADH is excluded, other possibilities include psychogenic polydipsia, hypothyroidism, primary adrenal insufficiency (Addison disease), and drugs with ADH-like (vasopressin-like) effect, including desmopressin, serotonin reuptake inhibitors (SSRIs), and tricyclic antidepressants. The recreational drug ecstasy (3,4-methylenedioxy-N-methylamphetamine or MDMA) is also thought to produce hyponatremia by this mechanism. One caveat with regard to the differential diagnosis: a misdiagnosis of SIADH may be made in the presence of recent diuretic use when there is a brief reflex water retention. The diagnosis of SIADH should be made only when hyponatremia exists prima facie, with a urine sodium >20 mmol/L, euvolemia, normal renal function, no recent use of diuretics, and normal adrenal function.

In patients who are hypervolemic, the differential diagnosis includes congestive heart failure, cirrhosis, and nephrotic syndrome. In this group of patients, urine sodium is usually <20 mEq/L.

Hypernatremia

Hypernatremia is most commonly seen in an individual with dehydration (due to diarrhea or insensible water losses) and the inability to respond to their thirst response; thus, hypernatremia tends to affect infants, ICU patients, and debilitated adults.

The cause of hypernatremia may be apparent in individual cases, where exposure or severe diarrhea, in the face of a scarcity of water, has led to hypernatremia. In other cases, the differential diagnosis is approached in a manner similar to hyponatremia, noting first the hydration status of the patient. Most patients with hypernatremia are hypovolemic; that is, there have been water losses in excess of sodium losses, resulting in a dehydrated but hypernatremic patient. Excess water losses in this context may be extrarenal losses (diarrhea, vomiting, burns) or renal (osmotic diuretics, loop diuretics, postobstructive diuresis, intrinsic medullary renal disease).

Some patients are euvolemic, and the differential is similar to that for hypovolemic patients with the caveat that diabetes insipidus must be considered (see below). Lastly, some patients are hypervolemic; this most often implies iatrogenic administration of sodium as part of intravenous fluid administration, sodium bicarbonate administration, or other intervention.

Diabetes insipidus (DI) results from insufficient antidiuretic hormone (ADH) activity. ADH is responsible for increasing water absorption in the renal collecting ducts. DI may be central (too little ADH made in the posterior pituitary) or nephrogenic (ADH is produced normally, but the collecting ducts are resistant to its action). Central DI has many causes, including damage to the hypothalamus or neurohypophysis related to surgery, space-occupying lesions in the region of the sella, head trauma, and infiltrative lesions such as eosinophilic granuloma and sarcoidosis.

Nephrogenic DI can be caused by renal diseases that affect the medullary space, where urine is concentrated, including sickle cell disease and tubulointerstitial nephritis. Certain electrolyte disturbances, notably hypokalemia and hypercalcemia, render the loop of Henle relatively incapable of concentrating urine. This renal compartment may also be affected in some types of renal tubular acidosis and in Fanconi syndrome. Lastly, a number of drugs result in nephrogenic DI, including lithium, demeclocycline, colchicine, amphotericin B, gentamicin, and furosemide.

Potassium

Potassium measurement

Potassium measurements are among the most notoriously spurious results in clinical chemistry. The most common scenario is spurious hyperkalemia attributed to in vitro hemolysis. Both the treatment of spurious hyperkalemia and the mistaken assumption that hyperkalemia is spurious can result in patient harm. Any unexpectedly abnormal potassium result, whether low or high, should be corroborated with an electrocardiogram and/or repeat sampling.

Pseudohyperkalemia is an elevated measured potassium in the absence of in vivo hyperkalemia. After blood is collected, potassium may be released from the cellular components of blood. Immediate centrifugation is among the most important ways to reduce this problem. When potassium is released from red cells as a result of in vitro hemolysis, the simultaneous release of hemoglobin serves as a visible warning that this has occurred. Correction formulas have been proposed for estimating the correct potassium in this setting, but their use is not recommended.

Pseudohyperkalemia may result from the release of potassium from platelets as a result of in vitro clot formation (serum has a higher potassium result than plasma for this reason); this effect is more pronounced in patients with thrombocytosis. Passive transmembrane potassium leak from leukocytes may be pronounced, particularly when there is marked leukocytosis. Thus a complete blood count should be part of the evaluation of suspected pseudohyperkalemia. A passive transmembrane leak of potassium from red cells, without concomitant hemolysis, has been associated with an autosomal dominant abnormal gene on chromosome 16 (familial pseudohyperkalemia).

Lastly, a variety of specimen collection issues can spuriously alter free potassium in a laboratory sample. Raised potassium may result from prolonged tourniquet time, excessive fist clenching, traumatic draw, inappropriate order of tubes drawn, venipuncture proximal to intravenous infusion, and small-gauge needles. The potassium may be raised by overly vigorous tube mixing, rough handling in the pneumatic tube system, and delays in transport or processing.

Hypokalemia

The differential diagnosis includes potassium loss through the gastrointestinal tract, potassium loss through the kidneys, and transcellular shifts of extracellular potassium to the intracellular space. Transcellular shifts occur in the setting of metabolic alkalosis, or in the correction of diabetic ketoacidosis. GI potassium loss is suggested when the urinary potassium is low (U_K<30 mEq/day); significant GI losses may be due to vomiting, nasogastric tube suction, diarrhea, or (theoretically) a large villous adenoma.

Renal loss of potassium is suggested by elevated urinary potassium (U_K>30 mEq/day); major urinary losses may result from diuretics, hypomagnesemia, antibiotics (carbenicillin, amphotericin-B), mineralocorticoid excess, renal tubular acidosis (RTA) types I & II, severe Cushing syndrome, congenital adrenal hyperplasia, Bartter syndrome, Liddle syndrome, Gitelmand syndrome, licorice (glycyrrhizin) consumption, and hyperreninism. Bartter syndrome and Liddle syndrome are inherited transmembrane channel defects in which potassium is lost in the urine. Gitelmand syndrome is a transmembrane channel defect caused by inactivating mutations in the *SLC12A3* gene encoding the thiazide-sensitive sodium-chloride cotransporter, characterized by renal loss of sodium and resulting hypovolemia, hypokalemia, and metabolic alkalosis. It is distinguished from Bartter and Liddle syndromes by the presence of low urinary calcium excretion. Historically, licorice was made from licorice root and contained glycyrrhizin, a compound capable of inhibiting the conversion of cortisol to cortisone by renal 11-β-hydroxysteroid dehydrogenase, thereby allowing cortisol to exert mineralocorticoid action on the renal tubule. Most commercially available licorice does not contain glycyrrhizin. However, products of black licorice oil may be found in some herbal supplements and have been linked to hypokalemia. Licorice induced hypokalemia can be supported by an increased urinary cortisol:cortisone ratio.

Note that in diabetic ketoacidosis, there is an initial hyperkalemia (as in most acidotic states), but correction of diabetic ketoacidosis results in a profound hypokalemia unless supplemental potassium is given.

Hyperkalemia

The differential diagnosis includes acidosis, renal failure, potassium-sparing diuretics (spironolactone, triamterene, amiloride, eplerenone), adrenal insufficiency, iatrogenic, and rhabdomyolysis. Nearly all cases of acidosis are associated with hyperkalemia. The main exception is renal tubular acidosis types I & II in which the potassium is low.

Calcium

Calcium measurement

When total calcium is reported, this must be interpreted in light of the serum albumin concentration. About 50% of serum calcium is bound to protein, mainly albumin, such that total calcium may be low in hypoalbuminemic patients, while free (ionized) calcium is normal. In hypoalbuminemic patients, an estimate of the expected total calcium if the serum albumin concentration were normal may be calculated by increasing the calcium level 0.8 mg/dL for each 1 g/dL that albumin is below the "normal" albumin level of 4 g/dL. For example, a calcium of 8.0 mg/dL in a patient with an albumin of 2.0 g/dL would result in a corrected calcium of 9.6 mg/dL. While this formula often provides a useful estimate, its use should be avoided in patients with acid-base disturbances, renal insufficiency, liver disease, and in neonates.

The free calcium fraction (ionized calcium) is biologically active and is a more accurate reflection of the clinical calcium status. The effect of protein binding is relevant, for example, in patients with significant paraproteinemia, especially in IgA and IgM-producing myeloma, or hypoproteinemia due to malnutrition or liver disease. Conditions such as these may be associated with an abnormal total calcium despite a normal ionized calcium. Acidosis decreases the binding of calcium to albumin and thus increases the proportion of free calcium. Likewise, alkalosis decreases free calcium.

The sample for ionized calcium must not be exposed to air (metabolism will change pH); it must not be drawn in calcium-chelating anticoagulants (EDTA, citrate); fist clenching and prolonged tourniquet application, capable of altering the local pH, are to be avoided; it must be kept cool and delivered to the laboratory rapidly. The measurement is usually performed on a blood gas analyzer.

Hypercalcemia

Hypercalcemia may present with nephrolithiasis, lethargy, hyporeflexia, slowed mentation, nausea, vomiting, constipation, depression, and high peaked T waves on ECG. Hypercalcemia increases the risk of both pancreatitis and peptic ulcer disease. When long term hypercalcemia is associated with concomitant hyperphosphatemia (increased calcium × phosphate product), there may be so-called metastatic calcification of vessel walls and soft tissue (calciphylaxis). This may be seen in skin and GI biopsies and often presents with pruritus.

The most common cause of hypercalcemia t1.10 is primary hyperparathyroidism. Excess parathyroid hormone (PTH) results in increased serum calcium with decreased serum phosphate; these abnormalities are accompanied by an increased chloride/phosphate ratio and an increased urinary cAMP. This is in contrast to many other forms of hypercalcemia in which the phosphate is high (leading to an increased calcium × phosphate product). This is because PTH has the dual effect on the renal tubules of increasing calcium reabsorption while increasing phosphate excretion. In 90% of cases, primary hyperparathyroidism is due to a solitary parathyroid adenoma; 9% of cases are caused by 4-gland hyperplasia, and <1% are caused by parathyroid carcinoma.

t1.10 Differential diagnosis of hypercalcemia

Etiology	Notes
Primary hyperparathyroidism	Parathyroid adenoma (most common), 4-gland hyperplasia, parathyroid carcinoma
Tertiary hyperparathyroidism	Post renal transplant
Malignancy	Squamous cell carcinoma, multiple myeloma, breast carcinoma, islet cell tumors, paraganglioma, renal cell carcinoma, hepatocellular carcinoma, T-acute lymphoblastic lymphoma, small cell carcinoma of ovary (hypercalcemic type)
Familial hypocalciuric hypercalcemia	CASR gene on 3q
Drugs	Thiazides, calcium-containing antacids or calcium supplements (milk-alkali syndrome), hypervitaminosis D
Other endocrine	Hyperthyroidism, Addison, acromegaly
Granulomatous disease	Sarcoidosis, primarily
Paget disease	Only if the patient is immobilized

Secondary hyperparathyroidism refers to the excessive secretion of PTH in response to hypocalcemia of any cause. Secondary hyperparathyroidism is most commonly seen in chronic renal failure but may also be seen in vitamin D deficiency. The calcium is low, while the PTH is normal to high.

Phosphate is retained by the kidneys in this setting, creating the potential for tissue deposition of calcium salts. This persistent hyperparathyroid state produces marked activation of osteoclasts in bone, leading to so-called brown tumors of bone (renal osteodystrophy). Persistent states of secondary hyperparathyroidism lead to hypertrophy of the parathyroids. Tertiary hyperparathyroidism may occur after long periods of secondary hyperparathyroidism. It is caused by the development of autonomous parathyroid function following a period of persistent parathyroid stimulation. It may occur in the post-renal transplant period.

Malignancy may produce hypercalcemia either with or without bone metastases; the latter phenomenon is often called humoral hypercalcemia of malignancy. A common mediator of this syndrome is PTH-related protein (PTHrP), which is secreted by some normal epithelia (squamous epithelium and lactating breast epithelium) and certain tumors (squamous cell carcinoma of lung, head & neck, skin, cervix, and esophagus, breast carcinoma, T cell lymphoma). It is responsible for many cases of so-called humoral hypercalcemia of malignancy. PTHrP is encoded by a gene on chromosome 12 and has homology with the amino-terminal, biologically active component of PTH. Current immunoassays for PTH do not detect PTHrP, and PTHrP must be specifically assayed.

Hypervitaminosis D results from long term ingestion of vitamin supplements (recall that A, D, E, and K are lipophilic vitamins that, when taken in excess, are not readily excreted). Vitamin D, unlike PTH, enhances reabsorption of both calcium and phosphate by the kidneys, potentially leading to calciphylaxis. The histiocytes of sarcoidal granulomas appear to have the capacity to activate vitamin D to the active form (1,25 di-hydroxy vitamin D) and this may result in hypercalcemia. This phenomenon is rarely seen in other types of granulomatous disease.

Milk-alkali syndrome seems to be making a resurgence, due to high dose calcium supplementation for the prevention of osteoporosis.

The laboratory evaluation of hypercalcemia can be made simple by remembering that the vast majority (80-90%) of cases are the result of hyperparathyroidism and malignancy. Distinguishing these 2 is easiest with clinical correlation and a PTH level, with elevated or "inappropriately" normal PTH associated with hyperparathyroidism and low PTH associated with malignancy.

Assays for PTH, which are immunoassays, are sensitive to particular portions of the PTH molecule. PTH is initially synthesized as an 84 amino acid protein which is subsequently broken down, both within the parathyroid and in the blood, into smaller fragments—amino terminal fragments (PTH-N), a midmolecule fragment (PTH-M), and carboxy terminal fragments (PTH-C) t1.11. N-terminal and intact PTH have biological activity and, like other biologically active hormones, there are mechanisms in place to rapidly clear them from the blood.

t1.11 Forms of parathyroid hormone (PTH)

	Biologic activity	Half life
Intact PTH	+	Short
N-terminal PTH	+	Short
Mid-region PTH	−	Long
C-terminal PTH	−	Long

The secreted 84 amino acid polypeptide, PTH(1-84) and the N-terminal fragments (PTH-N) have the ability to activate the PTH receptor (PTHR-1). These active forms have half lives of ~5 minutes, while the inactive forms, PTH-C and PTH-M, have half lives of 24-36 hours; thus, inactive fragments of PTH make up much of the circulating PTH; the effect is magnified in renal failure, because these inactive fragments are cleared by the kidneys. It has recently become clear that some PTH-C fragments may have biologic activity not mediated through the PTHR-1 receptor; in fact, the activity of these fragments, at high concentration, appears to antagonize those of PTH(1-84).

Thus, the ideal PTH assay would measure PTH(1-84) and PTH-N, without crossreacting with PTH-C and PTH-M. Early assays were somewhat indiscriminate and tended to include C-terminal and mid-fragments in their measurements. This is problematic, because the body makes no special effort to quickly clear these fragments from the blood. First-generation PTH assays displayed substantial crossreactivity. Second-generation of PTH assays are designed to detect PTH(1-84) only and are therefore called "intact" or "whole-molecule" PTH assays. Still, second-generation assays suffer from some crossreactivity with nonintact PTH, chief among which is the fragment, PTH(7-84). This crossreactivity is particularly problematic in patients with renal failure. Third-generation assays have been developed which demonstrate enhanced specificity for PTH(1-84). The clinical utility of third-generation assays appears to be highest in patients with renal failure.

Lastly, the rapid in vivo degradation of PTH(1-84) provides the opportunity for this assay to be used for intraoperative assessment of the adequacy of parathyroid gland resection. Baseline PTH is determined on the morning of surgery. Approximately 10 minutes after the surgeon has removed the abnormal parathyroid gland(s), blood is collected for PTH measurement. A decrease of 50% or more is thought to correlate with adequate surgical resection. If PTH levels fail to fall adequately, then this suggests residual hyperfunctioning parathyroid tissue.

Hypocalcemia t1.12

Hypocalcemia causes neurologic excitability, manifesting as perioral tingling (paresthesia), muscle spasms, and hyperreflexia. Classic findings include Chvostek sign and Trousseau sign. Chvostek sign is elicited by tapping on the face at a point just below the zygomatic arch and anterior to the ear (over the facial nerve), which produces ipsilateral facial twitching in hypocalcemia. Some patients normally express a Chvostek sign, so experienced surgeons will check for this preoperatively before thyroid or parathyroid surgery. Trousseau sign consists of carpopedal spasm elicited by inflating a blood pressure cuff for several minutes; it is painful for the patient. In the ECG, hypocalcemia produces lengthening of the QT interval, low voltage T waves, and dysrhythmias. Severe hypocalcemia may cause laryngeal spasm, tetany, and respiratory arrest.

t1.12 Differential diagnosis of hypocalcemia

Etiology	Notes
Hypoproteinemia	Due to low albumin; ionized calcium usually normal
Chronic renal failure	Hyperphosphatemia present
Drugs	Heparin, glucagon, osmotic diuretics, loop diuretics (eg, furosemide), aminoglycosides, mithramycin
Hypoparathyroidism	Post-surgical, hypomagnesemia, DiGeorge syndrome, autoimmune
Medullary thyroid carcinoma	Rarely affects serum calcium
Hyperphosphatemia	Calcium chelation
Vitamin D deficiency	Most patients with vitamin D deficiency have normal calcium levels
Pancreatitis	Extensive calcium deposition
Massive transfusion	Citrate

Primary hypoparathyroidism is most often iatrogenic, from surgical removal of the parathyroids. It is characterized by a low PTH and low calcium, with normal or increased phosphate. $1,25(OH)_2D$ levels are also low, due to the dependence upon PTH for production. Hereditary hypoparathyroidism can occur as an isolated anomaly or in association with the DiGeorge syndrome.

Hypomagnesemia is capable of suppressing PTH secretion by the parathyroid gland. In fact, mild transient decreases in serum magnesium actually cause increased PTH secretion, an attempt on the part of the parathyroids to maintain the balance of divalent cations. However, persistent or marked hypomagnesemia inhibits PTH secretion, leading to hypoparathyroidism.

Acid-base disorders
Definitions

- Acidemia: arterial pH <7.35.

- Alkalemia: arterial pH >7.45.

- Acidosis: a condition tending to lower the pH (the pH may not actually be lowered, because of compensation).

- Alkalosis: a condition tending to raise the pH (the pH may not actually be raised, because of compensation).

- Respiratory acidosis: insufficient elimination of CO_2 by the lungs (hypoventilation). The primary change is in CO_2. Compensation involves altered renal handling of bicarbonate (HCO_3^-).

- Respiratory alkalosis: excessive elimination of CO_2 by the lungs (hyperventilation). The primary change is in CO_2. Compensation involves altered renal handling of bicarbonate (HCO_3^-).

- Metabolic acidosis/alkalosis: excessive intake of, excessive production of, or too little renal elimination of an acid or a base. The primary change is in bicarbonate (HCO_3^-). Compensation involves alterations in pulmonary handling of CO_2.

- Simple acid/base disorder: a primary acid-base disturbance and associated compensation.

- Complex acid/base disorder: there is more than one primary acid-base disturbance.

Henderson-Hasselbalch equation

$$pH = pKa + \log(\text{base/acid})$$

In normal individuals

- pH = 7.4
- pKa = 6.1.
- The base, bicarbonate $(HCO_3^-) = 24$ mol/L
- The acid, carbonic acid $(H_2CO_3) = 0.03 \times PaCO_2 = 0.03 \times 40$ mm Hg = 1.2 mol/L

Thus,

$$pH = 6.1 + \log(\text{bicarb}/[0.03 \times PaCO_2])$$

While the equation looks complicated, note that what it expresses is a relatively simple dependence of pH upon the ratio of bicarbonate to $PaCO_2$. pH varies with the ratio of bicarbonate (in the numerator) to $PaCO_2$ (in the denominator). If bicarbonate is consumed, then pH falls, producing metabolic acidosis; in response, hyperventilation reduces the denominator by eliminating CO_2, bringing the pH back towards normal.

Methods

The pulse oximeter measures hemoglobin oxygen saturation directly, by measuring the absorbance of transdermally transmitted light. It emits 2 wavelengths of light, one that deoxyhemoglobin absorbs, and one that oxyhemoglobin absorbs.

A cooximeter is a spectrophotometric device that measures the absorbance of multiple wavelengths of light. It may be either a separate instrument or cooximetry functionality may be included in the blood gas analyzer. It is able to directly measure the proportions of oxyhemoglobin, deoxyhemoglobin, methemoglobin, and carboxyhemoglobin. Oxygen saturation is then computed as the ratio of oxyhemoglobin to total. Cooximetry has great utility in critical care settings, where pulse oximeters may fail for numerous reasons (not the least of which is poor peripheral perfusion at the location where the device is attached). Furthermore, when the patient has undergone red cell transfusion and levels of 2,3-DPG are low in the transfused cells, traditional ABG calculations of oxygen saturation can be misleading. Whenever oxygen variants (eg, methemoglobinemia) are present, cooximetry is superior to other modalities. Cooximetry is the method of choice for detecting carbon monoxide poisoning. It should be noted that even cooximetry may fail to detect sulfhemoglobinemia.

Traditional ABG (arterial blood gas) analyzers use a pH electrode, CO_2 electrode, and O_2 electrode to measure pH, PCO_2, and PO_2 directly. They usually also derive a percent saturation of oxygen through a calculation that *assumes a normal hemoglobin oxygen affinity*. Results of ABG testing must be interpreted with caution, particularly one is not certain of its source. At the bedside, an arterial source is generally assured by the rapid, pulsatile flow of arterial blood into the syringe. Otherwise, the PO_2 may be used to deduce the source; PO_2 in the range of 30-40 mm Hg is compatible with venous blood, except in the extremely hypoxemic patient.

Classifying an acid-base disorder

1. Determine the primary abnormality.

- Acidosis:
  - o Metabolic acidosis: pH and $[HCO_3]$ go in the same direction (bicarb usually <25 mEq/L)
  - o Respiratory acidosis: pH and $[HCO_3]$ go in opposite directions (PCO_2 usually >44 mm Hg)
- Alkalosis:
  - o Metabolic alkalosis: pH and $[HCO_3]$ go in the same direction (bicarb usually >25 mEq/L)
  - o Respiratory alkalosis: pH and $[HCO_3]$ go in opposite directions (PCO_2 usually <40 mm Hg)

2. Determine if the compensation is appropriate

- Metabolic acidosis: for each 1.3 mEq fall in $[HCO_3]$, the PCO_2 decreases by 1.0 mm Hg.
- Metabolic alkalosis: for each 0.6 mEq rise in $[HCO_3]$, the PCO_2 increases by 1.0 mm Hg.
- Respiratory alkalosis or acidosis:
  - o Acute: for each 1 mm Hg change in PCO_2, the $[HCO_3]$ changes by 0.1 in the same direction
  - o Chronic: for each 1 mm Hg change in PCO_2, the $[HCO_3]$ changes by 0.4 in the same direction

3. Differentials

- Metabolic acidosis: Disorders are categorized by presence or absence of anion gap t1.13 and osmolal gap t1.14.
  - o Calculate the anion gap

$$\text{Anion gap} = [Na] - [Cl] - [HCO_3]$$

  - o Normal is <12. In nonanion gap acidosis, the chloride level is often elevated (hyperchloremic metabolic acidosis). Note that a low anion gap is uncommon, but may be caused by hypoalbuminemia and paraproteinemia.

t1.13 Metabolic acidosis

Increased anion gap (≥12)	Normal anion gap (<12)
Methanol	Diarrhea
Uremia	Recovery phase diabetic ketoacidosis
Ketoacidosis (diabetic, EtOH, starvation)	Ureterosigmoidostomy
Paraldehyde	NH_4Cl
Lactic acidosis	Carbonic anhydrase inhibitors
Ethylene glycol	Total parenteral nutrition
Salicylate	Renal tubular acidosis

t1.14 Increased osmolal gap

With metabolic acidosis	Methanol
	Propylene glycol
	Ethylene glycol
	Paraldehyde
	Ethanol (sometimes)
Without metabolic acidosis	Isopropanol
	Glycerol
	Sorbitol
	Mannitol
	Acetone
	Ethanol (sometimes)

o Calculate the osmolal gap

Osmolal gap = $osm_{measured} - (2[Na] + [glucose]/18 + [BUN]/2.8)$

o In this form of the calculation, [Na] is in mEq/L, [glucose] is in mg/dL, and [BUN] is in mg/dL. When international units (mmol/L) are used, the osmolality is calculated by $osm_{measured} - 2[Na] - [glucose] - [BUN]$. Normal osmolal gap is <10.

- Metabolic alkalosis: Disorders are categorized by chloride responsiveness or resistance t1.15.

t1.15 Metabolic alkalosis

Chloride responsive (UCl<10)	Chloride resistant (UCl>10)
Diuretic therapy	Hyperaldosteronism
Vomiting	Cushing syndrome
Nasogastric tube suction	Exogenous steroids
Villous adenoma	Licorice (glycyrrhizin)
Carbenicillin	Bartter syndrome
Contraction alkalosis	Milk-alkali syndrome

- Respiratory acidosis results from any impairment to ventilation. Causes include those directly affecting the lungs (airway obstruction, alveolar infiltrates, perfusion defects) and those affecting the neuromuscular support of breathing.

- Respiratory alkalosis most often results from hypoxemia, in which compensatory hyperventilation leads to hypocapnia. A variety of other stimuli can lead to hyperventilation and hypercapnia, including anxiety, central nervous system insults, pregnancy, and a variety of medications.

Renal function
Renal function tests
Blood urea nitrogen (BUN)

There are several nonprotein nitrogenous compounds in the blood, collectively termed nonprotein nitrogen (NPN). These include urea, individual amino acids, urate, creatinine, and ammonia. These compounds are principally derived from the breakdown of protein and nucleic acids.

Urea, the end-product of the urea cycle, is the major component of NPN. Urea nitrogen is measured by first hydrolyzing urea to create ammonium ions with the enzyme urease, then quantifying the resulting ammonium ions by any one of a number of methods. The urea concentration is then calculated from the measured urea nitrogen. Methods to directly measure urea are also available.

Urea is freely filtered and partially reabsorbed by the nephron; this reabsorption has the consequence that BUN always slightly underestimates GFR. Reabsorption increases with hypovolemia; thus BUN underestimates GFR even more in hypovolemic states. An increase in BUN is called azotemia, and uremia refers to high BUN and its toxic effects.

Creatinine & GFR calculations

The creatinine concentration was classically determined, and is still often determined, by the Jaffe reaction—alkaline picrate forms a colored complex with creatinine. Alternative enzymatic (using creatinase) and colorimetric assays are available. The serum creatinine varies inversely with the GFR. Creatinine is an endogenously produced substance that passes freely through the glomerulus. A small amount is secreted by the tubules, and the quantity of tubular secretion increases with increasing serum creatinine concentration. Thus, at all serum concentrations, creatinine slightly overestimates GFR. The simplest way to calculate GFR is based upon the creatinine clearance:

$$Cl_{Cr} = \frac{U_{Cr}}{P_{Cr}} \times \frac{V_{Ur}}{time\ (minutes)}$$

U_{Cr} is urine creatinine (mg/dL), V_{Ur} is volume of urine (mL), typically collected for 24 hours or 1,440 minutes), and P_{Cr} is plasma creatinine (mg/dL). Units for Cl_{Cr} are in mL/min, with 80-120 mL/min being a typical normal range.

However, this formula is overly simplistic. While it is true that the greatest influence on serum creatinine is the GFR, and serum creatinine within an individual patient varies little from day to day, 2 phenomena conspire to weaken the suitability of the clearance formula for clinical use. First, the inverse relationship between GFR and creatinine is nonlinear. That is, mild to moderate degrees of GFR impairment do not cause appreciable increases in the creatinine concentration. At a certain point, however, when GFR is about half normal, creatinine rises precipitously and begins to linearly reflect changes in GFR. Second, there are nonglomerular influences upon creatinine. The serum creatinine concentration is increased by muscle mass, muscle activity, muscle injury (trauma, surgery), and protein intake. It tends to decrease with age, and it is influenced by race, sex, and numerous medications.

These considerations led to the development of formulas to calculate the estimated GFR (eGFR) from plasma creatinine, taking into account such factors as age and body weight. The Modification of Diet in Renal Disease (MDRD) Study equation is the most widely used formula. The MDRD equation has been studied and validated in adult Caucasian and African American populations with impaired kidney function (GFR <60) between the ages of 18 and 70 years. It has not been validated for use in pregnant women, children, the elderly, the acutely ill hospitalized patient, or those with essentially normal GFR. The MDRD equation requires knowledge of the serum creatinine (S_{cr}), patient age (in years), sex, and race (African American or not African American). The originally published MDRD equation is recommended for labs using a creatinine assay that has not been calibrated to be traceable to an isotope dilution mass spectrometry (IDMS) reference method. A different formula is recommended for labs with creatinine assays that have been calibrated to be traceable to IDMS (check package insert or contact manufacturer). Below are the MDRD equations:

Original (nontraceable), S_{Cr} in mg/dL

$$eGFR = 186 \times (S_{Cr})^{-1.154} \times age^{-0.203}$$

Traceable, S_{cr} in mg/dL:

$$eGFR = 175 \times (S_{Cr})^{-1.154} \times age^{-0.203}$$

The result is multiplied by 0.742 if the patient is female, and by 1.210 if African American. The units for eGFR are given as mL/min/1.73 m^2. The National Kidney Foundation recommends that eGFRs >60 mL/min/1.73 m^2 be reported simply as ">60 mL/min/1.73 m^2" rather than as a specific number.

A new equation, the Chronic Kidney Disease Epidemiology Collaboration (CKD-EPI) equation, has been recommended in several new guidelines and is increasingly used in place of the MDRD equation. It gives a more accurate eGFR, particularly at higher GFR levels. The CKD-EPI equation uses the same variables as the MDRD equation, and the result can be reported across the full range of eGFR.

BUN/creatinine ratio

Because of the ways that the renal handling of BUN and creatinine differ, useful information may be obtained by comparing these 2 analytes. The normal BUN/creatinine ratio is ~10:1. When the BUN/creatinine ratio is increased, frequently to >20:1, this is suggestive of renal hypoperfusion (due to, eg, hypovolemia, hypotension), and is termed *prerenal azotemia*. This occurs due to the increase in BUN reabsorption in states of decreased renal perfusion. A decreased BUN/creatinine ratio may be observed in some cases of intrarenal disease due to the decrease in BUN reabsorption occurring with renal tubular damage.

Cystatin C

Cystatin C is a cysteine protease inhibitor produced by nearly all cells in the body. It is freely filtered by the glomerulus and is completely reabsorbed by the proximal tubule. It has demonstrated superiority over serum creatinine for estimating the GFR and appears to be less dependant on age, sex, or muscle mass.

It has been known for some time that chronic kidney disease, as estimated by serum creatinine, is a risk factor for death from cardiovascular causes. In some studies, cystatin C has been found to be a stronger predictor of cardiovascular mortality than creatinine. Further, cystatin C elevation may be an early indicator of evolving chronic kidney disease.

Urine protein & urine albumin

Normal proteinuria does not exceed 150 mg/day. This consists mainly of Tamm-Horsfall protein and minute amounts of albumin. The normal glomerulus filters protein based on size and charge. Some proteins are small enough to be freely filtered by the glomerulus, but most of these filtered proteins are reabsorbed in the proximal tubules. Albumin, a small protein, does not normally freely cross the glomerular membrane.

Significant proteinuria is usually defined as exceeding 300 mg/day. Definitive assessment of proteinuria has traditionally been based upon a 24-hour urine collection. The urine protein concentration of a random urine sample ("spot urine") can be misleading, because protein handling by the kidney varies throughout the day. But when compared to a simultaneous creatinine determination, the spot urine protein measurement has greater meaning. In fact, the urine protein:creatinine ratio is a useful test for significant proteinuria and appears to be as good (if not better considering the host of practical problems with 24 hour urine collections) as the 24 hour urine for excluding significant proteinuria.

The urine dipstick result (1+ to 3+) typically demonstrates good correlation with the spot urine protein concentration; however, the urine dipstick test is most sensitive to albumin and relatively insensitive to other proteins. In addition, it is not sufficiently sensitive to detect microalbuminuria and it is not sensitive to globulins or Bence Jones proteins. The lower limit of detection of the urine dipstick test for albumin is ~30 mg/dL.

The microalbumin assay is capable of detecting as little as 0.3 mg/dL of albumin. Significant microalbuminuria is currently defined in terms of the albumin:creatinine ratio of a spot urine rather than a 24-hour timed urine collection. The albumin:creatinine ratio is reported in units of mg/g (protein:creatinine ratio is reported as mg/mg, a possible source of confusion). Microalbumin measurement is commonly performed to assess for the presence of early onset nephropathy in diabetic patients. It has also been demonstrated to be a generalized marker of cardiovascular disease.

The urine β_2-microglobulin and lysozyme assays can be used to detect tubular dysfunction. These proteins are freely filtered by the glomerulus and then completely reabsorbed by the normally functioning proximal convoluted tubule. Their presence in urine suggests tubular dysfunction. Urine lysozyme levels may also be elevated in a variety of myelomonocytic leukemias.

Laboratory screening for chronic kidney disease

The current recommendation of the National Kidney Foundation is annual testing for those at high risk for chronic kidney disease. High-risk individuals are those who have

- diabetes mellitus
- hypertension
- a family history of renal disease

Recommended screening for high risk groups includes an eGFR and a microalbuminuria screen (urine albumin:creatinine ratio), where albumin is measured by a microalbumin assay.

Chronic kidney disease is defined by either

1. GFR <60 mL/minute/1.73 m^2 of body surface area
2. albuminuria for 3 or more consecutive months

The degree (or stage) of chronic kidney disease is categorized as follows

- stage 1: kidney damage (albuminuria) without decreased GFR (GFR>90 mL/min/1.73 m^2)
- stage 2: kidney damage with a mild decrease in GFR (60-89 mL/min/1.73 m^2)
- stage 3: moderate decrease in GFR (30-59 mL/min/1.73 m^2)
- stage 4: severe decrease in GFR (15-29 mL/min/1.73 m^2)
- stage 5: renal failure (GFR <15 mL/min/1.73 m^2 or dialysis-dependence)

Laboratory evaluation in acute renal failure

There is no broadly accepted definition of acute renal failure (ARF), but the term implies a rapid and sustained decrement in renal function. One of the earliest problems encountered is the distinction of acute renal failure from an initial presentation of chronic renal failure in a patient with a poorly documented medical history. Patients with chronic renal failure may have hypocalcemia and accompanying secondary hyperparathyroidism and hyperphosphatemia from impaired phosphate clearance. In addition, they commonly demonstrate normocytic anemia, and broad waxy casts in their urine. Renal ultrasound usually demonstrates small kidneys with cortical atrophy.

The causes of ARF are categorized as prerenal, renal, or postrenal t1.16, t1.17. Prerenal ARF is the result of decreased renal perfusion, leading to a physiologic reduction in glomerular filtration rate (GFR). A sustained benefit by expansion of intravascular volume with colloid is characteristic; fluid replacement ("fluid challenge") is therefore both a therapeutic and a diagnostic maneuver in this setting. Postrenal ARF is caused by an obstruction of the renal collecting system. Intrarenal causes of ARF produce injury to the nephron (glomeruli, tubules, vessels, or interstitium). The most common cause of intrarenal ARF is acute tubular necrosis (ATN), and the most common causes of ATN are ischemia and nephrotoxins. Acute glomerulonephritis (AGN) may also cause intrarenal ARF.

t1.16 Acute renal failure (ARF): prerenal vs renal

Parameter	Prerenal ARF	Renal ARF
BUN/creatinine ratio	>20:1	<20:1
Urine specific gravity	High (>1.020)	Low (<1.010)
Urine osmolarity	High (>500 mOsm/kg)	Low (300-500)
FE Na	<1%	>2%
FE urea	<35%	>35%

t1.17 Causes of acute renal failure

Prerenal	Renal	Postrenal
Hypovolemia	Acute tubular necrosis (contrast media, aminoglycosides, amphotericin, tumor lysis syndrome, rhabdomyolysis)	Bladder outlet obstruction (prostatism)
CHF		Bilateral ureteral obstruction (tumor, retroperitoneal fibrosis)
Cirrhosis	Acute glomerular injury (penicillamine, cyclosporine, acute glomerulonephritis, thrombotic microangiopathy, malignant hypertension)	
NSAIDs		
ACE inhibitors		
Vasopressors	Acute tubulointerstitial nephritis (NSAIDs)	
	Vasculitis	

In addition to a battery of laboratory tests, a renal ultrasound may be performed to exclude hydronephrosis, which is indicative of postrenal ARF. Initial and serial measurements of serum BUN and creatinine are essential. In addition, there must be serial monitoring of variables that may indicate a need for dialysis initiation. Indications for dialysis include refractory volume overload, hyperkalemia, metabolic acidosis, end-organ damage due to uremia (eg, pericarditis), or BUN >100 g/dL. Urine volume is monitored.

Most cases of renal failure are oliguric (<400 mL/day of urine output). Nonoliguric renal failure may occur, especially in drug induced nephrotoxicity and interstitial nephritis, but rarely in prerenal ARF. BUN/Cr ratio, urine osmolarity, urine specific gravity, and fractional excretion of sodium (FENa) are helpful for distinguishing renal from prerenal causes. The FENa is almost always low (<1%) in prerenal ARF, the exception being the patient who has been given diuretics or who has glycosuria, in whom the fractional excretion of urea can be a useful alternative.

Urinalysis provides important information in renal failure. A lack of findings or isolated hyaline casts suggests prerenal ARF. Dysmorphic red blood cells and red blood cell casts suggest glomerulonephritis. Granular casts suggest acute tubular necrosis, glomerulonephritis, or interstitial nephritis. White blood cell casts are suggestive of pyelonephritis while the presence of eosinophils suggests acute allergic interstitial nephritis.

Hepatorenal syndrome

Hepatorenal syndrome (HRS) is the development of progressive renal impairment in patients with severe end-stage liver disease in the absence of another identifiable cause of renal disease (eg, shock, bacterial sepsis, nephrotoxin exposure). HRS has an incidence of ~5%/admission for decompensated cirrhosis, and ~50% over the course of cirrhosis. HRS in most instances is not present at admission but arises following profound fluid shifts such as occur in the treatment of ascites. It is thought to be due to dysregulation of renal blood flow.

Spontaneous bacterial peritonitis (SBP) is a common cause of renal failure in the cirrhotic patient, and must be excluded. Also common in hospital admissions for cirrhosis are the use of nephrotoxic agents (aminoglycosides, NSAIDs, radiocontrast dyes).

The renal biopsy is essentially normal in HRS, but an abnormal biopsy must be interpreted cautiously—many patients with cirrhosis due to hepatitis viruses have an associated glomerulonephritis, and cirrhosis can itself lead to an IgA-like nephropathy.

Nephrogenic systemic fibrosis

Nephrogenic systemic fibrosis is a systemic fibrosing disease affecting patients with renal failure, often in association with the administration of gadolinium-based radiocontrast agents. Initially described in the dermatology literature as "nephrogenic fibrosing dermopathy," the disorder is now known to be systemic, affecting the dura, heart, lungs, kidneys, and connective tissue. To prevent this disease, routine pregadolinium measurement of BUN and creatinine, at least in high risk patients (age >60, established renal disease, lupus, diabetes, myeloma), is recommended.

Laboratory tests in pregnancy
Amniotic fluid bilirubin (ΔOD 450)

The concentration of unconjugated bilirubin in amniotic fluid is used as a reflection of the severity of fetal hemolysis, especially in the setting of hemolytic disease of the fetus/newborn. The amniotic fluid bilirubin concentration can be assessed by scanning spectrophotometry. The maximal absorbance of bilirubin is at 450 nm.

Amniotic fluid should be obtained with minimal blood contamination, because the tail of the absorbance peak of oxyhemoglobin at 410 nm can affect the magnitude of the peak at 450 nm; a variable quantity of blood is nearly always present, however, and various means of correcting for its effect exist. The specimen should be protected from light (a brown plastic tube is usually provided in the amniocentesis tray), because bilirubin is rapidly degraded by it.

A scanning spectrophotometer is used to measure absorbances at intervals from 340-560 nm. On semilog paper, the absorbances are plotted against wavelength. A straight line is drawn from the point at 350 nm to the point at 550 nm. This line reflects the theoretical plot if there were no pigments in the fluid. The difference in optical density between the line and the actual absorbance at 450 nm is the "ΔOD 450" which reflects the bilirubin concentration.

The ΔOD 450 is then plotted against the estimated gestational age (EGA) on a Liley chart or similar nomogram to determine the degree of fetal hemolysis and assess fetal risk.

Human chorionic gonadotropin

Human chorionic gonadotropin (hCG) is a glycoprotein heterodimer composed of an α and a β chain. hCG is produced by the normal placenta and by certain tumors; a small quantity may be produced by the pituitary gland, particularly during menopause. The α subunit is identical to that found in thyroid stimulating hormone (TSH), follicle stimulating hormone (FSH), and luteinizing hormone (LH), while the β subunit is unique.

False negative hCG can occur with urine testing, especially if the urine is dilute. When there is a high suspicion of pregnancy, or when certainty is required, a negative urine hCG should be confirmed with a serum hCG test. In the presence of a negative serum test, pregnancy is exceedingly unlikely.

False positive hCG may be encountered. Most often this is the result of heterophile antibody interference. When heterophile interference is suspected, it can be helpful to repeat the measurement on a different analyzer, pretreat with heterophile binding reagent, or to run serial dilutions. Heterophile-associated false positive hCG is nonlinear when serially diluted. Lastly, urine hCG is usually negative in the presence of false positive hCG. A negative urine hCG, when the quantitative serum hCG is >50 IU/L, suggests false positive serum hCG.

True positive, low level hCG, not associated with heterophile antibody, pregnancy, or active gestational trophoblastic disease, is a recognized clinical phenomenon. Some of the patients in this group have been diagnosed as having so-called quiescent gestational trophoblastic disease; that is, despite having had an identified hydatidiform mole or other gestational trophoblastic disease that was appropriately treated with evacuation and/or chemotherapy, they are found to have persistent low levels of hCG for long periods of time. No demonstrable persistent lesion is found, and multiple rounds of chemotherapy and/or surgery do nothing to alter the hCG. Rarely, pituitary production is the source of the hCG; this may be found in 1 of 2 scenarios

1. the normal very low level pituitary production of hCG is increased somewhat in perimenopausal women

2. pituitary tumor

In perimenopausal women, an hCG >14 IU/L should raise strong suspicion of an actual pregnancy. In perimenopausal women with hCG <14 IU/L that does not change over time, serum FSH can be used to implicate pituitary hCG production and thereby exclude pregnancy; FSH >45 IU/L in this setting suggests pituitary hCG.

Certain investigations may be warranted to ensure the false nature of the hCG result, including imaging of the uterus, ovaries, lungs, mediastinum, retroperitoneum, and pituitary fossa. Some reports appear to support watchful waiting if no anatomic lesion is identified.

hCG in normal gestation

hCG becomes detectable ~6-8 days following conception (about the time of implantation), when levels are around 10-50 mIU/mL. The hCG concentration doubles roughly every 48 hours until ~10 weeks. It peaks near the end of the first trimester; thereafter it decreases gradually and by early second trimester plateaus. The quantity of hCG in normal pregnancy varies widely.

hCG may be higher than usual in pregnancies with multiple gestation, polyhydramnios, eclampsia, and erythroblastosis fetalis. After delivery, hCG normally remains detectable for 2 weeks. The disappearance of hCG after term pregnancy is best viewed as triphasic, with rapid, medium, and slow half lives of 3.6 hours, 18 hours, and 53 hours.

hCG in ectopic pregnancy

Ectopic pregnancy is the most common cause of maternal death in the 1st trimester. It usually presents with abdominal pain or mild vaginal bleeding (spotting) in a woman of childbearing age who may or may not know she is pregnant.

Ectopic pregnancy is defined as implantation outside the uterine cavity. The vast majority (>95%) occur in the fallopian tube, the remainder in the ovary, abdomen, or cornu. Heterotopic pregnancy, in which there is simultaneous intrauterine and ectopic implantation, was once exceedingly rare; however, in those treated with fertility-enhancing agents the incidence is approaching 1%.

A single β-hCG level alone cannot differentiate between ectopic and intrauterine pregnancy. However, if the normal hCG dynamic is not seen, this suggests an abnormal pregnancy. Specifically, if serum hCG does not rise ≥66% in 48 hours, or if the hCG falls during this time, this suggests an abnormal pregnancy (either ectopic pregnancy or nonviable intrauterine pregnancy). However, a normal rate of rise can be seen in 20% of ectopic pregnancies, and an abnormal rate of rise can be seen in 20% of normal intrauterine pregnancies (IUP).

Further elucidation relies on ultrasound demonstration of an intrauterine gestational sac. With transabdominal ultrasound, a gestational sac should be detectable when the hCG exceeds 6,000 mIU/mL. When the hCG is >1400 mIU/mL, the absence of an IUP detectable by transvaginal ultrasound is 90% specific for an ectopic. The detection of an IUP virtually excludes an ectopic, except in the case of heterotopic pregnancy which may be a consideration in the setting of fertility enhancement. The absence of an IUP beyond these hCG thresholds is highly specific for an ectopic pregnancy.

A useful adjunct can be the serum progesterone level. Serum progesterone >25 ng/mL virtually assures an IUP. Levels <5 ng/mL are strongly predictive of an abnormal pregnancy. However, many patients fall somewhere between these thresholds, reducing the utility of the measurement.

In summary, the combined clinical and laboratory approach is as follows. If a woman of childbearing age presents with abdominal pain, vaginal bleeding, or hemodynamic instability, a pregnancy test should be performed. The unstable patient may need rapid surgical intervention following a positive hCG and negative ultrasound for IUP. In this case, Rh status should be determined to guide Rho(D) immune globulin therapy. The stable patient with a positive hCG should then have a quantitative hCG performed while ultrasonography is performed. If an IUP is identified, then a threatened abortion is likely. If ultrasound evidence of an ectopic is found, then ablation with either surgical intervention or methotrexate is indicated. When neither definite IUP nor definite ectopic is found, what happens next depends upon the quantitative hCG level. If above the threshold where IUP should be visible, then the patient should be considered at high risk for ectopic pregnancy with the differential diagnosis including a completed spontaneous abortion.

After removal of an ectopic pregnancy, hCG normally remains detectable for several weeks. Levels must be monitored to exclude persistent trophoblastic tissue.

hCG in spontaneous abortion

Serial quantitative hCGs demonstrate an abnormal rate of change as in ectopic pregnancy. At this point, either an IUP is visible by transvaginal ultrasound, or spontaneous passage of tissue has occurred. After spontaneous abortion, hCG remains detectable for 4-6 weeks.

hCG in gestational trophoblastic disease (GTD)

Women with GTD usually produce a greater amount of hCG than normal gestations; and serial quantitative hCG shows an abnormal doubling time. Furthermore, average hCG levels are higher in complete moles than partial moles

In actual practice, most partial moles are diagnosed based upon the histological features of uterine contents. In contrast, most complete moles are diagnosed clinically. Complete moles have a characteristic clinical presentation, including uterine enlargement out of proportion for the gestational age, vaginal bleeding, hypertension, absence of fetal heart tones, and a characteristic ultrasound. Both types of molar pregnancy must be monitored for

1. persistence

2. the development of malignant trophoblastic disease

The risk of malignancy is <5% for partial moles and 20% for complete moles.

After evacuation of a molar pregnancy, hCG levels must be monitored weekly until undetectable for 3 consecutive weeks. hCG is then measured monthly for 1 year. After evacuation of an uncomplicated molar pregnancy, hCG remains detectable for up to 10 weeks. As long as hCG is falling, there is no need for intervention. If the hCG plateaus or rises, then persistent GTD is suspected. Most often this is an indication for chemotherapy following a metastatic workup.

Prenatal screening for trisomy & neural tube defects

An invasive procedure—amniocentesis or chorionic villus sampling—is required for confirmation of fetal trisomy. Unfortunately, such procedures carry a risk for fetal loss. Screening tests are used in an effort to limit invasive testing to only those women at high risk. When discussing these tests with clinicians and patients, the distinction between screening tests and confirmatory tests must be emphasized.

The original screening test for trisomy 21 and trisomy 18 was maternal age. The overall risk for having an affected neonate is 1:700, but the risk increases with maternal age, such that women who are 35 or older at the time of delivery have a risk of ~1:270. Nevertheless, the vast majority of pregnancies occur in younger women, such that most trisomies occur in women <35.

For decades, the approach consisted of offering invasive testing to all women over the age of 35 years and to offer non-invasive screening to younger women, with invasive testing offered to those with high risk serum findings. Based on 2007 ACOG recommendations, all women, regardless of age, should be offered noninvasive screening.

Initial panels, such as the "triple screen," consisted of hCG, AFP, & unconjugated estriol (uE) performed on maternal serum drawn during the 2nd trimester, ideally around 18 weeks. The sensitivity of this panel for Down syndrome is 70%, and the triple screen is no longer considered adequate for screening.

Available approaches to screening

The "quad screen" combines hCG, AFP, & uE with the dimeric inhibin A (DIA). Unlike the analytes of the triple screen, the concentration of DIA is fairly stable throughout the 2nd trimester. Risk is calculated based upon these analytes and maternal age. The improved performance of the Quad screen comes mainly from amelioration of the effects of inaccurate gestational age which plague the triple screen. The sensitivity of this panel for Down syndrome is ~78%.

The "first trimester test" is performed between 11-13 weeks. It consists of hCG, pregnancy associated plasma protein A (PAPP-A), and ultrasound assessment of nuchal fold translucency (NT) thickness (increased in Down syndrome). When combined with maternal age, the overall sensitivity of the first trimester test is 83%.

The "serum integrated screen" combines 1st and 2nd trimester serum testing. PAPP-A and hCG are measured in the 1st trimester, ideally between weeks 10-13; later, a 2nd trimester measurement of AFP, uE, and DIA is made, and the data combined. When combined with maternal age, the sensitivity for Down syndrome is ~85%. If combined with sonographic measurement of nuchal fold thickness (the "full integrated screen"), the sensitivity can be improved to 88%.

A "sequential screen" is essentially an integrated screen in which a risk is initially reported based upon the first trimester results if high (>1:25); if the first trimester results do not indicate high risk, then the risk is reported based upon the integrated results.

Analytes & risk calculation

Maternal age was the first parameter by which risk of Down syndrome was assessed. It is a powerful marker of Down syndrome risk, and maternal age remains a critical variable in the calculation of risk. The serum markers that are used in this context change with gestational age; the concentrations of these markers are often therefore expressed as multiples of median (MoM). The MoM values are combined with risk based upon maternal age to calculate combined risk.

The risk calculation begins with the risk based upon maternal age at delivery, derived from epidemiologic studies. Next, a likelihood ratio for each analyte's MoM is determined, based upon clinical studies. These are multiplied by the age-associated risk to arrive at an adjusted risk. Adjustments are made for maternal weight, race, and diabetes. Lastly, each laboratory applies a risk cutoff to report the screen as "positive"or "negative." Cutoffs vary, but most often are equal to the a priori risk of a 35 year old woman; ie, 1:270.

α-fetoprotein (AFP) is the most abundant plasma protein found in the fetus. Maternal serum AFP (MSAFP) rises progressively during the first and second trimesters. Adjustments to the MSAFP interpretation are routinely made for maternal weight, race, number of fetuses, and maternal diabetes. Increased maternal weight can have a dilutional effect on the AFP, providing a falsely low value. Levels tend to be higher in multiple gestations. MSAFP is >2.5 MoM) in >80% of pregnancies complicated by neural tube defect (NTD). Values >2.0 MoM are considered abnormal in maternal diabetes. In twin gestations, MSAFP is considered abnormal only above 4.5 MoM. Conditions associated with increased MSAFP include neural tube defects, omphalocele and gastroschisis, renal anomalies, sacrococcygeal teratoma, cystic hygroma, hydrops fetalis, Turner syndrome, bowel obstruction, twin gestations, wrong gestational age, fetal demise, and fetal-maternal hemorrhage. MSAFP is low in Down syndrome.

Maternal serum hCG is ~2× higher in fetal Down syndrome. Adjustments are typically made for maternal weight, multiple gestation, maternal diabetes, and race.

Fetal Down syndrome is associated with decreased maternal serum unconjugated estriol. uE is a somewhat weakly sensitive to Down syndrome pregnancies but is a very good indicator of trisomy 18 (Edward syndrome), Smith-Lemli-Optiz syndrome (SLOS), and inherited (fetal) deficiencies of steroid sulfatase.

Dimeric inhibin A (DIA) is increased to an average of 1.9 MoM in pregnancies complicated by Down syndrome. What makes DIA such a useful addition to the panel is that, unlike the other analytes in the triple screen, levels of DIA are relatively constant throughout the second trimester testing period, which minimizes the effect of erroneous gestational age estimates.

Estriol is a hormone produced by the placenta from precursors synthesized in the fetal adrenal gland. Throughout the pregnancy, it increases steadily in maternal blood, where it can be measured as unconjugated estriol (uE). Estriol is decreased in pregnancies associated with Down syndrome.

Pregnancy-associated plasma protein A (PAPP-A) levels increase steadily throughout pregnancy. PAPP-A concentrations are reduced in pregnancies complicated by Down syndrome.

Clinical considerations

In pregnant diabetic women, both the uE and hCG are decreased mildly. In pregnant smokers, AFP is increased, while uE and hCG are decreased. Twin gestations are problematic. Down syndrome occurs more frequently in twin than singleton pregnancies—both twinning and Down syndrome increase with maternal age. However, the sensitivity of routine screening in twin pregnancies is just under between 50-70% (better for monozygotic twins, both of which would have Down syndrome, than dizygotic, in which usually only one has Down syndrome).

Trisomy 21 (Down syndrome) has a characteristic pattern of low AFP, low uE, raised hCG, and raised DIA. Trisomy 18 (Edward syndrome) shows a low AFP, hCG, and uE.

Gestations with neural tube defect (NTD) show a pattern of elevated AFP, normal hCG, and low uE. Overall, AFP elevation is detected in 2-3% of gestations; of these, ~10% are due to an actual NTD. If an AFP is borderline elevated (2.5-3.0 MoM) and was obtained early (<18 weeks), there is value in repeating it. Otherwise, an ultrasound is required to confirm gestational age, exclude multiple gestations, look for overt anatomic abnormalities, and exclude fetal demise. Having excluded these possibilities, an amniocentesis may be performed to obtain amniotic fluid for AFP and acetylcholinesterase (AChE) to confirm the diagnosis of a NTD. The sensitivity of AFP screening is ~90%. The sensitivity is worse (~30%) for multiple gestations.

Assessing risk of preterm birth

Preterm labor is defined as regular contractions, with associated cervical change, prior to 37 weeks. Prematurity is the single most important cause of perinatal morbidity and mortality. A test that serves as a predictor of preterm labor would permit appropriate hospitalization and treatment of affected women. Markers which have demonstrated limited utility in this regard include serum estradiol and salivary estriol (both increase before the onset of labor) and screening for bacterial vaginosis (independently associated with preterm labor).

Fetal fibronectin is a protein found normally at the placental fetomaternal interface. Cervicovaginal fluid contains fetal fibronectin protein briefly during early gestation, after which time it is absent until just before labor. Several trials have demonstrated that the absence of fetal fibronectin has very high negative predictive value and can exclude impending preterm birth. A positive result suggests the onset of preterm labor, but the overall positive predictive value is low. Specimens for fetal fibronectin should be collected ideally >24 hours after the last cervical examination or intercourse. The only other test that shows similar performance is transvaginal cervical ultrasound to assess cervical length.

Determination of fetal lung maturity

Assuring fetal lung maturity (FLM) is necessary to avoid respiratory distress syndrome (RDS) in prematurely delivered infants. Fetal lung maturity is generally achieved at around 37 weeks gestation, but a fetus under the stress of a complicated pregnancy produces excess corticosteroid, which has the effect of accelerating FLM.

Assessment of fetal lung maturity is an issue for gestations between 32-38 weeks' gestation. Prior to this time, fetal lung maturity is unlikely. After this time the risk of RDS is low, and FLM testing is generally not indicated except in the presence of poorly controlled maternal diabetes (which has the effect of delaying FLM).

Mature type II pneumocytes produce surfactant, a mixture of phospholipids composed predominantly of lecithin. High lecithin-content surfactant is necessary to protect newborn lungs from RDS. The vast majority of lecithin is disaturated phosphatidylcholine (DSPC), with the remaining lecithin composed of phosphatidylglycerol (PG), phosphatidylinositol (PI), phosphatidylethanolamine (PE), and sphingomyelin.

Uncontaminated amniotic fluid obtained by amniocentesis is the optimal specimen for determination of FLM. Vaginal pool specimens from women with premature rupture of membranes (PROM) should be avoided as should specimens with blood or meconium contamination.

Most tests for FLM are better at predicting maturity than immaturity. Therefore, a mature result by any method is fairly reliable. If an initial result is below the maturity cutoff, therefore a second test by another technique may be warranted.

Lecithin/sphingomyelin (L/S) ratio

Lecithin increases with gestational age, while sphingomyelin remains at a relatively constant 2% of total surfactant phospholipid. Until ~26 weeks, the ratio is around 1:1. After 26 weeks, the L:S ratio increases. The ratio of 2.5:1 is generally taken to indicate fetal lung maturity. Above this threshold, <2% of premature infants will develop RDS.

In pregnancies complicated by maternal diabetes mellitus, a ratio of 2.5:1 is less predictive of fetal lung maturity. In this scenario, the phosphatidylglycerol concentration is a more reliable indicator of FLM. The presence of meconium falsely decreases the L:S ratio. Contamination by blood normalizes the L:S ratio to around 1.5; however, a mature result in the presence of blood is reliable.

The limitations of the L/S ratio include labor intensity, imprecision (CV >20%), and the interferences listed above. It is no longer generally considered the best first-line test.

Phosphatidylglycerol (PG) concentration

Phosphatidylglycerol is first detected around 35-36 weeks. Its presence is indicative of fetal lung maturity. The PG test is unique among the FLM tests in that neither blood nor meconium interfere with it; however PG is a late marker of pulmonary maturity which limits its utility in prematurity. Nevertheless, PG determination may be the best test in contaminated specimens.

Foam stability

When pulmonary surfactant is present in amniotic fluid in sufficient concentration, the fluid is able to form a highly stable film that can support the structure of a foam. The amniotic fluid is serially diluted with ethanol, and the highest concentration of ethanol at which a complete ring of bubbles is seen is the foam stability index (FSI). An FSI >0.47 is considered indicative of fetal lung maturity. This test is rarely used.

Lamellar body count (LBC)

Surfactant lamellar bodies are approximately the size of platelets, and the platelet channel of a cell counter may be used to quantify them. An LBC >50,000/mL is predictive of maturity, but instruments may vary and in-house validation is required.

This test is automated and precise and has become the initial FLM test of choice in many institutions. There are limitations, including blood and meconium contamination. Blood contamination decreases the LBC count, and meconium increases it.

Fluorescence polarization assay (S/A ratio)*

This test is rapid and precise, with a considerably lower coefficient of variation (<5%) than the L/S ratio. Fluorescent polarization measures the ratio of surfactant to albumin (S/A ratio). A fluorescence polarization value <40 mg/g is considered immature. Values >55 mg/g are considered mature.

The test is affected by blood and meconium contamination, and there is a wide grey zone between 40 and 54 mg/g. If there is <0.5% blood contamination, results are unaffected. Greater amounts tend to lower high values and raise low values.

*(The manufacturer no longer supplies reagents for this assay, and it is currently unavailable)

Laboratory evaluation of diseases in pregnancy

Physiologic changes & altered reference ranges in pregnancy

Expected laboratory test changes during pregnancy are listed in t1.18. Serum triglycerides are increased by ~40%, and a low level ketosis is often present. Hemodilution results in decreased albumin, total protein, hematocrit, and hemoglobin. Estrogen causes an increase in transport proteins such as thyroid binding globulin (TBG). GFR is increased; this is thought to be the result of increased blood volume, and it is reflected in decreased BUN and creatinine.

Relative insulin resistance emerges in the early 3rd trimester, reflected in prolonged elevations in serum glucose after meals. Perhaps the most important cause of this change is human placental lactogen (hPL) which has antiinsulin effects similar to growth hormone (GH).

Sodium and potassium remain relatively constant throughout pregnancy. Total calcium levels fall during pregnancy due to physiologic hypoalbuminemia. The ionized calcium level remains unchanged.

t1.18 Common laboratory values in pregnancy

Analyte	Change in pregnancy
Albumin	↓1 g/dL
Calcium (total)	↓10%
Creatinine	↓0.3 mg/dL
Fibrinogen	↑1-2 g/L
Albumin	↓0.5-1 g/dL
BUN	↓50%
Urine protein	Approximately doubles
Hct	↓4-7%
Hgb	↓1.5-2 g/dL

Medical conditions of particular importance in pregnancy

Autoimmune diseases

Though common among women of childbearing age, autoimmune diseases do not profoundly affect the course of most pregnancies. In fact, pregnancy seems to have a palliative effect on some autoimmune diseases, notably rheumatoid arthritis and Graves disease. Both Graves disease and myasthenia gravis are notorious for postpartum exacerbations.

In contrast, systemic lupus erythematosus (SLE) is often exacerbated by pregnancy. The risk of a SLE flare is highest early in pregnancy and during puerperium, with relative quiescence in the latter half of pregnancy. Renal deterioration that occurs in lupus during pregnancy is often irreversible. Mortality is increased in pregnant women with SLE, with deaths occurring as a result of pulmonary hemorrhage (lupus pneumonitis) or other lupus related complications (transverse myelitis, stroke, corticosteroid complications).

Pregnant women with SLE have an increased incidence of pregnancy induced hypertension (PIH). A lupus flare may be difficult to distinguish from pregnancy induced hypertension (PIH), as the features of hypertension, edema, and proteinuria are shared. The treatments are very different (delivery for PIH, corticosteroids for SLE). This distinction may be aided by complement levels (low in SLE flare, normal in PIH).

SLE is a cause of recurrent miscarriage, abortion, and pre-term labor. The lupus anticoagulant is thought to mediate these pregnancy loss effects, and these may occur without SLE. In this regard, the appropriate treatment is anticoagulation, not corticosteroids.

The neonate, too, may be affected by maternal SLE. There is increased incidence of intrauterine growth retardation and pre-term labor. Neonates born to mothers with SLE have a risk of congenital heart block. Transplacental passage of antibodies to SS-A and SS-B (Ro and La) are thought to mediate this complication.

In idiopathic thrombocytopenic purpura (ITP), antibodies can cross the placenta and lead to neonatal thrombocytopenia. It is important to distinguish this from neonatal alloimmune thrombocytopenia (NATP). Life threatening neonatal intracranial hemorrhages are a possible complication.

Genitourinary diseases

Chronic renal disease may be first detected during pregnancy (since proteinuria is routinely tested during pregnancy) or exacerbated by pregnancy. Pregnancy normally has the effect of increasing the creatinine clearance. In addition, a slight increase in normal urinary protein excretion is expected, up to 300 mg/day. This increase in GFR is somewhat protective early in pregnancy, with most profound exacerbations of underlying renal disease occurring during the third trimester. The greatest risk posed to the pregnant woman with chronic renal disease is significant hypertension.

Pregnant women are at increased risk for urinary tract infection (UTI), and UTIs developing during pregnancy have a high rate of progression to pyelonephritis. Therefore, asymptomatic bacteriuria is dealt with more aggressively in pregnant women. Asymptomatic bacteriuria is present in 10-20% of women and an equivalent proportion of pregnant women; however, while largely inconsequential in most women, it is associated with the development of urinary tract infection, with an attendant high risk of pyelonephritis, in 40% of pregnant women. Asymptomatic bacteriuria is diagnosed based upon a clean-catch voided urine specimen containing >100,000 colonies/mL. *Escherichia coli* is responsible for most cases. It is recommended that all pregnant women should undergo screening with urine culture at least once during pregnancy

Endocrine disorders

Sheehan syndrome (postpartum pituitary apoplexy) is due to the conspiring effects of pregnancy-associated pituitary enlargement and severe blood loss during delivery. It is considered to be the most common cause of hypopituitarism in women of childbearing age. 90% of affected women have a history of severe puerperal bleeding. Symptoms of Sheehan syndrome include the inability to lactate, amenorrhea, lethargy, weakness, and weight loss.

In normal pregnancy, there is increased demand placed upon the thyroid gland, due to an estrogen-driven increase in thyroid binding globulin (TBG) and the TSH-like stimulatory effect of hCG. Patients with borderline thyroid function or those with borderline availability of iodine will be unable to meet these demands. As a consequence, hypothyroidism is a more common problem in pregnancy than hyperthyroidism. The serum TSH is the single best test of thyroid status.

Hyperthyroidism must be distinguished from the syndrome of transient hyperthyroidism of hyperemesis gravidarum. It is thought that the high hCG levels associated with hyperemesis gravidarum may also stimulate the TSH receptor and cause transient hyperthyroidism.

Hepatic disease

Acute fatty liver of pregnancy is a rare but serious condition—a medical emergency usually complicated by disseminated intravascular coagulation (DIC). It affects ~1 in 10,000 pregnancies but has a case fatality rate as high as 30%. Acute fatty liver usually presents in the third trimester, with nausea, vomiting, and right upper quadrant tenderness. This is followed by jaundice and altered mental status. Several metabolic defects contribute to morbidity, including metabolic acidosis, renal failure, hypoglycemia, and a prolonged prothrombin time with or without DIC. Histologic examination of the liver shows widespread microvesicular steatosis, accentuated paracentrally (zone 3), with a paucity of inflammatory activity or hepatocellular necrosis. An oil-red-O stain (on frozen tissue) highlights the microvesicles. Immediate delivery is the treatment of choice.

Intrahepatic cholestasis may develop during pregnancy and presents with jaundice and pruritus, usually in the third trimester. While the jaundice is usually mild, the pruritus is distressing. Serum alkaline phosphatase levels are increased 5- to 10-fold (recall that alkaline phosphatase is normally increased in pregnancy due to the placental isoenzyme), with parallel increases in GGT and 5′ nucleotidase. Bilirubin is elevated, but usually remains below 5 mg/dL, and is composed largely of the direct (conjugated) form. Transaminase levels are usually normal or very mildly elevated. Serum bile acids (chenodeoxycholic acid, deoxycholic acid, and cholic acid) are increased, often to levels 10× the upper limit of normal, and this is considered the most characteristic laboratory finding. Histologically, the change is in the pericentral (zone 3) region, which shows dilated canaliculi containing bile plugs.

Recurrent pregnancy loss

Investigation is often undertaken following 2 or more spontaneous abortions. Laboratory evaluation usually involves parental karyotyping. Karyotyping of an abortus may be indicated as well. Endometrial biopsies may be obtained to exclude a luteal phase defect (endometrial histology that is 2 or more days discrepant with dates). Endometrial culture may be ordered to exclude subclinical infection with *Ureaplasma urealyticum* or *Chlamydia trachomatis*. Thyroid function tests, testing for inherited thrombophilic disorders (eg, factor V Leiden and prothrombin G20210 mutations), and testing for lupus antico-agulant may be indicated.

Toxicology

Clinical toxicology consists of 3 main applications: drugs of abuse screening, therapeutic drug monitoring, and management of overdose.

Pharmacokinetics

Half life

The half life (T½) is the time it takes for the concentration of drug to reach ½ of the starting concentration. Generally speaking, a drug is dosed according to its T½; that is, if a drug's half life is 12 hours, then doses are given every 12 hours. Drugs are eliminated by a limited number of mechanisms, including renal clearance, metabolism (usually in the liver), or both. Elimination of most agents follows so-called first-order (1°) kinetics, meaning that the concentration demonstrates exponential decay in time and asymptotically approaches 0.

An important concept in therapeutic drug monitoring is the steady state, which exists when the amount of drug leaving the body equals the amount entering. With many drugs, this point is reached after 5 half lives (ie, after 5 doses given at intervals of 1 half life each). When in the steady state, drug concentration is lowest right before a dose (trough), and highest shortly after a dose (peak).

Free vs bound

Like many small molecules, a variable fraction of the circulating drug is bound, usually to protein (such as albumin), and the remaining drug is free. The free drug is the therapeutically (and toxicologically) active component. When a drug's binding protein is decreased, more free drug is available for a given dose; conversely, when the binding protein is increased, less free drug is available for a given dose. Furthermore, small molecules compete for binding spots, and a second drug may displace the first, leading to increased free drug concentrations.

Volume of distribution (V_d)

The properties of a drug, in particular its size and solubility, influence how widely the drug is distributed in the body. Some drugs—that are extremely hydrophilic—remain confined within the vascular space. Others are capable of distributing within the vascular and extravascular aqueous (interstitial) spaces, and others (very hydrophobic) are primarily sequestered into adipose tissue.

The volume of distribution is defined as the theoretical volume in which the total amount of drug would need to be uniformly distributed to produce the measured plasma concentration of a drug. Hydrophilic drugs that remain confined within the vascular space have low V_d, while hydrophobic drugs that are sequestered in adipose tissue have high V_d. A drug's V_d is usually expressed in liters/kilogram body weight and can be calculated, based upon the quantity of an administered intravenous dose (D) and measured plasma concentration (C) following a period of distribution:

$$V_d = (D \div C) \div (\text{body weight in kg})$$

Drugs of abuse screening (forensic toxicology)

Forensic toxicology refers to testing in the workplace, as part of a drug treatment program, or in legal settings. Sometimes urine opiate screens are utilized to ensure that a prescribed opiate is being taken and not sold. Urine is the usual specimen for drug screening. In most cases, the urine is subjected to a panel of screening tests.

Screening drug tests are usually based upon immunoassay. These tests are designed for high sensitivity, and their specificity is fairly low. Crossreacting substances causing false positives are common in many of the assays and positive tests often require confirmation. If the screen is positive for a substance or if the history strongly implicates a particular substance, a confirmatory test can be ordered. Confirmatory assays are designed for high specificity, and gas chromatography/mass spectrometry is the typical method.

In some settings, a witnessed collection is required to ensure that the urine sample has not been altered. In addition, the specimen must be divided into 2 aliquots so that retesting can be performed if a positive result is obtained.

Numerous substances (adulterants) have been added to urine for the purpose of producing a false-negative result. Several products are commercially available for this purpose. To detect these substances, it is routine to check the specimen color, odor (eg, for bleach), temperature (suspicious if cool), pH (suspicious if <4.5 or >8.0), specific gravity (suspicious for dilution if <1.005), creatinine (suspicious if <20 mg/dL) and/or nitrite (suspicious if >500 µg/mL).

Chain of custody precautions are a requirement for any test that may have implications in criminal proceedings; eg, the specimens of a sexual assault kit or some instances of urine drug testing. Chain of custody requires that the specimen is always in the custody of someone and that all time periods from the point of collection until the time of testing are accounted for. A document accompanies the specimen that is first endorsed by both the person contributing the specimen and the person collecting, labeling, and sealing the specimen and subsequently signed with a note of time and date by both parties each time the specimen changes hands. The specimen cannot be left unattended unless in locked storage.

When drug screening is performed, questions are commonly asked regarding the duration that an agent may be detected (window of detection). While the answer to this question depends upon a range of variables including dose, methodology, and sample type, general guidelines are provided in t1.19.

t1.19 Approximate detection periods for urine drugs of abuse screening tests

Drug	Window of detection (in urine)
Cannabinoids (THC)	3 (single use) to 30 (chronic user) days
Benzodiazepines	2-10 days, depending on agent
Amphetamines, methamphetamines, opiates, cocaine	2-3 days
Barbiturates	3-15 days, depending on agent
Alcohol	1 day

Cocaine

The usual routes of administration are sniffing (the drug is absorbed across the nasal mucosa into the blood), injection, and smoking (crack, free-basing). Laboratory testing for cocaine is primarily applied to detecting abuse, but testing may support the evaluation of patients in the emergency setting who present with chest pain or acute intoxication.

Cocaine induced chest pain has coronary vasoconstriction as its basis. This effect is compounded by an increase in heart rate and arterial blood pressure, which, over time, leads to left ventricular hypertrophy. There appears to be an atherogenic effect of prolonged cocaine use. While vasospasm can produce chest pain without myocardial infarction, in many patients a full myocardial infarction occurs. Cocaine must therefore be considered in the differential diagnosis of chest pain, particularly in young patients with no risk factors for coronary artery disease. Chest pain usually arises within minutes of cocaine use, but may present many hours later. Patients are often not forthcoming with a history of cocaine use. Knowing that cocaine is involved influences both the immediate treatment and follow-up for chest pain, and thus a drug screen and confirmation may have considerable clinical utility.

The differential diagnosis of cocaine-associated chest pain is lengthy. In addition to myocardial infarction, considerations include pneumothorax (due to inhalational barotrauma), aortic dissection (due to hypertension), pulmonary embolus (due to clotting activation), and endocarditis (due to injection of cocaine). Because of cocaine's skeletal muscle effects, the specificity of both myoglobin and CK-MB is lower in cocaine induced acute myocardial infarction. The specificity of troponin is unchanged.

Acute intoxication with cocaine induces the sympathetic nervous system, leading to tachycardia, hypertension, diaphoresis, mydriasis, and agitation. Severe intoxication may present with altered mental status or seizures. Patients often have raised temperature, and on hot days may present with hyperthermia. Hypertension may be quite severe and lead to a hypertensive emergency (defined as hypertension with end-organ damage). Lastly, a life threatening arrhythmia may be induced.

Opiates

There are several abused opiates, including heroin, morphine, hydromorphone (Dilaudid), oxycodone (Oxycontin), and fentanyl (Duragesic). Acute intoxication with opiates produces sedation, pinpoint pupils, constipation, bradycardia, and hypotension. Severe intoxication can present with altered mental status and respiratory arrest. Naloxone (Narcan) and nalmefene are synthetic opioid antagonists that can be administered to treat opiate intoxication. Their use can be diagnostic as well as therapeutic, since failure to respond to an adequate dose essentially excludes opiate intoxication.

Symptoms of opiate withdrawal include increased lacrimation, rhinorrhea, diaphoresis, dilated pupils, tachycardia, irritability and restlessness. Withdrawal symptoms can be lessened by the use of clonidine or methadone in tapering doses. Methadone is a long-acting, orally administered, opioid agonist with fewer central nervous system effects and is less addictive than many opioids. However, methadone has itself become a substance of abuse. Clonidine does not interact with opioid receptors; rather, it antagonizes many of the sympathetic symptoms of opioid withdrawal.

Propoxyphene is an opioid which, in addition to producing the usual opioid related toxicities, can cause unusual toxicities, such as cardiac conduction abnormalities and seizures. This is because both propoxyphene and its major metabolite (norpropoxyphene) cause a quinidine-like interference with sodium channels.

Barbiturates

Barbiturates are CNS depressants which can be life threatening in both intoxication and withdrawal. They act through facilitating the effects of γ-aminobutyric acid (GABA), an inhibitor in the central nervous system. A large number of barbiturates are available, varying in onset and duration of pharmacologic effect. These include methohexital (Brevital), thiopental (Pentothal), pentobarbital (Nembutal), secobarbital (Seconal), and others.

Intoxication results in suppression of consciousness and respiratory suppression through direct action on the medulla. In addition, barbiturates impair myocardial function. Severe intoxication presents with altered mental status, hypotension, hypothermia, pulmonary edema, or respiratory arrest.

Amphetamines

Amphetamine and methamphetamine have stimulant properties mediated predominantly by the release of dopamine in the central nervous system. A consequence of long term use is destruction of the dopamine-secreting cells upon which amphetamines exert their effect, resulting in an irreversible Parkinsonian syndrome. Acute intoxication manifests with hyperpnea, hyperthermia, tachycardia, hypertension, anxiety and irritability. Severe intoxication may present with altered mental status, cerebral bleeds, or seizure.

Phencyclidine (PCP)

PCP may be ingested, injected, or smoked (by "dusting" tobacco or marijuana). It exerts its effects through blocking catecholamine re-uptake. The psychiatric effects of PCP (aggressive or paranoid) are the usual cause of an emergency room visit. The effects of intoxication include hyperpnea, hypertension, and tachycardia. Horizontal nystagmus is often present and provides a clue to PCP use. The behavioral effects include periods of remarkable calm and sedation interrupted by marked agitation, aggression, and incoordination. Many PCP-related emergencies, in fact, are trauma related. Severe intoxication, however, may present instead with hypoglycemia, hypotension, bradycardia, hypopnea, altered mental status, seizures, and/or life threatening hyperthermia. Rhabdomyolysis may be induced by PCP.

Ethanol

Ethanol is metabolized by hepatic alcohol dehydrogenase to acetaldehyde which is converted by aldehyde dehydrogenase to acetic acid.

The type of specimen required for testing depends on the clinical situation. Alcohol testing in an overdose evaluation is usually based upon serum or plasma. In forensic testing, either breath alcohol or whole blood alcohol is measured. Use of alcohol swabs on the venipuncture site should be avoided.

Blood alcohol level can be determined using serum, plasma, or whole blood. An enzymatic assay utilizing alcohol dehydrogenase is most often employed. This method is fairly specific for ethanol and does not measure other alcohols such as methanol.

Breath alcohol testing is based on the principle that blood alcohol diffuses across alveolar septa and is excreted in expired air. The ratio of blood:breath alcohol is 2100:1. Urine alcohol can be roughly correlated with blood levels and clinical effects; however, it is mainly useful as a qualitative test of alcohol consumption.

Most states define the legal limit for operation of a motor vehicle as 80-100 mg/dL (0.08-0.1%) in whole blood t1.20. Whole blood ethanol tends to run lower than serum or plasma ethanol concentration, and legal definitions are usually in terms of whole blood. One should not attempt to use a conversion formula, as conversion varies with hematocrit

t1.20 Clinical effects of blood alcohol

Blood alcohol concentration (%)	Clinical effects
<0.05	Sobriety
0.05-0.1	Euphoria
0.1-0.2	Excitement
0.2-0.3	Confusion
0.3-0.4	Stupor
>0.4	Coma & death

γ-glutamyl transferase (GGT) is increased in heavy consumers of alcohol (>4 drinks/day for >4 weeks). 4 or more weeks of abstinence are usually required for normalization of GGT.

Carbohydrate-deficient transferrin (CDT) has been investigated as a biological marker of heavy alcohol consumption. CDT was initially identified as transferrin isoforms with pI >5.7 found in the sera of alcoholics. CDT is a term that encompasses 3 types of glycan-deficient transferrin molecules: asialo-Fe2-transferrin, disialo-Fe2-transferrin, and monosialo-Fe2-transferrin. In general, CDT is at least as sensitive and probably more specific than γ-glutamyl transferase (GGT). CDT levels require only ~1-2 weeks of heavy consumption before levels are raised. Because the 2 analytes are not highly correlated, their use in parallel enhances the sensitivity of detection of heavy alcohol consumption, especially in clinical populations. Women produce more CDT under natural conditions and may produce less CDT in response to heavy drinking. In addition, there are some conditions such as severe liver disease in which higher than normal levels of CDT are produced, thereby reducing the specificity of this marker for detecting heavy drinking. CDT also appears to be a poor marker of alcohol consumption in obese patients and smokers. In the monitoring of alcoholics during treatment, changes in an individual's CDT baseline values appear to be more sensitive indicators of relapse drinking than the use of cutoff values.

Overdose

General aspects of laboratory evaluation

Laboratory evaluation of an apparent overdose may be guided by multiple considerations, including a history, when present, of exposure to a specific agent or the finding of a particular toxidrome. Toxidromes are constellations of findings that suggest a particular agent or group of agents t1.21, t1.22.

t1.21 Common toxidromes

Class	Signs	Agents
Anticholinergic	Hyperthermia, dry skin, flushing, altered mental status, psychosis ("hot as a hare, dry as a bone, red as a beet, mad as a hatter"), mydriasis, constipation	Atropine, antihistamines, tricyclic antidepressants, scopolamine
Cholinergic	Salivation, lacrimation, urination, diarrhea, GI cramps, emesis ("SLUDGE"); diaphoresis, miosis & wheezing	Organophosphates, pilocarpine, carbamate
Adrenergic	Hypertension, tachycardia, mydriasis, anxiety, hyperthermia	Amphetamines, cocaine, pseudoephedrine ephedrine, PCP
Sedative	Altered mental status, slurred speech, hypopnea/apnea	Barbiturates, alcohols, opiates
Narcotic	Altered mental status, hypopnea/apnea	Opiates
Hallucinogenic	Hallucinations, anxiety, hyperthermia	LSD, PCP, amphetamines, cocaine

t1.22 Signs or symptoms associated with toxic agents

Sign or symptom	Associated agents
Pinpoint pupils (miosis)	Cholinergics (organophosphates, pilocarpine, carbamate)
	Opiates
	Benzodiazepines
Dilated pupils (mydriasis)	Anticholinergics (atropine, antihistamines, tricyclics, scopolamine)
	Sympathomimetics (cocaine, amphetamines)
	Carbon monoxide
Note: A unilateral dilated pupil is indicative of an anatomic defect such as brain stem herniation, glaucoma, or cranial nerve palsy. It also may be caused by topical atropine.	
Diaphoresis	Sympathomimetics (cocaine, amphetamines)
	Organophosphates
Red skin	Carbon monoxide
	Cyanide
	Anticholinergics
Tremor	Lithium vs withdrawal
Dystonia	Neuroleptics (antipsychotics)
Bitter almond odor	Cyanide
Mothball odor	Camphor
Garlic odor	Organophosphates, arsenic

The National Academy of Clinical Biochemistry (NACB) has published guidelines for toxicology screening, in which so-called Tier 1 tests are advised for all laboratories that support emergency medicine departments t1.23. These include quantitative tests performed on serum/plasma and qualitative tests performed on urine. In emergency settings, a urine drug screen may be ordered to support the evaluation of patients with altered mental status, psychiatric presentations, certain metabolic disturbances, chest pain, and hypertension. Though widely available and often requested, the value of urine drug screening in acute management is debatable. Generally speaking, a positive drug screen has little or no impact on patient treatment, but may aid in decisions regarding the clinical severity of illness, patient disposition, and follow-up. The use of urine drug screening is further complicated by significant shortcomings in sensitivity and specificity. Furthermore, most assays rely on the monoclonal antibody detection of drug metabolites and may be positive for days after the clinical effects have abated.

t1.23 National Academy of Clinical Biochemistry tier 1 test recommendations

Testing category	Specific agents
Stat quantitative serum assays	Acetaminophen (paracetamol)
	Lithium
	Salicylate
	Theophylline
	Valproic acid
	Carbamazepine
	Digoxin
	Phenobarbital
	Iron
	Transferrin (or UIBC)
	Ethanol
	Methanol
	Ethylene glycol
	Cooximetry
Stat qualitative urine assays	Cocaine
	Opiates
	Barbiturates
	Amphetamines
	Propoxyphene
	Tricyclics
	PCP

Though qualitative in nature, urine drug screening assays are designed with quantitative screening cutoffs; screening cutoffs should be known and considered in test selection. For example, a THC screen with cutoff of 20 ng/mL may detect "passive" inhalation, whereas one with cutoff of 200 ng/mL will not. Benzodiazepine screening tests are usually optimized for one agent, such as nordiazepam and are variably sensitive for other benzodiazepines. Many assays are entirely insensitive to clinically relevant drugs, such as γ-hydroxybutyrate, fentanyl, and ketamine, and many are susceptible to false positives resulting from commonly used medications such as NSAIDs and antihistamines.

Laboratory evaluation of the apparently intoxicated patient may include urine toxicology screening, serum/plasma toxicology tests, and assessment of the anion gap, osmolar gap, and oxygen gap. An increase in the anion gap to >20 mEq/L is significant. It is important to note that some common conditions may lower the anion gap or mask a mildly increased anion gap. Chief among these is hypoalbuminemia; for every 1 g/dL decrease in albumin, there is a 2.5 mmol/L decrease in the anion gap. Specific toxins that cause an increased anion gap metabolic acidosis include acetaminophen, salicylates, ascorbate, hydrogen sulfide, ethylene glycol, propylene glycol, methanol, ethanol, formaldehyde, carbon monoxide, nitroprusside, epinephrine, and paraldehyde.

Sodium, glucose, and BUN normally account for all but ~5-10 mOsm of the serum osmolarity (normal 285-295 mOsm/L). The difference between the measured serum osmolarity and the osmolarity calculated from sodium, glucose, and BUN is the osmolal gap. The osmolarity is calculated as follows:

$$(2 \times Na) + (BUN \div 2.8) + (glucose \div 18)$$

Some agents t1.24 are capable of significantly altering the serum osmolarity, and when present, the sum of the contributions of sodium, glucose, and BUN will not approximate the serum osmolarity. Serum osmolarity is generally measured by freezing point depression osmometry, and this method will measure most alcohols (eg, ethanol, methanol, ethylene glycol). However, the less commonly used vapor pressure method does not detect ethanol and methanol; thus, these 2 agents will not give an osmolal gap if vapor pressure osmometry is used.

t1.24 Toxic alcohol poisoning

Alcohol	Source	Anion gap acidosis	Osmolal gap	Increased ketones	Metabolite
Ethanol		–/+	+	–/+	
Ethylene glycol	antifreeze	+	+	–	oxalate & glycolate
Isopropanol	rubbing alcohol	–	+	–	acetone
Methanol	windshield washer fluid	+	+	–	formate & formaldehyde

The oxygen saturation gap is the difference between the saturation given by cooximetry and the saturation given by pulse oximetry. Normally, the difference between these 2 determinations should be <5%. A cooximeter, which is incorporated into many arterial blood gas analyzers, measures the light absorption of blood at numerous wavelengths and is capable of determining the proportion of oxyhemoglobin and deoxyhemoglobin (in addition to carboxyhemoglobin and methemoglobin, if present) directly. Thus, if there is a species of hemoglobin that cannot bind oxygen (eg, carboxyhemoglobin, methemoglobin), the pulse oximeter is likely to give a falsely normal (falsely high) reading. Furthermore, in these circumstances there will be a difference between percent oxyhemoglobin given by the pulse oximeter and that given by the cooximeter. This difference is often called the oxygen saturation gap. Causes of an increased oxygen saturation gap include carbon monoxide poisoning (carboxyhemoglobin), methemoglobin, hydrogen sulfide poisoning (sulfmethemoglobin), and cyanide poisoning.

Confusingly, the term oxygen saturation gap is sometimes also used to refer to the difference between the percent oxyhemoglobin given by the ABG analyzer and that given by the pulse oximeter. The pulse oximeter measures transdermally by measuring absorption at 2 wavelengths. It measures oxyhemoglobin and deoxyhemoglobin directly, and does not differentiate carboxyhemoglobin and methemoglobin. When these abnormal hemoglobins are present, they will absorb light and give a falsely high reading to either the oxyhemoglobin or the deoxyhemoglobin, often in difficult to predict ways. For example, in the setting of methemoglobinemia, oxygen saturation by pulse oximetry may be falsely high in severe methemoglobinemia and falsely low in mild methemoglobinemia. Carboxyhemoglobin has a maximal absorption similar to oxyhemoglobin, leading to a falsely high oxyhemoglobin by pulse oximetry.

The difference between arterial and venous oxygen tension can be informative. An abnormally high venous oxygen content (arterialization of venous blood) is seen in cyanide and hydrogen sulfide poisoning.

Measurement or urinary pH may be required to monitor the efficacy of pH manipulation. Treating physicians commonly employ manipulation of the urinary pH to enhance drug excretion. Generally, the limits of urinary pH manipulation are 4.5-7.5 under conditions of enhanced acidification and alkalinization. Agents whose pKa are well outside this range (pKa<3 or >8) tend to be unaffected by these maneuvers.

Toxic alcohol (ethylene glycol, methanol & isopropyl alcohol) poisoning t1.24

A toxic alcohol ingestion is suspected if the osmolal gap exceeds 10 and suspected strongly if it exceeds 20. Ethylene glycol (found in antifreeze), methanol (windshield washer fluid, paint removers, wood alcohol) or isopropyl alcohol (rubbing alcohol) may be ingested accidentally, as readily available and cheap intoxicants, or in suicide attempts. Direct laboratory tests for methanol and ethylene glycol are not available in many settings, so the osmolal gap may be used as a surrogate marker.

Ethanol is often present in conjunction with toxic alcohol ingestion, and ethanol can itself widen the osmolal gap. It may be useful to calculate this effect, based upon the measured ethanol concentration, so that the toxic alcohol level can be more accurately estimated:

Calculated osmolality = 2[Na mEq/L] + [BUN mg/dL]/2.8 + [glucose mg/dL]/18 + [ethanol mg/dL]/4.6

Ethylene glycol or methanol ingestion is in the differential diagnosis of metabolic acidosis with an increased anion gap and increased osmolal gap. Isopropyl alcohol (like ethanol) does not cause acidosis but does cause an osmolal gap.

Ethylene glycol is metabolized to glycolaldehyde, glyoxal, glycolate, glyoxylate and oxalate under the action of alcohol dehydrogenase. Glycolate and glyoxylate cause spurious elevation in lactate levels on some brands of blood gas analyzer. Oxalate binds calcium to produce calcium oxalate, which is deposited in tissues. Glycolic acid is responsible for the CNS manifestations and for the anion gap acidosis. Calcium oxalate crystals can be found in the urine, where they appear envelope shaped, translucent, and birefringent. In renal biopsies, they may be found within renal tubules.

Methanol is metabolized to formaldehyde and then to formic acid by alcohol dehydrogenase. These metabolites result in ocular toxicity, anion gap acidosis, and an osmolal gap.

Isopropyl alcohol (isopropanol) is metabolized to acetone. Isopropyl alcohol ingestion is suspected when there is an increased osmolal gap, ketonemia/ketonuria, and neither acidosis nor an increased anion gap.

Treatment of methanol or ethylene glycol poisoning consists of inhibiting the activity of alcohol dehydrogenase, since metabolites cause the toxicity. In the case of isopropanol, its metabolite (acetone) is less toxic so this approach is not used. Traditionally, inhibition of alcohol dehydrogenase was accomplished with the administration of ethanol. Ethanol competitively inhibits the formation of glycolic acid, oxalate, formaldehyde, and formic acid. A clinically significant consequence of this is that, in methanol or ethylene glycol poisoning, concurrent ethanol use *delays the development of increased anion gap metabolic acidosis.* In such instances, the elevated osmolal gap may be the only clue to the diagnosis. Newer approaches include the administration of fomepizole (a strong competitive inhibitor of alcohol dehydrogenase) and, if needed, dialysis.

Lead poisoning (plumbism)

Sources of lead exposure include those found in the household (lead paint, lead pipes), the environment (lead gasoline), and in industry (manufacture of lead batteries, lead smelters, refurbishing lead-painted buildings). Lead enters the body through inhalation and ingestion. About 95% of ingested lead is distributed in erythrocytes and bone. In addition, a portion goes to the kidney where it is toxic to renal tubular cells. Lead is toxic to cells in 2 ways. First, it nonspecifically binds to and inhibits enzymes bearing sulfhydryl groups. Second, it is directly toxic to mitochondria.

Among the enzymes inhibited are many of the key enzymes involved in heme synthesis, particularly δ-ALA-dehydratase and ferrochelatase. This leads to an accumulation of the immediate precursor of heme, protoporphyrin (free erythrocyte protoporphyrin or FEP). FEP binds nonenzymatically to available zinc, yielding zinc protoporphyrin (ZPP). Both FEP and ZPP are also increased in iron deficiency. Lead inhibits sodium channel ATPases, leading to increased osmotic fragility and shortened red cell survival. Basophilic stippling results from the inhibition of 5' nucleotidase, an enzyme whose function is to break down RNA.

Iron deficiency and lead toxicity frequently coexist. The effect of iron deficiency is to enhance the toxic effects of lead in 2 ways. First, the final step in biosynthesis of heme, in which iron is incorporated into protoporphyrin, is further inhibited by iron deficiency. Second, in an attempt to upregulate intestinal absorption of iron, there is the unintended effect of increased lead absorption.

Manifestations are protean. Hematologic manifestations include a microcytic, hypochromic anemia with basophilic stippling. Neurologic manifestations range from mild cognitive impairment to encephalopathy. Severity correlates somewhat with the rate of lead toxicity and absolute lead level. Renal manifestations occur following long term lead toxicity. Mitochondrial toxicity leads to reduced ATP available to drive the numerous ATP-dependent channels involved in tubular epithelial function. The end-result is aminoaciduria, glycosuria, and phosphaturia (similar to Fanconi renal syndrome). Peripheral neuropathy results in a classic (though rarely observed) bilateral wrist drop. It is also thought that the common presentation of abdominal pain in lead toxicity is due at least in part to sensory neuropathy.

Nonspecific laboratory findings in lead poisoning include anemia, which is typically microcytic and hypochromic, with basophilic stippling. There is an elevated free erythrocyte protoporphyrin (FEP) and zinc protoporphyrin (ZPP). Lastly, there is usually mild to moderate proteinuria and glycosuria. Elevation of FEP or ZPP was used at one time to screen for lead exposure. However, these tests are insensitive at levels of lead below 35 μg/dL. Furthermore, they may be elevated in other conditions, most notably iron deficiency. Their advantage is that they can be performed on capillary blood samples and they easily detect moderate to severe lead toxicity. One further advantage is that blood lead levels tend to misleadingly "rebound" during treatment, so that the FEP and ZPP can be used to distinguish this phenomenon from a true increase in lead toxicity.

The CDC recommendation, made in 1978 and still upheld today, is that a blood lead level ≥10 µg/dL should be considered elevated. Thus, screening requires an assay capable of detecting lead levels this low. A blood lead level, determined by atomic absorption spectrophotometry, capable of detecting lead levels below the 10 µg/dL threshold, is the preferred screening method. A venous sample is necessary for this determination, as capillary blood obtained from heel- or finger-sticks can give erroneous results. Furthermore, repeat testing for the confirmation of any abnormal screening test is advised.

The calcium disodium ethylenediaminic acid (CaNa-EDTA) test is designed to assess the degree to which lead will be mobilized by chelation therapy. An intravenous dose of CaNa-EDTA is given followed by an 8-hour urine collection. The amount of lead excreted in the urine is determined. This test is sometimes administered prior to the initiation of chelation therapy.

At low levels (10-20 µg/dL), environmental interventions may be the only treatment indicated. Beyond that, both environmental interventions and chelation therapy are indicated. A level >70 µg/dL is considered an indication for inpatient monitoring and treatment. Chelators include dimercaprol (also known as British anti-Lewisite or BAL), CaNa-EDTA, D-penicillamine, and dimercaptosuccinic acid.

Carbon monoxide (CO) poisoning

CO binds tightly (with 200× the affinity of oxygen) to hemoglobin, forming carboxyhemoglobin (Hb-CO), thus reducing the available binding sites for oxygen. CO has even greater avidity for fetal hemoglobin, placing infants (and fetuses) at great risk. Furthermore, CO is directly toxic to intracellular oxidative mechanisms and appears to enhance production of nitric oxide (NO).

CO is produced in the environment when there is partial combustion of carbon-containing fossil fuels (complete oxidation leads to CO_2 production). It is produced endogenously from only one source: the breakdown of heme. Endogenous production usually results in Hb-CO levels ≤1%. Carbon monoxide is also generated in the hepatic metabolism of dichloromethane (methylene chloride), found in paint and varnish removers. Accidental poisoning results most often from house fires, engine exhaust, indoor heaters, and stoves. In fact, unventilated burning of charcoal or gas is a common source of poisoning during winter power outages. Intentional poisoning is a common means of suicide.

Hb-CO can be measured by the cooximeter, and venous blood is as good as arterial for this purpose. Hb-CO levels correlate well with clinical effects t1.25; however, there is some variability in the clinical effects of the 20-60% range. Models of blood gas analyzers lacking full co-oximetry do not measure hemoglobin variants and determine oxyhemoglobin by calculation. Pulse oximetry may give a falsely reassuring oxygen saturation. The oxygen gap (difference between pulse oximetry and cooximetry) reflects the level of Hb-CO.

t1.25 Clinical effects of carbon monoxide poisoning

Level of CO	Clinical findings
0.4-2%	Normal nonsmoker
2-6%	Normal smoker
10-20%	Mild symptoms: dyspnea on exertion
20-50%	Severe symptoms: intoxication, with headache, lethargy, loss of consciousness
>50%	Coma & death

Additional laboratory testing in support of the patient with CO poisoning may include measurement of lactate, anion gap, cardiac markers, and cyanide levels (smoke inhalation also poses a risk of cyanide inhalation, depending upon the materials present in the fire). In cases of intentional (suicidal) carbon monoxide poisoning, additional toxicology screening assays may be warranted.

CO is eliminated by slow replacement by oxygen on hemoglobin molecules. The half life of CO depends on the oxygen tension. The T½ on room air is ~6 hours, while the T½ on 100% O_2 is 1 hour.

Acetaminophen (Tylenol) poisoning

The clinical course of acute acetaminophen overdose is polyphasic. Initially (phase I), there may be mild nausea and abdominal discomfort, which is self limited and abates over a matter of hours. Often days later (usually >24 hours), there is progressive liver injury (phase II). This leads to fulminant hepatic failure (phase III), after which there is resolution (phase IV) in the form of complete recovery, liver transplant, or death.

The great danger is hepatic failure, but the majority of acetaminophen poisonings do not result in significant hepatic necrosis. For patients who present in the first phase, practitioners may utilize the Rumack-Matthew nomogram f1.14 to predict which patients are at risk. If the approximate time of ingestion is known, the initial blood samples should be drawn no earlier than 4 hours following ingestion (this is the time it takes for full absorption). The serum acetaminophen concentration and

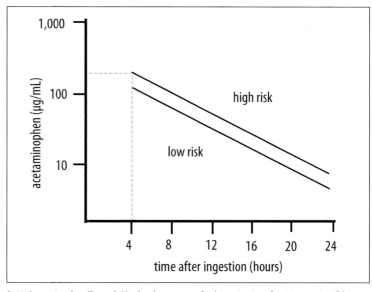

f1.14 Acetaminophen (Rumack-Matthew) nomogram for determination of toxicity severity; if the time of ingestion is known, plotting a single serum acetaminophen level, drawn >4 hours after ingestion, can triage the patient as being at high or low risk for toxicity

ISBN 978-089189-5985

time since ingestion can predict hepatic necrosis and whether ICU admission and N-acetyl cysteine treatment are indicated. The nomogram stratifies patients into 3 groups—probable hepatic toxicity, possible hepatic toxicity, and no hepatic toxicity. N-acetylcysteine is indicated for patients falling into the first 2 categories. ICU admission is indicated for those falling into the first category. The Rumack-Matthew nomogram should be used only in the setting of a single acute ingestion. In cases presenting late, samples drawn >2-3 hours apart can be used to estimate the elimination half life of acetaminophen in the patient. If the half life is >4 hours, then hepatic necrosis is likely. Furthermore, any single acetaminophen level >5 μg/mL places the patient at high risk.

In healthy individuals, the potentially toxic dose is any over ~150 mg/kg. The liver handles acetaminophen in 2 main pathways. Most of it is conjugated with glucuronide or sulfate to form *nontoxic* metabolites. A small amount is metabolized by the P_{450} system into the *toxic* metabolite N-acetyl-p-benzoquinone imine (NAPQI). NAPQI is normally detoxified by glutathione, but glutathione reserves are quickly overwhelmed in toxic ingestions. Furthermore, any agent that induces the P_{450} system increases the proportion of acetaminophen processed to NAPQI, enhancing toxicity. Chronic ethanol use, for example, has this effect. NAPQI is the primary cause of hepatotoxicity. This toxic metabolite induces centrilobular (zone 3) hepatic necrosis with periportal sparing. Its formation within hepatocytes makes the liver the primary target, but other organs may be affected.

N-acetylcysteine (Mucomyst) is the mainstay of treatment. Mucomyst promotes metabolism via the conjugation pathways, thereby decreasing the formation of the toxic metabolite NAPQI.

Cyanide poisoning

Cyanide poisoning may be due to inhalation of smoke from a fire (burning insulation), industrial exposure (present in pesticides and other industrial materials), or suicide/homicide attempt.

Cyanide binds to and inhibits cytochrome a3, thus uncoupling the electron transport system. This results in diminished oxygen-dependent metabolism and severe anion gap metabolic (lactic) acidosis. Oxygen accumulates in the blood, giving rise to the typical bright cherry-red skin color. Patients exposed to very high concentrations develop hyperpnea and loss of consciousness, followed within several minutes by apnea. Those exposed to smaller quantities may follow a slower course, complaining initially of headache, weakness, dyspnea, and altered mental status, but obtundation and death will usually occur even with small exposures. Due to the presence of HCN gas, an exposed patient's breath often has a bitter almond odor; however, only ~50% of the population is capable of detecting this odor.

Cyanide levels can be measured, but cyanide is rapidly metabolized to thiocyanate. Thiocyanate persists for a long period of time and is more reliable for the diagnosis of cyanide exposure. Neither test is commonly available acutely, however, so that a clinical suspicion in conjunction with surrogate markers are important in making the diagnosis. While nonspecific, all patients exposed to cyanide should have an elevated serum lactate and an anion gap metabolic acidosis.

Furthermore, the plasma lactate concentration correlates linearly with the cyanide concentration, and a normal lactate essentially excludes the diagnosis. Cyanide-poisoned patients usually have elevated serum glucose (due to decreased utilization). Blood gases, performed by cooximetry, can be informative. First, if compared to venous blood, a decrease in the arterial-venous oxygen gap (due to decreased utilization) is consistent with cyanide toxicity. Second, the cooximeter can specifically measure carboxyhemoglobin and methemoglobin, removing them from the differential diagnosis.

Treatment involves the administration of sodium nitrite and amyl nitrite, which leads to formation of methemoglobin, which binds available cyanide. Sodium thiosulfate is also given and enhances the conversion of cyanide to thiocyanate, which is renally excreted.

Salicylate (aspirin)

Aspirin exerts conflicting effects upon acid-base balance. First, it directly stimulates the respiratory center within the medulla, promoting respiratory alkalosis. Second, it uncouples oxidative phosphorylation and inhibits the Krebs cycle, shunting energy production towards anaerobic pathways with the development of a metabolic acidosis.

The acid-base disorder caused by salicylate is triphasic. Initially, direct stimulation of the respiratory center leads to hyperventilation and respiratory alkalosis. This effect is maximal between 3-8 hours following ingestion. The physiologic response creates a compensatory metabolic acidosis. It is in this stage, between 12-24 hours, that patients present. Alterations in metabolic pathways, in addition to a progressive loss of buffering capacity, finally combine to cause an increased anion gap metabolic acidosis. At this stage, CNS depression may contribute to hypoventilation and a compounding respiratory acidosis.

Mortality is best correlated with the 6-hour plasma salicylate concentration, with values of >130 mg/dL having a high fatality rate.

Chronic salicylate intoxication manifests as a chronic metabolic acidosis, hypoglycemia, and possible hearing loss. The latter relates to a presumed direct ototoxic effect. In fact, the earliest manifestations of salicylate toxicity include tinnitus and dizziness.

Arsenic

Though technically a metalloid, arsenic appears in the toxicology literature within the category of heavy metal toxicity (in addition to lead, mercury, and others). Arsenic has been linked to attempted homicide. It usually is acquired accidentally, however, through exposure to various pesticides, wood preservatives, and leather tanning. It occasionally contaminates water supplies. It is found in gaseous form (arsine gas) in certain industries, particularly the production of metal alloys and semiconductor manufacture. Arsine gas is the most toxic form of arsenic, capable of producing acute renal failure, hemolysis, and death within 24-48 hours.

Arsenic is largely excreted in urine, with most of the remainder distributed into skin, nails, and hair. Through a variety of mechanisms, arsenic inhibits oxidative production of ATP. Thus, initial toxicity is manifested in dividing tissue such as GI mucosa, with nausea, vomiting, bloody diarrhea, and abdominal pain. The marrow is affected, causing cytopenias (with erythrocyte basophilic stippling similar to that seen in lead toxicity). Chronic toxicity results in peripheral neuropathy, nephropathy, skin hyperpigmentation and hyperkeratosis (particularly palms and soles), and transverse Mees lines in the nails.

Samples for the diagnosis of chronic intoxication may include fingernails, hair, or urine. The most reliable test is a quantitative 24-hour urinary arsenic excretion; however, this result may be misleadingly elevated due to recent seafood ingestion. A blood arsenic level is highly unreliable, as the substance is rapidly cleared from circulation. Arsenic detection in hair and nails may reflect prolonged exposure.

Tricyclic antidepressants (TCAs)

TCAs exert their beneficial effect by blocking reuptake of dopamine and epinephrine from the synaptic space. There are also anticholinergic effects, more or less profound depending upon the particular agent (strongest for amitriptyline). Many of the adverse reactions within the therapeutic range (dry mouth, constipation, urinary retention), and some of the adverse effects in toxic ranges (pupillary dilation, hyperthermia, lethargy, confusion) relate to this effect.

The major adverse consequences of tricyclic overdose take place within cardiac conduction system and central nervous system. TCAs cause widening of the QRS complex (QRS prolongation) that can lead to ventricular arrhythmias. A QRS interval longer than 0.16 seconds is strongly associated with arrhythmia. Furthermore, the duration of the QRS is predictive of the likelihood of seizures, with a QRS interval longer than 0.1 seconds associated with a high seizure risk.

Organophosphates & carbamates

Organophosphates and carbamates are found in insecticides used in agriculture. These chemicals inhibit acetylcholinesterase, the enzyme involved in breakdown of the neurotransmitter acetylcholine at synaptic and neuromuscular junctions. This results in over stimulation of cholinergic processes.

The classic presentation is a farmer who presents with miosis (pinpoint pupils), diaphoresis, excess salivation, lacrimation, gastrointestinal hypermotility, bradycardia and bronchospasm. This constellation of symptoms is often referred to as the muscarinic toxidrome.

Laboratory testing involves the measurement of erythrocyte or plasma cholinesterase activity, which are decreased. Alternatively, organophosphate and carbamate metabolites can be detected in the urine up to 1 week after exposure.

Mercury

Mercury is an occupational hazard, most notorious for intoxication of hat makers ("mad hatter's disease"). Elemental mercury is a liquid at room temperature, and toxic exposure to mercury usually occurs through inhalation of the vapor. Ingestion of elemental mercury is largely inconsequential, as GI absorption does not occur to any significant degree. Recently, however, intoxication with organic mercury has been increasingly recognized, resulting from the ingestion of fish. Organic mercury is readily absorbed in the GI tract.

While acute elemental mercury toxicity manifests as respiratory distress and renal failure, chronic mercury toxicity takes the form of either 1 of 2 characteristic syndromes: acrodynia or erethism. Acrodynia (Feer syndrome) manifests with autonomic manifestations (sweating, hemodynamic instability) and a desquamative erythematous rash on the palms and soles. Feer syndrome is associated with increased urinary catecholamines and can in many ways mimic pheochromocytoma. Erethism is a central nervous system disorder manifesting as personality changes, irritability, and fine motor disturbances.

Organic mercury toxicity manifests as visual field constriction, peripheral neuropathy, tremor, and hearing loss. Importantly, organic mercury readily crosses the placenta, resulting in infants with severe neurologic impairment.

A 24-hour urine collection is essential for diagnosis or elemental mercury poisoning. Organic mercury, however, is not significantly excreted in urine. Whole blood or hair analysis is needed for the diagnosis of organic mercury toxicity.

Therapeutic drug monitoring (TDM)
Digoxin

Routine measurement of digoxin in patients stable on therapy is not widely recommended. Monitoring may be indicated, however, when there is a change in dose, a change in the patient's renal function, or a change in concomitantly administered medications. Digoxin is primarily excreted by the kidneys and has a long half life, around 36 hours. Samples for digoxin levels should be drawn ~8-12 hours after the last dose, ideally ~8-10 days after a dose change.

While serum samples are important, both the efficacy and the toxicity of digoxin may best measured by clinical parameters (eg, heart rate). Renal function tests should be performed initially to guide dosing.

Factors that increase digoxin toxicity include hypokalemia, hypercalcemia, hypomagnesemia, hypoxia, hypothyroidism, quinidine, and calcium channel blockers. Quinidine, in addition to enhancing end-organ effects of digoxin, frees digoxin from protein binding sites and impairs digoxin clearance.

Endogenous substances that cross react with digoxin, termed digoxin-like immunoreactive substances (DLIS), are found in the blood of some individuals who are not taking digoxin. This finding is particularly common in neonates, pregnant women, liver failure and renal failure.

Procainamide

Procainamide is cleared predominantly by the liver. Hepatic impairment leads to slower excretion. Procainamide is metabolized to N-acetylprocainamide (NAPA), which has pharmacologic activity of its own. The rate of conversion to NAPA is determined by the concentration of hepatic acetyltransferase, which is genetically determined. So-called fast acetylators, who have genetically high levels of acetyltransferase, will have higher levels of NAPA. Furthermore, NAPA is predominantly renally cleared. Thus, high levels of NAPA are found in renal insufficiency and in fast acetylators. Both procainamide and NAPA have biologic activity, and the levels of both should be measured. Usually the sum of procainamide and NAPA is considered for making dosing decisions.

Aminoglycosides (eg, gentamicin)

Aminoglycosides are mainly cleared by the kidneys. Patients with renal impairment require lower doses, less frequent doses, or both. Monitoring is advisable to ensure efficacy and to prevent toxicity. Toxicity is manifested primarily as nephrotoxicity and ototoxicity. Serum peaks are considered most useful for assessing efficacy, while troughs reflect the likelihood of toxicity.

In particular, patients who are anticipated to receive aminoglycosides for 7 or more days should be monitored. Monitoring involves not only serum drug levels, but attention to symptoms and renal function as well. For gentamicin, both peaks and troughs should be measured. Ideally, the gentamicin trough specimen is drawn immediately before a dose, and the peak is drawn 30 minutes after the completion of a dose. Levels should be drawn between the 3rd and 4th dose following initiation or dose adjustment, to reflect the steady state.

Vancomycin

For vancomycin, only troughs are routinely measured. Monitoring is generally recommended for patients who will be on vancomycin for 4 or more days. Trough levels should be obtained within 30 minutes before the 4th dose of a new regimen or of a dosage change.

Quinidine

Quinidine is a class IA antiarrhythmic agent that, like disopyramide, and procainamide, blocks sodium and potassium channels in cardiac conduction fibers. The typical manifestations of quinidine toxicity include altered mental status, cinchonism (tinnitus, vertigo, blurred vision), a widening of the QRS complex, a prolonged QT interval, and hypotension (without compensatory tachycardia). Conditions associated with a prolonged QT interval raise the likelihood of ventricular arrhythmias, particularly a polymorphic ventricular tachycardia called torsades de pointes. Quinidine is cleared by the liver. Quinidine levels are not routinely used to predict toxicity, and the ECG is more reliable in this regard. It is important to check and correct electrolyte levels.

Phenytoin

Routine monitoring of antiseizure drug levels is generally not indicated. This practice has not been shown to alter seizure control or the rate of adverse reactions. In certain circumstances, however, measurement of drug levels can be helpful, such as when drug toxicity is suspected. It may also be useful in noncompliant patients, patients with renal insufficiency, and pregnant patients. In regards to phenytoin, zero-order kinetics make it a special case that may deserve monitoring.

Early manifestations of phenytoin toxicity include ocular dysmotility (particularly horizontal gaze nystagmus), ataxia, and incoordination. More severe toxicity is associated with altered mental status and cardiac conduction disturbances. Interestingly, oral phenytoin overdose has not been associated with significant cardiac conduction abnormalities, whereas intravenous overdose often produces a prolonged PR interval (AV block), hypotension, and a risk of arrhythmia. It appears that this discrepancy and the arrhythmogenic effects of IV intoxication are due to the propylene glycol diluent in the IV preparation. In addition to overdose, phenytoin toxicity may result from concomitant use of agents that decrease clearance (inhibition of the cytochrome P_{450} system) or increase free drug concentrations (hypoalbuminemia, drugs that compete for albumin binding sites).

Fetal hydantoin syndrome is the result of intrauterine exposure to phenytoin. It is characterized by intrauterine growth retardation, microcephaly, mental retardation, midfacial hypoplasia, hypertelorism, a flattened philtrum, and shortened nose.

Lithium

The margin between therapeutic effect and toxicity is narrow for lithium. The therapeutic range is from 0.4–1.2 mmol/L. Above 1.5 mmol/L, the risk of adverse effects is high.

Several guidelines have been proposed for the routine monitoring of lithium therapy (patients who are stable on therapy). with a range of recommended monitoring intervals of 1-3 months. For routine monitoring, a sample should be measured 12 hours following the last dose.

The half life of lithium varies from 8-40 hours, depending largely upon age and renal function. Thus, following initiation of lithium or a change in dose steady state conditions would be expected in 2-8 days. Checking levels after a period of 3 days to 1 week is recommended.

Amiodarone

Amiodarone levels should not necessarily be routinely monitored in the stable patient. The major risks of amiodarone include pulmonary toxicity (incidence of 1% annually), thyroid toxicity (hypothyroidism 5-15%, hyperthyroidism 1-2%), hepatotoxicity (0.6%), and peripheral neuropathy (0.3%). Thus, at baseline and every 6 months it is recommended that there be thyroid function testing and liver function testing, in addition to an annual chest X-ray and ECG.

Amiodarone reduces the clearance of warfarin, and can thereby prolong the INR. This effect is usually fully manifest by 7 weeks of co-treatment with amiodarone and coumadin, so close INR monitoring need only be carried out for that period of time.

Amiodarone increases digoxin concentrations, and doses of digoxin must be reduced while closely monitoring digoxin concentrations.

Lipids & carbohydrates
Lipids
Brief review of lipids

The major lipids found in plasma are cholesterol, triglyceride (TG), and phospholipid. TG is composed of 3 fatty acids extending from a glycerol molecule by means of an ester linkage. Fatty acids are unbranched hydrocarbons that come in several lengths: short chain (4-6 carbons), medium chain (8-12 carbons), long chain (12-18 carbons), and very long chain (>18 carbons). In addition, some fatty acids have only single bonds between carbons and thus have the maximum number of attached hydrogens (saturated fatty acids), some have one double bond somewhere along their length and thus have 2 fewer hydrogens (monounsaturated), and some have several double bonds (polyunsaturated). In general, unsaturated fatty acids provide more fluidity than saturated fatty acids. Phospholipid is composed of 2 fatty acids extending from glycerol, with the third carbon (SN3) of glycerol occupied by a phosphatidyl group (such as phosphatidylcholine). Cholesterol is composed of 4 fused hydrocarbon rings incorporating one double-bond, a hydrocarbon side chain, and a hydroxyl group.

Lipids are insoluble in aqueous media such as plasma and therefore must be packaged into lipoprotein particles that have a hydrophilic exterior by virtue of a phospholipid coat. Embedded in the external phospholipid layer are the various apolipoproteins. In the core of the lipoprotein particle are cholesterol esters and TG. Every lipoprotein contains cholesterol, TG, phospholipids, and apolipoproteins. However, 5 different lipoprotein classes are identified based on the various proportions of these 4 constituents and the particular apolipoproteins they possess t1.26.

t1.26 Lipoprotein classes

Lipoprotein	Electrophoretic mobility	Average density (g/mL)	Major lipid	Protein (%)	Apolipoproteins
Chylomicrons	origin	0.95	TG	1	B-48, A-1, CII, E
VLDL	pre-β	1	TG	8	B-100, C, E
IDL	pre-β/β	1.02	Cholesterol	15	B-100, E
LDL	β	1.04	Cholesterol	20	B-100
HDL	α	1.1	Cholesterol	50	A-1, C, E

Ingested lipids are internalized by small bowel enterocytes and packaged into the first class of lipoproteins, called chylomicrons. These have low density due to a large TG component and, among others, contain the apolipoprotein B-48. The chylomicron transports lipid from enterocytes to other somatic cells, particularly hepatocytes, into which they are endocytosed via an apolipoprotein E-dependent process.

In the liver, cholesterol and TG undergo additional metabolism before being packaged, for secretion into the blood, into another class of lipoproteins called very low density lipoprotein (VLDL). VLDL has low density due to a large TG component and bears the apolipoproteins B-100, CII, and E. VLDL is the vehicle for transport of TG from the liver to the bloodstream.

In the blood, the TG in VLDL undergoes progressive hydrolysis by the endothelium-bound enzyme, lipoprotein lipase (LPL). Over time, enough TG is removed from VLDL to increase its density to that of intermediate density lipoprotein (IDL) and, eventually, low density lipoprotein (LDL). The typical LDL particle has lost most of its TG and the majority of its apolipoproteins CII and E, leaving predominantly phospholipid, cholesterol and apolipoprotein B-100. LDL is the main vehicle for transporting cholesterol from the bloodstream to somatic cells, where LDL particles undergo endocytosis mediated by the LDL receptor and apolipoprotein B-100.

The liver also produces a class of lipoproteins called high density lipoprotein (HDL) that contains a small amount of lipid, mainly phospholipid and cholesterol, the enzyme lecithin cholesterol acyl transferase (LCAT), and apolipoproteins, especially apolipoprotein A-1. The function of HDL is the scavenging of cholesterol from the periphery and returning it to the liver.

Methods

Since lipid levels are affected by diet, alcohol consumption, physical stress such as exercise, smoking, and posture, it is important that standard conditions, including a 12-hour fast (though many labs allow testing of nonfasting patients), surround the blood collection. Initially, the total cholesterol, HDL, and TG are determined, and LDL is usually calculated from these.

Total cholesterol and triglycerides are usually measured enzymatically. VLDL cholesterol is often estimated as TG ÷ 5 (when expressed in mg/dL) or TG ÷ 2.2 (when expressed in mmol/L). This estimation is valid in most circumstances but fails when TG is >400 mg/dL, when chylomicrons are present, or when there is β-VLDL characteristic of the very rare type III dyslipidemia.

HDL cholesterol is usually measured by an enzymatic sequence similar or identical to that for total cholesterol, after removal of non-HDL lipoproteins. This initial step may take the form of selective precipitation by physical or chemical pretreatment, followed by a cholesterol determination performed on the supernatant. Alternatively, in what are called homogeneous assays, a polymer, detergent, or enzyme is used to inactivate non-HDL cholesterol, followed by a cholesterol determination. The homogeneous assays are amenable to automation, without a manual step.

Separation of LDL from other lipoproteins, in order to directly measure LDL cholesterol, is difficult. Consequently, LDL is usually calculated, using the Friedewald equation (below). The Friedewald calculation is not considered valid for TG>400, if chylomicrons are present, in cholestasis, or in type III dyslipidemia.

Friedewald equation:

LDL cholesterol = total cholesterol − HDL cholesterol − TG ÷ 5

Direct methods for measuring the LDL cholesterol include ultracentrifugation, electrophoresis, and homogeneous assays. The homogeneous assays can be automated and these assays employ detergents to block or dissolve all lipoproteins except LDL, permitting the direct enzymatic measurement of LDL cholesterol.

The individual lipoproteins differ in density from one another, so that by ultracentrifugation, they can be separated into the various types and quantified. It is uncommon to have access to ultracentrifugation in routine laboratory practice; however, its use remains integral in reference methods for lipoprotein measurement. Lipoprotein electrophoresis is performed on a gel in a manner similar to protein electrophoresis, and stained with a fat stain such as oil red O or Sudan Black B. Chylomicrons do not move from the point of application. LDL migrates in the β region, VLDL in the pre-β region, and HDL in the α region. For these reasons, LDL is often referred to as β-lipoprotein and HDL is called α-lipoprotein. This method is employed as a basis for qualitative analysis of lipoprotein classes but is not suitable for quantitative analysis.

Overnight refrigeration produces characteristic patterns in plasma, depending upon the lipoprotein profile. The presence of a creamy layer atop the plasma indicates the presence of excess chylomicrons. Turbidity or opacity of the plasma below this indicates abundant VLDL. LDL and HDL, even when present in excess, do not visibly alter the plasma.

The apoproteins currently thought to be clinically relevant are apoB100, apoA1, and apolipoprotein(a), an apoprotein found on Lp(a). Immunoassays are available for the measurement of each. ApoB100 is the major apolipoprotein of LDL and VLDL. ApoA1 is the major apolipoprotein of HDL.

Lipid disorders

A confusing aspect of lipid disorders is that there are 2 major ways of classifying them. In the first, one looks at the lipoprotein profile, while the second is concerned more specifically with the serum concentrations of cholesterol and TG. If one recalls that VLDL and chylomicrons contain predominantly TG, while LDL contains predominantly cholesterol, the 2 concepts correlate fairly well.

Premature atherosclerosis is the most notorious consequence of hyperlipidemia t1.27. This complication may be observed in the setting of high LDL or IDL; that is, when the cholesterol is high. It is not a prominent feature when only TG is elevated. Eruptive xanthomas, presenting as crops of yellow, pruritic, papulonodules, are seen with elevated TG (chylomicrons or VLDL). Tendinous xanthomas are seen near the knees or elbows and appear when there are simultaneous elevations in TG and cholesterol (elevated IDL). Xanthelasma are yellow periorbital papules that are associated with high cholesterol (LDL). Acute pancreatitis is associated with elevated TG (chylomicrons or VLDL), particularly when TG exceeds 500 mg/dL.

t1.27 Classification of lipid disorders by predominant lipids

Disorder	Phenotype	Cholesterol	TG	Clinical features
Familial LPL deficiency	I	↑	↑↑↑	Eruptive xanthomas, pancreatitis
Familial apoC-II deficiency	I or V	↑	↑↑↑	Pancreatitis
Familial hypercholesterolemia	IIa	↑↑↑	→↑	Tendinous xanthomas, premature atherosclerosis
Familial dysbetalipoproteinemia	III	↑↑↑	↑↑↑	
Familial combined hyperlipidemia	IIb or IV	↑↑	↑↑	Premature atherosclerosis
Familial hypertriglyceridemia	IV or V	↑	↑↑↑	Eruptive xanthomas, pancreatitis

Predominant hypercholesterolemia

Generally considered to exist when the plasma total cholesterol exceeds 200 mg/dL, hypercholesterolemia is usually related to elevated LDL. In lipoprotein electrophoresis, it may fall into patterns II or III. Secondary causes of hypercholesterolemia are hypothyroidism, diabetes mellitus, nephrotic syndrome, cholestasis, cyclosporine, thiazide diuretics, or loop diuretics. The most common primary cause of hypercholesterolemia is familial hypercholesterolemia, an autosomal dominant deficiency of LDL receptors or LDL receptor activity.

Predominant hypertriglyceridemia

This is related to elevated chylomicrons or VLDL. Hypertriglyceridemia is not an independent risk factor for coronary artery disease when considered together with the LDL and HDL. A very common secondary cause of this is heavy alcohol consumption. It may also be secondary to: obesity, diabetes mellitus, hepatitis, pregnancy, renal failure, β-blockers, isotretinoin, corticosteroids, nephrotic syndrome, and gout. Primary causes include familial combined hyperlipidemia, familial LPL deficiency, familial apoC-II deficiency, and familial hypertriglyceridemia.

Mixed hypertriglyceridemia & hypercholesterolemia

This finding is most common in severe diabetes mellitus, hypothyroidism, or nephrotic syndrome. It may also be seen with thiazides, loop diuretics, and β-blockers. Primary causes include familial combined hyperlipidemia and type III hyperlipidemia (dysbetalipoproteinemia).

Low levels of HDL cholesterol

This, defined as HDL <35 mg/dL, is an independent risk factor for premature atherosclerosis. A high HDL, >70 mg/dL, is protective. Tangier disease is an autosomal recessive disorder of lipid metabolism characterized by low cholesterol, normal to increased TG, absent HDL, and absence of apoA1. Cholesterol esters deposit in the tonsils, lymph nodes, vasculature, and spleen, and corneal opacities develop. HDL cholesterol may also be reduced by smoking, obesity, sedentary lifestyle, and anabolic steroids.

Lipids in the assessment of coronary artery disease (CAD) risk

The National Cholesterol Education Program (NCEP) has been providing guidelines for cholesterol testing and treatment since 1988. Their most recent guidelines, the 3rd Adult Treatment Panel report (ATP III) reaffirms the traditional major risk factors for coronary artery disease: smoking, hypertension, low HDL, family history of premature CAD, and age (<45 years for men and <55 years for women). ATP III is also the first iteration to recognize the potential significance of the metabolic syndrome (syndrome X). Whereas ATP II recommended a screening measurement of TC and HDL-C (fasting not required) and a fasting lipoprotein profile only in those at increased risk, ATP III recommends a fasting lipoprotein profile (including total cholesterol (TC), LDL cholesterol, HDL cholesterol, and triglyceride) for all patients. In a nonfasting patient, the TGs and calculated LDL-C are not considered valid. ATP III further recommends specific cholesterol and LDL targets t1.28, t1.29.

t1.28 ATP III cholesterol classification

Total cholesterol (mg/dL)	Desirable <200
	Borderline 200-239
	High >240
LDL (mg/dL)	Optimal <100
	Near optimal 100-129
	Borderline 130-159
	High 160-189
	Very high >190
HDL (mg/dL)	Low <40
	High >60

t1.29 ATP III recommended LDL targets

Risk group	Notes	Target LDL
Presence of coronary heart disease (CHD) or CHD equivalents	CHD equivalents include: diabetes, noncoronary atherosclerotic vascular disease, Framingham risk of MI within 10 years of >20% (a complex formula determines this risk)	<100 mg/dL
2 or more major risk factors	Major risk factors include: smoking, hypertension (>140/90), HDL <40, family history of premature CHD (male 1st degree relative <55 or female 1st degree relative <65), age (men >45, women >55)	<130 mg/dL
0-1 major risk factors		<160 mg/dL

Carbohydrates

Insulin leads to an increase in cellular uptake of glucose from the blood and leads to an increase in overall intracellular anabolic activity including conversion of glucose to glycogen (glycogenesis) and increased conversion of carbohydrates to fatty acids (lipogenesis). This is noted in the peripheral blood as a decrease in blood glucose.

Several agents act counter to the effects of insulin, including glucagon, epinephrine, glucocorticoids, growth hormone, thyroxine, and somatostatin. In pregnancy, human placental lactogen (HPL), also called somatomammotropin, has antiinsulin properties and is responsible for the relative glucose intolerance of pregnancy.

Methods

Immunometric assays are available for the measurement of insulin and C peptide. Insulin is synthesized as proinsulin, a single amino acid chain 51 amino acids long. Though it is a single polypeptide chain, by convention the first (amino terminus) several amino acids are called the B chain, the next several amino acids are called the C peptide, and the carboxyterminal amino acids are called the A chain. Posttranslationally, disulfide bonds form between the A and B chains, and the C peptide is proteolytically cleaved to make insulin. When the β cells are induced to secrete, they secrete disulfide-linked A-B chains (insulin) and C peptides simultaneously. Although C peptide and insulin are produced in equimolar quantities, the ratio of C peptide:insulin is ~5-15:1. when both insulin and C peptide are expressed in SI units (pmol/L). This is because insulin is rapidly metabolized compared to C peptide.

Glucose measurement in the laboratory is an enzymatic assay, using glucose oxidase or hexokinase coupled with glucose-6-phosphate dehydrogenase, and measuring a reaction product. The latter method is considered more specific for glucose. The test is usually performed on plasma. Note that when blood is left in an un-separated test tube, glycolysis will reduce the glucose by ~5-10 mg/dL/hour depending on the temperature and white cell count. Sodium fluoride (NaF) added to the tube arrests this process for 24 hours; however, the initial arrest of glycolysis takes 1-2 hours to take effect. So an initial decrement of 5-10 mg/dL can be expected even in the presence of NaF.

Glucose is a frequent point of care analyte, and in this setting is usually performed on whole blood. Most are calibrated to give results that correlate with plasma, but un-calibrated whole blood glucose usually runs 10-15% lower than plasma glucose (depending upon the hematocrit). These measurements are inappropriate for the initial diagnosis of diabetes.

Interstitial glucose monitoring, using an electrochemical method, is a recent development with which continuous monitoring is possible. Changes in interstitial glucose lag changes in blood glucose by up to 30 minutes.

Glycosylated hemoglobin (GHb) is formed when hemoglobin undergoes nonenzymatic reaction with glucose. One type of glycosylated hemoglobin—HbA_{1c}—can be easily measured. The normal HbA_{1c} is <6%. The concentration of HbA_{1c} depends upon the concentration of serum glucose and, since glycosylation increases over time, the lifespan of the red cells (shortened red cell survival leads to relatively decreased HbA_{1c}). In patients with normal red cell survival, the concentration of HbA_{1c} is an indicator of glucose concentrations over the preceding 3 months (the red cell lifespan is 120 days; the average red cell is ~60 days old). In fact, the relationship is not quite linear with younger red cells disproportionately represented, and thus diabetic control over the past month has a disproportionate effect upon HbA_{1c}. There are several ways to measure HbA_{1c}, including affinity chromatography, immunoassay, high-pressure liquid chromatography (HPLC), and ion-exchange chromatography. HbA_{1c} can be translated into average blood glucose (AG) through the use of a formula:

$$AG \text{ (in mg/dL)} = (28.7 \times HbA_{1c}) - 46.7$$

Hypoglycemia

Symptoms of hypoglycemia are classified into 2 categories: neuroglycopenic and adrenergic. The first is related to the reliance of the brain upon glucose for metabolism, such that hypoglycemia directly leads to altered mental status. These symptoms predominate in so-called "fasting" hypoglycemia in which the drop in serum glucose is moderate and gradual. The adrenergic response leads to sweating, palpitations, tachycardia, and nervousness. These symptoms predominate in "reactive" hypoglycemia that tends to be more profound and rapid in onset.

Drug induced hypoglycemia may be caused by insulin, sulfonylureas (oral hypoglycemic agents), alcohol, and quinine.

Fasting hypoglycemia is the abnormal gradual-onset of hypoglycemia occurring following a prolonged fast or prolonged exercise. Causes include proliferations of islet β cells (nesidioblastosis or insulinoma), several inherited metabolic defects, certain large sarcomas, and end-stage liver disease. Insulinomas are tumors of the endocrine pancreas, consisting of neoplastic proliferations of β islet cells, resulting in high insulin levels. They present with the classic Whipple triad of: hypoglycemic symptoms, plasma glucose <45 mg/dL, and relief of symptoms with glucose administration. In patients with insulinoma, the absolute insulin concentration may be normal, but it is inappropriately high for the degree of hypoglycemia. Proinsulin normally represents <10% of circulating insulin; proinsulin exceeding 25% is typical of insulinoma. Note that serum calcium should be measured in patients diagnosed with insulinoma, because insulinomas may be a feature of MEN type 1.

Reactive hypoglycemia is the abnormal rapid-onset of hypoglycemia following a meal. Its causes include hereditary fructose intolerance, galactosemia, post-vagotomy states (dumping syndrome), and (sometimes) early type 2 DM.

The diagnostic approach to hypoglycemia involves first documenting hypoglycemia, then identifying a cause t1.30. Documenting hypoglycemia requires that a blood sample be obtained during a symptomatic period. This may require provocative testing such as fasting with or without exercise (when fasting hypoglycemia is suspected); or a carbohydrate-rich meal (when reactive hypoglycemia is suspected). The major clinical use of C peptide measurement is in the detection of exogenous insulin administration. In interpreting C peptide levels it must be considered that C peptide is cleared by the kidneys, and is therefore increased in renal impairment.

t1.30 Hypoglycemia, differential diagnosis

Insulinoma
Nesidioblastosis
Advanced malignancy
Antiinsulin receptor antibodies
Autoimmune insulin syndrome
Post-gastric surgery
Alcohol consumption
Drug induced (exogenous insulin, sulfonylureas, salicylates, quinine, haloperidol, β-blockers)
Hepatic failure
Inborn errors of metabolism (glycogen storage disease, hereditary fructose intolerance, galactosemia, carnitine deficiency)
Starvation

Antiinsulin antibodies can be raised in response to exogenous insulin but are rare in the era of human insulin administration. Antiinsulin antibodies may rarely occur in patients never exposed to exogenous insulin, and may cause reactive hypoglycemia (autoimmune insulin syndrome, AIS). Antiinsulin receptor antibodies (AIRAs) may cause either hyperglycemia or, more rarely, hypoglycemia.

An important concept is the distinction of hyperinsulinemic from hypoinsulinemic hypoglycemia: hyperinsulinemic hypoglycemia is (when not exogenous) most commonly due to insulinoma; while hypoinsulinemic hypoglycemia typifies most other causes. Hypoinsulinemic hypoglycemia is divided into ketotic (high β-hydroxybutyrate) and nonketotic (low β-hydroxybutyrate) types. Nonketotic hypoglycemia suggests the presence of insulin or insulin-like activity and may be seen in autoimmune hypoglycemia, liver failure, starvation, or defects in β-oxidation. All other causes of hypoglycemia are associated with ketosis.

Types of diabetes mellitus

Type 1 diabetes usually results from autoimmune islet β-cell destruction, causing a deficiency of insulin. This form of diabetes, previously called insulin-dependent or juvenile diabetes, accounts for 5–10% of diabetics. It most commonly presents in childhood. Autoantibodies can frequently be detected, in particular islet-cell antibodies (ICA), insulin autoantibodies (IAA), antibodies to glutamic acid decarboxylase (GAD), or insulinoma associated protein (IA-2, ICA512). There is a strong association with the HLA DR and DQ loci, with particular alleles having either predisposing or protective effects.

Type 2 diabetes results from progressive insulin resistance, compounded by a progressive defect in insulin secretion. This is the most common form of diabetes and typically presents in adulthood. Previously referred to as noninsulin dependent diabetes and adult-onset diabetes, affected individuals often do not require insulin treatment to survive.

Gestational diabetes mellitus (GDM) refers to the onset of diabetes during pregnancy, even if the condition persists beyond pregnancy.

Other forms of diabetes result from an assortment of genetic defects, exocrine pancreatic disease, other endocrinopathies, medications, and toxins. Many of the genetic defects affect the β cells and present as so-called maturity-onset diabetes of the young (MODY), presenting by adolescence or young adulthood. A second genetic mechanism affects the insulin receptor, causing insulin resistance; some of these are associated with acanthosis nigricans. The Rabson-Mendenhall syndrome is a form of this genetic defect. Furthermore, diseases of the exocrine pancreas, such as chronic pancreatitis and cystic fibrosis, if sufficiently severe, can secondarily involve the islets. Endocrinopathies, particularly those that result in the excess production of counter-regulatory hormones (cortisol, epinephrine, growth hormone, glucagon), can result in functional diabetes. Drugs that can induce or increase the risk of diabetes include pentamidine, glucocorticoids, β-agonists, and thiazide diuretics.

Diagnosis & monitoring

Current guidelines recognize 4 routes to the diagnosis of (nongestational) diabetes t1.31: fasting plasma glucose (FPG), 75 g oral glucose tolerance test (OGTT), HbA$_{1c}$, and random plasma glucose in patients with classic symptoms. The fasting plasma glucose (FPG) is the recommended test to diagnose diabetes in both children and adults. A FPG of 126 mg/dL (7.0 mmol/L) or higher is considered diagnostic, with fast defined as ≥8 hours with no caloric intake. Alternatively, in persons with classic symptoms of diabetes, a random nonfasting plasma glucose of 200 mg/dL (11.1 mmol/L) is diagnostic. In an oral glucose tolerance test (OGTT) with a 75 g glucose load, a 2-hour plasma glucose of 200 mg/dL (11.1 mmol/L) or higher is diagnostic. The HbA$_{1c}$ was recently accepted as a diagnostic test for diabetes, as a result of improved standardization across laboratories. Thus, HbA$_{1c}$ ≥6.5% may be used to diagnose diabetes. The caveat is that in certain hemolytic disorders, including some hemoglobinopathies (those that shorten red cell survival), glucose criteria should be used instead. Abnormal diagnostic tests should be repeated before a diagnosis is established;

alternatively, another of the tests that is concurrently beyond the threshold renders repeat testing unnecessary.

t1.31 Diagnostic criteria for diabetes

One of the following	Notes
HbA$_{1C}$ ≥ 6.5%	Test should be performed in a laboratory using a method certified by the National Glycohemoglobin Standardization Program (NGSP) & traceable to the Diabetes Control & Complications Trial (DCCT) reference assay; point of care HbA$_{1C}$ assays are not adequate at this time
FPG ≥126 mg/dL	Fasting = no caloric intake for ≥8 hours
OGTT 2 hour plasma glucose ≥200 mg/dL	75 g oral glucose load
Random plasma glucose ≥200 mg/dL	In a patient with classic symptoms of diabetes or in hyperglycemic crisis

In pregnancy, the ADA recommendations are as follows. First, women with risk factors are to be tested for type 2 diabetes at the first prenatal visit (standard criteria for type 2 diabetes applied). Second, pregnant women not previously known to have diabetes should be screened for gestational diabetes mellitus (GDM) at 24-28 weeks gestation using a 75 g 2-hour OGTT, after an overnight fast of at least 8 hours, applying the criteria listed t1.32.

t1.32 Diagnostic criteria for gestational diabetes, based upon 75 g oral glucose tolerance test

Time of collection	Plasma glucose
Fasting	≥92 mg/dL (5.1 mmol/L)
1 hour	≥180 mg/dL (10.0 mmol/L)
2 hours	≥153 mg/dL (8.5 mmol/L)

In many instances, the need for a 100 g test is determined by first performing a 50 g OGTT. A plasma glucose measurement at 1 hr that exceeds 140 mg/dL indicates the need for a 100 g oral glucose tolerance test. Some women, considered to be at very low risk, can avoid OGTT altogether; these patients have the following characteristics: age <25, normal prepregnancy weight, low-risk ethnic group, no family history of diabetes, and no prior obstetric complications. Women who have been diagnosed with GDM should be tested for (nongestational) diabetes at 6-12 weeks postpartum.

Conditions considered "prediabetic" include impaired glucose tolerance (IGT) and increased fasting glucose (IFG). IGT is diagnosed when an oral glucose tolerance test is abnormal but does not meet criteria for diabetes; that is, a 2-hour plasma glucose of 140 mg/dL (7.8 mmol/L) to 199 mg/dL (11.0 mmol/L). Increased fasting glucose (IFG) is diagnosed when a fasting glucose is abnormal but does not meet the criteria for diabetes; that is, a FPG of 100 mg/dL (5.6 mmol/L) to 125 mg/dL (6.9 mmol/L).

After the diagnosis of diabetes is made, initial and repetitive laboratory testing is performed to monitor disease status. The HbA$_{1c}$ is used to monitor glycemic control. The frequency of testing is often individualized. The American Diabetes Association (ADA) currently recommends HbA$_{1c}$ testing at least twice a year in stable patients and more frequently in others. The ADA-recommended goal of therapy is a HbA$_{1c}$ concentration of <7%. Adult patients with diabetes should be screened annually for lipid disorders. Annually, testing for microalbuminuria should be performed and the serum creatinine should be measured for calculation of the estimated glomerular filtration rate (eGFR). Hypomagnesemia is a common problem in diabetics. Furthermore, hypomagnesemia appears to complicate glycemic control. Magnesium levels should therefore be checked periodically.

Diabetic ketoacidosis (DKA)

DKA occurs in insulin-dependent diabetics. Patients with type 1 DM are far more prone to DKA than those with type 2. Generally, DKA follows some sort of provocation such as infection, trauma, or failure to take insulin. In early DKA, the patient experiences polyuria, polydipsia, nausea, and abdominal pain. Later there is the altered breathing pattern referred to as Kussmaul respiration, the onset of altered mental status progressing to coma and, if untreated, death.

Hyperglycemia, ketosis, and metabolic acidosis are the usual requirements for the diagnosis of DKA. Occasionally the diagnosis is made solely on the basis of the typical clinical presentation coupled with urine dipstick findings of glycosuria and ketonuria. More specifically, the glucose should be ≥200 mg/dL, and the venous pH <7.30 (or bicarbonate <15 mmol/L). Normoglycemic DKA is rare. Additional common, though nonspecific, findings include left-shifted neutrophilia, hyperamylasemia, and hyperlipasemia. The mechanism for these is unclear. Neutrophilia appears to directly result from DKA and does not necessarily imply underlying infection.

The major serum ketones are acetone, acetoacetic acid, and β-hydroxybutyrate. These are in a dynamic balance with one another and undergo continual interconversion, though the formation of acetone from acetoacetate is not a reversible reaction. Ketones may be measured by the nitroprusside technique, a semiquantitative method that is sensitive to acetoacetic acid but does not detect β-hydroxybutyrate. A discontinued tablet-based formulation of the nitroprusside test for ketones (Acetest) detected acetone weakly but the dipstick test (Ketostix) does not detect acetone in any reliable fashion. In normal circumstances, these are present in roughly equimolar concentrations. Due to an altered metabolic milieu, acetone and acetoacetic acid account for only around 20% of serum ketones in DKA, and the remaining 80% are β-hydroxybutyrate. Thus, it is important to understand that when you measure "ketones" you are only measuring a small fraction of serum ketones. In the treatment of DKA an initial apparent increase in "ketones" may be seen, which is due to β-hydroxybutyrate being converted to the other 2 forms as total serum ketones decrease.

Glucose is initially >200 mg/dL in typical DKA. The pH and bicarbonate are initially decreased and there is an increased anion gap.

The initial serum potassium is often elevated or normal, but total body potassium is usually severely depleted in DKA. The total body potassium deficit is due to transcellular shifts with loss of intracellular potassium combined with urinary potassium losses. Furthermore, insulin treatment of DKA leads to transcellular shifts of both glucose and hydrogen ions, taking potassium with them. This can result in rapid and profound hypokalemia in the treated DKA patient. Thus, both monitoring and supplementation of potassium during the treatment of DKA is crucial

Sodium is initially decreased due to urinary losses. The BUN is initially increased due to severe volume depletion resulting in prerenal azotemia.

Hyperglycemic hyperosmolar nonketotic coma (HHNC)

Patients with type 2 (noninsulin dependent) diabetes, especially the elderly, are particularly prone to this complication. It is rarely observed in insulin-dependent DM. HHNC is about one tenth as common as DKA but has a mortality rate 10× that of DKA.

HHNC presents with altered mental status, profound hyperglycemia, hyperosmolarity, dehydration, and essentially normal pH. Seizures and localizing neurologic deficits such as hemiplegia are common features, and the mortality rate varies from 15-50%.

Diagnosis relies on the typical clinical presentation in addition to extreme hyperglycemia (≥600 mg/dL, usually >1,000 mg/dL), hyperosmolarity (>330 mOsm/L), and essentially normal bicarbonate and ketones. Sodium and potassium tend to be elevated at presentation, but there is a profound total body potassium depletion as seen in DKA. The BUN is often markedly elevated, with an increased BUN:Cr ratio, reflective of profound dehydration.

The metabolic syndrome

Also known as syndrome X and the insulin resistance syndrome, this refers to a cluster of findings that appear together and that are risk factors for cardiovascular disease. These include a constellation of metabolic abnormalities, including impaired glucose tolerance, insulin resistance, central obesity, dyslipidemia (increased VLDL, increased TG, increased small dense LDL particles, decreased HDL), and hypertension. These individuals manifest accelerated atherosclerosis.

Tumor markers

Screening for cancer through the use of tumor markers is generally not cost-effective. The reason for this is the dependence of a test's positive predictive value (PPV) on the disease prevalence in the population. PPV is directly proportional to prevalence. Hence, the cost of evaluation of false positives can negate any cost-savings from early detection of true positives when no selection criteria are applied to the population. If, however, screening is applied to a selected population, then tumor marker screening may be cost-effective. A few examples exist, including the use of α-fetoprotein (AFP) to screen for hepatocellular carcinoma in China and the use of calcitonin to screen for medullary thyroid carcinoma in multiple endocrine neoplasia (MEN) kindreds. Detection of tumor recurrence can be thought of as an example of this application. The pretest probability of a positive result is high in this select group, and it is in this arena that serum tumor markers have enjoyed their greatest success.

A screening test is generally considered to be a good one if it is safe, highly sensitive, inexpensive, and capable of detecting a disease for which early treatment improves survival. Assays for tumor markers must have very high analytic sensitivity (defined as the lowest analyte concentration that will yield a result other than zero). Furthermore, they must have high between-run precision, since the time interval between measurements is often several months or a year. One strategy for dealing with assays lacking high between-run precision is to freeze samples, and thaw them to run parallel with later samples; thus, permitting direct comparisons to be made.

The Hook effect can be a problem in certain immunoassay formats, and immunoassays are heavily applied in tumor marker testing. In this scenario, a very high concentration of an analyte gives a falsely low result. If the sample is sufficiently diluted, the assay will give an appropriate result. In some patients with widely metastatic disease, serum tumor concentrations can be so high that they exceed the binding capacity of both the binding capture antibodies and the signal-bearing antibodies, preventing their association. This phenomenon, known as the high dose Hook effect, mostly affects one-step immunometric assays. It is for this reason that it is common practice to analyze samples at several different dilutions for assays known to be affected by the high dose Hook effect.

Heterophile antibodies can cause significant interference in any immunoassay. These are naturally occurring antibodies reactive against reagent components. So-called "sandwich" immunoassays are particularly susceptible to this interference. Heterophile antibodies may create false positives (by bridging the capture and signal antibody) or false negatives (by blocking one or the other). Both detecting and eliminating this interference is not straightforward. One option is to repeat the test using a different assay. Various heterophile blocking reagents, steps to remove immunoglobulins, and serial dilutions may also correct the problem.

Prostate-specific antigen (PSA)
Prostate cancer screening

PSA is a serine protease secreted by prostate epithelial cells. An annual PSA measurement, in addition to digital rectal examination (DRE), has been traditionally recommended for men over age 50. Abnormal DRE or PSA >4 ng/mL are considered indications for prostate needle biopsy.

However, the value of PSA as a screening test for healthy men has been recently questioned, with the US Preventive Services Task Force in 2012 recommending against routine PSA screening. This is because the PSA as a screening test is thought to fail the final criterion for a good screening test—that it detects a disease for which early treatment improves survival. This recommendation has met with considerable opposition and debate.

As a test, PSA also suffers from poor clinical accuracy. While PSA is organ-specific, it is not cancer-specific, and it may be elevated in benign prostatic hyperplasia, prostatitis, prostatic infarct, and following prostate needle biopsy. Small elevations following DRE are not large enough to be clinically relevant, but elevations following prostate needle biopsy may be. PSA undergoes significant physiologic variation within an individual, with great enough magnitude to be clinically significant, and serial measurements are recommended to support clinical decisions. PSA varies with race, with levels being significantly higher in blacks. In actual practice, only ~30-40% of men with elevated

PSA (>4.0 ng/mL) will be found to have prostate cancer, particularly when the PSA falls within the 4-10 ng/mL "gray zone," wherein the positive predictive value is only ~20%.

With regard to sensitivity, many men with prostate cancer have serum PSA levels <4.0 ng/mL. In the prostate cancer prevention trial, in which 18,886 men underwent biopsy regardless of PSA, the risk of cancer in men with PSA <4 ng/mL was found to be similar to that of men with PSA ≥ 4 ng/mL. An inference could be made from a variety of other data that high-PSA prostate cancer is more clinically aggressive.

In an effort to improve the performance of PSA, numerous derivative formulations have been studied, including age-specific PSA, PSA density, and PSA velocity. In addition, different molecular forms of PSA have been studied, including free PSA, pro-PSA, benign PSA, intact PSA, and complexed PSA.

Adjunctive PSA indices

PSA typically increases with age. Age-specific cutoffs increase sensitivity of PSA for younger men, while increasing specificity at older men. However, it appears that the latter effect is obtained at the expense of sensitivity in older men.

PSA density is defined as the PSA divided by the estimated prostatic volume (assessed by transrectal ultrasound). It was hoped that this might improve specificity by mitigating the effect of benign prostatic hyperplasia. A PSA density of >0.15 ng/mL/cc is considered abnormal. However, due to the difficulty in assessing prostatic volume or of knowing the gland to stroma ratio in any given prostate, this calculation does not perform significantly better than PSA.

PSA velocity refers to the rate of change in successive PSA determinations. A PSA velocity of >0.75 ng/mL/year is considered abnormal. While this appears to improve the sensitivity and specificity, the magnitude of improvement is limited by biologic variation in PSA.

Free PSA normally comprises a minority of total PSA. When released into circulation, PSA is quickly bound to protease inhibitors. In fact, most PSA (75-90%) circulates bound, mostly to α_1-antichymotrypsin (ACT). A *lowered* free PSA fraction (or elevated bound PSA fraction) correlates with the presence of prostate cancer. The likelihood of cancer is quite low in men with free PSA >25%, while it is high with free PSA <10%. The percent free PSA has proven to be more sensitive and specific than total PSA and has aided decision making, particularly in men with low PSA (<10 ng/mL) and in men with small-volume (<60 grams) prostates. Prostatic manipulation and instrumentation have been shown to significantly affect the ratio of free to total PSA. It has been recommended that these measurements be taken either before or several weeks after such manipulation. Specimen handling is of utmost importance in free PSA determinations. Free PSA is less stable than bound PSA, and specimens should be processed rapidly. Specimens that cannot be processed within 2 hours should be separated and frozen.

Prostate cancer prognosis & recurrence detection

Preoperatively, the serum PSA level roughly reflects tumor volume and stage. Following radical prostatectomy, serum PSA should drop to undetectable levels, and PSA can be used to screen for tumor recurrence or metastases. The correlation between PSA and tumor recurrence is somewhat weak in the first 5 years following treatment but improves thereafter.

While posttreatment PSA nadir appears to correlate with the likelihood of cancer cure, no specific value has been established which conclusively establishes disease eradication or treatment failure, particularly within the first 5 years. Various authors have placed the cutoff somewhere between 0.2 and 0.4 ng/mL.

Carcinoembryonic antigen (CEA) & colorectal carcinoma screening

In patients with average risk, screening for colorectal carcinoma is recommended beginning at age 50. The recommended tests include a combination of fecal occult blood testing, flexible sigmoidoscopy, barium enema, and colonoscopy. It appears that future recommendations will recognize the value of fecal DNA and computed tomography (CT) colonography.

Fecal occult blood testing comes in 2 varieties: guaiac-based testing and immunochemical testing. Hemoglobin has endogenous peroxidase activity that is capable of oxidizing guaiac (embedded in the test card) in the presence of hydrogen peroxide (present in the developer) to a blue colored product. False positive tests can result from a number of sources, including nonsteroidal antiinflammatory drug (NSAID) use, consumption of heme (in meat), and consumption of peroxidase (turnips and horseradish). Excessive vitamin C consumption can cause a false negative result. Immunochemical testing for fecal occult blood is based upon monoclonal antibodies to human hemoglobin, and no dietary or drug restrictions apply. The overall sensitivity of fecal occult blood testing for colon cancer ranges from 50-80%. Specificity ranges from 60-90%.

Carcinoembryonic antigen (CEA) is a glycoprotein produced normally in fetal gastrointestinal tissue. It is produced in only very low levels by the adult gastrointestinal tract, but its concentration is markedly increased in patients with colorectal carcinoma. CEA is not recommended for colon cancer screening. Instead, it plays a role in preoperative evaluation of patients with known colon cancer and in the postoperative monitoring of such patients.

In patients with colon cancer, high preoperative CEA concentration implies a worse overall outcome as compared to those with low concentrations. At presentation, the degree of CEA elevation is affected by tumor stage, tumor grade, tumor ploidy, tumor site, obstruction, liver function, and smoking. CEA varies inversely with grade, with well differentiated tumors producing more CEA than poorly differentiated tumors. CEA is elevated in only 25% of tumors confined to the colon, 50% with nodal metastasis, and 75% with distant metastases. Left-sided tumors generally have a higher CEA than right-sided tumors, and bowel obstruction produces a higher CEA. Aneuploid tumors produce higher concentrations of CEA than diploid tumors. Since the liver is the primary site for its metabolism, liver dysfunction can increase the CEA level. The median CEA value for smokers is higher than that for nonsmokers.

For posttreatment surveillance, serial CEA measurements can detect recurrence with a sensitivity of 80% and specificity of 70%. CEA is most sensitive to the presence of liver metastases (94% sensitivity) but is overall poorly sensitive to locoregional recurrences (~60%).

CEA elevations also occur with other malignancies, including gastric adenocarcinoma (particularly well differentiated intestinal type), breast cancer, lung cancer, pancreatic adenocarcinoma, medullary thyroid carcinoma, cervical adenocarcinoma, and urothelial carcinoma. Nonneoplastic conditions associated with elevated CEA include smoking, peptic ulcer disease, inflammatory bowel disease, pancreatitis, hypothyroidism, biliary obstruction, and cirrhosis. Levels exceeding 10 ng/mL are rarely caused by benign disease.

Thyroglobulin

Serum thyroglobulin is the mainstay for detection of tumor recurrence in so-called differentiated (follicular and papillary) thyroid carcinomas. Thyroglobulin is not produced by medullary or anaplastic thyroid carcinoma. Circulating thyroglobulin has a half life of ~65 hours, and it takes nearly a month before thyroglobulin becomes undetectable following total thyroidectomy.

In normal circumstances, thyroglobulin is cleared from the circulation by the catabolism in the liver and recycling in the thyroid. A thyroglobulin assay is only sufficiently specific if all functional thyroid tissue has been ablated (total thyroidectomy followed by radioactive iodine). Following ablation, a combination of serum thyroglobulin, cervical ultrasound, and nuclear medicine ^{131}I scans are used to assess the need for further ablation and subsequently serum thyroglobulin is measured serially to detect recurrence.

Because of inter-assay variation, it is important that serial thyroglobulin measurements be performed on identical assays, preferably within the same laboratory. To enhance sensitivity either TSH (thyrotropin) may be administered to the patient or thyroxine replacement therapy (generating an endogenous TSH response) can be withheld prior to testing.

Heterophile antibodies and antithyroglobulin antibodies are potential sources of interference in the thyroglobulin assay. Heterophile antibodies are present in ~3% of patients; antithyroglobulin antibodies are present in ~10% of normal adults and >20% of those with thyroid carcinoma. These antibodies usually result in underestimation but sometimes cause overestimation (in a macro-thyroglobulin type of mechanism) of the serum thyroglobulin. Assays are available to detect thyroglobulin antibodies such that the problem can be identified if suspected. Assessment of thyroglobulin in the presence of antibodies is challenging, since the effect of antithyroglobulin antibody upon the measurement of thyroglobulin is unpredictable. Serial quantitative serum antithyroglobulin antibody measurements may themselves serve as a surrogate tumor marker. Antibodies are expected to progressively diminish after thyroid ablation. Any increase is indicative of antigenic stimulation, suggesting recurrence.

Cancer antigen (CA) 125

CA 125 is elevated in nonmucinous epithelial ovarian neoplasms and has a major role in the monitoring of these patients. CA 125 has not proven useful in screening for ovarian neoplasms. This marker is elevated in only ~50% of patients with stage I disease, and CA 125 has a poor positive predictive value in unselected women. CA 125 may be elevated in a number of nonneoplastic abdominopelvic disorders (pregnancy, fibroids, benign ovarian cysts, pelvic inflammation, ascites, and endometriosis), and in some nonovarian neoplasms (endometrial, fallopian tube, pancreas, breast, and colon).

CA 125 <35 U/mL is considered normal. In post-menopausal women, levels tend to decrease. Normal values are lower for African American and Asian women. The level increases slightly during the follicular (proliferative) phase of the menstrual cycle. Values above 35 may be found in up to 2% of normal women.

CA 125 has utility in differentiating pelvic masses. In postmenopausal women with palpable adnexal masses, CA 125 levels >65 U/mL have a positive predictive value of >95% for ovarian malignancy.

It is in patients with known ovarian malignancy, whose presurgical CA 125 is elevated, that CA 125 finds its greatest utility. A fall in CA 125 during initial treatment suggests treatment efficacy, and the duration of disease-free survival seems to correlate best with the rate of fall. Conversely, an increase in CA 125 during treatment is indicative of treatment failure, and following treatment an increase is predictive of disease recurrence. A persistent elevation of CA 125 (>35 U/mL) predicts residual disease at the time of a second-look laparotomy with a specificity of >95%. Rising CA 125 suggests relapse. In fact, the rise often precedes clinical evidence of disease by a median interval of 3-6 months.

Prognosis relates to both the initial and posttreatment CA 125 value. A preoperative CA 125 >65 U/mL portends an unfavorable prognosis. Persistent elevations following chemotherapy indicate a poor prognosis. Furthermore, the half life of CA 125 after chemotherapy correlates with prognosis, with those patients demonstrating a CA 125 half life <20 days having improved survival. Lastly, the time to normalization of CA 125 impacts prognosis, with those patients whose levels normalized within 3 cycles of chemotherapy having improved survival.

CA 27.29 & 15-3

CA 27.29 (also called BR 27.29) and CA 15-3 measure different epitopes of a single antigen—the protein product of the breast cancer-associated *MUC1* gene. Both are elevated in ~60-70% of women with advanced-stage disease. Neither marker should be used to diagnose primary breast cancer since the overall incidence of elevation at presentation (20-25%) is low. Both markers demonstrate utility for monitoring recurrence and response to therapy.

Both CA 27.29 and CA 15-3 may also be elevated in patients with benign ovarian cysts, benign breast disease, and benign liver disease. They can be elevated in cirrhosis, sarcoidosis, and lupus. They may be elevated in nonbreast malignancies, including colon, stomach, pancreas, prostate, and lung. CA 27.29 levels >100 U/mL and CA 15-3 levels >25 U/mL are rare in benign conditions.

CA 19-9

CA 19-9 is a marker for pancreatic adenocarcinoma and is elevated in 80% of patients at presentation. In one study of patients with pancreatic lesions, a combination of a weight loss >20 lb, bilirubin >3 mg/dL, and CA 19-9 >37 U/L had a positive predictive value approaching 100% for pancreatic adenocarcinoma. With any 2 of these, the positive predictive value decreased to around 90%. CA 19-9 appears to be most useful in assessing the response to treatment. CA 19-9 is sometimes elevated in patients with hepatobiliary, gastric, colorectal, and breast cancer. It may also be elevated in benign conditions such as pancreatitis, cholestasis, cholangitis, and cirrhosis. Only ~3% of those with CA 19-9 >100 U/L have benign disease, however, and virtually no patients with CA 19-9 >1,000 U/L have benign disease. CA 19-9 is identical to the Lewis blood group antigen. It is thus not produced by Lewis-negative patients.

α fetoprotein (AFP)

AFP is a major component of fetal serum, having a physiologic role similar to albumin. It is synthesized in the yolk sac, fetal liver, and fetal gastrointestinal tract. After birth, it rapidly decreases to undetectable levels. Normal adults have AFP <5.4 ng/mL. While elevations may be seen in a number of benign conditions, values above 500 ng/mL are not seen in benign disease. AFP is elevated in normal pregnancy (usually not >100 ng/mL), cirrhosis, and hepatitis.

AFP has utility in detection of hepatocellular carcinoma and yolk sac tumors. It may also be elevated sporadically in other tumors, notably hepatoid variants of gastric carcinoma. In yolk sac tumors, the magnitude of AFP correlates with prognosis (AFP >10,000 ng/mL associated with poor prognosis). In hepatocellular carcinoma, most studies report AFP elevations in ~70% of patients.

Human chorionic gonadotropin (hCG)

hCG is elevated in pregnancy, trophoblastic disease, and choriocarcinoma. In the initial evaluation of germ cell tumors, the magnitude of elevation correlates with prognosis (hCG>50,000 mIU/mL associated with a poor prognosis). hCG may is elevated in ~15% of pure seminomas and in rare examples of tumors from numerous sites (GI tract, GU tract). By itself, this finding does not imply a choriocarcinoma.

The free β-subunit of hCG is elevated in up to 40% of patients with pure seminoma. It appears to be a better tumor marker in these patients than hCG. Using a combination of hCG and free β-subunit of hCG, ~57% of patients have elevation of one or both markers.

β₂ microglobulin (β₂M)

$\beta_2 M$ is a component of class I MHC molecules, and when cells die $\beta_2 M$ is released into the extracellular fluid. Thus, $\beta_2 M$ can be expected to be elevated whenever there is increased cell death, and has proven to be a good though nonspecific marker for several tumor types. It has been studied as a marker in both solid tumors and hematolymphoid neoplasms. It is an independent prognostic factor in multiple myeloma, with low levels associated with a good prognosis. It is cleared by the kidneys and may be nonspecifically elevated in renal insufficiency. Its level is raised in a number of inflammatory states (rheumatoid arthritis, lupus, inflammatory bowel disease).

Alkaline phosphatase

Alkaline phosphatase is a highly nonspecific tumor marker, but it has a place in certain settings. A raised alkaline phosphatase may be an indication of osteoblastic activity; thus, it may be elevated in osteogenic sarcoma or bone metastases. Alkaline phosphatase is the most sensitive liver function test to the presence of hepatic metastases. In some settings, such as primary intraabdominal carcinoids, the concentration of alkaline phosphatase correlates with prognosis. Some tumors, particularly when advanced, are associated with elevated alkaline phosphatase due to the Regan isoenzyme.

Markers of neuroendocrine tumors

Carcinoid tumors

Carcinoids are neoplasms of enterochromaffin cells, which are capable of producing *serotonin* (5-hydroxytryptamine, 5-HT). 5-HT is either stored (in the neurosecretory granules) or secreted. Most of the secreted 5-HT is taken up by platelets and stored in their secretory (dense) granules. A portion of the 5-HT enters the renal tubules, where it is converted into *5-hydroxyindoleacetic acid (5-HIAA)* by renal tubular monoamine oxidase and aldehyde dehydrogenase.

In addition to serotonin, carcinoids arising in the foregut (stomach, proximal duodenum, lung) often produce modest quantities of histamine, catecholamines, and 5-hydroxytryptophan (5-HTP). Midgut carcinoids (distal duodenum, jejunum, ileum, appendix, right colon) usually produce only serotonin; however, they tend to produce it in great quantity. The serotonin they produce is released largely into the portal circulation and is thus cleared by the liver. However, if there are metastases to or beyond the liver, serotonin may be present in the systemic circulation and carcinoid syndrome may result, characterized by diarrhea, flushing, nausea, and wheezing. Hindgut carcinoids are most often nonsecretory.

Both 5-HIAA and serotonin can be assayed in a urine sample. Urinary 5-HIAA and serotonin may be within normal limits in 20-30% of patients with a carcinoid tumor, particularly foregut and hindgut tumors. Furthermore, these analytes may be falsely elevated in patients with a tryptophan-rich diet. Platelets take up serotonin from the serum at a constant rate that is unaffected by serotonin in diet. Platelet serotonin appears to be the most accurate marker for the detection of a carcinoid tumor.

Other peptides that may be produced in excess include synaptophysin, neuropeptide K, pancreatic polypeptide (PP), and chromogranin A (CGA). CGA has been used as a measure of tumor burden and treatment response. In addition to carcinoids, elevated serum levels of chromogranin A have been found in pheochromocytoma, islet cell tumors, and small cell neuroendocrine carcinoma.

Markers of medullary thyroid carcinoma

Plasma calcitonin is useful to detect medullary thyroid carcinoma (MTC) and its recurrences. Mature, biologically active calcitonin is a 32 amino acid polypeptide that results from posttranslational modification of a larger 141 amino acid precursor called preprocalcitonin. Currently used assays are specific for the mature form of calcitonin. Normal individuals have calcitonin values <10 ng/L. Most patients with medullary thyroid carcinoma will have elevated calcitonin levels although up to 30% of those with familial MTC or MEN2 syndrome have normal levels. Provocative testing with calcium infusion is a more sensitive test that may be employed in MEN2 families. However, mutation screening of the *RET* gene has largely replaced calcium infusion testing in these patients. Note that calcitonin may also be increased in Hashimoto thyroiditis, C-cell hyperplasia, small cell lung carcinoma and breast carcinoma. It may be secondarily increased in chronic renal failure and Zollinger-Ellison syndrome.

CEA is very commonly elevated in medullary carcinoma. Higher CEA values correlate with greater de-differentiation in the tumor and suggest a worse prognosis.

Paraganglioma & pheochromocytoma

These are tumors of chromaffin cells, which are capable of secreting catecholamines. By convention, those arising in the adrenal medulla are called pheochromocytomas, and those arising extraadrenally are called paragangliomas. Chromaffin cells are nearly always capable of producing norepinephrine. Norepinephrine can be converted to epinephrine by the action of the enzyme PNMT (phenol ethanolamine-N-methyl transferase) and significant quantities of norepinephrine are converted to epinephrine in tumors of the adrenal medulla. Thus, adrenal tumors usually secrete both epinephrine and norepinephrine. In contrast, the majority of extra-adrenal tumors are either nonsecretory or secrete mainly norepinephrine.

Norepinephrine is metabolized to normetanephrine. Most normetanephrine is conjugated with sulfate and excreted in urine, and some is metabolized to vanillylmandelic acid (VMA). Epinephrine is metabolized to metanephrine. Most metanephrine is conjugated with sulfate and excreted in urine, but some is metabolized to VMA. Thus, VMA reflects both metanephrine and normetanephrine.

Available laboratory tests include urinary VMA, urinary metanephrines, urinary catecholamines, plasma metanephrines or plasma catecholamines. Certain antihypertensive and other medications can interfere with these assays including imipramine, reserpine, guanethidine, nitroglycerin, and monoamine oxidase (MAO) inhibitors. Among all these tests, plasma metanephrines are considered the most accurate for initial screening. The urine metanephrine and catecholamine tests perform only slightly worse. Due to the episodic nature of release, plasma catecholamines have poor sensitivity, with plasma metanephrines better reflecting long term catecholamine secretion. The clonidine suppression test may be used to clarify equivocal serum and urine tests.

Neuroblastoma

Urine vanillylmandelic acid (VMA) and homovanillic acid (HVA) are elevated in most cases. HVA is the final metabolic product of DOPA and dopamine, while VMA is the product of norepinephrine and epinephrine. Interestingly, the more poorly differentiated tumors make more HVA than VMA. A low VMA:HVA ratio portends a worse prognosis. Neuron-specific enolase (NSE), lactic dehydrogenase (LD), and ferritin are nonspecific markers that may be used to follow disease activity.

Urine markers for urothelial carcinoma

The NMP-22 (nuclear matrix protein 22) test detects a nuclear matrix protein, called NuMA (nuclear mitotic apparatus), that is released from the nuclei of tumor cells when they die. Elevated urinary levels of NMP-22 have been demonstrated in subjects with urothelial carcinoma. This test is mainly used for the monitoring of patients with a known history of bladder cancer. In this setting, it has proven quite sensitive but fairly nonspecific. When performed shortly (1-6 weeks) after tumor resection, >70% of patients with elevated NMP-22 have recurrent disease. >80% of patients with normal results have no evidence of disease. Other causes of rapid cell turnover (inflammation) may produce a positive test, and, in fact, leukocytes may be the source of these false positives.

The bladder tumor antigen (BTA) test detects complement factor H and complement factor H-related proteins (CFH-rp) in the urine. It demonstrates ~60% sensitivity and 70% specificity. False positives appear to be related to stone disease, inflammation, bladder or urinary tract trauma, and benign prostatic hyperplasia.

Endocrine
Thyroid chemistry
Thyroid function tests (TFTs) t1.33

Total T4 (thyroxine) is elevated in most hyperthyroid patients and decreased in hypothyroidism. Fewer than 5% of hyperthyroid patients have normal T4 but elevated T3 ("T3 toxicosis"), so measurement of total T3 can be useful in some instances. Fluctuations in serum proteins somewhat limits the value of total T4 and total T3 measurement, however. T3 and T4 are highly protein-bound, mainly to prealbumin (transthyretin) and thyroid binding globulin (TBG). Thus, total T3 and T4 are affected by levels of these serum proteins, and a patient may be clinically euthyroid but have abnormal total T4 and/or T3. TBG is increased by pregnancy, oral contraceptives, estrogen therapy, active hepatitis, and hypothyroidism. TBG is decreased by hypoproteinemic states, androgen therapy, and cortisol.

t1.33 **Thyroid function test patterns**					
	TSH	T3	T4 (total)	T4 (free)	rT3
Hyperthyroidism	↓	↑	↑	↑	→
Hypothyroidism	↑	↓	↓	↓	→↓
Euthyroid sick syndrome	→	↓	→↓	→↓	↑
Excess TBG	→	↑	↑	→	→

T3 resin uptake (T3RU) is a conceptually confusing test whose purpose is to circumvent the limitations of total T4 or T3 measurements. To perform this test, an excess of ^{125}I-labeled T3 is added to the serum to be tested; the ^{125}I-T3 binds to any available unoccupied sites on TBG. Next, a resin is added to the serum, which binds any unbound ^{125}I-T3. The amount of ^{125}I-T3 on the resin is measured. This amount is inversely proportional to the number of available binding sites on TBG and directly proportional to the amount of T3 present. In hypothyroidism, one would expect there to be more sites for ^{125}I-T3 to bind to TBG and less left over to bind to resin (low T3RU). In hyperthyroidism, the opposite occurs (high T3RU).

The free thyroxine index (fTI) is obtained by multiplying the T3RU by the total thyroxine.

Since the advent of fully automated chemiluminescent assays, the routine measurement of free T4 (fT4) and free T3 (fT3) has been practical. The fT4 level correlates well with the patient's clinical thyroid status. Measurement of fT3 is not commonly performed but may diagnose cases of "T3 thyrotoxicosis."

When T4 is metabolized in the peripheral blood, most of it is metabolized to T3. A smaller amount is metabolized to reverse T3 (rT3), an inactive metabolite. rT3 assays have little clinical utility other than to confirm the suspicion of euthyroid sick syndrome, in which rT3 is elevated.

Radioactive iodine uptake (RAIU) is a nuclear medicine test. The patient is given a dose of radioactive iodine then scanned for thyroid radioactivity. The expectation is that patients with Graves disease or functioning adenoma will have increased RAIU, while patients with hyperthyroidism caused by thyroiditis, struma ovarii, or exogenous thyroid hormone will have decreased uptake.

Thyroid stimulating hormone (TSH, thyrotropin) is the pituitary hormone whose function is to stimulate production and release of thyroxine from the thyroid gland. Through a tightly regulated feedback loop, TSH rises and falls in direct reflection of the patient's true thyroid status. As a result, TSH has become widely accepted as the best first-line test for diagnosing hypo- and hyperthyroidism.

Thyroid releasing hormone (TRH) is the hypothalamic hormone that stimulates production of TSH by the pituitary gland. Exogenous TRH is administered to a patient as part of the TRH stimulation test, which is used in the evaluation of hypothyroidism. In primary hypothyroidism (hypothyroidism due to intrinsic thyroid hypofunction), there is exaggerated secretion of TSH in response to TRH. An inappropriate TSH response to TRH stimulation suggests hypopituitarism. Note that normally TRH stimulates not only TSH but also GH and prolactin.

In summary, TSH is the screening test indicated for thyroid dysfunction in all contexts except in potential hypothalamic or pituitary dysfunction, and perhaps in neonatal screening. In these latter populations, a broader panel including fT4 may be indicated. Most of the other tests listed above are not commonly needed.

Hyperthyroidism

Hyperthyroidism is a generalized hypermetabolic state in which the patient experiences anxiety, tachycardia, palpitations, weight loss (without anorexia), diarrhea, and heat intolerance. Hyperthyroidism is found most commonly in women, attributed to the 5:1 female:male predominance of Graves disease, its most common cause.

Hyperthyroidism is diagnosed when there is suppressed TSH and high serum fT4. When fT4 is normal despite a low TSH, fT3 should be measured to assess for T3 thyrotoxicosis. When both fT4 and fT3 are normal, mild or subclinical hyperthyroidism is usually diagnosed. However, medication effect should be excluded in this latter setting.

The most common cause is Graves disease. Other causes are toxic multinodular goiter, toxic adenoma (Plummer syndrome), transient hyperthyroidism in various kinds of thyroiditis, exogenous thyroxine, and (rarely) pituitary adenoma & thyroid carcinoma.

Graves disease is further characterized by ocular retro-orbital soft tissue infiltration leading to exophthalmos, and pretibial myxedema. The serum of most patients (>95%) is found to contain thyroid-stimulating immunoglobulin (TSI), also called long-acting thyroid stimulating (LATS) antibodies, which are capable of acting upon TSH receptors as agonists. Anti-microsomal antibodies are found in 60% of cases, and antithyroglobulin antibodies in 30%.

Hypothyroidism

Hypothyroidism manifests as a generalized hypometabolic state, with symptoms of fatigue, cold intolerance, slowed mentation, reflexes and speech, and periorbital edema. Hypothyroidism is associated with mixed dyslipidemia, CK elevation in some patients, and a risk for spontaneous and statin-induced myopathy or rhabdomyolysis. Hypothyroidism is usually diagnosed with an elevated TSH and low fT4. Some patients have a normal fT4 in spite of a raised TSH, and these may be considered to have "subclinical" or "mild" hypothyroidism.

When a low fT4 is found with a normal or low TSH, this may indicate anterior pituitary pathology. In such cases, TSH is rarely the only deficient anterior pituitary product, and a complete evaluation of the pituitary gland is warranted.

The most common cause is Hashimoto thyroiditis. Others include thyroidectomy, ^{131}I therapy, exposure to certain drugs (iodine, amiodarone, lithium, IL-2, and α-IFN), and burn-out phase of lymphocytic and granulomatous (de Quervain) thyroiditis. A rare disease results in congenital resistance to TSH (Refetoff syndrome). Patients with this condition are typically euthyroid but have elevated TSH with normal fT4 levels.

Hashimoto thyroiditis is characterized by anti-tissue peroxidase (>90%) and antithyroglobulin (>90%) antibodies. TSI are not identified in Hashimoto thyroiditis. Secondary hypothyroidism (pituitary hypofunction with decreased TSH) and tertiary hypothyroidism (hypothalamic dysfunction with decreased TRH secretion) are both uncommon.

Neonatal hypothyroidism

The cause of neonatal hypothyroidism is most often the abnormal development of the thyroid gland (thyroid dysgenesis). Most cases are sporadic, and some familial (inherited mutations in *PAX8* or *TTF* genes). There may be complete (agenesis) or partial (dysgenesis) absence of thyroid tissue.

Other causes include familial thyroid dyshormonogenesis, peripheral hormone resistance (autosomal dominant Refetoff syndrome), hypopituitarism, and maternal factors (maternal autoantibodies, maternal medications) that may produce transient neonatal hypothyroidism.

Hypothyroidism in neonates manifests as dry skin, a hoarse cry, macroglossia, hypothermia, edema, neonatal jaundice, and inactivity. Many cases, however, are subclinical. If untreated, there is a high risk of mental and growth retardation. Early initiation of thyroid hormone replacement prevents sequelae.

Most commonly, the TSH assay alone is used to screen for this condition, with samples taken between 48-72 hours of age. However, numerous disparate approaches have been proposed for the detection of neonatal hypothyroidism, and some have advocated a second screening specimen at ~2-6 weeks of life. Test selection also varies, with some approaches including primary measurement of T4 with follow-up TSH, simultaneous T4 and TSH, and primary TSH-only screening methods. All of these detect congenital hypothyroidism cases at essentially similar rates but all suffer from false negatives. The TSH-only approach will miss cases of delayed TSH rise and central hypothyroidism. All methods are likely to miss mild hypothyroidism. Recent studies support the use of a second discretionary screening test in very low birth weight infants, infants with significant perinatal complications, and same-sex twins.

Nonthyroidal illness syndrome (euthyroid sick syndrome)

This is a "syndrome" consisting entirely of abnormal thyroid function tests in a euthyroid individual who is suffering from a nonthyroidal illness. The typical case involves a critically ill, elderly, hospitalized individual. Thyroid function tests in the euthyroid sick syndrome are typical and include decreased T3 and T4, increased rT3, and normal TSH. The TSH is decreased in 5-9% of cases.

Exogenous estrogens

A common problem in thyroid function test interpretation involves the patient taking exogenous estrogen, usually in the form of oral contraceptives. Such agents increase circulating thyroid binding globulin (TBG), thus elevating total thyroxine (T3 & T4). The free thyroxine and TSH remain normal.

Medications

Due to a combination of its direct thyroid toxicity and its large quantity of iodine, amiodarone exerts effects on thyroid function. The effect is unpredictable, but a general rule of thumb is that in the presence of a pre-existing state of iodine deficiency or multinodular goiter amiodarone causes hyperthyroidism, while in euthyroid iodine sufficient patients it causes hypothyroidism.

Lithium inhibits the release of thyroxine from the thyroid gland. Many patients on lithium therapy will therefore develop hypothyroidism with or without thyroid hyperplasia. Furthermore, it appears that lithium worsens preexisting antithyroid autoimmune conditions.

Adrenal cortex

Tests

Serum cortisol interpretation must be guided by knowledge of its physiology. First, it is essential to note that cortisol secretion normally undergoes diurnal variation. It is secreted in intermittent small surges throughout the day with a relative trough around midnight and a significant peak around 8 AM. Thus, interpretation of a single random serum cortisol depends upon a properly timed draw compared to appropriate reference intervals. Furthermore, the quantity of serum cortisol depends upon highly variable levels of cortisol binding globulin. Lastly, cortisol levels may be raised by stress. A single elevated midnight serum cortisol is highly suggestive of Cushing syndrome. Likewise, a single reduced 8 AM cortisol is consistent with adrenal insufficiency.

In the context of Cushing syndrome, the *urine free cortisol* test is more accurate than serum cortisol but requires a 24-hour urine collection. It is free (unbound) cortisol that passes into the urine, so this test reflects the amount of free cortisol. Furthermore, since measured in a 24-hour specimen, this test is independent of time of day considerations. An elevated urine free cortisol is highly suggestive of Cushing syndrome; however, like the serum test, false positive results may be seen in stress, depression, and chronic alcoholism. A negative test is incapable of excluding Cushing syndrome, and should be repeated. The test is invalid if there is renal insufficiency.

Dexamethasone is an agent capable of suppressing adrenocorticotrophic hormone (ACTH) without crossreacting with assays for cortisol and thereby forms the basis for the *dexamethasone suppression test* (DST). In patients with normal endocrine function, a dose of dexamethasone will suppress both ACTH and cortisol. A variety of abnormal suppression patterns are seen in Cushing syndrome.

There are 3 varieties of DST, 2 low dose tests and 1 high dose test. 2 main protocols are used for the low dose DST, the *rapid (overnight) DST* and the *standard (2-day) DST*. Both low dose DST tests are meant to answer the question: does the patient have Cushing syndrome (hypercortisolism)? In the rapid test, 1 mg of dexamethasone is administered at 11 PM, and the plasma cortisol is measured at 8 AM. In the standard low dose DST, 0.5 mg are given every 6 hours for 48 hours, followed by cortisol measurement. Normal individuals experience suppression of serum cortisol below 1.8 μg/dL (50 nmol/L) using modern analytically specific immunoassays for cortisol. Impaired suppression of plasma cortisol levels by these tests confirms the diagnosis of Cushing syndrome; however, abnormal suppression can also be seen in severe stress, alcohol abuse, and major depression (so-called pseudo-Cushing syndrome).

The *high dose DST* is used to answer the question: is Cushing syndrome caused by a pituitary corticotroph adenoma (Cushing disease), or is it caused by ectopic ACTH production? 2 mg dexamethasone every 6 hours for 48 hours should suppress pituitary adenoma related hypercortisolism (Cushing disease). Suppression is defined as 50% reduction in cortisol from baseline. Nonsuppression points to either ectopic ACTH production by tumor or primary adrenal hypercortisolism. It should be noted that suppression occurs in only ~80% of patients with Cushing disease; whereas ~20% of patients with ectopic ACTH production show suppression to <50% of baseline. The latter 2 possibilities can be distinguished by plasma ACTH measurement.

The *cortisol-releasing hormone (CRH) stimulation test*, like the high dose DST, is aimed at determining the cause of Cushing syndrome. After intravenous administration of CRH, a rise of 35% or more in ACTH suggests Cushing disease; with adrenal tumors or ectopic ACTH, no response is seen.

The *metyrapone stimulation test*, no longer used in clinical practice, was once used to determine whether the pituitary is to blame when a patient is deficient in cortisol. Metyrapone blocks the conversion of 11-deoxycortisol to cortisol. The decreased cortisol leads to increased ACTH production by the pituitary. In normal subjects, this increased ACTH can sufficiently increase the 11-deoxycortisol to overcome the metyrapone induced block, thus increasing serum cortisol. Patients who cannot overcome this block have impaired pituitary function.

With the improvement in immunoassay sensitivity and the advent of LC-MS/MS assays for cortisol it has become possible to measure salivary cortisol, the concentration of which is ~1% that of the serum. Saliva offers numerous advantages over blood, including ease of collection and low patient-stress induction; the latter is a critical feature in tests of the exquisitely sensitive endocrine system. The late night (11:00 PM to midnight) salivary cortisol is perhaps the best screening test for Cushing syndrome. It has a reported 100% specificity and 91-93% sensitivity for Cushing syndrome. It appears that salivary cortisol correlates well with serum cortisol, independent of salivary flow rates. Furthermore, it is free cortisol that crosses into the saliva; thus this assay reflects free serum cortisol and therefore does not have the problem of variation with changes in cortisol binding globulin that significantly hampers the interpretation of serum cortisol levels. Cortisol is stable in saliva for up to 1 week, so patients may collect the sample at home and then drop it off at the laboratory at their convenience.

Cushing syndrome (hypercortisolism)

Iatrogenic Cushing syndrome—administration of corticosteroids for the treatment of inflammatory disease—is the most common cause in the developed world. The underlying cause of spontaneous Cushing syndrome may be found in the pituitary (Cushing disease), adrenal gland, or ectopic sites. Overall, 70% of cases are caused by pituitary adenoma, 20% by adrenal cortical hyperplasia or neoplasia, and the rest are related to ectopic production of ACTH by neoplasia elsewhere.

The diagnosis of Cushing syndrome requires demonstration of persistent hypercortisolism. The recommended screening tests are the low dose DST, 24 hour urinary free cortisol, or midnight salivary or serum cortisol. A positive screening test should be confirmed by repeat testing.

The underlying cause of Cushing syndrome must then be determined, first by measuring ACTH to distinguish ACTH-dependent from ACTH-independent Cushing syndrome. ACTH-dependent Cushing is further evaluated with bilateral inferior petrosal sinus sampling (BIPSS), if available, or the high dose DST and/or CRH stimulation tests. Imaging of the pituitary provides corroborative information, but it lacks sensitivity and specificity for Cushing disease when used in isolation. ACTH-independent Cushing requires adrenal imaging, after the exclusion of surreptitious glucocorticoid administration.

Cushing disease is usually found in association with a pituitary microadenoma (<1.0 cm) of basophilic cells (corticotrophs). There is bilateral adrenal hyperplasia, and ACTH levels are elevated along with cortisol levels.

Ectopic ACTH is most commonly associated with bronchogenic neuroendocrine neoplasms. A variety of tumors account for the remaining cases, including pancreatic endocrine tumors, non-small cell lung carcinoma, thymic tumors, medullary thyroid carcinoma, and breast carcinoma.

Primary adrenal hypercortisolism may be due to adenoma, carcinoma, or bilateral adrenal hyperplasia. Bilateral adrenal hyperplasia may take the form of primary pigmented nodular adrenal dysplasia associated with Carney complex, or more commonly takes the form of nonpigmented macronodular hyperplasia or so-called ACTH-independent macronodular adrenal hyperplasia (AIMAH). In adults, adenomas and carcinomas have roughly equal incidence. In children, carcinomas actually outnumber adenomas. Carcinomas are associated with higher mean levels of serum cortisol than adenomas.

The biochemical effects of hypercortisolism include hyperglycemia, hypokalemia, protein catabolism, and osteoporosis. So-called centripetal fat deposition is seen in the face, supraclavicular, and posterior cervical adipose tissue, producing the classic "moon face" and "buffalo hump." Skin thinning is noted and results in visible striae. This reflects generalized protein loss that is also reflected in weakness of tendons and poor wound healing.

Lastly, it must be noted that non-Cushing hypercortisolic states exist, which can confound laboratory testing for Cushing syndrome. In general, these are not associated with the end-organ effects of hypercortisolism. Patients with major depression often exhibit biochemical findings indistinguishable from Cushing syndrome. Subtle differences of importance include that in depression the biochemical findings are relatively mild, that there is usually persistence of (sometimes reversed) diurnal variation, and that there is resolution with depression treatment. Anorexia nervosa, alcoholism, and pregnancy may be associated with a similar biochemical milieu. Apparent Cushing syndrome that is caused by a normal response to physiological stresses is commonly referred to as pseudo-Cushing syndrome.

Addison disease (primary adrenal insufficiency)

Historically, most cases of Addison disease were related to primary destruction of the adrenal gland by granulomatous disease (tuberculosis), a still common cause world-wide. Presently, the most common cause in developed nations is autoimmunity. Autoimmune adrenalitis may occur in isolation or as part of the autoimmune polyendocrinopathy syndrome. In type 1 autoimmune polyendocrinopathy syndrome, Addison arises in association with autoimmune hypoparathyroidism and chronic mucocutaneous candidiasis. In type 2 (Schmidt syndrome), Addison is found in association with autoimmune thyroiditis and type 1 diabetes mellitus. Both types may be associated with a wide variety of additional autoimmune conditions. Addison disease may also be caused by adrenal replacement with metastatic tumor, amyloid, or bilateral adrenal hemorrhage (Waterhouse-Friderichsen syndrome). Inherited diseases that cause Addison include congenital adrenal hyperplasia and adrenoleukodystrophy (accumulation of very long chain fatty acids in the adrenal gland and nervous system). Certain drugs are notoriously adrenostatic, including ketoconazole etomidate, and mitotane. Adrenal failure is frequent in severe sepsis, with a reported incidence as high as 61%. Liver failure is well recognized to cause renal (hepatorenal syndrome) and pulmonary (hepatopulmonary syndrome) disease; it has recently been recognized that patients with liver failure and patients undergoing liver transplantation have a very high rate (>70%) of adrenal failure (hepatoadrenal syndrome).

Addison disease may present abruptly (Addisonian crisis) with altered mental status. This is attended by hypotension and a characteristic set of biochemical abnormalities including hypoglycemia, hyponatremia (with high urine sodium and high urine osmolarity), and hyperkalemia with a metabolic acidosis.

Equally frequent is a more insidious presentation as fatigue, weakness, weight loss, and mood alteration. Postural hypotension, skin hyper-pigmentation, and hypoglycemia are clues to Addison in such a nonspecific form. Co-hypersecretion of melanocyte stimulating hormone (MSH) results in diffuse hyperpigmentation of the skin.

Diagnosis depends upon demonstration of a low 8 AM serum cortisol and/or a blunted increase in cortisol following cosyntropin stimulation. Cosyntropin is an ACTH analog whose administration should result in increased cortisol over 500 mmol/L. In patients with adrenal insufficiency, the ACTH level is used to guide further evaluation. Elevated ACTH indicates primary adrenal insufficiency, which may be further evaluated with autoantibody studies and/or adrenal imaging. Normal or low ACTH suggests secondary adrenal insufficiency, most likely related to pituitary pathology or exogenous glucocorticoid administration.

Secondary adrenal insufficiency

Most cases of secondary adrenal insufficiency are related to the administration of exogenous glucocorticoid that can lead to irreversible (or very slowly reversible) suppression of endogenous ACTH production by the pituitary.

Secondary adrenal insufficiency is not as severe as Addison disease, because mineralocorticoid production is maintained by the renin-angiotensin system. As a result, hyperkalemia is absent and hyponatremia mild. Hyperpigmentation is not a feature of secondary adrenal insufficiency.

Conn syndrome (hyperaldosteronism)

This is usually due to an adrenal adenoma (65% are caused by a bilateral adrenal hyperplasia, and 30% by solitary aldosterone-producing adenoma). Secondary hyperaldosteronism is seen in hyperreninemic states such as renal artery stenosis or the rare renin-producing juxtaglomerular cell tumor of the kidney.

The consequences of hyperaldosteronism may include hypertension, hypokalemia, and metabolic alkalosis. Some patients may develop mild hypernatremia. While the combination of hypokalemia and new-onset hypertension suggests hyperaldosteronism, about half of hyperaldosteronemic patients are normokalemic. When present, the hypokalemia is renal in origin, with 24-hour urinary potassium in excess of 30 mEq/day.

The ratio of the plasma aldosterone concentration (PAC) to plasma renin activity (PRA) is considered the best screening test. PAC/PRA ratio >20-30 (ng/dL)/(ng/mL/h) is consistent with primary hyperaldosteronism. This must be confirmed by one of several dynamic function tests, the most popular of which is the saline infusion test.

Congenital adrenal hyperplasia t1.34

At least 8 different inherited enzyme deficiencies of the adrenal cortex are known, all of which are autosomally and recessively inherited. 21-hydroxylase deficiency is the most common, accounting for 95% of cases, followed by 11-hydroxylase deficiency. The others are vanishingly rare.

t1.34 Congenital adrenal hyperplasia (CAH)

Enzyme deficiency	Adrenal hyperplasia	Virilization	Salt wasting	Hypertension
21-hydroxylase	+	+	+	–
11-hydroxylase	+	+	–	+

The incidence varies geographically, and in the US the disease is particularly common in Native Americans and Yupic Eskimos (incidence of 1/280). Among American Caucasians, the incidence is ~1/15000. A high rate of the disease is found on the island of La Réunion (1/2100), in Brazil (1/7500), and in the Philippines (1/7000).

The gene for 21-hydroxylase is found on 6p21.3, within the HLA complex. 21-hydroxylase deficiency results from a fairly unique sort of mutation. The gene consists of 2 highly homologous near-copies in series—an active gene (CYP21A), and an inactive pseudogene (CYP21P). Mutant alleles result from recombination between the pseudo and active genes in a process called gene conversion.

The severity of disease varies depending upon the nature of the mutation. In general, a compensatory increase in ACTH by the pituitary leads to increased production of steroid hormone precursors in the adrenal cortex. The resulting adrenal hyperplasia and altered hormonal milieu results in some degree of salt wasting, hypertension, and virilization. Affected individuals have increased 17-hydroxyprogesterone, decreased cortisol, increased ACTH, increased androgens, increased 17-ketosteroids, and decreased aldosterone. The effect on serum electrolytes is an increase in potassium and decrease in sodium.

Female infants with classic CAH have ambiguous genitalia because of exposure to high concentrations of androgens in utero, and CAH due to 21-hydroxylase deficiency is the most common cause of ambiguous genitalia in 46,XX infants. Less severely affected girls can present with early pubarche, or as young women with acne, hirsutism and irregular menses.

Boys have no signs of CAH at birth, except subtle hyperpigmentation and possible penile enlargement. If they have the classic salt-wasting variety of the disease, then they may present with severe shock in the second week of life. Thus, the age at diagnosis in boys varies according to the severity of aldosterone deficiency. Boys with the non-salt-wasting form present with early virilization at age 2-4 years.

A very high concentration of 17-hydroxyprogesterone (>3,470 ng/dL) in a randomly timed blood sample is diagnostic of classic 21-hydroxylase deficiency. Typically, salt-wasting patients have higher 17-hydroxyprogesterone concentrations than non-salt losers. False-positive results from neonatal screening are common with premature infants, and many screening programs have established reference ranges that are based on weight and gestational age. A corticotrophin stimulation test can be used in borderline cases. Genetic analysis is not generally necessary to confirm the diagnosis but may be useful in the evaluation of borderline cases. Treatment involves replacement of glucocorticoids and mineralocorticoids.

Renal artery stenosis

In renal artery stenosis there is diminished blood flow to the affected kidney, causing the juxtaglomerular (JG) apparatus to sense hypotension. The result is increased production of renin (and subsequently of aldosterone), producing hypertension. Most cases of renal artery stenosis are caused by atherosclerotic peripheral vascular disease, resulting in stenosis at the origin of the renal artery. A small group of cases are caused by fibromuscular dysplasia, wherein women are more commonly affected and stenosis usually affects the mid to terminal segment of artery. Historically, the diagnosis of renal artery stenosis was based upon selective renal vein renin measurements. Imaging modalities (Doppler ultrasound, magnetic resonance angiography, computed tomographic angiography) now permit diagnosis noninvasively.

Pituitary

The anterior pituitary (adenohypophysis) houses a heterogeneous population of cells, some of which are acidophilic with acridine orange while others are basophilic with this stain. The acidophils consist of 2 cell types: growth hormone-secreting cells and prolactin-secreting cells. The basophils include 4 cell types that secrete follicle-stimulating hormone (FSH), luteinizing hormone (LH), ACTH, and TSH. Hypersecretion of any of the anterior pituitary hormones is nearly always the result of a pituitary adenoma. Prolactinomas are the most common secretory tumors of the pituitary. Most prolactinomas are so-called microadenomas (measuring <1 cm). Physiologic control of anterior pituitary hormone secretion is dually mediated by feedback acting directly on the anterior pituitary as feedback mediated through hypothalamic hormones.

The posterior pituitary (neurohypophysis) contains the axon-termini of neurons that originate in the supraoptic and paraventricular nuclei in the hypothalamus and produce oxytocin and antidiuretic hormone (ADH; vasopressin).

Because of this communal living arrangement, pituitary hypofunction rarely involves a single hormone. Instead, pituitary insults generally manifest as global hyposecretion (panhypopituitarism). Causes include tumors impinging on the pituitary gland (nonsecretory pituitary adenomas, craniopharyngiomas), infarction (Sheehan syndrome, sickle cell anemia), sarcoidosis, histiocytosis X, hemochromatosis, irradiation, and autoimmune destruction.

Hypothalamic disorders and interruption of the pituitary stalk may produce a distinct pattern in which all anterior pituitary hormones except prolactin are suppressed. This pattern of prolactin-sparing hypopituitarism is called the "stalk effect."

Growth hormone (GH)

GH is secreted by acidophils (called somatotrophs) in the anterior pituitary. GH release is stimulated by growth hormone releasing hormone (GHRH) from the hypothalamus. Stimulants of GHRH and GH release are stress, hypoglycemia, and increased amino acid levels, particularly the amino acid arginine. GH release is inhibited by somatostatin (SS) from the pancreas.

GH may be undetectable in normal adult individuals. Small increases in the level of GH are noted during sleep—particularly the first 2 hours—and with exercise, hypoglycemia, and stress.

In children, GH deficiency causes dwarfism. In adults, it is relatively asymptomatic. Undetectable GH levels occur frequently in healthy subjects and are not diagnostic of hyposecretion. Thus, provocative testing is required, performed by measuring GH in the fasting state, during sleep, following exercise, or following insulin or arginine administration. An insulin tolerance test is performed by injecting insulin then serially measuring GH every 15 minutes. The hypoglycemia that results should cause a GH rise of >20 ng/mL. Similar provocative tests can be carried out with exercise, arginine injection, or oral clonidine.

GH hypersecretion causes gigantism in children and acromegaly in adults. GH hypersecretion cannot be excluded with a single normal GH level. A good test for GH excess is IGF-1. As it does not undergo diurnal variation and is consistently elevated in GH hypersecretion, a single normal IGF-1 determination is reliable for excluding GH excess. GH hypersecretion can also be diagnosed by a markedly elevated GH from a random blood sample or a relatively normal level that fails to suppress with glucose administration.

FSH & LH

Secretion of FSH and LH is stimulated by hypothalamic gonadotropin releasing hormone (GnRH), also called luteinizing hormone releasing hormone (LHRH). A unique property of GnRH activity is that when GnRH receptors are continuously stimulated, GnRH soon becomes inhibitory. This is the principle exploited by therapeutic GnRH agonists.

FSH assays can be useful in younger women (eg, <45 years) presenting with possible early menopause. The finding, on 2 separate determinations taken >4 weeks apart, of FSH >40 IU/L suggests ovarian failure.

Prolactin

Prolactin is unique among the anterior pituitary hormones in that it does not have a dedicated stimulator for its release; instead, the hypothalamus produces a potent inhibitor, dopamine. If connections between the hypothalamus and pituitary are severed, all anterior pituitary hormones decrease (due to lack of stimulation) except prolactin which markedly increases (due to lack of inhibition). In fact, this constellation of endocrine findings is often referred to as the "stalk effect," referring to its frequent relation to some kind of impingement upon the pituitary stalk.

In women, hyperprolactinemia produces the so-called amenorrhea-galactorrhea syndrome. In men, testicular atrophy, impotence, and gynecomastia are the result. Hyperprolactinemia is usually due to a prolactin-secreting pituitary adenoma. Other causes include pregnancy, lactation, stalk compression, macroprolactinemia, and phenothiazine therapy. Hypoprolactinemia is rare.

ACTH

Corticotrophin-releasing hormone (CRH) stimulates secretion of ACTH. ACTH is the product of posttranslational cleavage of a large precursor molecule called pro-opiomelanocortin (POMC). POMC is cleaved into ACTH, melanocyte-stimulating hormone (MSH), and β-endorphin. MSH is the reason that patients with excess ACTH production undergo hyperpigmentation.

Antidiuretic hormone (ADH)

ADH is secreted from the posterior pituitary in response to increased serum osmolarity and volume depletion.

Diabetes insipidus (DI), the condition that results from inadequate ADH activity, is characterized by polyuria and polydipsia. Patients produce a large quantity of very dilute urine. The condition arises when either ADH secretion is inadequate (central DI) or renal tubules are unresponsive to ADH (nephrogenic DI). Causes of central DI include head trauma, mass lesions involving the pituitary, and an X-linked recessive familial form. Nephrogenic DI may be due to hypercalcemia, hypokalemia, a very low-protein diet, demeclocycline therapy, lithium therapy, relief of longstanding obstruction, and familial causes. Normal aging may by itself be associated with partial nephrogenic DI.

The diagnosis of DI is suspected in any hypernatremic individual who has low urine osmolarity. It is confirmed by an overnight water deprivation test followed by administration of ADH (vasopressin). In healthy individuals, urine osmolarity progressively increases during water deprivation, and administration of exogenous ADH has no additional effect on urine concentration. In central DI, there is failure to appropriately concentrate the urine in response to dehydration and a rise in urine osmolarity in response to administered ADH. In nephrogenic DI, urine cannot be concentrated in either case.

The syndrome of inappropriate ADH (SIADH) is suspected in the hyponatremic individual who is relatively normovolemic with a urine sodium >20 mmol/L and a urine osmolarity >100 mOsm/kg. It may be caused by tumors (especially small cell carcinoma of the lung, pancreatic adenocarcinoma, and intracranial tumors), interstitial lung disease, cerebral trauma, and the drug chlorpropamide. Direct measurement of ADH is not widely available, such that SIADH is usually made as a diagnosis of exclusion, after ruling out diuretic use and Addison syndrome.

Postmortem chemistries
Samples

There are significant differences in glucose, insulin, pH, oxygen tension, LD, alkaline phosphatase, and many drugs between specimens taken from the left and right sides of the heart and between central (cardiac) and peripheral blood. The exact source of blood submitted is therefore important to know, and blind cardiac puncture is to be avoided. Up to 3 mL of vitreous humor can be obtained from the typical adult. It is important to obtain as much vitreous as can be extracted, as there is variation in the concentrations of many solutes between the vitreous next to the retina and the central vitreous.

Analytes
Glucose

Serum glucose tends to increase after death, due to postmortem hepatic glycogenolysis. Samples from the right heart or inferior vena cava (IVC) will usually have extremely high glucose, but even peripheral vessels cannot be relied upon to give useful measurements. The postmortem diagnosis of diabetes mellitus should not be made on the basis of postmortem blood glucose alone. Adjunctive tests include the HbA_{1c}, glycosuria, ketonuria, and serum acetone. Vitreous glucose falls after death, due to glycolysis. Vitreous is preferred for the postmortem diagnosis of diabetic ketoacidosis (DKA) which is diagnosed by the presence of high vitreous glucose and ketones. Hypoglycemia cannot be reliably diagnosed in the postmortem state.

BUN & creatinine

Both BUN and creatinine are remarkably stable after death. In addition to its value in diagnosing renal insufficiency, mild nitrogen retention in conjunction with hypernatremia is useful to diagnose dehydration.

Sodium & chloride

Sodium and chloride levels begin to decrease immediately after death, both at a rate of ~0.9 mEq/L/hour. Individual variation precludes their use in determining the postmortem interval. Vitreous sodium and chloride are very stable. Both reflect antemortem electrolyte status, and can be used in conjunction with BUN and potassium to categorize the patient into one of several patterns t1.35.

t1.35 Postmortem chemistry patterns

Pattern	Sodium	Chloride	Potassium	BUN	Creatinine
Dehydration	↑	↑	→	↑	↑
Uremic	→	→	→	↑	↑
Decomposition	↓	↓	↑	→	→

Potassium

Serum and CSF potassium rise abruptly after death. Vitreous potassium rises more linearly after death and is probably the most reliable chemical test for postmortem interval. Normal vitreous potassium is <15 mEq/L.

Digoxin

Digoxin is a lipophilic drug in vivo. After death, digoxin is released from tissues and reenters the serum. Thus, postmortem digoxin levels rise progressively, and the postmortem diagnosis of digoxin toxicity should not be made on this basis alone. Another source of error is the presence of endogenous digoxin-like substances (EDLS). EDLS are found in patients with volume overload, hepatorenal failure, pregnancy, hypertension, and in normal infants.

Tryptase & the postmortem diagnosis of anaphylaxis

The postmortem anatomic findings reported in anaphylaxis are numerous and somewhat nonspecific, including pulmonary and laryngeal edema. The postmortem serum tryptase has been advocated as a means to establish a diagnosis of anaphylaxis. Tryptase appears to be stable in serum for several days after death. An elevated serum tryptase is not an entirely specific finding, and has been reported in nonanaphylactic deaths. However, a normal postmortem serum tryptase has a high negative predictive value. The overall sensitivity of postmortem serum tryptase is ~85-90%. Specific IgE assays may be of some use if a particular stimulus is suspected.

Body fluids
Urine

Macroscopic examination

The color of urine is usually clear to yellow. A foam forms when urine is shaken—the color of the foam is yellow when excess bilirubin is present, but it is white under normal conditions or when only excess urobilinogen is present. Red urine is observed when there is hematuria (red blood cells in urine), hemoglobinuria (free hemoglobin in urine), or myoglobinuria; all 3 will produce a positive hemoglobin result on the urine dipstick test. If the dipstick is negative for hemoglobin, then additional causes of red urine to be considered include porphyria and the ingestion of rifampin, pyridium, L-dopa (Aldomet), or beets.

Urine chemistry
Glucose

The 2 methods widely employed for detecting glucose in urine (glycosuria) are the dipstick and the copper sulfate method (eg, Clinitest). Glucose begins to spill over into urine when the "renal threshold" for serum glucose is reached, at around 180 mg/dL. In pregnancy, this threshold is lower. If there is tubular dysfunction (impaired reabsorption), then glucose appears in the urine even when the serum glucose is normal.

The dipstick method relies on the enzymes glucose oxidase and peroxidase to convert glucose to gluconate with the resulting hydrogen peroxide byproduct reacting with a chromogen. This method is sensitive mainly to glucose, and other "reducing substances" do not tend to give a positive reaction. In a standing urine specimen, glucose progressively diminishes as a result of metabolism. Ascorbate inhibits several dipstick tests, including glucose, hemoglobin, bilirubin, nitrite, and leukocyte esterase.

The copper sulfate method (Benedict reaction) underlies the Clinitest procedure. The Clinitest reaction detects all reducing substances (substances that will reduce copper salts), including glucose, lactose, fructose, galactose, and pentose. A positive result, in the absence of glucosuria, may suggest a carbohydrate metabolic disorder, such as galactosemia.

Protein

Normal urine protein amounts to ~150 mg/day of predominantly Tamm-Horsfall (tubular) protein. Greater amounts of protein may be seen following vigorous exercise, dehydration, and fever. Benign types of proteinuria include postural and intermittent proteinuria, which together occur in up to 5% of the population. Patterns of pathologic proteinuria are discussed with urine protein electrophoresis.

Only albumin is detected by the dipstick reagent. Although semi quantitative, trace positive reactions correspond to around 15-30 mg/dL and 4+ positives correspond to around 2.0 g/dL. The dipstick reagent is essentially a pH indicator that responds to the alkalinization that proteins induce as a result of their net negative charge; thus, highly alkaline urine may produce a false positive.

Other methods for detecting proteinuria rely upon the tendency of proteins to precipitate in various environments (eg, in the presence of sulfosalicylic or trichloroacetic acid). Unlike the dipstick, these methods are sensitive to globulins and albumin. Precipitation techniques may be qualitative (precipitate is present or absent, graded 1+ to 4+) or quantitative (precipitate subjected to measurement by photometry or colorimetry). None of these methods are adequate for detection of microalbuminuria.

Ketones

There are 3 major ketones in blood and urine. The predominant ketone is β-hydroxybutyrate (80%), with acetoacetic acid and acetone comprising the remaining 20%.

The dipstick test for ketones is sensitive mainly to acetoacetic acid, but not β-hydroxybutyrate or acetone. Since the 3 major ketones exist in equilibrium in serum and urine, this provides a reliable means of detecting them. The dipstick result is semiquantitative and roughly reflects serum ketones; 3+ results can be diluted to provide a semiquantitative result (2+ at dilution 1:X) that can be serially followed. False positive dipstick ketones can be caused by ingestion of captopril or methyldopa.

It is important to note that patients undergoing appropriate treatment for ketoacidosis may appear initially to have an increase in ketonuria, as a result of the conversion of the β-hydroxybutyrate to acetoacetic acid.

The tablet test (Acetest) can be used instead of the dipstick; it is somewhat more sensitive overall but remains sensitive primarily to acetoacetic acid and is liable to false positive results with certain agents.

In standing urine, acetoacetic acid progressively diminishes, so fresh samples should be tested when possible, refrigerated samples in other circumstances.

Hemoglobin

Hemoglobinuria must be distinguished from hematuria and myoglobinuria, all of which produce a positive test for hemoglobin on dipstick. Hematuria, the presence of red blood cells in the urine, is the most common cause of hemoglobinuria. This is confirmed by microscopic examination of the urine; however, red cells may undergo lysis in a specimen that has been left standing, so a fresh sample should be requested if no erythrocytes are seen. Asymptomatic hematuria may be found in up to 15% of adults and often results from a pathologic process. Hematuria without serious underlying pathology may follow strenuous exercise.

Uncommonly free hemoglobin may be present in the urine, indicating intravascular hemolysis. In such cases, there is usually pink-tinged serum (a finding absent in hematuria and myoglobinuria). Free hemoglobin in serum is bound to haptoglobin, which prevents its filtration through the glomerulus; however, the store of haptoglobin is quickly depleted, at which time free hemoglobin appears in urine. A quantity of the hemoglobin is reabsorbed by proximal tubular cells and converted into hemosiderin; when these cells slough, they appear in urine as hemosiderin-laden mononuclear cells. Thus, the finding of intracellular hemosiderin on Prussian blue-stained urine indicates intravascular hemolysis within the past several days.

The best way to distinguish myoglobinuria from hemoglobinuria is by history and additional lab tests. Specifically, myoglobinuria is accompanied by a history of severe muscle tenderness, with elevated creatine kinase, in the presence of a provocative event t1.36. The presence of myoglobinuria in this setting supports a diagnosis of rhabdomyolysis but does not predict resultant renal failure. Laboratory findings supportive of myoglobinuria include elevated serum creatine kinase and normal haptoglobin.

t1.36 Causes of rhabdomyolysis

Trauma (crush injury)
Strenuous exercise
Seizure
Heat injury
Infection (Influenza, HIV, bacterial myositis)
Electrolyte disturbance (hypocalcemia, hypokalemia)
Drug (statins, cocaine, amphetamine)
Inherited (eg, glycogen storage disease, mitochondrial myopathy)

Bilirubin & urobilinogen

Since unconjugated bilirubin does not pass through the glomerulus, urinary bilirubin is indicative of conjugated hyperbilirubinemia.

Urobilinogen, on the other hand, is a more complicated matter. Urobilinogen is the product of hydrolysis of bilirubin by intestinal bacteria. In the usual course of events, a certain amount of the conjugated bilirubin that is excreted into the intestine via the bile is converted into urobilinogen by bacterial flora. A fraction of this urobilinogen is absorbed by the enterocytes and passed into the portal circulation where most of it goes to the liver to be re-excreted, and a small amount is excreted in urine. Whenever there is either liver disease that prevents the re-excretion step or increased bilirubin excretion leading to increased urobilinogen formation thus exceeding the capacity of the re-excretion step, one sees increased urobilinogen in the urine.

In the jaundiced patient, the interpretation of urinary bilirubin and urobilinogen is shown in t1.37.

t1.37 Urine bilirubin interpretation

Test	Normal	Unconjugated hyperbilirubinemia	Conjugated hyperbilirubinemia
Urine bilirubin	−	−	+
Urine urobilinogen	±	−	+++

Nitrite

Most bacterial agents that cause urinary tract infection are nitrite producing organisms such as *E coli*. Thus, this test will be positive in the presence of most urinary tract infections. Urine must have been standing in the bladder for 4 hours to give a positive test. Nitrite negative organisms that may cause urinary tract infection include enterococci, *N gonorrhea*, and *M tuberculosis*.

Leukocyte esterase

Also useful to screen for urinary tract infection, this test is a reflection of the number of urinary neutrophils. Trichomonads and eosinophils are possible sources of esterases giving false positive results.

Specific gravity

The urine specific gravity is increased when the urine is concentrated, either as a result of fluid retention by the kidney or added solutes in the urine. Increased specific gravity is therefore a feature of dehydration, diabetes mellitus, proteinuria, congestive heart failure, Addison disease, and the syndrome of inappropriate antidiuretic hormone (SIADH).

Specific gravity is decreased when the urine is dilute. Conditions in which specific gravity is reduced include polydipsia, diuretic therapy, and diabetes insipidus (DI).

The specific gravity is fixed at around 1.010 in isosthenuria, in which tubular damage results in the urine specific gravity equaling that of the glomerular filtrate. Isosthenuria results from renal medullary dysfunction and is a common finding in sickle cell disease.

Urine specific gravity is most often measured by the dipstick method. This method is based upon an indirect measurement that is most sensitive to small solutes (eg, salt, urea) and relatively insensitive to large solutes such as glucose and radiologic contrast agents. Refractometry, also an indirect measurement of specific gravity, is sensitive to such agents.

pH

Normal urinary pH varies between 4.6 and 8.0. Under normal conditions, metabolic activities result in the net production of hydrogen ions; these are removed from the body by the lungs (respiration of CO_2) and kidneys (reclamation of bicarbonate), such that urine is typically mildly acidic (pH 6.0).

In general, patients with acidosis (metabolic or respiratory) should be producing urine with pH <6, while those with alkalosis (metabolic or respiratory) usually produce urine with pH >6. In renal tubular acidosis (RTA) the urine is inappropriately alkaline relative to the blood pH, and the kidneys cannot acidify the urine beyond pH 6.5.

Urine pH is most often measured with the dipstick, and care should be taken to test the specimen quickly (standing urine becomes more alkaline over time) and without allowing carryover of buffers from other portions of the dipstick.

Nephrolithiasis (kidney stones)

The majority (70%) of kidney stones are composed of calcium oxalate. In decreasing order of incidence, the remaining stones are composed of calcium phosphate, struvite (magnesium ammonium phosphate stones or triple phosphate stones), urate, and cystine.

Stone formation requires a nidus; thus, not all patients with a predisposing metabolic state will form a stone. One regularly sees crystals in the urine of people without a history of stones t1.38 f1.15. Nonetheless, knowing the chemical composition of a stone helps to illuminate treatable underlying metabolic conditions. The chemical composition of stones is most often studied by crystallography or infrared spectroscopy.

t1.38 Urine crystals

Crystal	Comments
Calcium oxalate	"Envelopes"
Uric acid	Pleomorphic crystals, most often diamond, square, or rod shaped, which polarize in a variety of colors
Triple phosphate (magnesium ammonium phosphate; struvite)	"Coffin lids"
	Form in alkaline pH, related to urea-splitting organisms (*P mirabilis*)
	May cause "staghorn calculi" (75% of staghorn calculi are struvite)
Ammonium biurate	"Thorn apples"
Cystine	Hexagonal crystals, related to cystinuria
Tyrosine	"Silky" or "sheaves of wheat" crystals
Cholesterol	"Broken panes of glass"
Sulfa	"Fans"
Bilirubin	Yellow-brown needles

The routine laboratory can be of significant aid in the evaluation of stone disease, however. Routine urine microscopy can support the diagnosis of nephrolithiasis with the finding of hematuria (without red cell casts), crystals, and clusters of reactive urothelial cells (which may be indistinguishable from clusters of low grade papillary urothelial carcinoma). The measurement of pH, calcium, phosphate, urate, and oxalate in a 24 hour urine collection specimen can predict, with relative accuracy, the composition of the stone.

The most common stone, calcium oxalate, is promoted by low urine volumes (a factor common to all stone types), low urinary citrate, hypercalciuria, and oxaluria. Hypercalciuria is present in about half of patients who form calcium stones; most such cases do not demonstrate hypercalcemia and, in fact, have idiopathic hypercalciuria. Oxaluria is increased in patients with Crohn disease, who have undergone small bowel resection or small bowel bypass, or who ingest excessive amounts of oxalate (rhubarbs, spinach, and nuts). Urinary pH has little effect on calcium oxalate crystallization. Primary hyperoxaluria is a rare autosomal recessive condition which results in a very high oxalate excretion with stone formation that begins in childhood. Tubulointerstitial nephritis develops, ultimately leading to renal failure.

Calcium phosphate stones are promoted by low urinary volumes, hypercalciuria, and elevated (alkaline) pH. Many types of stones are promoted by systemic hypercalcemia, and this should be diagnosed and treated. X linked nephrolithiasis (Dent disease) is a very rare condition caused by a mutation in the voltage-gated chloride channel 5 (*CLCN5*) gene, leading to a renal calcium leak, hypercalciuria, and stone formation. Formers of calcium-containing stones who demonstrate hypercalciuria may benefit from thiazide diuretics (which increase calcium reabsorption). Citrate functions as a stone inhibitor because it binds calcium.

Struvite stones are promoted by urinary infection by urea-splitting organisms (eg, *Proteus mirabilis*) which contribute to a markedly elevated (alkaline) urine pH.

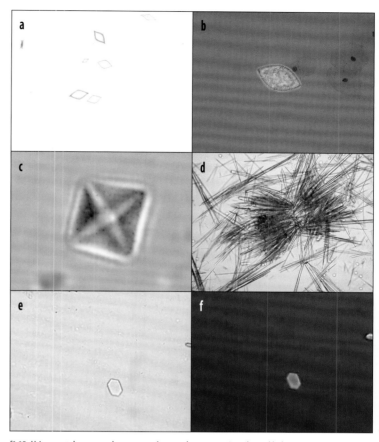

f1.15 Urine crystals: a amorphous urates, b amorphous urates in polarized light, c oxalate crystal resembling a sealed envelope, d tyrosine crystals resembling "sheaves of wheat, e cystine crystals appearing as hexagons, f cystine crystals in polarized light

Urate stones are promoted by acidic pH and hyperuricosuria. While patients with chronic ulcerative colitis and Crohn disease tend to develop hyperoxaluria and oxalate stones, up to 30% of stones identified in these patients are urate stones. Urate stones are particularly common in patients after colectomy. Hyperuricosuria can be treated with allopurinol (xanthine oxidase inhibitor) that reduces the endogenous formation of urate. Urine alkalinization is also helpful.

Cystine stones are seen in the setting of the inherited disease cystinuria (not cystinosis), an autosomal recessive disease characterized by defective renal and intestinal dibasic amino acid transport, affecting cystine, ornithine, lysine, and arginine (COLA). Of these, cystine is the least soluble and the most likely to precipitate as a stone. Cystine stone formation can be inhibited by urine alkalinization and dietary protein restriction.

2,8-Dihydroxyadenine stones are extremely rare, representing ~1 in 1,000 stones, and are due to an autosomal recessive deficiency of adenine phosphoribosyl transferase, which is necessary for purine metabolism. In its absence, 2,8-dihydroxyadenine appears in urine resulting in stone formation. Treatment is with allopurinol.

ISBN 978-089189-5985

Urine microscopy

Red blood cells (hematuria)

Insight into the source of urinary red blood cells can be gained by observing the red blood cell morphology. In glomerular pattern bleeding, the red cells are polymorphous, with various shapes and hemoglobin concentrations. Furthermore, there are often red blood cell casts and erythrophagocytosis. In nonglomerular pattern bleeding, the red cell morphology is relatively uniform, red cell casts are absent, and no erythrophagocytosis is seen.

Casts

Hyaline casts are clear, colorless casts that are difficult to see and are relatively nonspecific. Though they may be seen in renal disease, they may also be the consequence of dehydration, heat related trauma, or vigorous exercise. The hyaline cast may be pigmented as a result of pigments in the urine (eg, bilirubin, hemoglobin).

Red cell casts are relatively specific for glomerulonephritis, these casts have lumpy edges and are composed of anucleate, slightly reddish, pale discs.

White cell casts are typical of tubulointerstitial nephritis, particularly pyelonephritis. The casts are composed of nucleated cells with the typical lobated nuclei of neutrophils.

Tubular casts are composed of renal tubular cells characterized by their mononuclear, cuboidal, cells and generally indicate acute tubular necrosis.

Granular casts are somewhat nonspecific but are typically present when there is significant renal disease. They are acellular and characterized by a rough, granular, surface. The granules may be fine or coarse. Granular casts are often found accompanying hyaline casts and may be seen following vigorous exercise, dehydration, heat related trauma, or renal disease.

Waxy casts are indicative of severe renal disease, these casts are acellular and characterized by blunt ends, a pale yellow color, and cracks along their length. Their diameter is typically at least twice that of nonspecific casts (granular and hyaline).

Broad casts are hyaline, granular, or waxy casts that are unusually broad and indicate end-stage renal disease. They correspond to the widely dilated collecting ducts seen in advanced atrophy.

Fatty casts are indicative of nephrotic syndrome, in which lipiduria is a common feature. They consist of cellular casts in which lipid droplets are absorbed. With polarized light, the absorbed lipid has a Maltese-cross appearance. Fatty casts may contain oval fat bodies and/or fat globules and can be highlighted by stains for lipid (eg, Sudan black).

Bacterial casts are rarely identified but when present may be indicative of pyelonephritis. Morphologically, these may be mistaken for granular casts. A Gram stain can easily differentiate bacterial casts from granular casts.

Crystals (crystalluria) t1.38 f1.15

Conditions supporting crystal formation include solute concentration, pH, and temperature. The effect of pH differs depending upon the solute, but in general organic solutes (eg, urate, cysteine) precipitate in acidic urine, and inorganic solutes (eg, magnesium, ammonium, phosphate) precipitate in alkaline urine. With regard to temperature, cold favors precipitation; thus, crystals may not be present immediately upon voiding but may form as urine cools.

Amorphous crystals (amorphous sediment) are crystals that have no consistent shape or size; they are usually clinically insignificant. In alkaline urine, one sees amorphous phosphate, magnesium, and/or calcium crystals. In acidic urine, one sees amorphous urate crystals; these appear yellow-brown in various shapes, eg, footballs, diamonds, needles, cubes, dumbbells. A second type of urate crystal, the sodium urate crystal, is more monomorphous, colorless, and rodlike (or resembling slender prisms). Like other urate crystals, these are usually clinically insignificant.

Calcium oxalate forms clear crystals that resemble envelopes, forming in acidic urine. Calcium oxalate crystals are found in association with oxaluria, which may be indicative of high oxalate intake (rhubarbs, cabbage, asparagus), small bowel disease (eg, Crohn disease), renal failure, diabetes mellitus, ethylene glycol poisoning, or acetazolamide therapy.

Cystine crystals are colorless hexagonal plates observed in cystinuria; they are not pathognomonic, however, since they may also be seen in pyelonephritis and renal tubular disorders. Fresh urine is preferable as cystine is metabolized by urinary bacteria.

Triple phosphate (magnesium ammonium phosphate) crystals resemble coffin lids and form preferentially in alkaline urine. They are usually clinically insignificant.

Biurate crystals are described as resembling thorn apples; they are yellow-brown rounded structures with thorn-like excrescences. They form in alkaline urine and are usually clinically insignificant.

Tyrosine crystals appear as thin, delicate needles, often arranged in clumps, resembling sheaves of wheat. Tyrosine crystals are seen in tyrosinosis, hyperbilirubinemia, and liver disease (in which context they may be seen with leucine crystals).

Cholesterol crystals appear as broad plates, often with a notched corner, resembling damaged plates of glass. They are often seen in nephrotic syndrome. Some radiocontrast dyes can mimic cholesterol crystals, so it is helpful to confirm that the urine shows other features of nephrotic syndrome.

Urine microscopy in the patient with acute renal failure

Urine microscopy can be helpful in the differential diagnosis of acute renal failure. Several of the key etiologies to be distinguished include acute tubular necrosis (ATN), rapidly progressive (crescentic) glomerulonephritis (RPGN), and acute interstitial nephritis (AIN) t1.39.

t1.39 Urine microscopy in acute renal failure

Finding	ATN	RPGN	AIN
Red blood cells	Normal numbers or slightly increased with nonglomerular pattern	Increased with glomerular pattern	Normal numbers or slightly increased with nonglomerular pattern
Casts	Granular & waxy; tubular casts	Granular & waxy; red cell casts	Granular & waxy; tubular casts
Erythrophagocytosis	–	+	–
Granulocytes	Scant	Scant	Numerous, including neutrophils & eosinophils

Cerebrospinal fluid (CSF)

CSF chemistry

Xanthochromia is defined as pink or yellow-tinged fluid following centrifugation. Pink xanthochromia is due to free hemoglobin and is detected following sub-arachnoid hemorrhage. Yellow xanthochromia is due to bilirubin derived from hemoglobin metabolism and begins around 12 hours after a bleed, peaking at 72 hours, and disappearing in 2-4 weeks. Artifactual xanthochromia may be due to: hyperbilirubinemia, CSF protein >150 mg/dL, carotinoids, melanin, rifampin, or delay of >1 hour prior to examination.

When bloody or xanthochromic CSF is encountered, the challenge is distinguishing truly bloody from traumatic taps. If the fluid becomes progressively clearer from tube 1 to tube 4, then it is likely traumatic. If xanthochromia is present, then it is probably truly bloody. Erythrophagocytosis and hemosiderin-laden macrophages also provide evidence for a truly bloody tap.

CSF protein is normally 15-45 mg/dL. Increased CSF protein is seen in the presence of nearly any central nervous system pathology, including inflammatory states, hemorrhage, and CSF obstruction. Albumin permits assessment of the integrity of the blood-brain barrier; when intact, the ratio of CSF:serum albumin is <1:230.

CSF leak, such as when a patient has post-traumatic rhinorrhea or otorrhea, may be diagnosed by glucose measurement or electrophoresis. Glucose, which is very nonspecific, looks for the typically lowered glucose content of CSF. Protein electrophoresis looks for the typical twin transferrin peak and prealbumin bands of CSF. Lastly, detection of asialated transferrin (β_2 transferrin) is suggestive of CSF.

CSF glucose levels are normally 60% of serum levels (ie, somewhere around 60 mg/dL), varying from 40-80%. Hypoglycorrhachia (<30%) is seen in bacterial meningitis.

CSF glutamine is elevated in hepatic encephalopathy.

Multiple sclerosis

Examination of the CSF is important for supporting the diagnosis of multiple sclerosis (MS). In particular, the 2 cerebrospinal fluid findings that support a diagnosis of MS include intrathecal IgG synthesis and oligoclonal bands.

The ratio of CSF to serum IgG is elevated whenever there is intrathecal immunoglobulin production or increased permeability of the blood-brain barrier. One can exclude the effect of increased permeability by using the albumin CSF:serum ratio as a control; thus, the IgG index is obtained by dividing the CSF IgG/serum IgG ratio by the ratio of CSF albumin/serum albumin. Intrathecal IgG synthesis (CSF IgG index) has a sensitivity of ~90% for MS.

Oligoclonal bands (several distinct bands in the γ region) by agarose gel electrophoresis has a sensitivity of 50-75% and a specificity of 95-97% for MS. Isoelectric focusing (IEF) appears to be more sensitive for the detection of oligoclonal bands, with a reported sensitivity of 90% and specificity of 95%. Recall that in simple electrophoresis, after voltage has been applied to the sample for a period of time, the gel is fixed and stained, whereas in IEF anti-IgG antibody is added prior to staining. This step amplifies any bands that may be present. In simple electrophoresis, 2 or more bands are typically considered positive, whereas in IEF, 4 or more bands are considered positive. The CSF banding pattern must be compared to simultaneous serum protein electrophoresis; if similar bands are identified in the serum, then the CSF bands are discounted.

CSF microscopy

The normal cell count is 0-5/mL for adults and 0-20/mL for neonates. In a traumatic tap, some WBCs may be from peripheral blood, as may be some protein. For normal individuals, ~1 WBC can be expected for every 700 red cells, and ~8 mg/dL protein for each 10,000 RBC/mL. The differential cell count t1.40, t1.41 is important for patient classification.

t1.40 Normal cerebrospinal fluid differential counts

Cell type	Adults	Neonates
Lymphocytes	30-90%	10-40%
Monocytes	10-50%	50-90%
Neutrophils	0-6%	0-10%
Ependymal	Rare	Rare
Eosinophils	Rare	Rare

t1.41 Cerebrospinal fluid differential counts in meningitis

Type of infection	Leukocyte count	Protein	Leukocyte differential	Glucose	Comment
Bacterial	1,000-10,000	>100	Polys predominate	<40	Partially treated infections may be lymphocyte predominant
Viral	50-500	20-100	Polys early, lymphs late	Normal	Decreased glucose is characteristic of HSV encephalitis
Fungal & mycobacterial	50-500	20-100	Lymphs predominate	<50	

Pleural fluid

Pleural fluid chemistry

Exudate vs transudate

Light criteria t1.42 help to classify effusions as exudative or transudative. Besides Light criteria, additional features that have been demonstrated to correlate with the presence of an exudate include specific gravity >1.016, pleural fluid protein >3 g/dL, pleural fluid cholesterol >45 mg/dL, and pleural fluid bilirubin:serum bilirubin ratio >0.6.

t1.42 Light criteria

Pleural fluid:serum protein ratio >0.5
Pleural fluid:serum LD ratio >0.6
Pleural fluid LD >2/3 of the upper limit of normal for serum LD

The presence of any criterion is indicative of exudate

Generally speaking, most transudates are due to alterations in the balance between venous blood pressure and serum osmotic pressure; thus, transudates are typical of congestive heart failure, cirrhosis, and nephrotic syndrome.

Nearly all other causes of pleural effusions result in exudative effusions. Causes of exudative pleural effusions include bacterial pneumonia, malignancy (usually bloody), tuberculosis, pulmonary embolus, collagen vascular diseases (especially rheumatoid arthritis), pancreatitis (classically left-sided), esophageal perforation, chylothorax, asbestos exposure, post-myocardial infarction (Dressler syndrome), uremia, and ovarian fibromas (Meigs syndrome).

Chylous vs pseudochylous

Both chylous and pseudochylous effusions are usually exudates, and both are uncommon. True chylous effusion (chylothorax) is caused by lymphatic (thoracic duct) obstruction. In older studies, over half of cases were due to malignancy. Lymphoma was the most common malignancy, followed by bronchogenic carcinoma. In more recent series, trauma and surgery are the most common causes. Other cases are due to lymphangioleiomyomatosis (LAM) of the lung, sarcoidosis, and infection. A creamy top layer of chylomicrons may form if the fluid is allowed to stand.

Pseudochylous effusions result from the gradual accumulation of lipids from cellular breakdown in conditions such as tuberculosis, rheumatoid pleural effusion, and myxedema t1.43.

t1.43 Chylous vs pseudochylous effusions

	Chylous	Pseudochylous
Gross appearance	Milky	Milky
Microscopic appearance	Lymphocytes	Mixed leukocytes, cholesterol crystals
Triglycerides	>110 mg/dL	<50 mg/dL
Chylomicrons (by electrophoresis)	+	−

CHF is the most common cause of transudative pleural effusions. In treated congestive heart failure, a transudate may be "converted" into an exudate when progressive reabsorption of effusion fluid leads to increased specific gravity and increasingly concentrated solutes such as protein and LD. Effusions due to CHF tend to be larger on the right or, when unilateral, are usually right-sided.

Parapneumonic pleural effusions refer to effusions that develop in association with bacterial pneumonia. Generally these effusions are sterile or contain few bacteria and are associated with low numbers of neutrophils. If a frank bacterial infection arises as a complication of bacterial pneumonia, this is called an empyema. Empyema is diagnosed when the pleural fluid contains >100,000 neutrophils/mL, pH <7.2, and bacteria on Gram stain.

Tuberculosis-associated pleural effusions are noted for being lymphocyte-predominant and for containing a paucity of mesothelial cells. Adenosine deaminase (ADA) may be used to support a diagnosis of tuberculous pleural effusion, with ADA >40 U/L being consistent with, though not entirely specific for, tuberculosis.

Up to 50% of patients with pulmonary embolus (PE) have an associated, usually small, pleural effusion. Most are exudates. PE-associated effusions tend to be bloody and may contain increased neutrophils, giving way to lymphocytes as they mature. Marked mesothelial cell hyperplasia, often with variable atypia, is common.

Nearly any systemic collagen vascular disease may cause a pleuritis and an exudative pleural effusion. The one most likely to do so is rheumatoid arthritis. The pleural fluid chemistries are distinctive: pH <7.2, LD >700, and glucose <30. In addition, rheumatoid factor (RF) is often elevated. Cytologically, an abundance if fibrin, relative paucity of mesothelial cells, and occasional histiocytes, some multinucleated, are often seen.

Amylase is elevated in pleural effusions related to esophageal perforation, pancreatitis, and malignancy. Pleural effusions associated with pancreatitis are classically left-sided.

The combination of low pH (<7.30) and low glucose (<60 mg/dL) indicates empyema, malignancy, or rheumatoid pleuritis. A low pH alone, often <6.0, is seen in esophageal perforation.

Pleural fluid microscopy

Neutrophils, when numerous, suggest empyema, but they often predominate early in the course of PE-associated effusion. Lymphocytic pleural effusions, particularly when mesothelial cells are sparse, are suggestive of tuberculous effusions. Lymphocytic pleural effusion may also result from involvement of the pleural space by lymphoma, a common finding in chronic lymphocytic leukemia. Mesothelial cells are conspicuously decreased or absent in rheumatoid pleuritis, tuberculous pleuritis, and post-pleurodesis pleuritis. Eosinophils are common if there has been prior instrumentation or introduction of air into the pleural space.

Peritoneal fluid (ascites fluid)

Peritoneal fluid chemistry

In peritoneal fluid, using criteria similar to Light criteria is unreliable for determining the cause of ascites. The serum-ascites albumin gradient is perhaps the most useful index and can distinguish portal hypertension related ascites from others. The serum-ascites albumin gradient is simply the arithmetic difference between the albumin measured in serum and that measured in ascites fluid. In portal hypertension, the serum-ascites albumin gradient is >1.1 g/dL. In ascites from other causes, it is <1.1. Causes of ascites with high albumin gradient include cirrhosis, Budd-Chiari syndrome, portal vein thrombosis, hepatic veno-occlusive disease, myxedema, and right heart failure.

Peritoneal fluid microscopy

The differential count is quite variable in the variety of pathologic conditions causing ascites. Infection is suggested if there are >250 neutrophils/mm^3; in such cases, neutrophils usually comprise >70% of all nucleated cells. In spontaneous bacterial peritonitis, the ascites Gram stain is often negative, because of overall low bacterial counts; a floridly positive Gram stain indicates secondary bacterial peritonitis (eg, from bowel perforation).

Synovial fluid

Synovial fluid chemistry

In general, inflammation in synovial fluid reduces its viscosity because of degradation of hyaluronic acid. The mucin clot test is an outdated approach for determining whether there is inflammation in synovial fluid. Acetic acid is added to the synovial fluid which normally should lead to congealing of the hyaluronic acid, forming a "mucin clot." In the presence of ongoing inflammation, the fluid's hyaluronic acid is largely degraded, leading to a poor mucin clot.

In septic arthritis, the synovial fluid demonstrates low glucose, low pH, and high lactate levels; however, there is considerable overlap with rheumatoid arthritis and gout. Serologic testing of synovial fluid (eg, for rheumatoid factor, ANA, and complement levels) has been shown to be diagnostically ineffective; serum testing should be sufficient for this purpose.

Synovial fluid microscopy

The cell count and differential t1.44 is useful for distinguishing between inflammatory and noninflammatory conditions, but the utility ends there. In the presence of significant neutrophilic inflammation, immediate treatment decisions depend largely upon the presence or absence of crystals; for this reason, technical proficiency in this analysis is of paramount importance. The synovial fluid Gram stain is positive in only ~50% of cases of septic arthritis.

t1.44 Synovial fluid

Condition	WBC count	Neutrophils (%)	Glucose difference*	Other
Normal	0-150	<25	0-10	Clear-straw colored
Noninflammatory effusion	0-3,000	<25	0-10	Clear-straw colored
Inflammatory effusion	3,000-75,000	30-75	0-40	Turbid & opaque
Septic joint, gout & rheumatoid arthritis	>100,000	>90	30-100	Yellow & purulent

*between plasma and synovial glucose

Monosodium urate crystals f1.16 are found in gout. These are seen as needle shaped rods, varying from 2-20 μm in length and manifesting strong negative birefringence. Negative birefringence refers to a crystal that appears yellow when parallel to the compensator and blue when perpendicular.

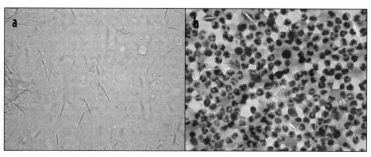

f1.16 Synovial fluid urate crystals
a urate crystals in direct light, in which they appear as translucent needle shaped crystals
b urate crystals in polarized light, in which they appear as negatively birefringent crystals, those parallel to the compensator being yellow, and those perpendicular being blue; note the abundance of neutrophils

Calcium pyrophosphate crystals are found in pseudogout, also called calcium pyrophosphate deposition disease (CPPD). These are seen as rods or rhomboids, varying from 2-20 μm, and demonstrate weak positive birefringence, appearing blue when parallel to the compensator and yellow when perpendicular.

Methods in enzymology

Enzyme activity

Measurement of enzyme activity is based upon Michaelis-Menten kinetics which holds, in brief, that the rate of enzyme activity varies linearly with substrate concentration up to the substrate concentration when the enzyme is fully saturated with substrate. At this saturation point, the enzyme is working as fast as it can (V_{max}), and the rate of reaction, all things being equal, varies only with the enzyme concentration. Thus, by using an excess of substrate, the enzyme concentration can be determined.

Measurement of enzyme activity requires a way to measure that the reaction has taken place. Some reaction products can themselves be measured. In other instances, NADH or NAD is utilized in the reaction. Since *NADH absorbs light at 340 nm* (and NAD does not) the formation or disappearance of NADH can be measured. If this is not the case, a reaction that does utilize NAD/NADH can be coupled to the reaction (coupled enzyme assay).

For example, AST, which converts aspartate (Asp) and α-ketoglutarate (αKG) to oxaloacetate (OAA) and glutamate, does not utilize NADH. So in addition to an excess of NADH and α-ketoglutarate, malate dehydrogenase (MD) is added to the reagents. The following reactions occur, the first catalyzed by AST and the second by MD:

$$Asp + \alpha KG \rightarrow OAA + glutamate + NADH \rightarrow malate + NAD$$

Thus, the disappearance of NADH (absorbance at 340 nm) can be used as a reflection of the activity of AST. This is a coupled enzyme assay.

An assay that does not utilize NADH/NAD is that used to measure alkaline phosphatase. When an excess of p-nitrophenyl phosphate is added at pH 10, the following reaction is catalyzed by alkaline phosphatase:

$$p\text{-nitrophenyl phosphate} \rightarrow p\text{-nitrophenol} + phosphate$$

p-nitrophenyl phosphate has little absorbance at 405 nm, where p-nitrophenol has its peak absorbance. The absorbance of p-nitrophenol at 405 nm is measured as a reflection of alkaline phosphatase activity. Note that if this same assay is run at pH 5.0, acid phosphatase is measured.

Enzyme antigen

Immunoassays are routinely employed for measurement of enzyme antigen concentration. For the most part, the quantity of enzyme determined by immunoassay corresponds with the enzyme activity. Discordance between these 2 measurements usually takes the form of the immunoassay result overestimating the activity. This effect may be seen in the presence of serum enzyme inhibitors, in a deficiency of a necessary cofactor, macroenzymes, defective enzyme, and proteolytically inactivated enzymes.

Cofactors are substances that bind to an enzyme and enhance its activity. There are inorganic cofactors (eg, zinc, calcium, magnesium, iron and organic cofactors (also called coenzymes). Coenzymes include NAD, protein S (a cofactor for protein C), and pyridoxine (vitamin B$_6$).

Macroenzymes are ordinary enzymes bound to antibodies. Being bound to an antibody has 2 effects upon an enzyme: it usually makes it incapable of functioning, and it prevents it from being cleared from the blood.

References

ACOG Committee on Practice Bulletins and the SGO Education Committee [2004] Diagnosis and treatment of gestational trophoblastic disease. *ACOG Practice Bulletin 53* PMID:15196847.

ADAG Study Group [2008] Translating the hemoglobin A1c assay into estimated average glucose values. *Diab Care* 31:1473-1478. PMID:18540046.

Alpert JS, Thysegen K, Antman E, Bassand JP, et al [2000] Myocardial infarction redefined—a consensus document of the Joint European Society of Cardiology/American College of Cardiology. *J Am Coll Cardiol* 36:959-969. PMID:10987628.

American College of Cardiology/American Heart Association Task Force on Practice Guidelines [2001] ACC/AHA guidelines for the evaluation and management of chronic heart failure in the adult. *Circulation* 104:2996-3007. PMID:11739319

American Diabetes Association [2005] Diagnosis and classification of diabetes mellitus. *Diab Care* 28Suppl1:S37-S42 PMID:15618111

American Diabetes Association [2006] Standards of medical care in diabetes *Diab Care* 29(5):1192 PMID:16373931

American Diabetes Association [1997] Report of the expert committee on the diagnosis and classification of diabetes mellitus. *Diab Care* 20:1183-1197. PMID:9203460

Amiodarone Trials Meta-Analysis Investigators [1997] Effect of prophylactic amiodarone on mortality after acute myocardial infarction and in congestive heart failure: meta-analysis of individual data from 6500 patients in randomised trials. *Lancet* 350:1417-1424. PMID:9371164

Ammar KA, Heckerling PS [1996] Ethylene glycol poisoning with a normal anion gap caused by concurrent ethanol ingestion: importance of the osmolal gap. *Am J Kidney Dis* 27:130-133. PMID:8546127

Anderson RJ, Chung HM, Kluge R, Schrier RW [1985] Hyponatremia: a prospective analysis of its epidemiology and the pathogenetic role of vasopressin. *Ann Intern Med* 102(2):164-168. PMID:3966753.

Apple FS, Wu AH [2001] Myocardial infarction redefined: role of cardiac troponin testing. *Clin Chem* 47(3):377-379. PMID:11238285.

Apple FS, Wu AHB, Mair J, et al [2005] Future biomarkers for detection of ischemia and risk stratification in acute coronary syndrome. *Clin Chem* 51(5):810-824. PMID:15774573.

Apple FS, Pearce LA, Smith SW, et al [2009a] Role of monitoring changes in sensitive cardiac troponin I assay results for early diagnosis of myocardial infarction and prediction of risk of adverse events. *Clin Chem* 55(5):930-937. PMID:19299542.

Apple FS, Smith SW, Pearce LA, Murakami MM [2009b] Assessment of the multiple-biomarker approach for diagnosis of myocardial infarction in patients presenting with symptoms suggestive of acute coronary syndrome. *Clin Chem* 55(1):93-100 PMID:19028826.

Arndt T [2001] Carbohydrate-deficient transferrin as a marker of chronic alcohol abuse: a critical review of preanalysis, analysis, and interpretation. *Clin Chem* 47:13-27. PMID:11148172.

Bachorik PS, Ross JW [1995] National cholesterol education program recommendations for measurement of low-density lipoprotein cholesterol: executive summary. *Clin Chem* 41(10):1414-1420. PMID:7586510.

Balk EM [2001] Accuracy of biomarkers to diagnose acute cardiac ischemia in the emergency department. *Ann Emerg Med* 37(5):478-494. PMID:11326184.

Balk SP, Ko Y-J, Bubley GJ [2003] Biology of prostate-specific antigen. *J Clin Oncol* 21(2): 383-391. PMID:12525533.

Banks PA [1997] Practice guidelines in acute pancreatitis. *Am J Gastroenterol* 92(3):377-386. PMID:9068455.

Bar-Or D, Winkler JV, VanBenthuysen K, Harris L, Lau E, Hetzel FW [2001] Reduced albumin-cobalt binding with transient myocardial ischemia after elective percutaneous transluminal coronary angioplasty: a preliminary comparison to creatine kinase-MB, myoglobin, and troponin I. *Am Heart J* 141:985-991. PMID:11376314.

Basaria S, Cooper DS [2005] Amiodarone and the thyroid. *Am J Medicine* 118:706-714. PMID:15989900.

Baskin L, Jialal I [1998] Detection of oligoclonal bands in cerebrospinal fluid by immunofixation electrophoresis. *Am J Clin Pathol* 109:585-588. PMID:9576577.

Basturk O, Coban I, Adsay NV [2009] Pancreatic cysts: pathologic classification, differential diagnosis, and clinical implications. *Arch Pathol Lab Med* 133:423-438. PMID:19260748.

Baud FJ, Borron SW, Megarbane B, et al [2002] Value of lactic acidosis in the assessment of the severity of acute cyanide poisoning. *Crit Care Med* 30(9):2044- 2050 PMID:12352039.

Begg EJ, Barclay ML, Kirkpatrick CJM [1999] The therapeutic monitoring of antimicrobial agents. *Br J Clin Pharmacol* 47:23-30. PMID:10073735.

Bender TM, Stone LR, Amenta JS [1994] Diagnostic power of lecithin/sphingomyelin ratio and fluorescent polarization assays for respiratory distress syndrome compared by relative operating characteristic curves. *Clin Chem* 40:541-545. PMID:8149607.

Benn PA, Fang M, Egan JF, Horne D, Collins R [2003] Incorporation of inhibin-A in second trimester screening for Down syndrome. *Obstet Gynecol* 101:451-454. PMID:12636947.

Bertholf RL, Johannsen LM, Bazooband A, Mansouri V [2003] False-positive acetaminophen results in a hyperbilirubinemic patient. *Clin Chem* 49(4):695-698. PMID:12651837.

Bhatnagar J, Tewari H, Bhatnagar M, Austin GE [1999] Comparison of carcinoembryonic antigen in tissue and serum with grade and stage of colon cancer. *Anticancer Res* 19:2181-2188. PMID:10472328.

Bidart JM, Thuillier F, Augereau C, Chalas J, Daver A, Jacob N, Labrousse F, Voitot H [1999] Kinetics of serum tumor marker concentrations and usefulness in clinical monitoring. *Clin Chem* 45(10):1695-1707. PMID:10508114.

Bornstein SR [2009] Predisposing factors for adrenal insufficiency. *New Engl J Med* 360:2328-2339. PMID:19474430.

Brent J [2009] Fomepizole for ethylene glycol and methanol poisoning. *New Engl J Med* 360(21):2216-2223. PMID:19458366.

Bruns DE, Knowler WC. Stabilization of glucose in blood samples: why it matters. *Clin Chem* 2009;55(5):850-852. PMID:19282352.

Bussmann C, Bast T, Rating D [2001] Hyponatraemia in children with acute CNS disease: SIADH or cerebral salt wasting? *Childs Nerv Syst* 17(1-2):58-62. PMID:11219625.

Buyon JP, Cronstein BN, Morris M, Tanner M, Weissmann G [1986] Serum complement values (c3 and c4) to differentiate between systemic lupus activity and preeclampsia. *Am J Med* 81(2):194-200. PMID:3740078.

Canto EI, Slawin KM [2002] Early management of prostate cancer: how to respond to an elevated PSA. *Annu Rev Med* 53:355-368. PMID:11818479.

Caragher TE, Fernandez BB, Barr LA [2000] Long term experience with an accelerated protocol for diagnosis of chest pain. *Arch Pathol Lab Med* 124:1434-1439. PMID:11035571.

Carter AB, Howanitz PJ [2003] Intraoperative testing for parathyroid hormone: a comprehensive review of the use of the assay and the relevant literature. *Arch Pathol Lab Med* 127:1424-1442. PMID:14567726.

Carvounis CP, Nisar S, Guro-Razuman S [2002] Significance of the fractional excretion of urea in the differential diagnosis of acute renal failure. *Kidney Int* 62:2223-2229. PMID:12427149.

Catalona WJ, Hudson MA, Scardino PT, Richie JP, Ahmann FR, Flanigan RC, et al [1994] Selection of optimal prostate specific antigen cutoffs for early detection of prostate cancer: receiver operating characteristic curves. *J Urol* 152(6):2037-2042. PMID:7525995.

Centers for Disease Control [1978] *Prevention of Lead Poisoning in Children* Atlanta: US Department of Health.

Centers for Disease Control and Prevention [2005] *Preventing Lead Poisoning in Young Children* Atlanta: US Department of Health and Human Services.

Chiriboga DE, Ma Y, Li W, et al [2009] Seasonal and sex variation of high-sensitivity C-reactive protein in healthy adults: A longitudinal study. *Clin Chem* 55(2):313-321. PMID:19179270.

Clark PM. Laboratory services for thyroglobulin and implications for monitoring of differentiated thyroid cancer. *J Clin Pathol* 62:402-406. PMID:19398593.

Clerico A, Fontana M, Zyw L, et al [2007] Comparison of the diagnostic accuracy of brain natriuretic peptide (BNP) and the N-terminal part of the propeptide of BNP immunoassays in chronic and acute heart failure: A systematic review. *Clin Chem* 53(5):813-822. PMID:17384013.

Coe JI [1993] Postmortem chemistry update: emphasis on forensic application. *Am J Forensic Med Pathol* 14(2):91-117. PMID:8328447.

Cole LA, Shahabi S, Butler SA, Mitchell H, Newlands ES, Behrman HR, Verrill HL [2001] Utility of commonly used commercial human chorionic gonadotropin immunoassays in the diagnosis and management of trophoblastic diseases. *Clin Chem* 47:308-315. PMID:11159780.

Compton CC, Fielding LP, Burgart LJ, Conley B, Cooper HS, Hamilton SR, Hammond MEH, Henson DE, Hutter RVP, Nagle RB, Nielsen ML, Sargent DJ, Taylor CR, Welton M, Willett C [2000] Prognostic factors in colorectal cancer. *Arch Pathol Lab Med* 124:979-994. PMID:10888773.

Connolly SJ [1999] Evidence-based analysis of amiodarone efficacy and safety. *Circulation* 100:2025-2034. PMID:10556230.

Cook DS, Braithwaite RA, Hale KA [2000] Estimating antemortem drug concentrations from postmortem blood samples: the influence of postmortem redistribution. *J Clin Pathol* 53:282-285. PMID:10823124.

Cooper LT [2009] Myocarditis. *New Engl J Med* 360:1526-1538. PMID:19357408.

Cowper SE, Robin HS, Steinberg SM, et al [2000] Scleromyxoedma-like cutaneous disease in renal dialysis patients. *Lancet* 356:1000-1001. PMID:11041404.

Dagher L, Moore K [2001] The hepatorenal syndrome. *Gut* 49:729-737. PMID:11600480.

Dalal BI, Brigden ML [2009] Factitious biochemical measurements resulting from hematologic conditions. *Am J Clin Pathol* 131:195-204. PMID:19141380.

Dawson AH, Whyte IM [1999] Therapeutic drug monitoring in drug overdose. *Br J Clin Pharmacol* 48: 278-283. PMID:10510137.

Delanghe JR, DeBuyzere ML, Casneuf V, Peeters M [2008] Unusual serum electrophoresis pattern in a woman with pancreatic carcinoma. *Clin Chem* 54(9):1572-1575. PMID:18755907.

Derksen RH, Meilof JF [1992] Anti-Ro/SS-A and anti La/SS-B autoantibody levels in relation to systemic lupus erythematosus disease activity and congenital heart block. *Arthritis Rheum* 35(8):953-959. PMID:1642661.

Dervenis C, Johnson CD, Bassi C [1999] Diagnosis, objective assessment of severity, and management of acute pancreatitis. *Int J Pancreatol* 25:195-210. PMID:10453421.

Doerr CH, Allen MS, Nichols FC III, Ryu JH [2005] Etiology of chylothorax in 203 patients. *Mayo Clin Proc* 80(7):867-870. PMID:16007891.

Dolci A, Dominici R, Cardinale D, et al [2008] Biochemical markers for prediction of chemotherapy induced cardiotoxicity. *Am J Clin Pathol* 130:688-695. PMID:18854260.

Dombrowski RA, Mackenna J, Brame RG [1981] Comparison of amniotic fliud lung maturity profiles in paired vaginal and amniocentesis specimens. *Am J Obstet Gynecol* 140:461-464. PMID:6894668.

Dorin RI, Qualls CR, Crapo LM [2003] Diagnosis of adrenal insufficiency. *Ann Int Med* 139:194-204. PMID:12899587.

Doumas BT, Peters T [2009] Origins of dye binding methods for measuring serum albumin. *Clin Chem* 55(3):583-584.

Dubin SB [1998] Assessment of fetal lung maturity. *Am J Clin Pathol* 110:723-732. PMID:9844584.

Duffy MJ [2001] Carcinoembryonic antigen as a marker for colorectal cancer: is it clinically useful? *Clin Chem* 47:624-630. PMID:11274010.

Duffy MJ [2005] Predictive markers in breast and other cancers: a review. *Clin Chem* 51:94-503. PMID:15637130.

Dufour DR [1999] Laboratory evaluation of renal function. In: *Professional Practice in Clinical Chemistry, a Companion Text,* 1999 ed. Washington, DC: American Association for Clinical Chemistry.

Dufour DR, Lott JA, Nolte FS, Gretch DR, Koff RS, Seeff LB [2000] Diagnosis and monitoring of hepatic injury: I. performance characteristics of laboratory tests. *Clin Chem* 46: 2027-2049. PMID:11106349.

Dworkin LD, Cooper CJ [2009] Renal artery stenosis. *New Engl J Med* 361:1972-1978. PMID:19907044.

Eckel RH, Grundy SM, Zimmet PZ. The metabolic syndrome. *Lancet* 2005; 365: 1415-1428. PMID:15836891.

Edston E, van Hag-Hamsten M [1998] Beta-tryptase measurements postmortem in anaphylactic deaths in controls. *Forensic Sci Int* 93:135-142. PMID:9717264.

Edston E, Gidlund E, Wickman M [1999] Increased mast cell tryptase in sudden infant death syndrome: anaphylaxis, hypoxia, or artifact? *Clin Exp Allergy* 29:1648-1654. PMID:10594541.

Emancipator K [1999] Laboratory diagnosis and monitoring of diabetes mellitus. *Am J Clin Pathol* 112: 665-674. PMID:10549254.

Erickson JA, Ashwood ER, Gin CA [2004] Evaluation of a dimeric inhibin A assay for assessing fetal Down syndrome. *Arch Pathol Lab Med* 128:415-420. PMID:15043467.

Esson ML, Schrier RW [2002] Diagnosis and treatment of acute tubular necrosis. *Ann Intern Med* 137:744-752. PMID:12416948.

Eustatia-Rutten CFA, Smit JWA, Romijn JA, van der Kleij-Corssmit EPM, Pereira AM, Stokkel MP, Kievit J [2004] Diagnostic value of serum thyroglobulin measurements in the follow-up of differentiated thyroid carcinoma, a structured meta-analysis. *Clin Endocrinol* 61:61-74. PMID:15212646.

Federle MP, McGrath KM [2007] Cystic neoplasms of the pancreas. *Gastroenterol Clin N Am* 36:365-376. PMID:17533084.

Fleisher M [2003] Criteria for tumor marker evaluation and utilization. *MLO Med Labs Obs* April:16-18. PMID:12705209.

Flynn SD, Seifer DB [1996] Clinical application of human chorionic gonadotropin. In: *Clinical Diagnosis and Management by Laboratory Methods,* 19th ed. Philadelphia: WB Saunders Company.

Fortgens P, Pillay TS [2011] Pseudohyponatremia revisited. *Arch Pathol Lab Med* 135:516-519. PMID:21466372.

Fortini AS, Sanders EL, Weinshenker BG, Katzmann JA [2003] Cerebrospinal fluid oligoclonal bands in the diagnosis of multiple sclerosis: isoelectric focusing with IgG immunoblotting compared with high-resolution agarose gel electrophoresis and cerebrospinal fluid IgG index. *Am J Clin Pathol* 120:672-675. PMID:14608891.

Freedland SJ, Partin AW [2005] Detecting prostate cancer with molecular markers: uPM3. *Rev Urol* 7(4):236-238. PMID:16985837.

Fritsche HA, Bast RC [1998] CA125 in ovarian cancer: advances and controversy. *Clin Chem* 44:1379-1380. PMID:9665412.

Gabay C, Kushner I [1999] Acute-phase proteins and other systemic responses to inflammation. *N Engl J Med* 340: 448-454. PMID:9971870.

Gabow PA, Kaehny WD, Fennessey PV, Goodman SI, Gross PA, Schrier RW [1980] Diagnostic importance of an increased serum anion gap. *N Engl J Med* 303:854-858. PMID:6774247.

Gabow PA [1985] Disorders associated with an altered anion gap. *Kidney Int* 27:472-483. PMID:2581012.

Gadducci A, Cosio S, Fanucchi A, Negri S, Cristofani R, Genazzani AR [2004] The predictive and prognostic value of serum CA125 half life during paclitaxel/platinum-based chemotherapy in patients with advanced ovarian carcinoma. *Gynecol Oncol* 93:131-136. PMID:15047226.

Gama R, Teale JD, Marks V [2003 Clinical and laboratory investigation of adult spontaneous hypoglycaemia. *J Clin Pathol* 56:641-646. PMID:12944543.

Gambino R, Piscitelli J, Ackattapathil TA, et al [2009] Acidification of blood is superior to sodium fluoride alone as an inhibitor of glycolysis. *Clin Chem* 55:1019-1021. PMID:19282354.

Ganguly A [1998] Primary aldosteronism. *N Engl J Med* 339: 1828-1834. PMID:9854120.

Gao P, Scheibel S, D'Amour P, John MR, Rao SD, Schmidt-Gayk H, Cantor TL [2001] Development of a novel immunoradiometric assay exclusively for biologically active whole parathyroid hormone 1-84: implications for improvement of accurate assessment of parathyroid function. *J Bone Miner Res* 16:605-614. PMID:11315988.

Gimovsky ML, Montoro M, Paul RH [1984] Pregnancy outcome in women with systemic lupus erythematosus. *Obstet Gynecol* 63(5):686-692. PMID:6717873.

Glynn RJ, MacFadyen JG, Ridker PM [2009] Tracking of high-sensitivity C-reactive protein after an initially elevated concentration: the JUPITER study. *Clin Chem* 55(2):305-312. PMID:19095726.

Görögh T, Rudolph P, Meyer JE, Werner JA, Lippert BM, Maune S [2005] Separation of beta2-transferrin by denaturing gel electrophoresis to detect cerebrospinal fluid in ear and nasal fluids. *Clin Chem* 51(9):1704-1710. PMID:16020492.

Grenspan JS, Rosen DJO, Roll K, et al [1995] Evaluation of lamellar body number density as the initial assessment in a fetal lung maturity test cascade. *J Reprod Med* 40:260-266. PMID:7623354.

Grobner T [2006] Gadolinium—a specific trigger for the development of nephrogenic fibrosing dermopathy and nephrogenic systemic fibrosis? *Nephrol Dial Transplant* 21:1104-1108. PMID:16431890.

Gronowski AM, Fantz CR, Parvin CA, et al [2008] Use of serum FSH to identify perimenopausal women with pituitary hCG. *Clin Chem* 54(4):652-656. PMID:18258666.

Gröschl M [2008] Current status of salivary hormone analysis. *Clin Chem* 54(11):1759-1769. PMID:18757583.

Groskopf J, Aubin SM, Deras IL, Blase A, Bodrug S, Clark C, Brentano S, Mathis J, Pham J, Meyer T, Cass M, Hodge P, Macairan ML, Marks LS, Rittenhouse H [2006] APTIMA PCA3 molecular urine test: development of a method to aid in the diagnosis of prostate cancer. *Clin Chem* 52(6):1089-1095. PMID:16627561.

Grundy SM and the Expert Panel on Detection, Evaluation, and Treatment of High Blood Cholesterol in Adults [2001] Executive summary of the third report of the National Cholesterol Education Program (NCEP) expert panel on detection, evaluation, and treatment of high blood cholesterol in adults (adult treatment panel III). *JAMA* 285(19): 2486-2497. PMID:11368702.

Hadley AG [2002] Laboratory assays for predicting the severity of haemolytic disease of the fetus and newborn. *Transpl Immunol* 10: 191-198. PMID:12216949.

Harris KR, Dighe AS [2002] Laboratory testing for viral hepatitis. *Am J Clin Pathol* 118:S18-25. PMID:14569810.

Harrison LE, Guillem JG, Paty P, Cohen AM [1997] Preoperative carcinoembryonic antigen predicts outcome in node negative colon cancer patients: a multivariate analysis of 572 patients. *J Am Coll Surg* 185:55-59. PMID:9208961.

Heeschen C, Hamm CW, Bruemmer J, Simoons ML [2000] Predictive value of C-reactive protein and troponin t in patients with unstable angina: a comparative analysis. *J Am Coll Cardiol* 35(6):1535-1542. PMID:10807457.

Heffner JE.[2006] Discriminating between transudates and exudates. *Clin Chest Med* 27:241-252. PMID:16716816.

Henry JB, Lauzon RB, Schumann GB [1996] Basic examination of urine. In: *Clinical Diagnosis and Management by Laboratory Methods.* Philadelphia: WB Saunders Company; Chapter 18.

Hessels D, Klein-Gunnewiek JMT, van Oort I, Karthaus HFM, van Leenders GJL, van Balken B, Kiemeney LA, Witjes JA, Schalken JA [2003] DD3^PCA3-based molecular urine analysis for the diagnosis of prostate cancer. *Eur Urol* 44(1):8-15. PMID:15245824.

Hjiyiannakis P, Mundy J, Harmer C [1999] Thyroglobulin antibodies in differentiated thyroid cancer. *Clin Oncol* 11(4):240-244. PMID:10473720.

Holland L, Blick K [2009] Implementing and validating transcutaneous bilirubinometry for neonates. *Am J Clin Pathol* 132:555-561. PMID:19762533.

Holstege CP, Dobmeier SG, Bechtel LK [2008] Critical care toxicology. *Emerg Med Clin N Am* 25:715-739. PMID:18655942.

Ibrahim D, Froberg B, Wolf A, Rusyniak DE [2006] Heavy metal poisoning: clinical presentations and pathophysiology. *Clin Lab Med* 26:67-97. PMID:16567226.

John MR, Goodman WG, Gao P, Cantor TL, Salusky IB, Juppner H [1999] A novel immunoradiometric assay detects full-length human pth but not amino-terminally truncated fragments: implications for pth measurements in renal failure. *J Clin Endocrinol Metab* 84:4287-4290. PMID:10566687.

Joint ESC/ACCF/AHA/WHF Task Force for the Universal Definition of Myocardial Infarction [2012] Third universal definition of myocardial infarction. *European Heart Journal* 33(18):2551-2567. PMID:22922414.

Jones JH, Weir WB [2005] Cocaine-associated chest pain. *Med Clin N Am* 89:1323-1342. PMID:16227065.

Jürgens G, Graudal NA, Kampmann JP [2003] Therapeutic drug monitoring of antiarrhythmic drugs. *Clin Pharmacokinet* 42:647-663. PMID:12844326.

Kallemuchikkal U, Gorevic PD [1999] Evaluation of cryoglobulins. *Arch Pathol ab Med* 123:119-125. PMID:10050784.

Kaplan AA, Kohn OF [1992] Fractional excretion of urea as a guide to renal dysfunction. *Am J Nephrol* 12:49-54. PMID:1415365.

Kapoor AK, Ravi A, Twomey PJ [2009] Investigation of outpatients referred to a chemical pathologist with potential pseudohyperkalemia. *J Clin Pathol* 62:920-923. PMID:19783721.

Katzmann JA, Clark R, Sanders E, Landers JP, Kyle RA [1998] Prospective study of serum protein capillary zone electrophoresis and immunotyping of monoclonal proteins by immunosubtraction. *Am J Clin Pathol* 110(4):503-509. PMID:9763037.

Keffer JH [1996] Myocardial markers of injury. Evolution and insights. *Am J Clin Pathol* 105:305-319. PMID:8602612.

Keifer MC [1998] The clinical laboratory in the diagnosis of overexposure to agrochemicals. *Lab Med* 29:689-695.

Keller T, Zeller T, Peetz D, et al [2009] Sensitive troponin I assay in early diagnosis of acute myocardial infarction. *New Engl J Med* 361:868-877. PMID:19710485.

Kellermann AL, Fihn SD, LoGerfo JP, et al [1987] Impact of drug screening in suspected overdose. *Ann Emerg Med* 16(11):1206-1216. PMID:3662178.

Kelley WE, Januzzi JL, Christenson RH [2009] Increases of cardiac troponin in conditions other than acute coronary syndrome and heart failure. *Clin Chem* 55(12):209-2012. PMID:19815610.

Kemppainen EA, Hedstrom J, Puolakkainen P [1997] Rapid measurement of urinary trypsinogen-2 as a screening test for acute pancreatitis. *N Engl J Med* 336:1788-93. PMID:9187069.

Keren DF, Alexanian R, Goeken JA, Gorevic PD, Kyle RA, Tomar RH [1999a] Guidelines for clinical and laboratory evaluation of patients with monoclonal gammopathies. *Arch Pathol Lab Med* 123:106-107. PMID:10050781.

Keren DF [1999b] Procedures for the evaluation of monoclonal immunoglobulins. *Arch Pathol Lab Med* 123: 26-132. PMID:10050785.

Keren DF [2012] *Protein Electrophoresis in Clinical Diagnosis.* Chicago: ASCP Press. ISBN:978-0891895916.

Khan AI, Cimo M, Hashim IA, Wians FH [2006] Hyperammonemia in a 20 year old woman. *Lab Med* 37(4):226-228.

Kjos SL, Walther FJ, Montero M, Paul RH, Diaz F, Stabler M [1990] Prevalence and etiology of infants of diabetic mothers: predictive value of fetal lung maturation tests. *Am J Obstet Gynecol* 163: 898-903. PMID:2144951.

Klee GG [1994] Human chorionic gonadotropin. *Mayo Clin Proc* 69:391-392. PMID:8170184.

Koenig W, Sund M, Fröhlich M, et al [1999] C-reactive protein, a sensitive marker of inflammation, predicts future risk of coronary heart disease in initially healthy middle-aged men. Results from MONICA (Monitoring Trends And Determinants In Cardiovascular Disease) Augsburg Cohort Study, 1984 to 1992. *Circulation* 99(2):237-242. PMID:9892589.

Koenig W, Twardella D, Brenner H, Rothenbacher D [2005] Plasma concentrations of cystatin c in patients with coronary heart disease and risk for secondary cardiovascular events: more than simply a marker of glomerular filtration rate *Clin Chem* 51:321-327. PMID:15563478.

Koenig W, Khuseyinova N, Baumert J, Meisinger C [2008] Prospective study of high-sensitivity C-reactive protein as a determinant of mortality: Results from the MONICA/KORA Augsburg cohort study, 1984-1998. *Clin Chem* 54(2):335-342. PMID:18156284.

Kohorn EI [2001] The new FIGO 2000 staging and risk factor scoring system for gestational trophoblastic disease: description and clinical assessment. *Int J Gynecol Cancer* 11:73-77. PMID:11285037.

Koreishi AF, Nazarian RM, Saenz AJ, et al [2009] Nephrogenic systemic fibrosis: a pathologic study of autopsy cases. *Arch Pathol Lab Med* 133:1943-1948. PMID:19961249.

Korhonen J, Alfthan H, Ylöstalo P, Veldhuis J, Stenman UH [1997] Disappearance of human chorionic gonadotropin and its a- and b-subunits after term pregnancy. *Clin Chem* 43:2155-2163. PMID:9365402.

Krishnamurthy S, Korenblat KM, Scott MG [2009] Persistent increase in aspartate aminotransferase in an asymptomatic patient. *Clin Chem* 55(8):1573-1577. PMID:19638492.

Kumpel BM [2000] Quantification of anti-D and fetomaternal hemorrhage by flow cytometry. *Transfusion* 40:6-9. PMID:10644805.

Kushner I, Rzewnicki D, Samols D [2006] What does minor elevation of C-reactive protein signify? *Am J Med* 119:166.e17-166.e28 PMID:16443421.

Lameire N, Van Biesen W, Vanholder R [2005] Acute renal failure *Lancet* 365:417-30. PMID:15680458.

Larsen LC, Fuller SH [1996] Management of acetaminophen toxicity. *Am Fam Physician* 53:185-190. PMID:8546045.

Lempiainen A, Stenman U, Blomqvist C, Hotakainen K [2008] Free beta-subunit of human chorionic gonadotropin in serum is a diagnostically sensitive marker of seminomatous testicular cancer. *Clin Chem* 54(11):1840-1843. PMID:18787014.

Levey AS, Bosch JP, Lewis JB, Greene T, Rogers N, Roth D [1999] A more accurate method to estimate glomerular filtration rate from serum creatinine: a new prediction equation. *Ann Intern Med* 130:461-70. PMID:10075613.

Lieb JG, Draganov PV [2008] Pancreatic function testing: Here to stay for the 21st century. *World J Gastroenterol* 14(20):3149-3158. PMID:18506918.

Lim PO, Young WF, MacDonald TM [2001] A review of the medical treatment of primary aldosteronism. *J Hypertens* 19:353-361. PMID:11288803.

Linder M, Keck PE [1998] Standards of laboratory practice: antidepressant drug monitoring. national academy of clinical biochemistry. *Clin Chem* 44:1073-1084. PMID:9590392.

Litovitz TL, Felberg L, White S, Klein-Schwartz W [1996] 1995 annual report of the American Association of Poison Control Centers: toxic exposure surveillance system. *Am J Emerg Med* 14:487 PMID:8765118.

Livingston EG, Herbert WNP, Hage ML, Chapman JF, Stubbs TM [1995] Use of the TDx-FLM assay in evaluating fetal lung maturity in an insulin-dependent diabetic population. *Obstet Gynecol* 86:826-829. PMID:7566857.

Løvås K, Husebye ES [2005] Addison's disease. *Lancet* 365:2058-61. PMID:15950720.

MacRae AR, Kavsak PA, Lustig V, et al [2006] Assessing the requirement for the 6-hour interval between specimens in the American Heart Association classification of myocardial infarction in epidemiology and clinical research studies. *Clin Chem* 52:812-818. PMID:16556688.

Madison LD, LaFranchi S [2005] Screening for congenital hypothyroidism: current controversies. *Curr Opin Endocrinol Diabetes Obes* 12:36-41.

Mahoney JD, Gross PL, Stern TA, et al [1990] Quantitative serum toxic screening in the management of suspected drug overdose. *Am J Emerg Med* 8(1):16-22. PMID:2293827.

Maisel A [2001] B-type natriuretic peptide levels: a potential novel "white count" for congestive heart failure. *J Card Fail* 7:183-193. PMID:11420771.

Maisel A, Krishnaswamy P, Nowak RM, et al [2002] Rapid measurement of B-type natriuretic peptide in the emergency diagnosis of heart failure. *New Engl J Med* 347:161-167. PMID:12124404.

Malaty W, Stigleman S [2008] FPIN's clinical inquiries. Antiepileptic drug level monitoring. *Am Fam Physician* 78(3):385-386. PMID:18711955.

Malkasian GD Jr, Knapp RC, Lavin PT, Zurawski VR Jr, Podratz KC, Stanhope CR, et al [1988] Preoperative evaluation of serum CA 125 levels in premenopausal and postmenopausal patients with pelvic masses: discrimination of benign from malignant disease. *Am J Obstet Gynecol* 159:341-346. PMID:2457318.

Mansour MMH, Azzary HME, Kazmierczak SC [2009] Correction factors for estimating potassium concentrations in samples with in vitro hemolysis: A detriment to patient safety. *Arch Pathol Lab Med* 133:960-966. PMID:19492890.

Marik PE, Zaloga GP [2003] Adrenal insufficiency during septic shock. *Crit Care Med* 31(1):141-145. PMID:12545007.

Marik PE, Gayowski T, Starzl TE [2005] The hepatoadrenal syndrome: a common yet unrecognized clinical condition. *Crit Care Med* 33(6):1254-1259. PMID:15942340.

Marsik C, Kazemi-Shirazi L, Schickbauer T, et al [2008] C-reactive protein and all-cause mortality in a large hospital-based cohort. *Clin Chem* 54(2):343-349. PMID:18156283.

Marton KI, Gean AD [1986] The spinal tap: a new look at an old test. *Ann Int Med* 104:840-848. PMID:3518565.

Marx SJ [2000] Hyperparathyroid and hypoparathyroid disorders. *N Engl J Med* 343:1863-1875. PMID:11117980.

Matull WR, Pereira SP, O'Donohue JW [2006] Biochemical markers of acute pancreatitis. *J Clin Pathol* 59:340-344. PMID:16567468.

McPherson RA [1996] Specific proteins. In: *Clinical Diagnosis and Management by Laboratory Methods,* 19th ed. Philadelphia: WB Saunders Company.

Meijer WG, Kema IP, Volmer M, Willemse PHB, de Vries EGE [2000] Discriminating capacity of indole markers in the diagnosis of carcinoid tumors *Clin Chem* 46(10):1588-1596. PMID:11017936.

Merke DP, Bornstein SR [2005] Congenital adrenal hyperplasia *Lancet* 365:2125-2136. PMID:15964450.

Miller WG, Bruns DE, Hortin DE, et al [2009] current issues in measurement and reporting of urinary albumin excretion. *Clin Chem* 55(1):24-38. PMID:19028824.

Mitchell PB [2000] Therapeutic drug monitoring of psychotropic medications. *Br J Clin Pharmacol* 49:303-312. PMID:10759685.

Miyanaga N, Akaza H, Tsukamoto S, et al [2003] Usefulness of urinary NMP22 to detect tumor recurrence of superficial bladder cancer after transurethral resection. *Int J Clin Oncol* 8:396-373. PMID:10759685.

MMWR [2008] Carbon monoxide related deaths—United States 1999-2004. *JAMA* 299(9):1011-1012.

Moniz CF, Nicolaides KH, Bamforth FJ Rodeck CH [1985] Normal reference ranges for biochemical substances relating to renal, hepatic, and bone function in fetal and maternal plasma throughout pregnancy. *J Clin Pathol* 38:468-472. PMID:3988961.

Morocco AP [2005] Cyanides. *Crit Care Clin* 21:691-705. PMID:16168309.

Morrison LK, Harrison A, Krishnaswamy P, Kazanegra R, Clopton P, Maisel A [2002] Utility of a rapid B-natriuretic peptide assay in differentiating congestive heart failure from lung disease in patients presenting with dyspnea. *J Am Coll Cardiol* 39:202-209. PMID:11788208.

Mueller C, Scholer A, Laule-Kilian K, Martina B, Schindler C, Buser P, Pfisterer M, Perruchoud AP [2002] Use of b-type natriuretic peptide in the evaluation and management of acute dyspnea. *N Engl J Med* 350:647-654. PMID:14960741.

Munoz SJ [1991] Prothrombin time in fulminant hepatic failure. *Gastroenterology* 100:1480-1481. PMID:2013397.

Murphy SC, Agger S, Rainey PM [2009] Too much of a good thing: A woman with hyptertension and hypokalemia. *Clin Chem* 55(12):2093-2097. PMID:19946064.

Nauck M, Warnick R, Rifai N [2002] Methods for measurement of LDL-cholesterol: a critical assessment of direct measurement by homogeneous assays vs calculation. *Clin Chem* 48(2): 236-254. PMID:11805004.

O'Grady JG, Alexander GJM, Hayllar KM, Williams R [1989] Early indicators of prognosis in fulminant hepatic failure. *Gastroenterology* 97:439-445. PMID:2490426.

Oelkers W [1996] Adrenal insufficiency. *N Engl J Med* 335:1206-1212. PMID:8815944.

Ogedegbe HO, Brown DW [2001] Lipids, lipoproteins, and apolipoproteins and their disease associations. *Lab Med* 7:384-388.

Ojomo EO, Coustan DR [1990] Absence of evidence of pulmonary maturity at amniocentesis in term infants of diabetic mothers. *Am J Obstet Gynecol* 163:954-957. PMID:2403174.

Ottani F, Galvani M, Nicolini FA, Ferrini D, Pozzati A, Di Pasquale G, Jaffe AS [2000] Elevated cardiac troponin levels predict the risk of adverse outcome in patients with acute coronary syndromes. *Am Heart J* 140(6):917-927. PMID:11099996.

Owen WE, Roberts WL [2003] Performance characteristics of 4 immunonephelometric assays for the quantitative determination of IgA and IgM in cerebrospinal fluid. *Am J Clin Pathol* 119:689-693. PMID:12760287.

Pajak TF, Clark GM, Sargent DJ, McShane LM, Hammond ME [2000] Statistical issues in tumor marker studies. *Arch Pathol Lab Med* 124:1011-1015. PMID:10888777.

Papachristou GI, Whitcomb DC [2005] Inflammatory markers of disease severity in acute pancreatitis. *Clin Lab Med* 25:17-37. PMID:15749230.

Pass HI, Lott D, Lonardo F, Harbut M, Liu Z, Tang N, Carbone M, Webb C, Wali A [2005] Asbestos exposure, pleural mesothelioma, and serum osteopontin levels. *N Engl J Med* 353:1564-1573. PMID:16221779.

Pateron D, Ganne N, Trinchet JC, Aurousseau MH, Mal F, Meicler C, et al [1994] Prospective study of screening for hepatocellular carcinoma in caucasian patients with cirrhosis. *J Hepatol* 20:65-71. PMID:7515408.

Peacock F, Morris DL, Anwaruddin S, Christenson RH, Collinson RO, Goodacre SW, Januzzi JL, Jesse RL, Kaski JC, Kontos MC, Lefevre G, Mutrie D, Sinha MK, Uettwiller-Geiger D, Pollack CV [2006] Meta-analysis of ischemia-modified albumin to rule out acute coronary syndromes in the emergency department. *Am Heart J* 152:253-262. PMID:16875905.

Pearce EN, Farwell AP, Braverman LE [2003] Thyroiditis. *N Engl J Med* 349:2646-2655. PMID:12826640.

Pearson TA, Mensah GA, Alexander RW, Anderson JL, Cannon RO 3rd, Criqui M, Fadl YY, Fortmann SP, Hong Y, Myers GL, Rifai N, Smith SC Jr, Taubert K, Tracy RP, Vinicor F [2003] Markers of inflammation and cardiovascular disease application to clinical and public health practice: a statement for healthcare professionals from The Centers for Disease Control and Prevention and The American Heart Association. *Circulation* 107(3):499-511. PMID:12551878.

Peddy SB, Rigby MR, Shaffner DH [2006] Acute cyanide poisoning. *Pediatr Crit Care Med* 7(1):79-82. PMID:16395080.

Petersen JR, Okorodudu AO, Mohammad A, Fernando A, Shattuck KE [2005] Association of transcutaneous bilirubin testing in hospital with decreased readmission rate for hyperbilirubinemia. *Clin Chem* 51:540-544. PMID:15738516.

Pezzilli R, Billi P, Plate L, Barakat B, Bongiovanni F, Miglioli M [1994] Human pancreatic secretory trypsin inhibitor in the assessment of the severity of acute pancreatitis. A comparison with C-reactive protein. *J Clin Gastroenterol* 19:112-117. PMID:7963355.

Piehler AP, Gulbrandsen N, Kierulf P, Urdal P [2008] Quantitation of serum free light chains in combination with protein electrophoresis and clinical information for diagnosing multiple myeloma in a general hospital population. *Clin Chem* 54(11):1823-1830. PMID:18801937.

Pincus MR, Brandt-Rauf PW, Nostro D [1996a] Cell biology and early tumor detection. In: *Clinical Diagnosis and Management by Laboratory Methods*, 19th ed. Philadelphia: WB Saunders Company; Chapter 15.

Pincus MR, Schaffner JA [1996b] Assessment of liver function. In: *Clinical Diagnosis and Management by Laboratory Methods*, 19th ed. Philadelphia: WB Saunders Company.

Pincus MR, Zimmerman HJ, Henry JB [1996c] Clinical enzymology. In: *Clinical Diagnosis and Management by Laboratory Methods*, 19th ed. Philadelphia: WB Saunders Company.

Piomelli S, Rosen JF, Chisolm Jr JJ, et al [1984] Management of childhood lead poisoning. *J Pediatr* 105:523-532. PMID:6481529.

Piomelli S [2002] Childhood lead poisoning. *Pediatr Clin N Am* 49:1285-1304. PMID:12580366.

Piper JM, Langer O [1993] Does maternal diabetes delay fetal pulmonary maturity? *Am J Obstet Gynecol* 168:783-786. PMID:8456880.

Pratt DS, Kaplan MM [2000] Evaluation of abnormal liver-enzyme results in asymptomatic patients. *N Engl J Med* 342:1266-1271. PMID:10781624.

Price CP, Newall RG, Boyd JC [2005] Use of protein:creatinine ratio measurements on random urine samples for prediction of significant proteinuria: a systematic review. *Clin Chem* 51:1577-1586. PMID:16020501.

Pumphrey RSH, Roberts ISD [2000] Postmortem findings after fatal anaphylactic reactions. *J Clin Pathol* 53:273-276. PMID:10823122.

Qiu LL, Levinson SS, Keeling KL, Elin RJ [2003] Convenient and effective method for removing fibrinogen from serum specimens before protein electrophoresis. *Clin Chem* 49(6):868-872. PMID:12765981.

Rabb H [1998] Evaluation of urinary markers in acute renal failure. *Curr Opin Nephrol Hypertens* 7:681-685. PMID:9864665.

Raff H, Findling JW [2003] A physiologic approach to diagnosis of the Cushing syndrome. *Ann Int Med* 138:980-991. PMID:12809455.

Rajmkumar SV, Kyle RA, Therneau TM, Melton LJ III, Bradwell AR, Clark RJ, Larson DR, Plevak MF, Dispenzieri A, Katzmann JA [2005] Serum free light chain ratio is an independent risk factor for progression in monoclonal gammopathy of undetermined significance. *Blood* 106:812-817. PMID:15855274.

Ramsey PS, Andrews WW [2003] Biochemical predictors of preterm labor: fetal fibronectin and salivary estriol. *Clin Perinatol* 30(4):701-733. PMID:14714920.

Randall D, Butts J, Halsey J [1995] Elevated postmortem tryptase in the absence of anaphylaxis. *J Forensic Sci* 40:208-211. PMID:7602279.

Reichlin M [1998] Systemic lupus erythematosus and pregnancy. *J Reprod Med* 43(4):355-360. PMID:9583068.

Reichlin T, Hochholzer W, Bassetti S, et al [2009] Early diagnosis of myocardial infarction with sensitive cardiac troponin assays. *New Engl J Med* 361(9):858-867. PMID:19710484.

Reid LD, Horner JR, McKenna DA [1990] Therapeutic drug monitoring reduces toxic drug reactions: a meta-analysis. *Ther Drug Monit* 12:72-78. PMID:2137650.

Repke JT [1998] Hypertensive disorders of pregnancy: differentiating preeclampsia from active systemic lupus erythematosus. *J Reprod Med* 43(4):350-354. PMID:9583067.

Reyes CA, Stednitz DR, Hahn C, et al [2008] Evaluation of the BiliChek being used on hyperbilirubinemic newborns undergoing home phototherapy. *Arch Pathol Lab Med* 132:684-689. PMID:18384220.

Ridker PM, Danielson E, Fonseca FA, et al [2008] Rosuvastatin to prevent vascular events in men and women with elevated C-reactive protein. *N Engl J Med* 359:2195-207. PMID:18997196.

Rifai N, Ridker PM [2001] High-sensitivity C-reactive protein: a novel and promising marker of coronary heart disease. *Clin Chem* 47:403-411. PMID:11238289.

Rodman JS [1999] Struvite stones. *Nephron* 81(suppl1):50-59. PMID:9873215.

Rodriguez-Capote K, Balion CM, Hill SA, et al [2009] Utility of myoglobin for the prediction of acute renal failure in patients with suspected rhabdomyolysis: a systematic review. *Clin Chem* 55(12):2190-2197. PMID:19797717.

Romero-Candeira S, Hernández L, Romero-Brufao S, Orts D, Fernández C, Martin C [2002] Is it meaningful to use biochemical parameters to discriminate between transudative and exudative pleural effusions? *Chest* 122:1524-1529. PMID:12426248.

Rumack BH, Matthew H [1975] Acetaminophen poisoning and toxicity. *Pediatrics* 55(6):871-876. PMID:1134886.

Runyon BA, Montano AA, Akriviadis EA, Antillon MR, Irving MA, McHutchison JG [1992] The serum-ascites albumin gradient is superior to the exudate-transudate concept in the differential diagnosis of ascites. *Ann Int Med* 117:215-220. PMID:1616215.

Saeed BO, Beaumont D, Handley GH, Weaver JU [2002] Severe hyponatraemia: investigation and management in a district general hospital. *J Clin Pathol* 55:893-896. PMID:12461050.

Sands JM, Bichet DG [2006] Nephrogenic diabetes insipidus. *Ann Intern Med* 144:186-194. PMID:16461963.

Sanoski CA, Bauman JL [2002] Clinical observations with the amio-darone/warfarin interaction: dosing relationships with longterm therapy. *Chest* 121:19-23. PMID:11796427.

Sardana G, Dowell B, Dimandis EP [2008] Emerging biomarkers for the diagnosis and prognosis of prostate cancer. *Clin Chem* 25(12):1951-1960. PMID:18927246.

Sarnak MJ, Levey AS, Schoolwerth AC, Coresh J, Culleton B, Hamm LL, McCullough PA, Kasiske BL, Kelepouris E, Klag MJ, Parfrey P, Pfeffer M, Raij L, Spinosa DJ, Wilson PW [2003] Kidney disease as a risk factor for development of cardiovascular disease. *Circulation* 108:2154 PMID:14581387.

Sassoon CS, Light RW [1985] Chylothorax and pseudochylothorax. *Clin Chest Med* 6:163-171. PMID:3847300.

Schieneman SJ [1998] X-linked hypercalciuric nephrolithiasis: clinical syndromes and chloride channel mutations. *Kidney Int* 53:3-17. PMID:9452994.

Scouller K, Conigrave KM, Macaskill P, Irwig L, Whitfield JB [2000] Should we use carbohydrate-deficient transferrin instead of g-glutamyltransferase for detecting problem drinkers? A systematic review and metaanalysis. *Clin Chem* 46:1894-1902. PMID:11106319.

Seaman E, Whang M, Olsson CA, Katz A, Cooner WH, Benson MC [1993] PSA density (PSAD). Role in patient evaluation and manage-ment. *Urol Clin North Am* 20(4):653-663. PMID:7505973.

Seifter JL [2004] Acid-base disorders. In: *Cecil Textbook of Medicine,* 22nd ed. Philadelphia: WB Saunders Company.

Sellebjerg F, Christiansen M, Nielsen PM, Fredericksen JL [1998] Cerebrospinal fluid measures of disease activity in patients with multiple sclerosis. *Mult Scler* 4:475-479. PMID:9987755.

Sevastos N, Theodossiades G, Efstathiou S, Papatheodoridis GV, Manesis E, Archimandritis AJ [2006] Pseudohyperkalemia in serum: the phenomenon and its clinical magnitude. *J Lab Clin Med* 147:139-144. PMID:16503244.

Shannon M [2000] Ingestion of toxic substances by children. *N Engl J Med* 342:186-191. PMID:10639545.

Sherman M, Peltekian KM, Lee C [1995] Screening for hepatocellular carcinoma in chronic carriers of hepatitis B virus: incidence and prevalence of hepatocellular carcinoma in a North American urban population. *Hepatology* 22:432-438. PMID:7543434.

Shlipak MG, Sarnak MJ, Katz R, Fried LF, Seliger SL, Newman AB, Siscovick DS, Stehman-Breen C [2005] Cystatin C and the risk of death and cardiovascular events among elderly persons. *N Engl J Med* 352(20):2049-2060. PMID:15901858.

Skowasch D, Jabs A, Andrié R, Lüderitz B. Bauriedel G [2005] Progression of native coronary plaques and in-stent restenosis are associated and predicted by increased preprocedural C-reactive protein. *Heart* 91:535-536. PMID:15772225.

Slev PR, Williams BG, Harville TO, et al [2008] Efficacy of the detec-tion of the a₁-antitrypsin "Z" deficiency variant by routine serum protein electrophoresis. *Am J Clin Pathol* 130:568-572. PMID:18794049.

Smotkin J, Tenner S [2002] Pancreatic and biliary disease: laboratory diagnostic tests in acute pancreatitis. *J Clin Gastroenterol* 34:459-462. PMID:11907364.

Soldin SJ [1999] Free drug measurements: when and why? An overview. *Arch Pathol Lab Med* 123:822-823. PMID:10458831.

Soloway MS, Briggman J, and Carpinito GA, et al [1996] Use of a new tumor marker, urinary nmp-22 in the detection of occult or rapidly recurring transitional cell carcinoma of the urinary tract following surgical treatment. *J Urol* 156:363-367. PMID:8683680.

Speiser PW, White PC [2003] Congenital adrenal hyperplasia. *N Engl J Med* 349:776-788. PMID:12930931.

Spencer CA, Takeuchi M, Kazarosyan M, Wang CC, Guttler RB, Singer PA, et al [1998] Serum thyroglobulin autoantibodies: prevalence, influence on serum thyroglobulin measurement, and prognostic significance in patients with differentiated thyroid carcinoma. *J Clin Endocrinol Metab* 83(4):1121-1127. PMID:9543128.

Stenman U [2002] Tumor-associated trypsin inhibitor. *Clin Chem* 48(8):1206-1209. PMID:12142374.

Stevens LA, Levey AS [2005] Chronic kidney disease in the elderly—how to assess risk *N Engl J Med* 352:2122-2124. PMID:15901867.

Stevens LA, Coresh J, Greene T, Levey AS [2006] Assessing kidney function—measured and estimated glomerular filtration rate. *N Engl J Med* 354:2473-2483. PMID:16760447.

Stowasser M, Gordon RD [2004] The aldosterone-renin ratio in screening for primary aldosteronism. *Endocrinologist* 14:267-276.

Taglieri N, Koenig W, Kaski JC [2009] Cystatin C and cardiovascular risk. *Clin Chem* 55(11):1932-1943. PMID:19713275.

Tate JR, Gill D, Cobcroft R, Hickman PE [2003] Practical consider-ations for the measurement of free light chains in serum. *Clin Chem* 49(8):1252-1257. PMID:12881439.

Tessler DA, Catanzaro A, Velanovich V, Havstad S, Goel S [2006] Predictors of cancer in patients with suspected pancreatic malignancy without a tissue diagnosis. *Am J Surg* 191:191-197. PMID:16442944.

The Diabetes Control and Complications Trial Research Group [1993] The effect of intensive treatment of diabetes on the development and progression of long term complications in insulin-dependent diabetes mellitus. *N Engl J Med* 329:977-979. PMID:8366922.

Thompson IM, Pauler DK, Goodman PJ, et al [2004] Prevalence of pros-tate cancer among men with a prostate specific antigen level ≤ 4.0 ng/milliliter. *N Engl J Med* 350:2239-2246. PMID:15163773.

Thygesen K, Mair J, Giannitsis E [2012] How to use high-sensitivity cardiac troponins in acute cardiac care. *Eur Heart J* 33(18):2252-2257. PMID:22723599.

Todd DJ, Kagan A, Chibnik LB, Kay J [2007] Cutaneous changes of nephrogenic systemic fibrosis: Predictor of early mortality and asso-ciation with gadolinium exposure. *Arthritis Rheum* 56:3433-3441. PMID:17907148.

Usta IM, Barton JR, Amon EA, Gonzalez A, Sibai BM [1994] Acute fatty liver of pregnancy: an experience in the diagnosis and manage-ment of fourteen cases. *Am J Obstet Gynecol* 171(5):1342-1347. PMID:7977544.

Valdes R Jr, Jortani SA, Gheorghiade M [1998] Standards of labora-tory practice: cardiac drug monitoring. *Clin Chem* 44:1096-1109. PMID:9590394.

Valentine VG, Raffin TA [1992] The management of chylothorax. *Chest* 102:586-591. PMID:1643953.

Van Der Cruijsen-Koeter IW, Wildhagen MF, DeKoning HJ, Schröder FH [2001] The value of current diagnostic tests in prostate cancer screening. *BJU International* 88:458-466. PMID:11589658.

Van der Hoek J, Hoorn EJ, de Jong GMT, et al [2009] Severe hypo-natremia with high urine sodium and osmolality. *Clin Chem* 55(11):1905-1909. PMID:19864513.

Verbalis JG, Goldsmith SR, Greenberg A, et al [2007] Hyponatremia treatment guidelines 2007: expert panel recommendations. *Am J Med* 120(11A):S1-S21 PMID:17981159.

Vicini FA, Vargas C, Abner A, Kestin L, Horwitz E, Martinez A [2005] Limitations in the use of serum prostate specific antigen levels to monitor patients after treatment for prostate cancer. *J Urol* 173:1456-1462. PMID:15821460.

Wald NJ, Watt HC, Hackshaw AK [1999] Integrated screening for Down's syndrome based on tests performed during the first and second trimesters. *N Engl J Med* 341:461-467. PMID:10441601.

Ward JF, Moul JW [2005] Biochemical recurrence after definitive prostate cancer therapy. Part I: defining and localizing biochemical recurrence of prostate cancer. *Curr Opin Urol* 15(3):181-186. PMID:15815195.

Weaver LK [2009] Carbon monoxide poisoning. *New Engl J Med* 360(12):1217-1225. PMID:19297574.

Weetman AP [2000] Graves disease. *N Engl J Med* 343:1236-1248. PMID:11071676.

Wenk RE, Rosenbaum JM [2011] Examination of amniotic fluid. In: *Clinical Diagnosis and Management by Laboratory Methods,* 22nd ed. Philadelphia: WB Saunders Company. ISBN:978-1437709742.

Wenzel JJ, Rossmann H, Kullmer U, et al [2009] Chronic diarrhea in a 5 year old girl: pitfall in routine laboratory testing with potentially severe consequences. *Clin Chem* 55(5):1026-1031. PMID:19395441.

Whitfield JB, Dy V, Madden PAF, et al [2008] Measuring carbohy-drate deficient transferrin by direct immunoassay: Factors affecting diagnostic sensitivity for excessive alcohol intake. *Clin Chem* 54(7):1158-1165. PMID:18487284.

Williams RH, Erickson T [1998] Evaluating toxic alcohol poisoning in the emergency setting. *Lab Med* 29:102-108.

Williams RH, Leikin JB [1999] Medicolegal issues and specimen collection for ethanol testing. *Lab Med* 30:530-536.

Wilson JW [1979] Inherited elevation of alkaline phosphatase activity in the absence of disease. *N Engl J Med* 301:983 PMID:492229.

Wolf SJ, Heard K, Sloan EP, Jagoda AS [2007] Clinical policy: critical issues in the management of patients presenting to the emergency department with acetaminophen overdose. *Ann Emerg Med* 50:292-313. PMID:17709050.

Woodrum DL, Brawer MK, Partin AW, Catalona WJ, Southwick PC [1998] Interpretation of free prostate specific antigen clinical research studies for the detection of prostate cancer. *J Urol* 159(1):5-12. PMID:9400426.

Wu AH, Broussard LA, Hoffman RS, et al [2003] National Academy of Clinical Biochemistry Laboratory Medicine Practice guidelines: recommendations for the use of laboratory tests to support the impaired and overdosed patients from the emergency department. *Clin Chem* 49:357-379. PMID:12600948.

Wu AHB, Branch J, Schafer AI, Murphy EJ [2009] Mild positive human chorionic gonadotropin in a perimenopausal female: normal, malignancy, or phantom? *Lab Med* 40(8):463-468.

Wu JT [2011] Diagnosis and management of cancer using serologic tumor markers. In: *Clinical Diagnosis and Management by Laboratory Methods,* 22nd ed. Philadelphia: WB Saunders Company; Chapter 45 ISBN:978-1437709742.

Wu SL, Li W, Wells A, Dasgupta A [2001] Digoxin-like and digitoxin-like immunoreactive substances in elderly people. *Am J Clin Pathol* 115:600-604. PMID:11293909.

Yadav D, Agarwal N, Pitchumoni CS [2002] A critical evaluation of laboratory tests in acute pancreatitis. *Am J Gastroenterol* 97:1309-1318. PMID:12094843.

Yamashita H, Gao P, Cantor T, Noguchi S, Uchino S, Watanabe S, Ogawa T, Kawamoto H, Fukagawa M [2004] Comparison of parathyroid hormone levels from the intact and whole parathyroid hormone assays after parathyroidectomy for primary and secondary hyperparathyroidism. *Surgery* 135:149-156. PMID:14739849.

Yeast JD, Lu G [2005] Biochemical markers for the prediction of preterm labor. *Obstet Gynecol Clin N Am* 32:369-381. PMID:16125038.

Yilmaz A, Tunaboyu İK, Akkaya E, Bayramgürler B [2000] A comparative analysis of the biochemical parameters used to distinguish between pleural exudates and transudates. *Respirology* 5:363-367. PMID:11192547.

Zaninotto M [1999] Strategies for the early diagnosis of acute myocardial infarction using biochemical markers. *Am J Clin Pathol* 111:399-405. PMID:10078116.

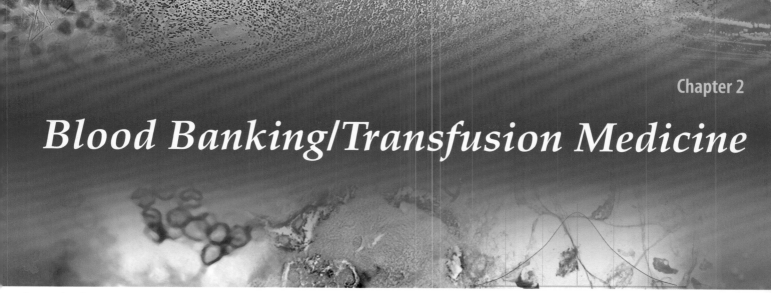

Chapter 2

Blood Banking/Transfusion Medicine

Blood donation

Donor history & physical examination

Registration & donor identification

All donors are required to provide some form of acceptable identification. Most donor centers require a government issued photo identification such as a state issued driver's license or passport. Blood centers require an address or telephone number for follow-up counseling if infectious disease serology is positive.

Timing

The following assessments must occur on the day of donation and before collection.

History

In addition to demographic and medical information, donors should be asked to report any illness developing within a few days after donation and to report a new positive HIV or hepatitis result within 12 months after donation t2.1. Unless cleared by the medical director, the donor must be free of major disease (heart, liver, lung disease), must be free of cancer, and have no abnormal bleeding tendency. Donors must be volunteers; use of paid donors is associated with an increased risk of transfusion transmitted infection, especially hepatitis. The "Uniform Donor Health Questionnaire" is an FDA-sanctioned questionnaire, developed by the AABB that is widely used but not required.

Required donor information includes name, home address, date of birth or age (donors must be ≥16 years of age or in accordance with state law), reasons for any previous deferral, and date of last donation. The allowable minimum donor interval is ≥8 weeks or 56 days after whole blood donation. For 2-unit RBC donations by apheresis, the interval is 16 weeks. The allowable minimum donor interval is ≥2 days for apheresis (plasma, platelet, or leukocytes). For plasmapheresis programs that do not meet criteria for "frequent plasmapheresis" (see below), the interval is 4 weeks.

t2.1 Donor deferrals

Reason for deferral	Deferral
Viral hepatitis after 11th birthday	Indefinite
Family history of Creutzfeldt-Jakob disease	Indefinite
Travelers who have spent >3 months in the United Kingdom or 5 years total in Europe due to risk of variant Creutzfeldt-Jakob areas	Indefinite
Used a needle to administer nonprescription drugs	Indefinite
Male who has had sex with another male since 1977	Indefinite
Receipt of dura mater or pituitary growth hormone of human origin	Indefinite
Confirmed positive test for HbsAg or repeatedly reactive test for anti-HBc	Indefinite
Laboratory evidence of HCV infection	Indefinite
Laboratory evidence of HTLV-1 infection	Indefinite
Have donated the only unit of blood to a patient who developed HIV or HTLV & had no other probable cause of infection	Indefinite
Use of bovine insulin manufactured in UK	Indefinite
Etretinate (Tegison)	Indefinite
History of babesiosis	Indefinite
History of Chagas disease	Indefinite
Obvious stigmata of parenteral drug use or use of a needle to administer nonprescription drugs	Indefinite
Receiving money or drugs for sex	Indefinite
Acitretin (Soriatane)	3 years after last dose
Malarial infection (after becoming asymptomatic)	3 years
Lived for >5 years in malaria-endemic areas (after departure, if symptom free), regardless of prophylaxis	3 years
Paying for sex	12 months
History of syphilis or gonorrhea, treatment for syphilis or gonorrhea, or positive syphilis screening test (after completion of therapy)	12 months
Receipt of blood products, human tissue, or plasma derived clotting factors	12 months
Hepatitis B immune globulin administration	12 months
Any other unlisted vaccine	12 months
Mucous membrane exposure to blood	12 months
Nonsterile skin penetration, including tattoos or permanent makeup, unless applied by a state-regulated entity with sterile needles & ink that has not been reused	12 months
Residing with or having sexual contact with an individual with viral hepatitis	12 months
Sexual contact with an individual with HIV or at high risk for HIV	12 months
Incarceration >72 consecutive hours	12 months
Travelers to malaria-endemic areas (after departure, if symptom free) regardless of prophylaxis	12 months
Dutasteride (Avodart)	6 months after last dose

(continued on next page)

t2.1 Donor deferrals (continued)

Reason for deferral	Deferral
Pregnancy	Defer until 6 weeks postpartum/posttermination (exceptions for transfusion to the infant with physician approval)
Live attenuated vaccines: German measles (rubella) & chicken pox (varicella zoster) vaccines	4 weeks
Finasteride (Proscar, Propecia)	1 month after last dose
Isotretinoin (Accutane)	1 month after last dose
Clopidogrel (Plavix) & Ticlopidine (Ticlid) (donor excluded as sole source of platelets)	14 days
Live attenuated vaccines: measles (rubeola), polio (Sabin oral), mumps, typhoid (oral) & yellow fever vaccines	2 weeks
Smallpox vaccine	In those with no complications of vaccine, 21 days or until scab falls off, whichever is longer. In those with severe complications, 14 days after resolution. Asymptomatic contacts of vaccine recipients need not be deferred
West Nile virus	14 days after resolved or 28 days after onset, whichever is longer. Positive West Nile antibody test, without illness, is not grounds for deferral
Warfarin (Coumadin)	7 days (donor excluded as source of plasma products
Aspirin & piroxicam (Feldene)	48 hours (donor excluded as sole source of platelets)
Toxoids, synthetic or killed vaccines: anthrax, cholera, diphtheria, hepatitis A, hepatitis B, influenza, Lyme, paratyphoid, pertussis, plague, pneumococcal polysaccharide, polio (Salk injection), rabies, Rocky Mountain spotted fever, tetanus, typhoid (injection), recombinant HPV vaccine	None (if donor is afebrile & symptom-free)
Stigmata of alcohol intoxication or habituation	Exclude donor, no specific period of time stated
Other travel	Refer to www.cdc.gov/travel
Antibiotics	As defined by medical director

Physical examination

The prospective donor must be checked for general appearance, temperature, weight, blood pressure, pulse, hemoglobin or hematocrit, and venipuncture sites t2.2

t2.2 Physical examination requirements

General appearance	Must appear in good health
Temperature	Temperature: ≤37.5°C (99.5° F), measured orally
Pulse	Should be regular & between 50-100 beats/minute Donor with heart rate <50 may be accepted if an otherwise healthy athlete
Blood pressure	No higher than 180 systolic & 100 diastolic
Skin of venipuncture site	Venipuncture site must be free of lesions Both arms must be examined for evidence of repeated parenteral entry (IV drug use)
Hemoglobin or hematocrit	The hemoglobin or hematocrit must be ≥12.5 g/dL or ≥38%, respectively Must be determined by blood sample taken at the time of donation & cannot be obtained by earlobe puncture

Autologous donors

The requirements of autologous donors are not as stringent as those for allogeneic donation, the minimum requirements including a physician order, hemoglobin ≥11.0 g/dL or hematocrit ≥33%, and no condition that places the autologous donor at

risk for bacteremia. Blood must be collected >72 hours prior to anticipated surgery or transfusion. Note that the unit can only be used for autologous donation, if the unit is not transfused to the patient it is destroyed.

Apheresis donors

The requirements of apheresis donors are the same as allogeneic donors with the exception of donation intervals. For plasmapheresis, donations must be 4 weeks apart, and the donor must weigh ≥50 kg (110 lb). A "frequent" donor plasmapheresis program is one in which donations occur more frequently than every 4 weeks. In such a scenario, donations must be limited to 2/week, each ≥2 days apart. In manual separation procedures, no more than 500 mL of whole blood should be removed from a donor during the procedure at one time unless the donor weighs ≥80 kg (175 lb), in this case as much as 600 mL can be removed at any time. For automated instruments, the allowable volume has been predetermined by the FDA. For plateletpheresis, donations must be limited to 2/week, ≥2 days apart, and not >24 in a 12-month period. If there is a whole blood donation by a donor, or if RBCs cannot be returned to a donor during apheresis, then 8 weeks must elapse before repeat apheresis. A platelet count of ≥150,000/μL is required for plateletpheresis. For red blood cell (RBC) apheresis and multicomponent donations, if the donor is giving a single unit of RBCs with platelets and/or plasma they are deferred for 8 weeks. If a donor gives a double RBC donation by apheresis, they are deferred for 16 weeks.

Blood obtained from therapeutic phlebotomy

Blood obtained from therapeutic phlebotomy should not be used for allogeneic transfusion unless the donor meets all requirements for allogeneic transfusion. Potential donors with myeloproliferative disorders such as polycythemia vera or hemoglobin synthesis disorders such as porphyria cutanea tarda are not acceptable donors, and their blood is destroyed after phlebotomy. Since 1999, the FDA has allowed blood centers to obtain variances to collect blood from donors with hemochromatosis. If the donor has no other medical conditions, the medical director of the blood center may allow these units to "cross-over" into the general blood supply as long as these units are clearly labeled with the donor's disease. Blood centers that provide phlebotomy service for free regardless of donor eligibility status are listed on the FDA website (http://www.fda.gov/BiologicsBloodVaccines/BloodBloodProducts/RegulationoftheBloodSupply/Variances/ucm164649.htm).

Collecting blood from donor
Information given to donor

Blood centers must give potential donors educational material informing them of the risks associated with phlebotomy and information regarding infections transmitted by transfusion, the signs and symptoms of AIDS, the importance of giving accurate information, the importance of refraining from donating blood if they believe they have an increased risk of infection and the reporting requirements of positive results to federal or state health authorities. Donors may contact the blood collection center and request their unit is not used. In this scenario, the blood is still subjected to screening procedures, and donors informed of abnormal results. Donors must be given an opportunity to ask questions before providing written consent for donation. Parental consent is required in states collecting blood from 16 year old donors. Donors must be notified of any significantly abnormal test results; in the case of autologous donation, both the donor and physician are notified.

Blood collection system

Blood must be collected in an aseptic manner and drawn into a closed sterile system; that is, a preattached group of bags and integral tubing that, following blood collection, can be manipulated without ever entering the system again. If platelets are prepared from a whole blood collection, a diversion pouch must be used to divert the first 30-45 mL of blood which contains the skin plug from phlebotomy. Diversion pouches have decreased bacterial contamination in blood components by as much as 50%. If at any point in the life of this closed sterile system it is penetrated ("spiked") the shelf-life is shortened. Sterile connection devices (docking devices) exist that allow access into the unit without compromising sterility. At the time of collection, a certain amount of blood is left in the integral tubing which is then pinched (by a heat sealer) in several places to create several sealed segments of blood-filled tubing. These segments can be separated, without entering the unit, at any time for lab testing.

Volume drawn

The maximum blood drawn from the donor is 10.5 mL/kg of donor weight, including samples for testing. Most samples for testing are collected from the diversion pouches. The total volume collected amounts to nearly 15% of the whole blood volume (whole blood volume being ~70 mL/kg), and the maximum allowable volume collected is 15% of the donor's whole blood volume. This volume must be collected within 10-15 minutes if platelets or plasma are to be made from the unit. The typical collection bag has a volume of anticoagulant that is appropriate for 450±45 cc of whole blood (some are made with anticoagulant sufficient for 500±50 cc). When 300-404 cc whole blood is collected in a 450 cc bag (or 333-449 cc is collected in a 500 cc bag), it must be labeled as "RBCs Low Volume;" such a unit cannot be used for preparation of other components.

After collection

The unit must be processed into components within 8 hours of collection in order to create fresh frozen plasma and platelets. If transported from collection facility, the whole blood donations should be transported at 1-10°C if the unit will be used only to create RBCs. If platelets are to be made from whole blood, units are allowed to cool to room temperature, 20-24°C.

Donor adverse reactions

Donors must be observed during donation and for an appropriate length of time thereafter. Vasovagal reactions are recognized by a slow heart rate in addition to dizziness, sweating, pallor, nausea, vomiting, hypotension, syncope and convulsions. To treat vasovagal reactions, begin by elevating the feet, loosening clothes, and applying cold compresses to the donor's head or back of neck while continuing to monitor the donor. Hypovolemia is recognized by a fast heart rate with hypotension and possible nausea and syncope. In this case, the donor

must be given fluids, often intravenously. Hyperventilation is characterized by an altered, rapid and shallow, respiratory pattern that results in hypocapnia. The donor may also manifest facial twitching and seizures. The donor should be assisted with breathing into a paper bag. Citrate effect is only seen in apheresis donors in whom citrate must be used as an anticoagulant. Sometimes the citrate returning to the donor's circulation results in hypocalcemia manifested by perioral tingling possibly progressing to nausea, vomiting, arrhythmias and seizures. The initial treatment, for mild symptoms, is to simply slow the infusion rate, as well as provide oral calcium carbonate. Hematoma may occur during or after phlebotomy. Remove the tourniquet and needle from the donor's arm and use sterile gauze to apply digital pressure. Ice may also be helpful to decrease pain and swelling.

Laboratory testing of donor blood
ABO & Rh testing

Determinations of the ABO group and Rh type must be made on donor blood. ABO antigen testing of patient RBCs must be done with anti-A and anti-B reagents (RBC or forward grouping) and A1 and B reagent RBCs to detect the patient's serum/plasma ABO antibodies (serum or reverse grouping) t2.3, f2.1. The Rh type is determined with anti-D. If the anti-D test is negative, then testing must be performed for weak D, including extended incubation and addition of anti-human globulin (AHG). Only when both of these are negative can a unit be labeled Rh–. If either is positive, it is labeled Rh+. Note: at the receiving blood bank, there must be a method to confirm that the ABO/Rh label on the blood is correct. At final labeling, the ABO/Rh must be compared to prior records (historical group), if available, and any discrepancies must be resolved before the unit is issued.

t2.3 ABO forward & reverse grouping

Forward grouping		Reverse grouping		
Anti-A	Anti-B	A cells	B cells	Group
0	0	4+	4+	0
4+	0	0	4+	A
0	4+	4+	0	B
4+	4+	0	0	AB

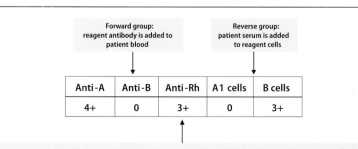

	Forward group: reagent antibody is added to patient blood			Reverse group: patient serum is added to reagent cells	
Anti-A	Anti-B	Anti-Rh	A1 cells	B cells
4+	0	3+	0	3+

Strength of reaction is graded 0 to 4+ and mf+ (mixed field). The term mixed field reaction means some cells are reacting and others are not; it is best seen microscopically. It implies that 2 populations of red cells are present, as in recent transfusion or following stem cell/bone marrow transplant. In ABO grouping, 3+ or 4+ reactions are expected. Weaker reactions (2+) may be seen, or example, if the cell group is a subgroup of A or there has been transfusion of group O cells.

f2.1 Initial blood group; in this example, the patient tests as blood group A, Rh+, with the expected anti-B antibody

Antibody screen

Blood from donors with a history of transfusion or pregnancy must be screened for unexpected antibodies to RBC antigens. RBCs may be processed from donors testing positive for alloantibodies and sent only to accepting medical centers.

Infectious disease screening

Tests currently required on donor blood include HBsAg, anti-HBc, anti-HCV, HCV nucleic acid (HCV RNA), anti-HIV-1/2, HIV-1 nucleic acid (HIV-1 RNA), anti-HTLV-I/II, serologic testing for syphilis (RPR), and West Nile virus (WNV RNA) during times of geographic activity of the virus. In January 2007, licensing of the first screening test for *Trypanosoma cruzi* became available in the US. Currently many centers test all donors for *Trypanosoma cruzi* either at the first time of donation or with each donation. Prepared units of platelets must be tested for bacterial contamination. The units are incubated for 24 hours prior to sampling for culture. All tests must be performed on each distinct donation, and all results must be negative.

Certain exceptions should be noted. A positive test for syphilis, that has been demonstrated to be a false positive in a particular donor, may be permitted. Infectious disease screening tests can be bypassed in an emergency or critical blood shortage, but this omission must be indicated on the label. The medical directors of the blood center and the medical center must sign releases before the units are transported to the medical center. Testing must still be completed as soon as it is possible. Lastly, directed apheresis donors (for a specific recipient) and autologous donors may be tested initially and at 30-day intervals thereafter.

Pretransfusion procedures t2.4
Routine pretransfusion procedures
Blood collection from recipient

Patient identification must be affixed to blood samples. Clerical errors cannot be tolerated in any part of the process. Mislabeled specimens should be discarded and a new sample requested. In the event of an emergency, group O RBC units may be issued. Blood samples from potential recipients must be labeled at the bedside with the following information: ≥2 unique identifiers (eg, name, medical record number, date of birth or unique armband number), date of collection, and information identifying the phlebotomist.

The AABB standards require a new sample for pretransfusion testing every 3 days. If the patient has no pregnancy or transfusion history within 3 months, samples may be drawn earlier for elective surgeries. In such cases, ABO testing, Rh testing and antibody screening must be performed and no discrepancies or alloantibodies must be detected to use this sample for crossmatching blood prior to elective surgery.

Either serum or plasma is acceptable for traditional tube testing; plasma is preferred for newer platforms (gel or solid phase testing). Hemolysis may interfere with interpretation of tube testing.

The blood sample, as well as a tube segment from any transfused blood, must be retained for 7 days after transfusion.

t2.4 Routine pretransfusion procedures

Procedure	Notes
Blood sample(s) obtained from intended recipient	Labeled at bedside with 2 unique identifiers, date, time & identity of phlebotomist
	Drawn within 3 days of transfusion (longer under certain circumstances) & retained for 7 days after
ABO & Rh testing of recipient	ABO: Forward & back group
	Rh: Do not need to test for weak D
Antibody screen of recipient	Antibody panel if positive
Comparison with prior records on recipient	If any
Testing of donor blood	ABO & Rh, determined initially at collection facility, must be confirmed at the transfusion facility; repeat testing for weak D is not required
	Granulocytes must be ABO compatible with the recipient's plasma & require crossmatching because of large numbers of RBCs in the component
	Platelets may be transfused outside of ABO compatibilities unless the units are visibly bloody
Visual inspection of donor blood	Labeled with 2 unique identifiers of the intended recipient, the donation identification number (DIN) & interpretation of compatibility tests, if applicable
	Bacterial contamination should be suspected if units are discolored (purple), if there is a visible zone of hemolysis, or if clots can be seen
	Visibly lipemic units should not be transfused
Proper identification of recipient at bedside	2 unique identifiers

ABO & Rh testing of recipient blood

Anti-A and Anti-B antisera are used to determine which antigens are present on the recipient's RBCs (forward grouping). In a typical forward grouping, one drop of recipient washed RBCs is added to one drop of anti-A and anti-B in separately labeled test tubes. These are centrifuged for 15 seconds, and the resulting button is resuspended. The tubes are then examined visually for agglutination; agglutination is graded 0-4+. Reagent A1 and B test cells are used to determine which antibodies are present in the serum (reverse typing). 2 drops of recipient serum/plasma are added to A1 test cells and B test cells in separately labeled test tubes. These are centrifuged for 15 seconds, resuspended, examined visually and agglutination is graded. If there is an ABO discrepancy, only group O blood may be issued pending resolution.

Rh testing is carried out with anti-D sera. Unlike donor blood, recipient blood need not be tested for weak D.

The antibody screen

The purpose of the antibody screen is to detect unexpected RBC alloantibodies in the recipient. These are antibodies, other than ABO, that are capable of causing hemolysis or hemolytic disease of the newborn. These are acquired through a sensitizing event, such as prior transfusion or pregnancy. The antibody screen is performed using 2-4 reagent group O test cells that have differential expression of antigens. It is required that 18 clinically significant antigens are represented.

Patient plasma/serum is added to the test cells, followed by immediate spin, 37°C incubation, and addition of anti-human globulin (AHG). See f2.2. The immediate spin phase consists of adding patient serum/plasma to the test cells at room temperature, then briefly centrifuging; the resultant button is

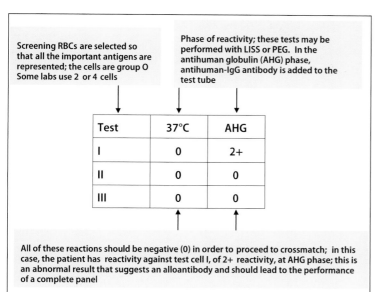

Test	37°C	AHG
I	0	2+
II	0	0
III	0	0

Screening RBCs are selected so that all the important antigens are represented; the cells are group O Some labs use 2 or 4 cells

Phase of reactivity; these tests may be performed with LISS or PEG. In the antihuman globulin (AHG) phase, antihuman-IgG antibody is added to the test tube

All of these reactions should be negative (0) in order to proceed to crossmatch; in this case, the patient has reactivity against test cell I, of 2+ reactivity, at AHG phase; this is an abnormal result that suggests an alloantibody and should lead to the performance of a complete panel

f2.2 An antibody screen; this test is abnormal & should be followed by a full antibody panel which uses between 10-14 test cells

resuspended and examined visually for clumping or hemolysis. If using automated methods, the immediate spin phase is omitted to decrease the detection of clinically insignificant cold reacting antibodies. The 37°C incubation phase consists of incubating the resuspended cells for a period of time at 37°C; the duration of incubation may be up to 60 minutes, depending upon whether or not enhancing agents (eg, LISS or polyethylene glycol PEG) are added. In the AHG phase, the cells are first washed, then mixed with AHG, briefly centrifuged, resuspended, and visually examined for agglutination. An autocontrol may be run in parallel with the test cells. Patient plasma and patient RBCs are incubated then washed to remove the plasma. AHG is then added to the patient cells; in many labs the autocontrol is run only when an antibody panel is performed and is used to detect possible autoantibodies. Room temperature incubation is omitted by many labs, since it mainly detects clinically insignificant, alloantibodies such as anti-M, N, Lewis, I, and P.

If no reactions take place with any of the test cells, then the antibody screen is negative and one may proceed to crossmatch. If any of the cells react in the antibody screen, then the responsible antibody must be identified with an antibody panel.

An antibody panel is required if the antibody screen is positive. The antibody panel is similar to an expanded antibody screen, except more test cells are used. Usually 10-14 different donor test cells are used in the panel, all group O, which have known antigenic composition. An autocontrol is run in parallel, in which recipient serum/plasma is added to recipient RBCs. Panel interpretation is discussed more fully below, under "Investigating a positive antibody screen or unexpected crossmatch incompatibility."

While many laboratories perform these studies in traditional test tubes, with macroscopic and microscopic inspection by a technologist, other methods exist. New methods such as testing in microplates, solid-phase enzyme linked immunosorbent assays, and column agglutination (gel techniques) are being used more commonly. Several automated "walk away" testing platforms are now available. These systems perform all steps in the testing process from initial sample aliquoting, testing, to result reporting. These automated systems allow for multiple patient samples to be tested in parallel. Solid phase, gel-column, and microtiter technology may be employed in any one system. Ideally, these testing systems are interfaced with the blood bank information system. The use of barcode technology further enhances these systems by ensuring excellent efficiency without sacrificing accuracy.

Comparison with prior transfusion records

Current results must be compared with prior pretransfusion testing results, if any exists, on each patient. One looks for concurrence between current and previous ABO groups and Rh types and for previous alloantibodies that are currently undetectable. Certain alloantibodies, notoriously Kidd, fall below the threshold of detection and yet remain clinically significant. If the previous and current blood group does not match, this suggests a patient identification problem or sample mix-up (wrong blood in tube). The first step is to repeat the ABO and Rh testing; if these remain inconsistent with prior records, obtain a new sample.

ABO & Rh testing of donor blood

Donor blood is tested at the donation facility for ABO, D, and weak D. This must be confirmed at the transfusion facility prior to issue. Repeat testing for weak D is not required.

The crossmatch

The purpose of the crossmatch is to serve as a final check for ABO incompatibility. Low incidence alloantibodies can be detected as well, particularly if the antibody screen is carried out at 37°C, and low titer alloantibodies (eg, Kidd) may be detected. Currently, either an immediate spin (IS) serologic or computer crossmatch is allowed in patients with negative antibody screens.

The IS crossmatch is performed as follows. At room temperature, recipient serum/plasma is mixed with a sample of the donor RBCs obtained from one of the segments of integral tubing, followed by centrifugation. This is the usual type of routine crossmatch performed. When a clinically insignificant, cold reacting, antibody is present, the crossmatch may be prewarmed to prevent interference by this antibody. If known clinically significant alloantibodies are present, then a complete or full crossmatch with AHG phase testing is required.

A computer crossmatch is permissible in patients with no detectable clinically significant alloantibodies. Certain conditions must be met for this to be an acceptable alternative to the serologic crossmatch, including, but not limited to: "validating" the computer system, 2 separate determinations of the recipient's ABO/Rh, the computer system contains donor identification number, component type, ABO/Rh of unit and has the logic to alert when a unit and patient are ABO/Rh incompatible.

Infant blood, up to 4 months old, need not be crossmatched if no clinically significant maternal antibodies are detected. The ABO/Rh is determined as for adult recipients, but it need only be determined once and may be omitted for the remainder of the hospitalization, unless lasting beyond the age of 4 months or if the infant leaves the hospital and is readmitted. The serum of the neonate or the mother may be used to test for clinically significant antibodies.

What a crossmatch will not accomplish must also be borne in mind. The crossmatch will not detect errors in patient identification (wrong blood in tube); this limitation is part of the reason for comparison with prior transfusion records, if they exist. The crossmatch will not detect Rh typing errors, since most recipients have not formed anti-D antibodies. Lastly, the crossmatch will not always detect (or prevent) alloimmunization, since it is sensitive primarily to incompatibility to preformed (ABO) antibody.

Compatible products t2.5–t2.13

When transfusing RBC products and granulocytes (because they contain a significant quantity of RBCs) the transfused RBCs must be ABO compatible with the intended recipient and must be subjected to crossmatch. If whole blood is transfused, blood must be ABO identical.

Due to the limited shelf life and shortages of platelets, both apheresis and random donor platelets may be transfused outside of ABO compatibilities unless the units are visibly bloody. Most random donor unit platelets contain <0.5 mL RBCs and apheresis platelets contain <2 mL of donor RBCs. Neither platelets nor cryoprecipitate have strict compatibility requirements; still, it is preferable that the plasma in these products be compatible with the recipient's RBCs. Furthermore, avoidance of Rh+ platelets in Rh– recipients is advisable. If this is unavoidable Rh immune globulin (RhIg) should be offered to the patient's physician.

When transfusing plasma, the plasma must be compatible with the intended recipient, because it contains sufficient donor ABO antibody to be clinically significant.

t2.5 Compatible products overview

Product	Requirement
Whole Blood	ABO identical to recipient
Packed Red Blood Cells	ABO compatible with recipient plasma
Granulocytes	ABO compatible with recipient plasma
Plasma	ABO compatible with recipient RBCs
Platelets	No specific requirement; preferred: ABO compatible with recipient RBCs
Cryoprecipitate	ABO compatible with recipient RBCs

t2.6 Compatible RBC components

Component	Recipient group	Compatible donor group
Whole Blood	Any	ABO identical
Red Blood Cells; see t2.8 & t2.9	O	O
Red Blood Cells	A	A or O
Red Blood Cells	B	B or O
Red Blood Cells	AB	AB, A, B, or O

t2.7 Compatibility of components containing Plasma (Platelets & Plasma/FFP)

Recipient blood group	Donor blood group			
	A	B	AB	O
A	compatible	incompatible	compatible	incompatible
B	incompatible	compatible	compatible	incompatible
AB	incompatible	incompatible	compatible	incompatible
O	compatible	compatible	compatible	compatible

If group compatible platelets are not available, any group can be given to a patient >2 years of age
See **t2.10–t2.13**

t2.8 Recommended RBC product selection for recipients >4 months old

Patient group	First choice	Second choice	Third choice	Last choice
A+	A+	A–	O+	O–
B+	B+	B–	O+	O–
O+	O+	O–		
AB+	AB+	AB–	A+ B+ O+	A– B– O–
A–	A–	O–		*A+ *O+
B–	B–	O–		*B+ *O+
O–	O–			*O+
AB–	AB–	A– B– O–		*AB+ *A+ *B+ *O+

*If there are no Rh– RBC units available, and there is an emergent need for blood, then Rh+ units of the same blood group or group O may be issued, with the consent of the treating physician

t2.9 Recommended RBC product selection for recipients <4 months old

Patient group	First choice	Second choice	Third choice
A+	O+ CMV– & irradiated	O–, CMV– & irradiated	A+ or A– CMV– & irradiated
B+	O+ CMV– & irradiated	O– CMV– & irradiated	B+ or B– CMV– & irradiated
O+	O+ CMV– & irradiated	O– CMV– & irradiated	
AB+	O+ CMV– & irradiated	O– CMV– & irradiated	AB+ or AB– CMV– & irradiated
A–	O– CMV– & irradiated	A– CMV– & irradiated	
B–	O– CMV– & irradiated	B– CMV– & irradiated	
O–	O– CMV– & irradiated	O– CMV– & irradiated	
AB–	O– CMV– & irradiated	AB– CMV– & irradiated	

t2.10 Recommended Plasma (or FFP) product selection for recipients > 4 months of age

Patient group	First choice	Second choice	Third choice
A+/A–	A+/A–	AB+/AB–	
B+/B–	B+/B–	AB+/AB–	
0+/0–	0+/0–	AB+/AB–	A+/A– B+/B–
AB+/AB–	AB+/AB–		

t2.11 Recommended Plasma (or FFP) product selection for recipients <4 months of age

Patient group	First choice	Second choice
A+/A–	AB+/AB–	A+/A–
B+/B–	AB+/AB–	B+/B–
0+/0–	AB+/AB–	0+/0–
AB+/AB–	AB+/AB–	

t2.12 Recommended Platelet apheresis product selection for recipients >4 months of age

Patient group	First choice	Second choice	Third choice
A+	A+	A–	AB+ AB–
B+	B+	B–	AB+ AB–
0+	0+	0–	AB+, AB–, A+, A–, B+, B–
AB+	AB+	AB–	
A–	A–	AB–	
B–	B–	AB–	
0–	0–	AB–	A– B–
AB–	AB–	A– B–	

Rh– patients should receive Rh– platelets, when possible; if Rh+ platelets are administered to Rh– patients, RhIg should be considered within 3 days of transfusion, especially for women of childbearing potential

t2.13 Recommended Platelet product selection for neonates <4 months old

Patient group	First choice	Second choice
A+	AB+ AB– Irradiated & CMV–	A+ A– Irradiated & CMV–
B+	AB+ AB– Irradiated & CMV–	B+ B– Irradiated & CMV–
0+	AB+ AB– Irradiated & CMV–	0+ 0– Irradiated & CMV–
AB+	AB+ AB– Irradiated & CMV–	
A–	AB– Irradiated & CMV–	A– Irradiated & CMV–
B–	AB– Irradiated & CMV–	B– Irradiated & CMV–
0–	AB– Irradiated & CMV–	0– Irradiated & CMV–
AB–	AB– Irradiated & CMV–	

Visual inspection of blood prior to issue

The blood or component must be inspected prior to issue. The units must be labeled with 2 unique identifiers of the intended recipient, the donation identification number (DIN), and interpretation of compatibility tests, if applicable. The contents of the unit must also be visually inspected. Blood contamination should be suspected if units are discolored (purple), if there is a visible zone of hemolysis, or if clots can be seen. Also, visibly lipemic units should not be transfused.

Transfusion

Transfusion procedures are usually contained in nursing policies, but the blood bank medical director should be involved in their formulation, periodic review and assistance with ensuring compliance of the hospital staff. Transfusion requires a physician order. Informed consent should be performed by a physician, should precede the transfusion and include a thorough explanation of the risks of transfusion, alternatives to transfusion, and the patient's right to refuse transfusion.

The person administering the transfusion must confirm, at the bedside, the identity of the recipient (with 2 unique identifiers) and ensure that the unit label matches the recipient. Blood must be transfused through a sterile transfusion set with an inline filter (such filters are not capable of leukocyte reduction). If a leukocyte reduction filter is used, the inline filter may be omitted.

Neonatal transfusions are usually performed through a syringe. Only one filtration is required and may be performed by the blood bank staff if the aliquot is filtered during removal from the original unit into the syringe. Manufacturers now offer inline filters with aliquoting systems.

Only normal saline can run in the same line as the unit; use of lactated ringers may cause blood clotting, while dextrose solutions may cause hemolysis.

The transfusion must be started within 30 minutes of issue and completed within 4 hours of spiking the unit. A baseline set of vital signs should be recorded prior to transfusion. The patient should be observed for the first 15 minutes of transfusion and a second set of vital signs is obtained at 15 minutes after starting transfusion. The recipient should be observed throughout the transfusion and for an appropriate length of time thereafter. At the completion of the transfusion the licensed health care provider should document the following: time the transfusion was completed, another set of vitals and if the patient experienced any adverse symptoms.

Reactivity (0-4+) is recorded at 3 separate phases. In the IS (immediate spin) serum is mixed with cells at room temp, then centrifuged and examined. In the 37°C phase, the same is done at 37°C. In AHG (antihuman globulin) phase, also called IAT (indirect agglutination test), the same is done followed by addition of AHG

Test cell antigen expression is known and expressed in tabular form

Test cells are group O

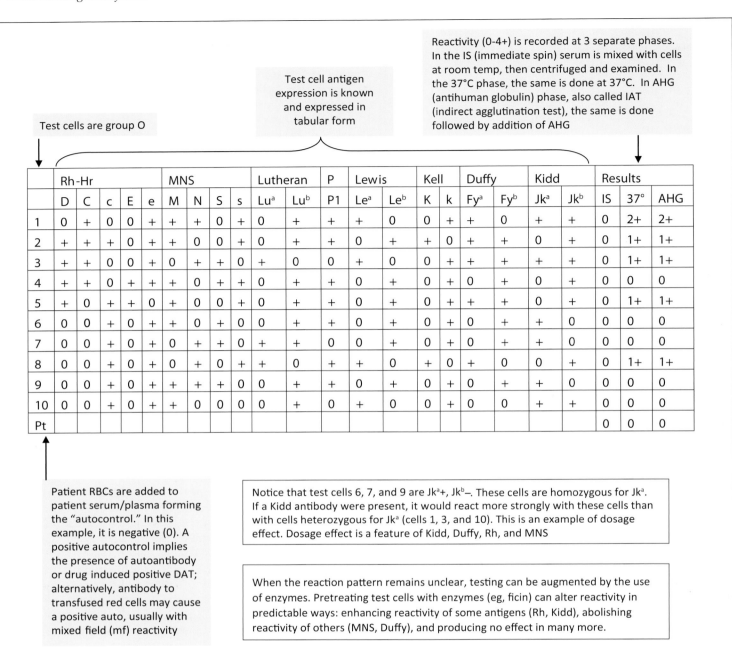

	Rh-Hr					MNS				Lutheran		P	Lewis		Kell		Duffy		Kidd		Results		
	D	C	c	E	e	M	N	S	s	Lu^a	Lu^b	P1	Le^a	Le^b	K	k	Fy^a	Fy^b	Jk^a	Jk^b	IS	37°	AHG
1	0	+	0	0	+	+	+	0	+	0	+	+	+	0	0	+	+	0	+	+	0	2+	2+
2	+	+	+	0	+	+	0	0	+	0	+	+	0	+	+	0	+	+	0	+	0	1+	1+
3	+	+	0	0	+	0	+	+	0	+	0	0	+	0	0	+	+	+	+	+	0	1+	1+
4	+	+	0	+	+	+	0	+	+	0	+	+	0	+	0	+	0	+	0	+	0	0	0
5	+	0	+	+	0	+	0	0	+	0	+	+	0	+	0	+	+	+	0	+	0	1+	1+
6	0	0	+	0	+	+	0	+	0	0	+	+	0	+	0	+	0	+	+	0	0	0	0
7	0	0	+	0	+	0	+	+	0	+	+	0	0	+	0	+	0	+	+	0	0	0	0
8	0	0	+	0	+	0	+	0	+	+	0	+	+	0	+	0	+	0	0	+	0	1+	1+
9	0	0	+	0	+	+	+	+	0	0	+	+	0	+	0	+	0	+	+	0	0	0	0
10	0	0	+	0	+	+	0	0	0	0	+	0	+	0	0	+	0	0	+	+	0	0	0
Pt																					0	0	0

Patient RBCs are added to patient serum/plasma forming the "autocontrol." In this example, it is negative (0). A positive autocontrol implies the presence of autoantibody or drug induced positive DAT; alternatively, antibody to transfused red cells may cause a positive auto, usually with mixed field (mf) reactivity

Notice that test cells 6, 7, and 9 are Jk^a+, Jk^b–. These cells are homozygous for Jk^a. If a Kidd antibody were present, it would react more strongly with these cells than with cells heterozygous for Jk^a (cells 1, 3, and 10). This is an example of dosage effect. Dosage effect is a feature of Kidd, Duffy, Rh, and MNS

When the reaction pattern remains unclear, testing can be augmented by the use of enzymes. Pretreating test cells with enzymes (eg, ficin) can alter reactivity in predictable ways: enhancing reactivity of some antigens (Rh, Kidd), abolishing reactivity of others (MNS, Duffy), and producing no effect in many more.

f2.3 Antibody panel

Nonroutine pretransfusion procedures: investigation of a positive antibody screen or unexpected crossmatch incompatibility

The reagent RBC panel f2.3

If an antibody screen is positive, a RBC panel is used to determine the antibody responsible. The identity of the antibody is the key to knowing

1. whether it is clinically significant

2. the best strategy for finding antigen-negative blood

A panel is essentially an expanded antibody screen. Recipient serum is tested against a panel of group O blood cells, usually 10-14 different cells, which have been selected so that it is possible to identify the antibody in question. Reagent cells licensed by the FDA must express the following 18 antigens: D, C, E, c, e, M, N, S, s, P1, Le^a, Le^b, K, k, Fy^a, Fy^b, Jk^a and Jk^b. Usually panel reactions are carried out using some type of enhancement media, designed to make antibody-antigen reactions more obvious. Enhancement media include such solutions as low ionic strength saline (LISS) or polyethylene glycol (PEG). Panels typically involve both a 37°C incubation phase and an AHG phase using either polyspecific reagent or monospecific anti-IgG reagent. The particular phase during which reactivity is seen is important to note. IgM antibodies can directly agglutinate RBCs, whereas IgG antibodies usually require addition of AHG. Furthermore, IgM antibodies are reactive at room temperature, but some (the clinically significant ones) have a broad thermal range and react at 37°C. Panels usually are run in parallel with an autocontrol. This helps recognize reactivity due to RBC autoantibodies.

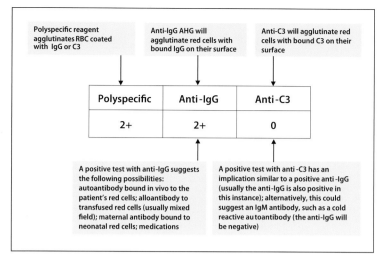

Polyspecific	Anti-IgG	Anti-C3
2+	2+	0

Polyspecific reagent agglutinates RBC coated with IgG or C3

Anti-IgG AHG will agglutinate red cells with bound IgG on their surface

Anti-C3 will agglutinate red cells with bound C3 on their surface

A positive test with anti-IgG suggests the following possibilities: autoantibody bound in vivo to the patient's red cells; alloantibody to transfused red cells (usually mixed field); maternal antibody bound to neonatal red cells; medications

A positive test with anti-C3 has an implication similar to a positive anti-IgG (usually the anti-IgG is also positive in this instance); alternatively, this could suggest an IgM antibody, such as a cold reactive autoantibody (the anti-IgG will be negative)

f2.4 DAT (direct antiglobulin test)

Types of reaction

As in the antibody screen, a positive test is indicated either by agglutination or hemolysis. Agglutination is characterized by RBC clumps seen either grossly or microscopically and is usually graded m+ (microscopic agglutination) to 4+. Hemolysis is identified by the presence of a pink supernatant.

Phases of testing

This refers to the conditions under which a test is run. For example, if serum/plasma is mixed with test RBCs and centrifuged at room temperature, this is said to be the immediate spin (IS) phase. Antibodies active at this phase are called "cold reacting." If this is preheated before performance, then it is the 37° phase, and antibodies detected in this phase are called "warm reacting." If serum and RBCs are mixed in the presence of AHG, then this is the indirect antiglobulin test (IAT). Warm reacting antibodies are usually IgG antibodies and are considered at least potentially clinically significant. Cold reacting antibodies are usually IgM and are likely to be clinically insignificant. Notable exceptions are ABO antibodies that are IgM but react over a broad thermal range and are, obviously, clinically significant, and the anti-P antibody of paroxysmal cold hemoglobinuria (PCH) is a clinically significant, cold reacting, IgG antibody. As a general rule of thumb, antibodies that are reactive at 37°C and/or reactive in the AHG phase are more likely to be clinically significant.

Direct antiglobulin test (DAT) & indirect antiglobulin test (IAT)

In the direct antiglobulin test f2.4, also known as the direct Coombs test, AHG is added to washed patient RBCs. If the RBCs therein are coated with IgG antibodies or complement in vivo, then there will be agglutination.

In the indirect antiglobulin test, also called the indirect Coombs test or antibody screen, antibodies that may be present in the patient's plasma are added to known reagent RBCs, followed by the addition of AHG. If the patient's sample contains an IgG antibody to an antigen present on the reagent RBCs, then there will be agglutination.

Thus, the DAT can be used to detect in vivo coating of RBCs with antibody, while the IAT is used to detect in vitro coating of reagent RBCs with antibodies. In the addition of AHG, one may select either polyspecific (contains both anti-IgG and anti-C3d) or monospecific (contains either anti-IgG or anti-C3d) anti-human globulins.

Clinical significance of detected antibodies

An antibody has "clinical significance" when it has the potential to cause hemolysis or hemolytic disease of the fetus or newborn. As a general rule of thumb, cold reacting IgM antibodies are usually clinically insignificant unless the antibody is high in concentration (titer >1,000) or reacts at temperatures close to 37°C. Warm reacting or AHG-reacting IgG antibodies are considered significant. Alloantibodies that are nearly always insignificant include: anti-Lewis, Lutheran, and I. Alloantibodies that are nearly always significant include Kell, Kidd, Rh, and Duffy.

How to interpret the routine panel f2.5, f2.6

Look at the autocontrol. When patient plasma is reactive with panel cells and is nonreactive with the autocontrol, then an alloantibody is present. When both the panel cells and autocontrol are positive, this may be due to autoantibody alone; however, an underlying alloantibody needs to be excluded especially in a patient with a transfusion or pregnancy history. (see section IV)

In the usual scenario where only a single antibody is present, one sees a few cells positive and some negative. For each cell with which the patient is nonreactive, cross out all the antigens for which that cell is positive. For example, if the recipient serum is nonreactive with cell #1, which expresses the C antigen, then anti-C specificity can be tentatively excluded. Usually this simple process will leave one antigen that fits best with the reactivity seen. In actual practice, reactivity with 3 positive cells and nonreactivity with 1 negative cell, preferably homozygous, is required to statistically establish a specific antibody.

If the reactivity is still not clear-cut, then consider the possibility of more than one antibody, a single antibody showing dosage, antibodies to high-incidence antigens, antibodies to low-incidence antigens, antibodies to reagents, or polyagglutination. In confusing cases, it may be helpful to phenotype the recipient blood cells. Antigens borne on recipient cells can be excluded as alloantibodies.

Once the alloantibody is identified, this should be noted in the transfusion record for future transfusions. The recipient should be antigen grouped, and he/she should be negative for this antigen. The crossmatch, because an alloantibody now exists, must be carried through the antiglobulin phase.

The nonroutine panel

Multiple antibodies are suspected when all or nearly all cells are positive but with differing strengths of reaction or at different phases. Various techniques can assist in clarifying the antibodies present, including the use of enzymes, adsorption, and neutralization.

	Rh-Hr					MNS				Lutheran		P	Lewis		Kell		Duffy		Kidd		Results		
	D	C	c	E	e	M	N	S	s	Lu^a	Lu^b	P1	Le^a	Le^b	K	k	Fy^a	Fy^b	Jk^a	Jk^b	IS	37°	AHG
1	0	+	0	0	+	+	+	0	+	0	+	+	+	0	0	+	+	0	+	+	0	0	2+
2	+	+	+	0	+	+	0	0	+	0	+	+	0	+	+	0	+	+	0	+	0	0	2+
3	+	+	0	0	+	0	+	+	0	+	0	0	+	0	0	+	+	+	+	+	0	0	2+
4	+	+	0	+	+	+	0	+	+	0	+	+	0	+	0	+	0	+	0	+	0	0	2+
5	+	0	+	+	0	+	0	0	+	0	+	+	0	+	0	+	+	+	+	0	0	0	0
6	0	0	+	0	+	+	0	+	0	0	+	+	0	+	0	+	0	+	+	0	0	0	0
7	0	0	+	0	+	0	+	+	0	+	+	0	0	+	0	+	0	+	+	0	0	0	0
8	0	0	+	0	+	0	+	0	+	+	0	+	+	0	+	0	+	0	0	+	0	0	0
9	0	0	+	0	+	+	+	+	0	0	+	+	0	+	0	+	0	+	+	0	0	0	0
10	0	0	+	0	+	+	0	0	0	0	+	0	0	0	0	+	0	+	+	+	0	0	0
Pt																					0	0	0

f2.5 Panel 1. The autocontrol is negative, suggesting that the reactions are due to alloantibody (not autoantibody). All the reactions are of similar strengths & at similar phases, suggesting that only one antibody is present. All antigens can be crossed out due to nonreactivity, except C. Even antigens known to show dosage (MNS, Kidd, C/c, E/e, & Duffy) can be excluded by nonreactivity with homozygous cells. The remaining specificity, C, fits perfectly with the observed reactions. Panel interpretation: anti-C

	Rh-Hr					MNS				Lutheran		P	Lewis		Kell		Duffy		Kidd		Results		
	D	C	c	E	e	M	N	S	s	Lu^a	Lu^b	P1	Le^a	Le^b	K	k	Fy^a	Fy^b	Jk^a	Jk^b	IS	37°	AHG
1	0	+	0	0	+	+	+	0	+	0	+	+	+	0	0	+	+	0	+	+	0	2+	2+
2	+	+	+	0	+	+	0	0	+	0	+	+	0	+	+	0	+	+	0	+	0	1+	1+
3	+	+	0	0	+	0	+	+	0	+	0	0	+	0	0	+	+	+	+	+	0	1+	1+
4	+	+	0	+	+	+	0	+	+	0	+	+	0	+	0	+	0	+	0	+	0	0	0
5	+	0	+	+	0	+	0	0	+	0	+	+	0	+	0	+	+	+	+	0	0	1+	1+
6	0	0	+	0	+	+	0	+	0	0	+	+	0	+	0	+	0	+	+	0	0	0	0
7	0	0	+	0	+	0	+	+	0	+	+	0	0	+	0	+	0	+	+	0	0	0	0
8	0	0	+	0	+	0	+	0	+	+	0	+	+	0	+	0	+	0	0	+	0	2+	2+
9	0	0	+	0	+	+	+	+	0	0	+	+	0	+	0	+	0	+	+	0	0	0	0
10	0	0	+	0	+	+	0	0	0	0	+	0	0	+	0	+	0	+	+	+	0	0	0
Pt																					0	0	0

f2.6 Panel 2. The autocontrol is negative, suggesting that the positive reactions are due to alloantibody. The observation that there are different strengths of reactivity clues us in to the possibility that there may be more than one antibody or there is one manifesting dosage, or both. After the process of crossing-out, only K & Fy^a remain. In this case the reactions match both anti-Fy^a (showing dosage) & anti-K. Panel interpretation: anti-Fy^a & anti-K.

Antibodies showing dosage should be suspected when

1. there is less reactivity with some cells, but the process of crossing-out has eliminated all specificities

2. there is variable strength of reactivity

Dosage means that an antibody's strength of binding is influenced by the number of antigens on the RBC surface. Thus, antibodies with dosage react more strongly with cells from individuals homozygous for an antigen. Looking at the phenotype of the test cells on f2.6 Panel 2, one notes that some of the cells are homozygous and some heterozygous; eg, cell #1 which is Fy^a positive and Fy^b negative is considered homozygous for Fy^a. Cell #2 is positive for Fy^a and Fy^b antigens and is therefore heterozygous. If anti-Fy^a were present, one might see reactivity with cell #1 and weaker or no reactivity with cell #2, even though both bear the antigen. Antigens that display dosage include MNS, Kidd, C/c, E/e, Duffy. The dosage phenomenon is a reason to routinely employ a slight alteration in the strategy for "crossing out" antigens. Fully cross out, nonreactive antigens that do not manifest dosage, while only crossing out nonreactive homozygous antigens that do display dosage. Place an "X" through dosage-manifesting antigens only if a homozygous cell is nonreactive. Only then can one confidently exclude MNS, Kidd, C/c, E/e, and Duffy.

Antibodies to high incidence antigens or high-titer, low avidity (HTLA) antibodies. An HTLA antibody is suspected when there is weak reactivity in the AHG phase to all cells in the antibody panel. The antibody continues to react at dilutions >1:64. HTLA antibodies are a group of antibodies which

1. are directed against high incidence antigens (present in >99.9% of population)

2. usually show weak reactivity to all cells in an antibody panel at the AHG phase

3. continue to react at high dilutions (high titer, usually >1:64)

The significance of HTLA antibodies is that they mask other alloantibodies. Some HTLA antibodies may be clinically significant themselves. These include Cartwright (Yt[a]), Holley (Hy), and Gregory (Gy). HTLA antibodies that are usually not clinically significant include: Chido/Rogers (Ch/Rg), Sd[a], Cs[a], Kn[a], McC[a] and York (Yk[a]).

Antibodies to test reagents are suspected when the auto-control is negative (because the reagents in question are in the diluent for the test cells) and there is across-the-board reactivity in the panel. The test cells can be washed to remove these substances. Another phase of testing or enhancement media may be required in these cases. This occurs most frequently with gel and solid phase systems; however, when testing is performed using the tube method, the panreactivity disappears. When lot numbers of reagent systems change this panreactivity may also disappear.

Antibodies to low-incidence antigens (Wr[a] and Kp[a]) may be suspected when only one test cell is reactive within a panel of test cells. Typically these antigens are not indicated on the panel, but the package insert for the test cells delineates a longer list of antigens for which the cell is positive or contact the manufacturer.

Polyagglutination

Adult sera contain naturally occurring IgM antibodies to T, Tn, Tk, and Cad. Some of these crypt antigens (T, Tn, and Tk) exist only when bacterial neuraminidase enzymatically alter RBC antigens by removing the sialic acid residues, a process known as T-activation. Bacteria such as *Streptococcus pneumoniae*, *Clostridia* species and influenza viruses are responsible for this activation in infants with necrotizing enterocolitis and pneumonia. All adult plasma contains some amount of naturally occurring anti-T antibodies and infants with activated T RBCs can develop intravascular hemolysis due to passive infusion of this antibody. Therefore, infants should receive RBCs with additive solutions containing minimal plasma or washed RBCs. This effect is transient and abates following resolution of the infection. Cad is a rare inherited antigen. The test for polyagglutination: polyagglutinable RBCs are agglutinated by adult but not cord serum.

Elution

An antibody may be removed or eluted from RBCs by several techniques such as freeze-thaw, heat, acid or digitonin elution. The eluate contains the concentrated antibody, and can then be tested against a panel of RBCs to determine its specificity. When a patient who has a positive DAT, for example, has been transfused in the past 3 months, the specificity of the presumed alloantibody can be determined in this fashion. When a patient who has not been transfused recently has a positive DAT, the presumed autoantibody usually is broadly reactive with all cells tested; however, some autoantibodies have narrow specificity which can be determined by performing a panel.

Autoadsorption

Autoadsorption is a useful technique when there are autoantibodies potentially masking underlying alloantibodies. The masking autoantibody can be adsorbed by using the patient's own (autologous) RBCs which are pretreated with ZZAP to remove bound autoantibody. ZZAP is a mixture of DTT and papain or ficin which can remove autoantibodies in one step. The sulfhydryl component makes the IgG molecules more susceptible to the proteolytic enzymes so the antibody dissociates from the cell. Adsorbed plasma or serum, which will contain any alloantibodies that were present, can then be tested against a panel of RBCs. Autoadsorption cannot be used if the patient has recently been transfused or pregnant in the past 3 months since they potentially have donor or fetal cells present in circulation.

Allogeneic adsorption

Allogeneic adsorption is used for patients who have been transfused within 3 months or pregnant patients with autoantibodies. RBCs are selected from 3 different donors who have different Rh phenotypes (R1R1, R2R2 and rr) and an extended phenotype is performed. The 3 donor RBCs are selected so that one donor is negative for each clinically significant antigen. Aliquots of the patient's plasma are incubated with each donor RBC to remove autoantibody and leave alloantibody within the adsorbed plasma if the adsorbing cell is negative for this antigen. If the adsorbing cell is positive for the antigen it will adsorb out both the autoantibody and alloantibody. The aliquots of adsorbed plasma are then reacted against panel cells to confirm the presence of an underlying alloantibody. For example, if the plasma is adsorbed with an E negative allogenic cell and the adsorbed plasma reacts with panel cells that are E positive, then you can infer the presence of an alloanti-E is present.

Hemagglutination inhibition (neutralizing substances)

Hemagglutination inhibition is a term that refers to the use of a substance [12,14] that is known to contain or mimic a particular antigen. If a serum sample is thought to contain an antibody with specificity for this antigen, this suspicion can be confirmed by the abolition of (neutralization of) reactivity. Alternatively, neutralization of a particular antibody can assist in detecting additional antibodies that may be masked. Hemagglutination inhibition is also used to determine the secretor status (by detecting H substance in saliva).

Lectins

Lectins t2.14 are reagents derived from plants that will bind to specific antigens on RBCs and agglutinate them (causing hemagglutination). 2 lectins that are commonly used to resolve ABO discrepancies include *Ulex europaeus* to detect the H antigen and *Dolichos biflorus* to detect A1 antigen.

t2.14 Neutralizing substances & lectins

Neutralizing substance	Antigenic activity
Guinea pig urine	Sda
Hydatid cyst fluid	P1
Saliva	H, Le^a
Breast milk	I
Pigeon eggs	P1
Plasma	Chido, Rodgers

Lectin	Binds to
Dolichos biflorus	A1 (used to distinguish A1 phenotype from A subgroups)
Bandeiraea simplicifolia	B
Ulex europaeus	H (agglutinates group O erythrocytes); useful in determination of secretor status
Lotus tetragonolobus	H
Arachis hypogaea	T
Vicea graminea	N

Enzymes

Proteolytic enzymes such as ficin, papain, and trypsin, when added to serologic tests, act to enhance the antigenicity of some antigens, while suppressing the antigenicity of others. Antigens enhanced by enzymes: AB, Le, I/i, P, Rh, Kidd. Some Kidd antibodies can only be detected following enzyme enhancement. Antigens destroyed by enzymes: MNS, Fy^a, Fy^b, Lutheran, Chido, Rodgers, and Yt^a. Antigens unaffected by enzymes: most remaining antigens, notably Kell.

Recipient phenotype

The recipient RBC phenotype for the antigen in question should be determined. The recipient should lack the antigen corresponding to the suspected alloantibody. Recently transfused patients may be difficult to phenotype.

Recipient genotype

Enough is known about the molecular basis of RBC antigen expression and about genotype-phenotype relationships, that prediction of phenotype from genotype is now possible. Furthermore, most alleles in the major blood groups are the result of single nucleotide polymorphisms (SNPs), which lend themselves to differential hybridization of PCR-amplified SNP-flanking regions. While the widespread application of genotyping to blood bank testing is a possibility, currently it is most commonly available at donor centers and reference labs. Genotyping can be helpful in patients with the following clinical situations: autoantibodies, multiple alloantibodies, confusing or conflicting serologic results, transfusion dependent patients such as those with sickle cell anemia, hemolytic transfusion reactions (HTRs) and pregnant women with alloantibodies. Molecular assays can be applied to material obtained from chorionic villus sampling, amniocentesis, or free fetal DNA in maternal plasma, to determine the genotype of the fetus.

Likelihood of finding compatible blood

When blood is needed for a patient with an alloantibody, the likelihood of finding blood is equal to the likelihood of antigen-negative blood in the population. The likelihood of antigen-negative blood is equal to 100-antigen frequency. So, for example, if the patient has an anti-Jk^a t2.15, then the likelihood of finding an antigen-negative unit is 100 minus 75% or ~25%. This has some practical relevance, as it guides the laboratorian in deciding how many units to pull from the shelf in order to attempt to find a crossmatch compatible unit. In this case, to find one antigen negative unit, one should test 4 units.

When blood is needed for a patient with 2 or more alloantibodies, the calculation is similar; except the frequencies of antigen-negatives are multiplied. For example, if the patient has anti-Jk^a (frequency of antigen negative = 100–75% = 25%) and anti-E (frequency of antigen negative = 100–70% = 30%), then the frequency of Jk^a and E-negative blood is 0.25 × 0.3 = 0.075 × 100 = 7.5%. So 1/7.5 × 100 = 13; ~13 units will have to be crossmatched to find one compatible.

t2.15 Approximate frequency of antigens in US donor population

Antigen	Frequency
D	85%
C	70%
c	80%
Cw	2%
E	30%
e	98%
G(CD)	84%
f(ce)	65%
V	1%
K	10%
k	98%
Kpa	2%
Jk^{a*}	75%
Jk^{b*}	75%
Js^a	0.1% whites, 20% blacks
Fy^{a†}	65% in whites, 10% in blacks
Fy^{b†}	83% in whites, 20% in blacks
M	80%
N	72%
S	55%
s	90%
U	99.9% whites, 99% blacks
P1	80%

*Jk(a−b−) rare, except in Pacific Islanders
†Fy(a−b−) rare in whites, 68% in blacks

The positive crossmatch

An incompatible crossmatch mandates a halt to the process. If the antibody screen was negative and the crossmatch reaction is strong (4+) at immediate spin, then ABO incompatibility should be suspected. ABO testing of recipient and donor should be repeated. If the antibody screen was negative and weaker reactions occur, then consider anti-A1 in a blood group A or AB recipient. Other possibilities include passively acquired ABO antibodies from prior transfusion of plasma containing products (eg, group O platelets). Lastly, an expanded panel may be considered to detect alloantibodies to low incidence antigens.

If the antibody screen was positive, then the most likely explanation is that antigen positive blood has been selected. Other possibilities include autoantibody and antibodies to test reagents.

Illustrative nonroutine cases t2.16, t2.17

t2.16 Unusual findings in forward & reverse grouping

Case	Forward grouping			Reverse grouping			Antibody screen
	Anti-A	Anti-B	Anti-RH	A cells	B cells	D+ cells	All cells
1	0	0	4+	4+	4+	1-2+	Negative
2	1-2+	4+	0	4+	0	0	Negative
3	4+	1-2+	0	0	4+	0	Negative
4	4+	4+	0	1-2+	0	0	Negative
5	0	0	0	4+	4+	0	4+

Case 1 t2.16 illustrates an O+ patient with apparent anti-D antibody. This may have one of several explanations. The first is autoantibody in warm autoimmune hemolytic anemia (WAIHA). When WAIHA autoantibodies demonstrate specificity, the most common is anti-Rh. Another explanation is the alloantibody anti-LW. The LW antigen is expressed more strongly on D+ cells than D–. If anti-LW antibodies are present, they may appear to be reacting with only D+ cells, thus simulating anti-D antibodies. Lastly, a patient with partial D may have these findings. Such individuals lack epitopes of the D antigen and therefore develop antibodies to the D antigen after exposure during transfusion or pregnancy.

Case 2 t2.16 is a group B individual manifesting the B(A) phenotype. Certain blood group B individuals have such high levels of glucosyltransferase that a small amount of A antigen is produced, and their RBCs react weakly with anti-A reagent. These patients have a β glycosyltransferase with an increased ability to use UDP-N-acetyl galactosamine and UDP-galactose that causes production of A antigen in small amounts.

Case 3 t2.16 shows a group A patient with acquired B phenotype. In acquired B phenotype, the RBCs of a blood group A individual acquire reactivity with anti-B reagent and thus group as AB, despite having serum anti-B antibodies. This phenomenon occurs in A1 individuals when the A1 antigen is acted upon by bacterial deacetylases which will deacetylate the A antigen (N-acetyl-galactosamine) to the B antigen (galactose). Thus, the acquired B phenotype is associated with conditions that give rise to transient or persistent bacteremia such as colon cancer, colonic obstruction, and Gram– sepsis. Due to the presence of anti-B in serum, this can also result in a positive DAT. To confirm acquired B, several avenues are available. A different manufacturer's monoclonal anti-B typing reagent can simply be used to resolve this discrepancy. The altered A1 antigen with B antigenic activity can be re-acetylated in vitro with acetic anhydride. Further, the patient's own anti-B will agglutinate these RBCs. Acidified human anti-B does not react with acquired B antigen. If the patient is a secretor, their saliva will not contain the B antigen.

Case 4 t2.16 illustrates a group AB patient who has anti-A1 antibodies. This is commonly identified in individuals with A2B blood group. Approximately 1-8% of A2 patients will have anti-A1 antibodies and 22-35% of A2B individuals have anti-A1 antibody. Anti-A1 is usually a clinically insignificant

IgM antibody reacting at room temperature or below; compatible blood can be found with a prewarmed crossmatch. Any anti-A1 antibodies reacting at 37°C are clinically significant and patients should receive O or A2 compatible blood.

Case 5 t2.16 shows the Bombay phenotype. These patients have anti-H in their plasma and therefore react with all group O screening cells.

t2.17 Unusual findings in antibody screen and/or panel

Case	Finding
6	All cells in panel & autocontrol positive at AHG only
7	All cells in panel, except autocontrol, positive at AHG only, weak (1+ to 2+)
8	All cells in panel & autocontrol positive at IS only
9	All cells in panel & autocontrol positive at IS & 37°C, not at AHG
10	Antibody screen negative, but transfusion records show previous alloantibody

Case 6 t2.17 describes the typical reaction pattern of a warm autoantibody. Warm autoantibodies may also be positive at 37° phase. An adsorption technique may succeed in removing these antibodies, permitting further testing.

Case 7 t2.17 is the typical pattern of a high-titer, low avidity antibody to a frequently occurring antigen (eg, Chido, Rodgers). These can often be neutralized with serum.

Case 8 t2.17 shows the usual reaction pattern of a cold autoantibody. If the antibody has broad thermal amplitude, it may also be positive in the 37° phase. Since usually these are IgM antibodies, they are not reactive at AHG (IAT) phase. A prewarmed antibody screen and prewarmed crossmatch may be used so these clinically insignificant antibodies do not interfere with pretransfusion testing.

Case 9 t2.17 describes the way an antibody to enhancement media or other reagents, such as LISS, PEG, gel or solid phase media, may react.

Case 10 t2.17 describes a common scenario in which a previously identified alloantibody is not detected in the present screen. This is the result of reduced titer of alloantibody below the level of detection of the antibody screen; the alloantibody remains clinically significant, however. In such cases, antigen-negative units should be selected, and the crossmatch must be carried through the antiglobulin phase. Moreover, if the current screen does detect alloantibody and transfusion records show a previously identified antibody, then a modified antibody panel can be utilized, one that consists entirely of cells that are negative for antigen corresponding to the known alloantibody. This way, only newly formed alloantibodies will be detected. One must still select antigen negative blood, and the crossmatch must still be carried through the antiglobulin phase.

Other unusual findings

In patients with hematolymphoid neoplasms, there is often weakened expression of A or B antigens with mixed-field agglutination.

In patients with gastric adenocarcinoma, excess free A or B antigens may be present in the serum. This may have the effect in vitro of binding anti-A or anti-B reagents thereby neutralizing them and thus giving the false impression that the patient has group O RBCs.

Autoantibodies, a common cause of nonroutine findings
When to consider autoantibody

Autoantibodies are suspected in one of several scenarios:

1. when there is unexplained anemia with a reticulocytosis or microspherocytosis

2. when there is a positive DAT

3. when there is a positive autocontrol in antibody panel (a positive autocontrol should prompt a DAT to ensure that the reaction is immune mediated)

A+ DAT is very common, affecting ~1% of outpatients and up to 15% of hospitalized patients. If the laboratory's standard DAT uses a polyspecific reagent (C3 and IgG), then a positive DAT should be followed by incubation with specific anti-IgG and anti-C3 antisera, called monospecific DAT. This may result in one of 3 findings

1. a DAT reactive only with anti-IgG

2. a DAT reactive with both anti-IgG and anti-C3

3. a DAT reactive only with anti-C3

The first 2 results are consistent with the presence of a warm autoantibody. The last result is consistent with the presence of a cold autoantibody, in which IgM has activated and fixed complement to the RBC membrane, since IgM is not detectable by DAT reagents. A+ DAT on cord blood is most likely the result of maternal alloantibody, but passively acquired antibody from RhIg is also a possibility. Lastly, a positive DAT could be examined microscopically to determine whether there are clumped and unclumped cells (a so-called "mixed-field" pattern); this finding may be caused by recently transfused blood, wherein the clumped RBCs are presumably the allogeneic RBCs. An elution should be performed for all positive IgG DAT results.

Whenever an autoantibody is suspected, several questions should be considered. First, is the patient hemolyzing? If there is evidence of hemolysis (elevated lactate dehydogenase [LD], depressed haptoglobin, elevated bilirubin, or anemia) with a positive IgG DAT, then the patient most likely has WAIHA. If there is no hemolysis, then the main significance of these antibodies has to do with their potential to complicate pretransfusion testing. Second, is there an obvious explanation, such as a history of recent transfusion? This may be the cause of the positive DAT or autocontrol. Typically this gives a mixed-field reaction. The patient may be experiencing a delayed serologic or delayed hemolytic transfusion reaction. If the antibody responsible is not detectable in the serum it may be coating the transfused RBCs and an elution may be needed to characterize the antibody. What drugs is the patient taking? Drugs classically associated with a positive DAT (see below) are penicillin, cephalosporins, procainamide, and methyldopa (Aldomet). Other uncommon causes of a positive DAT include patients who have received ABO incompatible bone marrow transplants and patients receiving antithymocyte globulin (ATG) after solid organ transplants. If all these have been excluded, then one of the primary autoimmune conditions described below must be considered.

Warm reacting autoantibodies

Warm reacting antibodies react optimally at 37°C. Typically, they react with the patient's own RBCs (produce a positive autocontrol/DAT) and are pan-reactive with all cells tested in the screen, panel, and crossmatch. Warm reacting antibodies are usually IgG, uncommonly IgA or IgM. The AHG phase is positive with polyspecific antisera and monospecific anti-IgG antisera. In some cases (30-50%), anti-C3 is also positive. The presence and strength of C3 correlates with the likelihood of hemolysis. RBC autoantibodies may demonstrate anti-Rh specificity.

The significance of warm reacting antibodies reside, first, in their capacity to cause WAIHA, the most common type of autoimmune hemolytic anemia. However, not all warm reacting antibodies cause hemolysis; in fact, most do not. The other major significance of warm reacting antibodies is their potential to interfere with pretransfusion testing. Transfusions are best avoided, if possible, as there is a greater than usual risk of transfusion related complications in these patients, and transfusion may exacerbate the underlying hemolytic anemia. When transfusion is required, the major challenge is to identify underlying alloantibodies. This may require an autoadsorption procedure (to clear the autoantibody from the serum) followed by an antibody screen using the adsorbed serum/plasma to detect underlying alloantibodies. Autoadsorption usually is performed using the patient's (autologous) RBCs, after pretreatment with ZZAP, at 37°C (warm autoadsorption). Autoadsorption is performed only on patients who have not been transfused within the last 3 months. If the patient has been recently transfused, an alloadsorption may be attempted using cells of known phenotypes.

Cold reacting autoantibodies

Benign cold agglutinins are the most commonly encountered autoantibodies Benign cold agglutinins react most strongly at 4°C, but they have variably wide thermal amplitudes and may react up to 22°C. They usually do not interfere with routine tests, but they may do so when they react at or near room temperature, making CBCs unreliable. The only reliable CBC index in the presence of cold agglutinins is the hemoglobin. The titer of benign cold agglutinins is usually <64 at 4°C. Most are IgM and can activate complement in vitro, thus reactions may be seen at the AHG phase using polyspecific antisera. If monospecific reagents are used, the cells are agglutinated by anti-C3d but not anti-IgG. The antibody specificity of benign cold agglutinins is most commonly anti-I. The I antigen is strongly expressed on virtually all adult RBCs but only weakly on cord RBCs. Adult levels are reached at around 2 years of age. The less common anti-i reacts with cord blood but not with adult blood. Anti-H reacts best with group O and A2 RBCs, because they have the most H substance. A1 RBCs have the least H substance and react weakly. It is important not to confuse this with the anti-H in Oh (Bombay) individuals that is a potent alloantibody reacting at 4-37°C and causing severe, life threatening, hemolysis.

Pathologic cold agglutinins are reactive over a broad thermal range, up to 32-37°C, and cause spontaneous autoagglutination in anticoagulated blood at room temperature. As with benign cold agglutinins, CBCs may be unreliable. The DAT is 2+ to 3+ with polyspecific reagent, positive with monospecific anti-C3d, but negative with monospecific anti-IgG. The titer is often >1,000 when tested at 4°C. There are several types of pathologic cold agglutinins, based upon clinical features. *Idiopathic cold autoimmune hemolytic anemia* (CAIHA) or *cold agglutinin syndrome* (CAS) is a chronic idiopathic condition found predominantly in older individuals complaining of acrocyanosis and Raynaud phenomenon with a moderate hemolytic anemia. The responsible antibody is almost always an IgM with anti-I, anti-i, or rarely anti-Pr specificity, which is often monoclonal. The antibody causes agglutination in the extremities and fixing of complement, leading to intravascular hemolysis. *Secondary CAIHA* is a transient cold agglutinin, IgM anti-I, is seen in 50% of patients with *M pneumonia* infection. This usually resolves within 2-3 weeks. A more persistent anti-I may be associated with lymphoproliferative disorders. Some of these are clinically significant. Epstein-Barr viral infection less frequently causes the emergence of IgM anti-i.

Mixed type autoantibodies

As the name implies, these patients have both cold reacting IgM and warm reacting IgG autoantibodies. Most often, they show reactions with both IgG and C3 at the AHG phase. No particular antigen specificity has been consistently shown. Clinically, these patients present with an acute-onset hemolytic anemia, usually idiopathic or associated with lupus. It is markedly responsive to corticosteroid therapy, a fact that may help to avoid transfusion.

Paroxysmal cold hemoglobinuria (PCH)

The least common type of AIHA, PCH is responsible for ~1-2% of cases. It most commonly affects children with bacterial infections (otitis media) or viral infection (upper respiratory viral infections, measles, mumps, chickenpox, and infectious mononucleosis). PCH was originally described in patients with congenital or tertiary syphilis. It presents with paroxysmal episodes of hemoglobinuria provoked by cold exposure. These attacks are characterized by sudden fever, chills, abdominal and back pain, hemoglobinuria, and jaundice. The resultant anemia is usually severe (eg, Hgb<5 g/dL). Treatment consists of keeping the patient warm and transfusions as necessary.

The responsible antibody is an IgG biphasic hemolysin with anti-P specificity (Donath-Landsteiner antibody). It is called a biphasic hemolysin because of its capacity to produce hemolysis only when incubated at 2 different temperatures in vitro. Like CAIHA, the DAT is positive with polyspecific AHG, negative with anti-IgG, and positive with anti-C3. To confirm the diagnosis, the Donath-Landsteiner (DL) test is performed. The direct DL test may be performed on adults using 2 vials of blood at 2 different temperatures: 4°C and 37°C. A positive test is obtained if only incubation of the patient's RBCs at 4° then 37° leads to hemolysis. The indirect DL test uses patient plasma with reagent RBCs. Series of tubes are incubated at 90 minutes at 0°C, 37°C and one set is incubated for 30 minutes at 0°C and transferred to 37°C for 60 minutes. If positive for the DL antibody, hemolysis should be observed only in the set of tubes incubated at 0° then transferred to 37°C.

Blood banking considerations with a cold autoantibody

The first objective is to determine whether the autoantibody is pathologic, based on its titer and thermal amplitude. Most pathologic examples have high titer (>1,000) and react over a broad temperature range, including temperatures >30°C. The second is to find a way to carry out the search for alloantibodies in spite of the cold autoantibody. The first and most straightforward way to do this is to keep blood at 37°C and perform all tests at 37°C (prewarmed antibody screen and panel). Second, the use of monospecific anti-IgG AHG reagent will allow circumvention of the often C3-only positivity of the cold antibody. Lastly, the cold autoantibody can be adsorbed in the cold by autologous RBCs.

Drugs may induce a positive DAT by several mechanisms

The *drug adsorption (hapten) mechanism* refers to the noncovalent coating of RBCs with drug to which the patient has antibodies, leading to coating of the RBC with antibody. Penicillin is the prototypic agent. 3% of patients on penicillin develop a positive DAT; 5% of those with a positive DAT experience hemolysis. The effect is dose-dependent. The drug becomes adsorbed to the RBC membrane and the RBC subsequently becomes coated with antipenicillin antibodies. RBCs are destroyed *extravascularly* since they are coated with antibodies. Lab confirmation involves demonstrating that the serum and eluate react with drug-treated RBCs but not with untreated RBCs.

In the *drug dependent antibody mechanism*, the drug becomes adsorbed to the RBC membrane and subsequently becomes coated, with antibody and complement. Complement is activated to cause *intravascular* hemolysis. This only takes a small dose to initiate this reaction and upon re-exposure brisk hemolytic reactions can be seen. Piperacillin and other second and third generation cephalosporins are the prototype. Lab confirmation involves demonstrating a positive DAT, with C3 and possibly IgG, and that the drug must be present in the specimen to demonstrate the reactive antibody. The patient experiences intravascular hemolysis with hemoglobinemia and hemoglobinuria. Renal failure commonly occurs in these patients.

The *autoimmune induction mechanism* implies that the drug induces RBC auto-immunity that persists after withdrawal of the agent (drug independent); though drug withdrawal is often associated with abatement over time. Methyldopa, levodopa, procainamide, fludarabine, second and third generation cephalosporins are typical causes. In this mechanism, the drug stimulates formation of an autoantibody directed against an innate component of the RBC membrane. In the laboratory, an autoantibody is detected that is indistinguishable from those that cause idiopathic warm autoimmune hemolytic anemia. The antibody screen and panels are panreactive, DAT IgG is positive and the eluate is panreactive. When the drug is withdrawn, hemolysis gradually improves. If the drug is reintroduced, the hemolysis recurs.

The *nonimmune protein adsorption mechanism* refers to drug induced nonspecific, nonimmune, binding of immunoglobulin to the RBC surface. Cephalothin (Keflin) is the prototype. Other medications that are capable of causing this reaction include piperacillin, tazobactam sodium, cisplatin, and amoxicillin. These medications cause the nonspecific adsorption of albumin, IgG, IgA, IgM and complement onto the RBC membrane. There is no antibody production that occurs. Antibody screens and DATs are positive, but eluates are negative even when drug coated RBCs are used.

Transfusion in special clinical circumstances

Transfusion in SCD

While in most respects transfusion in sickle cell disease (SCD) does not differ from transfusion in other circumstances, there are some unique considerations. First, multiple transfusions pose a risk of iron overload and alloimmunization. Second, in both emergency and elective transfusion, exchange vs simple transfusion should be considered in SCD patients since this lessens the risk of iron overload, hyperviscosity, and volume overload. Lastly, whereas transfusion in ordinary circumstances is aimed at achieving a certain hemoglobin level, the end-point in SCD is a certain proportion of HbS, usually <30%.

Strong indications for emergency transfusion in SCD include stroke, retinal artery occlusion, splenic sequestration crisis, acute chest syndrome, and aplastic crisis. Some advocate emergency transfusion for priapism and severe acute pain crises. Priapism is treated initially with supportive therapy consisting of hydration with intravenous fluids, pain control, and consultation with a urologist. When priapism does not resolve within 48 hours, simple or exchange transfusion may be considered, although there are no studies comparing simple vs exchange transfusion therapy, an adverse reaction after exchange transfusion has been associated with a syndrome of neurologic changes known as ASPEN syndrome (*a*ssociation of *S*CD, *p*riapism, *e*xchange transfusion, and *n*eurologic events). This syndrome presents as headache, seizures, altered mental status, and/or hemiparesis within 11 days of exchange transfusion.

Elective chronic transfusion is indicated in children with abnormal blood flow velocities detected by transcranial Dopplers (TCD) for stroke prevention, for patients with progressive renal or cardiopulmonary disease, and for complicated pregnancies. With regard to stroke prevention, ~3.75% of SCD patients will experience one or more strokes over their lifetime. For practical purposes, 70% of children who have suffered a first stroke will have a recurrent stroke within 2-3 years. Most frequently, stroke is caused by occlusion of the internal carotid or middle cerebral arteries. High velocity blood flow caused by these blockages can be detected by TCDs and therefore screening SCD children with TCD can identify children at high risk. The STOP trial demonstrated that starting chronic simple or exchange transfusions in children with high risk TCD helped reduce strokes by 91%.

Some practitioners, though, liberally apply exchange transfusion to all SCD patients. The desired endpoint after exchange transfusion is for a HbS concentration <30%. With regard to pregnancy, there is no convincing evidence at this time of a benefit to prophylactic transfusion in uncomplicated pregnancies. In surgical patients, it is recommended that patients be transfused to a target hemoglobin of 10 g/dL prior to surgery. One study compared exchange vs simple transfusion prior to surgery and found that preoperative exchange transfusion is unnecessary.

Alloimmunization rates in multiply transfused SCD patients receiving nonphenotypically matched blood are between 19-47%. The most common alloantibodies are anti-K, C, E, Fy[a] and Jk[b]. In large centers where it is possible to transfuse SCD patients with donor blood matched for Cc, D, Ee, and Kell antigens, the alloimmunization rate/unit transfused can be reduced from 3% to 0.5%.

With improved donor screening and testing, the risk of transfusion transmitted infection is low, and the risk of iron overload is ameliorated somewhat with exchange transfusion and improved oral chelation therapy, which has increased compliance and resulted in more continuous chelation.

Shock: fluid resuscitation, emergency release & massive transfusion

Shock

Shock caused by hemorrhage may require treatment with fluid resuscitation, emergency release of blood, and/or massive transfusion. Acute blood loss is categorized clinically into 4 classes t2.18.

t2.18 **Classes of acute hemorrhage**	
Class I hemorrhage	Loss of <15% of blood volume (<750 cc), usually asymptomatic or manifests as mild tachycardia
Class II hemorrhage	Loss of 15-30% of blood volume (750-1,500 cc) may manifest as tachycardia, tachypnea, anxiety & clammy skin In most cases, only fluid resuscitation is required, depending upon the underlying health of the patient
Class III hemorrhage	Loss of 30-40% of blood volume (1,500-2,000 cc), may manifest as hypotension, tachycardia, tachypnea, pallor & alteration in mental status Transfusion is usually necessary, depending upon the response to fluid resuscitation
Class IV hemorrhage	Loss of >40% of blood volume (>2,000 cc), results in severe manifestations of shock, including thready pulse & the risk of imminent death Fluid resuscitation is the first priority, but transfusion will be necessary

Fluid resuscitation

A principle of resuscitation is the priority of fluid resuscitation. Fluid resuscitation with crystalloids should precede transfusion of blood products, a fact that gives the blood bank time to prepare in the properly orchestrated resuscitation. A rule of thumb states that transfusion of RBCs should be initiated once administered fluids exceed 30 mL/kg of body weight (around 2 L). Resuscitation fluids for volume expansion do not carry oxygen, of course, but their role in maintaining blood volume and blood pressure assists in delivery of RBCs to target tissue. The term crystalloid refers to asanguineous aqueous solutions of inorganic ions and small organic molecules. These usually include NaCl and/or glucose and may be isotonic, hypotonic or hypertonic. Colloids may be human derived or synthetic and include albumins, gelatins, dextrans, or hydroxyethyl starch (HES). These may be presented dissolved in a crystalloid solution, most commonly normal saline. The various fluids differ in the degree to which they expand intravascular volume and the duration of this expansion. ~20% of crystalloids will remain within the intravascular space, for example, 1 L infusion of normal saline will expand intravascular volume by ~250-350 mL, the other 650-750 mL contributing to tissue and pulmonary edema. The attractive feature of colloid solutions is that they persist in the intravascular space for ~24 hours and their lesser tendency to produce tissue edema; however, the exact duration of intravascular retention is a function of

1. the rate of colloid molecule metabolism

2. the integrity of the endothelium, which may be compromised due to vascular injury, sepsis and other conditions

All fluids have some capacity to impair hemostasis, at least through hemodilution, with many having direct effects upon clotting factors as well. Furthermore, all colloidal solutions have been associated with a small risk of anaphylactic or anaphylactoid reactions. Controversy over the best type of resuscitation fluid to use and in particular over the issue of colloid vs crystalloid permeates the medical literature. Crystalloids are favored for their relative safety—low risk of hemostatic anomalies, adverse drug reactions, and intravascular fluid overload. Nevertheless, controlled clinical trials have not shown a benefit of one over the other.

Emergency release

Emergency release of RBC products, implying that transfusion is required immediately to prevent patient mortality, involves the release of blood without completion of recipient blood typing or testing. There are differing levels of immediacy, though, and in general routine practices should be followed when possible.

When possible (ie, a 45 minute delay is acceptable), recipient blood should be grouped and screened, with ABO/Rh-matched and crossmatch compatible blood released. Note that 2% of recipients harbor alloantibodies which may delay matched blood by much longer.

When greater urgency exists (blood needed now), uncrossmatched O– blood can be released to females of childbearing years. Rh+ blood can be released to males and older females. The practice of releasing ABO/Rh-compatible blood with ABO/Rh testing only, omitting the crossmatch, is discouraged in routine settings. The practice of releasing ABO/Rh-compatible blood based solely upon historical ABO/Rh typing should be strictly forbidden.

Whenever emergency release is undertaken, the treating physician must sign within 24 hours, a statement indicating that he/she is aware of the nature of the blood released; ie, that it has not been fully tested for compatibility. This is not required prior to release of blood. The blood product label must indicate that compatibility testing was not completed. In some cases, due to inventory considerations, the patient whose blood group is known must be given ABO-Rh compatible but uncrossmatched blood. This switch requires medical director approval.

When Rh+ blood products must be given to an Rh– recipient, Rh immune globulin (Ig) should be considered to prevent Rh immunization in women of childbearing potential t2.19. When a patient who requires emergency release RBCs has a known anti-E or anti-C antibody, then Rh– blood should be given. Most Rh– blood is from patients with ce/ce genotype. When a patient who requires emergency release RBCs with

a known anti-c and is Rh+, then Rh+ blood should be given, because of the lower likelihood of c expression.

t2.19 **Principles of Rh immune globulin administration for Rh-incompatible blood products**
RhIg should be given within 72 hours of transfusion
IV RhIg dosage: 90 IU/1 mL of transfused Rh+ RBCs or/2 mL of transfused whole blood
Administer entire dose of IV RhIg into suitable vein >3-5 minutes; if dilution is preferred prior to IV administration use only normal saline as diluent
IV RhIg is discouraged for transfusion of a quantity of Rh+ blood that exceeds 20% of blood volume, as this may cause severe hemolysis

Massive transfusion

Definitions of massive transfusion vary, including when

1. the patient is transfused total blood volume (10-15 units of RBCs in a 70 kg patient)

2. half of the patient's blood volume is replaced within 3 hours

3. >4 units of RBCs are transfused within 4 hours with continued bleeding

The point of defining massive transfusion is that certain potential complications attend transfusion of a large volume of blood.

1. Transfused blood does not immediately have the oxygen-carrying capacity of innate blood, because of depletion of 2,3-DPG and ATP. This results in a shift of the oxygen dissociation curve to the left (impaired release of oxygen from hemoglobin).

2. Transfusing massive amounts of blood may lower pH and raise potassium, lower the body temperature and raise the free hemoglobin.

3. There is the potential for developing coagulopathy due to coagulation factor and platelet consumption, dysfunction, or dilution.

Preparation of RBCs involves the removal of most plasma and platelets, and whatever plasma is present in stored blood is rapidly depleted of multiple coagulation factors (especially the labile factors V and VIII). Patients experiencing massive hemorrhage are rapidly consuming coagulation factors and platelets, are transfused with asanguineous fluids and blood components that lack coagulation factors or platelets and develop hypothermia or acidosis from massive bleeding causing platelet or coagulation factor dysfunction, all of which contribute to coagulopathy.

Massive transfusion protocols (MTPs) have been implemented in trauma centers to prevent the development of coagulopathies which increases the rate of mortality from 40-75% in the setting of massive transfusion. MTPs use predetermined ratios of RBC, plasma and platelets for transfusion to prevent development of coagulopathies. Although there is no consensus on the optimal ratio, some ratios that are utilized include 1:1:1, 1:2:1, or 1:3:1 of RBCs, plasma and random donor platelets units.

Therapeutic apheresis

Definition

Apheresis means that whole blood is removed from the patient, a component of the blood is separated, and the remainder of the blood is returned to the patient along with a replacement fluid. For example, erythrocytapheresis implies removal of RBC with return of the patient's plasma and a replacement fluid consisting of donor RBC. In plasmapheresis the patient's plasma is removed with the return of the patient's RBC with replacement fluid of either albumin or donor plasma.

Indications

The American Society for Apheresis has established category indications for therapeutic apheresis and cytapheresis in clinical conditions based on evidence reported in the literature t2.20, t2.21.

Replacement fluid

3 replacement fluids may be used in therapeutic apheresis: Normal (0.9%) saline, 5% albumin, and allogeneic plasma (eg, FFP or cryo-poor FFP). Sometimes these are used in combination. Albumin has the advantage over saline of returning serum osmolytes. In TTP, it is necessary to use plasma as replacement fluid, as this provides both normal von Willebrand factor (vWF) multimers and the protease ADAMTS-13. Saline or a mix of saline and albumin may be used in hyperviscosity syndromes.

Vascular access

A large bore stiff walled dialysis type catheter is required for apheresis. For patients who will require frequent apheresis over a short period of time a central line, usually placed into the internal jugular vein, is desirable.

Medication interactions

It is important to note that some medications may be removed by apheresis, especially those with high protein binding, >80%, and low volume of distribution (V_d) properties, V_d <0.2 L/kg. Dosing immediately after apheresis should be considered for such medications. Furthermore, ACE inhibitors (eg, captopril, lisinophril, ramipril) should be discontinued for the 24 hours preceding apheresis, since they pose a significant risk of severe hypotension during apheresis.

t2.20 Cytapheresis with category indications

Marked leukocytosis with leukostasis (cytapheresis)	Category I
SCD, acute stroke	Category I
SCD, acute chest, stroke prophylaxis or prevention of iron overload	Category II
Thrombocytosis, symptomatic	Category II

t2.21 Categorical indications for apheresis

Category	Definition	Indications
Category I	Apheresis is standard & acceptable as a primary therapy or first-line adjunct therapy. This designation does not imply that apheresis is mandatory in all cases	Acute inflammatory demyelinating polyneuropathy (Guillain-Barré syndrome). Antineutrophil cytoplasmic antibodies (ANCA)-associated rapidly progressive glomerulonephritis. Antiglomular basement membrane disease (Goodpasture syndrome). Chronic inflammatory demyelinating polyneuropathy (CIDP). Cryoglobulinemia: severe or symptomatic. Focal segmental glomerulosclerosis, recurrent. Hyperviscosity due to monoclonal gammopathies (best results when hyperviscosity is caused by IgM paraprotein). Myasthenia gravis (apheresis generally reserved for severe exacerbations with respiratory difficulty; apheresis may significantly reduce pyridostigmine, causing paradoxical respiratory depression following treatment). Paraproteinemic polyneuropathies. Pediatric autoimmune neuropsychiatric disorders associated with streptococcal infections (PANDAS) & Sydenham chorea. Renal transplantation, antibody mediated rejection. Thrombotic thrombocytopenic purpura (TTP)
Category II	Apheresis is generally accepted but considered to be supportive or adjunctive to other, more definitive treatments, rather than a primary first-line therapy	Renal transplantation: HLA densensitization or ABO incompatible transplant. Catastrophic antiphospholipid syndrome. Chronic focal encephalitis (Rasmussen encephalitis). Multiple sclerosis: acute CNS inflammatory demyelinating disease refractory to steroids. Mushroom poisoning. Phytanic acid storage disease (Refsum disease). Neuromyelitis optica (Devic syndrome). Systemic lupus erythematosus: cerebritis, diffuse alveolar hemorrhage
Category III	Apheresis may be beneficial; however, there is insufficient evidence to establish the efficacy or to clarify the risk or benefit	Heart transplantation antibody mediated rejection. Acute hepatic failure. Posttransfusion purpura. Multiple sclerosis, chronic progressive
Category IV	Controlled trials have not shown benefit, or anecdotal reports have been discouraging. Apheresis for these disorders should be carried out only in the context of an Institutional Review Board (IRB) approved research protocol, if at all	Immune thrombocytopenia purpura. Diarrhea-associated hemolytic uremic syndrome. Systemic lupus erythematosus nephritis

Neonatal & intrauterine transfusion

Special blood requirements neonatal & intrauterine transfusion

RBCs for intrauterine or neonatal exchange transfusion should be fresh (<5 days old), irradiated, group O, and negative for any maternal antibody (eg, anti-D) that is active. Preferably serologically tested CMV– or CMV risk-reduced (leukoreduced) blood products should be used in intrauterine transfusion or in neonates <1,200 g who are CMV–.

RBC products do not ordinarily need to be washed (eg, to remove potassium or anti-A/anti-B antibodies); however, if fresh (<5 day old) blood is not available and transfusion with

2: Blood Banking/Transfusion

large volumes of RBCs are needed, the neonatologist may request this. Washing adds ~1 hour to the preparation time and results in product loss during the procedure. Plasma or plasma containing products (platelets) must be compatible with the neonate's RBCs.

Routine volume reduction of platelets for neonates is not routinely warranted, for a variety of reasons. First, there is very little volume involved to begin with, and volume reduction only decreases it on average ~10-20%. In the case of platelets, centrifugation causes potential platelet loss, platelet activation and/or platelet functional defects. Lastly, volume reduction introduces a potential for bacterial contamination and an inherent time delay.

Dosing must be calculated on the basis of weight t2.22.

t2.22 Doses for neonatal & intrauterine transfusion

RBCs	15 mL/kg
FFP	10 mL/kg
Platelets	5 mL/kg (for a 10 kg infant, this is ~1 random donor unit or 1/6 of an apheresis unit)
Cryoprecipitate	10-20 mL/kg

Maternal immune thrombocytopenic purpura (ITP)

ITP is the immune-mediated destruction of platelets, usually on the basis of autoantibodies directed against platelet surface antigens such as HPA-1a (formerly known as PLA1). In women with a history of ITP who become pregnant, or in women who have the onset of ITP during pregnancy, there is a risk of neonatal thrombocytopenia caused by autoantibodies crossing the placenta. There is a low risk of severe neonatal thrombocytopenia (<50,000) and a low but definite risk of serious hemorrhage (intracranial hemorrhage in <1%, confined to neonates with platelets <20,000).

There is no lab test that is a reliable predictor of neonatal thrombocytopenia. The risk of neonatal thrombocytopenia is highest with previous maternal splenectomy for ITP, previous infant with ITP, and gestational (maternal) platelet count <100,000. It is recommended that serial neonatal platelet counts be monitored for a few days after delivery.

Supportive platelet transfusions are sparingly given, typically in the cases of active bleeding. During pregnancy mothers with significant thrombocytopenia, petechiae or hemorrhage should be started on steroids and if thrombocytopenia persists IV immunoglobulin (IVIG) may be necessary. After delivery, the neonatal platelet count will begin to rise early, due to cessation of maternal autoantibody infusion.

Neonatal alloimmune thrombocytopenic (NAIT)

NAIT is caused by maternal antiplatelet alloantibodies that cross the placenta and cause destruction of fetal platelets. Most commonly the maternal alloantibodies are directed against the platelet antigen, HPA-1a. In the general population, 2% of individuals are HPA-1a negative, and they can develop anti-HPA-1a antibodies if exposed to the antigen such as through transfusion or pregnancy. In contrast to the analogous situation of hemolytic disease of the fetus/newborn (HDFN), NAIT can affect the first pregnancy.

There is a 12% incidence of fatal intracranial hemorrhage and a 20% incidence of intracranial hemorrhage overall. About half of serious hemorrhages occur in utero, so treatment should begin as soon as the diagnosis is suspected. Unfortunately, the diagnosis can only be suspected in a woman with a previously affected infant, but the likelihood of recurrence in subsequent pregnancies is high. In fact, fetal/neonatal thrombocytopenia is more severe with each successive pregnancy.

Lab testing may involve maternal and paternal platelet antigen phenotyping and screening of maternal serum for antiplatelet antibodies. Neonatal platelet counts are commonly <20,000.

In cases that are suspected in utero, maternal treatment with high dose IVIg and/or corticosteroids should be considered. Intrauterine platelet transfusion is sometimes undertaken, and should always be strongly considered if diagnostic cordocentesis (PUBS) is performed, as this poses a risk of serious bleed. Intrauterine platelet transfusion may begin at 18-20 weeks gestation, with antigen-negative platelets. Maternal platelets may be used if they have been washed and irradiated. If compatible platelets are not available, platelets from the blood bank inventory should be used if transfusion is urgent. Delivery by C-section is recommended, if possible. After birth, the risk of hemorrhage is greatest during the first 24-36 hours of life, so expedient platelet transfusion is desirable. Platelet counts usually rise above 50,000 by 2-3 weeks.

Hemolytic disease of the fetus & newborn (HDFN)

HDFN results from maternal alloantibodies crossing the placenta, entering the fetal circulation, and causing hemolysis. This, depending on the severity, can lead to the appearance of bilirubin in the amniotic fluid, progressive fetal anemia, and eventual hydrops fetalis. To be significant, the maternal alloantibody must be of the IgG1, IgG3, or IgG4 class, since IgA, IgG2 and IgM do not cross the placenta.

Rh HDFN, the classic form of HDFN, is caused by maternal anti-D antibodies. Since anti-D antibodies are not naturally occurring, this indicates the woman has been exposed to D+ erythrocytes, either through prior pregnancy or transfusion. Thus, anti-D HDFN is usually not seen with the first pregnancy. In the course of a normal pregnancy, there is usually entry of fetal blood cells into the maternal circulation (fetomaternal hemorrhage), most often at the time of delivery. However, sensitization may occur as a result of other events t2.23 and without the carriage of a pregnancy to term; at the very least, the second trimester must be reached, as this is when the fetus begins to produce circulating RBCs.

Prior to the introduction of RhIg, the incidence of sensitization in an Rh– woman bearing an Rh+ fetus was around 15%. The incidence is actually somewhat lower if the mom and fetus are also ABO incompatible. Prevention of Rh HDFN begins with checking every pregnant woman's D status. D– women should be checked for anti-D antibodies. In D– women without antibodies, interventions are aimed at preventing the development of anti-D antibodies. This is achieved through prophylactic doses of Rh immune globulin (RhIg), given at set intervals and whenever a fetal-maternal hemorrhage occurs

ISBN 978-089189-5985   **87**

t2.23, t2.24. The idea is that the RhIg coats any fetal RBCs that enter the maternal circulation, thus preventing maternal immune sensitization. The half life or RhIg is ~24 days.

t2.23 Sources of fetomaternal hemorrhage & Rh(D) sensitization

Normal pregnancy
Chorionic villus sampling
Amniocentesis
Cordocentesis
Abortion, threatened or completed (spontaneous or elective)
Placental abruption
Trauma

t2.24 Prevention of Rh HDFN is achieved by the administration of RhIg

Scenario	Recommendation	Notes
D– women bearing D+ or D-unknown fetus	Prophylactic 300 µg (1 full dose vial) at 28 weeks & at term	Without RhIg, the risk of developing anti-D is 16%; with RhIg at 28 weeks & term, the risk is 0.1%
	Fetal-maternal hemorrhage of unknown quantity due to ectopic pregnancy, trauma, amniocentesis, chorionic villus sampling, spontaneous abortion, delivery	In the first 12 weeks of gestation, if available, a mini-dose (50 µg) or a full dose (300 µg) can be administered After 12 weeks, a full dose (300 µg) vial is given The quantity of fetomaternal hemorrhage should be determined & additional doses of RhIg given as indicated (see t2.25)
D+ women	RhIg not indicated	No benefit
D– women who have already formed anti-D antibodies	RhIg not indicated	No benefit

In D– women with anti-D antibodies (previously sensitized), management is aimed at minimizing the effect on the fetus. A maternal antibody titer is first determined. If this titer is <16, then severe hemolysis is considered unlikely. However, once the titer reaches or exceeds 16, monitoring the degree of fetal hemolysis (discussed in Chapter 1) becomes the chief concern. Fetal hemolysis can be monitored in 1 of 2 ways:

1. amniotic fluid sampling with plotting of OD450 on a Liley curve

2. noninvasive Doppler ultrasound measurement of middle cerebral artery (MCA) flow

The latter is a reflection of fetal anemia, with MCA flow increasing in proportion to the degree of anemia. If anemia is severe, then intrauterine transfusions and early delivery may be necessary to minimize the harm to the fetus.

Intrauterine transfusion may be carried out by 1 of 2 methods: direct cannulation of the umbilical cord or intraperitoneal transfusion. Transfused RBCs should be <5 days old or washed, irradiated, CMV serologically negative, leukocyte reduced, and compatible with the mom (in this case D–). While not entirely necessary, it is helpful to know the phenotype of the fetal blood. This can be achieved through cordocentesis (PUBS), molecular (PCR) testing of amniotic fluid cells, or molecular (PCR) analysis of free fetal DNA (ffDNA) in maternal blood. After delivery, management is aimed at treating severe anemia and preventing kernicterus.

t2.25 Calculating the dose of RhIg

Step	
1	Maternal whole blood volume is often assumed to be around 5,000 mL Otherwise, it is calculated as the mother's body weight (kg) times 70 mL/kg (assuming a weight of 70 kg & a blood volume of 5,000 mL may cause under-dosing)
2	The proportion of fetal cells is determined by a Kleihauer-Betke (or other) test In the Kleihauer-Betke, fetal & maternal cells are counted separately for a total of 2,000 cells Percentages are converted into decimals (if, for example, fetal cells comprise 3% of maternal blood, then substitute 0.03 into the formula)
3	Calculate dose (number of vials) according to formula Dose (vials) = (maternal blood volume in mL) × (proportion fetal cells in maternal blood) ÷ 30 Why divide by 30? Each full dose vial (300 µg) protects against 30 mL whole blood or 15 mL of RBCs
4	**Always add 1 vial to dosage** If the number after the decimal is <5 round down & add 1 vial; if the number after the decimal is >5 round up & add 1 vial For example, if the result is 3.3, then round down to 3 & add 1 vial; the patient will receive 4 vials If the result is 3.6, then round up to 4 & add 1 vial so the patient will receive 5 vials
5	No more than 5 vials should be given IM at one time; larger doses may be divided or given IV

A group and screen is performed on the maternal blood upon admission to labor and delivery. Furthermore, cord blood from each newborn should be subjected to ABO/Rh testing and a DAT. ABO testing in this case omits the reverse grouping, and Rh testing should include testing for weak D since weak D fetal RBCs can sensitize D– mothers. Noting that cord RBC should be washed thoroughly to remove umbilical cord matrix, Wharton jelly, which is a cause of false positive DAT. Next, a confirmed positive DAT should be compared with the maternal antibody screen. If the latter is positive, then the identity of the maternal antibody can be determined by RBC panel. If the maternal antibody screen is negative, then several possibilities should be considered: ABO HDFN, prior RhIg administration, and fetal low-incidence antigens that are not present on the screen cells, extended panel may be necessary. Next, the neonatal bilirubin should be checked serially. A high (>20 mg/dL) or rapidly rising (>0.5 mg/dL/hour) bilirubin is an indication for phototherapy or, in severe cases, exchange transfusion. The rosette test is a qualitative test for fetomaternal hemorrhage. Maternal blood is incubated with anti-D antibody and D+ indicator cells which form rosettes around D+ fetal cells. The incubated mixture is examined microscopically for rosettes. The rosette test will detect as little as 10 cc of fetal blood, but the result is qualitative. If this test is negative, then the single 300 µg dose of RhIg is adequate. If this test is positive, then a quantitative test (Kleihauer-Betke, ELAT, or flow cytometry) is indicated. The Kleihauer-Betke (acid elution) test works on the principle that fetal hemoglobin (HbF) is resistant to acid elution, unlike adult hemoglobin. Thus when maternal blood is subjected to acid elution then eosin stained and examined under the microscope, any cells that take up stain (rather than appearing "ghosted") represent RBCs containing HbF. A cell count is performed to determine the percentage of fetal RBCs (see below). The enzyme linked antiglobulin test (ELAT) is another quantitative assay for fetal-maternal hemorrhage. Flow cytometry is now commonly used to calculate the quantity of HbF.

Determining the fetal Rh type may sometimes be undertaken. This can be achieved through percutaneous umbilical blood sampling (cordocentesis); alternatively, the Rh type can be determined by PCR of amniocentesis (by PCR), chorionic villus sampling (by PCR), or free fetal DNA (ffDNA) in maternal blood (by PCR).

Non-Rh HDFN now is more common than Rh HDFN. HDFN due to ABO is the most common type of HDFN overall, but it is clinically mild. ABO HDFN is predominantly seen in blood group O mothers bearing blood group A or B fetuses.

Hemolysis is caused by an IgG anti-A,B antibody. Since ABO antibodies are naturally occurring, this may be seen in the first pregnancy. HDFN due to Kell is now the most common cause of severe HDFN. Anti-c is second. Kell HDFN differs in that Kell is established early in erythroid maturation; thus, there is destruction of marrow precursors as well as destruction of circulating erythrocytes. A maternal critical titer for anti-Kell antibody is 8. In contrast a critical titer for Rh antibodies is 16.

Blood components t2.26

t2.26 Summary of blood products

Blood product	Composition	Volume	Indications (I) & contraindications (CI)	Storage	Storage time
Whole Blood	RBCs (Hct 40%), plasma, WBC, platelets	500 cc	I: Need for increase in both RBC mass & plasma volume Relative CI: volume overload	1-6°C	Varies with preservative t2.27
RBCs	RBCs (Hct 55-80%), minimal plasma, WBC, platelets & preservative solution	300 cc	I: Symptomatic anemia Relative CI: AIHA or hyperhemolysis in SCD patients	1-6°C	Varies with preservative t2.27
Frozen RBC	RBCs & 40% glycerol (deglycerolized when thawed)	250 cc	Same as RBCs, usually rare blood groups are frozen	≤ -65°C	10 years (24 hours following thawing/deglycerolization)
Irradiated RBC	RBCs	250 cc	Same as RBCs, irradiate to prevent TA-GVHD	1-6°C	28 days or original expiration, whichever comes first
Platelets (random donor)	Platelets ($>5.5 \times 10^{10}$), minimal plasma, WBC, RBC (<0.5 mL), pH>6.2	50 cc	I: Bleeding in thrombocytopenic patient or prophylactic transfusion for severely thrombocytopenic patients Relative CI: ITP Absolute CI: HIT & TTP	20-24°C (constant gentle agitation; may go without agitation for 24 hours)	5 days (max time without agitation: 24 hours) 4 hours after pooling
Apheresis platelets (platelets pheresis)	Platelets ($>3 \times 10^{11}$) reduced amount of plasma, WBC, RBC (<2 mL)	300 cc	Same as platelets (random donor) Use of single donor minimizes alloimmunization	20-24°C (constant gentle agitation; may go without agitation for 24 hours)	5 days (max time without agitation: 24 hrs)
FFP	Plasma separated within 8 hours of collection (all coagulation factors)	200 cc	I: Multiple coagulation factors deficiency, PT/PTT $>1.5\times$ mid-range of normal Relative CI: IgA deficient patient	≤ -18°C	1 year (if stored at ≤ -65°C, then 7 years)
Cryoprecipitated AHF (cryoprecipitated antihemophilic factor)	Cold insoluble portions of plasma; must contain ≥ 150 mg fibrinogen & 80 IU of factor VIII; also contains factors XIII, vWF	15 cc	I: Deficient fibrinogen or factors VIII, XIII or VWf when safer coagulation factors not available	≤ -18°C	1 year
Apheresis granulocytes (granulocytes pheresis)	Granulocytes ($>1 \times 10^{10}$)	200 cc	I: Neutropenic patients with documented infection unresponsive to standard medical therapy	22-24°C	24 hours

RBC components

How prepared & stored

In most instances, RBCs are administered in the form of concentrated RBCs with a hematocrit ranging from 55-80%, depending on the preservative. This is obtained by separating most of the plasma and platelets from the original bag of whole blood (see below).

Anticoagulant-preservative solutions t2.27 are required for prolonged blood storage. Blood is collected into bags containing ~60 mL of an anticoagulant-preservative solution. The different anticoagulant-preservative solutions vary in composition and in the duration over which RBCs are considered acceptable for donation. These solutions are intended to maximize posttransfusion viability and all contain dextrose as a carbohydrate source for the glycolytic production of ATP. Post-storage levels of ATP correlate with posttransfusion RBC viability. CPDA contains adenine (a substrate for the production of ATP), citrate (an anticoagulant that chelates calcium), and sodium phosphate (a pH buffer). The additive solutions, known as AS-1 (Adsol), AS-3 (Nutricel), AS-5, contain different concentrations of additional dextrose, adenine, buffer, and sodium chloride. Only AS-1 and AS-5 contain mannitol which has diuretic effects and may have possible side effects on intracerebral pressure if transfused in large quantities to neonates. Allowable storage time is the maximum time after which 75% of transfused RBCs will be viable in the circulation 24 hours after transfusion.

t2.27 RBC preservatives

Solution	Allowable storage	Usual hematocrit	Comments
Citrate phosphate dextrose (CPD), ACD, CP2D	21 days	70%	Whole blood or RBC
Citrate phosphate dextrose adenine-1 (CPDA-1)	35 days	70%	Whole blood or RBC
Additive solutions (AS-1, AS-3 or AS-%), added to CPD	42 days	60%	Must be added within 72 hours of collection Used for RBC only

Storage lesion

Storage "lesion" refers to progressive changes that occur within stored RBCs. Continued intracellular metabolism cause levels of 2,3-DPG (2,3-diphosphoglycerate) to fall linearly. RBCs leak potassium into the plasma, the pH decreases, and ATP levels fall. Decreased pH causes a shift in the hemoglobin saturation curve to the right; that is, decreased pH enhances release of oxygen from hemoglobin and inhibits oxygen binding. Decreased 2,3-DPG shifts it to the left and increases oxygen binding. Both of these shifts in the hemoglobin saturation curve inhibit oxygen delivery to tissues. After transfusion, normal 2,3-DPG, ATP, and pH are completely restored within 24 hours. There is always a slight degree of hemolysis in a bag of RBCs, and some free hemoglobin is present in every unit. In the plasma contained in the unit, there is progressive diminution of clotting factors, particularly the labile clotting factors V and VIII. The platelets contained in the unit become rapidly dysfunctional and should not be considered therapeutic after the first few days.

Transport & reissue

Transport and reissue must be tightly controlled. RBCs must be transported in a monitored, refrigerated, device. Units that have left the blood bank and have been returned unused may be reissued for transfusion if

1. the unit has not been "spiked" (entered)
2. the blood has been maintained continuously between 1-10°C in a monitored storage device and has not been outside a monitored storage device for >30 minutes
3. at least 1 segment of sealed tubing remains

Whole Blood

Whole Blood is the unit of blood immediately drawn from the donor before any processing is performed. Although this is an ideal treatment for the patient with extreme blood loss, it must be ABO identical to the patient and therefore is not routinely used. Currently, RBCs, transfused concurrently with asanguineous fluids or other blood components, have supplanted whole blood in most cases. Whole blood contains ~450-525 mL of RBCs, plasma and platelets; however, the coagulation factor activity diminishes over time particularly labile factors V and VIII as well as platelet function.

RBCs

RBCs (or PRBCs) refers to the product that results after removing most of the Plasma and Platelets via slow centrifugation of Whole Blood. Standards requires that the final hematocrit shall be ≤80%. RBCs are stored at 1-6°C within 8 hours of collection and for the duration of their storage. For transport, they must be kept between 1-10°C. They expire in 21 days if stored in CPD, 35 days if stored in CPDA, and 42 days if AS is added to CPD. If the system is opened ("spiked"), then the product expires in 24 hours when refrigerated and in 4 hours at room temperature. Rejuvenating solutions, which contain additional pyruvate, inosine, phosphate, and adenine, can extend the expiration date by a few days. The total volume of a bag of RBCs is around 250 mL. This is composed of ~200 mL

of RBCs, 50 mL plasma and anticoagulants. Note that each mL of RBCs contains ~1 mg of iron; thus, a bag of RBCs contains ~200 mg iron.

Apheresis RBCs

Apheresis RBCs should contain ≥60 g of hemoglobin/unit (or ~180 mL RBC volume). At least 95% of units sampled must contain >50 g of hemoglobin (or ~150 mL RBC volume).

RBC manipulations

RBCs, Leukocyte Reduced (leukoreduced RBCs) is the most common RBC product in use today, with leukoreduction occurring at the time of blood donation. The typical nonleukoreduced unit of RBCs contains around 5×10^9 white cells. To qualify as leukoreduced, it must have $<5 \times 10^6$ (a 3-log reduction). The leukoreduced unit must retain ≥85% of the original RBCs (whole blood derived units) or ≥51 g of hemoglobin (pheresis units). Leukoreduction is generally achieved through filtration and can occur at the time of collection or at the time of transfusion, but prestorage filtration is thought to be more effective. Note that washed RBCs and RBCs that have been frozen, thawed, and deglycerolized (because extensive washing is involved) are considered leukoreduced. Note also that leukoreduction is not effective for the prevention of transfusion associated graft vs host disease.

Washed RBCs are the product of RBCs washing and resuspension in normal saline for the purpose of removing the plasma. Since washing requires an open system, the shelf-life of washed RBCs is 24 hours t2.28. Washed RBCs are used to prevent severe or recurrent allergic reactions, such as anaphylaxis in the IgA-deficient recipient.

t2.28 Some hard to remember shelf lives (outdates)

RBCs, saline washed or thawed & deglycerolized	24-hour shelf life, refrigerated
Thawed FFP	24-hour shelf life, refrigerated (after 24 hours, re-labeled as "thawed plasma")
Thawed Plasma	5-day shelf life, refrigerated
Pooled Platelets in open system	4-hour shelf life, room temperature
Pooled Platelets in closed system	5 days or shortest outdate of RDP in pool, room temperature
Thawed cryoprecipitated AHF, unpooled	6-hour shelf life, room temperature
Thawed & pooled cryoprecipitated AHF in open system	4-hour shelf life, room temperature

RBCs Irradiated are required in some instances, for the prevention of transfusion associated graft vs host disease (TA-GVHD). Once irradiated, RBCs are good for 28 days post-irradiation, or the original outdate, whichever comes first.

Frozen RBCs are sometimes prepared to preserve rare donor groups or blood for autologous donation. The cells must be frozen within 6 days if no additive solution is present; with additive solution, they must be frozen before the expiration date appropriate for the additive solution. Freezing RBCs can result in serious damage to the cells, unless so-called cryoprotective agents are used. Glycerol is a commonly used cryoprotective. After the slow addition of 40% glycerol, RBCs can be placed in a −80°C freezer and kept at <65°C for up to 10 years. When thawed, the RBCs must be immediately washed in a series of progressively more hypotonic solutions to remove the glycerol while preventing hemolysis. Once thawed, washed, and stored at 1-6 °C, the RBCs must be transfused within 24 hours. Frozen and deglycerolized RBCs are considered both leukoreduced and washed (free of IgA, for example).

Indications

The main indication for RBCs is decreased oxygen-carrying capacity. Transfusion "triggers" vary, but generally healthy individuals can tolerate a hematocrit as low as 20% (hemoglobin 7 g/dL) without severe symptoms, while those with moderate cardiopulmonary insufficiency may need to be transfused at higher rates between 24-30% (hemoglobin 8-10 g/dL). A large-scale study of critical care patients showed no difference in outcome between patients whose hemoglobin was maintained between 7-9 g/dL and those maintained between 10-12 g/dL, irrespective of cardiopulmonary status.

The expected effect of a unit of RBCs is a 1 g/dL increase in hemoglobin and 3% increase in hematocrit. A pediatric dose of around 4 mL/kg will achieve the same effect. All RBC products must be transfused through a filter, most commonly a 170-260 μm filter. In pediatric patients, a 20-40 μm microaggregate filter can remove fibrin strands and degenerated cellular elements; however, this is not commonly used. The only fluid that may be transfused simultaneously through the infusion line is isotonic saline (0.9% saline). No medications may be added to the infusion.

Contraindications

There are no absolute contraindications; however, crystalloids are a better choice for patients whose blood loss is <20% of blood volume (about a liter) or whose hematocrit is >30% in the absence of complicating factors. Additionally, some consider autoimmune hemolytic anemia or hyperhemolysis syndrome in SCD patients, a relative contraindication to blood transfusion, and at the very least other means of increasing oxygenation should be attempted first.

Platelets

How prepared & stored

When whole blood is slow-centrifuged, it separates into RBCs and platelet-rich plasma. When the platelet-rich plasma is fast-centrifuged, it separates into platelet concentrate and plasma. Platelets may also be collected by apheresis. The platelets are removed and stored at 20-24°C with gentle agitation. They expire in 5 days; platelets function for up to 7 days, but the shorter 5 day shelf-life was mandated in order to reduce the incidence of transfusion transmitted bacterial infection. If the system is opened (such as for pooling), the unit expires in 4 hours. As with RBCs, one may prepare leukoreduced platelets & irradiated platelets. Leukoreduced platelets must contain $\leq 8.3 \times 10^5$ leukocytes (leukoreduced whole blood derived platelets and leukoreduced pheresis platelets must contain $\leq 5 \times 10^6$ leukocytes).

What it contains

Each single donor derived unit has a volume of ~50 mL consisting of some plasma, a few white cells, ~80 mg fibrinogen, and a minimum of 5.5×10^{10} platelets (in ≥75% of units tested). Pheresis platelets have a volume of ~100 mL, consisting of plasma, white cells, fibrinogen (~150 mg), and a minimum of 3.0×10^{11} platelets. Thus, a pheresis platelet unit has ~6× the number of platelets in a single donor derived unit.

Indications

In the nonbleeding patient with thrombocytopenia, the aim is to prevent bleeding with prophylactic platelet transfusions whenever the patient falls below a certain threshold. Traditionally, this transfusion "trigger" was between 15,000 and 20,000/μL. However, a trigger of 10,000/μL appears equally safe, in the absence of fever, sepsis, coagulopathy, hypersplenism, and lesions that pose a risk of bleeding.

In the bleeding patient with thrombocytopenia, platelets are often administered for platelet counts below 50,000/μL. For the thrombocytopenic patient undergoing an invasive surgical procedure, a target platelet count of 50,000/μL is desirable. For patients with central nervous system (CNS) bleeding or CNS surgery the threshold is 100,000/μL.

There is some role for platelets in patients with Glanzmann thrombasthenia, Bernard-Soulier syndrome, aspirin ingestion, and renal failure. In the latter, a trial of DDAVP or cryoprecipitate is first indicated.

Contraindications

Relative contraindications include immune thrombocytopenic purpura (ITP), in which platelet transfusion is usually ineffective at raising the platelet count and may actually enhance platelet destruction. When patients with ITP experience significant bleeding, co-administration of platelets with IVIg may enhance platelet recovery. Absolute contraindications include heparin induced thrombocytopenia (HIT) and thrombotic thrombocytopenic purpura (TTP), in which platelet transfusion may induce intravascular thromboses.

Dosing

Adults are given 4-6 pooled random donor platelets (RDP) or 1 single donor apheresis platelet (SDP) at a time. Neonates are given 10-15 mL/kg or 1 unit/10 kg. The expected result, in adults, of transfusing 1 unit (5.5×10^{10}) of platelets is an increase in the platelet count of ~5,000/μL. Hence, the average platelet dose will increase the platelet count around 30-60,000 μL. The average platelet life span is 9.5 days. Like RBCs, platelets must always be transfused through at least a 170 μm filter. Platelets need not be crossmatched unless they contain >2 mL of RBCs; such units are visibly bloody. It is desirable that the plasma contained in the platelet unit be compatible with the recipient.

Prevention of platelet-transmitted infection

It is required by the AABB that methods be employed to limit and detect platelet contamination by bacteria. See discussion under transfusion complications.

Compatibility

It is desirable to use ABO identical or compatible platelets when possible but some centers will transfuse platelets without regard to ABO compatibility for certain patient groups. Platelets carry AB antigens and are potentially targeted by the recipient's isoagglutinins which may result in a poor rise in platelet count after transfusion. The greater danger is ABO incompatible plasma within the platelet dose, which could cause hemolysis in the recipient. Many patients do not experience any symptoms after receiving the ABO incompatible platelets. The following situations present the greatest risk for hemolysis

1. recipients with small blood volumes, such as infants

2. single donor apheresis units with high titer isohemagglutinins

3. multiply transfused recipients

Several approaches may be used to prevent hemolysis in high risk patients. The platelets can be centrifuged and most of the plasma may be removed, reducing but not eliminating the risk; however, centrifugation can cause platelet activation. Another approach is to perform A and B titers on apheresis platelets to identify donors with dangerously high titers and restrict these products to ABO identical patients; however, this approach lacks standardization of both titration methods and the critical isohemagglutinin titer. The last approach is to avoid ABO incompatible platelets for high risk patients. In bone marrow transplant patients there is some literature to suggest that transfusion with ABO incompatible platelets can increase the rate of alloimmunization, platelet refractoriness and reduce survival after marrow transplant.

Rh matching is recommended for Platelets, since a small volume of contaminating RBCs can cause formation of anti-D antibody. This risk is higher in Whole Blood derived Platelets than apheresis Platelets, since they have a greater amount of RBC contaminants. Therefore if an Rh– individual must receive Rh+ Platelets, administration of RhIg should be considered, especially for females of child bearing potential.

Granulocyte concentrates

How prepared & stored

Granulocytes are often obtained by apheresis. They are stored without agitation at 20-24°C for up to 24 hours. The product should be administered without a leukoreduction filter.

What it contains

Each unit contains a certain amount of contaminating RBCs, a large number of platelets, and around 10^{10} white blood cells.

Indications & contraindications

Granulocytes are usually employed for neutropenic sepsis or fungal infections that are unresponsive to standard therapy.

Dosing

There is no agreed-upon dose, but several days of granulocyte therapy are generally required. As with all cellular blood products, a filter is required, but a leukoreduction filter is must not be used. Units should be ABO crossmatch compatible with the recipient and should be irradiated.

Plasma products

How prepared & stored

When whole blood is slow-centrifuged, it separates into RBCs and Platelet-rich Plasma. This latter product, when fast-centrifuged, can be separated into Platelet concentrate and Plasma. The Plasma must be placed into a –18°C or colder freezer within 8 hours of blood collection to make FFP. Plasma not frozen within 8 hours may be frozen within 24 hours and labeled as "Plasma frozen within 24 hours after phlebotomy" or "FP24"; these units are relatively depleted of factors V and VIII but are useful for most of the indications for FFP. FFP expires in 1 year at ≤–18 °C, and expires in 7 years if stored at ≤–65°C. For administration, it must be thawed at 30-37°C. After thawing it expires in 24 hours.

What it contains

A unit of Plasma has a volume of ~200 mL and it usually contains ~1 IU/mL of all coagulation factors (by definition, an IU of coagulation factor is that amount contained in 1 mL normal plasma). The reason for freezing is to preserve the function of coagulation factors, particularly the so-called labile factors V and VIII. Units usually contain 2-4 mg of fibrinogen/mL.

Indications & contraindications

Plasma is given for coagulopathies caused by multiple factor deficiencies. In this scenario, a PT or PTT that is 1.5× normal (or INR that is 2× normal) are generally considered a transfusion "trigger"; administration of Plasma is unlikely to lower an INR <1.8. Multiple factor deficiencies often arise in the setting of disseminated intravascular coagulation (DIC), warfarin therapy, coagulopathy of prematurity, or massive transfusion ("dilutional" coagulopathy). In DIC, both Plasma and cryoprecipitate are usually indicated, but this decision should be based on measurements of PT, PTT, and fibrinogen. In cases of single factor deficiencies (eg, factor VIII), recombinant factor or factor concentrates are preferred, and if that is not available, then cryoprecipitate is the second choice. For warfarin reversal, the American College of Chest Physicians has published specific guidelines (see chapter 5). Plasma is also indicated as the replacement solution in plasma exchange for thrombotic thrombocytopenic purpura (TTP) and for treatment of antithrombin (AT) deficiency. In TTP, plasma exchange must be performed immediately; if this is delayed, transfusion of plasma should be instigated in the interim. Note that plasma is not useful for the reversal of heparin and may actually worsen heparinization by providing additional AT.

Dosing

Usually 2 units are given at a time for adult patients; more precisely, 10 mL/kg for both adults and neonates. When given prior to invasive procedure, the transfusion should be given no >2 hours before incision. Each unit is expected to increase factor activities by around 20%. Plasma must be given through a standard 170 μm filter.

Compatibility

The plasma, which contains ABO antibodies, should be compatible with the recipient's RBC phenotype. Type AB is the universal plasma donor; however, the first choice should be plasma that is ABO identical with the patient. Donor Rh type should not affect product choice, and there is no need to give RhIg in association with plasma transfusion.

Cryoprecipitated anti-hemophilic factor (cryoprecipitate or cryo)

How prepared & stored

When FFP is thawed to 1-6°C then centrifuged, a precipitate (the so-called cold-insoluble portion of plasma) forms. After removal of the thawed plasma, the precipitate must be replaced, within 1 hour, in a –18°C or colder freezer to make cryoprecipitate. It expires in 1 year. After thawing, pooled units of cryo expire in 4 hours.

What it contains

Each unit of cryoprecipitate contains ~15 mL of total volume. It must have a minimum of 150 mg fibrinogen and 80 IU of factor VIII in all units tested. Cryo also contains factor XIII and vWF but does not contain appreciable quantities of factor V. Note that each unit of cryo contains the amount of factors present in 1-2 units of FFP, but in a significantly smaller volume (1 unit of FFP has the volume of ~20 units of cryo).

Indications & contraindications

The treatment of choice for hemophilia A (factor VIII deficiency) is factor VIII concentrate or recombinant factor VIII. In unusual situations, cryoprecipitate may be used. The dose can be calculated (see below). The T½ of factor VIII is 12 hours, and this dose will be repeated in 12 hours. Alternatively, a continuous infusion to run >12 hours may be administered. Recombinant factor VIIa has demonstrated efficacy in hemophilia complicated by acquired inhibitors against factor VIII or fIX. The half life of recombinant factor VIIa is ~3.5 hours. In patients with factor VIII or fIX inhibitors, the dose is 90 μg/kg q 2-3 hours until hemostasis is obtained, after which doses are titrated for bleeding. Cryoprecipitate may be used to treat fibrinogen deficiency, which is most often seen in the setting of DIC. Cryoprecipitate should not be used alone to treat DIC, as it lacks certain factors, notably factor V. FFP should be given as well. A rule of thumb is that 1 unit of cryo can raise the fibrinogen level by around 7 mg/dL; thus, a dose of 10 pooled cryo units is expected to raise the fibrinogen by 70 mg/dL. Other indications include bleeding in uremic patients and factor XIII deficiency. While cryo can be employed in the treatment for von Willebrand disease, the initial treatment of choice is usually DDAVP.

Dosing

The usual dose for adults is 6-10 bags.

Calculating the dose of cryo for factor VIII deficiency

$$\text{Bags of cryo} = (\text{weight in kg} \times 70 \text{ mL/kg}) \times (1-\text{Hct})$$
$$\times (\text{target} - \text{actual factor VIII activity level}) \div 80$$

Note that the number 80 is the amount of factor VIII (IU) in each bag of cryoprecipitate

Plasma derivatives

Plasma derivatives are sources of particular plasma proteins. Plasma derivatives are made from pools of donor plasma that are processed for the elimination of transmissible diseases and purified. The donors are usually paid, and the pooled plasma is subjected to virus inactivation by heat, solvent, and/or filtration. The desired protein is then purified.

Albumin is a plasma derivative that may be used as a plasma expander or as plasma exchange replacement fluid; in this latter indication, albumin is particularly useful for its ability to bind bilirubin in neonates with severe hyperbilirubinemia. RhIg is a plasma derivative. It is available in forms for intramuscular and intravenous administration for prevention of hemolytic disease of the newborn and for treatment (intravenous form only) of immune thrombocytopenic purpura. Antithrombin (AT) concentrate can be used for treatment of inherited or acquired AT deficiency. Protein C concentrate can be used for treatment of protein C deficiency and severe sepsis. In sepsis, protein C concentrate has been shown to significantly reduce mortality. Factor VII concentrate is used in patients with factor VII deficiency and in patients with anti-factor VIII or anti-fIX inhibitors. "Off-label" use in trauma patients has been undertaken but not extensively studied. Factor VIII (factor VIII) concentrate is used in the treatment and prophylaxis of hemophilia A. Humate-P contains sufficient von Willebrand factor to be used in the treatment of von Willebrand disease. The dose of factor VIII depends upon the patient's actual starting factor VIII activity and target factor VIII activity. To calculate the dose, the following should be understood:

1. 1 international unit (IU) of factor VIII is defined as the activity of factor VIII in 1 mL of normal plasma (the plasma of someone with factor VIII activity of 100%), and is the expected activity of 1 mL of pooled plasma

2. the intravascular recovery of factor VIII is nearly 100%

3. the half life of factor VIII is ~12 hours

The dose can be estimated or calculated. Factor IX concentrate is used in patients with hemophilia B. Dose calculation is similar to factor VIII, but some of the assumptions differ. First, the half life of factor IX is around 24 hours. Second, the intravascular recovery of factor IX is only ~50%. Lastly, it is notable that some of the less-purified forms of factor IX, such as AlphaNine-SD, have variable quantities of other vitamin K-dependent factors (II, VII, and X) and are also called "prothrombin complex concentrates." This should be distinguished from the next product. Factor IX complex, also called anti-inhibitor coagulant complex (AICC), under the brand name FEIBA-VH, contains factor IX, factor II, factor X, and activated factor VII (factor VIIa). This can be used in patients with high dose anti-factor VIII or anti-factor IX inhibitors.

Estimating the dose of factor VIII

- 30% activity desired: 15 IU/kg
- 50% activity desired: 25 IU/kg
- 100% activity desired: 50 IU/kg

Calculating the dose of factor VIII

$$Dose = (patient\ weight\ in\ kg \times 70\ mL/kg) \times (1\text{–}Hct) \times (target - actual)$$

Example

An 80 kg patient with actual starting factor VIII of 1%, target activity of 50%, Hct of 35%

$$Dose = (80\ kg \times 70\ ml/kg) \times 0.65 \times 0.49 = 1784\ mL$$

Irradiated products

How prepared & stored

AABB Standards stipulate that 25 Gy (2,500 cGy) are delivered to the mid-plane of the product. The minimum dose to any portion of the product shall be 15 Gy (1,500 cGy). A method must be used to ensure that irradiation has occurred. For RBCs, the storage time becomes 28 days or the original outdate, whichever is sooner.

Indications

Irradiation is carried out solely for the purpose of preventing TA-GVHD, an often fatal complication of transfusion of cellular products to immunocompromised recipients. TA-GVHD is mainly a risk in bone marrow transplant recipients, neonates, fetuses receiving intrauterine transfusions, recipients of blood from blood relatives, Hodgkin and non-Hodgkin lymphoma, patients receiving purine analogs, and patients with congenital T cell defects (such as DiGeorge syndrome and severe combined immunodeficiency [SCID]) but not in B cell or macrophage defects. Irradiation is not effective in preventing CMV transmission.

Leukoreduced products

How prepared & stored

Filtration is the usual method of leukoreduction. RBC leukoreduction filters contain multiple layers of woven synthetic fibers that will retain both platelets and leukocytes. To be labeled as leukoreduced, the product must contain $<5 \times 10^6$ white cells (RBCs and apheresis derived Platelets) or $<8.3 \times 10^5$ (Whole Blood derived Platelets). Note that washed RBCs and frozen, deglycerolized, RBCs are considered leukoreduced. Blood banks differ on whether filtration is accomplished at the bedside (during transfusion) or at the time of collection. Pre-storage leukocyte reduction is more effective than bedside leukocyte reduction, since it is performed in a controlled environment, but it is not yet mandatory in the United States.

Indications

Prevention of HLA alloimmunization is an issue in patients who are anticipated to require multiple transfusions, such as a leukemic patient undergoing induction chemotherapy. The acquisition of HLA alloimmunization is a cause of platelet refractoriness. Prevention of HLA alloimmunization requires $<5 \times 10^6$ white cells/unit.

Febrile, nonhemolytic, transfusion reactions are thought to be largely due to white cells and their secreted cytokines. When a patient is experiencing refractory febrile reactions with every transfusion, filtering to reduce white cells is indicated. This requires a reduction only to 5×10^8 white cells to be effective.

It has been shown that leukoreduction is effective in reducing the risk of transmission of CMV by CMV+ blood products given to CMV– recipients. Nonetheless, it is still considered less effective than transfusion of CMV serologically negative units. This, still somewhat controversial, indication requires a reduction to $<5 \times 10^6$.

Leukoreduction is effective in preventing variant Creutzfeldt-Jakob disease (vCJD). vCJD is detected in high concentration in lymphoid tissue and therefore prestorage leukocyte reduction was mandated in Canada and the United Kingdom to minimize the risk of transfusion transmission. However, there has been insufficient evidence to support leukoreduction as a way to decrease transmission of vCJD.

Leukoreduction is effective in preventing transfusion related immune modulation (TRIM).

Leukoreduction is not effective in preventing transfusion associated graft vs host disease. Only irradiation of cellular products can prevent it.

Washed RBCs

How prepared & stored

RBCs are washed to remove plasma proteins. It is rarely indicated, and it can delay transfusion by hours. RBCs that have been washed represent an open system and expire in 24 hours.

Indications

The primary indication for washed RBCs is the prevention of recurrent or severe allergic reactions, particularly in IgA-deficient recipients who may suffer anaphylactic reactions to transfusion of IgA-containing products. Rarely, washed RBCs may be used in patients suffering recurrent severe febrile nonhemolytic transfusion reactions. Since these reactions are largely due to cytokines, washing can prevent them, though it is usually not be worth the time and expense. Lastly, washed RBCs may be indicated when transfusing neonates with RBCs from a parent or with RBCs bearing ABO incompatible plasma.

Blood substitutes

Many putative hemoglobin substitutes have been studied and found to be limited mainly by their inability to persist in circulation and continue to carry oxygen for a sufficient length of time. Other major problems have included severe toxicities, mainly related to renal toxicity and vasoconstriction, in addition to profound effects on laboratory tests.

Synthetic oxygen carriers

A hemoglobin-based oxygen carrier (HBOC) is a cell-free product derived from hemoglobin, either through purification of human or bovine hemoglobin or from recombinant production. HBOCs offer the advantage of long shelf-life with no concern for compatibility testing. One problem has been toxicity. Hemoglobin tetramers in solution quickly dissociate into free globin chains that

1. are freely filtered by the kidney, reducing their half lives and causing renal damage
2. quickly bind nitric oxide (a natural vasodilator), causing vasoconstriction

Polymerization and "cellular" liposome-enclosure of hemoglobin led to products that were less prone to these toxicities; however, none has yet been approved for use in humans by the FDA. Perfluorocarbons have been investigated as hemoglobin substitutes, but they have significant toxicity.

Blood avoidance strategies

There are a number of strategies that can be employed to reduce the need for allogeneic blood transfusion. At the moment, these are the only real "blood substitute" available.

Autologous blood

As discussed elsewhere in this chapter, autologous blood donation has been used as a means of avoiding allogeneic blood transfusion. It is arguable, though, that autologous donation is of no benefit, given the level of safety that has been achieved with allogeneic blood. Putting aside the higher cost of autologous donation, the practice is associated with a higher rate of postoperative anemia and may actually increase the rate of postoperative transfusion. Since every transfusion, allogeneic or autologous, poses the same deadly risk of patient misidentification, the practice may place autologous donors at higher risk.

Iron supplementation and/or erythropoietin

Autologous transfusion may be avoided by simply repleting iron stores in iron deficient patients. Erythropoietin (EPO), given days to weeks before surgery, has been demonstrated to reduce the need for allogeneic blood transfusion. A significant lag in the onset of action precludes the use of EPO in emergency situations. EPO should always be given with supplemental iron.

Acute normovolemic hemodilution

Acute normovolemic hemodilution (ANH) offers many of the advantages of autologous donation, without the added cost and risk. In ANH, 1 to several units of blood are drawn from the patient intraoperatively, before incision, and replaced with equal volume of crystalloid. The blood is kept, anticoagulated, at the bedside and reinfused within 4 hours.

Intraoperative cell salvage

Intraoperative cell salvage is particularly useful in highly bloody procedures, such as cardiac, vascular, orthopedic surgeries and liver transplantation. In cell salvage, blood that has been suctioned from the surgical field is anticoagulated, washed, filtered and returned to the patient. Cell salvage is contraindicated for patients undergoing surgery for malignancy or bowel contamination of surgical field.

Blood group antigens
ABO & the carbohydrate antigens
ABO, Lewis, H, I & i

ABO and the related carbohydrate antigens (Lewis, H, I, and i) are carbohydrate antigens, in contrast to most relevant RBC antigens that are proteins t2.29. Carbohydrate antigens are affected by genes that encode enzymes, in contrast to protein antigens that are typically the result of genes that encode structural proteins. The carbohydrate antigens are built upon a precursor substance, H antigen. H antigen, in turn, is made from type 1 and type 2 precursor carbohydrate chains. In secretions (saliva, tears) and in plasma, type 1 chains are converted into H antigen by the enzymatic action (fucosylation) of the Se gene product. On the surfaces of RBCs, type 2 chains are converted to H antigen by the enzymatic action (fucosylation) of the H gene product.

t2.29 Comparison of carbohydrate & protein antigens

Carbohydrate antigens	Protein antigens
ABO, Le, I, M, N, P1	All others, including Rh, Kidd, Kell, S, s & Duffy
Naturally-occurring antibodies	Antibodies acquired only after exposure to products containing antigen
Antibodies usually IgM	Antibodies usually IgG
Antibodies usually reactive at room temperature	Antibodies usually reactive at 37°C
"Agglutinating" antibodies	"Coating" antibodies
React at immediate spin (IS)	React at AHG phase

The Lewis antigens result from the complex interplay of Lewis and Secretor genes (see below). Secreted Le^b and type 1 H antigens are receptors for both Norwalk virus and *Helicobacter pylori*. This seems to explain the prevalence of *H pylori*-associated gastric disease among group O secretors. Le^a is the CA 19-9 epitope, a serum and immunohistochemical marker of pancreatobiliary adenocarcinoma.

The genes related to carbohydrate antigens encode specific enzymes (glycosyltransferases) that catalyze the transfer of specific saccharides to specific carbohydrate chains. The *ABO* gene on chromosome 9 is responsible for A, B and O blood groups. The A and B alleles encode enzymes that catalyze addition of saccharide groups to H antigen. When the A gene product (N-acetyl-galactosaminyltransferase) acts enzymatically on the H antigen, resulting in the addition of N-acetyl galactosamine (NAG), the A antigen results. When the B gene product (galactosyltransferase) acts on the H antigen, D-galactose (GAL) is added, and B antigen results. The O allele does not encode a functional enzyme, usually due to a frame shift mutation, and group O RBCs contain abundant unaltered H antigen.

The I and i antigens are epitopes within the ABH antigens. Unbranched type 1 and 2 oligosaccharides represent i antigen. Branched type 1 and 2 oligosaccharides are I antigens. In the neonate, unbranched (i antigen) oligosaccharides predominate; thus, cord blood RBCs are rich in i antigen. The activity of the glycosyltransferase responsible for oligosaccharide branching increases with age. Adults have mostly branched oligosaccharides, thus having little i antigen and much I antigen. In high red-cell turnover states, a resurgence of the i phenotype is sometimes observed; furthermore, retention of i expression is characteristic of congenital dyserythropoietic anemia (CDA) type II (HEMPAS).

ABO phenotypes

The O blood group is the result of inheriting neither A nor B genes, resulting in production of only H antigen. Group O persons have naturally-occurring IgM anti-A and anti-B. They also have IgG anti-AB. The IgG antibody can be the cause of ABO-related hemolytic disease of the newborn, which is typically mild.

The A blood group results from the AA or AO genotype t2.30. Inheritance of A transferases of varying efficiencies results in subgroups of A that differ primarily in the quantity of A antigen on RBCs. There are also small qualitative differences in the A1 and A2 antigen with A1 antigen possessing slightly different chains (type 3 and 4) that are not found on A2 and weaker subgroups of A. The 2 principal subgroups are A1 and A2. A1 cells express more A substance than A2 cells. 80% of blood group A individuals have the A1 phenotype, and most of the remaining 20% are A2. A1 and A2 cells can be distinguished by the strength of their reactions with anti-A1 reagent prepared from the serum of blood group B individuals or with *Dolichos biflorus* lectin which has anti-A1 activity. Clinically significant anti-A1 can be found in the serum of 5% of blood group A2 and 35% of group A2B individuals. The B blood group results from the BB or BO genotype. B subgroups are rare. The AB blood group results from the AB genotype. It is the least frequent ABO phenotype.

t2.30 Distribution of blood groups by ethnicity

Group	White (%)	Black (%)	Hispanic (%)
O	45	50	55
A	40	25	30
B	10	20	10
AB	5	5	3
D+	82	92	92
D−	18	8	8

The Bombay phenotype is so-named because it was initially discovered in people living in Bombay, India. It is extremely rare, even in this demographic, but it has been seen in all populations. When the *h* gene (an amorph) is inherited instead of H, no H substance can be produced in blood (although H can be produced in secretions if the *Se* gene is present), and the person has the Bombay phenotype. Such individuals, who are extremely rare, produce a dangerous anti-H.

The relationship of Le, Se, H, I, i & ABO

There are 2 precursor oligosaccharides: type 1 precursor substance and type 2 precursor substance. Type 1 (historically called Le^c) is unbound and is found in secretions and in plasma, while type 2 is found only on the RBC surface. Unbranched type 1 and 2 oligosaccharides represent i antigen. Branched type 1 and 2 oligosaccharides are I antigens.

The *H* (*FUT1*) gene encodes a fucosyl transferase that adds fucose to type 2 precursor substance on the surfaces of RBCs, to make H antigen (also called 2H antigen, when built upon type 2 precursor). The *h* gene is an amorph; ie, it encodes no functional enzyme. When no further modifications are made on the H antigen, the blood cells are group O. When the A gene product acts on the H antigen, adding N-acetyl galactosamine, the A antigen results. When the B gene product acts on the H antigen to add galactose, the B antigen results. H antigen can be detected by *Ulex europaeus* lectin. The relative amount of H antigen in blood groups is as follows:

$$O \gg A2 > B > A2B > A1 > A1B$$

The *Se* (*FUT2*) gene encodes a fucosyl transferase that adds fucose to type 1 precursor, resulting in H (1H). It acts upon both secretory type 1 precursor and plasma type 1 precursor; thus, it produces the secretion and plasma equivalent of H substance and is responsible for the appearance of A, B, and H substances in secretions. The *se* gene is an amorph. 80% of the population has the *Se* (*FUT2*) gene and are secretors; 20% are homozygous for se/se and are nonsecretors.

The *Le* (*FUT3*) gene encodes a fucosyl transferase enzyme that can do 2 things. First, it can add fucose to type 1 precursor (in a different linkage than that catalyzed by FUT2 [Se]) to make Le^a antigen. Second, it can add fucose to 1H antigen to make Le^b antigen. However, when 1H (the product of Se [FUT2]) is present, *Le* (*FUT3*) prefers it as a substrate over type 1 precursor. Note that Le^a can be made if *Le* (*FUT3*) is present, but Le^b is made only if both the *Se* (*FUT2*) and *Le* (*FUT3*) are present. Put another way, persons with Le(a+b−) phenotype have inherited an *Le* gene but not an *Se* gene. In Le(a−b+) individuals, a minute amount of Le^a is still made, such that anti-Le^a antibodies do not form. Though Lewis antigen is synthesized on free type 1 precursor substance, it becomes passively adsorbed onto RBC surfaces. The Lewis substances are thought to be synthesized in the gut and salivary glands; it is from these origins that plasma Lewis antigen is derived.

Lewis gene expression increases with age, and the Lewis type cannot be reliably determined until the 2nd birthday. Those persons destined to be Le(a−b+) are as neonates Le(a−b−) then Le(a+b−) then Le(a+b+) and finally Le(a−b+). Lewis antigen expression is decreased on RBCs during pregnancy and the Le(a−b−) phenotype is transiently expressed. Lewis phenotype frequencies t2.31 are notable for the presence of Le(a−b−) mainly in blacks and the rarity of Le(a+b+). t2.32 and f2.7 summarize the relationships among ABH, Le, H and Se genotypes and phenotypes.

t2.31 Lewis phenotypes

Phenotype	Whites (%)	Blacks (%)
Le(a−b+)	72	55
Le(a+b−)	22	22
Le(a−b−)	6	23
Le(a+b+)	0	0

t2.32 Lewis & secretor genotypes & phenotypes

Lewis genes	H gene	Secretor genes	ABO genes	RBC phenotype	Substances in saliva
Le	H	*Se*	O	H, Le(a−b+)	H, ↓Le^a, Le^b
le	H	*Se*	O	H, Le(a−b−)	H
Le	H	*se*	O	H, Le(a+b−)	Le^a
le	H	*se*	O	O, Le(a−b−)	None
Le	H	*Se*	A1	A1, Le(a−b+)	↓↓H, A, ↓Le^a, Le^b
le	H	*Se*	A1	A1, Le(a−b−)	↓↓H, A
Le	H	*se*	A1	A1, Le(a+b−)	Le^a
le	H	*se*	A1	A1, Le(a−b−)	None
Le	H	*Se*	B	B, Le(a−b+)	↓H, B, ↓Le^a, Le^b
le	H	*Se*	B	B, Le(a−b−)	↓H, B
Le	H	*se*	B	B, Le(a+b−)	Le^a
le	H	*se*	B	B, Le(a+b−)	None

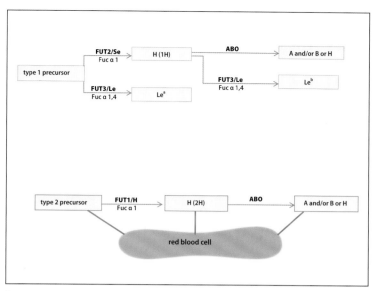

f2.7 H gene product fucosyltransferase (FUT1), secretor gene product (FUT2), Lewis gene product (FUT3) & N-acetylgalactosyltransferase (NAG)

Antibodies

ABO antibodies are naturally occurring (do not require antigen exposure for their formation). They are detectable in infants by 3-6 months of age, but they may not reach adult titers until 2 years old. ABO incompatibility results in complement activation and brisk intravascular hemolysis. Severe reactions can accompany transfusion of incompatible RBCs (so-called major incompatibility) and transfusion of incompatible plasma (minor incompatibility). Anti-H antibodies are usually clinically insignificant, with the exception of the anti-H of Bombay phenotype.

Lewis antibodies are naturally occurring antibodies found almost exclusively in Le(a–b–) individuals who are commonly Black. Le(a–b+) persons do not make anti-Le^a antibodies. Lewis antibodies are nearly always IgM and insignificant. During pregnancy, women can acquire the Le(a–b–) phenotype, and they can develop anti-Le^a or Le^b antibodies. These antibodies cannot harm the baby, since fetal cells do not express Le antigens. The rare significant Lewis antibody is always anti-Le^a. These antibodies are usually inconsequential, because

1. transfused RBCs shed their Lewis antigens and acquire the Lewis phenotype of the recipient and

2. Lewis antibodies are quickly adsorbed by free serum Lewis antigens

Anti-I and anti-i antibodies are autoantibodies that are usually clinically insignificant. They are associated with infections. Anti-I antibodies are associated with *Mycoplasma pneumoniae* infections and anti-i antibodies are associated with Epstein-Barr viral infections.

P/GLOB blood group

Antigens & phenotypes

The P blood group consists of the antigen P1. The antigens P (globoside), Pk, and LKE have been reclassified into the globo-antigen (GLOB) group. The P antigen serves as the receptor for parvovirus B19 (fifth disease); P– persons are relatively resistant to B19 infection. The P group phenotypes are defined by reactivity with the antibodies anti-P1, anti-P, anti-Pk, and anti-PP1Pk which reacts with the whole P complex of antigens.

80% of whites and 95% of blacks have the P1 phenotype and demonstrate reactivity with these antisera: anti-P1+, P+, Pk– and PP1Pk+. ~20% of whites and 5% of blacks have the P2 phenotype and demonstrate reactivity with these antisera: anti-P1–, P+, Pk–, PP1Pk+. The rare p phenotype is characterized by absence of P antigens (anti-P1–, P–, PP1Pk– and Pk–).

Antibodies

Individuals with p phenotype make a potent anti-PP1Pk. This antibody can be broken into its 3 component antibodies through adsorptions. Anti-PP1Pk may be associated with delayed hemolytic transfusion reaction and hemolytic disease of the newborn. There is also an association between both anti-P1 and anti-PP1Pk antibodies and first trimester spontaneous abortion.

Antibodies to P antigens are most commonly anti-P1, produced by P2 phenotype individuals. These are usually IgM anti-P1 that are reactive at 4°C and are not clinically significant. Anti-P1 can be agglutinated by hydatid cyst fluid and by egg whites from pigeon eggs and turtledove eggs.

The P antigen is the target of antibodies in paroxysmal cold hemoglobinuria (PCH). Auto-anti-P IgG antibodies act as a biphasic hemolysin. The cold reacting IgG anti-P binds as blood passes through the cool (acral) portions of the body and activates complement, leading to hemolysis upon recirculation to the warm core of the patient. This antibody is not usually detected in routine antibody screens, but can be detected with the Donath-Landsteiner test.

Rh

Rh antigens & phenotypes

Rh antigens are polypeptide antigens encoded by closely linked gene loci C, D, and E. *RHD* and *RHCE* gene loci are found on chromosome 1. The *RHAG* gene which encodes the Rh associated glycoprotein (RhAG) is found on chromosome 6. The polypeptides produced from *RHD* and *RHCE* genes form a large complex on the RBC membrane with the Rh associated glycoprotein; furthermore, several additional proteins associate with the Rh complex, including LW and Duffy (Fy5).

The size and intricacy of the Rh complex result in a multitude of epitopes and antigens composed of compound epitopes; for example, RBCs that bear c and e are antigenic for c, e, and the compound antigen ce (also called f or RH6). Furthermore, C, D, and E are "multi-pass" proteins with several extracellular domains—the D antigen is composed of several amino acids from different extracellular domains, creating the possibility of "partial D" phenotypes.

The most common Rh– genotype, in both blacks and whites, is r/r (cde/cde) t2.33. Overall, ~10-15% of blood donors are Rh–. The highest incidence of Rh negativity is found in the Basques (25%), a phylogenetically ancient population found on the border of France and Spain. The most common Rh+ genotype (Weiner nomenclature) is R1/R1 or R1/r in whites and R0/R0 or R0/r in blacks. R0 is uncommon in whites. The prevalence of R0 in blacks and R1 in whites explains the high likelihood of black Rh+ recipients developing anti-C. Furthermore, the prevalence of r/r in Rh– blood explains why recipients with anti-c or anti-e should not be given Rh– blood.

t2.33 Rh nomenclature & incidence

Weiner	Antigens	White (%)	Black (%)
R1	DCe	40	15
R2	DcE	10	10
R0	Dce	5	45
Rz	DCE	rare*	rare
r'	dCe	3	3
r"	dcE	2	rare
r	dce	40	30
ry	dCE	rare	rare

6% of Native Americans

The D– phenotype, while sometimes written as "d," merely denotes the absence of the D antigen. There is no d antigen. D negativity results from a gene deletion in most cases; however, in about half of D– blacks an altered *RHD* gene is inherited which is a noncoding pseudogene called *RHD*Ψ. In these individuals the D polypeptide never reaches the RBC surface.

Rh null individuals have no Rh antigens (no Rh or RhAG). The absence of the Rh complex results in diminished expression of LW, Fy5, S, s, and U. RBCs lacking Rh/RhAG proteins have structural abnormalities. This results in enhanced osmotic fragility, chronic hemolysis, and stomatocytosis. Patients who have Rh null should only receive Rh null RBCs. If they receive Rh– RBCs they will form an anti-total Rh antibody (anti-Rh29).

Weak expression of D was formerly called Du antigen, a term no longer used. Patients with weak D possess the D antigen, only in smaller quantities; therefore, they do not form an anti-D antibody. Weak expression of D antigen is defined historically by weak reactivity with anti-D reagent, typified by the following reactions

1. negative at IS with anti-D reagent

2. negative after 37°C incubation with anti-D reagent

3. positive at AHG phase with anti-D reagent

Modern monoclonal anti-D reagents can detect most weak D RBCs at the IS phase, such that weak D cells simply looks like typical D+ cells. Decreased quantity of D may come about in several ways. One is an alteration in the nonepitope sequence of the *D* gene that results in reduced D transport to or insertion into the cell membrane. A less common form of weak D is that relating to the position effect. In persons with the Dce/Ce genotype, there is weakened D antigen expression due to the presence of the C allele situated trans (on the other homologous chromosome) to D (the Ceppelli effect). The C allele in the trans position has a suppressive effect on the D antigen on the opposite chromosome. Currently available reagents detect weak D expression as normal expression of D, and this is largely of historical interest.

Partial D is the term used for alterations in one of the epitope sequences of the *D* gene, resulting in a D antigen with some, but not all, epitopes. In the past, this was referred to as "D mosaic" or "D variant." Partial D phenotypes can be defined in terms of their D epitopes. Over 30 have been described. The importance of this is that persons with partial D are capable of making alloantibody against the D epitopes they lack, and partial D women are at risk for forming anti-D antibodies with D+ pregnancies. For this reason, partial D female recipients should be treated as D–. In fact, partial D is frequently identified because of an apparent discrepancy—the coexistence of D expression and anti-D antibodies.

About 1-2% of individuals from European ethnicity carry RHD alleles for weak D or partial D phenotypes, but the frequency is higher in those of African descent. Transfusion of weak or partial D cells into D– recipients can cause sensitization, which is most important to avoid in women of childbearing years. Therefore, AABB Standards require that donor samples be tested for weak D and labeled D+ if found. The recipient need not be tested for weak D.

Rh antibodies

Rh antibodies are IgG antibodies that are acquired through exposure, unlike the naturally occurring ABO antibodies. D antigen is the most immunogenic of all the non-ABO antigens. Historically, the rate of development of anti-D in D– individuals exposed to a single D+ unit was reported as 80%. More recently, in a study of transfusion in emergency settings, this rate was reported as nearer to 30%. This may be due to the release of endogenous steroids in trauma settings decreasing the rate of sensitization.

All Rh antibodies except anti-D display dosage. This refers to an antibody that reacts more strongly with RBCs homozygous for an antigen (such as CC or EE) than with RBCs heterozygous for the antigen (such as Cc or Ee). All Rh antigens are enhanced by enzymes. This means that the test RBCs react more strongly with the patient's serum in vitro after treatment with enzymes such as ficin or papain. Rh antibodies may result in HTR with extravascular hemolysis and a severe form of hemolytic disease of the fetus or newborn (HDFN).

If anti-E is detected in the serum, then the additional presence of anti-c should be suspected. This is because most individuals who have anti-E have the R1R1 phenotype (CDe/CDe), and have been transfused with R2 blood, which has the phenotype cDE. Such individuals develop anti-E and too-weak to detect anti-c as well. Anti-c is a common cause of delayed hemolytic transfusion reactions (DHTR). It is common practice to select c– and E– blood for recipients with anti-E.

G antigen is found on all D+ RBCs and most C+ RBCs. Clinically, Anti-G antibodies mimic anti-D and anti-C antibodies; however, multiple absorption and elution studies are performed using D–C+e (r') and D+C–E+(R2) RBCs to distinguish anti-G from anti-D and anti-C antibodies. Transfuse patients who have anti-G antibodies with D–C– RBCs. In pregnant women, it is important to distinguish between anti-D, anti-C antibodies and anti-G antibody since they will need RhIg to prevent formation of anti-D antibodies for future pregnancies.

Anti-f (antibody against the compound antigen ce) is the most common alloantibody directed against compound Rh antigens. It is found primarily in persons with DCe/DcE (R1R2).

Kidd blood group system

Kidd antigens

Race has a major impact on Kidd antigen frequencies t2.34. The Jk^b− phenotype is twice as common in blacks as whites. The Jk(a−b−) phenotype is rare, being encountered primarily in Finns and Polynesians.

Kidd is a urea transport protein; Jk(a−b−) cells are resistant to hemolysis in 2M urea. Individuals with this phenotype have a mild urine concentrating defect.

t2.34 Kidd phenotypes

Phenotype	Whites (%)	Blacks (%)
Jk(a+b−)	30	60
Jk(a+b+)	50	30
Jk(a−b+)	20	10
Jk(a−b−)	rare	rare

Kidd antibodies

Kidd antibodies are warm reacting IgG antibodies that are acquired only through exposure. Kidd antibodies are clinically significant. They are common causes of transfusion reactions, both immediate and delayed, and both intravascular and extravascular. Kidd antibodies are notorious for being difficult to detect ("tricky Kidd") for many reasons, not the least of which is that they tend to fall below the threshold of detection over time. A strong antibody may be detected today that is undetectable in a few months. This is one of the main reasons to check blood bank records prior to transfusion. Historical Kidd antibodies, despite the absence of currently detectable antibody, is reason enough to give Kidd antigen-negative blood. Lastly, Kidd antibodies do not store well (eg, when serum is sent to a reference lab).

Kidd antibodies display dosage; that is, RBCs from homozygous [Jk^{a}Jk^a or Jk(a+b−)] individuals express more antigen than heterozygous [Jk^{a}Jk^b or Jk(a+b+)] individuals. Among the test cells in a panel some RBCs may be homozygous and others heterozygous. Kidd antibody may only react with homozygous cells. In addition, dosage effect may result in a false-negative crossmatch. Type all crossmatch compatible units with commercial antisera to make sure they are antigen negative. Kidd antibodies most often react only at the AHG phase, and Kidd antigens are enhanced by enzymes.

Clinically, Kidd antibodies are a common cause of immediate HTRs. They are capable of binding complement and can produce intravascular hemolysis, but most often they produce acute extravascular hemolysis. Furthermore, Kidd antibodies are the most common cause of DHTRs. Kidd antibodies very rarely cause hemolytic HDFN due to weak antigen expression by the fetus and neonate.

Duffy

Duffy antigens

2 antigens, Fy^a and Fy^b, comprise the Duffy system. Duffy antigens are present on DARC (Duffy-associated receptor for chemokines), which is also a receptor for *Plasmodium vivax*. Note that Duffy is expressed on multiple tissue types in addition to erythrocytes. 2 additional epitopes, Fy3 and Fy5, are high-incidence antigenic components of DARC. Fy5 expression depends upon the presence of the Rh complex.

Fy(a+b−) is more common than Fy(a−b+). Fy(a−b−) is rare in whites, but common in blacks (68%). This phenotype confers resistance to *Plasmodium vivax* malaria. Of some clinical significance is the differing mechanisms of Duffy negativity in whites and blacks. In blacks, there is a mutation in the RBC-specific DARC promoter region. This mutation disrupts the binding site for the GATA-1 transcription factor and therefore prevents the expression of the Duffy antigens on erythroid cells; however, expression of Duffy antigens on other tissues is unaffected. Therefore, most Fy(a−b−) blacks do not form anti-Fy antibodies. In contrast, loss of Duffy in whites is caused by a mutation in the *DARC* gene that affects all tissues equally; thus, Fy(a−b−) whites can, and do, form antibodies.

Duffy antibodies

Duffy antibodies are warm reacting IgG antibodies acquired through exposure. Duffy antibodies show dosage effect, and Duffy antigens are destroyed by enzymes. Duffy antibodies are capable of causing HTR, with extravascular hemolysis, and severe HDFN.

MNS system

MNS antigens

MNS antigens are found on RBC surface glycophorin A and glycophorin B molecules. The antigens M and N reside on glycophorin A. ~25% of the population is M+N−, 25% is M−N+, and 50% is M+N+. The M−N− phenotype is rare.

The S, s, and U antigens reside on glycophorin B. Both s and U are high frequency antigens, present in 98% and nearly 100% of the population, respectively. S is more variable, being present in 50% of whites and 30% of blacks. It may be very difficult to find compatible blood for rare S-s-U-negative recipients, who are usually black.

The MN and SsU genes display genetic linkage. The most frequent haplotypes are Ns and Ms.

MNS antibodies

MNS antibodies display dosage, and M and N antigenicity is destroyed by enzymes.

Anti-M antibodies are naturally occurring, cold reacting, IgM antibodies that are clinically insignificant. Because an epitope on glycophorin B usually has N-like antigenicity, anti-N antibodies are rare. Anti-M or N antibodies reactive at 37°C are capable of causing acute or delayed hemolytic transfusion reactions and there are case reports of some anti-M antibodies responsible for severe HDFN.

Anti-N is usually a cold reacting antibody. Anti-Nf antibodies may be formed in dialysis patients who were exposed to formaldehyde used in cleaning dialysis machines and induced formation of Nf antigen on RBCs.

Anti-S, anti-s, and anti-U antibodies are acquired following exposure and are warm reacting IgG antibodies that are clinically significant.

Kell blood group

Kell antigens

The Kell group includes the antigens K, k, Kp^a, Kp^b, Js^a, and Js^b. Kell antigens are expressed on mature RBCs and erythroid precursors; thus, alloantibodies are capable of suppressing erythropoiesis. The Kell antigens are expressed in covalent association with the Kx antigen, encoded by the *XK* gene. The *XK* gene is on the X chromosome, and the *KEL* gene is on chromosome 7.

The k antigen (also called Cellano or KEL2), Kp^b, and Js^b are high-frequency antigens, each present in 99% of donors. K (KEL1), Kp^a and Js^a are present in 9%, 2% and 0.1% of Caucasian donors, respectively.

Kell antigens are unaffected by enzymes (neither enhanced nor destroyed) but are reliant on disulfide bonds and therefore destroyed by ZZAP and DTT.

The McLeod phenotype t2.35 results from mutations in the Kx-encoding (*XK*) gene; it is an X-linked recessive disorder. Affected RBCs express Kell antigens very weakly. Lack of this Kx protein depresses the expression of Kell antigens and is associated with shortened RBC survival, reduced deformability, hemolytic anemia, acanthocytosis, elevated serum creatine kinase and various muscular and neurological defects. This phenotype is frequently associated with coexisting chronic granulomatous disease (CGD), a late-onset type of muscular dystrophy ("neuro-acanthocytosis"), and retinitis pigmentosa. Note that patients with McLeod phenotype would be incompatible with both normal and Kell null blood (which expresses plenty of Kx antigen).

The Kell null phenotype results from homozygous inheritance of the amorph K$_0$, such that RBCs have no Kell antigens but an abundance of Kx.

Kell antibodies

Most commonly these are anti-K and are acquired through exposure. They are warm reacting IgG antibodies. Kell antigen expression is diminished by agents that dissolve sulfhydryl bonds; thus, they are very sensitive to 2-mercaptoethanol (2-ME), ZZAP, and dithiothrietol (DTT). Kell antibodies are associated with HTRs with extravascular hemolysis and hemolytic disease of the fetus and newborn (HDFN). Kell related HDFN is characterized by suppression of erythropoiesis.

Lutheran

Lutheran antigens

Lu^b is a high-incidence antigen, present in 99% of the population. Lu^a is present in 7% of the population. Thus, ~93% of people are Lu(a-b+), and ~7% are Lu(a+b+). Lutheran antigens are destroyed by enzymes and destroyed by 2-ME and DTT. Lutheran antigen expression is increased on the surface of sickle cells.

Lutheran antibodies

Lutheran antibodies usually have anti-Lu^a specificity and are usually clinically insignificant cold reacting IgM antibodies. Mixed-field reactions are a typical feature. When a significant warm reacting IgG is identified, compatible blood is relatively easy to find.

t2.35 RBC antigen associations

Phenotype or antibody	Association
Fy(a-b-)	Duffy antigen is the receptor for P vivax Duffy- confers resistance to P vivax & is more common in blacks
McLeod	Chronic granulomatous disease Acanthocytosis Late onset muscular dystrophy-like syndrome, lab values: elevated creatine kinase (CK)
Anti-P1	Paroxysmal cold hemoglobinuria (PCH), viral infections in children, syphilis
Anti-I	*Mycoplasma pneumoniae* infection, lymphomas
Anti-i	EBV infection (infectious mononucleosis)
Anti-Nf	Renal dialysis
Acquired B phenotype	Colorectal carcinoma Intestinal obstruction Gram- sepsis
Rh null	Hereditary stomatocytosis (HS)
Diego negative	Diego is an epitope on band 3 protein; Band 3 deficiency causes some cases of HS, acanthocytosis & hereditary elliptocytosis (HE)
Gerbich negative (Leach phenotype)	Gerbich is an epitope on glycophorin C; a cause of HE

Human leukocyte antigens (HLA)

HLA is encoded on the major histocompatibility complex (MHC), a complex of several gene loci found on chromosome 6p. The loci are closely linked and inherited en bloc from each parent, with little to no crossing over. Each locus has a multitude of possible alleles distributed through the population, making HLA genes the most polymorphic in the human genome.

The MHC encodes MHC class I, class II, and class III proteins. Class III genes encode complement proteins. Also embedded in the MHC region are the *HHF* gene (hemochromatosis), the 21-hydroxylase gene, and the gene for tumor necrosis factor (TNF). Class I genes encode HLA class I antigens that are found on the surfaces of all nucleated cells and platelets.

Class I genes are distributed among 3 loci, termed HLA-A, HLA-B, and HLA-C. For each locus there are several possible alleles, termed, eg, HLA-A1, HLA-A2. Class I genes encode a single polypeptide chain that has 3 domains very similar to the domains of an immunoglobulin heavy chain, in addition to a transmembrane domain. The class I molecules are embedded as a transmembrane protein in the cell membrane, and each is noncovalently associated with a single molecule of α_2-microglobulin. All nucleated cells have MHC class I antigens. RBCs progressively lose class I MHC antigens as they age, such that mature RBCs have very little class I antigen expression. The exception is a group of residual HLA class I antigens collectively referred to as Bg (Bennett-Goodspeed) antigens, which are rarely the cause of alloantibody-mediated hemolytic transfusion reactions. The 3 major Bg antigens are Bga (HLA-B7), Bgb (HLA-B17), and Bgc (HLA-A28/A2).

Platelets have generous amounts of class I antigens, particularly HLA-A and HLA-B antigens.

Class II genes encode HLA class II antigens that are found on 3 cell types: B cells, macrophages, and dendritic cells. Class II genes are distributed among 3 loci, termed HLA-DR, HLA-DP, and HLA-DQ. For each locus, there are several possible alleles, termed, eg, HLA-DR3, HLA-Dw2. The class II genes encode 2 polypeptide chains, α and β, each with 2 domains similar to the immunoglobulin light chains, in addition to a transmembrane domain. Class II antigens are expressed on neither RBCs nor platelets.

HLA plays a small role in RBC compatibility, but it is pivotal in platelet refractoriness, solid-organ compatibility, and some transfusion reactions (febrile nonhemolytic reactions, transfusion related acute lung injury [TRALI], and TA-GVHD).

Since each MHC complex is closely linked and inherited en bloc, each parental chromosome can be thought of as a haplotype. One haplotype in inherited from each parent. Thus, the chance that 2 siblings are HLA-identical is 25%. The chance of having an HLA-identical sibling goes up with the number of siblings: with 1 sibling, the chance is 25%, with 2 it is around 45%, and with 3 it is nearly 60%.

Some hard to remember antigen/ antibody facts

- Naturally occurring antibodies: I, i, ABO, Le, Lu, M, N, P.

- Antigens that display dosage: MNS, Kidd, C/c, E/e, Duffy.

- Antibodies that react at room temperature: Anti-M, N, P1, Le^a, and Le^b.

- Antibodies that are nearly always clinically insignificant: Anti-M, N, P1, Lewis, Lutheran, and I.

- The 4 most common antibodies implicated in immediate HTR: anti-A, anti-Kell, anti-Jk^a, and anti-Fy^a.

- The 4 most common antibodies implicated in delayed HTR: anti-Jk^a, anti-E, anti-D, anti-C.

- The 4 most common antibodies implicated in HDFN: anti-AB, anti-D, anti-Kell, anti-c.

- Antigens that are enhanced by enzymes: AB, I/i, P1, Le, Rh, Kidd.

- Antigens that are destroyed by enzymes: MNSs, Fy^a, Fy^b, Lutheran, Chido.

- Mixed field reactions are expected with: Lutheran, Sid, A3, (and post-bone marrow transplant).

- Antibodies that commonly produce intravascular hemolysis: ABO, Kidd, P (paroxysmal cold hemoglobinuria).

Transfusion complications
Suspected transfusion reaction
Clinical signs & symptoms

A transfusion reaction is suspected whenever the patient experiences unusual signs or symptoms temporally related to transfusion. Procedures should delineate which signs and symptoms should prompt suspicion of a transfusion reaction and under what circumstances a transfusion should be stopped and a work-up initiated.

What to do

1. *Stop the transfusion.*

2. *Leave IV open.* The intravenous line should be left open with a saline infusion.

3. *Notify physician.* The treating physician must evaluate the patient, provide supportive care, and determine whether to proceed with a transfusion reaction workup. If the reaction consists solely of a mild allergic reaction or mild circulatory overload, then the transfusion may be re-started and the reaction need not be reported to the laboratory. If a transfusion reaction workup t2.36 is initiated, then further transfusions should ideally await its completion.

t2.36 Transfusion reaction workup

Clerical check	Paperwork & bag check to detect obvious clerical errors; the most common cause of severe hemolytic transfusion reaction is clerical error
Inspection for hemolysis	Check patient serum/plasma for hemolysis (visually) & check urine for hemoglobin (dipstick)
	Blood drawn too late after the event (>8 hours) may be negative visually for significant hemolysis but may be icteric; in this event, a serum bilirubin will be elevated for up to 24-36 hours
	Free serum myoglobin may give a false positive visual inspection; in this event there should be a clinical history of severe trauma
	If a urine dipstick is positive, then examine the urine microscopically for hematuria; in an intravascular hemolytic transfusion reaction, there is hemoglobinuria without hematuria; myoglobinuria is another cause of a false positive urine dipstick
Recheck ABO	Repeat the recipient ABO group determination on a posttransfusion sample
DAT	Perform a direct antiglobulin test (DAT) & compare results to a pretransfusion sample; in a hemolytic transfusion reaction, the DAT is usually positive due to the presence of antibody on transfused RBCs
	If the hemolysis was quite severe, the DAT may be negative due to acute destruction of transfused cells

4. *Transfusion service physician review.* A physician from the transfusion service must review the workup and determine the nature of the reaction and whether additional testing is required. If the reaction is deemed to be nonhemolytic, then additional transfusions can be administered with crossmatch compatible blood. If, on the other hand, there is evidence of hemolysis, then additional workup, including repeat ABO and Rh typing and tests similar to the pretransfusion antibody panel must be carried out to identify the responsible antibody. Then antigen-negative, crossmatch compatible blood can be given for transfusion.

5. *Notification.* When a transfusion fatality or transfusion related serious morbidity occurs, this must be reported within 24 hours by telephone to the FDA and within 7 days in writing. When a transfusion fatality or transfusion related serious morbidity occurs that appears to be related to a single donor, then the collecting facility must be notified immediately, followed and by notification in writing. When a transfusion related infection is confirmed or cannot be excluded, then the identity of the donor units must be conveyed to the collecting facility, any other recipients of blood components from the donor, and the recipient's physician.

6. *Written report by transfusion service physician.* Lastly, a written report should be entered into the chart. This should include an interpretation of the transfusion reaction workup (ie, what is the nature of the transfusion reaction, if any) and a recommendation regarding further transfusion.

Febrile, nonhemolytic transfusion reactions (FNHTR)

This is the most common type of transfusion reaction, with an incidence of around 1 in 200 transfusions, and is defined as an increase in temperature of 1°C or 2° F with no other explanation (such as hemolytic transfusion reaction, bacterial contamination of the unit, or concurrent infection). Therefore, it is essentially a diagnosis of exclusion. The fever is often accompanied by rigors and tachycardia, but hypotension is not a typical feature of febrile reactions.

FNHTR is likely mediated by cytokines released by white blood cells in the stored unit of blood. This theory is supported by the observation that the incidence of febrile reactions can be reduced by prestorage leukoreduction or post-storage washing of cellular blood products prior to transfusion. Washing cellular blood products may be considered in patient with recurrent or severe FNHTR. FNHTR can be diminished by prestorage leukocyte reduction.

Treatment is as for any suspected transfusion reaction; the transfusion must be stopped and not restarted. The usual transfusion reaction workup is completed. In a patient with repeated FNHTR, pretreatment with antipyretics and/ or transfusion with leukocyte reduced products is recommended. Prevention may be possible with prestorage leukocyte reduction or washed blood products.

Allergic transfusion reactions

These range from mild reactions with urticaria (hives) and pruritus to severe, life threatening, anaphylactic reactions. The incidence of allergic transfusions reactions, most of which are mild, is ~1:300 transfusions.

Etiologically, allergic reactions are related to plasma proteins to which the recipient is allergic. In the classic scenario with anaphylaxis, the recipient may be IgA-deficient and has a reaction to IgA in the donor plasma. IgA deficiency affects around 1 in 700 recipients, but only a minority of these patients will react adversely to IgA exposure. Furthermore, a normal total serum IgA does not exclude the possibility of IgA subclass deficiency.

Clinical findings depend on the severity and range from trivial reactions with pruritus to severe, life threatening anaphylactic reactions with hemodynamic collapse. Usually there are no findings on the transfusion reaction workup.

Treatment, as usual, begins with stopping the transfusion. For mild and focal urticarial reactions, administer antihistamines and, if symptoms remit, then the transfusion can be restarted within 30 minutes. A slower rate of infusion may ameliorate some reactions. Transfusion should not be restarted if there is a generalized urticarial reaction or upper airway involvement (perioral or laryngeal). The reaction is unlikely to be repeated with subsequent transfusions.

For anaphylaxis, parenteral epinephrine is indicated. In the usual IgA-deficient scenario, either washed or IgA-deficient blood or platelets must be given. For plasma, only that obtained from IgA-deficient donors can be used.

Acute HTRs

This is among the most feared transfusion reactions and may be fatal. The incidence is thought to be between 1/6,000 and 1/30,000 transfusions [2.38]. HTRs may be acute or delayed, intravascular or extravascular. It is the acute intravascular type that is very dangerous, and this is nearly always related to ABO incompatibility that most often results from clerical error. Rarely, non-ABO antibodies, most notoriously Kidd, may be responsible for acute intravascular hemolytic reactions. Most commonly, though, non-ABO alloantibodies are associated with either acute extravascular hemolysis or delayed extravascular hemolysis. These latter reactions are also called DHTRs. There are really no examples of delayed intravascular hemolysis.

Importantly, not all hemolysis is immune-mediated. Nonimmune hemolysis may be due to prolonged storage, storage at inappropriate temperatures, the use of mechanical devices to infuse blood, blood warmers, needles of too small caliber, or the addition of anything other than normal saline to the infusion. In addition, bacterial contamination of the product, particularly with *Clostridia* species, may cause hemolysis. Lastly, the donor may have an unrecognized intrinsic RBC defect causing hemolysis.

Clinically, intravascular hemolysis is accompanied by fever, chills, back pain, pain at infusion site, hypotension, and DIC. Extravascular hemolysis is often asymptomatic or may present with pallor or hyperbilirubinemia. Laboratory findings may include a positive DAT (both intra- and extravascular hemolysis), pink serum (intravascular hemolysis), hyperbilirubinemia (extravascular hemolysis), hemoglobinuria (intravascular hemolysis), coagulation abnormalities (intravascular hemolysis), schistocytes (intravascular hemolysis), and/or spherocytes (extravascular hemolysis).

Treatment begins with stopping the transfusion, leaving the line open with a saline infusion. Support the patient hemodynamically. Also note that fatalities related to blood transfusion must be reported to the FDA as soon as possible by phone and in writing within 7 days.

DHTR & delayed serologic transfusion reaction (DSTR)

DHTR presents as progressive anemia, with or without fever and jaundice, occurring days to weeks after transfusion. DSTR presents as a newly detectable alloantibody following transfusion, without hemolysis. DSTR is more common than DHTR by ~3:1. The overall incidence of DHTR/DSTR is around 1 in 1500 transfusions.

Historically, alloantibodies directed against Kidd (especially anti-Jk^a) accounted for 1 in 3 cases of DHTR/DSTR. In a recent study of cases at the Mayo Clinic, Rh antigens (especially anti-E) were more commonly implicated than Kidd. Commonly, multiple specificities are found. The vast majority of cases are related to Kidd, E, c, Kell, and Duffy.

Onset is typically between 5 and 14 days after transfusion. The presentation varies from symptomatic anemia to an inadequate increase in hematocrit to serologic findings only. Findings include a positive DAT (often with a mixed field reaction), icteric serum, anemia, spherocytosis, and absence of free hemoglobin (extravascular hemolysis). Some cases are not associated with hemolysis and present only as the finding of a new alloantibody or positive DAT; such reactions are called DSTRs.

Usually no treatment is indicated except to identify the responsible antibody and avoid further exposure to it.

Bacterial contamination

Transfusion transmitted bacterial infection (septic transfusion reaction) is now considered the most common cause of transfusion related fatality in the United States. It is by far the most common transfusion transmitted infection. It is estimated that between 1/1,000 and 1/4,000 units are contaminated, but the incidence of septic transfusion reaction is much lower: 1/25,000 platelet transfusions and 1/250,000 RBC transfusions.

The bacteria are thought to originate primarily from donor skin; less commonly, donor blood is the source (transient bacteremia). Bacterial proliferation is most often a problem with platelets that are stored at room temperature, but cold-stored products (containing psychrophilic organisms) can also transmit bacteria. Platelets are most likely to be associated with infection by Gram+ cocci. Mortality rates with platelet derived sepsis is around 25%. With RBCs, the most commonly implicated organisms are psychrophilic Gram− bacilli, especially *Yersinia enterocolitica, Serratia liquifaciens, Citrobacter* and *Pseudomonas* species. Mortality rates are much higher with RBC derived sepsis, approaching 70%.

Clinically, bacterial contamination is suspected whenever the transfusion recipient experiences high fever and shock. Of course, a hemolytic reaction is also considered in this scenario and must be excluded. Bacterial contamination is equally grave, however. Upon inspection, the blood product may be visibly discolored, hemolyzed, or contain clots, all evidence of bacterial contamination. Generally, the patient's serum and urine will contain free hemoglobin, but the DAT is negative.

Treatment begins with stopping the transfusion. Administer broad spectrum antibiotics, and provide hemodynamic support. A Gram stain, though of low yield, must be performed on the unit of blood, and the blood product must be cultured.

The recipient's blood should also be cultured. The blood supplier must be notified. Prevention includes methods to detect bacterial contamination and efforts to reduce bacterial contamination.

The AABB requires that the blood bank have methods to limit and detect bacterial contamination in platelet components. Methods to limit bacterial contamination include attention to donor history, scrupulous cleansing of the donor venipuncture site, and discarding the first (15-30 cc of) blood drawn into a diversion pouch. In addition, there is some evidence that preferential use of apheresis platelets may reduce the risk.

The blood bank must have a methods to detect bacterial contamination. Several methods are available, including culture, microscopy, immunoassay, flow cytometry, and nucleic acid tests. The most commonly used method is culture, in which units are sampled early and cultures are incubated for the shelf-life of the unit; platelets are released if culture is "negative to date." Several rapid culture systems are commercially available, which detect bacteria through measurement of CO_2 emission or O_2 consumption. Limitations include the failure to detect slow growing organisms, with the frequent occurrence of cultures turning positive after the unit has been administered. Metabolic detection systems, including monitoring of pH, are relatively insensitive and must be applied in a late-sampling strategy. More sensitive applications to a late-sampling strategy include flow cytometry, nucleic acid tests (NAT), and immunoassay. NAT, using PCR, is attractive because a single primer, for bacterial 16S ribosomal RNA, is sensitive to all bacteria; however, turnaround time is slow, and infrastructural demands are high.

TA-GVHD

TA-GVHD is a highly (>90%) fatal complication of transfusion of cellular blood products. Etiologically, immunocompetent T lymphocytes from the donor engraft in the immunocompromised recipient, permitting HLA-guided reactions between donor lymphocytes and recipient tissues. A peculiarity of this reaction is that in order for the donor cells to survive the recipient's defenses, the recipient must be immunocompromised or the donor white cells must be compatible with the recipient (while the recipient is not compatible with the donor). This latter circumstance arises in the case of HLA-similar individuals. As a very simplified example, if the donor is homozygous HLA-A1/HLA-A1 and the recipient is heterozygous HLA-A1/HLA-A2, then the recipient is not able to recognize the donor cells as foreign, while the donor does recognize the recipient tissues as foreign.

TA-GVHD presents with the classic tetrad of dermatitis (periauricular, palmar and plantar erythroderma), enterocolitis (watery diarrhea), hepatitis (aminotransferase elevation), and bone marrow suppression (pancytopenia).

Preventive measures should be directed at those at risk for TA-GVHD, including

1. transplant recipients

2. patient with hematologic malignancies

3. intrauterine transfusion recipients and infants with prematurity, low birth weight, or hemolytic disease of the newborn

4. patients with congenital or T cell immunodeficiency, eg, Wiskott-Aldrich

5. recipients of granulocyte concentrates

6. patients receiving nucleoside analogs

7. recipients of donations from related donors

Irradiation of blood products renders white cells incapable of proliferation. All cellular blood products (FFP has not been implicated in TA-GVHD) transfused among relatives must be irradiated, even if the recipient is immunocompetent. The dose required by the AABB Standards is 2,500 cGy to the center of the bag and a minimum of 1,500 cGy to any part of the bag. Leukoreduction has no role in prevention of TA-GVHD, and irradiation has no role in preventing CMV transmission.

There is no effective treatment and most cases are fatal, therefore the emphasis is placed on prevention.

Transfusion related acute lung injury (TRALI)

TRALI is noncardiac pulmonary edema that follows transfusion of plasma containing blood products. The incidence is estimated at 1/5,000 transfusions. It is the cause of ~15% of fatal transfusion reactions, with a 5-10% mortality overall. There is no readily available test that confirms the diagnosis of TRALI. Furthermore, there is no universally accepted definition. Criteria have been proposed t2.37.

t2.37 Criteria for the diagnosis of TRALI

Acute onset during or within 6 hours of transfusion
Hypoxemia (eg, PaO$_2$:FiO$_2$ ratio <300 or O$_2$ saturation <90% on room air)
Bilateral pulmonary infiltrates on chest x-ray
No preexisting acute lung injury, no competing risk factors for acute lung injury & no evidence of circulatory overload (eg, elevated pulmonary arterial wedge pressure)

Regarding etiology, the leading hypothesis is that donor antibodies against granulocytes or HLA class I/II antigens react with recipient granulocytes to produce white cell microaggregates in the pulmonary circulation. While TRALI is possible in any recipient, 2 groups seem to be at increased risk: patients undergoing induction therapy for hematologic malignancies and patients undergoing cardiac bypass surgery. Furthermore, it appears that both multiparous donors and prolonged blood storage raise the likelihood of TRALI. Plasma containing blood components pose the greatest risk, with platelet concentrates and plasma being the most commonly implicated since they contain the HLA antibodies.

The presentation consists of tachypnea, cyanosis, dyspnea, fever (1°C or more increase), hypoxemia, and diffuse bilateral fluffy infiltrates on chest x-ray (resembling pulmonary edema). TRALI presents within 6 hours of transfusion, but most cases present during or just after transfusion. The differential diagnosis in a patient with pulmonary insufficiency following transfusion includes volume overload (transfusion associated circulatory overload [TACO]), anaphylaxis, bacterial contamination, hemolytic transfusion reaction, and acute respiratory distress syndrome (ARDS). Volume overload typically presents within minutes to hours of transfusion and responds just as rapidly to diuresis. The B-type natriuretic peptide (BNP) is elevated in volume overload. Anaphylactic reactions are often characterized by wheezing, edema of the face and trunk, and urticaria, respond rapidly to epinephrine, and usually do not produce lung opacity. Serum tryptase may be elevated following anaphylactic reactions. Transfusion related sepsis manifests as pronounced fever and vascular collapse, with or without and usually out of proportion to respiratory distress. Cultures of blood units and/or recipient blood would support this diagnosis. Lastly, evidence of hemolysis should accompany a hemolytic transfusion reaction. The distinction from ARDS is a bit arbitrary, as the histopathologic findings at autopsy resemble ARDS, with leukocyte infiltration, pulmonary edema, hyaline membranes, and destruction of the normal lung parenchyma. However, the ARDS-like change in TRALI has a significantly better prognosis than ARDS generally, with 90-95% of patients recovering with adequate support. TRALI is confirmed by finding antigranulocyte, anti-HLA class I, or anti-HLA class II antibodies in the donor plasma; the diagnosis is buttressed if the corresponding antigens are present on donor leukocytes or there is an incompatible lymphocyte crossmatch. TNF-α has been noted to increase following TRALI, but this is a nonspecific marker.

Treatment, as for other reactions, begins with stopping the transfusion. Support the patient with ventilation and pressor agents as needed while the evaluation proceeds. Though there is a 5-10% mortality rate, most patients recover clinically within 72 hours, with infiltrates resolving within 2-4 days. The risk of a second episode of TRALI is exceedingly low, so additional transfusion, if needed, should not be withheld. Prevention strategies include

1. exclusion of implicated donors from future transfusion

2. restriction of all female plasma products or at least exclusion of multiparous women

Donors are considered "implicated" if they are

1. "associated" with an episode of TRALI—a plasma containing product from the donor was infused within 6 hours of the onset of TRALI

2. found to have an antigranulocyte or anti-HLA class I/II antibody that reacts with the recipient with TRALI

Posttransfusion purpura (PTP)

PTP presents as profound thrombocytopenia that develops 2-14 days following RBC or platelet transfusion. Thrombocytopenia is severe, often <10,000. Affected recipients are almost always multiparous women.

PTP is caused by platelet alloantibodies, most commonly anti-HPA-1a, that are responsible for destruction of donor and, mysteriously, native recipient platelets. This is analogous to hyperhemolytic transfusion reactions in sickle cell patients. About 98% of the population is HPA-1a+. This reaction is a risk in the 2% of HPA-1a– individuals when they receive HPA-1a+ platelets.

PTP is usually a self limited process that resolves within ~3 weeks. Treatment with intravenous γ globulin usually results in rapid platelet recovery within 3-5 days.

Platelet refractoriness

Platelet refractoriness presents as a progressive diminution in the quantity of platelet increase following platelet transfusion. It arises in patients who require repeated platelet transfusions.

Platelet refractoriness has many causes, most of which are forms of secondary platelet refractoriness, including systemic infection, splenomegaly, drugs such as amphotericin, and ongoing platelet consumption (eg, DIC). After all of these have been excluded, primary platelet refractoriness, due to HLA alloimmunization, must be considered.

In patients with AML, the incidence of platelet refractoriness (on any basis, including alloimmunization) arising during treatment is ~25%. Factors associated with refractoriness include a positive lymphocytotoxic antibody test, multiple ($\geq$2) pregnancies, male gender, heparin exposure, fever, bleeding, larger numbers of platelet transfusions, and a palpable spleen.

In one large study looking at posttransfusion platelet increments (instead of formal refractoriness), the status of the spleen was the most important factor. Splenectomized patients had the largest posttransfusion increments, followed by patients with clinically normal spleens, followed by those with palpable spleens. Other factors that adversely affected increments included $\geq$2 pregnancies in a female, male sex, increasing weight and height (presumably reflecting greater volumes of distribution), amphotericin, heparin, fever, bleeding, and infection. Note that only a subset of these patients developed true primary refractoriness. While DIC did not affect posttransfusion increments, it did decrease the time to next platelet transfusion.

Primary platelet refractoriness is due to HLA alloimmunization on the basis of HLA class I antigens (primarily HLA-A and HLA-B) present on platelet surfaces. It is the transfused white cells that elicit this response. Definitions of refractoriness vary. A lower-than-expected posttransfusion platelet increment (platelet count posttransfusion minus platelet count pretransfusion) on 2 consecutive occasions is considered by many to be an acceptable definition. Expected platelet increment depends upon the dose. A quad-pack of single-donor unit of platelets would be expected ~5,000/μL/unit transfused. Thus, a quad-pack would be expected to produce an increment of ~20,000/μL. A 6-pack of single-donor platelets or a single pheresis unit should produce an increment of around 30,000. A more accurate assessment of response is the platelet count increment (CI), calculation shown below. A normal CI is $\geq$ 7,500.

The timing of the posttransfusion platelet count is critical. A sample must be drawn within 10-60 minutes after transfusion. <10,000 rise in platelet count for a 1-hour post platelet count is typical of immune mediated platelet refractoriness, while a substantial immediate increment with diminished 4-hour increment suggests secondary refractoriness.

$$\text{platelet count increment (CI)} = \frac{\text{increment} \times \text{body surface area}}{\text{\# platelets transfused}/10^{11}}$$

An example: A patient with BSA of 1.9 m^2 has a pretransfusion platelet count of 12,000 and posttransfusion platelet count of 21,000 after a 6-pack of platelets (5.5$\times$ 10^{10} $\times$ 6 = 3.3 $\times$ 10^{11} platelets).

$$CI = 9,000 \times 1.9 = 5,182/3.3$$

This result is <7,500 and suggests refractoriness.

In patients undergoing chemotherapy who are expected to require repeated platelet transfusions, prevention of HLA alloimmunization is essential, though not always possible. The first step is to minimize transfusions, possibly by using a conservative transfusion trigger. Second is to minimize donor exposures by using pheresis products instead of pooled whole blood derived platelets. Third, leukoreduction filtration (to below 5 $\times$ 10^6 leukocytes/unit) can help prevent HLA alloimmunization. In a large study of AML patients it was demonstrated that UV-B irradiation and leukoreduction were equally effective in preventing the development of lymphocytotoxic antibodies and platelet refractoriness due to alloimmunization. Although UV-B irradiation is effective in preventing alloimmunization, it is not licensed in the United States. Following alloimmunization, a PRA assay can help determine extent of immunization. Treatment may require HLA crossmatching, often with relatives or random pheresis donors.

Infections t2.38

t2.38 Approximate risk of transfusion complications

Complication	Risk
HIV	1/2.3 million
HTLV-1	1/2.9 million
HCV	1/1.8 million
HBV	1/220,000
EBV	Unknown, rare
CMV	Unknown, rare given leukoreduced cellular blood products
ABO-Rh incompatibility	ABO mismatch: 1/6,000-1/30,000 Fatal reactions: 1/100,000-600,000
TRALI	1/5,000-190,000
DHTR	1/3,000
Allergic reaction	Allergic:1/100 Anaphylactic: 1/20,000-50,000
Septic reactions with platelets	1/75,000
Septic reactions with RBC	1/500,000
Febrile reaction	1/100

Cytomegalovirus (CMV)

CMV is transmitted by mononuclear white blood cells in which it is carried intracellularly. Most individuals are already CMV+, and most of those who are not will suffer no ill effects from its acquisition; however, it is particularly important to reduce the transmission of CMV in CMV– transplant candidates/recipients and low birth weight neonates.

This is accomplished by administering CMV– blood products, when available. If no CMV– blood is available, then leukoreduction (to <5 $\times$ 10^6 WBCs) is generally considered an acceptable alternative.

West Nile Virus (WNV)

Most infections with WNV are asymptomatic or mild. Severe infection occurs in ~1 in 150 cases, with ~1 in 1,000 cases proving fatal. Both symptoms and serologic evidence of disease, though, arise after a several-week-long period of viremia. Currently, in the United States, NAT testing is performed during outbreaks, and donors are deferred if they have had symptoms consistent with WNV. The risk of transfusion transmitted WNV is low but may occur despite NAT testing.

Syphilis (*Treponema pallidum*)

Treponema pallidum is transmitted by transfusion only very rarely, due to a very brief period of bacteremia. No new transfusion transmitted cases have been reported in >30 years. The RPR test that is required testing for all donated blood is not very useful to screen for syphilis, since RPR is usually not positive while individuals are experiencing the brief period of bacteremia. Furthermore, most positive RPRs are false positives. Thus, screening for syphilis is not the main reason to perform RPRs on donor blood. RPR is used as a surrogate marker for high risk behavior for other transfusion transmitted infections such as HIV.

Chagas disease (*Trypanosoma cruzi*)

Chagas disease can be transmitted by transfusion and is prevalent in Central and South America. In Mexico, nearly 1 in 100 donors are positive for Chagas disease. Currently, donors are tested initially for the first donation or with each donation.

Malaria (*Plasmodium* species)

The risk of transfusion transmitted malaria is 1/4 million transfusions. Malaria is screened for by history.

Babesiosis (*Babesia microti*)

In endemic areas, the risk of transfusion transmitted babesiosis is around 1/1,000 transfusions. Babesiosis is screened for by history. Persons with a history of babesiosis are permanently deferred.

Creutzfeldt-Jakob disease (CJD)

This prion mediated disease has never been documented to be transmitted by transfusion. However, variant CJD (vCJD) can be transmitted by transfusion. Where it is prevalent, such as in the UK, universal prestorage leukoreduction was undertaken to reduce this risk; however, there has been insufficient evidence that leukoreduction significantly reduces the risk of transfusion transmitted vCJD. In the United States, individuals at risk for vCJD by virtue of history (those who have traveled to or lived in BSE-endemic areas) are excluded from donation, as are those who have received dural transplants, pituitary derived growth hormone or bovine insulin. Relatives of patients with classic CJD are deferred.

Transfusion associated metabolic derangements

Transfusion-associated circulatory overload (TACO)

TACO is a common event, manifesting essentially as congestive heart failure, which is often mistaken for a possible HTR or TRALI. TACO, unlike TRALI, is associated with elevated BNP. TACO is particularly common in neonates and elderly recipients and may be prevented by slow or diuretic-assisted transfusion.

Hypocalcemia (citrate toxicity)

With large volumes of products, sufficient citrate can be infused to cause hypocalcemia.

Hypothermia

With large volumes of unwarmed products, the recipient's core body temperature can be reduced. Hypothermia exacerbates the effects of other metabolic derangements such as hypocalcemia and hyperkalemia. Prewarming is recommended for massive transfusion; however, standards requires that the temperature not exceed 42°C.

Hyperkalemia

With every cellular blood product, there is a certain degree of unavoidable hemolysis upon storage of RBCs, resulting in high extracellular potassium levels. The problem is proportional to the age of the product. Most patients can handle the extra potassium, but neonates and those who suffer from impaired renal function may not.

Hypokalemia

Some patients may experience hypokalemia due to transfusion of cells that are intracellularly potassium depleted, leading to transcellular shifts of serum potassium.

Iron overload

This is mainly a problem in chronically transfused patients. Each unit of RBCs contains around 200 mg of iron. When the whole body iron burden reaches ~500 mg/kg, clinical iron overload can develop, affecting the heart and liver function primarily. Iron chelation with desferoxamine can be helpful to prevent this complication; however, compliance is poor because it requires a painful subcutaneous overnight infusion with neurotoxicity as a side effect. More recently, an oral iron chelator, deferasirox, has become available and has improved compliance.

Immunomodulation

Transfusion of cellular blood products appears to have a dampening effect on the immune system. This has been exploited for some time in renal transplantation recipients, in whom pretransplant transfusion promotes graft survival. However, there is ongoing investigation into the question of whether there is an increased risk of infection or malignancy recurrence in transfused patients.

Medical directorship considerations unique to blood banking: Hospital Transfusion Committee, Process Control & Blood Bank Equipment

Hospital Transfusion Committee

Regulatory requirements

Regulatory agencies, including the Joint Commission, AABB, and CAP, require that a hospital ensure appropriate use of blood products. This is most commonly implemented through the conduct of a hospital transfusion committee or similar body.

Transfusion Committee purpose

This committee forms policy and conducts audits to ensure compliance, particularly in the following areas

1. proper patient identification, sample collection, and labeling,

2. blood ordering practices, utilization review, and compliance with ordering criteria

3. proper blood administration and monitoring

4. blood wastage

5. adverse events

6. alternatives to allogeneic transfusion

Conduct of the transfusion committee

Most utilization review actually occurs in real time, through the prospective review of blood orders by the medical director or designee. Medical directors differ in the degree to which they become involved in medical decision making. At the very least, the medical director must advise against contraindicated transfusions; the degree to which the medical director becomes involved in halting nonindicated transfusions or in minimizing marginally indicated transfusions; however, is a matter of philosophy. The transfusion committee is a body that provides objective retrospective review of transfusions, usually through review of the charts of transfused patients. How chart review is conducted varies; in general, it is most efficient to have charts screened by a knowledgeable staff member, for transfusions that appear out of compliance t2.39. Charts that fail to pass the screener are submitted for review by a committee member. If the committee member finds that, indeed, a variance occurred, then the case is submitted to the committee for opinion. The committee may choose at this point to contact the ordering physician for clarification. If this fails to provide the needed justification, then a formal letter is sent and filed, informing the physician of the committee's findings. The matter may then be submitted to a credentialing committee.

t2.39 Measures of compliance

Criteria for transfusion were met & documented
Written informed consent & opportunity to refuse transfusion were provided
Written physician order was given
Appropriate transfusion procedure was followed, including confirmation of patient identification, documentation of blood issue & appropriate patient monitoring during & after transfusion
Measures of posttransfusion increments or clinical benefit were documented

Documentation of transfusion committee proceedings

As a quality control instrument, the proceedings (minutes) of the transfusion committee may be protected from legal discovery. Nonetheless, these documents should be available for review by hospital wide clinical practices councils or equivalent bodies.

Other regulatory requirements

Component identification & traceability

At the blood collection facility, donor identity must be confirmed (proof of ID required). The donor must be linked, if a repeat donor, to existing records.

For every critical step in the transfusion process (eg, sample collection from recipient, blood collection from donor, testing, transport) it must be possible to retrospectively ascertain who performed the step and when was it performed.

All critical materials and equipment used in the processing of a blood product must be uniquely identified and traceable.

The process by which the blood bank labels blood, blood components, and derivatives must ensure that they can be traced back to their origin.

Labeling must be in accordance with the "Industry Consensus Standard for the Uniform Labeling of Blood and Blood Components Using ISBT 128."

The label must be subjected to a second check to ensure the correctness of the donation identification number (DIN), ABO/Rh, expiration date, product name, and product code.

Storage

Blood products must be segregated, according to, eg, type of product, ABO group, autologous, or banked donor blood.

The storage temperature must be continuously monitored or monitored at least every 4 hours.

For those storage units that utilize liquid nitrogen, one may monitor either the level of liquid nitrogen or the temperature.

Storage units must be equipped with alarms, and alarms must be set to activate before critical temperatures are reached; ie, so that action can be taken before harm comes to the stored products.

The temperatures of warming devices must also be monitored and alarmed.

Records t2.40

All donor and unit records must be retained for a minimum of 10 years. The exception is records pertaining to permanently deferred donors, which must be maintained indefinitely. For patient (recipient) records, required retention times are 5 or 10 years, depending upon the nature of the record. The exception is records pertaining to difficulty typing, clinically significant antibodies, adverse reactions, special transfusion requirements, and investigation/resolution of discrepancies, which must be maintained indefinitely.

t2.40 Retention of patient records

Patient records	Retention period
Quality control documents	5 years
Quality management reviews	
Proficiency testing	
Instrument quality control/maintenance including irradiation dose delivery & control systems for patient testing	
Retyping of donor units upon receipt	
Inspection of blood & critical materials	
Annual review of procedures & discontinued procedures	
Patient pretransfusion testing results	10 years
Transfusion records	
Immediate evaluation/interpretation of transfusion reactions	
Therapeutic apheresis/phlebotomy records	
Final unit disposition	
Employee signatures, initials & identification codes	
Transfusion problems including transfusion reactions, unexpected antibodies & special transfusion requirements	

Blood bank regulatory authority

The FDA Center for Biologics Evaluation and Research (CBER) has authority to regulate blood collection and blood processing. FDA guidance and mandates may be found at www.fda.gov. AABB accreditation is voluntary.

Common calls

Transfusion reactions

Evaluate the reaction in light of the workup, determine its nature, and decide whether additional testing is needed and, finally whether it is safe to administer additional transfusions.

The most important things to exclude are the potentially dangerous reactions: acute HTR, transfusion transmitted bacterial infection, TRALI, and anaphylaxis. HTR is essentially excluded by a clerical check, negative (or unchanged) DAT, negative urine hemoglobin, and yellow serum. At times it seems that all hospitalized patients have positive urine hemoglobin, but this is related usually to RBCs in urine, not free hemoglobin; urine microscopy can confirm this. If not sure whether there is hemolysis, consider ordering serum haptoglobin, LD, and bilirubin. If hemolysis is suspected, then it may help to repeat the ABO and Rh determinations on a pretransfusion specimen and perform extended crossmatches on a posttransfusion specimen. Transfusion transmitted bacterial infection should be suspected if there is high fever especially with hypotension and the transfusion involved platelets, bearing in mind that RBCs may also be suspect. There is no quick way to exclude bacterial infection. Both the units and the patient should be cultured to identify the causative organism. TRALI is considered if the patient experiences acute-onset respiratory distress without any cardiovascular disease, especially if requiring ventilator support with radiographic bilateral lung opacification. Assess the history and request a BNP to exclude cardiogenic pulmonary edema. It may then be necessary to consider this a suspected TRALI and ask for testing of the associated donor blood for HLA and neutrophil antibodies. Anaphylactic reactions should be considered in the appropriate clinical context, whenever a component with significant plasma was administered. If suspected, then recipient IgA levels should be determined. If confirmed or suspected (pending workup), washed RBCs may be administered.

When a transfusion fatality or transfusion related serious morbidity occurs, this must be reported immediately to the FDA and within 7 days in writing. When a transfusion fatality or transfusion related serious morbidity occurs that appears to be related to a single donor, then the collecting facility must be notified—immediately followed and by notification in writing. When a transfusion related infection is confirmed or cannot be excluded, then the identity of the donor units must be conveyed to the collecting facility, any other recipients of blood components from the donor, and the recipient's physician.

Lastly, in any instance in which a transfusion reaction workup has occurred, a written report by transfusion service physician must be charted, but this can be done the next day.

Platelet shortage

Prospectively, it is important to have a process in place that enables technologists to reorder platelets before the blood bank is completely depleted. The blood bank medical director or on call pathologist should be notified when this threshold is reached. Despite these efforts, regional platelet shortages may at times leave the blood bank with few or no platelet units.

Determine the likely duration of the shortage. Your supplier should be able to give an estimate of expected delivery time.

Triage the need for platelets. Actively bleeding patients should supersede elective surgical cases, and outpatient oncology patients can often have their transfusions delayed for a limited period of time. If there are no platelets available in the blood bank or the anticipated urgent need exceeds the current supply, then the operating room should be informed and asked to delay or cancel certain elective cases.

Incoming platelet orders should be handled on an individual basis, by contacting the ordering physician and discussing the urgency of their order in light of the shortage.

Compatible blood cannot be found for an anemic patient

This is a common circumstance when dealing with multiply transfused patients or patients with autoantibodies. Patients with new autoantibodies or unexpectedly positive crossmatches with positive autocontrols demonstrating the same level of reactivity may be transfused with least-incompatible blood if all significant alloantibodies have been excluded by adsorption techniques. Even if a particular antibody cannot be excluded, antigen-negative blood may be given. If particular alloantibodies cannot be excluded and corresponding antigen-negative blood is unavailable, then the specimen must be sent to a reference laboratory for further evaluation.

The blood bank medical director or on call pathologist should discuss the situation with the ordering physician. Often it is not possible to confidently estimate the length of time required for finding compatible blood, especially if samples need to be sent to a reference laboratory. In urgent situations, group O least-incompatible blood can be offered.

Mislabeled specimen

Specimens that are not labeled according to blood bank standards (eg, 2 unique identifiers without misspellings) cannot be used for pretransfusion testing. Expect to be assailed for this policy, but be firm. The patient can be given emergency release group O, Rh– blood if the need is urgent.

References

Adams RJ, McKie VC, Hsu L, et al [1998] Prevention of a first stroke by transfusions in children with sickle cell anemia and abnormal results on transcranial Doppler ultrasonography. *N Engl J Med* 339(1):5 11 PMID: 9647873.

Ansell J, Hirsh J, Hylek E, et al [2008] Pharmacology and management of the vitamin K antagonists: American College of Chest Physicians Evidence-Based Clinical Practice Guidelines (8th ed). *Chest* 133:166-98. PMID: 18574265.

Avent ND [2008] Large-scale blood group genotyping—clinical implications. *Br J Haematol* 144:3-13. PMID: 19016734.

Aygun B, Padmanabhan S, Paley C, Chandrasekaran V [2002] Clinical significance of RBC alloantibodies and autoantibodies in sickle cells patients who received transfusions. *Transfusion* 42:37-43. PMID: 11896310.

Benjamin RB, Antin JH [1999] ABO-incompatible bone marrow transplantation: the transfusion of incompatible plasma may exacerbate regimen related toxicity. *Transfusion* 39:1273-4. PMID: 10604259.

Blanchette VS, Kühne T, Hume H, Hellmann J [1995] Platelet transfusion therapy in newborn infants. *Transfus Med Reviews* IX:215-230. PMID: 7549233.

Branch DR, Petz LD [1999] Detecting alloantibodies in patients with autoantibodies. *Transfusion* 39:6-10. PMID: 9920160.

Brand A [2002] Immunologic aspects of blood transfusions. *Transpl Immunol* 10:183-190. PMID: 12216948.

Brecher ME, Ed [2005] *Technical Manual*, 15th ed. Bethesda: American Association of Blood Banks.

Burns KH, Werch JB [2004] Bacterial contamination of platelet units. *Arch Pathol Lab Med* 128:279-281. PMID: 14987162.

Carr R, Hutton JL, Jenkins JA et al [1990] Transfusion of ABO-mismatched platelets leads to early platelet refractoriness. *Br J Haematol* 75:408-413. PMID: 2201403.

Carson TH, Ed [2011] *Standards for Blood Banks and Transfusion Services*, 27th ed. Bethesda: American Association of Blood Banks.

Castro O, Sandler SG, Houston-Yu P, Rana S [2002] Predicting the effect of transfusing only phenotype-matched RBCs to patients with sickle cell disease: theoretical and practical implications. *Transfusion* 42(6):684-690. PMID: 12147019.

Choi PT, Yip G, Ouinonez LG, Cook DJ [1999] Crystalloids vs colloids in fluid resuscitation: a systemic review. *Crit Care Med* 27:200-210. PMID: 9934917.

Code of Federal Regulations [2010] *Title 21 CFR Part 640—Additional standards for human blood and blood products*. Washington, DC: US Government Printing Office (revised annually).

Daniels G, Poole J, deSilva M, Callaghan T, MacLennan S, Smith N [2002] The clinical significance of blood groups antibodies. *Transfus Med* 12:287-295. PMID: 12383334.

Domen RE [2000] Policies and procedures related to weak D phenotype testing and Rh immune globulin administration. *Arch Pathol Lab Med* 124:1118 1121 PMID: 10923069.

Domen RE, Hoeltge GA [2003] Allergic transfusion reactions: an evaluation of 273 consecutive reactions. *Arch Pathol Lab Med* 127:316-320. PMID: 12653575.

Dreier J, Vollmer T, Kleesiek K [2009] Novel flow cytometry-based screening for bacterial contamination of donor platelet preparations compared with other rapid screening methods. *Clin Chem* 55(8):1492-1502. PMID: 19498052.

Dzik WH, Anderson JK, O'Neill EM, Assmann SF, Kalish LA, Stowell CP [2002] A prospective, randomized clinical trial of universal WBC reduction. *Transfusion* 42:1114-1122. PMID: 12430666.

Eder AF, Manno CS [2001] Does red-cell T activation matter? Annotation. *Br J Haematol* 114:25-30. PMID: 11472340.

Fridberg MJ, Hedner U, Roberts HR, Erhardtsen E [2005]A study of the pharmacokinetics and safety of recombinant activated factor VII in healthy Caucasian and Japanese subjects. *Blood Coagul Fibrinolysis* 16(4):259-266. PMID: 15870545.

Frohn C, Dumbgen L, Brand JM, et al [2003] Probability of anti D development in D- patients receiving D+RBCs. *Transfusion* 43(7):893-8. PMID: 12823749.

Gajic O, Moore SB [2005]Transfusion related acute lung injury. *Mayo Clin Proc* 80(6):766-770. PMID: 15945528.

Garratty G, Petz LD [2000a] Approaches to selecting blood for transfusion to patients with autoimmune hemolytic anemia. *Transfusion* 2000; 42:1390-1392. PMID: 12421209.

Garratty G, Dzik W, Issitt PD, Lublin DM, Reid ME, Zelinski T [2000b] Terminology for blood group antigens and genes—historical origins and guidelines in the new millennium. *Transfusion* 40:477-489. PMID: 10773062.

Garratty G, Glynn SA, McEntire R [2004] ABO and Rh(D) phenotype frequencies of different racial/ethnic groups in the United States. *Transfusion* 44:703-706. PMID: 15104651.

Goodnough LT, Brecher ME, Kanter MH, AuBuchon JP [1999] Transfusion medicine: first of 2 parts. *N Engl J Med* 340:438-447. PMID: 9971869.

Goodnough LT, Lublin DM, Zhang L, Despotis G, Eby C [2004] Transfusion medicine service policies for recombinant factor VIIa administration. *Transfusion* 44:1325-1331. PMID: 15318856.

Grocott MPW, Hamilton MA [2002] Resuscitation fluids. *Vox Sang* 82:1-8. PMID: 11856460.

Hebert PC, Wells G, Tweeddale M, et al [1999] A multicenter, randomized, controlled clinical trial of transfusion requirements in critical care. *N Engl J Med* 340:409-17. PMID: 9971864.

Hebert PC [2002] Transfusion requirements in critical care: the TRICC trial—a focus on the sub-group analysis. *Vox Sang* 83(S1):387-396. PMID: 12617174.

Hess JR [2004] Update on alternative oxygen carriers. *Vox Sang* Suppl2:S132-S135 PMID:.

Holland LL, Brooks JP [2006] Toward rational fresh frozen plasma transfusion: the effect of plasma transfusion on coagulation test results. *Am J Clin Pathol* 126:133-139. PMID: 16753596.

Hübel K, Dale DC, Engert A, Liles WC [2001] Current status of granulocyte transfusion therapy for infectious diseases. *J Infect Dis* 183:321-328. PMID: 11112098.

Josephson CD, Su LL, Hillyer KL, Hillyer CD [2007] Transfusion in the patient with sickle cell disease: a critical review of the literature and transfusion guidelines. *Transfus Med Rev* 21:118-33. PMID: 17397762.

Klein HG, Anstee D [2005] ABO, Lewis and P group and Ii antigens. In: *Mollison's Blood Transfusion in Clinical Medicine*. 11th ed. Oxford: Blackwell 114-62. PMID:.

Kleinman S, Caulfield T, Chan P, et al [2004] Toward an understanding of transfusion related acute lung injury: statement of a consensus panel. *Transfusion* 44:1774-1789. PMID: 15584994.

Koshy M, Burd L, Wallace D, et al [1998] Prophylactic red-cell transfusions in pregnant patients with sickle cell disease: a randomized cooperative study. *N Engl J Med* 319:1447-1452. PMID: 3054555.

Larson LG, Welsh VJ, Ladd DJ [2000] Acute intravascular hemolysis secondary to out of out of group platelet transfusion. *Transfusion* 40:902-6. PMID: 10960514.

Laupacis A, Brown J, Costello B, Delage G, Freedman J, Hume H, King S, Kleinman S, Mazzulli T, Wells G [2001] Prevention of posttransfusion CMV in the era of universal WBC reduction: a consensus statement. *Transfusion* 41:560-569. PMID: 11316911.

Manci EA, Culberson DE, Yang Y-M, Gardner TM, Powell R, Haynes J Jr, Shah AK, Mankad VN [2003] Causes of death in sickle cell disease: an autopsy study. *Br J Haematol* 123:359-365. PMID: 14531921.

McCane AV, Ward N, Senn C, et al [2009] Analysis of bacterial detection in whole blood derived platelets by quantitative glucose testing at a university medical center. *Am J Clin Pathol* 131:542-551. PMID: 19289590.

McDonald CP, Roy A, Mahajan P, et al [2004] Relative values of the interventions of the diversion and improved donor-arm disinfection to reduce the bacterial risk from blood transfusion. *Vox Sang* 86(3):178-82. PMID: 15078252.

Midathada MV, Mehta P, Waner M, Fink LM [2004] Recombinant factor VIIa in the treatment of bleeding. *Am J Clin Pathol* 121:124-137. PMID: 14750250.

Moise KJ [2002] Management of Rhesus alloimmunization in pregnancy. *Obstet Gynecol* 100:600-611. PMID: 12220785.

Myhre BA, McRuer D [2000] Human error—a significant cause of transfusion mortality. *Transfusion* 40:879-885. PMID: 10924620.

Palfi M, Berg S, Ernerudh J, Berlin G [2000] A randomized controlled trial of transfusion related acute lung injury: is plasma from multiparous blood donors dangerous? *Transfusion* 41:317-322. PMID: 11274583.

Pantanowitz L, Telford III SR, Cannon ME [2002] Tick-borne diseases in transfusion medicine. *Transfus Med* 12:85-106. PMID: 11982962.

Pineda AA, Vamvakas LD, Gorden JL, et al [1999] Trends in the incidence of delayed hemolytic and delayed serologic transfusion reactions. *Transfusion* 39:1097-1103. PMID: 10532604.

Price TH, Ed [2009] *Standards for Blood Banks and Transfusion Services.* 26th ed. Bethesda, MD: AABB.

Przepiorka D, LeParc GF, Stovall MA, Werch J, Lichtiger B [1996] Use of irradiated blood components. *Am J Clin Pathol.* 106:6-11. PMID: 8701934.

Rackoff WR, Ohene-Frempong K, Month S, et al [1992] Neurologic events after partial exchange transfusion for priapism in sickle cell disease. *J Pediatr* 120:882-885. PMID: 1593347.

Ramasethu J, Luban MLC [2001] T activation. *Br J Haematol* 112:259-263. PMID: 11167817.

Ramsey G [2009] Inaccurate doses of Rh immune globulin after Rh-incompatible fetomaternal hemorrhage: survey of laboratory practice. *Arch Pathol Lab Med* 133:465-469. PMID: 19260751.

Rebulla P [2001] Revisitation of the clinical indications for the transfusion of platelet concentrates. *Rev Clin Exp Hematol* 5.3:288-310. PMID: 11703819.

Rood IGH, Pettersson A, Korte D, Savelkoul PHM [2008] Reducing the risk of transfusion transmitted bacterial infections in platelet concentrates: current status and developments. *Lab Med* 39(9):553-557. PMID:.

Sacher RA, Kickler TS, Schiffer CA, Sherman LA, Bracey AW, Shulman IA [2003] Management of patients refractory to platelet transfusion. *Arch Pathol Lab Med* 127:409-414. PMID: 12683867.

Sazama K, DeChristopher PJ, Dodd R, Harrison, CR Shulman IA, Cooper ES, Labotka RJ, Oberman HA, Zahn CM, Greenburg G, Stehling L, Lauenstein KJ, Price TH, Williams LK [2000] Practice parameter for the recognition, management, and prevention of adverse consequences of blood transfusion. *Arch Pathol Lab Med* 124:61-70. PMID: 10629134.

Schierhout G, Roberts I [1998] Fluid resuscitation with colloid or crystalloid solutions in critically ill patients: a systematic review of randomised trials. *BMJ* 316:961-964. PMID: 9550953.

Schiffer CA [2001] Management of patients refractory to platelet transfusion. *Leukemia* 15:683-685. PMID: 11368381.

Schroeder ML [2002] Transfusion associated graft vs host disease. *Br J Haematol* 117:275-287. PMID: 11972509.

Siegel JF, Rich MA, Brock WA [1993] Association of sickle cell disease, priapism, exchange transfusion, and neurologic events: ASPEN syndrome. *J Urol* 150:1480-1482. PMID: 8411432.

Silberman S [1999] Platelets: preparations, transfusion, modifications, and substitutes. *Arch Pathol Lab Med.* 123:889-894. PMID: 10506440.

Silliman CC, Boshkov LK, Mehdizadehkashi Z, Elzi DJ, Dickey WO, Podlosky L, Clarke G, Ambruso DR [2003] Transfusion related acute lung injury: epidemiology and a prospective analysis of etiologic factors. *Blood* 101:454-462. PMID: 12393667.

Silliman CC, Ambruso DR, Boshkov LK [2005] Transfusion related acute lung injury. *Blood* 105:2266-2273. PMID: 15572582.

Simpson J, Kinsey S [2001] Paediatric transfusion. *Vox Sang* 81:1-5. PMID: 11520408.

Slichter SJ, and the Trial to Reduce Alloimmunization to Platelets Study Group [1997] Leukocyte reduction and ultraviolet B irradiation of platelets to prevent alloimmunization and refractoriness to platelet transfusions. *N Engl J Med* 337:1861-1869. PMID: 9417523.

Slichter SJ, Davis K, Enright H, Braine H, Gernsheimer T, Kao K-J, Kickler T, Lee E, McFarland J, McCullough J, Rodey G, Schiffer CA, Woodson R [2005] Factors affecting posttransfusion platelet increments, platelet refractoriness, and platelet transfusion intervals in thrombocytopenic patients. *Blood* 105(10):4106-4114. PMID: 15692069.

Smith JW, Weinstein R, Hillyer KL [2003] Therapeutic apheresis: a summary of current indication categories endorsed by the AABB and the American Society for Apheresis. *Transfusion* 43:820-822. PMID: 12757535.

Stowell CP, Levin J, Spiess BD, Winslow RM [2001] Progress in the development of RBC substitutes. *Transfusion* 41:287-299. PMID: 11239237.

Task Force of the College of American Pathologists [1994] Practice parameter for the use of fresh-frozen plasma, cryoprecipitate, and platelets. *JAMA.* 271:777-781. PMID: 8114215.

Toy P [1999] Guiding the decision to transfuse: interventions that do and do not work. *Arch Pathol Lab Med* 123:592-240. PMID: 10388913.

Toy P, Popovsky MA, Abraham E, et al [2005] Transfusion related acute lung injury: definition and review. *Crit Care Med* 33:721-726. PMID: 15818095.

Smith JW, Weinstein R, Hillyer KL et al [2003] Therapeutic apheresis: a summary of current indications categories endorsed by the AABB and the American Society for Apheresis. *Transfusion* 43:820-822. PMID: 12757535.

Spiess BD [2004] Risks of transfusion: outcome focus. *Transfusion* 44:4S-14S PMID: 15585000.

Stainsby D, Williamson L, Jones H, et al [2004] 6 years of SHOT reporting: its influence on UK blood safety. *Tranfus Apheresis Sci* 31:123-131. PMID: 15501416.

Szczepiorkowski Z, Winters JL, Bandarenko N, et al [2010] Guidelines on the use of therapeutic apheresis in clinical practice—evidence-based approach from the Apheresis Applications Committee of the American Society for Apheresis. *J Clin Apher* 25:83-177. PMID: 20568098.

Vichinsky EP, Haberkern CM, Neumayr L, et al [1995] A comparison of conservative and aggressive transfusion regimens in the perioperative management of sickle cell disease. *N Engl J Med* 333:206-213. PMID: 7791837.

Vichinsky E, Luban N, Wright E, et al [2001] Prospective RBC phenotype matching in a stroke-prevention trial in sickle cell anemia: a multicenter transfusion trial. *Transfusion* 41:1086-1092. PMID: 11552063.

Wanko SO, Telen MJ [2005] Transfusion management in sickle cell disease. *Hematol Oncol Clin N Am* 19:803-826. PMID: 16214645.

Wheeler CA, Calhoun L, Blackall, DP [2004] Warm reactive autoantibodies: clinical and serologic correlations. *Am J Clin Pathol* 122:680-685. PMID: 15491963.

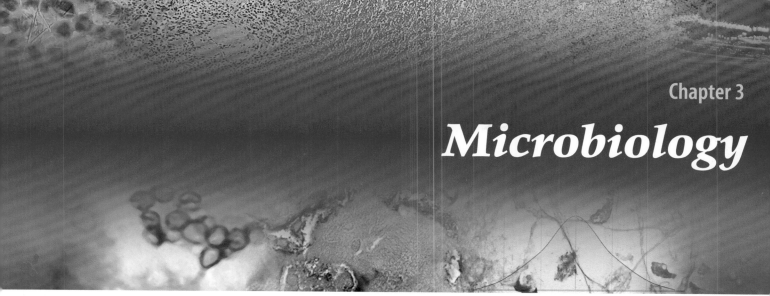

Microbiology

Clinical syndromes & causative agents
Urinary tract infection (UTI)
Differential diagnosis

The term UTI encompasses asymptomatic bacteriuria, urethritis, cystitis, and pyelonephritis. UTIs are categorized clinically as complicated and uncomplicated, although agreement on the definition of these terms is not universal. Uncomplicated UTI often refers to those cases of cystitis that arise in essentially healthy young adult (nonpregnant) females without anatomic genitourinary anomalies. Essentially, the term is meant to imply a UTI that will not result in serious sequelae and that will go away with treatment. Thus, complicated UTI often refers to one arising in association with pregnancy, diabetes, stone, structural genitourinary anomalies, spinal injury, as well as in children and males. The implication is an increased risk of complications such as sepsis, chronic pyelonephritis, and treatment failure.

In the neonatal period, UTI is in the differential for fever of unknown etiology. Boys are most often affected. In children and adults, UTI is much more common in females. After ~50 years of age, men and women are affected equally.

Cystitis presents with dysuria, frequency, urgency, and, sometimes, hematuria. These symptoms, however, can be produced by noninfectious causes, such as stone, tumor, and upper tract bleeding. Vaginitis can also be mistaken by the patient as a UTI; thus, documenting infection is necessary prior to instigating treatment.

Pyelonephritis presents with flank pain, fever, nausea, and vomiting, often in association with the symptoms of cystitis. Again, this presentation may be produced by stone or papillary necrosis, and documentation of infection is important.

Bacterial colonization of urine without clinical symptoms (asymptomatic bacteriuria) usually requires no treatment. The exceptions are pregnant women and patients undergoing urologic instrumentation. Asymptomatic bacteriuria is diagnosed on the basis of:

- In asymptomatic women, 2 consecutive voided urine specimens with isolation of the same bacterial strain in quantitative counts of $\geq 10^5$ colony-forming units (cfu) per mL.

- In asymptomatic men, a single voided urine specimen with isolation of a single bacterial species in a quantitative count of $\geq 10^5$ cfu/mL.

- In men and women, a single catheterized specimen with a single bacterial species in a count of $\geq 10^2$ cfu/mL.

Purple urine bag syndrome is a rare and still somewhat perplexing phenomenon, in which urine is noted to have a purple color that it also imparts upon the bag in which it collects. To form, it appears to require the coincidence of bacteriuria, an indwelling catheter, alkaline urine, and a diet high in tryptophan. Partial or complete colonic obstruction appears to contribute in some way. Furthermore, the bacteria must be capable of producing sulfatase and phosphatase, in order to metabolize dietary tryptophan into indigo and indirubin which combine to produce the purple color. The associated organisms have included *Providencia stuartii*, *Providencia rettgeri*, *Klebsiella pneumoniae*, *Proteus mirabilis*, *Pseudomonas aeruginosa*, *Escherichia coli*, and enterococcus species.

Laboratory approach

There are numerous surrogate markers for UTI. Hematuria, detected microscopically or by positive urine dipstick for hemoglobin, is a nonspecific but sensitive marker for UTI. A positive urine dipstick leukocyte esterase, reflective of pyuria, has a sensitivity of 70-95% and, though more specific than red cells, has a specificity of only 70%. The dipstick nitrite test is positive whenever an organism capable of reducing nitrate to nitrite, such as a coliform, is present. In this test the specificity is quite high, 95%, but sensitivity is only ~50%. The nitrite test is negative in the presence of *Staphylococcus saprophyticus* and enterococci. In combination, the nitrite and leukocyte esterase tests perform better; that is, if either leukocyte esterase or nitrite positivity is considered a positive result, then the sensitivity is 75% and the specificity is 82%. A bioluminescence assay is available that has a very high negative predictive value, thus permitting one to rapidly dispense with negative specimens. False negatives are mainly seen in candidal and enterococcal infections. Microscopic detection of pyuria or bacteriuria is highly suggestive of UTI; however, numerous causes of sterile pyuria are recognized. Recall that eosinophiluria is suggestive of acute interstitial nephritis and not of UTI.

The most direct and informative test, however, continues to be culture. A sterile calibrated loop (1, 2, or 10 μL) is used to inoculate the agar plate. The bacterial count is calculated from the number of cfu on the plate after overnight incubation and the quantity of urine originally inoculated. In early studies validating the midstream urine, it was demonstrated that >95% of patients with acute pyelonephritis had >10^5 cfu/mL, whereas <6% of asymptomatic patients had this degree of bacteriuria. This was accepted as the defining criterion for significant bacteriuria for many years. More recently, it has been suggested that lower bacterial counts may be important in particular circumstances, particularly in men and symptomatic women, when unusual organisms are present (fungi, fastidious bacteria), and in the so-called urethral (frequency-dysuria) syndrome. Patients with this syndrome may show no growth in routine media and should be investigated for other agents that cause nonspecific urethritis, such as *Chlamydia trachomatis*. Lastly, almost any bacterial count from specimens obtained directly from the bladder (suprapubic aspiration), ureter, or kidney must be considered clinically significant. The Infectious Disease Society of America (IDSA) has revised its definition of cystitis to >10^2 cfu/mL for symptomatic females.

Specific agents

Escherichia coli is the most common cause of UTI. About 85% of all community acquired UTIs are due to *E coli*, particularly so-called UPEC (uropathogenic) strains.

Staphylococcus saprophyticus is a particularly common cause of UTI in young sexually active women, and is responsible for ~10% of all community acquired UTIs.

Other Enterobacteriaceae—especially *Klebsiella* species and *Enterobacter* species—cause a significant number of the remaining cases.

Enterococcus increases in prominence in older males with obstructive uropathy.

Many UTIs are culture negative; such cases are often due to *Ureaplasma urealyticum*, *Chlamydia* species, or *Mycoplasma hominis*.

Fungal UTI is mainly caused by *Candida* species and associated with indwelling catheters or recent antibiotic therapy.

Hemorrhagic cystitis due to adenoviruses, especially types 11 and 21, is most often seen in bone marrow transplant recipients and children.

Infectious diarrhea

Differential diagnosis

The most common cause of acute infectious diarrhea is a virus, especially noroviruses (calicivirus, Norwalk-like virus), enteric adenoviruses, and rotavirus. These agents account for ≥50% of community acquired acute infectious diarrhea. In fact, if there is nothing unusual in the history, such as hospitalization, antibiotic use, or travel, these agents cause 80-90% of cases. Viral agents tend to produce a brief (< 5 days) diarrheal illness, often accompanied by vomiting, at most mild fever, mild abdominal pain, no neutrophilic exudate in stool, and minimal blood. These patients often do not see a physician and when they do are treated supportively.

Bacterial agents are significantly less common than viruses, the most common being *E coli*, *Salmonella*, *Shigella*, and *Campylobacter*. Bacteria may cause inflammatory (colitic, dysenteric) or noninflammatory (watery) diarrhea. The typical causes of noninflammatory bacterial diarrhea are *Vibrio cholera*, *E coli* (especially enterotoxigenic *E coli* [ETEC]), *C perfringens*, *S aureus*, and *B cereus*. Features that suggest a bacterial cause of noninflammatory diarrhea, as opposed to the more common viral causes, include prolonged (>5 days) illness and fever. Clinical features of bacterial inflammatory diarrhea are fever, bloody stool, severe abdominal pain, tenesmus, and neutrophils in stool. Patients who seek medical care represent a select group of patients who are more likely to have inflammatory diarrhea. In descending order of frequency, inflammatory bacterial diarrhea is caused by *Shigella*, *Campylobacter*, *Salmonella*, *E coli*, *C difficile*, *Aeromonas*, *Yersinia*, and *Vibrio* (noncholera). *C difficile*, long recognized as a cause of diarrheal illness in hospitalized patients, is an increasingly recognized cause of community acquired inflammatory diarrhea in outpatients. Diarrhea with blood, especially *without* fecal neutrophils, suggests enterohemorrhagic (EHEC) *E coli* (O157:H7). This may also be seen with amebiasis (capable of destroying leukocytes). Foreign travel alters the picture considerably. Most cases associated with travel to South and Central America are due to varieties of *E coli* (ETEC, enteroinvasive *E coli* [EIEC]), whereas travel to the far East is more often associated with *Campylobacter*, *Shigella*, and *Salmonella*.

Parasites (with the exception of *Giardia* and *Cryptosporidium*) are an uncommon cause of acute infectious diarrhea in developed countries.

Specific agents

Escherichia coli is a major cause of bacterial diarrhea, but in speaking about *E coli*, the strain must be specified.

- EHEC, otherwise known as Shiga-toxigenic *E coli* (STEC), or verotoxin-producing *E coli* (VPEC) is usually acquired through the ingestion of undercooked processed (ground) beef and contaminated milk, fruit, and vegetables. About 15% of cases result from person to person spread and another 15% from water sources. *E coli* O157:H7 is the most common strain. Infection may result in uncomplicated watery diarrhea, but in some cases it causes acute colitis with cramps, abdominal pain, and bloody diarrhea. Fever is usually at most mild, and often there are no fecal leukocytes. The reason this bacterium has been the subject of much attention is its association with the hemolytic uremic syndrome (HUS). This appears to result from the presence in circulation of Shiga toxins and presents as the triad of microangiopathic hemolytic anemia, renal failure, and thrombocytopenia. HUS predominantly affects children under the age of 5; in fact, it represents a major cause of renal failure in this age group. The mortality rate is ~5%. The laboratory diagnosis (see "Bacteriology," p 177) requires the use of sorbitol-MacConkey agar, but there are enzyme linked immunosorbent assay (ELISA) and polymerase chain reaction (PCR) assays for the Shiga toxin that can be performed on stool. Positive cases should be reported and referred to a reference laboratory for serotyping.

- ETEC causes severe watery diarrhea without dysenteric features, by elaboration of a cholera-like toxin. It is the most common cause of traveler's diarrhea. Detection is discussed in the bacteriology section.

- EIEC causes a similar syndrome to EHEC but does not produce toxins. Colitis is caused by the ability of the organism to use adhesion proteins to invade the bowel wall.

Salmonellae (nontyphoidal species) are often contracted in association with animal contact—either live or in the form of food (milk, chicken, eggs). Recent cases of infections associated with reptile pets (turtles, iguanas) have also been reported. *Salmonella* is the most common cause of death from food borne illness in the United States. Most infections produce only mild watery diarrhea, while others may take the form of a severe colitis. The real morbidity derives from a tendency to produce bacteremia, with a potential for seeding of bone, joints, vascular walls, heart, or brain. The very young and very old are at greatest risk for bacteremia, in addition to those with immunodeficiency, malignancy, diabetes, HIV infection, and indwelling prostheses. *Salmonella* is diagnosed with routine stool culture or PCR.

Campylobacter jejuni is the most common cause of bacterial enteritis in the US. Infection most often results from ingestion of contaminated food (chicken) or water. Diarrhea often lasts for >1 week. While usually not severe, complications such as bacteremia and severe colitis may occur. Furthermore, *C jejuni* is the most commonly identified cause of the Guillain-Barré syndrome, implicated in ~30% of cases. Type O:19 is most commonly associated with Guillain-Barré. Another important complication of *C jejuni* is the development of a reactive arthropathy (so-called enteropathic arthritis), noted in persons with HLA-B27. *Campylobacter* can be diagnosed with routine stool culture or PCR techniques.

Clostridium perfringens spores may be found within food that is inadequately cooked or improperly stored. After consumption, sporulation within the small bowel and enterotoxin production produces a typical syndrome of vomiting and watery diarrhea that, like *S aureus* food poisoning, may present within 8 hours of consumption and resolves quickly, within 24-48 hours.

Diarrhea that develops during or shortly after hospitalization is most commonly due to *Clostridium difficile*. Increasingly, *C difficile* is being identified as a cause of community acquired diarrhea, such that it is now a serious consideration in the differential diagnosis. It is the most common cause of antibiotic-associated diarrhea, being found in ~25% of cases (most of the remaining cases have no identified cause). *C difficile* may lead to severe colitis with toxic megacolon and death, with an overall mortality rate of ~10%. There is a range of illness severity, however, varying from asymptomatic carriage to fulminant colitis. Asymptomatic carriage is found in ~3% of all adults, 50% of neonates, and up to 30% of hospitalized adults. Most symptomatic patients manifest only watery diarrhea, without hematochezia or systemic symptoms. Only ~30% of infected patients develop inflammatory colitis (pseudomembranous colitis), and this group of patients experience abdominal pain, fever, and bloody stool. Recently, there has been a noted increase in the virulence of *C difficile*, attributed to the emergence of the BI/NAP1/027 strain. This strain has undergone deletion of a regulatory gene, such that it produces increased amounts of toxins A and B. Uncomplicated cases of *C difficile* colitis present with watery diarrhea, but if there is progressive colitis there may be systemic manifestations such as fever and neutrophilia. Patients who are at particular risk for *C difficile* include patients with a history of antibiotic use, especially elderly patients, patients receiving proton pump inhibitor therapy, and patients with inflammatory bowel disease. The most commonly implicated antibiotics in antibiotic-associated *C difficile* are clindamycin, cephalosporins, penicillins, and the fluoroquinolones. Testing for *C difficile* may include antigenic assays for stool toxin, culture, or PCR. Culture may give misguiding results, since hospitalized inpatients are rapidly colonized with *C difficile*; it is toxin production that is diagnostic of *C difficile* colitis. The reference method for the detection of *C difficile* is the cytotoxicity assay, in which either stool or cultured bacteria is incubated with a cell culture, looking for cytotoxic activity that can be neutralized by antisera. Antigenic toxin assays (eg, by ELISA or immunochromatography) provide rapid results with high specificity, but they have limited sensitivity, varying from 60-80%. An assay that detects both toxin A and toxin B is required. There is an ELISA for glutamate dehydrogenase, an enzyme produced by *C difficile*; while relatively sensitive, the enzyme is produced by other bacteria, limiting its specificity, and it is uninformative with regard to toxin production. PCR, using real time assays for toxin genes (*tcdA* for toxin A, *tcdB* for toxin B & *tcdC* toxin A/B regulator gene), has emerged as a substitute for ELISA, with sensitivity and specificity of 95-100%. This permits one-time testing for each patient and rapid exclusion or confirmation of clinically significant *C difficile* infection; therefore it is rapidly becoming the gold standard. Endoscopy and biopsy are sometimes undertaken, particularly when the clinical picture is unclear and in patients with *C difficile* related acute exacerbations of chronic colitis. Most patients with *C difficile* colitis (patients with more than just watery diarrhea) have pseudomembranes (~90%), and most patients with pseudomembranes have *C difficile* colitis (~95%). The histologic appearance is highly characteristic but not entirely specific, consisting of sharply bordered foci of superficial mucosal necrosis from which emanates, in "volcano-like" manner, a discharge of mucinopurulent debris.

A presentation similar to antibiotic-associated *C difficile* colitis may be caused by another cytotoxin-producing bacteria, *Klebsiella oxytoca*. Instead of causing pseudomembranes, however, *K oxytoca* causes antibiotic-associated hemorrhagic colitis. The distinction is important, because *K oxytoca* related hemorrhagic colitis appears to resolve quickly with the discontinuation of antibiotics. Antibiotic-associated hemorrhagic colitis involves the right colon predominantly, and biopsies show features suggesting ischemic colitis. Crypt abscesses, the usual hallmark of infectious colitis, are notably absent. Culture for *K oxytoca* should be considered in *C difficile*-negative cases of suspected antibiotic-associated diarrheal illness.

Cholera is a severe epidemic form of voluminous watery diarrhea with flecks of white mucus (rice-water stool) that is very rare in the United States. The syndrome is caused principally by 2 serogroups of *V cholerae*: serogroup O1 (*V cholerae*

O1) and serogroup O139. Noncholera (non-01 and non-139) strains may cause less severe gastroenteritis and/or wound infections. Cholera tends to occur in pandemics, related to a particular strain of *V cholerae* (eg, El Tor from south and central Africa). *Vibrio* species, including cholera and noncholera species, are commonly acquired in the United States from shellfish (especially oysters from the Gulf Coast). Clinically, cholera strains may produce illness ranging from very mild to very severe watery diarrhea of sufficient quantity to cause dehydration and death. Laboratory diagnosis requires plating on selective media such as thiosulfate citrate bile salt sucrose (TCBS) agar.

Vibrio parahaemolyticus, like non-01, non-139 strains of *V cholerae*, can cause gastroenteritis and wound infections related to seafood or seawater. In fact, *V parahaemolyticus* is the most common cause of food borne illness in Japan. *V parahaemolyticus* wound infection is seen when wounds are exposed to or acquired within seawater and can lead to severe septicemia, particularly in diabetics and alcoholics.

Vibrio vulnificus can cause fatal food borne infection in hosts with hepatic disease or immunodeficiency as well as wound infections, again related to seafood and seawater, respectively.

Yersinia enterocolitica has been associated with infectious diarrhea and distal ileitis resembling acute appendicitis. Pathogenicity appears to relate to the presence within the bacterium of a particular plasmid (the pYV virulence plasmid) for which DNA-based assays are available. *Y enterocolitica* is not among the more common causes of infectious diarrhea in the United States, but is very common in northern Europe. Infection frequently results from consumption of contaminated pork, but contaminated drinking water may also transmit infection. An HLA-B27-linked postinfectious arthritis may occur as with *Campylobacter* infection.

Whereas most agents of bacterial diarrhea are food borne, *Shigella* is known for person to person spread and spread by insects (houseflies). It is an agent that can spread quickly among close contacts, for example in daycare centers, nursing homes, and military barracks, due to the very small inoculum required for infection. While some infections may be mild, *Shigella* is a major cause of dysentery, with bloody stool, fever, and tenesmus.

Entamoeba histolytica should be considered in prolonged diarrhea or in a recent traveler (or immigrant) who presents with bloody diarrhea. The organisms invade the colonic mucosa to produce the characteristic flask shaped ulcers, especially within the right colon. Colonic biopsies that contain ulcers or pronounced neutrophilic inflammation should be scoured for organisms, typically seen at the leading edge of the ulcer. Stool microscopy has only ~50% sensitivity for *E histolytica* (and specificity is limited by the morphologically identical but nonpathogenic *E dispar*), but stool EIA has very high sensitivity and specificity. Organisms are rarely recognizable in extraintestinal *E histolytica* infections (eg, amebic liver abscess).

Viruses are the most common cause of infectious diarrhea in all age groups in the United States. Causes of pediatric viral gastroenteritis, in order of frequency, include rotavirus (most common), norovirus, enteric adenoviruses (serotypes 40, 41), coronavirus, and astroviruses. The laboratory diagnosis of viral gastroenteritis is influenced by the fact that as a group these agents grow poorly in cell culture. Electron microscopy (of stool) has traditionally been used for diagnosis, with each virus having distinctive morphology; however, this modality is rarely used today. Rotavirus infection is especially common between 6-12 months of age. It is responsible for over half of cases of watery diarrhea in infants and very young children in the United States, and, worldwide, is a common cause of death in this age group. Nursing home outbreaks are an increasingly recognized problem. Rotavirus outbreaks tend to occur during the cold weather months (hence the nickname "winter vomiting disease"). Caliciviruses that cause gastroenteritis include noroviruses (Norwalk-like virus) and sapoviruses (Sapporo-like viruses). Norovirus is food borne but can be transmitted from person to person and requires a very small inoculum. It tends to occur in outbreaks affecting large numbers of children and adults simultaneously; in fact, norovirus is the most common cause of epidemic gastroenteritis in all age groups, in all parts of the world, accounting for about half of outbreaks worldwide. It is a common cause of cruise-ship acquired diarrhea. Infection with norovirus is characterized by a prominent component of nausea and vomiting in addition to diarrhea. Real time PCR (RT-PCR) assays have been developed for detection of norovirus in stool, water, and food. EIA detection methods are also available. Both assays suffer from low sensitivity but have high specificity; therefore, positive tests for norovirus in a few patient samples from an outbreak implicate the others as being norovirus related. Astroviruses get their name from a star-like appearance on electron microscopy. Diarrheal illness due to astrovirus affects primarily children younger than 4 years of age and has a seasonal—winter—peak. Adenovirus serotypes 40 and 41 (enteric adenoviruses) are the cause of ~20% of pediatric viral gastroenteritis. There is no distinct seasonality, and the virus primarily afflicts children <4 years of age.

Infectious diarrhea in AIDS

AIDS (and other forms of immunodeficiency) is characterized by infection with the common agents of infectious diarrhea as well as unique agents. With regard to the common agents, infection tends to be more severe, more prolonged, and require antibiotics.

Agents somewhat unique to or more severe in immunodeficient patients include *Cryptosporidium* species, *Cyclospora cayetanensis*, microsporidia, *Cystoisospora belli*, CMV and *Mycobacterium avium* complex (MAC).

Laboratory evaluation

In those presenting for laboratory evaluation, the approach includes stool examination and selective application of specialized techniques including EIA and culture.

Stool microscopy has 2 purposes

1. to determine whether leukocytes are present

2. to look for parasite ova and larvae

Assays for stool lactoferrin (a product of neutrophils) can substitute for a microscopic search for leukocytes.

Routine stool culture is capable of isolating a limited range of organisms: *Salmonella* species, *Shigella* species, *E coli*, *Campylobacter* species, *Yersinia enterocolitica*, and *Vibrio* species (TCBS agar). Most labs routinely test for *E coli* O157:H7 by culture, EIA, and or PCR-based tests, and many labs now routinely test for *C difficile* in community acquired diarrhea (and always in hospital acquired cases) using EIA or PCR-based tests.

Pneumonia
Differential diagnosis

The probable microbial agents differ with the circumstances—especially important are the underlying condition of the host (alcoholism, smoking, COPD, age, overall health) t3.1 and whether acquired in or out of the hospital. The most common causes of community acquired pneumonia in immunocompetent, healthy, adults are *Mycoplasma pneumoniae*, *Chlamydia pneumoniae*, *Streptococcus pneumoniae*, and *Haemophilus influenzae*.

The distinction of typical pneumonia from atypical pneumonia is an idealized dichotomy that nonetheless holds some value. Typical pneumonia, which presents abruptly with fever, productive cough, and a distinct, usually lobar, infiltrate on chest x-ray, is usually caused by pyogenic bacteria (*Streptococcus pneumoniae* being the prototype). Atypical pneumonia classically presents with a dry cough of prolonged duration and diffuse bilateral pulmonary infiltrates. It is caused by "atypical" agents, prototypically *Mycoplasma pneumoniae*.

In elderly nursing home tenants, mycoplasma and chlamydia fall away from the list; *S pneumoniae*, *H influenzae*, aerobic Gram− bacilli, and anaerobes become more common.

AIDS patients are particularly susceptible to bacterial and mycobacterial pneumonia when CD4 counts are moderately depressed. At very low CD4 counts, opportunistic infections due to *Pneumocystis jiroveci* (formerly *P carinii*) and *Cryptococcus neoformans* are common.

In hospitalized ventilated patients, the most common agents are *S aureus*, *S pneumoniae*, *P aeruginosa*, *K pneumoniae*, *Serratia* species, *Enterobacter* species, *E coli*, and fungi.

Aspiration pneumonia must be distinguished from aspiration pneumonitis (Mendelson syndrome). The latter is a sterile form of pulmonary injury that results from aspiration of gastric contents, with acid mediated pulmonary injury ensuing. As in the original description by Mendelson, aspiration pneumonitis is most commonly encountered in young patients undergoing general anesthesia. Aspiration pneumonitis may be eventually complicated by infection and pneumonia, especially in patients with bacterial colonization of the stomach, as happens when the gastric pH is raised (eg, proton pump inhibitor therapy). Aspiration pneumonia, on the other hand, results from aspiration of oropharyngeal material, including oropharyngeal flora, which results in lung infection. The factors that increase the risk of aspiration pneumonia, therefore, are those factors that either increase the number of oropharyngeal bacteria or decrease the natural barriers to aspiration (effective swallowing, cough reflex, ciliary motility). Elderly patients, especially those with a history of stroke and/or poor dentition, are at highest risk. The most commonly implicated organisms are *Streptococcus pneumoniae*, *Staphylococcus* aureus, *H influenzae*, Enterobacteriaceae, and *P aeruginosa*. *P aeruginosa* is the most common organism isolated in hospital acquired aspiration pneumonia. Anaerobes are only rarely encountered.

t3.1 Risk factors for agents of pneumonia

Host factor	Agents suggested
COPD	*Haemophilus influenzae*, *Moraxella catarrhalis*, *Legionella pneumophila*
Alcoholism	*S pneumoniae*, *Klebsiella pneumoniae*, anaerobes (aspiration), Gram− aerobic bacilli
Neutropenia	Aerobic Gram− bacilli
Animal exposure	*Coxiella burnetii* (cattle, cats), *Chlamydophila psittaci* (birds), *Cryptococcus neoformans* (birds), *Histoplasma capsulatum* (bat or bird droppings, especially pigeons), Hantavirus (mouse urine & feces), *Francisella tularensis* (rabbits)
Sandstorm exposure	*Coccidioides immitis/posadasii*
Bronchiectasis, cystic fibrosis	*Pseudomonas aeruginosa*, *Burkholderia cepacia*, *Staphylococcus aureus*

Specific agents

Streptococcus pneumoniae (pneumococcus) is the most common cause of community acquired pneumonia and a very common cause of hospital acquired pneumonia. The typical case presents as lobar pneumonia. An increased risk is associated with extremes of age, chronic alcoholism, dementia, HIV, and stroke. Pneumococcus is isolated in ~1/3 of community acquired pneumonia requiring hospitalization, and >1/2 of pneumonia associated with bacteremia. In fact, blood culture often provides the diagnosis of pneumococcal pneumonia. Since ~5-10% of adults have pharyngeal colonization by *S pneumoniae*, sputum cultures produce an unacceptably high false positive rate. Ideally, the culture diagnosis relies upon a specimen that bypasses the upper aerodigestive tract (ie, an invasive specimen or blood culture). A urinary antigen test has been developed that can be used in cases of invasive disease. There have been increasing rates of penicillin-resistant pneumococci.

Staphylococcus aureus is an uncommon cause of community acquired pneumonia, producing ~5% of cases, but a major cause of hospital acquired pneumonia. *S aureus* pneumonia is typically severe, tending to produce cavitary disease. Risk factors include prolonged hospitalization, old age, preexisting lung disease, and recent antibiotic therapy. Methicillin-resistant strains should be suspected, particularly when the infection is hospital acquired.

Haemophilus influenzae is isolated in ~10% of patients with community acquired pneumonia. Most isolates are nontypeable strains. *H influenzae* typically presents with a bronchopneumonia pattern consisting of patchy segmental infiltrates. Patients with COPD (airway type more than emphysematous) are at particular risk for *H influenzae* pneumonia. Other risk factors include the recent use of antibiotics or corticosteroids.

Moraxella catarrhalis is found to colonize the upper airways of ~5% of healthy adults, and lung disease promotes lower respiratory tract infection. Severe infection is seen predominantly in elderly patients with COPD, risk factors for aspiration, or congestive heart failure. Together, *H influenzae* and *M catarrhalis* are major causes of acute exacerbation in patients with COPD.

Legionella pneumophila causes ~15% of community acquired pneumonia, but a much larger proportion of fatal community acquired pneumonia, with 1 in 5 infected patients requiring admission to the ICU and a 15-50% mortality rate.

The infection is often acquired in association with an unusual exposure to aerosolized particles—construction associated dust, hot tub, cooling systems. Severely affected patients usually have unhealthy lungs, due to smoking or COPD, or systemic illness such as diabetes, hepatic insufficiency, renal insufficiency, hematolymphoid neoplasms, or immunodeficiency. Legionellosis encompasses 2 clinical syndromes: Legionnaires disease and Pontiac fever. Legionnaires disease is an atypical pneumonia with characteristic clinical features, including high fever, hyponatremia, renal dysfunction, diarrhea, and neurologic abnormalities. Pontiac fever is a flu-like illness without pneumonia. The laboratory diagnosis of *L pneumophila* is usually based upon culture on specialized charcoal media (BCYE: buffered charcoal-yeast extract agar with cysteine). More rapid tests include direct fluorescence antibody (DFA), which, when performed on sputum or respiratory specimens, has a reported 70% sensitivity and 97% specificity. The *Legionella* urinary antigen assay plays an important role in the diagnosis of *L pneumophila* serogroup 1 which accounts for ~80% of all *Legionella* infections. In addition, PCR assays are becoming an increasingly more common component of *Legionella* diagnostics.

Aerobic Gram– bacilli, such as **Pseudomonas aeruginosa**, are uncommon causes of community acquired pneumonia, but they tend to be quite severe and to afflict those with underlying disease such as bronchiectasis, cystic fibrosis, and advanced malignancy. They are significant causes of hospital acquired pneumonia, particularly ventilator-associated pneumonia. *P aeruginosa* produces severe necrotizing pneumonia, often associated with ARDS. In patients successfully treated, the organism is rarely actually eradicated, and most patients become chronic carriers, reinfecting themselves over time. *Serratia marcescens* and *Acinetobacter baumannii* have clinical and epidemiologic features similar to *Pseudomonas* species

Anaerobes are generally acquired through aspiration. They often produce cavitary disease, abscess, and empyema. Since anaerobes are common in the oral cavity, the diagnosis of anaerobic lung infection must circumvent the upper airway; thus, the diagnosis relies upon transtracheal aspirates, transthoracic aspirates, or pleural (empyema) fluid. As a result, anaerobic lung infections are usually diagnosed and treated based upon clinical findings.

Mycoplasma pneumoniae and *Chlamydia pneumoniae* cause atypical pneumonia, together causing the majority of community acquired pneumonia that does not require hospitalization. These agents should be considered strongly in outbreaks amongst groups of young healthy adults, such as military recruits. *M pneumoniae* and *C pneumoniae* produce patchy, sometimes bilateral, infiltrates, a prolonged (weeks) dry cough, and extra-pulmonary manifestations; eg, cold agglutinins and bullous myringitis. The diagnosis of *C pneumoniae* is facilitated by serology: detection of IgM in a titer of >1:16 or a 4-fold increase in IgG. The gold standard is culture, but this is not widely available. Serology for *M pneumoniae* is limited by a commonly delayed antibody response. Nucleic acid based techniques such as PCR are becoming more common for diagnosis of these organisms.

Viral pneumonia

Acute viral lower respiratory tract infection may take the form of bronchitis, bronchiolitis, or pneumonia. The major viral pathogens are influenza viruses, respiratory syncytial virus (RSV), parainfluenza viruses, rhinovirus, adenovirus, and the recently described agents hantavirus, metapneumovirus, severe acute respiratory syndrome (SARS)-associated coronavirus, coronavirus NL63, coronavirus HKU1, bocavirus, and HPV viruses KI and WU. The traditional methods of respiratory virus detection, cell culture and direct fluorescent assays (DFA) are capable of detecting the first 5 agents, but the recently described agents, which were discovered by molecular techniques, are not routinely detected. Multiplex PCR assays for numerous bacterial and viral pathogens are increasingly used for diagnosis.

Hantavirus pulmonary syndrome (HPS) was initially identified as an ARDS-producing illness in the 4 Corners region of New Mexico. HPS was caused by a member of the Bunyaviridae family, a hantavirus that came to be named Sin Nombre virus. The virus is carried by the deer mouse (different than the white-footed mouse that is a reservoir for Lyme disease), which sheds virus into the environment, mainly in the form of infected urine and feces. Humans are exposed to the virus through contact with this material and, in 1-2 weeks, develop a flulike illness, a prodrome in which thrombocytopenia is commonly noted. Pulmonary edema develops, followed by hypotension, and additional peripheral blood findings: persistent thrombocytopenia, neutrophilia without toxic granulation, erythrocytosis (a reflection of hemoconcentration), and a population of immunoblastic lymphocytes that exceed a proportion of 10%. Eventually, a clinicopathologic picture of acute respiratory distress syndrome (ARDS) with diffuse alveolar damage (DAD) develops within the lungs. There is at present a fatality rate of 30-40%. A definitive diagnosis requires serologic detection of IgG and IgM anti-hantavirus antibodies. The most recent outbreak of hantavirus in the US occurred in the summer of 2012 and was associated with travel to Yosemite National Park in California.

Parainfluenza virus type 3 is predominantly an affliction of spring and summer, while types 1 and 2 occur in the fall. Parainfluenza viruses affect mainly children, producing cases of croup, bronchitis, bronchiolitis, and pneumonia. Parainfluenza viruses, especially type 1, are the most common cause of croup.

Respiratory syncytial virus (RSV) peaks in winter, especially in January and February, with nearly all cases falling between November and May. RSV is the most common cause of bronchiolitis in children, in which initial infections may be quite severe and require hospitalization.

Human metapneumovirus overlaps RSV, occurring in winter and spring, and turns out to be the second most common cause of bronchiolitis in children after RSV. The 2 viruses produce a very similar clinical picture.

Severe acute respiratory syndrome (SARS) emerged in the Guangdong province of China and spread to Hong Kong, from where travelers carried it to the world. SARS is attributed to a coronavirus which is now called the SARS coronavirus (SARS-CoV), a virus that is efficiently spread from person to person and carries a 10% mortality. Following an incubation period of 2-10 days, the infection produces a flulike syndrome that leads to respiratory compromise clinicopathologically resembling ARDS with DAD. While SARS-CoV appears to grow well in specialized cell culture (Vero E6 cell lines), real time PCR, performed on a nasopharyngeal specimen, is the preferred means of laboratory diagnosis.

There are a number of tests available for the detection of respiratory viruses, with varying performance characteristics. A handful of rapid, nonimmunofluorescent, tests are available, including enzyme immunoassay (EIA) and optical immunoassay (OIA), that can provide results within 30 minutes. Nonimmunofluorescent tests are sensitive to a limited variety of agents (usually only influenza and RSV) and provide low analytic sensitivity (require a large number of viral particles for a positive result) but provide good specificity in season (70-100%). In nonpeak seasons, specificity is low, and positives should be confirmed by another method. Direct fluorescent antibody (DFA) testing panels may be performed directly on respiratory specimens. Panels commonly include influenza A, influenza B, RSV, parainfluenza 1-3, and adenovirus. The preferred specimen is a nasopharyngeal aspirate or swab; specimen adequacy is assessed based upon the number of ciliated epithelial cells. Spots are made upon slides from the swab or aspirate, and fluorescence tagged monoclonal antibody is added to each. DFA provides results within 90 minutes. The sensitivity depends upon the virus: DFA is more sensitive for RSV than culture (because of the lability of RSV); for adenovirus it is significantly less sensitive than culture (50%); for all others the sensitivity of DFA is ~80% compared to culture. Many laboratories are also currently testing for metapneumovirus by DFA which can also be grown, albeit slowly, in culture. Traditional respiratory viral tube cultures are incubated at 37°C for 14 days and inspected daily for viral cytopathic effect (CPE). Clues to the identity of the viral agent are given by the morphology of the cytopathic effect (CPE) and the types of cells in which it is shown; presently, fluorescent-tagged monoclonal antibodies are used to aid in identification. A hemadsorption test is performed to detect influenza. A rapid cell culture is performed by incubating specimens in shell vials, microtubes, or other support, and adding fluorescence tagged monoclonal antibodies at 24-72 hours. Lastly, nucleic acid tests (NAT), which are largely in development, offer numerous advantages. These include rapidity, high sensitivity, and minimization of risk to laboratory personnel. Multiplex molecular assays for the detection of viral respiratory pathogens are the future of viral pneumonia diagnostics.

Laboratory approach to the diagnosis of pneumonia

The peripheral blood leukocyte count and differential are provide limited assistance in differentiating bacterial from viral infections. More importantly, a total leukocyte count may reveal evidence of immunodeficiency, in the form of neutropenia or lymphopenia; however, it is useful to remember that neutropenia may be a manifestation of overwhelming sepsis in very young and very old patients. The serum lactate dehydrogenase (LD) is characteristically quite high in *Pneumocystis* pneumonia (PCP).

Direct examination and culture of sputum specimens has unclear value, depending largely upon the quality of the specimen, and is not currently recommended as a routine test by the Infectious Disease Society of America and American Thoracic Society (IDSA/ATS). There has been much controversy over the issue of what constitutes adequate sputum for culture. Generally speaking, yield improves with more neutrophils and fewer squamous cells, but there is a range of what is considered acceptable. Nonetheless, many laboratories apply microscopic examination criteria to prescreen sputum specimens for adequacy, most commonly requiring <5 squamous cells and >25 neutrophils per high power field. Standard culture media for routine respiratory pathogens include 5% sheep blood agar, MacConkey, and chocolate agar. Chocolate agar is incubated in a hypercapnic environment to encourage the growth of *H influenzae*. Special media are required when *Legionella* or pertussis is suspected.

Blood culture is positive in ~30% of patients with pneumonia but is, like sputum, not currently recommended (IDSA/ATS) for all patients. Blood culture is generally reserved for patients admitted to the intensive care unit and are ideally obtained before the administration of antibiotics.

Infective endocarditis (IE)
Differential diagnosis

The microbial differential diagnosis of infective endocarditis depends largely upon the status of the underlying valve. Endocarditis should thus be viewed as 3 major clinical syndromes, each with its own differential diagnosis: infection of a previously normal native valve, infection of a previously abnormal native valve, and infection of a prosthetic valve.

Native valve endocarditis affecting a previously normal valve is due to infection by highly virulent organisms that rapidly destroy the valve, causing the clinical picture of acute bacterial endocarditis. The responsible agent is most often *S aureus*. Less common causes of acute bacterial endocarditis include enterococci and certain streptococci, especially *Streptococcus milleri*. Tricuspid endocarditis due to *S aureus* may be seen in IV drug abusers. Pneumococcal endocarditis is not seen much anymore, but it is a virulent form of acute bacterial endocarditis that historically formed part of Austrian syndrome—the triad of endocarditis, meningitis, and pneumonia—seen in alcoholics.

Native valves with underlying structural damage can be infected by less virulent organisms. These organisms do not cause valve destruction; instead, they tend to form vegetations. The resulting syndrome is known as subacute bacterial endocarditis (SBE). In most cases, the underlying valvular anomaly is due to rheumatic heart disease, most often affecting the mitral valve. Other cases are related to mitral valve prolapse, nodular dystrophic (age related) calcification of the aortic valve, and congenital heart disease (eg, atrial septal defect, ventricular septal defect, patent ductus arteriosus, idiopathic hypertrophic subaortic sclerosis, and coarctation of the aorta). The clinical features derive from: infection itself (fever, constitutional symptoms); valve dysfunction (hemodynamic instability); emboli from the vegetation (Janeway lesions, Roth spots, strokes, renal dysfunction; Osler nodes); and immune stimulation (rheumatoid factor, circulating immune complexes leading to, eg, glomerulonephritis). These infections are predominantly due to viridans streptococci (*Streptococcus sanguis*, *Streptococcus mutans*, and *Streptococcus mitis*), group B streptococci, group D streptococci (*Streptococcus bovis*), enterococci (*Enterococcus faecalis*) and HACEK organisms.

The microbiology of very early (within 2 months) and early (within the 1st year) prosthetic valve endocarditis differs from that of late (>1 year) prosthetic valve endocarditis. Very early infection is caused by *S aureus*, *S epidermidis*, and Gram– bacilli, reflecting their basis in hospital/surgical contamination. Early infection of prosthetic valves is most often due to *Staphylococcus epidermidis* and *S aureus*. Late infection has a microbial differential diagnosis resembling that of SBE involving native valves. Very early infection (<2 months) of all types of prosthetic valve, and infection of mechanical valves regardless of timing, centers upon the valve suture ring, leading to the possibility of dehiscence, fistula, dysrhythmia, and stenosis. Infections of bioprosthetic valves is likely to affect the leaflets, with manifestations similar to native valve endocarditis.

~5-10% of cases of endocarditis are associated with negative blood cultures. The most common cause of blood culture-negative endocarditis (BCNE) is prior antibiotic therapy. Furthermore, causes of noninfectious endocarditis must be considered (Libman-Sacks endocarditis, nonbacterial thrombotic (marantic) endocarditis, carcinoid heart syndrome). The infectious agents that cause BCNE include *Coxiella burnetii*, *Bartonella*, *Chlamydia*, *Legionella*, *Tropheryma whipplei*, and the highly fastidious "HACEK" organisms.

Specific agents

While coagulase– staphylococci (eg, *S epidermidis*) are uncommon causes of native valve endocarditis, they are a major cause of prosthetic valve and nosocomial endocarditis.

S aureus is the most common cause of acute bacterial endocarditis in native valves, and it is a major cause of prosthetic valve and nosocomial endocarditis. Furthermore, it causes the majority of right-sided (tricuspid) endocarditis in IV drug abusers. *S aureus* causes rapid destruction of the valve leaflets and the formation of abscesses in the valve ring and underlying myocardium. This produces a fulminant clinical picture with high fever, prostration, and in many cases hemodynamic collapse. Urgent surgical valve replacement is often required.

Streptococci, especially the viridans streptococci, are the most common causes of subacute bacterial endocarditis (SBE); however, *S anginosus* group is known for its ability to cause acute endocarditis. As discussed later in this chapter, the α-hemolytic streptococci include *S pneumoniae* (not currently a common cause of endocarditis) and the viridans streptococci (including such common causes of SBE as *S sanguis*, *S mutans*, and *S salivarius*). Group D organisms, including the enterococci and *S bovis*, follow slightly in incidence and tend to affect an older age group. Isolation of *S bovis* should generate interest in lower GI endoscopy, because of a strong correlation with colorectal pathology, especially colorectal carcinoma. In series conducted in the first half of the 20th century, *S pneumoniae* was a major consideration in infective endocarditis, causing 10-20% of cases, and usually running a fulminant (acute endocarditis) course. Currently it is found in ~1% of cases. Many patients with pneumococcal infective endocarditis have traditionally been alcoholics, with concurrent meningitis and pneumonia (Austrian syndrome), and a very high rate of mortality. *Enterococci* represent the third most common cause of infective endocarditis (after *Staphylococcus* and *Streptococcus*), responsible for 10-15% of cases.

HACEK organisms, including members of the genera *Haemophilus*, *Aggregatibacter* (formerly *Actinobacillus*), *Cardiobacterium*, *Eikenella*, and *Kingella* are known for producing SBE with large friable vegetations with frequent embolic complications. The main HACEK species among *Haemophilus* are *H parainfluenzae*, *H aphrophilus*, and *H paraphrophilus* (the latter 2 have been grouped together under a new name, *Aggregatibacter aphrophilus*). *Aggregatibacter* (formerly *Actinobacillus*) actinomycetemcomitans, *Cardiobacterium hominis*, *Eikenella corrodens*, and *Kingella kingae*.

Bartonella species, especially *B quintana* and *B henselae*, account for ~1% of all infective endocarditis cases and 10% of blood culture negative endocarditis (BCNE). The clinician must seek epidemiological clues when cultures turn up negative, such as homelessness and chronic alcohol use for *B quintana* infection and cat (kitten, usually) exposure for *B henselae*. Serology is probably the most useful confirmatory test for *Bartonella* endocarditis. High-titer (>1:800) IgG has a high predictive value (IgM is usually gone by the time of presentation). Culture is difficult but should be attempted. PCR testing on blood or excised heart valves may also be attempted.

Coxiella burnetii, the causative agent of Q fever, is thought to cause up to 3% of cases of infective endocarditis. *C burnetii* does not produce vegetations or other macroscopic clues to endocarditis. Microscopic sections may only show fibrosis, calcification, and a sparse mononuclear infiltrate. The aortic valve is involved in >80% of the cases. While the organisms can be demonstrated histologically in most cases, serology is the mainstay of clinical diagnosis. The presence of antibodies against so-called phase I antigen of *C burnetii* are indicative of remote or chronic infection; a high IgG titer (>1:200) of antibody against phase II antigen has high positive predictive value for current active infection. Furthermore, a 4-fold rise in antibodies against phase II antigen is indicative of active infection.

Tropheryma whipplei, like *Coxiella*, is likely to be missed clinically and pathologically. Histological findings, while including histiocytes, are not the classic findings of Whipple disease seen in other organs. Microbial staining can highlight the organisms, however. PCR of heart valve tissue can be used to confirm the diagnosis.

Fungal endocarditis is unusual and largely restricted to certain susceptible groups:

1. patients who are immunodeficient

2. patients who have undergone long-term antibiotic therapy

3. patients who have received total parenteral nutrition

4. intravenous drug abusers

5. patients who have undergone open heart surgery

Candida species are the most common cause of fungal endocarditis, most commonly *C parapsilosis* in intravenous drug abusers and *C albicans* in heart surgery related cases. *Candida* glabrata and *Aspergillus* species are responsible for a significant portion of the remaining cases.

Laboratory approach to diagnosis

The diagnosis of endocarditis is based upon the Duke criteria which encompasses numerous clinical parameters and blood cultures. The proposed St Thomas modifications, seeking to detect atypical cases of bacterial endocarditis, include serologic and molecular assays for fastidious organisms. Nonspecific inflammatory markers, such as C-reactive protein and procalcitonin, may be measured initially as a way to follow the progress of treatment. In relatively stable patients (most of those with SBE), it is preferable to identify an organism prior to instigating antibiotic therapy; whereas in acute presentations empiric antibiotics are initiated immediately following the collection of blood for cultures.

It is advised that multiple blood cultures be performed: 3 sets of blood cultures, drawn at separate times (1-8 hours apart), each paired and of adequate volume (ideally 20-30 cc).

It is traditional teaching that blood cultures should optimally be drawn in the hour preceding a fever spike; most patients spike fever at about the same time every day, so that this is not as absurd as it might at first appear. However, the bacteremia in IE is relatively continuous, and culture timing does not appear to alter yield for most organisms; furthermore, in acute endocarditis, a delay in obtaining cultures prior to initiating antibiotics is unacceptable.

Paired cultures should be obtained (2 separate sites, ideally opposite arms, with 1-2 aerobic bottles and 1 anaerobic bottle at each site).

There are several reasons to obtain more than 1 set of cultures when possible:

1. more cultures increase the likelihood of a positive culture

2. positive cultures >2 or more separate times documents the continuous bacteremia that typifies endocarditis

3. positive cultures >2 or more separate times helps to justify that an organism is not a contaminant (especially important in prosthetic valve endocarditis where *S epidermidis* is common).

In modern automated blood culture systems using highly supportive media, most etiologic agents (including fastidious ones such as HACEK, *Brucella,* and *Francisella*) should produce a positive culture within 5 days.

Fungal endocarditis is most commonly due to *Candida* species. Fortunately, most blood cultures will support the growth of *Candida*. Recovery of other agents, including *Aspergillus,* requires special media, and many fungal agents are only diagnosed upon examination of the excised valve (or excised thromboemboli).

The identification of organisms such as *Bartonella* may require prolonged (>4 weeks) incubation. Identification of *C burnetii, T whipplei,* and *Chlamydophila psittaci* require special cell culture techniques that are not typically available in the microbiology lab.

There has been an increase in demand for molecular assays in the diagnosis of bacterial endocarditis, particularly in 2 clinical circumstances:

1. culture negative endocarditis

2. *S aureus* endocarditis with possible methicillin resistant strains

PCR amplification of the universal bacterial gene that encodes 16S ribosomal RNA, 16S rDNA, provides a useful means of confirming bacterial infection in a wide range of circumstances. Either peripheral blood or excised valve tissue may be the subject of amplification.

The pathologist is likely to become involved directly in the case only upon examination of the excised valve. Gram staining of this material, particularly after a course of antibiotic therapy, can be somewhat misleading as antibiotic therapy can significantly alter the morphology of stained organisms (eg, elongated and enlarged cocci). Nonetheless, in blood-culture negative cases, histologic examination may be fruitful. Microbial stains (Gram, PAS, GMS, Steiner or Warthin-Starry) should be scrutinized; in some cases, immunohistochemical staining or PCR can facilitate the diagnosis of a suspected organism.

Meningitis
Differential diagnosis

There are ≥3 major clinical syndromes produced by infection of the central nervous system: bacterial meningitis, "aseptic" (usually viral) meningitis, and encephalitis. Meningitis refers to inflammation of the meninges, whereas encephalitis refers to inflammation of the brain parenchyma. There are, of course, overlapping presentations (meningoencephalitis). The presentation of encephalitis is dominated by altered mental status. Bacterial and aseptic meningitis have similar clinical presentations (meningismus): headache, stiff neck, photophobia, fever, altered mental status, positive Brudzinski and Kernig signs. By definition, they are distinguished by microbial cultures, but they may be distinguished prospectively by the chemical and microscopic CSF findings.

CSF in aseptic meningitis (viral) shows low level leukocytosis (often <250 leukocytes/mL) with a predominance of mononuclear cells (especially lymphocytes). While the protein is moderately increased, the glucose is in the normal range.

In bacterial meningitis, there is marked leukocytosis with a predominance of neutrophils. The glucose is markedly depressed.

In encephalitis the CSF can vary between normal and findings typical of viral meningitis. The major exception is herpes encephalitis, which can present with a bloody CSF, very high protein, and low glucose.

Encephalitis is usually a viral illness but can be caused by other agents, notably the amebic organisms *Naegleria fowleri* (primary amebic meningoencephalitis), *Acanthamoeba* species, and *Balamuthia mandrillaris* (granulomatous amebic encephalitis). The most common viral causes are herpes simplex type 1 (HSV-1), arboviruses (St Louis encephalitis, California encephalitis, West Nile virus, western equine encephalitis, eastern equine encephalitis), HHV-6, mumps virus, measles virus, and varicella zoster virus.

Aseptic meningitis is more common than bacterial meningitis and is most often due to a virus; however, it may be caused by mycoplasma, rickettsiae, mycobacteria, and parasites. The enteroviruses (coxsackie A and B, echoviruses, poliovirus) are the most common cause of aseptic meningitis in all age groups, causing up to 70% of cases. Summer/fall outbreaks are typical. Other viral causes of aseptic meningitis include herpes simplex virus type 2 (HSV-2), mumps virus, human immunodeficiency virus (HIV), and lymphocytic choriomeningitis virus (LCM).

Traditionally, the list of most common agents causing bacterial meningitis was topped by *H influenzae* type B; immunization has led to a major decline in *H influenzae* meningitis, and *S pneumoniae* is now the most common agent overall. Furthermore, since *H influenzae* was a major cause of childhood meningitis, the average age of patients afflicted has changed; previously a disease mainly of infants and young children, meningitis now peaks in young adults. The causes of meningitis vary with demography.

- Worldwide and for all age groups, the most common causes of meningitis are *Streptococcus pneumoniae*, *Haemophilus influenzae*, and *Neisseria meningitidis*.

- In neonates, group B streptococci, Gram– aerobic bacilli (*E coli*, *Klebsiella*), and *Listeria monocytogenes* are the most common causes of meningitis.

- In infants and young children, *Neisseria meningitidis*, *S pneumoniae*, and *H influenzae* type B (nonimmunized patients) are the most common causes.

- In adults, *S pneumoniae* is the most common cause, followed by *N meningitidis*.

- In elderly adults, *N meningitidis* is replaced by *L monocytogenes* in second place, followed by Gram– aerobic bacilli.

- *Streptococcus suis* is the most common cause of meningitis in Southeast Asia, but it is rare elsewhere.

- In HIV infection, *S pneumoniae* is the most common cause of meningitis, but one must consider *Mycobacterium tuberculosis* (a cause of basilar meningitis) and *Cryptococcus neoformans*.

- In endemic regions, cerebral malaria must be distinguished from bacterial meningitis.

Specific agents

Herpes simplex virus type 1 causes a form of encephalitis that is associated with necrosis and hemorrhage within the anterior temporal lobes. The presence of particular neurologic abnormalities—aphasia, olfactory and gustatory hallucinations, abnormal behavior—suggests HSV encephalitis, as does the finding of red cells in the cerebrospinal fluid. HSV encephalitis has a high fatality rate as well as a high rate of long-term neurologic deficits in survivors. When HSV-1 encephalitis is suspected, a rapid and reliable way to make the diagnosis is PCR, performed upon the cerebrospinal fluid.

Herpes simplex virus type 2 causes aseptic (viral) meningitis. CSF PCR is the best way to confirm this diagnosis.

HHV-6, the virus that causes exanthem subitum, is a common cause of viral encephalitis in children, and it is thought to contribute to many cases of febrile seizures in children. A rash that develops upon the breaking of a several-days-long high fever characterizes exanthem subitum. Most children recover without long-term sequelae.

The arboviruses, especially St Louis and California (especially La Crosse) encephalitis viruses, are the most common causes of viral encephalitis in the United States. These agents are transmitted by mosquito and most commonly affect children. Characteristic clinical features include vomiting, hyponatremia, altered mental status, nystagmus, ataxia, and seizures.

West Nile Virus, an arbovirus of the family Flaviviridae, causes encephalitis with the characteristic findings of weakness, paresis, and peripheral neuropathy. The virus, not found in the US prior to 1999, is found primarily in birds. Mosquitoes transmit it from infected birds to humans. The best way to diagnose all of these arboviruses is by serology.

Enteroviruses are the most common cause of aseptic (viral) meningitis. In particular, enterovirus meningitis occurs in the summer and fall. CSF PCR for enterovirus can help confirm the diagnosis.

Lymphocytic choriomeningitis (LCM) virus is the most common cause of aseptic (viral) encephalitis in the winter and spring. LCM is acquired through exposure to the saliva, urine, and feces of an infected house mouse. Infection with LCM during pregnancy may lead to serious visual or brain dysfunction in the fetus. The mumps virus used to be the most common cause of winter/spring aseptic meningitis, but immunization has altered this pattern in the United States. Occasional cases still arise in adolescents.

Haemophilus influenzae was once the most common cause of bacterial meningitis, before the advent and wide application of immunization. Prior to immunization, it caused nearly 50% of cases; now it is responsible for ~5%. *H influenzae* is broadly divided into strains that do not possess an outer capsule (nontypeable strains) and strains that are encapsulated (typeable, based upon capsular proteins). The typeable strains are further divided into 6 serotypes, with type b being responsible for most cases of meningitis (prior to the widespread application of immunization). Nontypeable *H influenzae* strains are the cause of an increasing proportion of meningitis, particularly in adults. The organism gains entry into the meninges usually following an untreated upper respiratory infection—otitis media, sinusitis. The fatality rate is ~5%.

Neisseria meningitidis, especially serotypes C and Y, cause a large number of cases of bacterial meningitis and remains the most common cause of bacterial meningitis in infants, children, and young adults. The bacterium is easily spread from person to person, leading to localized outbreaks—eg, in schools, barracks, and dormitories. Persons with terminal complement deficiencies (C5, C6, C7, C8, C9 and properdin) are at high risk for *N meningitidis* infection (and infection with *Neisseria* species generally). The case fatality rate is between 10 and 15%. In addition to the usual findings of bacterial meningitis, *N meningitidis* infection is often associated with a petechial rash, first appearing on the trunk and lower extremities. In some patients the lesions coalesce, forming large ecchymoses (purpura fulminans); this finding is associated with a poor outcome. Meningococcal septicemia is a fulminant form of *N meningitidis* infection, in which a nonspecific febrile illness rapidly, within 12-24 hours, leads to deterioration and death; bilateral adrenal destruction and hemorrhage (Waterhouse-Friderichsen syndrome) may occur as part of this illness. Meningococcal septicemia may occur with or without manifestations of bacterial meningitis.

S pneumoniae is now the most common cause of bacterial meningitis overall, causing ~50% of cases. Furthermore it has for some time represented the most serious form of bacterial meningitis—producing the highest rates of mortality and long-term neurologic deficits. Mortality from pneumococcal meningitis ranges from 16-37% and neurological sequelae are estimated to occur in 30-52% of survivors.

Listeria monocytogenes is responsible for ~10% of cases of bacterial meningitis overall, with a fatality rate of 15-30%. It is especially common at the extremes of age: younger than 1 month or older than 70 years of age. Other risk factors are corticosteroid therapy, transplant, diabetes mellitus, HIV infection, and iron overload.

Cryptococcus neoformans is the most common cause of fungal meningitis. The organism is found mainly in dirt and bird (eg, pigeon) droppings. Cryptococcal meningitis is common in patients with HIV infection.

Group B streptococcus (*S agalactiae*) is a common cause of meningitis in neonates, especially because asymptomatic carriage in the vagina is common in pregnant women.

Aerobic Gram– bacilli (*Klebsiella* species, *Escherichia coli*, *Serratia marcescens*, *Pseudomonas aeruginosa*, *Salmonella* species) are important causes of bacterial meningitis in neonates, the elderly, and those with head trauma.

Naegleria fowleri, the etiologic agent of primary amebic meningoencephalitis (PAM), is a free living ameba acquired from fresh water sources, usually after swimming or diving in bodies of fresh water. Death generally occurs within 2-3 days from the onset of symptoms. Children are most commonly affected. In contrast, *Acanthamoeba* species and *Balamuthia mandrillaris* are opportunistic free living amebae capable of causing granulomatous amebic encephalitis (GAE), typically in immunocompromised hosts, following infection through the skin or lungs.

Laboratory evaluation

Blood and cerebrospinal fluid (CSF) should be obtained for culture. In endemic areas, peripheral blood should be examined for malaria, particularly *Plasmodium falciparum* which may be associated with cerebral malaria; even if malaria is found in the peripheral blood, concomitant malaria and bacterial meningitis cannot be excluded without evaluation of the CSF.

Both C-reactive protein (CRP) or procalcitonin (PCT) have proved useful to distinguish bacterial from nonbacterial causes in patients with signs and symptoms of meningitis; this is particularly true of procalcitonin, especially when the CSF Gram stain is negative.

Chemistry and cell count studies, performed on CSF, should be used to guide the differential diagnosis. Findings in the CSF that are typical of bacterial meningitis include a low glucose concentration (< 45 mg/dL), a high protein concentration (> 500 mg/dL), and a high white blood cell count (> 1,000/mL), predominantly composed of neutrophils. CSF lactate, procalcitonin, and CRP have shown promise in distinguishing bacterial from viral meningitis. Several studies have demonstrated the capacity of urine dipstick reagents (glucose, protein, and leukocyte esterase) to reliably assess for bacterial meningitis, a finding of interest in resource poor settings.

Gram stain of the CSF may quickly reveal the type of organism present. CSF Gram staining, when the more common organisms are involved, has a sensitivity of 70-80%. The sensitivity falls below 50% for Gram– bacilli and *L monocytogenes*.

Latex agglutination tests are available for performance on CSF. These tests are based upon reagents containing antibodies to specific bacteria and can be performed quickly.

Assays are available for *H influenzae* type B, *S pneumoniae*, *Streptococcus agalactiae* (group B streptococcus), *N meningitidis*, and *Cryptococcus neoformans*.

Prosthetic joint infections

Definition

Studies on the topic of prosthetic joint infection have applied the following criteria for the diagnosis: growth of the same microorganism in 2 or more cultures of synovial fluid or periprosthetic tissue, purulence of synovial fluid or periprosthetic tissue, acute inflammation on histological examination of periprosthetic tissue, or presence of a sinus tract.

Causative agents

The most commonly involved organisms are coagulase–staphylococci (30-40%), *S aureus* (10-20%), mixed flora (10%), streptococci (10%), Gram– bacilli (5%), enterococci (5%), and anaerobes (2-4%). *Propionibacterium acnes* is a relatively common agent in infected shoulder prostheses.

Some organisms (coagulase– staphylococci) can represent either contaminants or pathogens and may have to be interpreted in the light of other laboratory findings.

Infections can be classified as early (developing <3 months after implantation), delayed (3-24 months), or late (>24 months), each representing roughly a third of cases.

- Early infections are typically related to organisms implanted at the time of surgery. Early infections present in fairly pronounced fashion—abrupt onset of joint pain, effusion, erythema and warmth over the implant site, fever, and, sometimes, overlying cellulitis or sinus tract formation—and are usually related to more virulent organisms such as *S aureus* and Gram– bacilli.

- Delayed infection also is caused by organisms implanted during surgery, but less virulent ones—such as coagulase– staphylococci and *P acnes*. Delayed infection presents more subtly with implant loosening or persistent joint pain, symptoms that are difficult to distinguish from noninfectious joint failure.

- Late infections are usually the result of hematogenous spread of organisms from skin, respiratory tract, teeth, or urinary tract.

Laboratory evaluation

While some prosthetic joint infections present as obvious infection, most present a diagnostic dilemma. Joint failure is the most common presentation, but both infectious and noninfectious causes of joint failure exist. The overall incidence of infection is low, affecting ~1% of prosthetic joints overall.

Radiographic studies may be helpful in diagnosing joint infection, including serial plain radiographs (looking for subperiosteal new bone and sinus tracts), arthrography (to detect implant loosening), nuclear scintigraphy (detects inflammation), and PET.

The CRP has a sensitivity of 75-90% and specificity of 80-85% when a cutoff of 13.5 mg/L is used. CRP returns to baseline within 2 months of joint replacement, in the absence of other systemic inflammatory conditions.

With regard to synovial fluid leukocyte count and differential analysis, criteria differ for the knee and hip. In the knee, a synovial fluid leukocyte count and differential, using cutoffs of 1,700/mL and 65% neutrophils, has a sensitivity of 95% and specificity of ~90%, whereas in the hip, cutoffs of 4,200/mL and 80% neutrophils gives roughly equivalent performance.

Culture of synovial fluid, optimally placed directly into blood culture bottles at the bedside, has a sensitivity of only ~60-70%, with a specificity of 95%. Draining sinuses should not be cultured, because of a high rate of contamination with skin flora. Intraoperative culture of periprosthetic tissue, optimally from 5-6 periprosthetic sites, provides sensitivity ranging from 65-95%. Multiple site culture not only increases sensitivity but also increases specificity, if the same organism is found in 2 or more sites. The yield from intraoperative culture is further enhanced if antibiotics are discontinued 2 weeks prior to surgery. Culture of intraoperative swab is discouraged because of low sensitivity. The seemingly low yield of intraoperative cultures is ascribed to the notion that microorganisms occupy a space—the biofilm—between the prosthesis and the surrounding tissue. A technique to culture this biofilm has been described, in which the prosthetic device is subjected to vortexing and sonication after being immersed in Ringer lactate within a sterile container. This technique is reported to provide high sensitivity, especially in patients who have received antibiotics within the 2 weeks preceding surgery, but it has not been widely adopted.

Cultures do not address the need for intraoperative decision making, however; so a great deal of hope has been placed in intraoperative consultation with frozen section examination. Surgical management may include debridement with retention of the prosthesis, 1-stage exchange (single surgical procedure to remove old and insert new prosthesis) or 2-stage exchange (removal of old prosthesis and periprosthetic tissue with cultures, postsurgical antibiotics, and second surgery to implant new prosthesis). Intraoperative histologic examination of periprosthetic tissue, in studies using cutoffs varying from 1-10 neutrophils per high power (400×) field, has demonstrated variable sensitivity and specificity, probably because of high interobserver variability and the patchy nature of the infiltrate. The largest study to date applied the following criteria for a positive frozen section: >5 neutrophils per high power field in 5 different high power fields, excluding surface exudate and fibrin. With this definition, the study found a sensitivity of 29% and specificity of 95%. Gram staining of synovial fluid and periprosthetic tissue has a high specificity (>95%) but a fairly low sensitivity (<30%).

Intraoperative testing of synovial fluid for leukocyte esterase, using colorimetric strip (urine dipstick) has been studied prospectively. This was found to be a highly accurate predictor of periprosthetic joint infection. One limitation of this technique is its unsuitability for testing bloody specimens.

Sepsis

Does this patient have sepsis?

Early sepsis detection and intervention are clearly related to survival. In view of this, the microbiology of sepsis shrinks in relevance to the monitoring for entry into the septic pathophysiologic state, particularly in patients at risk for sepsis.

Many of the early indicators of sepsis, and indicators of sepsis severity, are laboratory parameters.

With regard to the definition of sepsis, there have been many promulgated, beginning with the definition of "sepsis syndrome" in 1989. This was defined as clinical evidence of infection in the presence of hypothermia or hyperthermia, tachycardia, tachypnea, and end-organ dysfunction. In 1991, the American College of Chest Physicians and the Society of Critical Care Medicine proposed the "systemic inflammatory response syndrome (SIRS)," defined as the presence of any 2 of the following criteria:

1. temperature >38°C or <36°C

2. heart rate >90 beats per minute

3. respiratory rate >20 per min or $PaCO_2$ <32 mm Hg

4. WBC >12,000/mL or < 4,000/mL with >10% immature neutrophils

"Sepsis" in their formulation was defined as SIRS with a documented infection. "Severe sepsis" was defined as sepsis with hypotension, hypoperfusion, or end-organ dysfunction unresponsive to fluid challenge. In 2001, the terms were updated to include sepsis, severe sepsis (sepsis with organ dysfunction), and septic shock (severe sepsis with recalcitrant hypotension). In the 2001 formulation, sepsis was defined as an infection with "several" markers of systemic inflammation: fever, hypothermia, tachypnea, respiratory alkalosis, hypoxemia, fluid overload, tachycardia, hypotension, increased cardiac output, decreased systemic vascular resistance, altered skin perfusion, oliguria, altered mental status, abnormal WBC count, increased CRP, increased interleukin 6 (IL-6), increased procalcitonin (PCT), increased lactate, hyperglycemia, altered coagulation parameters, thrombocytopenia, hyperbilirubinemia.

In the evaluation of a patient at risk for sepsis, certain laboratory tests have become routine. These include a CBC with differential, coagulations studies, D-dimer, lactate, and a chemistry panel that includes bicarbonate, creatinine, and liver function tests. In the CBC and differential, indicators of possible sepsis include neutrophilia or neutropenia, immature granulocytes, toxic changes (Döhle bodies, toxic granulation, toxic vacuolization), and thrombocytopenia (which may indicate evolving disseminated intravascular coagulation). The main purpose of the chemistry panel is to detect metabolic acidosis, especially lactic acidosis. However, lactate, without associated acidosis, serves as an early marker of sepsis (and sepsis severity) and should be measured directly. Lactate is best assessed on an arterial sample; the peripheral blood (peripheral venous) lactate corresponds well with central (arterial or central venous) lactate when normal, but a high peripheral vein lactate should be confirmed with a central venous or arterial sample. The most important aspect of the liver function tests, in assessing severity, is the bilirubin. Currently, the focus of research into additional markers of sepsis and sepsis severity is on CRP, IL-6, protein C, and PCT. PCT, the most recent of these markers, becomes elevated within 6-12 hours of systemic infection and rapidly normalizes upon resolution.

Catheter related sepsis

Where there is an indwelling catheter to consider, there is an added level of complexity. In addition to determining whether the patient has sepsis, one must determine whether the catheter is the source. Thus, in addition to the 2 or more peripheral blood cultures, additional cultures proximate to the catheter should be considered. Some advocate the use of simultaneous culture from peripheral venipuncture sites and culture of blood drawn from the catheter. In this scenario, catheter related sepsis is supported by a quantitative colony count from the catheter specimen that is 5× higher than that obtained from peripheral venipuncture. Catheter related sepsis is also supported by a time to positivity that is earlier, by 2 or more hours, in the catheter specimen; the time to positivity criterion has been demonstrated to have high sensitivity and specificity but requires a well staffed and attentive laboratory. Probably the most widely applied approach is to remove the catheter and culture the tip; sensitivity can be increased by sonication, but in most instances the tip is simply rolled on the surface of the agar. Isolation of an identical isolate from the culture tip and peripheral blood is supportive evidence of catheter related sepsis, but isolation of an organism only from the catheter tip or of an organism different from that obtained from the peripheral blood may indicate only catheter colonization.

The most common agents of catheter related sepsis are skin-derived organisms such as coagulase– staphylococci (*S epidermidis*), followed by *S aureus*, Gram– bacilli (*Klebsiella pneumoniae*, *Enterobacter* species, *Pseudomonas* species), and *Candida albicans*. *S aureus* is associated with a high (10%) mortality and a high (70%) rate of venous thrombosis in the catheterized vessel.

Neonatal sepsis

The issue of laboratory testing for sepsis in the neonate is complicated. The patient in this case has a rapidly changing physiology, such that normal ranges vary significantly with time/age; furthermore, time/age-sensitive normal ranges for most analytes have not been well defined. Likewise, the literature pertaining to laboratory testing in neonatal sepsis has not been rigid in this regard. Many such studies have been based upon patients with a wide range of postnatal ages, some including patients from 24 hours to 6 weeks old. One study, evaluating the CRP in neonates at specified postnatal ages sheds light upon the folly of this approach: it found that at the times of birth (0 hours), 24 hours, and 48 hours, the 95th percentile for CRP was 5.0 mg/L, 14.0 mg/L, and 9.7 mg/L, respectively. Newer analytes, such as IL-6 and PCT, have been elucidated even less.

The continued reliance upon the band count is nowhere more prevalent than amongst neonatologists. Nonetheless, it has been well documented that this fraction is heavily influenced by postnatal age and can be significantly altered by vigorous crying. Furthermore, the precision of the test is very low, with tremendous interobserver variation. The distinction of bands from neutrophils is highly subjective, so much so that the College of American Pathologists no longer tests proficiency in this distinction.

Causative agents t3.2, t3.3

Neonatal sepsis, especially sepsis with early onset (within the first 7 days of postnatal life), is most commonly caused by *Escherichia coli* and Group B streptococcus. A recent study of early onset sepsis confirmed that this is still the case. The most common cause remains Gram– bacteria (61%), with *Escherichia coli* and *Haemophilus* influenzae dominating. Gram+ organisms are responsible for ~37% of cases, largely attributable to Group B streptococci, other staphylococci and streptococci, and *Listeria monocytogenes*. *Candida albicans* is responsible for 2-3% of cases. When compared with older data, the findings were similar, with the exception that the contribution of group B streptococcus has been reduced, probably because of screening and treatment interventions. Neonatal sepsis with later onset (7-28 days) raises additional possibilities, including *S pneumonia*, *Salmonella*, *N meningitidis*, and *S aureus*.

The causes of postneonatal sepsis include Gram+ bacteria (52%), Gram– bacteria (38%), polymicrobial infection (5%), fungi (5%), and anaerobes (1%). In decades past, Gram– bacilli accounted for most cases of sepsis, but this has steadily changed such that Gram+ cocci now predominate.

Rapid deterioration and massive hemolysis are characteristics of sepsis caused by *C perfringens*, the agent traditionally associated with post-abortion sepsis. Currently, clostridial sepsis is most often associated with penetrating wounds, liver abscess, or pathology in the gastrointestinal tract.

Establishing the microbial agent responsible for sepsis depends upon the collection of appropriate cultures before the initiation of antimicrobial treatment, if possible, and thereby requires close collaboration with the emergency department with regard to obtaining adequate samples in which contaminants are minimized. The rate of positive blood culture, even in patients with sepsis, is only 50%, partially because of low volume samples; ideally, 10-20 mL of blood are added to each blood culture vial, 2 vials inoculated from each venipuncture site (1 aerobic, 1 anaerobic). Multiple samples, from different sites and/or at different times, increase the yield moderately; importantly, multiple samples aid in distinguishing a true pathogen from a contaminant. Next, attention is turned towards microbiologic culture of suspected sources of infection; the most common sources are lung (pneumonia), genitourinary (urosepsis), intraabdominal (GI-related abscess), skin, and indwelling catheters. Thus, it is reasonable to collect cultures from the bronchial tree (BAL specimens or sputum), urine cultures, cultures of any excess peritoneal or pleural fluid, cultures of any festering skin or soft tissue lesions, and cultures of any suspicious catheter tips.

t3.2 **Clinical syndromes & causative agents**

Syndrome		Causative agents (most common)
Bacteremia in patients with colon cancer		*C septicum, S bovis*
Bacterial meningitis	Neonates	*S agalactiae* (group B *streptococcus*), *E coli, L monocytogenes*
	Infants & young children	*S pneumoniae, N meningitidis, H influenzae*
	Young adults	*S pneumoniae, N meningitidis, H influenzae*
	Elderly adults	*S pneumoniae, N meningitidis, H influenzae, L monocytogenes*
Fungal meningitis		*Cryptococcus*
Viral (aseptic) meningitis		Enteroviruses (*Coxsackie, Echovirus, Enterovirus*)
Viral encephalitis		α-viruses (eastern & western equine encephalitis; flaviviridae (WNV, St Louis encephalitis); Herpes simplex virus type 1
Impetigo (infection of epidermis)		*S aureus, S pyogenes*
Furunculosis (infection of skin adnexa, boils)		*S aureus, S pyogenes*
Carbunculosis (draining sinuses from multiple confluent infected skin adnexa)		
Skin infection associated with whirlpools		*P aeruginosa*
Skin infection following dog-bite		*Capnocytophaga canimorsus, Pasteurella multocida, Staphylococcus intermedius*
Mycobacterial skin infection		*M fortuitum, M chelonae, M marinum, M haemophilum, M ulcerans, M leprae*
Toxic shock syndrome		*S aureus*
Scalded skin syndrome (Lyells or Ritters syndrome)		*S aureus, S pyogenes*
Erythrasma		*Corynebacterium minutissimum*
Pseudomembranous colitis		*C difficile*
Botryomycosis		*S aureus, P aeruginosa*
Juvenile periodontitis		*Aggregatibacter* (formerly *Actinobacillus*) *actinomycetemcomitans*
Ulceroglandular fever		*Francisella tularensis*
Glanders		*Burkholderia mallei*
Melioidosis		*Burkholderia pseudomallei*
Rocky mountain spotted fever		*Rickettsia rickettsii*
Visceral larva migrans (VLM)		*Toxocara canis/cati*
Cutaneous larva migrans (CLM)		*Ancylostoma braziliense*
Bacterial cellulitis	Most common overall & the cause of erysipelas	*S pyogenes* (group A *streptococci*)
	Erysipeloid	*Erysipelothrix rhusiopathiae*
	Animal bite-associated	*Pasteurella multocida*
	Fresh water-associated	*Aeromonas hydrophila*
	Salt water-associated	*Vibrio vulnificus*
Bacterial pharyngitis		*S pyogenes* (group A *streptococci*), *C diphtheriae*
Whooping cough		*Bordetella pertussis*
Acute epiglottitis		*H influenzae* type B (HITB)
Chancroid		*Haemophilus ducreyi*
Lymphogranuloma venereum (LGV)		*C trachomatis*
Bacterial ("septic") arthritis	Children & adults, monoarticular	*S aureus, Streptococci*
	IV drug abusers	*Pseudomonas*
	Young adults, polyarticular	*N gonorrhoeae*
Croup (acute laryngotracheobronchitis)		*Parainfluenza virus, serotypes 1-3*
Viral pneumonia	Infants/children	*Respiratory syncytial virus (RSV)*
	Adults	*Influenza A (orthomyxovirus)*
Bacterial pneumonia	Community-acquired	*S pneumoniae, L pneumoniae, H influenzae, S aureus, M pneumoniae*
	Chronic alcoholics	*K pneumoniae*
	Cystic fibrosis	*P aeruginosa*
	"Atypical" or "walking" pneumonia	*Mycoplasma pneumoniae, Chlamydia pneumoniae*
	Nosocomial pneumonia	*E coli, P aeruginosa, S aureus, L pneumoniae*
Otitis media		*S pneumoniae, H influenzae, M catarrhalis*
Bacterial peritonitis	Spontaneous (cirrhosis with ascites)	*S pneumoniae*
	Secondary (ruptured bowel)	Mixed: *E coli*, enterococci, *B fragilis*, other anaerobes
Gastroenteritis	With short incubation period (1-8 h)	*S aureus, B cereus*
	Fried rice	*B cereus*
	Traveler's diarrhea	*E coli* (ETEC)
	Hamburgers in fast food restaurants	*E coli* (EHEC)
	Antibiotic-associated colitis	*C difficile*
	Viral	Rotavirus, Norwalk virus, enteric adenoviruses
	Causing blood diarrhea	*Salmonella enteriditis, Shigella* species, *Campylobacter jejuni*, EHEC, EIEC, *K oxytoca, Entamoeba histolytica, Balantidium coli*, CMV
	Diarrhea with systemic disease	*Salmonella typhi*, other *Salmonella* species, *Yersinia enterocolitica, Campylobacter* species
Osteomyelitis		*S aureus*
Necrotizing fasciitis	Usually polymicrobial	*Streptococcus pyogenes* & anaerobes such as *Bacteroides fragilis*

(continued on next page)

t3.2 Clinical syndromes & causative agents (continued)

Syndrome		Causative agents (most common)
Undulant fever	Pig-associated	*Brucella suis*
	Goat-associated	*Brucella melitensis*
	Dog-associated	*Brucella canis*
Rabbit fever or deer-fly fever (tularemia)		*Francisella tularensis*
Plague		*Yersinia pestis*
Carrion disease or verruga peruana (Bartonellosis)		*Bartonella bacilliformis*
Uterine infection following septic abortion		*Clostridium perfringens*
Leprosy (Hansen disease)		*Mycobacterium leprae*
Rat-bite fever		*Streptobacillus moniliformis*
San Joaquin Valley fever		*Coccidioides immitis*
Superficial (noninvasive) mycoses	Dermatophytes (causing tinea capitis, tinea cruris)	*Epidermophyton, Microsporon,* & *Trichophyton* species
	Black piedra	*Piedraia hortae*
	White piedra	*Trichosporon beigelii* & other *Trichosporon* species
	Tinea versicolor	*Malassezia furfur*
	Tinea nigra palmaris/plantaris	*Hortaea* (formerly *Phaeoannelomyces*) *werneckii*
Cutaneous & subcutaneous mycoses	Chromoblastomycosis	*Phialophora verrucosa, Fonsecaea pedrosoi*
	Lobomycosis	*Lacazia* (formerly *Loboa*) *loboi*
	Phaeohyphomycosis	*Exophiala jeanselmei, Phialophora verrucosa, Wangiella dermatitidis, Alternaria* species, many others
	Sporotrichosis	*Sporothrix schenckii*
	Eumycotic mycetoma	*Exophiala jeanselmei, Madurella* species, *Pseudallescheria boydii* (*Scedosporium*)
	Rhinosporidiosis	*Rhinosporidium seeberi*
Rhinoscleroma		*Klebsiella rhinoscleromatis*
Actinomycotic mycetoma (Madura foot)		*Actinomyces, Nocardia, Streptomyces*
Measles		Rubeola virus
Erysipelas		*S pyogenes* (group A streptococci)
German measles		Rubella virus
Chicken pox		Varicella zoster virus
Labial herpes		Herpes simplex virus type 1 (majority)
Genital herpes		Herpes simplex virus type 2 (majority)
Roseola infantum (exanthem subitum)		Human herpesvirus 6
Fifth disease (erythema infectiosum, slapped-cheek disease)		Parvovirus B19
Chagas disease		*Trypanosoma cruzi*
African sleeping sickness		*Trypanosoma brucei*
Adiaspiromycosis		*Emmonsia* (formerly *Chrysosporium*) *parvum*
Fungal external otitis		*Aspergillus niger*
Subacute sclerosing panencephalitis (SSPE)		Measles virus (reactivation)
Hand-foot-mouth disease		Coxsackie A
Viral myocarditis		Coxsackie B
Progressive multifocal leukoencephalopathy (PML)		JC virus
Scarlet fever		*S pyogenes* (Group A streptococci)
Acute mastitis		*S aureus*
Q fever		*Coxiella burnetii*
Primary amebic meningoencephalitis (PAM)		*Naegleria fowleri*
Granulomatous amebic encephalitis (GAE)		*Acanthamoeba* species & *Balamuthia mandrillaris*
Postsplenectomy sepsis		*S pneumoniae*

t3.3 Vectors

Vector	Disease	Organism
Mosquitoes		
Anopheles species	Dog heartworm	*Dirofilaria immitis*
	Malaria	*Plasmodium* species
	Lymphatic filariasis	*Brugia malayi*
	Lymphatic filariasis	*Wuchereria bancrofti*
Aedes species, most commonly *A aegypti* & *A albopictus*	Arboviral disease	Including: dengue virus, yellow fever virus & Chikungunya virus
Culex species	Arboviral disease	Including: WNV, SLE, Japanese encephalitis virus
	Lymphatic filariasis	*Wuchereria bancrofti*
	Lymphatic filariasis	*Brugia malayi*
Ticks		
Ixodes species	Lyme disease	*Borrelia burgdorferi*
Most common:	Babesiosis	*Babesia* species
Eastern US: *I scapularis*	Anaplasmosis	*Anaplasma phagocytophilum*
Western US: *I pacificus*	Tick-borne encephalitis	Tick-borne encephalitis virus (TBEV)
Europe: *I ricinus*		
Lone Star tick—*Amblyomma americanum*	Ehrlichiosis	*Ehrlichia* species
	Tularemia	*Francisella tularensis*
	Southern tick-associated illness (STARI)	Unknown etiology
Dermacentor species	Rocky Mountain spotted fever	*Rickettsia rickettsii*
Most common:	Tularemia	*Francisella tularensis*
Southern & western US: *D andersoni*	Colorado tick fever	Colorado tick fever virus
Southern & eastern US: *D variabilis*		
Ornithodoros species (soft ticks)	Relapsing fever	*Borrelia* species
Flies		
Deer fly—*Chrysops* species	Tularemia—"deer fly fever"	*Francisella tularensis*
	Loiasis	*Loa loa*
Dung fly—*Musca sorbens*	Trachoma	*Chlamydia trachomatis*
Sandfly—(*Phlebotomus* & *Lutzomyia* species)	Leishmaniasis	*Leishmania* species
	Bartonellosis; carrion disease	*Bartonella bacilliformis*
	Arboviral disease	Vesicular stomatitis virus, toscana & sicilian virus
Black fly—*Simulium* species	Onchocerciasis; river blindness	*Onchocerca volvulus*
Tsetse fly—*Glossina* species	African trypanosomiasis	*Trypanosoma brucei*
Fleas		
Rat fleas	Plague	*Yersinia pestis*
	Murine typhus	*Rickettsia typhus*
Dog and cat fleas	Double-pored dog tapeworm	*Dipylidium caninum*
Lice		
Body lice—*Pediculus humanus*	Epidemic typhus	*Rickettsia prowazekii*
	Lice-borne relapsing fever	*Borrelia recurrentis*
	Trench fever	*Bartonella quintana*
Mites		
Mite (*Liponyssoides sanguineus*)	Rickettsial pox	*Rickettsia akari*
Chigger (Trombiculid mite)	Scrub typhus	*Orientia tsutsugamushi*
Others		
Midges—*Culicoides* species	Filariasis	*Mansonella* species
Reduviid Bug—*Triatominae*	American trypanosomiasis; Chagas disease	*Trypanosoma cruzi*

Virology
Laboratory methods
Cell culture

The gold standard method for diagnosing most viruses is viral isolation in cell culture. Exceptions are many and include EBV, arboviruses, and rubella for which serology is the primary method, and rotavirus and rhabdovirus for which antigen detection is the primary method. Not all viruses can replicate in cell lines used in routine cell culture, and turnaround time (TAT) is not ideal. Consequently, molecular methods have become an important addition to viral diagnostics improving TATs.

Cell cultures are of 3 types. Primary cell cultures are the result of culture of a minced organ; the proliferating cells can be maintained for a limited time with repetitive changes of the supporting fluid. Examples are primary monkey kidney (PMK; eg, rhesus monkey kidney/RMK). Since they contain a mixture of cell types, they have a pleomorphic microscopic appearance. Once cells are transferred or subcultured, a primary cell culture becomes a secondary cell culture or cell line. These are usually diploid cell lines derived from fibroblasts. After a limited number of transfers (usually ~50), cell lines become exhausted and will no longer replicate. A commonly used diploid cell line is human diploid fibroblasts (HDF, eg, MRC-5/Medical Research Council-5). Since most diploid cell lines are morphologically fibroblastic, uninfected cell sheets consist microscopically of long slender parallel cells. In some cell lines, individual cells may acquire an unlimited ability to replicate, and cell lines that continue to proliferate after having been transferred ≥70 times are considered established cell lines (and are often heteroploid). Established cell lines are often obtained from human malignancies; eg, HEp-2 is derived from laryngeal carcinoma, and HeLa is derived from cervical adenocarcinoma. Uninfected established cell lines morphologically appear as polygonal epithelioid cells. Cell cultures vary in their susceptibility to become infected by different viruses, which is a helpful feature for determining the identity of the infecting virus t3.4. Specimens should be inoculated onto 2 or more cell lines, selected according to the source of the specimen and the most likely agents for that source.

Contamination of culture media is most commonly due to *Mycoplasma* species or simian viruses. *Mycoplasma* contamination results in poor cell growth and inhibition of viral infection. Simian viral contamination may result in a false positive hemadsorption; this problem is the reason for running parallel control hemadsorption tests on uninoculated tubes.

In routine cell culture, a virus is detected by visual examination of cultures for viral cytopathic effect (CPE) with a phase-contrast microscope. CPE is the characteristic degenerative changes of cells associated with the intracellular multiplication of certain viruses. Viruses t3.4, t3.5 can be provisionally identified based on

1. the morphology of the CPE

2. the types of cells displaying CPE

3. the time from inoculation to detection of CPE

For example, HSV shows CPE usually within 3 days of inoculation, while RSV, CMV, and VZV may require 2 weeks. Influenza and parainfluenza viruses do not always induce CPE;

however, they express hemagglutinins with which they can adsorb guinea pig RBCs to the surface of the culture cells. This forms the basis for the hemadsorption/hemagglutination tests.

t3.4 Routine cell culture

Virus	PMK	Hep2/HeLa	HDF	CPE	Time to CPE
Enteroviruses (including coxsackie A & B, echovirus, poliovirus)	+++	+	+++	Angular, tear shaped, cells, focal swollen or glassy cells	1-7 days
Rhinovirus	+	-	+++	Focal granular & swollen cells	
Influenza, mumps & parainfluenza	+++	±	±	None or focally enlarged & granular cells; parainfluenza may have focal multinucleated giant cells. If minimal to no CPE, confirm with hemadsorption/hemagglutination	2-5 days 3-10 days 3-10 days
Adenovirus	++	+++	+	Grapelike clusters on Hep2	2-7 days
RSV	++	+++	+	Syncytia in Hep2 cells (syncytia can be produced in various cell types by measles, parainfluenza & mumps viruses)	~14 days
VZV	++	-	++	Focal shrunken or enlarged cells, advancing in a slow contiguous manner; grows poorly in culture	~14 days
CMV	-	-	+++	Slow, focal clusters of CPE (plaques) on HDF only	~14 days
HSV1 & 2	++	++	+++	Rapid (1-3 days), shrunken or enlarged cells starting at the edge of the cell sheet, sweeping CPE, occasional giant cells	1-3 days

t3.5 Viral CPE

Enterovirus	CMV	Adenovirus	RSV	HSV
Tear shaped cells	Focal plaques in HDF	Grapelike clusters	Syncytial cells	Sweeping, globular cells

A modification of the cell culture is the *shell vial technique*. This method is most commonly employed in respiratory virus panels and for CMV. The general procedure involves the inoculation of shell vials containing a monolayer of cells on a circular cover slip at the base of the vial. Specimen is inoculated into the shell vial and infection of the cells is enhanced by low speed centrifugation. After a short incubation (<3 days) the coverslip is removed and stained with antiviral antibody tagged with a fluorescent dye directed to early antigens of the replicating virus to stain viral specific foci. Thus, early antigens of viral infection can be recognized rapidly in the shell vial technique by immunologic detection several days earlier than most viruses are able to produce recognizable CPE in conventional tube cell cultures. *It is the combination of centrifugation and immunologic detection that make this a more rapid test than traditional tube culture for some viruses.* The rapid turnaround time is a key advantage of this method over traditional cell culture.

Other methods
Serology

Serology (detection of circulating antibody) is helpful in the detection of current or past viral infection, particularly when isolation of the pathogen is difficult. A single positive IgM antibody can be considered diagnostic in many circumstances, although false positive results may be common for some assays. Paired sera taken 7-10 days apart are recommended for diagnosis based upon IgG, although a single sample is acceptable for screening purposes. With paired samples, a fourfold or greater rise in IgG titer, between the acute and convalescent samples, is considered diagnostic of infection. Thus, the diagnostic usefulness of serologic tests is limited and often retrospective. In general elevated IgM titers or rising IgG titers (4-fold) are definitive of *seroconversion*, indicative of acute infection. In the typical scenario, virus-specific *IgM* is detectable shortly after the first week of a primary infection and becomes undetectable within 1-4 months. However, in certain instances, IgM can remain elevated for up to a year. Virus-specific IgG begins to emerge 1-2 weeks into a primary infection and peaks between 4-8 weeks; subsequently, it declines continually but usually remains detectable for life. In secondary infection (reactivation or new infection with the same virus), there may be a re-emergence of IgM, and IgG increases for the next 4-8 weeks.

Direct antigen detection

Enzyme linked immunosorbent assay (EIA), latex agglutination, and direct fluorescent antibody (DFA) techniques are available. DFA provides the opportunity to directly observe the specimen and thereby determine that cells are present in the sample and which cells display reactivity (analogous to FISH).

Histology

Conventional light microscopy is useful for the detection of certain viruses, particularly those with characteristic inclusions t3.6. 2 important exceptions that do not cause formation of inclusions are EBV and influenza. Ultrastructural morphology (electron microscopy) allows recognition of several viral types and were used for detection of viral agents causing diarrhea that do not grow in routine cell culture (rotavirus, enteric adenovirus, norovirus (Norwalk-like virus), astrovirus, and other caliciviruses). However, EM is rarely used today for this purpose, and has been replaced with antigen or molecular detection methods.

t3.6 Viral histology

Virus	Nuclear inclusions	Cytoplasmic inclusions	Syncytia	Notes
RSV	-	-	+	
HSV	+	-	+	Cowdry type A ("owl eye") bodies in *m*ultinucleated cells; nuclei are *m*olded & chromatin is *m*arginalized (3 Ms of HSV infection)
Adenovirus	+	-	-	"Smudge cells"
CMV	+	+	-	"Owl eye" inclusion, not multinucleated
Measles	+	+	+	Warthin-Finkeldey giant cells
Rabies	-	+	-	Negri bodies

Molecular techniques

Polymerase chain reaction (PCR) and in-situ hybridization (ISH) may be used for direct detection of viral nucleic acid. ISH is often applied to the histologic identification of HPV (cervical biopsies), CMV (lung biopsies), HSV (skin biopsies), and parvovirus B19 (marrow). Direct DNA (genomic) sequencing with PCR and branched (bDNA) amplification is commonly employed in the monitoring of patients with HIV and HCV infection.

Classification t3.7

t3.7 Virus classification

| | DNA viruses | | RNA viruses | |
	Single stranded	Double stranded	Single stranded	Double stranded
Nonenveloped	*Parvoviridae* *Bocavirus*	*Adenoviridae* *Papillomaviridae* *Polyomaviridae*	*Picornaviridae* (Poliovirus, Enteroviruses), Hepatitis A, Rhinovirus) *Calciviridae* (Norovirus) *Hepeviridae* (Hepatitis E)	*Reoviridae*: Rotavirus
Enveloped		*Herpesviridae* *Hepadnaviridae* (HBV) *Poxviridae*	*Flaviviridae* (HCV, yellow fever, dengue, WNV, St Louis & Japanese encephalitis) *Togaviridae* (rubella, EEE, WEE) *Retroviridae* (HIV, HTLV) *Orthomyxoviridae* (influenza) *Paramyxoviridae* (RSV, hMPV, parainfluenza, mumps, measles) *Rhabdoviridae* (rabies) *Coronaviridae* *Arenaviridae* *Bunyaviridae* (hantavirus, California encephalitis) *Deltavirus* (hepatitis D)	

Human herpesviruses (HHV) t3.8

t3.8 Human herpesviruses

| Herpes virus | Latency | Clinical disease | |
		Acute	Reactivation
HSV 1	Dorsal root ganglia	Acute gingivostomatitis Pharyngitis Skin infection (herpetic whitlow) Genital herpes (less commonly)	Herpes labialis Herpes encephalitis Less likely to cause recurrent genital herpes lesions than those caused by HSV 2
HSV 2	Dorsal root ganglia	Genital herpes Skin infection (herpetic whitlow) Acute gingivostomatitis (less commonly)	Genital herpes Herpes meningitis
CMV	Histiocytes, endothelial cells, T lymphocytes	Mononucleosis-like syndrome; disseminated infection in neonates & immunocompromised hosts	Disseminated infection
VZV	Dorsal root ganglia	Varicella (chicken pox)	Zoster (shingles)
EBV	B cells	t3.9	t3.9
HHV-6	T cells	Roseola (exanthem subitum)	Reactivation in immunocompromised hosts
HHV-7	Lymphocytes	Roseola (occasionally)	Reactivation in immunocompromised hosts
HHV-8	B lymphocytes, endothelial cells	Unknown	Kaposi sarcoma Primary body cavity lymphoma

t3.9 Clinical syndromes caused by EBV

Disease	Stage of infection	Notes
Infectious mononucleosis	Primary	Mainly in adolescents & young adults
X-linked lymphoproliferative disease (Duncan disease)	Primary	Mainly males affected (usually boys); patients with this disorder mount an overactive immune response to EBV, resulting in fulminant infectious mononucleosis, B cell lymphoma, aplastic anemia & dysgammaglobulinemia
Burkitt lymphoma	latent	Endemic, sporadic & immunodeficiency-associated forms; nearly 100% of endemic BL in African children & 25% of sporadic & immunodeficiency associated cases
Hodgkin lymphoma	Latent	EBV in 50% of cases
Primary effusion lymphoma	Latent	EBV in 70% of cases (HHV8 in 100%)
Lymphomatoid granulomatosis	Latent	Systemic angiodestructive lymphoproliferative disease
Posttransplant lymphoproliferative disorder (PTLD)	Latent	>95% EBV+
Oral hairy leukoplakia	Latent	In HIV infection; EBER−
Nasopharyngeal carcinoma	Latent	Nearly 100% EBV+ in Chinese & Inuit populations; 75% EBV+ in US

Herpes simplex virus (HSV)

HSV type 1 is associated with gingivostomatitis, pharyngitis, keratoconjunctivitis, herpes labialis (cold sores), occasional skin infections (herpetic whitlow), and herpes encephalitis. Less commonly, HSV-1 causes genital lesions. Immunocompromised persons are at risk for herpetic esophagitis, tracheobronchitis, pneumonia, and hepatitis. Herpes encephalitis, accounting for 15% of all viral encephalitides, is characterized by bilateral hemorrhagic necrosis of the anterior poles of the temporal lobes. The CSF usually shows a pleocytosis, elevated protein, and numerous red blood cells. HSV-1 is most often transmitted by saliva. Most primary infections occur before puberty. Some primary infections are asymptomatic, while others produce a painful gingivostomatitis, affecting the oral cavity diffusely, associated with fever and constitutional symptoms. The virus ultimately infects and achieves dormancy within the nuclei of trigeminal ganglia. Occasionally there is reactivation leading to localized lesions of the mouth or lips. Although HSV-1 is generally associated with oral lesions, it has become a common cause of genital infection in certain populations.

HSV type 2 is the cause of genital herpes, occasional skin infections, and herpes meningitis (does not typically cause encephalitis). Less commonly, HSV-2 causes oral lesions. HSV type 2, like HSV-1, produces primary, latent, and recurrent infection, with dormancy being established in sacral ganglia. Interestingly, HSV-2 seropositivity can be found in ~20% of the population, but only ~2% of the population suffers from genital herpes. HSV type 2 is also the cause of congenital and neonatal herpes. Congenital herpes, implying in utero infection resulting from transplacental viremia, is rare in comparison with neonatal herpes. Neonatal herpes results from HSV transmission from mother to child during passage through an infected birth canal. In nearly half of these cases, there is no maternal history of genital herpes. The severity of neonatal HSV-2 ranges from a few skin lesions to encephalitis, chorioretinitis, and sepsis. The American Congress of Obstetricians

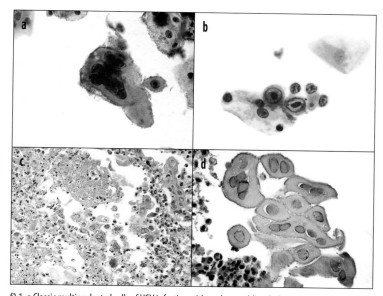

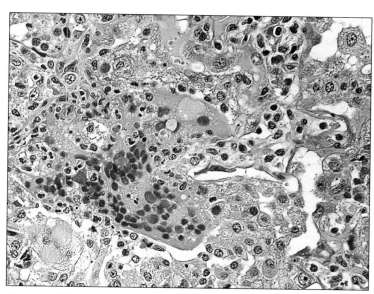

f3.1 a Classic multinucleated cells of HSV infection with nuclear molding & chromatin margination and b Cowdry type A inclusions seen in Pap stained preparations c Necrotizing pneumonitis with d typical cytopathic effect seen in H&E stained sections

f3.2 Neonatal VZV pneumonitis, showing multinucleated cells with viral cytopathic effect

and Gynecologists (ACOG) recommends cesarean delivery for pregnant women with prodromal symptoms or active genital HSV lesions.

While cell culture is still considered the definitive method for the diagnosis of HSV-1 and HSV-2, direct DNA probes are becoming more widespread. HSV-1 and HSV-2 characteristically grow rapidly in almost any cell culture. CPE that sweeps across the culture monolayer is usually detectable by day 2 or 3. The cells display rounded enlargement (ballooning) with occasional syncytia. An FA test (culture cells are transferred to a glass slide and stained with fluorescent-tagged HSV antibodies) is confirmatory. An increasingly popular alternative is the shell vial technique, in which centrifugation is used to promote virus-culture cell interaction. This technique does not result in visible CPE; however, a DFA stain will usually be positive after one day. A Tzanck smear is prepared by directly smearing material obtained from a lesion onto a glass slide, followed by Giemsa staining. If typical HSV CPE is observed, the diagnosis can be made. The technique has a sensitivity of 60-70%. Negative Tzanck smears should therefore be followed by culture or PCR. PCR techniques now make up an important component of HSV diagnostics. Serology has limited utility in the diagnosis of HSV-1 and HSV-2.

Viral cytopathic effect may be observed in esophageal brushings or Pap smears. In tissue sections, herpetic mucocutaneous lesions demonstrate ulcer, often with a bed of fibrinopurulent debris. HSV CPE can be found in the keratinocytes f3.1.

Varicella-zoster virus (VZV)

Varicella-zoster virus (VZV) is the cause of childhood varicella (chicken pox). Though chicken pox in childhood is generally benign, it may be complicated by life threatening pneumonia in healthy adolescents and adults. Pregnant women and immunocompromised individuals are at risk for serious disseminated infection. Furthermore, infected pregnant women can transmit the virus transplacentally, leading to congenital varicella. Congenital varicella is diagnosed when there is

evidence of maternal varicella infection during pregnancy, skin lesions on the newborn that have a dermatomal distribution, and serologic evidence of infection in the newborn (either IgM or persistent IgG beyond 7 months). The incidence and severity of congenital varicella depend upon the timing of maternal infection. When a woman is infected during pregnancy, the overall incidence of congenital varicella is ~1-5%. The incidence is lowest when maternal infection occurs in the 1st trimester, higher in the 2nd, and highest in the 3rd. So-called perinatal varicella arises when maternal infection occurs within a few days of delivery. The likelihood of perinatal varicella in this instance is ~50-60%. Perinatal varicella can be quite severe f3.2, and before the availability of antiviral agents, the mortality was 15-30%. The CDC recommends the administration of varicella zoster immunoglobulin (VZIG) to infants born to a mother who develops a rash attributable to varicella between 5 days before and 2 days after delivery. VZIG may be augmented by intravenous acyclovir. Reactivation of VZV is the cause of zoster (shingles). Herpes zoster presents as a dermatomal vesicular rash that is often quite painful. Pain can be present for long after the rash clears (post herpetic neuralgia). Reactivation of latent infection in the geniculate ganglion of the facial nerve is the cause of Ramsay Hunt syndrome—presenting as otalgia, unilateral facial paresis, vertigo, hearing loss, and tinnitus. This syndrome is rare in the United States. The diagnosis of VZV may be made by serology (positive IgM or 4-fold rise in IgG), direct antigen detection (DFA of skin scrapings), PCR (especially useful for diagnosis of CNS involvement), histology, or culture (long TAT; up to 2 weeks for CPE).

Cytomegalovirus (CMV)

Primary CMV infection, in the immunocompetent older child or adult, is either asymptomatic or causes a mononucleosis-like syndrome. The rate of seropositivity (seroprevalence) of CMV infection increases with age, but rates differ substantially worldwide. In some parts of Africa, the seropositivity rate can reach 90% by the age of 10; whereas in the United

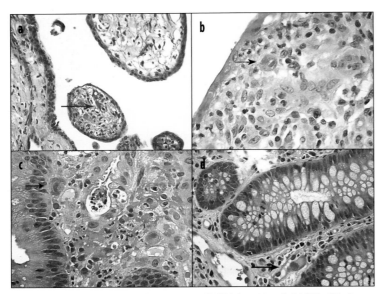

f3.3 H&E stained histologic sections demonstrating a & b CMV placentitis and c & d CMV colitis; the infected cells are markedly enlarged endothelial cells with cytoplasmic inclusions & nuclear Cowdry type A inclusions

States, the seropositivity rate at age 10 is ~20%. Even within the US rates differ with socioeconomic status.

CMV colitis is common in patients with idiopathic inflammatory bowel disease (Crohn disease or ulcerative colitis). This is thought to be related to immunosuppressive therapy. In these patients, CMV colitis presents as a typical colitis exacerbation. Identification of viral CPE by light microscopy is usually possible f3.3, but immunohistochemistry may be requested when clinical suspicion is high and the H&E is negative.

In immunocompromised persons and neonates, primary CMV infection can cause pneumonia, hepatitis, retinitis, or disseminated disease. In allograft recipients, CMV infection commonly presents as a mononucleosis-like syndrome with fever and leukopenia. This may lead to infection within particular organs, especially the lungs, GI tract (CMV colitis), liver, or kidneys. Interestingly, CMV tends to set up infection within the transplanted organ. In fact, CMV is thought to contribute to chronic rejection. In HIV infection, CMV becomes a major problem when CD4 counts are quite low (<100-200 cells per mL). CMV retinitis, encephalitis, and nephritis, while reported in transplant recipients, are much more common in HIV patients.

CMV is the most common congenital infection in the United States. Neonatal CMV results from transplacental infection and is most likely to occur when a pregnant woman experiences primary CMV infection during gestation. In its most severe form (cytomegalic inclusion disease—CID) it manifests with low birth weight, microcephaly, intracerebral calcifications, hepatosplenomegaly, jaundice, chorioretinitis, thrombocytopenia, petechial rash, and purpura. Only 30% of pregnancies with *primary* CMV infection result in congenital CMV, and only 10% of congenital CMV is severe as described above. In survivors of congenital CMV, the most common long-term problem is *sensorineural hearing loss*. Reactivation infection during pregnancy results in a much lower incidence (<1%) of transplacental transmission.

The diagnosis of CMV may be made by serology (positive IgM or 4-fold rise in IgG), pp65 antigenemia (DFA on peripheral blood leukocytes for detection of the pp65 matrix protein antigen), PCR (on any body fluid or tissue), histology (characteristic inclusions), or culture (long TAT; up to 2 weeks for CPE).

Epstein-Barr virus (EBV)

Epstein-Barr virus (EBV) is transmitted mainly by salivary or sexual contact. Uncommonly, it may be transmitted through blood transfusion or solid-organ transplantation. About 90% of people worldwide are infected with EBV. There are 2 genomic types of EBV: EBV1 and EBV2. It seems that these do not differ in disease association, but EBV1 is the predominant type in the West, whereas EBV1 and EBV2 are evenly distributed elsewhere. EBV enters the body through the pharyngeal or genital mucosa and subsequently infects B lymphocytes via the C3d receptor (CD21). Reacting to the virus, CD8+ T lymphocytes are responsible for the peripheral blood atypical lymphocytosis that is seen. The site of EBV latency is the B lymphocyte. The EBV genome persists in episomal form within a small population of B cells, where it usually causes no additional effects. Persistent viral shedding may occur, and in some cases latency and reactivation are associated with clinical disease t3.9.

Primary infection with EBV is usually subclinical but may take the form of infectious mononucleosis (IM). Early asymptomatic childhood infection is common; in affluent populations, EBV infection tends to occur in late childhood or adolescence. Liver function tests (LFTs) are frequently (50%) elevated in EBV infectious mononucleosis. The classic IM presentation, seen primarily in adolescents, includes sore throat (pharyngitis), lymph node enlargement, tonsillar enlargement, and fever. In primary infection of older adults these findings are less likely; instead, hepatitis and jaundice become more common. As in other herpesvirus infections, latency ensues.

X-linked lymphoproliferative disorder (Duncan disease) is a manifestation of acute disease and refers to fulminant primary EBV infection that is frequently fatal and appears confined to males of rare kindreds. The mechanism of death is usually hepatic necrosis, associated with a pronounced T/NK cell infiltrate. In other cases, affected individuals have manifested hemophagocytosis, agammaglobulinemia, and B cell lymphoma. The underlying genetic defect is found in the *SH2D1A* (aka SAP) gene that is normally expressed in T and NK cells. The SAP protein is a transmembrane signaling protein that becomes involved in the usual course of the immune reaction to viral infection. In those harboring this mutation, for as yet unknown reasons, EBV in particular results in uncontrolled activation of T/NK cells.

The traditional diagnostic criteria for infectious mononucleosis are Hoagland criteria: a leukocytosis consisting of >50% lymphocytes and >10% atypical lymphocytes, fever, pharyngitis, and adenopathy, and a positive serologic test. These criteria are quite restrictive, and many patients routinely diagnosed with infectious mono do not qualify. However, numerous other causes of sore throat with fever and adenopathy must be

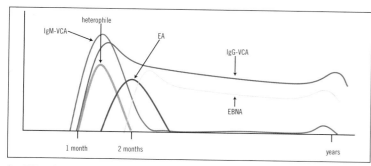

f3.4 EBV serology in primary infection & reactivation

considered: streptococcal pharyngitis, pharyngitis due to other viruses (eg, CMV and acute HIV). Other causes of a mononucleosis syndrome must be considered, eg, toxoplasmosis, CMV, phenytoin. The laboratory diagnosis of EBV is primarily serologic t3.10, f3.4, based on the fact that EBV induces production of antibodies including anti-i, rheumatoid factor, ANA, and the Paul-Bunnell heterophile antibodies. Heterophile antibodies are IgM antibodies that have an affinity for sheep and horse red cells. They emerge during the first week of symptoms, 3-4 weeks after infection, and return to undetectable levels by 3-6 months. Antibody with strong affinity for beef erythrocyte antigens, uninhibited by adsorption with guinea pig kidney antigen (the differential absorption test), is specific for acute EBV infection. This test was developed into a rapid latex agglutination test (monospot test). Heterophile antibody is fairly specific but insensitive, being present in 80% of infected teens and adults, 40% of all infected children, and only 20% of infected children <4. Sometimes heterophile antibodies arise in non-EBV infections, such as the Forsmann antibody, therefore making this test less specific for EBV infection. In addition, conditions such as HIV, lupus, rheumatoid factor, pregnancy, and lymphoma can cause false positive results. Subsequently, multiple specific EBV serologic markers were developed, including the IgG/IgM anti-viral capsid antigen (anti-VCA), EBV early antigen (EBV-EA), and EBV nuclear antigen (EBNA). These have very high sensitivity (>94%) and specificity (>95%) for EBV infectious mononucleosis and can be used when the monospot result does not fit the clinical picture. Following infection, the first marker t3.10 to appear is IgM anti-VCA. IgM anti-VCA becomes undetectable after acute infection but re-emerges with reactivation. IgG anti-VCA emerges shortly after the IgM and slightly before the heterophile antibody. IgG anti-EBNA and IgG anti-VCA persist indefinitely.

t3.10 EBV serology

Stage	Heterophile	IgM anti-VCA	IgG anti-EA	IgG anti-VCAgG	anti-EBNA
Uninfected	–	–	–	–	–
Early acute	–/+	+	–	+	–
Acute	±	+	+	+	–/+
Convalescent	–	–	+	+	+
Remote	–	–	+	–/+	+

Since EBV does not form recognizable inclusions, there are other ways to demonstrate EBV cellular infection in tissue.

- In situ hybridization with EBV-encoded RNA (EBER) can be performed on histologic sections or cytologic preparations, permitting determination of the EBV status

in cells of interest. For example, in Hodgkin lymphoma EBER is localized to the nuclei of Reed-Sternberg cells, with little to no expression in the background small lymphocytes. EBER is positive in all EBV-related tumors (oral hairy leukoplakia is the only EBV-related lesion that is negative for EBER by ISH). In hyperplastic lymphoid tissue during infectious mononucleosis, EBER is expressed in a large number of lymphocytes. In the lymph nodes of patients with latent EBV infection, EBER is expressed in a very small percentage (~0.1%) of lymphocytes. EBER is used to support the diagnosis of posttransplant lymphoproliferative disorder (PTLD). It is expressed in ~50% of Hodgkin lymphomas and a large percentage of nasopharyngeal carcinomas, T/NK lymphomas of the nasal type, and endemic-type Burkitt lymphoma.

- In situ hybridization with the BamHIW sequence of EBV DNA. This provides excellent sensitivity, since the BamHIW sequence is repeated 11 times throughout the EBV genome; thus, it is preamplified.

- LMP1 immunohistochemistry performs nearly as well as EBER in situ hybridization in many settings—Hodgkin lymphomas, infectious mononucleosis, and PTLD; however, there continues to be discordance between the results of the 2 assays in other EBV-associated lesions. LMP1 staining is cytoplasmic and membranous. LMP1 IHC rarely produces a false positive result; false positives may result from nonspecific staining in plasma cells and eosinophils. However, when positive in the cells of interest, there is excellent correlation with EBER ISH. Thus a positive LMP1 is useful, but a negative one may need to be confirmed with EBER ISH.

HHV6

HHV6 is the common collective name for HHV6A and HHV6B. These viruses cause disease that is clinically significant primarily in small children and in immunocompromised hosts (transplant recipients and HIV patients). HHV6B primary infection typically occurs within a matter of months of the waning maternal antibodies, with transmission likely being via saliva. Little is known of HHV6A transmission. HHV6 (mostly HHV6B) is the etiologic agent of roseola infantum (sixth disease, exanthem subitum) in infants and toddlers. Fully-developed roseola manifests in only ~10% of those with acute HHV6 infection; however, the remaining children displaying a nonspecific febrile illness. HHV6 has been found to be highly neurotropic and is one of the causes of viral encephalitis due to its combined propensity to produce fever and CNS infection. It is also responsible for a significant proportion of childhood febrile seizures. In addition, HHV6 (more commonly HHV6A) is an important cause of infection in immunocompromised hosts where HHV 6 can reactivate and cause disease. Reactivation occurs in ~1/2 of bone marrow transplant recipients and 1/3 of solid organ transplant recipients. Interestingly, HHV6 is unique as it is the only human herpesvirus that can become chromosomally integrated (0.5-1% of individuals harbor germ line-integrated HHV6 genomes). A more recently described herpesvirus, HHV7, appears to have clinicopathologic features similar to HHV6 and is an occasional cause of roseola infantum.

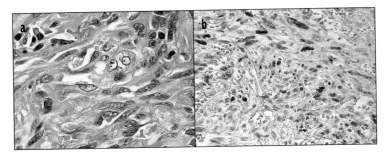

f3.5 Malignant spindled cells of Kaposi sarcoma
a H&E stained section
b HHV8 immunohistochemically stained section

HHV8 has come to be known as the Kaposi sarcoma-associated herpesvirus (KSHV). It is associated with all clinical variants of Kaposi sarcoma f3.5, in addition to primary effusion lymphoma (PEL) and the subset of multicentric Castleman disease seen in HIV+ patients. The diagnosis of KSHV relies on molecular methods (either FISH or PCR), immunohistochemical staining (LANA-1 expression, in a speckled nuclear pattern, is the hallmark of cells harboring KSHV), or serology (IFA, ELISA, or western Blot).

Adenovirus

Adenoviruses are grouped into >50 types (initially based on serologic reactions, but now based on molecular data). Most of the respiratory infections are caused by the lower-numbered serotypes (1-14 & 21). Types 4 & 7 are associated with epidemic outbreaks of respiratory disease. Types 11 & 21 are associated with hemorrhagic cystitis. Types 40 & 41 are associated with childhood gastroenteritis. The diagnosis of adenovirus may be made by serology (positive IgM or 4-fold rise in IgG), direct antigen detection, PCR, or culture (CPE: grapelike clusters in 1-7 days). Histologically, one sees cells with basophilic nuclear inclusions referred to as "smudge cells."

Parvovirus

Parvoviruses include parvovirus B19 and the recently discovered human bocavirus. Parvovirus B19 is the cause of erythema infectiosum (slapped cheek disease; fifth disease), but it is also capable of infecting erythroid marrow precursors and causing aplastic anemia. Primary maternal infection during gestation can lead to hydrops fetalis, and infection in persons with chronic hemolytic anemia (eg, sickle cell disease) can cause an aplastic crisis. Characteristic smudgy nuclear inclusions are seen in bone marrow biopsies. PCR is the most sensitive technique for detecting B19-specific DNA within a specimen and is considered the test of choice for diagnosing infection in hosts with limited ability to produce antibodies (immunocompromised, in the fetus or neonate) for whom serologic tests are not advised. Serologies detecting B19-specific antibodies to viral capsid antigen remain the cornerstone in determining the immune status of immunocompetent individuals. Immunocytochemical or immunohistochemical techniques can be performed on specimen detecting the presence of B19-specific capsid antigens using commercially available antibodies to this virus. Parvovirus culture is not readily available, since it requires nucleated red blood cells. Human bocavirus is a respiratory virus that, at this time, is detectable only by PCR.

Polyomaviruses

JC virus and BK virus, named for the initials of the patients in whom they were first isolated, are initially associated with asymptomatic infection. Both are acquired in childhood and enter latency, especially within epithelia of the urogenital tract and cells of the lymphoid system. Most adults are seropositive. If immunosuppression occurs, viral reactivation may occur. Progressive multifocal leukoencephalopathy (PML) is caused by reactivation of JC virus and infection of oligodendroglia, most often in the setting of AIDS. Reactivation of BK virus causes both hemorrhagic cystitis and polyomavirus nephropathy, usually in the setting of transplant related immunosuppression. In urine cytologic specimens, BK virus causes the appearance of so-called decoy cells, urothelial cells with a very high nuclear to cytoplasmic ratio that mimic the cells of urothelial carcinoma in situ (CIS). Attention to the slight degeneration in these cells, the characteristic smudgy nuclear inclusions, and lack of the usual chromatin detail seen in CIS are the helpful clues to avoid this pitfall. Similar inclusions are seen within oligodendroglial cells in the demyelinative lesions of PML. PCR is the test of choice for diagnosis of both JC and BK virus infections.

The Merkel cell polyomavirus (MCPyV) has been associated with merkel cell carcinoma (MCC) and chronic lymphocytic leukemia (CLL). Clonally integrated and mutated MCPyV DNA can be found in 80% of MCC. MCPyV can be found in ~15% of normal skin samples, but such skin is free of integrated and mutated forms. More recently, mutant MCPyV has been found in ~25% of CLL clones.

Papillomavirus

Human papillomavirus (HPV) causes proliferative epithelial lesions (eg, warts) in various locations t3.11. The incubation period after primary exposure is between 2-4 months.

t3.11 Lesions related to HPV

Lesion	HPV types (order of frequency)
Plantar wart	1,2
Common wart	2,1,4 (HPV 7 in handlers of fish & meat)
Flat (juvenile) wart	3, 10
Oral squamous papilloma	6, 11
Oral focal epithelia hyperplasia (Heck disease)	13, 32
Epidermodysplasia verruciformis	2, 3, 10, 5, 8
Laryngeal papillomas	6, 11
Condyloma acuminatum (genital warts)	6, 11
Low grade cervical squamous intraepithelial lesions (LSIL)	6, 11
High grade cervical squamous intraepithelial lesions (HSIL)	16, 18, 31, 33, 35
Cervical adenocarcinoma in situ (AIS)	18, 16, 45
Invasive cervical adenocarcinoma	

Common, plantar, and flat (juvenile) warts are acquired by direct contact; although, local abrasion or other trauma appears to enhance infectivity. Many forms of HPV (cervical, anal, and vulvar lesions) are sexually transmitted. In benign lesions, HPV DNA is episomal (extra-chromosomal), whereas in malignant lesions, it is integrated into the host cell DNA. The viral E6 & E7 genes are crucial for subsequent oncogenesis.

Epidermodysplasia verruciformis is the condition in which the oncogenic potential of HPV was first noted. This is an autosomal recessive condition associated with a gene locus on chromosome 17 which seems to impair defenses against several specific HPV types. The lesions are found on the trunk and upper extremities, tend to be exophytic, and usually appear in the first decade of life. In young adulthood the lesions may undergo malignant transformation, invading as squamous cell carcinomas. Unlike other types of warts, epidermodysplasia verruciformis does not appear to be transmissible by contact with healthy subjects. Some of the implicated HPV types (especially HPV 5) have been associated with psoriasis. Furthermore, lesions resembling epidermodysplasia verruciformis are sometimes seen in organ transplant recipients.

Recurrent respiratory papillomatosis (RRP) is caused by HPV 6 and HPV 11. There are 2 main clinical types: a juvenile-onset form, in which HPV is thought to be acquired during passage through the birth canal, and is more aggressive; and an adult form, thought to be sexually transmitted, in which papillomas are fewer. The papillomas arise most often on the true vocal cords. Malignant transformation is quite rare, but the lesions can be life threatening because of airway obstruction, particularly in children. The juvenile form of RRP usually presents between the ages of 2-4 years. It is characterized by multiple papillomas that arise synchronously and serially. Affected children often require numerous, sometimes monthly, endoscopic resections. Adult-onset RRP is diagnosed most commonly between the ages of 20 and 40 years. Sometimes an HPV subtype is requested, as HPV 11 is associated with more aggressive disease than HPV 6.

Anogenital HPV

Benign squamous lesions (condyloma acuminata) of the anogenital region are usually associated with HPV 6 or HPV 11.

Bowenoid papulosis is a condition that presents as multiple small (2-3 mm) pearly papules on the anogenital skin. Histologically, it resembles squamous cell carcinoma in situ (Bowen disease), but Bowenoid papulosis rarely results in invasive carcinoma. While histologically difficult or impossible to distinguish, true squamous cell carcinoma in situ (Bowen disease and erythroplasia of Queyrat) is usually easy to distinguish clinically. Bowenoid papulosis is caused by HPV 16.

Together, HPV 16 and HPV 18 account for >70% of all malignancies in the anogenital region. The correlation is tightest with high grade dysplasia and squamous cell carcinoma of the cervix, in which >98% of cases have detectable HPV. In fact, HPV is present in >95% of cervical adenocarcinomas and adenocarcinoma in situ. Outside the cervix, the rate of HPV detection in high grade and invasive squamous lesions varies from 80-95% for anal lesions to 30-40% for vulvar and penile lesions.

Verrucous carcinoma (giant condyloma of Buschke and Lowenstein) is nearly always associated with HPV 6 or HPV 11.

Poxviruses

Poxviruses cause vesicular skin eruptions.

Variola causes smallpox, the last endemic case of which was in 1977. Eradication was officially declared in 1980; however, stocks of the virus are maintained in labs throughout the world. Recently, there has been concern about smallpox as an agent of bioterrorism t3.12. The potential is significant, as variola can be easily acquired through aerosolized material, requires only a very small inoculum, and widespread immunization has not been practiced for some time. Many febrile illnesses with rash may be confused with smallpox; especially similar are chickenpox and monkeypox. The latter is mostly confined to

parts of western and central Africa, although a recent outbreak in the US was caused by exposure to pet prairie dogs who had contracted infection when exposed to exotic African rodents in the pet shop. Nonetheless, suspected smallpox is reportable, and the diagnosis should be confirmed in a Biological Safety Level (BSL) 4 laboratory by technologists who have been vaccinated. A patient suspected of having smallpox should be isolated and vaccinated (even after infection, vaccination can ameliorate the illness). Samples should preferably be collected by someone who has been immunized. The best samples are scrapings, biopsy, or fluid from a skin lesion, in addition to tonsillar swabs and blood. Samples should be submitted to a specialized laboratory (eg, the CDC) that not only has the means for making the diagnosis but also has BSL 4 capabilities. While there are characteristic light microscopic (viral inclusions called Guarnieri bodies) and electron microscopic findings, these lack specificity. Specific tests, including viral isolation in cell culture, DFA testing, and PCR are available at the CDC.

t3.12 CDC classification of agents of bioterrorism

Category A (highest priority)	Category B (second priority)	Category C (third priority; emerging threat agents)
Variola (smallpox)	Encephalitis viruses (α-viruses)	Influenza viruses
Hemorrhagic fever viruses	*Brucella* species (brucellosis)	Nipah virus
Bacillus anthracis (anthrax)	*Burkholderia mallei* (glanders)	Hantavirus
Yersinia pestis (plague)	*Burkholderia pseudomallei* (melioidosis)	Rabies virus
Clostridium botulinum (botulism)	*Chlamydophila psittaci*	Yellow fever virus
Francisella tularensis (tularemia)	*Coxiella burnetii* (Q fever)	Drug-resistant TB
	Clostridium perfringens toxin	*Rickettsia conorii*
	Foodborne bacteria (eg, *Salmonella* species, *E coli* O157:H7, *Shigella*)	
	Waterborne bacteria (eg, *Vibrio cholerae*, *Cryptosporidium* species)	
	Rickettsia prowazekii (typhus fever)	
	Staphylococcus aureus enterotoxin B	

Vaccinia virus is a lab derived virus closely related to cowpox and variola virus that is used in the small pox vaccine.

Molluscum contagiosum virus causes a vesicular eruption characterized by small waxy papules with central umbilication, single or multiple, located anywhere on the body but classically on the perineal skin in sexually active individuals or face, neck, and arms in children. The lesions are quite characteristic histologically f3.6, with prominent eosinophilic cytoplasmic inclusions seen in lesional keratinocytes. If clinically confused with HSV, this confusion can carry over to the laboratory where in cell culture the virus can mimic the CPE of herpes. Unlike HSV, molluscum cannot be subcultured to subsequent cell cultures.

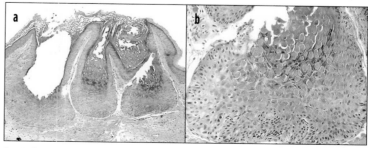

f3.6 Molluscum contagiosum
a H&E stained sections demonstrate a craterlike papilliferous lesion
b Characteristic intracytoplasmic molluscum bodies

Hepatitis viruses t3.13

Hepatitis A virus (HAV)

Hepatitis A virus (HAV) is an RNA virus (Picornavirus) that causes hepatitis associated with food related outbreaks. It causes acute disease with relatively short incubation period and chronicity does not occur. However, a relapse of HAV occurs, usually proximate to the acute infection by no more than a few months, in ~5% of cases. Diagnosis of acute infection depends on demonstrating IgM anti-HAV which emerges early, slightly before the onset of symptoms. The presence of IgG anti-HAV may indicate acute or past infection, as it also emerges early but persists for life.

t3.13 Hepatitis viruses

Virus	Transmission	Incubation	Chronicity	Comments
HAV	Fecal-oral	15-30 days	0%	Most common viral hepatitis in US; Abrupt onset
HBV	Parenteral	15-150 days, average 60-90	2-10% of everyone 30-90% of children < 5 years	Usually insidious; mortality: ~1%
HCV	Parenteral	30-150 days	60-85%	~10,000 deaths annually
HDV	Parenteral	21-49 days	5% of coinfections ≤80% of superinfections	Exists as a co-infection with HBV
HEV	Fecal-oral	15-60 days, average 40	0%	20-30% fatality rate in pregnancy
HGV	Parenteral	Unknown	Unknown	Significance of infection unknown

Hepadnavirus (hepatitis B virus, HBV)

HBV virus is a DNA virus whose intact virion is called the Dane particle. Important HBV viral markers include:

- Hepatitis B surface antigen (HbsAg; Australia antigen), whose presence in serum *indicates active disease*; HBsAg would be expected to clear if infection is resolved and persist if infection is chronic. HbsAg positivity indicates acute infection or chronic carriage

- Hepatitis B e antigen (HBeAg) *indicates active viral replication*. In the hepatocyte, the genome of HBV can be present in 2 forms: as replicating virus or integrated into the host genome as a nonreplicating form. HBeAg is only produced when the virus is in replicating form; thus, it can be used as a surrogate for HBV DNA production.

- Antibody against hepatitis B core antigen (IgM and IgG anti-HBc) is present throughout the lifetime of somebody who has been infected with HBV. Generally, hepatitis B core IgM antibody is only present during the acute infection (but may persist for up to a year or appear in acute flares), whereas the hepatitis B core total antibodies (IgM & IgG) are present in both acute and past infection.

- Antibody against hepatitis B e antigen (anti-HBe) is found when HBe becomes negative. The presence of anti-HBe does not imply resolved infection or immunity. Anti-HBe positivity indicates chronic carrier without active viral replication.

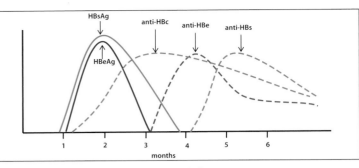

f3.7 Serologic patterns in acute HBV with resolution of infection

- Antibody against surface antigen (HBsAb) *indicates resistance to infection*. It is found in immunized persons and those who have successfully cleared HBV infection. HBsAb positivity indicates recent or past infection or immunization.

- Note: there is no circulating core antigen.

In acute hepatitis B infection f3.7 t3.14 serologic markers begin to emerge between 2-10 weeks following exposure. *HBsAg appears first,* followed by HBeAg and IgM anti-HBc. *HBV DNA is detectable in serum before HBsAg.* HBsAg becomes detectable before clinical symptoms appear. The development of antibodies (anti-HBs, anti-HBc) roughly coincides with the development of clinical symptoms. In the majority of patients, there is complete resolution of acute HBV infection. This is heralded by the emergence of anti-HBe and anti-HBs. Usually the latter developments somewhat follow the disappearance of HBsAg and HBeAg from serum. Anti-HBs therefore is indicative of resolved HBV hepatitis and implies lifelong immunity.

t3.14 HBV serology

Clinical status	HBsAg	Anti-HBc	Anti-HBs
Neither prior infection nor immunization	–	–	–
Prior immunization	–	–	+
Acute HBV	+	+ (IgM)	–
Chronic HBV	+	+	–
Resolved HBV	–	+ (IgM & IgG)	+

With older less sensitive assays, there was a brief interval between disappearance of HBsAg and appearance of HBsAb, termed the "window" period. The possibility of a false negative serologic diagnosis of HBV infection existed during this period, unless IgM anti-HBc was measured. With present more sensitive assays, this window has narrowed considerably.

IgM anti-HBc emerges shortly after HBsAg and persists for many months. It is eventually replaced by IgG anti-HBc, sometimes 18-24 months after infection. Thus, IgG anti-HBc indicates past infection, either resolved (anti-HBs+) or in the chronic phase (HBsAg+). In patients who develop chronic HBV infection, IgM anti-HBc may re-emerge during acute flares.

There is a small group of patients who are found to have only anti-HBc, without HBsAg or anti-HBs. This may be seen in 4 scenarios: the "window" period; chronic HBV infection in which levels of HBsAg have fallen to undetectable levels; remote resolved HBV infection in which levels of anti-HBs have fallen to undetectable levels (common in HIV infection); and nonspecific false positives. The presence of circulating

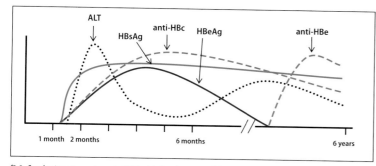

f3.8 Serologic patterns in acute HBV with development of chronic infection

The response to therapy is monitored in several ways

1. in the liver biopsy, a decrease in the histologic activity index (HAI) of ≥2 is considered a histologic response

2. normalization of serum ALT is definitive of a biochemical response

3. either a negative HBeAg or an undetectable HBV DNA level (< 10^5 copies/mL) is considered a virologic response

Circulating HBV DNA can be found by PCR in a high percentage of patients with negative HBsAg and positive anti-HBs, anti-HBe, and anti-HBc. The significance of this is unclear at this time.

HBV DNA in this setting is consistent with chronic HBV infection (with undetectably low HBsAg).

Chronic hepatitis B infection is defined by persistence of HBsAg after the acute phase (for >6 months) f3.8, t3.14. Persistent HBsAg without clinical hepatitis is called the chronic "carrier" state. Chronicity develops in ~5% of healthy infected adults, 10% of immunocompromised adults, and up to *90% of neonates who have become infected transplacentally*. Chronic HBs antigenemia can be associated with polyarteritis nodosum (PAN). Hepatitis D virus (HDV) is capable of infecting hepatocytes with HBV DNA but not uninfected hepatocytes.

The HBV genome has several major gene regions: pre-S, S, C, P, and X. The pre-S genes encode the hepatocyte receptor–binding site. The S gene encodes surface antigen (HBsAg), a component of the viral envelope. The C gene encodes core antigen (HBcAg) and e antigen (HBeAg). The P gene encodes a DNA polymerase. The HBV genome can undergo mutation, altering the clinical features. One such mutation takes the form of so-called HBeAg– chronic hepatitis B. This is characterized by circulating HBV DNA, fluctuating aminotransferases, and a tendency towards fulminant hepatitis with liver failure. This form of hepatitis B results from mutations in the C or pre-C region, the most common mutation being an adenosine (A) for guanine (G) substitution at nucleotide position 1896 ($G_{1896}A$), leading to a premature stop codon that impairs synthesis of HBeAg. Mutations in the DNA polymerase gene often arise during treatment with lamivudine, resulting in decreased binding of lamivudine. These mutations may lead to abrupt progression of chronic hepatitis B in patients previously stable on treatment.

Molecular assays

There are 3 major applications of molecular assays in HBV: making the initial diagnosis, particularly when serology is equivocal; distinguishing replicative from nonreplicative chronic HBV infection; and monitoring therapy.

With regard to diagnosis, HBV DNA can be detected ~3 weeks before HBsAg becomes detectable in serum. This lead-time is particularly useful to evaluate patients after an exposure (eg, a needle stick).

The HBe antigen status is the traditional way to classify chronic HBV carriers as replicative or nonreplicative. Certain limitations in this approach—a tendency of HBe antigen to be undetectable in reactivation disease or to never appear in precore mutations—have made HBV DNA a more attractive analyte for this purpose. Currently, those with >10^5/mL copies of HBV DNA are considered replicative.

Hepatitis C virus (HCV)

HCV is an RNA virus from the Flavivirus family. It causes the vast majority of transfusion associated viral hepatitis and the vast majority of what was previously called non-A, non-B hepatitis. ~60-85% people infected develop chronic HCV infection. ~10-15% of those with chronic HCV will develop cirrhosis, usually after an illness of ~20 years. Those with cirrhosis due to HCV have a ~5% chance of developing hepatocellular carcinoma. The most powerful predictor of progression to cirrhosis is the finding of more than portal fibrosis (Ishak 3) on a liver biopsy. Extrahepatic manifestations of HCV infection include mixed cryoglobulinemia, glomerulonephritis, and aplastic anemia.

HCV infection has traditionally been diagnosed with EIA-based assays for anti-HCV antibodies, their presence indicative of infection. It is important to note that IgM and IgG anti-HCV cannot be reliably used to distinguish acute from chronic HCV infection; in fact, there is no reliable way to distinguish acute from chronic HCV infection and, for that matter, no compelling reason to do so. Most patients diagnosed with HCV, it is believed, are diagnosed with HCV in the chronic phase. The anti-HCV antibody test is now augmented by molecular assays for HCV RNA. While either a qualitative or quantitative HCV RNA test will suffice for this purpose, many clinicians request the quantitative test. A third test, the recombinant-immunoblot assay (RIBA), may be used to determine whether a positive anti-HCV but negative HCV RNA assay is significant for past infection or a false positive screen. RIBA is an enzyme immunoblot assay for the detection of Abs to multiple individual proteins encoded by HCV. Possible results are summarized in t3.15.

t3.15 Possible HCV results

Anti-HCV EIA	RIBA	HCV RNA	Interpretation
–	–	+	Very early HCV infection (<3 months)
+	+	+	Current HCV infection, acute or chronic
+	–/indeterminate	–	False positive anti-HCV EIA
+	+	–	Cleared/resolved prior HCV infection

Chronic HCV develops in >60% of infected patients. In some patients, the decision is made to treat, and the standard treatment presently is a combination of peginterferon α with ribavirin (PEGIFNa/RBV). The desired endpoint of treatment is a sustained virologic response (SVR), defined as undetectable HCV RNA *for a period of 24 weeks (6 months) after the end of treatment*. The most significant predictor of treatment response is the viral genotype: genotypes 2 and 3 have a high (90%) rate of response; genotype 1 has a low (~70%) rate of response. Recently 2 FDA approved direct acting antivirals, the protease inhibitors Telaprevir and Boceprevir, have been approved for the treatment of genotype 1 HCV infections in combination with PEGIFNa/RBV. The addition of the protease inhibitor to the combination treatment of genotype 1 infections has improved the SVR to >75% for primary infections with genotype 1. Furthermore, the nature and duration of treatment is influenced by the genotype. The other genotypes—4 through 9—have not been sufficiently studied due to low prevalence.

HCV genotyping may be performed on the basis of either molecular or serologic assays. The molecular assays involve direct sequencing of portions of the HCV genome (eg, the 5' noncoding region), hybridization with genotype-specific sequences, RFLP analysis or more recently using multiplex real time PCR assays. Serologic assays detect serum antibodies against genotype-specific antigens. In the United States, the most common HCV genotype is 1 (~70% of patients). Genotype 1 is further subdivided into 1a (~60%) and 1b (~40%). The significance of sub-genotypes 1a and 1b lies in the development of resistance to the protease inhibitors. Genotype 1a has a lower threshold to develop resistance than 1b as it requires fewer nucleotide substitutions to achieve resistances. Genotype 2 represents ~20% of all infections, and genotype 3 ~5%.

Qualitative assays for HCV RNA are based upon conventional PCR or transcription mediated amplification (TMA) platforms. *Quantitative* assays for HCV RNA can be performed by real time PCR (RT-PCR), transcription mediated amplification (TMA), or branched DNA (bDNA). These techniques must be capable of detecting as little as 50 IU/mL, since this is the definition of a sustained virologic response. Furthermore, they must be equally sensitive to RNA from the different genotypes. The same testing platform should be used throughout treatment, since quantitative results are not directly comparable between methods.

The liver biopsy remains important, particularly in making treatment decisions in patients infected with HCV genotype 1 or 4-9. Furthermore, the quantitative HCV RNA reflects neither the degree (grade) of hepatic inflammation nor the extent (stage) of hepatic fibrosis. And while HCV RNA is the best predictor of treatment response, it does not correlate, as histology does, with the likelihood of progressing to cirrhosis. Serial ALT measurements are only slightly better at predicting liver histology. Most clinicians, therefore, continue to rely on the liver biopsy for assessing severity of liver disease, predicting prognosis, and deciding whether to treat.

Other hepatitis viruses

Hepatitis E virus (HEV) is an RNA virus with some clinical similarities to HAV, including fecal-oral spread and the rarity of chronic infection. One major difference is that HAV causes infection predominantly in children, usually before their 11th birthday, whereas HEV usually affects young adults, peaking between 15 and 35 years of age. HEV infection is more common in males, but it is more virulent in pregnant women, with a mortality rate approaching 30%. Overall mortality is ~1%. Chronicity is rare, but it is common in immunosuppressed transplant recipients who become infected with HEV. Infection is rarely seen in the United States but is common in many tropical and subtropical pockets of the developing world, including India, southeast Asia, northern Africa, and Mexico. Most cases in the US are found in travelers, but true autochthonous cases have been documented. The diagnosis is made by detecting IgM anti-HEV in serum. IgM is usually detectable at presentation, its elevation coinciding with the elevation of liver function tests and the onset of symptoms. IgM disappears within 1-3 months. IgG anti-HEV also rises early and persists for years. Lastly, HEV RNA can be detected by PCR during acute illness, disappearing within 4 weeks.

Hepatitis G virus, also called GBV-C virus, is an RNA virus belonging to the Flaviviridae family. Like HCV, it is transmitted by parenteral routes and leads to long-term chronic infection. Since its discovery, however, there has been no convincing evidence of it causing hepatitis. While the virus is present in 1-2% of the population and is known to infect hepatocytes for a very long time, it is not clear that it causes clinical disease.

Other viruses may secondarily involve the liver as part of systemic infection causing hepatitis including EBV, CMV, HSV, VZV, and yellow fever.

Orthomyxovirus

Influenza viruses cause annual outbreaks, usually during cold weather, and undergo regular antigenic changes that prevent the development of lifelong immunity. Influenza is usually heralded by the abrupt onset of fever, with myalgias, headache, sore throat and cough. Influenza B typically produces milder symptoms than influenza A. In the usual course of events, influenza resolves within 1 week; however, several complications may ensue, including influenza pneumonia, secondary bacterial pneumonia (*S aureus*, *S pneumonia*, and *H influenza* most commonly), Reye syndrome, myositis, myocarditis, and Guillain-Barré syndrome. Most influenza related deaths are the result of secondary bacterial pneumonia.

The virions have a lipid envelope containing several surface antigens. The dominant antigen is hemagglutinin. Hemagglutinin binds to sialic acid-containing receptors on respiratory epithelial cells and becomes expressed on the surface of infected cells. This expression forms the basis for the hemadsorption test. Only influenza A & B viruses and parainfluenza and mumps viruses are hemadsorption positive; such viruses are said to be "hemagglutinating viruses." Hemagglutinin (H) and neuraminidase (N) glycoprotein antigens form the basis for influenza virus identification (an isolate may be characterized H1N1, for example). H and N undergo periodic major antigenic changes and more frequent minor changes, while the other antigens are stable. Antigenic drift (minor changes) are the result of point mutations in the H and N genes; these drifts result in new strains of virus, producing annual outbreaks and epidemics. Antigenic shifts (major changes) are the result of genetic reassortment between distinct strains; shifts result in worldwide outbreaks (pandemics) that occur about every 10-20 years. Currently, there are 16 H subtypes and 9 N subtypes. For the past several years, the major strains in circulation have been influenza A (H1N1), influenza A (H3N2), and influenza B. Birds, especially aquatic birds, serve as reservoirs for all subtypes, and avian strains have been responsible, historically, for most pandemics.

The most recent avian influenza (H5N1) has been responsible for scattered pandemics in chickens, most recently in southeast Asia. Hundreds of humans have become infected with H5N1, with a ~50% mortality rate. Unlike the more common influenza strains, H5N1 has affected predominantly children and young adults, with a median age of ~15 years. Infection rapidly produces patchy then diffuse lung opacity and an increased oxygen requirement; histologic findings of acute and organizing DAD have been found in autopsies. Lymphopenia is characteristic, without significant changes in the neutrophil count, erythrocytes, or platelets. The high mortality rate seems to be related to complete naivety to the H5 antigen and its tropism for nonciliated epithelial cells of the lower respiratory tract. Tropism for the distal airways leads to an ARDS/DAD-like clinicopathologic picture and may explain the low rate of human to human transmission. Almost all human cases appear to result from exposure to sick birds (epizoonotic).

The 2009 pandemic was related to an H1N1 strain that was briefly called "Swine flu," because it was thought to be derived from genetic reassortment between distinct strains of swine-origin H1N1. This strain has now replaced the previously circulating H1N1 virus.

Diagnosis

Specimens for diagnosis of influenza are ideally obtained from the respiratory tract within the first 1-2 days of illness. Preferred specimens include throat swabs, nasopharyngeal swabs and bronchoalveolar lavages, placed directly into viral transport medium.

Culture is traditionally considered the gold standard diagnostic test, but is rapidly being replaced by PCR. Conventional cell culture may require a week, but shell-vial techniques can provide a diagnosis within 2-3 days. The presence of virus in the culture may be confirmed by cytopathic effect, hemadsorption, immunofluorescent staining, or EIA. Culture is important for strain identification.

Rapid antigen tests are capable of providing a result within 30 minutes. However, these tests are traditionally much less sensitive than culture, with overall sensitivity of ~50%, though their specificity is generally high during influenza season. Newer rapid antigen tests have improved sensitivities to >80%. Rapid antigen tests are generally incapable of strain identification. Direct fluorescent antibody (DFA) staining is more sensitive and specific than other rapid antigen tests, though still significantly less than culture. DFA staining of nasopharyngeal secretions has a sensitivity of ~80%. DFA may also be performed on BAL fluid, sputum, or incubated cell-culture cells.

Nucleic acid detection (NAT), detection of influenza viral RNA, can be performed using reverse transcriptase PCR and has sensitivity and specificity comparable to culture. This can be done alone or as part of a multiplex PCR assay capable of detecting multiple viruses, and in some cases bacteria, that cause respiratory disease. Amplification targets are selected from the conserved sequences found in the matrix or nucleoprotein genes, rather than the often-mutated H and N genes, to avoid false negatives. In contrast, subtyping assays generally target the H gene. PCR assays have mostly replaced culture as the test of choice due to increased sensitivity and rapid turnaround time.

Serology can confirm influenza infection retrospectively, after study of acute and convalescent sera. The most commonly used serologic test to document influenza virus infection is hemagglutination inhibition (HI). This assay allows determination of the virus subtype and strain based upon specific antibody. As in other scenarios, the utility of serology is limited by the need to test acute and convalescent sera.

The treatment for severe cases of influenza A are the neuraminidase inhibitors oseltamivir (Tamiflu; most effective when given in the first 48 hours of illness) and zanamivir (Relenza). The ion channel inhibitor, Amantadine, is rarely used today due to widespread resistance.

Paramyxoviruses

Parainfluenza virus 1 and parainfluenza virus 2 cause most cases of croup in children between the ages of 2 and 6, while parainfluenza virus 3 is the second most common cause (after RSV) of respiratory bronchiolitis ("viral pneumonia") in infants under age 2. Parainfluenza viruses are spread by large droplet aerosols and by contact with contaminated surfaces. Infections with parainfluenza virus generally occur in spring, summer and fall. The viruses can be detected via cell culture (see t3.4; little to no CPE after 3-10 days, detection is made possible by hemabsorption/hemagglutination), antigen detection (immunofluorescent assays), and PCR.

Measles (rubeola) is the cause of classic measles, atypical measles (teenage patients who have received only one vaccination), and subacute sclerosing panencephalitis (SSPE). Measles is characterized by the classic prodrome of cough, coryza and conjunctivitis with or without Koplik spots, followed by a descending rash beginning on the head. The complications of measles include otitis media, pneumonia, myocarditis, and subacute sclerosing panencephalitis—SSPE (rare). The first 2 of these complications are often due to bacterial superinfection. Measles virus may directly involve the appendix, resulting in a form of appendicitis; more often, measles-induced mesenteric adenitis causes an appendicitis-like presentation. Progressive fatal measles giant cell pneumonia occurs in immunocompromised hosts or in nutritionally deficient hosts. The characteristic histologic findings in lungs and other organs infected with measles include multinucleated cells with nuclear and cytoplasmic inclusions (Warthin-Finkeldey giant cells). The risk of SSPE is ~0.001% with a higher risk if measles is acquired at an early age, with an average incubation period of 7 years. Vaccines have an SSPE risk of 0.0001% with an incubation period of 3 years.

Mumps virus is best known as a cause of parotitis in the prevaccine era. However, neither the rate of vaccination nor the efficacy of vaccination is 100%, and recent outbreaks have occurred in the United States and United Kingdom. Furthermore, the manifestations of mumps are not confined to the parotid glands. In fact, only ~60% of infected individuals have overt parotitis, while 10% will have clinical meningoencephalitis, 15% orchitis, and 5% pancreatitis. 13% of

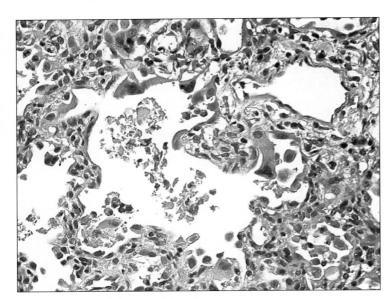

f3.9 RSV pneumonitis with classic syncytia formation

the rule, though infections are progressively less severe with bronchiolitis uncommon after 12 months. RSV is also a cause of croup. Rapid diagnosis is important so that appropriate isolation precautions can be taken and so that aerosolized ribavirin can be initiated, the treatment of choice for severe RSV infection. Diagnosis can be made by rapid DFA or EIA techniques, performed on swab or secretion samples, or viral culture, with the highly characteristic formation of syncytia in Hep2 cells. The difficulty in diagnosing RSV by culture is its extreme fragility; specimen transport must be expeditious. Furthermore, RSV grows slowly in cell culture, often requiring over a week. Shell-vial techniques have ameliorated this somewhat. Nonetheless, as a result of these difficulties direct (DFA and EIA) techniques have proven as sensitive as culture for the diagnosis of RSV. PCR is the preferred method for detection.

Human metapneumovirus (hMPv) is a recently identified virus that appears to be responsible for a significant proportion (up to 20%) of viral lower respiratory tract infections. It is capable of causing upper respiratory tract infections, lower respiratory tract infections (both bronchiolitis and pneumonia), and a flulike illness. Growth has been slow on standard cell culture media, but both shell-vial techniques and RT-PCR offer more rapid diagnosis.

Picornaviruses (small [pico-] RNA viruses)

Enteroviridae include poliovirus, coxsackie A, coxsackie B, echovirus, and enterovirus. They enter the body via the GI tract and are capable of causing a flulike illness which may be accompanied by gastroenteritis and aseptic meningitis. Enteroviruses are the most common cause of viral meningitis (aseptic meningitis). RT-PCR is currently considered the gold standard for making the diagnosis of enterovirus in CSF. It demonstrates excellent sensitivity and same-day turnaround time. Cell culture can be performed as well, in case the PCR test is negative.

- Poliovirus causes the well known neurologic infection poliomyelitis, which causes destruction of spinal ventral horn motor neurons.

- Coxsackie A virus causes herpangina (a painful oral infection) and hand-foot-mouth disease. Hand-foot-mouth disease is most often caused by Coxsackie A16.

- Coxsackie B virus causes epidemic pleurodynia (the grippe), myocarditis, and pericarditis.

Rhinovirus is considered the most common cause of the common cold. Culture is possible, but requires incubation at 32°C. RT-PCR methods are much more sensitive than culture for the diagnosis of rhinovirus.

Hepatitis A virus (see p 134).

Arboviruses

Transmitted by arthropods, the following group was historically classified as arboviruses (arbo being short for *ar*thropod-*bo*rne). They had in common bird reservoirs and arthropod vectors. These viruses have now been dispersed into 4 families: bunya-, toga-, reo-, & rhabdoviruses. Not all the viruses within these families are arthropod-borne.

adults with mumps have myocarditis with S-T changes; some develop endocardial fibroelastosis. Pre-vaccine cases arose in young children and young adults, especially military recruits; however, recent outbreaks have occurred mainly in young adult college students; some of these cases could be attributed to incomplete vaccination, but most patients had been fully vaccinated as children, suggesting waning immunity. Mumps virus has an affinity for various epithelia. Viral replication in the ductal epithelium of the parotid gland, pancreas, and testes leads to marked periductal chronic inflammation and edema, leading to obstruction and pressure-induced atrophy. Orchitis is almost exclusively a feature of mumps in post-pubertal males. Despite its reputation for causing infertility, this outcome is in fact rare. CSF pleocytosis occurs in 50-60% of all mumps infections, and clinical evidence of meningoencephalitis in ~10%, with permanent sensorineural hearing complicating ~1% of cases. The laboratory diagnosis of mumps may be based upon viral culture, nucleic acid testing (NAT), or serology. Virus can be isolated in culture from saliva, CSF, or urine, but yield diminished rapidly after the first week. The presence of virus in culture can be detected by immunofluorescence staining, since the formation of viral cytopathic effect is slow and unreliable. NAT by RT-PCR can be performed directly upon clinical specimens. Timing substantially impacts the sensitivity of serologic testing for mumps IgM, with frequent false negative tests in blood obtained in the first week of infection; specimens are ideally obtained between 7-10 days after the onset of symptoms.

Respiratory syncytial virus (RSV) is the most common cause of lower respiratory tract infection (pneumonia & respiratory bronchiolitis) in infants and toddlers. RSV causes 90% of respiratory bronchiolitis in infants and almost half of lower respiratory tract infections in children f3.9. It is responsible for localized outbreaks, such as in daycare centers, where the attack rate can reach nearly 100%. Immunity to RSV is short-lived, and recurrence throughout childhood is

Bunyaviridae

Family Bunyaviridae includes hantaviruses (Sin Nombre, Black Creek, and Prospect Hill Hantaviruses), California encephalitis, and several hemorrhagic fever viruses (Crimean-Congo hemorrhagic fever virus, Rift Valley fever virus, LaCrosse virus).

- **Hantavirus** is not acquired through an arthropod vector but rather through aerosolized rodent excreta. Hantavirus pulmonary syndrome is a cause of often fatal (30-40%) acute respiratory failure characterized by histologic changes indistinguishable from diffuse alveolar damage.

- **Hemorrhagic fever viruses** are numerous and not limited to the bunyavirus family. They share common manifestations including the sudden onset of fever, chills, severe epigastric pain, and the development of disseminated intravascular coagulation (DIC). The hemorrhagic fever viruses are
  - **Bunyaviruses,** including Crimean-Congo Hemorrhagic Fever (CCHF) virus, Rift Valley Fever virus, and LaCrosse virus, are noteworthy for causing so-called hemorrhagic fever with renal syndrome (acute tubular necrosis).
  - **Togaviruses** include Flaviviruses (Dengue & Yellow Fever virus) and Togaviruses (Chikungunya virus).
  - **Arenaviruses** include the Lassa fever virus
  - **Filoviruses** include Marburg & Ebola viruses

Togaviridae

Family Togaviridae includes the genus α-virus (eastern equine, western equine, & Venezuelan encephalitis), flavivirus (WNV, St Louis encephalitis, dengue, yellow fever), and rubivirus (rubella virus). With the exception of yellow fever (viral hepatitis) and rubella (viral exanthema), this family causes arthropod-borne encephalitis.

- **Rubella virus** is biologically different from the others in this family. It is transmitted by person to person spread and causes a febrile illness with rash (German measles) which is only really consequential in pregnancy. *First-trimester infections* have the most serious fetal implications. Defects in first-trimester-infected neonates include sensorineural deafness, cataracts, glaucoma, microphthalmia, congenital heart disease (PDA), intrauterine growth retardation, and microcephaly. Hepatosplenomegaly, radiolucent bone lesions, and thrombocytopenia may occur. In affected adults, rubella is acquired by respiratory secretions and manifests as posterior cervical or suboccipital lymphadenopathy with a rash that first appears on the face and spreads down the body. Vaccination is given in childhood, usually in combination with measles and mumps (MMR vaccine). Because of the possibility of waning immunity, the IgG titer of women of childbearing age should be tested prior to anticipated pregnancy, when possible. A booster vaccination is usually recommended in nonimmune women of childbearing age. In a patient with suspected rubella, serologic testing for rubella IgG and IgM can provide the diagnosis. IgM antibodies are indicative of acute infection; in the absence of IgM, IgG seroconversion (4-fold increase of convalescent over acute titer) also confirms, retrospectively, the diagnosis of rubella. In newborns with suspected congenital rubella, neonatal IgM can provide the diagnosis; any IgG is presumed to be maternal.

- **Dengue & yellow fever** are transmitted most commonly by *Aedes* species mosquitos (*Aedes aegypti* or *Aedes albopictus*). Dengue fever (breakbone fever) and yellow fever cause fever, chills, backache, jaundice, and hemorrhage in severe cases. Dengue hemorrhagic fever (DHF) is seen more commonly in children than adults and is more common after prior infection with another dengue virus serotype (of which there are 4). Yellow fever is viscerotropic for the heart, kidney, GIT, and liver. The most characteristic lesion of yellow fever is in the liver: extensive *midzonal* necrosis, Councilman bodies, microvesicular fatty metamorphosis, and absence of an inflammatory component.

- **West Nile virus (WNV)** is maintained in a bird-mosquito-bird cycle where humans are incidental hosts. Transmission occurs through the bite of an infected female *Culex* species mosquito. It can also occur via transplanted organs and blood transfusion. Infection with WNV has 3 clinical presentations: 1) asymptomatic (~80%), 2) West Nile fever (~20%) or 3) CNS disease (<1%). Serology is the primary diagnostic test. However, PCR plays an important role in diagnosis of CNS disease and early infection (within 10 days of infection when a transient viremia occurs) prior to the development of detectable antibodies.

Reoviridae

Family Reoviridae contains orbivirus and rotavirus. Rotavirus is the most common cause of viral gastroenteritis, other cases being due to norovirus, enteric (serotypes 40 & 41) adenoviruses, calicivirus, and astrovirus.

Rhabdoviridae

Family Rhabdoviridae includes rabies and vesicular stomatitis virus. In poorly controlled areas, dogs and cats transmit 90% of rabies. In areas with good control of domestic rabies, most cases are the result of exposures to bats, wolf, coyote, foxes, skunk, and raccoon. Rare cases have been transmitted by aerosol or organ transplant. The bite of an infected animal deposits virus into soft tissues where it can enter the axon terminus of nerve cells at the neuromuscular junction. The virus is then transported via retrograde fast axonal transport to the central nervous system (CNS). While it is causing neuronal damage in the CNS, the virus is transmitted to the periphery along autonomic and sensory neurons. This peripheral dissemination is the basis for infection of the salivary gland (permitting transmission to other animals) and infection of the neural tissue that surrounds hair follicles (permitting diagnosis by skin biopsy). Antirabies antibodies in serum are useful for diagnosis in patients who have not been given prophylaxis, but they emerge only after about the first week of infection. In skin biopsies, rabies virus antigen can be detected by immunofluorescence (usually at state health laboratories); the samples are most often taken from the nape of the neck, wherein antigen is found in

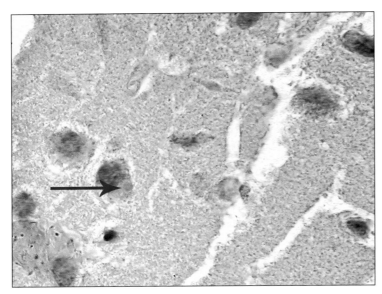
f3.10 Classic intracytoplasmic inclusion of rabies virus in the brain

perifollicular nerves. Histologic findings in the brain consist of cytoplasmic Negri bodies within Purkinje cells f3.10 of the cerebellum and hippocampus and Babes nodules, which are essentially microglial nodules.

Arenavirus

Arenaviruses include Lassa fever virus, lymphocytic choriomeningitis (LCM) virus, machupo virus, & sabia virus. Of these, only LCM virus is located in the United States, and it causes the least severe form of infection. Virus particles contain host cell ribosomes in their interior, giving them a granular appearance. Arenaviruses are parasites of rodents which shed virus in their urine and feces—hamsters and house mice are the hosts to LCM virus. Human infection is characterized by a viral prodrome followed by: hemorrhagic manifestations in all of them, hepatitis and myocarditis in Lassa fever, and meningitis in LCM. Serology is the most commonly used diagnostic technique.

Retroviridae

Family Retroviridae comprises the human T-lymphotrophic viruses (HTLVs) and human immunodeficiency virus (HIV)

HTLV-1

HTLV-1 is a retrovirus endemic in southern Japan, the Caribbean, southern Africa, and Brazil. There is a pocket of relative prevalence in the southeastern United States. The virus is transmitted parenterally (intravenous drug use, transfusion, sexual contact) and transplacentally. Like HIV, the HTLV-1 virus infects CD4+ T lymphocytes; the diagnostic strategy is similar to HIV—a screening ELISA followed by confirmatory western blot or PCR. The proviral load (see below) appears to correlate with the likelihood of neurologic disease. While acute infection may be asymptomatic, after a variably prolonged incubation period, the virus may cause late neurologic (tropical spastic paraparesis) or hematologic (adult T cell leukemia) disease.

Tropical spastic paraparesis (HTLV-1-associated myelopathy, Jamaican neuropathy) affects women ~3 times as often as men. The incubation period is much shorter than for ATLL, with some cases arising during acute infection. The disease tends to progress for 1-2 years then arrest, leaving affected individuals with a set of irreversible neurologic deficits. Histopathologically, demyelinating lesions are found in association with perivascular lymphocytic infiltrates, predominantly within the upper thoracic and lower cervical cord.

Adult T cell leukemia/lymphoma (ATLL) is the most common type of non-Hodgkin lymphoma in many HTLV-1-endemic parts of the world. The lifetime risk of ATLL is ~5% in people infected before the age of 20 years, with a mean incubation period of 20-30 years. It presents with hepatosplenomegaly, jaundice, and weight loss. Peculiar features are hypercalcemia, a skin rash, high serum concentrations of free IL-2 receptor, and a pronounced sense of thirst. The neoplastic cells, having the characteristic "flower cell" morphology, express CD4 and CD25 (the IL-2 receptor).

HIV-1 & HIV-2

The Centers for Disease Control and Prevention (CDC) makes the following recommendations with regard to screening and diagnostic testing; wherein screening is defined as testing of all members of a particular population, and diagnostic testing refers to testing patients in whom there is a clinical suspicion of HIV infection.

The CDC recommends that "opt out" screening be offered to all patients aged 13-64 years, all patients newly diagnosed with TB, and all patients seeking treatment for sexually transmitted diseases. Opt-out screening means that the patient is informed that the test will be performed, and the test is indeed performed if the patient does not object; ie, acquiescence is taken to imply assent. Repeat screening should be offered to all high risk persons on an annual basis; high risk applying to intravenous drug users, sexual partners of intravenous drug users, persons who exchange sex for money or drugs, sexual partners of HIV-infected persons, men who have sex with men, and heterosexual persons who themselves or whose sex partners have had more than one sex partner since their most recent HIV test.

Diagnostic testing refers to testing when there is clinical suspicion of HIV. The CDC recommends that diagnostic testing be offered to all patients with signs or symptoms of HIV infection, including having an opportunistic illness characteristic of AIDS. When the acute phase of HIV infection, acute retroviral syndrome, is considered, then the CDC recommends that both an HIV RNA test and an HIV antibody test be offered. In this instance, the CDC considers a general consent for treatment to be adequate, so long as the patient is informed that testing is being undertaken and offered the opportunity to opt out.

With regard to pregnancy, the CDC recommends screening all women prior to conception, when possible. Screening early in pregnancy is recommended if preconception status is unknown. Lastly, the CDC urges consideration of repeat testing in the third trimester (at <36 weeks) for all pregnant women and recommends repeat testing in the third trimester for the following groups

1. women in states with increased incidence of HIV or AIDS among women aged 15-45 years (Alabama, Connecticut, Delaware, the District of Columbia, Florida, Georgia, Illinois, Louisiana, Maryland, Massachusetts, Mississippi, Nevada, New Jersey, New York, North Carolina, Pennsylvania, Puerto Rico, Rhode Island, South Carolina, Tennessee, Texas, and Virginia)

2. women being treated in facilities that identify at least one HIV-infected pregnant woman per 1,000 women screened

3. women who are known to be at high risk for HIV (injection drug users and their sex partners, women who exchange sex for money or drugs, women who are sex partners of HIV-infected persons, and women who have had a new or more than one sex partner during this pregnancy)

4. women who have signs or symptoms of acute HIV infection

Women who present in labor with an unknown HIV status should undergo opt out screening, in this case using a rapid HIV test, and antiretroviral prophylaxis should be initiated in patients screening as positive. Women who deliver before their HIV status is known should likewise undergo opt out screening; in these women, rapid testing of the newborn is recommended so that antiretroviral prophylaxis can be given to the newborn. The benefits of neonatal antiretroviral prophylaxis diminish when initiated >12 hours after birth.

In all instances, screening should be performed only with the knowledge of the patient. Patients may decline (opt out), but neither written informed consent nor special handling of HIV results, aside from the usual diligence attached to confidential patient information, is required.

ELISA

ELISA, a test for anti-HIV-1/-2 antibodies to recombinant antigens and peptides, is the principal method for HIV screening. The sensitivity for current HIV ELISA tests is > 99%. Anti-HIV antibodies are detectable within 6-8 weeks of infection; however, some patients seroconvert only after many months. So it is in these first weeks to months that most false negative ELISA tests occur (the window period). To decrease the window period, 4th generation screening tests include the detection of p24 antigen. The p24 protein is expressed very early in HIV infection, capable of reducing the duration of the serologic "window" by more than half. Because of passive transfer of maternal antibodies, the serologic diagnosis of neonatal HIV infection is not reliable.

Western blot

Confirmatory testing for HIV is based generally upon the western blot f3.11. In this assay, a sample containing known HIV proteins is subjected to gel electrophoresis. The gel is then transferred (blotted) onto nitrocellulose paper, to which patient serum is added. After staining, visible bands reflect antibodies within patient serum. *The CDC has defined a positive HIV-1 western blot as the presence of any 2 of the following bands: p24, gp41, gp120/160.* If no bands are present, the test is considered negative. If one or more bands are present but not in a combination that meets criteria for positivity, then the test is considered indeterminate. The specificity of western blot, when these criteria are rigorously applied, approaches 100%. Conventional western blot results can give a false negative result in HIV subtype O.

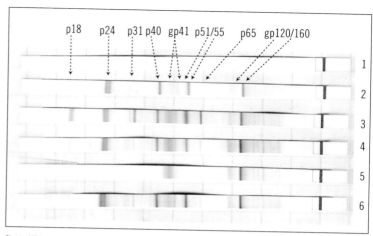

f3.11 HIV western blot
Lane 1 is negative control
Lane 2 is weak positive control & lane 6 is the strong positive control
Lanes 3-5 are positive patient samples

False positive western blots have been reported in patients with hyperbilirubinemia, HLA antibodies, autoantibodies, and polyclonal hypergammaglobulinemia. Patients who test as indeterminate should have a repeat test within 6 months. Those who are repeatedly indeterminate >6 months and who have no risk factors can be considered negative. If there are risk factors and repeatedly indeterminate results, a nucleic acid based test is advised.

CD4 count

The CD4 count, determined by flow cytometry, was the earliest index of disease progression. Counts of circulating CD4+ T lymphocytes undergo pronounced diurnal variation, so specimens should be obtained at a consistent time of day. Furthermore, the CD4 count should be compared to age-appropriate reference ranges. Counts are monitored approximately every 6 months while the disease is stable and more frequently when treatment is being altered or there is illness. While CD4 counts are still instrumental in making treatment decisions (eg, the decision to instigate PCP prophylaxis or define AIDS), the quantitative HIV RNA (viral load) is the preferred means of assessing response to antiretroviral therapy.

Proviral DNA

Detection of proviral DNA can be used to confirm the diagnosis of HIV infection. Proviral DNA is the result of HIV RNA reverse transcription into cDNA, which then integrates into the host cell genome. Its presence can be detected by PCR; however, the sensitivity of this assay is ~95% and the specificity 98%, both low by HIV-diagnosing standards.

HIV RNA

Quantification of circulating HIV RNA (viral load) has become a mainstay in HIV management.

Long-term outcome correlates extremely well with the viral load. The viral load has been found to be superior to the CD4 count for predicting disease progression; however, it appears that the combination of the 2 is superior to either in isolation. Furthermore, while viral load correlates very well with long-term (>10 years) prognosis, the CD4 count correlates better with short term (6 months) prognosis and susceptibility to infection.

Results of viral load testing are often expressed in log units. For example, a viral load of 1,000 would be 3 log units, and a change in viral load from 1,000-10,000 would be expressed as a 1 log change. A change from 1000-3000 would be expressed as a 0.5 log change. Generally speaking, a change in viral load of >0.5 log is considered significant in most assays, since this exceeds the technical variation of the assay and exceeds the patient's expected day to day variation. Transient increases in the quantitative HIV RNA (viral load) may occur following immune provocation, eg, following immunization. Up to a 0.3-0.4 log change can be attributed to nonspecific alteration in the quantitative HIV RNA; thus, changes >0.5 log are considered significant.

The viral load is the primary variable used to determine when to initiate highly active antiretroviral therapy (HAART), and it is the viral load that determines the efficacy of this treatment. The anticipated duration of viral suppression relate to both the rate of decline in viral load and the magnitude of the nadir.

3 methods are currently available for measuring the HIV RNA (viral load): real time PCR (RT-PCR), branched DNA (bDNA), and nucleic acid sequence-based amplification (NASBA). These methods have comparable analytic sensitivity and precision, but quantities cannot be directly compared between methods. An individual patient should be followed with a single method. In the RT-PCR assay, HIV-1 RNA and known standard RNA (a control of known copy number) compete for amplification within the same reaction chamber. First, the RNA is converted to cDNA by adding reverse transcriptase. Then a specific portion of the cDNA—within the *gag* gene—is amplified by PCR. Enzyme linked oligonucleotide probes are added, one complementary for the HIV gag sequence and one for the RNA standard, and reaction product is measured. The ratio of reaction products determines the quantity of HIV RNA that is present. In the bDNA assay, complementary oligonucleotide is fixed to a solid substrate (microplate). The patient sample is added, capturing any HIV RNA present. Then a chemiluminescent enzyme linked probes are added which are complementary to additional sequences of HIV RNA. The chemiluminescent signal is measured and compared to a known standard. The NASBA method is similar in concept to RT-PCR, except RNA is amplified instead of DNA.

Detection of HIV infection shortly after a presumed exposure may be very important, as there appears to be significant merit in the early administration of highly active antiretroviral therapy (HAART). Serology (ELISA and western blot) are not useful in this setting, since antibodies do not reliably appear for many weeks. The p24 antigen seems to wane at various times during acute infection, leading to a suboptimal sensitivity of 89%. The best test in this setting may be HIV RNA quantification. HIV DNA detection may be just as good but has not been studied in the acute stage. The sensitivity of HIV RNA in acute infection is essentially 100%. However, the specificity is not 100%, and some false positives occur; as soon as feasible, a positive HIV RNA should be confirmed with ELISA and western blot.

Detection of HIV infection in neonates and infants is sometimes difficult. ELISA and western blot are not useful due to the persistence of transplacentally-acquired maternal antibodies. Furthermore, p24 antigen has a poor sensitivity in neonates and young infants, as low as 20% in the first month of life. PCR testing for HIV proviral DNA is the recommended test in this setting, but HIV RNA may be equally good. Umbilical cord blood should not be tested.

Parasitology
Laboratory methods
Direct examination

Diagnosis of parasitic infection most commonly depends upon macroscopic and microscopic examination. Microscopic examination makes up the bulk of parasite diagnostics, although macroscopic examination is important for certain nematodes (round worms) and cestodes (tapeworms). The use of an eyepiece micrometer is essential, since the size of the observed forms is often the key to identification.

Specimens

Stool and blood are by far the most common specimens submitted for examination of parasites. Body sites and possible parasites recovered are summarized in t3.16

t3.16 Most common parasites by body site

Body site	Parasites
Intestinal tract	*Entamoeba* species, *Iodamoeba butschlii*, *Endolimax nana*, *Blastocystis hominis*, *Giardia intestinalis*, *Chilomastix mesnili*, *Dientamoeba fragilis*, *Pentatrichomonas hominis*, *Balantidium coli*, *Cryptosporidium* species, *Cyclospora cayetanensis*, *Cystoisospora belli*, microsporidia, *Ascaris lumbricoides*, *Enterobius vermicularis*, hookworm, *Strongyloides stercoralis*, *Trichuris trichiura*, *Hymenolepis nana*, *Hymenolepis diminuta*, *Taenia saginata*, *Taenia solium*, *Diphyllobothrium latum*, *Dipylidium caninum*, *Schistosoma* species (eggs only), *Fasciolopsis buski*
Blood	Erythrocytes: *Plasmodium* species & *Babesia* species
	Leukocytes: *Leishmania* species & *Toxoplasma gondii*
	Whole blood/plasma: *Trypanosoma* species, microfilariae
Bone marrow	*Leishmania* species, *Plasmodium* species
Central nervous system	*Taenia solium* (neurocysticercosis), *Echinococcus* species, *Naegleria fowleri*, *Acanthamoeba* species, *Balamuthia mandrillaris*, *Toxoplasma gondii*, microsporidia species & *Trypanosoma brucei*
Cutaneous ulcer	*Leishmania* species, *Acanthamoeba* species
Liver, spleen	*Echinococcus* species, *Entamoeba histolytica*, *Leishmania* species, microsporidia, *Schistosoma mansoni* & *japonicum* (eggs only), *Fasciola hepatica*, *Clonorchis sinensis*
Muscle	*Trichinella* species, *Taenia solium* (cysticerci), *Trypanosoma cruzi*, microsporidia
Lungs	*Cryptosporidium* species, *Echinococcus* species, *Paragonimus* species, *Toxoplasma gondii*, *Strongyloides stercoralis* larvae, microsporidia
Skin & subcutaneous tissue	*Leishmania* species, *Onchocerca volvulus*, microfilariae, *Sarcoptes scabei*, *Loa loa* (adult worm)
Urogenital system	*Trichomonas vaginalis*, *Schistosoma* species (eggs only), microsporidia, microfilariae
Eyes	*Acanthamoeba* species, *Toxoplasma gondii*, *Loa loa*, *Onchocerca volvulus*, microsporidia

Stool

This mainstay of parasitology is typically referred to as the "ova and parasite" test or "stool O&P." The test requires the acquisition of solid to liquid stool, examination of direct (unfixed) wet mounts (when fresh stool is submitted), stool concentration and examination of permanent stains with examination of a "wet prep" using a fixed stool specimen. 3 separately obtained specimens ≥24 hours apart are required as a minimum to exclude infection with any confidence as many parasites (especially *Giardia intestinalis* and *Strongyloides stercoralis*) are shed intermittently in stool. The components of a complete stool exam are:

Fresh specimen

Fresh specimens should be examined within 1 hour of collection, before disintegration of protozoan trophozoites can occur. The direct wet mount, wherein fresh unconcentrated specimen is mixed with saline and examined, allows observation of motile protozoan trophozoites and helminth larvae. If fresh specimens cannot be examined within 1 hour of collection, preservatives such as formalin or alcohol should be used. Preservatives maintain protozoan morphology and help prevent the continued development of helminth eggs and larvae.

Concentrate

From fixed stool, concentration (by either sedimentation or flotation) enhances detection of protozoan cysts and helminth eggs.

Permanent preparation

Permanent stains are performed on the fixed specimen for confirmation and enhanced detection of protozoan trophozoites and cysts. The most commonly used stains are the Wheatley trichrome and iron hematoxylin stains.

Protozoa that are likely to be missed with routine O&P stains include microsporidia (fungi detected in the parasite lab) *Cryptosporidium* species, *Cyclospora cayetanensis*, and *Cystoisospora* (formerly *Isospora*) *belli*. The latter 3 require modified acid-fast (Kinyoun, DMSO, or auramine-O) or modified safranin stains, while the microsporidia are detected by a Modified Trichrome (chromotrope 2R) stain.

Duodenal contents

For the detection of duodenal infections such as *Giardia intestinalis* or *Strongyloides stercoralis*, duodenal contents may need to be collected. These can be collected using direct aspiration during endoscopy or by the Beale string technique, wherein one end of a string in a gelatin capsule is swallowed while the other end is taped to the patient's cheek; after several hours the string is pulled back, and the attached mucus is examined microscopically.

Cellophane tape preparation

Stool is a poor specimen for the detection of *Enterobius vermicularis* (pinworm). Instead, a strip of clear (not frosted) cellophane tape is applied to the perianal area in the early morning, before the patient gets out of bed and defecates. The adult female worm migrates to the anus to deposit eggs during the night and these eggs will adhere to the tape. The tape can then be removed and applied to a slide for microscopic examination.

Blood

Parasites that may be detected in blood include: *Plasmodium* species and *Babesia* species within erythrocytes, *Leishmania* species amastigotes and *Toxoplasma gondii* tachyzoites in leukocytes, and extracellular *Trypanosoma* species and the microfilariae (*Wuchereria bancrofti*, *Brugia malayi*, *Loa loa*, *Mansonella*

species) in whole blood/plasma. Giemsa-stained thick and thin blood films are the gold standard method for *Plasmodium/ Babesia* detection. Thin films are the same as those used in routine hematology blood smear review, while thick films are prepared by concentrating blood in a small portion of the slide and lysing the red cells. Thick films are the best for screening, as they provide more blood per microscopic field, whereas thin films are good for species identification. Sometimes buffy coat preparations are examined for the detection of *Leishmania* species, trypanosomes, and microfilariae. Microfilariae detection can also be enhanced by filtration or concentration techniques.

Respiratory specimens

Respiratory specimens (eg, sputum, BAL) may be examined for the detection of *Paragonimus* species (lung fluke) eggs, *Strongyloides stercoralis* larvae and hooklets of *Echinococcus* species from ruptured hydatid cysts.

CSF

CSF is examined in the case of suspected primary amebic meningoencephalitis (PAM).

Serology

There is a limited role for serology in parasitology, especially in acute disease, in which it should almost never be considered the test of choice. Exceptions where serology testing is routinely used include prenatal and postnatal toxoplasmosis screening, toxocariasis, schistosomiasis, echinococcosis, cysticercosis, schistosomiasis, trichinellosis, and Chagas disease. Serology is also the test of choice for diagnosis of amebic liver abscess due to *E histolytica*. Otherwise, the main application for serology is epidemiologic studies.

Culture

Parasites are usually not cultured. Some exceptions **t3.17** in clinical practice are the free living amebae (*Acanthamoeba* species, *Naegleria fowleri*), *Trichomonas vaginalis*, and less commonly, *Leishmania* species. There is also a "culture" method for *Strongyloides stercoralis* even though it does not involve actual replication of the organism. Culture for other organisms (eg, *Entamoeba* species, *Blastocystis hominis*, *Trypanosoma* species) is performed primarily in the research setting.

t3.17 Parasites in culture

Free living amebae	Tap water agar on a bed of *E coli* (for nutrient source)
Leishmania species & *Trypanosoma* species	Novy-MacNeal-Nicolle (NNN) medium
Trichomonas vaginalis	Diamond media

Molecular methods

There is a limited role for molecular methods in parasite diagnostics, with most tests being developed in individual laboratories and not approved by the Federal Drug Administration (FDA). The few commercially available tests include a newly FDA approved nucleic acid amplification test (NAAT) for *Trichomonas vaginalis*, and new stool multiplex PCR panels that include *Giardia intestinalis*, *Cryptosporidium* species, and *Entamoeba histolytica*.

Parasites

Parasites are traditionally divided into 2 groups: the protozoa and the metazoa. The protozoa are unicellular eukaryotic organisms whereas the metazoa are complicated multicellular organisms (worms).

Protozoa

The protozoa are traditionally divided into: Sarcodina (the amebae), Mastigophora (flagellates), Ciliophora (ciliates), and Apicomplexa (formerly Sporozoa; a diverse group including plasmodia, coccidia, and piroplasms). More recently, *Blastocystis hominis* has been recognized as a potential human pathogen belonging to the *Stramenopiles*. The microsporidia were also previously grouped with the protozoa but they are now considered to be highly specialized fungi. However, microsporidia testing is still widely performed in parasitology labs and therefore they will be covered in this section.

Amebae

Amebae (Sarcodina) are unicellular organisms that are motile by pseudopodal extension f3.12

Intestinal amebae include the 3 main genera: *Entamoeba, Endolimax*, and *Iodamoeba*. The nucleus is the key structure for identification along with the size of the organism.

Entamoeba histolytica

Entamoeba histolytica is the primary pathogen in this group. Unfortunately, *E histolytica* is morphologically indistinguishable from more common nonpathogen, *E dispar* (usual ratio 1:9). The other amebae are mostly considered to be nonpathogenic for humans but may mimic *E histolytica* by microscopy. In particular, *E histolytica/E dispar* must be distinguished from *E coli* and *E hartmanni*, the closest mimics t3.18. Although most other intestinal amebae are considered nonpathogenic commensals, their presence is still reported by the laboratory, because they serve as an indicator of exposure to fecally contaminated water or food.

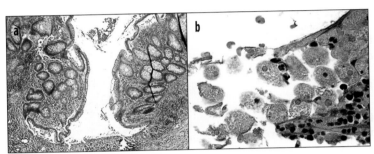

f3.12 Amebae

f3.13 H&E stained sections of amebic colitis
a Low magnification shows classic flask shaped ulcer
b Higher magnification reveals trophozoites with ingested RBCs

t3.18 Amebae that resemble *E histolytica/E dispar*

Form	Characteristic	E coli	E histolytica/ dispar	E hartmanni
Trophozoite	Size	20–25 μm	15–20 μm	5–10 μm
	Motility	Nondirectional	Unidirectional	Nondirectional
	Ingested erythrocytes	Absent	Present (*E histolytica* only)	Absent
	Karyosome	Large, eccentric	Small, central	Small, central
	Nuclear chromatin	Clumped along nuclear membrane	Fine, evenly distributed along nuclear membrane	Fine, evenly distributed along nuclear membrane
Cyst	Size	15–25 μm	12–15 μm	5–8 μm
	Nuclei	Up to 8	Never >4	Never >4
	Chromatoidal bars	Frayed ends	Rounded ends	Rounded ends

E histolytica/dispar trophozoites measure ~15-20 μm. The nucleus is characterized by a small, central karyosome and fine evenly distributed peripheral chromatin which is applied evenly to the inner nuclear membrane. The cytoplasm has a "ground glass" appearance and may contain ingested red cells. Although rarely seen, erythrophagocytosis is the only morphologic feature that can be used to presumptively differentiate *E histolytica* from the nonpathogenic *E dispar* and other intestinal amebae. Under direct examination in wet mounts, the trophozoites display progressive unidirectional motility. Cyst forms have up to (and no more than) 4 nuclei and may contain chromatoidal bodies with smooth, rounded, ends. Microscopic identification of cysts and trophozoites in the stool is the most common method for diagnosing *E histolytica*. Stool antigen and molecular methods have been used to differentiate *E histolytica* and *E dispar*.

E histolytica is acquired through ingestion of cysts in fecally contaminated food or water. Its distribution is worldwide. Although most infections are asymptomatic, it can cause intestinal amebiasis, a syndrome of protracted diarrhea, dysentery, and abdominal pain due to infection of the colon. Rarely, the trophozoites can invade the intestinal wall and disseminate to the liver (*most common site of extraintestinal amebiasis*), lung, or brain. Amebic abscesses are described as containing anchovy paste-like material. The lesion of intestinal amebiasis is the "flask shaped" ulcer in the colon, usually the *cecum*, named because the base of the ulcer is broader than the apex f3.13. Protracted infection may eventually lead to a proliferative "napkin ring" lesion (ameboma) mimicking colonic adenocarcinoma.

Entamoeba coli

The main features permitting distinction of *E coli* from *E histolytica* are its larger size, nondirectional motility, larger eccentric karyosome, clumped peripheral nuclear chromatin, frayed (splintered) chromatoidal bodies, and the presence of up to 8 nuclei in cyst forms.

Entamoeba hartmanni

Entamoeba hartmanni closely resembles *E histolytica*. The main feature distinguishing *E hartmanni* from *E histolytica* is its small size.

Endolimax nana

Endolimax nana is easily recognized by its large knobby "ball & socket" central karyosome. The cyst form has the same nuclei and lacks chromatoidal bodies and lack of peripheral nuclear chromatin.

Iodamoeba butschlii

The quickest way to recognize *I butschlii* is the cyst's prominent iodine-staining vacuole (when present). The trophozoite and cyst form, like *E nana*, have a large "ball & socket" central karyosome, and the nuclear membrane is inconspicuous.

Free living amebae

These amebae are found widely in the environment where they exist as free living organisms. Only rarely do they become opportunistic pathogens in humans.

Naegleria fowleri

Naegleria fowleri does not form cysts in human tissues. Its trophozoites (10-35 µm), which can be found in CSF or in meninges and surrounding brain tissue, appear as typical amebae with a single small nucleus with a large dense central karyosome and no peripheral chromatin. *Naegleria fowleri* can be cultured on solid agar medium using a lawn of bacteria (*E coli*) as the nutrient source. The fragile trophozoites do not survive in colder temperatures and therefore CSF specimens should not be refrigerated.

Infection with this organism causes primary amebic meningoencephalitis (PAM), typically seen in children who have been swimming or diving in warm stagnant fresh water sources. The organism enters through the nasal cavity and travels to the frontal lobe of the brain via the olfactory nerve running through the cribriform plate. The infection is usually fatal within a matter of days.

Acanthamoeba species & Balamuthia mandrillaris

Diagnosis can be made from identification of both cysts and amebic trophozoites in brain tissue, skin, lung and corneal (*Acanthamoeba* species only) specimens. The cysts (10-25 µm) of *Acanthamoeba* species have 2 walls (inner wall may be star shaped) and contain only 1 nucleus with a large karyosome. Cysts of *B mandrillaris* have a similar appearance. Trophozoites (15-45 µm) of both *Acanthamoeba* and *Balamuthia* are pleomorphic and contain a small nucleus with a large, centrally-located karyosome but no peripheral chromatin. Like *Naegleria*, *Acanthamoeba* can be cultured on solid agar medium using a bacterial nutrient source. *Balamuthia mandrillaris* can only be cultured using cell culture. PCR-based techniques have been developed to distinguish between the free living amebae directly from specimen.

Both *Acanthamoeba* and *Balamuthia mandrillaris* cause granulomatous amebic encephalitis (GAE), a subacute and often fatal granulomatous brain infection. Infection begins in a cutaneous or pulmonary f3.14 source, followed by hematogenous dissemination to the brain, where organisms are found in perivascular locations. *Acanthamoeba* species can also cause amebic keratitis, usually in contact lens wearers.

Flagellates (Mastigophora) f3.15

Giardia intestinalis (previously G duodenale or G lamblia)

Giardia trophozoites (10-20 µm in length) may be seen in stool specimens or small bowel biopsies. When viewed from the top, they are kite shaped organisms that have a central axoneme running along their length, and a comma shaped median body f3.16. The flagella are not easily seen on standard trichrome stain. From the side, the organisms are curved or "spoon shaped." Cysts (10-14 µm) are oval, thick-walled, and contain 4 nuclei when mature (2 nuclei in immature cysts) located along a central axoneme. In a direct unfixed stool preparation, trophozoites demonstrate characteristic falling-leaf

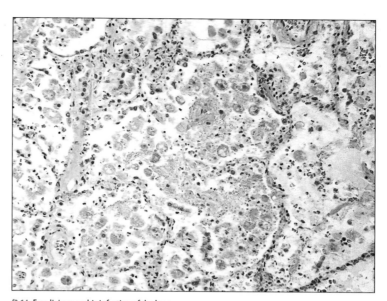

f3.14 Free living amebic infection of the lung

	Giardia intestinalis	Chilomastix mesnili	Dientamoeba fragilis	Trichomonas vaginalis
trophozoites				Giemsa stain
cysts			none known	none known

scale: ⊢——————⊣ = 10 µm

f3.15 Common intestinal & genitourinary flagellates (modified trichrome stain unless indicated)

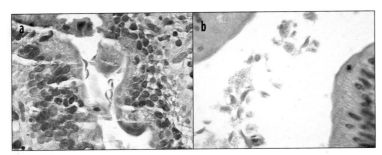

f3.16 *Giardia* trophozoites

	Leishmania species promastigote	*Trypanosoma cruzi* trypomastigote	*Trypanosoma brucei* trypomastigote
flagellated form			
nonmotile form (amastigote)			none known

f3.17 Hemoflagellates; images not shown to scale

motility. In stool samples, *G intestinalis* must be distinguished from nonpathogenic flagellate, *Chilomastix mesnili*. The preferred method of *Giardia* diagnosis is via antigen detection, which is more sensitive than stool exam.

Giardia is the most common cause of protozoal gastroenteritis; it causes a spectrum of disease ranging from asymptomatic carriage to severe watery diarrhea and malabsorption. It has worldwide distribution and is most prevalent in warm climates and in children. In developed countries, infection is associated with daycare centers, ski resorts & backcountry hiking/camping.

Chilomastix mesnili

Chilomastix mesnili is a nonpathogenic organism that lacks an obvious central axoneme, has rotary motion, and has only anteriorly located flagella. The cyst (6-10 μm) form is lemon shaped with a single nucleus at the anterior end.

Dientamoeba fragilis

Dientamoeba fragilis is actually an ameboflagellate, and is sometimes grouped with the amebae. Trophozoites appear as a round binucleate structure whose nuclei have a "fractured" (fragile) central karyosome. Another characteristic feature is the single internalized flagellum which appears attached to the wall of the organism at several points. There is no known cyst form. It has a worldwide distribution and is an occasional cause of diarrhea and anal pruritus, particularly in children. *Dientamoeba* and *Enterobius vermicularis* (pinworm) co-infection is common.

Trichomonas vaginalis is the most common pathogenic protozoan in industrialized countries and is the cause of the sexually transmitted trichomoniasis (the most common nonviral STI). Trophozoites (7-30 μm long) are vaguely pear shaped with a large nucleus located at the anterior end of a central axostyle. It characteristically has an undulating membrane that extends about halfway down the organism. Microscopic examination of wet mounts of vaginal, prostatic or urethral secretions may establish the diagnosis by detecting its characteristic jerky nondirectional motility. *Pentatrichomonas* (formerly *Trichomonas*) *hominis* is a closely related nonpathogenic gastrointestinal organism.

Leishmania species f3.17

Leishmania infection is best diagnosed by biopsy of infected tissue, most often skin f3.18, bone marrow, or spleen. Careful scrutiny of Giemsa-stained smears or H&E-stained sections from infected tissue reveal multiple tiny 2-5 μm intracellular amastigotes within histiocytes f3.19. The organisms appear as oval structures with a small nucleus adjacent to the distinct rod shaped kinetoplast (a kinetoplast is also found in *Trypanosoma* species and *Crithidia luciliae*, the organism that forms the substrate for ANA screening). *The amastigote is the only stage seen in the human host*; it lacks an external flagellum and proliferates exclusively intracellularly within histiocytes. Other small intracellular organisms must be considered in the morphologic differential diagnosis (histoplasmosis, toxoplasmosis, trypanosomes). The organism may be cultured using Novy-MacNeal-Nicolle (NNN) medium; culture is more sensitive than visual detection and permits subsequent speciation by PCR or isoenzyme analysis. In culture (as well as within the insect vector), the motile flagellated promastigote form is observed. It is traditionally classified as a hemoflagellate (along with the trypanosomes) since the promastigote stage is flagellated and the parasite may be found in blood.

t3.19 Differential diagnosis for multiple tiny 2-5 μm intracellular organisms f3.19

Organism	Differentiating features	Cell type infected
Leishmania species	Amastigotes with a small, bar-like kinetoplast, GMS negative	Histiocytes
Histoplasma capsulatum	Small oval yeasts with narrow-based budding, pseudocapsule on H&E, GMS positive	Histiocytes
Toxoplasma gondii	Somewhat curved tachyzoites, mostly extracellular, some in cysts, GMS negative	Multiple cells types
Trypanosoma cruzi	Amastigotes with a large prominent kinetoplast, GMS negative	Multiple cell types including heart muscle (classic)

Leishmania infection is acquired from the bite of an infected sandfly (*Phlebotomus* and *Lutzomyia* genera). While leishmaniasis is found throughout the tropical and subtropical world, most cases are found in Algeria, Afghanistan, Saudi Arabia,

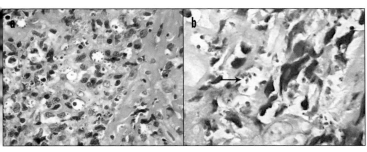

f3.18 Cutaneous leishmaniasis; small amastigotes are visible within histiocytes (arrow) although the detail of the kinetoplast is not easily appreciated in formalin fixed paraffin embedded tissue

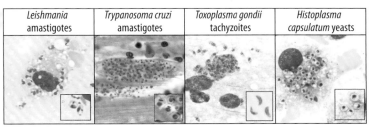

Leishmania amastigotes	*Trypanosoma cruzi* amastigotes	*Toxoplasma gondii* tachyzoites	*Histoplasma capsulatum* yeasts

f3.19 Intracellular objects

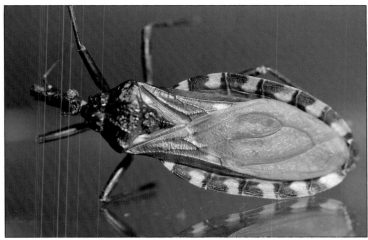

f3.20 Reduviid bug, vector of *Trypanosoma cruzi*

Syria, Pakistan, Peru, and Brazil. There are 3 main forms of disease: cutaneous, mucocutaneous and visceral leishmaniasis. The factors determining the form of disease include leishmanial species and immune response of the host. There are >20 morphologically indistinguishable species that cause human disease.

Cutaneous disease, associated most often with *L tropica, L major, L aethiopica* (Old World) and *L mexicana* and *L braziliensis* (New World), results in a solitary self-limiting cutaneous lesion at or near the insect bite f3.18. *L aethiopica* may disseminate to other cutaneous sites, producing multiple lesions. Cutaneous leishmaniasis is seen principally around the Mediterranean (southern Europe, northern Africa, Middle East), and it was seen in troops returning from deployment in Kuwait. In this latter setting, visceral dissemination was often noted. It is also common in central and south America.

Mucocutaneous leishmaniasis is most often caused by members of the *L braziliensis* complex. Primary infection begins as a cutaneous lesion, but when left untreated, disseminates to the oral and nasal mucosal membranes causing persistent and highly destructive lesions.

Visceral leishmaniasis (kala-azar) is usually caused by *L donovani* which results in widespread systemic disease associated with hepatosplenomegaly and bone marrow infection. *L donovani* infections are found in Africa, India, Asia, and the Middle East.

Trypanosoma species

Trypomastigotes are the motile forms of *Trypanosoma* species that are can be found in the peripheral blood. In African trypanosomiasis, they may also be found in lymph node aspirates or CSF. In American trypanosomiasis, they may be seen in aspirates of chagomas, lymph nodes, or infected tissue. Trypomastigotes are slender, extraerythrocytic forms with a flagellum that is attached along its length as an undulating membrane until reaching the anterior end where it emerges as a free flagellum (contrary to common belief, the flagellum is at the *anterior* end of the organism). Trypomastigotes of *T cruzi* measure ~20 μm and are often C-shaped f3.17, with a large posterior kinetoplast. Those of *T brucei* appear as 30 μm delicately curved structures with a smaller posterior kinetoplast. *The size of the round or dot-like kinetoplast is the most important feature for differentiating the 2 species.* Finding peripheral blood trypomastigotes is more common in the acute phase than in chronic infection and can be aided by examination of the buffy coat. Organisms can be cultured using Novy-MacNeal-Nicolle (NNN) medium. In chronic *T cruzi* infection, biopsy of the heart or other affected organ may reveal the nonmotile amastigote form with an associated mononuclear inflammatory infiltrate and interstitial fibrosis. More commonly, the diagnosis of *T cruzi* infection is based upon clinical presentation in conjunction with serology.

Trypanosoma cruzi

T cruzi is the cause of Chagas disease (American trypanosomiasis) and is the most common fatal parasitic disease in the Americas. *T cruzi* can infect the muscularis of the distal esophagus, resulting in achalasia. It also infects the myocardium and is a leading cause of congestive heart failure in South and Central America. Chagas disease is typically acquired from the blood sucking reduviid (kissing) bug f3.20, a member of the Triatominae family. When the reduviid takes a blood meal it releases trypomastigotes in its feces near the site of the bite wound. Inoculation of the wound with the contaminated feces results in infection. The inoculation site (chagoma) is often on the face, the reason for the "kissing bug" appellation; when conjunctival contamination with the vector's feces occurs, Romaña sign (unilateral palpebral and periocular swelling) may develop. The reduviid bugs are typically found in homes constructed of mud, adobe, and/or thatch (straw). The bugs acquire the organism from infected animals, including raccoon, armadillo, opossum, and dogs. *T cruzi* can also be transmitted in other ways, however, including from mother to child during gestation, through ingestion of food

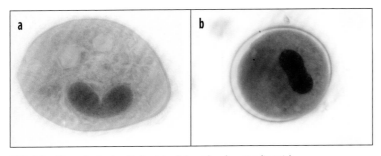

f3.21 *Balantidium coli*; a trophozoite (unstained), b cyst (iron hematoxylin stain)

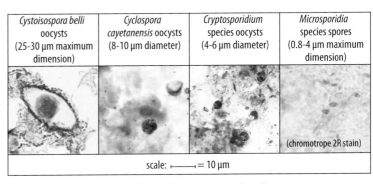

Cystoisospora belli oocysts (25-30 μm maximum dimension)	*Cyclospora cayetanensis* oocysts (8-10 μm diameter)	*Cryptosporidium* species oocysts (4-6 μm diameter)	*Microsporidia* species spores (0.8-4 μm maximum dimension)
			(chromotrope 2R stain)

scale: ⊢———⊣ = 10 μm

f3.22 Coccidia & microsporidia (modified acid fast stain unless indicated)

and beverages contaminated with reduviid feces, and through blood transfusion. Donor blood units are now screened for *T cruzi* antibodies in the US. Most infections are asymptomatic but acute disease is associated with constitutional symptoms and parasitemia. A latent phase follows, characterized only by seropositivity. Chronic disease typically begins 10 or more years after initial infection, the most serious manifestation of which is cardiac disease that may present as congestive heart failure, conduction abnormalities, or sudden cardiac death.

Trypanosoma brucei

T brucei is the cause of African sleeping sickness (African trypanosomiasis), which is a potentially fatal febrile illness with neurologic manifestations, including extreme somnolence. It is acquired from the bite of a tsetse (*Glossina*) fly. Cases in western Africa are caused by *T brucei gambiense*, while cases in eastern Africa are caused by *T brucei rhodesiense*, with the latter being more severe and rapidly progressive. Neurologic manifestations are more frequent in late stages, and the WHO defines CNS involvement by CSF findings, including increased white blood cell count, increased protein, or the finding of trypanosomes.

Ciliates (Ciliophora)

There is only 1 ciliate that infects humans, *Balantidium coli* f3.21, an organism whose trophozoite form is characterized by cilia uniformly covering its surface. Diagnosis is based on detection of trophozoites in stool specimens or in tissue collected during endoscopy. Trophozoites measure ~40-200 μm, making this the largest protozoan to infect humans. It has a kidney bean shaped macronucleus and a smaller less conspicuous micronucleus. Cysts (50-70 μm) are seen less frequently and also have the characteristic kidney bean shaped macronucleus.

Microspora (microsporidia) f3.22

The microspora constitute a phylum of spore-forming unicellular organisms. Microsporidia were once thought to be protists but are now thought to be fungi. The microsporidia known to infect humans include *Enterocytozoon bieneusi* (intestinal hepatobiliary microsporidiosis), *Encephalitozoon hellem* (eye infections), and *Encephalitozoon* (formerly *Septata*) *intestinalis* (intestinal and disseminated infections, including the lungs and bladder). Infection is thought to occur following ingestion or inhalation of infective spores. The spore's coiled

polar tubule is then extruded and injects its infective material into the host cells (much like a syringe).

In small intestinal biopsies, microsporidia appear as numerous tiny oval intracellular organisms within the apical aspect of enterocytes. In stool samples, 1-3 μm spores stain deep red with a modified (chromotrope 2R) trichrome stain (different than the traditional stool trichrome stain). Often a transecting bar is seen in the center of the spore running perpendicular to the long axis. Traditionally, electron microscopy was used to determine the infecting species, using characteristic features such as the number of rows and coils of a polar tubule and other ultrastructural elements. Molecular methods (mainly PCR) provide an alternative method for the laboratory diagnosis of microsporidiosis in specialized labs.

Apicomplexa

Apicomplexa is a diverse group that includes coccidia, plasmodia, and piroplasms.

Coccidia f3.22

Cryptosporidium species

Cryptosporidium (*C parvum* and *C hominis*) are recognized in small intestinal biopsies as rounded or dome shaped, 8-15 μm, basophilic structures at the apical surface of enterocytes. Even though they appear to be adherent to the enterocyte brush border, they are actually located inside the enterocyte within an apical vacuole. In stool samples, the small, 4-6 μm oocysts are difficult to detect with traditional concentrates or permanently stained preparations; instead a modified acid-fast stain is recommended which stains the round oocysts a deep pink/red. Antigen detection methods are commercially available and have a greater sensitivity than special stains. *Cryptosporidium* is a major cause of protracted watery diarrhea in immunocompromised hosts, especially those with AIDS (in whom disease can be life threatening). In developed countries, *Cryptosporidium* is responsible for ~2% of diarrheal illness in immunocompetent persons; ~15% in AIDS. In developing countries, it causes ~10% of cases in immunocompetent persons, and ~25% in AIDS. *Cryptosporidium* species may also ascend the biliary tree to cause strictures, and less commonly, can infect the respiratory tract. Infection is associated with ingestion of contaminated food or water (including inadvertent swallowing of water at recreational water parks and swimming pools). Waterborne outbreaks are common.

Cyclospora cayetanensis

Small bowel biopsies show active inflammation and different stages of the organism inside enterocytes. Diagnosis is traditionally by microscopy using concentrated stool wet preps, by a modified acid-fast stain, or via autofluorescence. On acid-fast stain, the round pink/red staining 8-10 µm *Cyclospora* oocytes must be differentiated from the similar appearing but smaller *Cryptosporidium* oocysts. Infection is found principally in Nepal, Peru, Haiti, and Guatemala, but has been identified as a source of food borne disease in the United States from imported soft fruits and vegetables. The organism is acquired from ingestion of oocysts in contaminated food and water. It infects the small bowel and produces a highly characteristic syndrome: several days of fever accompanied by severe watery diarrhea, followed by an extended period of anorexia and fatigue associated with significant weight loss.

Cystoisospora (formerly Isospora) belli

In small intestinal biopsies, *Isospora* appears as large oval structures within enterocytes. Infected mucosa demonstrates atrophic villi and sometimes tissue eosinophilia. In stool samples, the oocysts are large (25-30 µm) and have a typical ellipsoidal shape with one (unsporulated) or 2 (sporulated) sporocysts. They are easily seen on wet prep or modified acid-fast stain. Like the other coccidia, *Cystoisospora belli* causes watery diarrhea in immunocompetent and immunocompromised individuals, with more severe disease in the latter.

Sarcocystis

Human sarcocystosis involves either the intestinal or muscular systems, depending on the infecting species. Diagnosis of intestinal sarcocystis is made by identification of oocysts (15-20 µm long by 15-20 µm wide) containing 2 sporocysts or the individual sporocysts that have been released from the oocysts in stool. Sporocysts will autofluoresce under ultraviolet (UV) microscopy but are not acid fast like the other coccidia. Sarcocystis can also infect striated (skeletal or cardiac) muscle, and diagnosis is typically by finding sarcocysts containing many bradyzoites in tissue specimens. In cases of intestinal sarcocystosis (*S hominis* and *S suihominis*), when humans serve as the definitive hosts, infections may asymptomatic or associated with fever, diarrhea, and vomiting. Infection is usually self limited. Muscular infections present with myalgia, edema, and muscle weakness.

Toxoplasma gondii

The diagnostic forms are found in touch preparations and sections of infected tissue such as brain, retina, or lymphoreticular tissue f3.23, f3.24. The tachyzoite is a small (3-5 µm), curved, actively replicating form of the organism with a large eccentric nucleus. Unlike amastigotes of *Leishmania* or *T cruzi*, tachyzoites have no kinetoplast. Tachyzoites are usually seen free (extracellular) but may also be in seen in small cysts. The bradyzoite is the slowly replicating, dormant stage of the organism, found within pseudocysts of nucleated host cells. This intracellular form must be distinguished from other small intracellular organisms (histoplasmosis, leishmaniasis). Serology, based usually upon an EIA platform, is the most common way to make the diagnosis of toxoplasmosis. IgM antibodies to *Toxoplasma gondii* establishes the diagnosis of

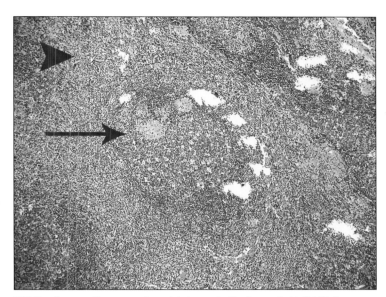

f3.23 *Toxoplasma gondii*; acute toxoplasmosis is characterized by clusters of epithelioid histiocytes (arrow) that impinge upon germinal centers & monocytoid B cell expansion (arrowhead)

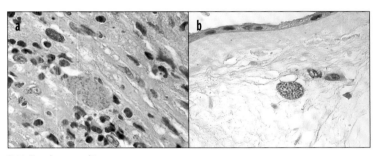

f3.24 *Toxoplasma gondii* cysts

congenital and acute infection, but false positive reactions and a tendency for IgM to persist for months limit the specificity. Since exposure to toxoplasma is relatively widespread, IgG antibodies to *Toxoplasma gondii* are very common. Still, rising or very high (>1:1,024) IgG titers suggest recent infection. Furthermore, the presence of low level IgG suggests prior infection and suggests that a pregnant woman is at little risk of experiencing neonatal complication associated with a new infection. Antibody avidity studies may be used to determine if the antibodies present were recently formed (they would have relatively low avidity) or were formed long ago (high avidity). Less commonly, PCR is used for diagnosis of CNS, intrauterine and systemic infections. *Toxoplasma gondii* infects most species of warm blooded animals, including humans, and can cause the disease toxoplasmosis. The cat is the definitive host. Infection is acquired through ingestion of food or water contaminated with cat feces containing oocysts, eating undercooked meat of animals harboring tissue cysts, blood transfusion or organ transplantation and transplacentally from mother to fetus. The recently infected child or adult may develop a mononucleosis-like syndrome characterized by fever and posterior cervical lymphadenopathy. ~15% of women of childbearing age have been previously infected with toxoplasmosis, and are therefore protected from acute, intrauterine toxoplasmosis infection. However, when primary infection is acquired during pregnancy, there may be transplacental spread. When maternal infection occurs in the first trimester, there is a risk of fetal loss. If infection occurs in late pregnancy, there is a risk of fetal CNS infection. CNS infection centers on the fetal retina and brain, with the residual effect of periventricular calcification and chorioretinitis. Immunocompromised patients are also at great risk for potentially fatal, primary or reactivated, CNS toxoplasmosis.

Plasmodium species (malaria)

There are 4 major species that cause malaria: *P falciparum, P vivax, P ovale, & P malariae*. Human cases of *Plasmodium knowlesi*, a monkey parasite, have also been reported with some frequency in South East Asia. Malaria is found in many parts of the tropics and subtropics worldwide. All except *P ovale* are widely distributed, with most cases of *P ovale* being acquired in western Africa. Malaria can be a life threatening disease. Most malaria related deaths are recorded in sub-Saharan Africa, where most of the victims are young children. Outside of Africa, malaria is endemic in nations along the southern third of Asia; in the Americas, malaria is found in abundance in the Amazon basin. Although malaria in the United States is usually found in travelers returning from endemic areas, cases are rarely found in nontravelers; such cases have been traced to blood transfusion, contaminated needles, congenital infection, and transmission by American mosquitoes from infected persons (so-called airport malaria). In endemic areas, young children and pregnant women are at greatest risk, with relative immunity developing in those who survive childhood; outside of endemic areas, all age groups are nonimmune and equally susceptible. In returning travelers, malaria usually presents within the first month; however, it may present >6 months after returning.

There are several inherited red cell anomalies that are relatively protective against malaria and are thought to have persisted in the population on that basis. Hemoglobin S, alone or in combination with any other hemoglobin variant, offers some protection against *P falciparum*. It is thought that in the presence of HbS the preparasite cannot complete its life cycle due to sickling and red cell destruction. It is also thought, though the data are not quite as strong as for HbS, that thalassemia, HbC, HbE, and hereditary persistence of HbF are protective against malaria. Duffy blood group antigens mediate attachment of *P vivax*; thus, Duffy negative individuals are protected from *P vivax*. Glucose-6-phosphate dehydrogenase (G6PD) deficiency, in both males and heterozygous females, protects against all *Plasmodium* species. Lastly, it is thought that hereditary ovalocytosis prevents cerebral malaria in patients infected with *P falciparum*, by preventing microvascular obstruction.

All malarial species are spread by the female Anopheles mosquito, making her the deadliest animal in the world. Sporozoites are injected into a host through the bite of an infected mosquito and go directly to the liver where they proliferate (this phase is called exoerythrocytic schizogony).

Schizonts then rupture and release merozoites into the bloodstream. These infect red cells to initiate the phase of erythrocytic schizogony. The first week after inoculation is asymptomatic. The initial stages of erythrocyte schizogony and hemolysis are relatively disorganized, and the associated symptoms somewhat vague, but within weeks schizogony becomes synchronized and produce *characteristic fever cycles*. Malaria infection initially presents with low grade fever, anemia, and splenomegaly. Eventually, symptoms are *paroxysmal*, with symptomatic periods lasting 6-12 hours and correlating with intermittent intravascular hemolysis. A paroxysm begins with shaking chills, followed by high fever, followed by profuse sweating and defervescence. Leukopenia is a common finding during paroxysms.

Some clinical features are species-specific. Fever spikes every 48 hours (tertian fever) characterize *P ovale, P vivax,* and *P falciparum*. Because of its lethality and every other day fever, *P falciparum* is also called "malignant tertian malaria." *P vivax & P ovale* are known as "benign tertian malaria" since they are rarely deadly. *P malariae* produces febrile spikes every 72 hours (quartan fever). Nephrotic syndrome is associated primarily with *P malariae*, whereas CNS involvement is seen mainly in *P falciparum*. Hemosiderinuria and hemoglobinuria with *P falciparum* infection result in "blackwater fever" associated with high fever, dark urine and kidney failure. True disease relapse or recurrence, referring to reinvasion of the red blood cells by liver merozoites (from hepatic hypnozoites), after complete clearing of the blood stream by therapy or immunity, is seen only with *P vivax & P ovale*. Recrudescence, in which a parasitemia rendered low by treatment or immunity increases again, is possible with any of the species. Importantly, relapse is not seen in transfusion transmitted or transplacental infection, since the sporozoite component of the life cycle is not present and therefore no liver stage occurs. *P vivax* and *P ovale* infect younger erythrocytes. This is the reason infected erythrocytes appear enlarged. *P malariae* infects older erythrocytes (smaller erythrocytes), and *P falciparum* infects erythrocyte of any age.

The role of the pathologist in malaria consists of detecting it, identifying the species, and quantifying the degree of parasitemia. With regard to detection, there are several options: direct microscopic examination of peripheral blood (Wright or Giemsa stains or fluorescent stains such as acridine orange and rhodamine 123), flow cytometry, antigen detection, and antibody detection. In most instances, malaria is diagnosed by direct examination of Giemsa-stained peripheral blood thick and thin blood films f3.20, f3.25, f3.26. The thick smear is used for screening and the thin smear is best used to speciate. The ideal time to obtain a specimen is immediately preceding the next anticipated fever spike. Examination of ≥100 oil-immersion thick film fields or 300 thin-film fields is required to achieve the reported sensitivity of direct examination (5 parasites per microliter), and it is after this has been completed that a smear may be reported as negative. Furthermore, a single negative smear is insufficient to exclude malaria; 2-3 smears over a 24-hour period are preferred.

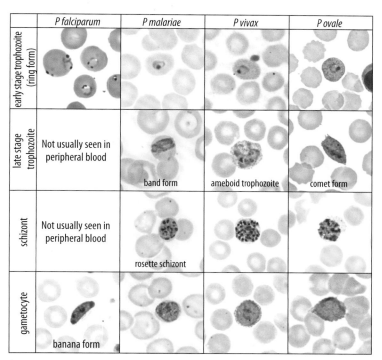

	P falciparum	*P malariae*	*P vivax*	*P ovale*
early stage trophozoite (ring form)				
late stage trophozoite	Not usually seen in peripheral blood	band form	ameboid trophozoite	comet form
schizont	Not usually seen in peripheral blood	rosette schizont		
gametocyte	banana form			

f3.25 Malaria forms

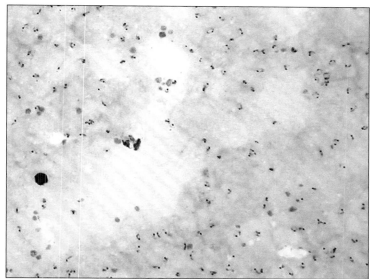

f3.26 Thick blood film showing numerous early trophozoite (ring) forms of *Plasmodium falciparum*

t3.20 *Plasmodium* species

	P vivax/P-ovale	*P malariae*	*P falciparum*
Infected red cell	Enlarged (reticulocyte), may be fimbriated (*P ovale*)	Small to normal size	All sizes
Ring form trophozoite	≥1/3 the size of red cell, multiple infection not uncommon	Thick, small (1/3 the size of the red cell), bird's eye forms (chromatin dot appears to be detached in center of ring, forming an "eye")	Delicate, small (<1/3 the size of the red cell), may have 2 chromatin dots, appliqué forms, multiply-infected RBCs common
Mature trophozoite	*P vivax*: Large amoeboid form that fills red cells. *P ovale*: More compact than *P vivax*	Band & basket forms, do not fill red cell, prominent hematin pigment	Rare in peripheral blood
Schizont	*P vivax*: 12-24 merozoites. *P ovale*: 6-14 merozoites	6-12 merozoites, often surrounding a clump of hematin pigment ("rosette" form)	Rare in peripheral blood
Gametocytes	Large, oval	Oval, often fills red cell	Banana shaped, distorts red cell
Inclusions	Schüffner dots	–	Maurer clefts
Hematin pigment (brown-black)	+, delicate	+, coarse	+, delicate

There are several forms of the organism that can be readily appreciated on the thin blood film. Early trophozoites (ring forms), often the most numerous form to be seen in peripheral blood films and in the early stages, consist of a ring like structure occupying <½ the red cell with 1 or at most 2 nuclei. The trophozoite is the growing form of the organism. Ring forms enlarge as they mature and may take on characteristic forms for different species. The trophozoites then divide into multiple merozoites which make up the schizont stage, where multiple nuclei are seen. Eventually the schizont ruptures and releases the merozoites into the blood to infect other RBCs. Some trophozoites also form a gametocyte; a solid mononuclear structure occupying >½ the red cell that is the infective stage for the mosquito. All mature stages of the organism may contain hematin (brown-black) pigment, a heme breakdown product formed by *Plasmodium* metabolism.

P falciparum is potentially lethal and must be identified when present. The overall mortality is between 1 and 3%; lethal cases of nonfalciparum malaria are rare and most often caused by splenic rupture. Morphologic features allow the distinction of falciparum from nonfalciparum malaria. Except in very severe disease, only ring forms and gametocytes are seen within peripheral blood erythrocytes. This is because erythrocytes infected with intermediate forms are sequestered in capillaries, especially within those of the liver, brain, heart, and kidneys, due to parasite-derived endothelial binding proteins inserted into the infected RBC membrane. *P falciparum* ring forms may have double chromatin dots ("headphone forms"), and multiple ring forms are commonly seen in a single erythrocyte, often appearing as appliqué (aka accolé or marginal) forms. Maurer clefts may be seen in some cases when the Giemsa stain with a 7.2 pH is used, appearing as large round to comma shaped red cytoplasmic dots. They are rarely seen on a Wright stain (commonly used in hematology; pH 6.8). Schizonts are not usually seen in the peripheral blood, and gametocytes are banana shaped. Infected red cells may be of any size, although most are seen in normal sized cells. If these features are seen in the blood smear, alert the clinician immediately that you suspect *P falciparum*. Patient management is typically guided by clinical assessment and the estimate of parasitemia (percentage of infected red cells); >2% parasitemia is considered severe. Patients with severe *P falciparum* malaria may be considered for ICU admission, parenteral quinine or artemisinin therapy, or exchange transfusion (parasitemia ≥10%). The presence of more mature ring forms, pigment, and schizonts in peripheral blood is associated with severe disease, and should be communicated to the clinician. Furthermore, when malarial pigment is seen within neutrophils, severe or prolonged (chronic) disease is suggested. Peripheral blood smears should be examined to monitor treatment, as reflected by the degree of parasitemia. An initial increase in parasitemia is expected, followed by progressive diminution. Additional laboratory support of the patient with severe *P falciparum* infection includes monitoring for severe anemia, coagulopathy, hypoglycemia, abnormal hepatic and renal function, hypocalcemia, hypomagnesemia, lactic acidosis, myocardial damage, and, in some cases, the exclusion of HIV infection.

P vivax and *P ovale* are morphologically very similar to one another, and their distinction is not of major clinical importance. When one is asked to distinguish them, the travel history is often useful, since *P ovale* is fairly rare and confined to limited regions of western Africa. *P vivax* and *ovale* are found in erythrocytes that are slightly enlarged compared to uninfected erythrocytes in the same smear, since they tend to infect younger red cells. Schüffner dots (stippling) may be present, especially on Giemsa stain, which are smaller and more numerous than Maurer clefts of *P falciparum*. All stages of developing organism are seen—early rings, developing (enlarging) rings, large gametocytes, and schizonts. Morphologically they may be differentiated as follows

1. schizonts of *P ovale* and *P vivax* have 6-14 and 12-24 merozoites, respectively

2. *P vivax* tends to have more ameboid forms whereas *P ovale* is more compact

3. ~1/3 of the erythrocytes infected by *P ovale* are oval (hence the name)

P malariae forms are found within erythrocytes of small to normal size, since they infect older erythrocytes. There are no Schüffner dots. Like *P vivax/ovale*, all stages of developing organism are seen. Schizonts have 6-12 merozoites. Coarse malarial pigment may be present. Most useful is the finding of occasional band, basket, and bird's eye form trophozoites.

P knowlesi infection resembles *P falciparum* (including multiplicity of rings and chromatin dots) in early stages, and in late stages resembles *P malaria* (including band forms). Fever periodicity is every 24 hours. Like *P falciparum*, infection may be fatal.

Lastly, mixed infections are encountered in up to 5% of cases, most often *P falciparum* and *P vivax*.

Other detection methods include fluorescent microscopy, which may be applied to blood smears or cytocentrifuged red cell layers, flow cytometry, antigen detection, and antibody detection. Antigen detection methods usually involve a solid phase (eg, membrane strip) containing bound antibody to malarial antigens such as pLDH, HRP2, and aldolase. Blood is applied, with a colorimetric result typically indicating presence of *Plasmodium* antigens. Some tests detect all *Plasmodium* species, while others only detect *P falciparum*. All are more expensive and less sensitive than conventional microscopy, and are therefore seen as an adjunct to the thick and thin smears. Detection of antibody by serology (IgG malarial antibodies) is useful only for the retrospective diagnosis of malaria in a previously nonimmune individual. If persistent infection is suspected, then a Wright or Giemsa stained smear is required for confirmation and species identification. False positive results are common, particularly in patients with autoantibodies.

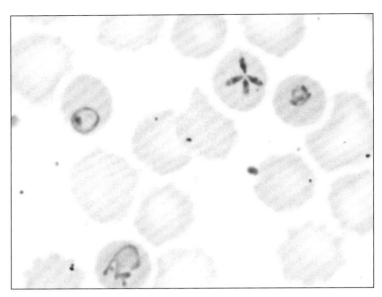

f3.27 *Babesia*

Molecular approaches, such as PCR, are especially useful for species identification and differentiation of *P falciparum* trophozoites from the similar appearing *Babesia* parasites. PCR may also be useful for detecting very low parasitemia and mixed infections, depending on the design and sensitivity of the assay.

Babesiosis

Babesia trophozoites (ring forms) are usually multiple within red cells in peripheral blood f3.27, occasionally forming diads, or rarely, tetrads (Maltese cross arrangements). They appear as round to oval light blue ring forms with red chromatin dots. Unlike malaria, extraerythrocytic ring forms are often present, and neither pigment nor nonring forms are seen. Ring forms closely resemble those of *P falciparum* but are often much more pleomorphic in size and shape. Babesiosis occurs in expanding locations across the United States, Europe, Asia, and Africa. In the United States, it is encountered mainly in the northeastern states, including Connecticut, Massachusetts, Rhode Island, and New York and the midwest (Minnesota and Wisconsin) due to *B microti*. Less commonly, cases are seen in the West (Oregon and northern California) due to *Babesia duncani* (WA-1). Most recently, an un-named strain designated MO-1 from Missouri has been described. *Babesia divergens* is the most prevalent species in Europe. The organism is transmitted by ticks of the genus *Ixodes*. In the Northeastern US, *Ixodes scapularis* (formerly *I dammini*) is the most common vector, where the primary reservoirs are the white-tailed deer and the white-footed mouse. It is important to note that the white-footed mouse may also harbor *Borrelia burgdorferi* (Lyme disease) and *Anaplasma phagocytophilum* (human granulocytic ehrlichiosis); thus, the *I scapularis* tick may transmit all 3. Coinfection with flavivirus has also been noted. Babesiosis is transmitted by *Ixodes pacificus* in the western US, and *Ixodes ricinus* in Europe. Infection results in a nonperiodic fever and hemolysis. The severity varies from asymptomatic to fatal, with fatal disease occurring mainly in splenectomized and immunodeficient individuals. As a result of hemolytic anemia, laboratory findings include decreased serum haptoglobin,

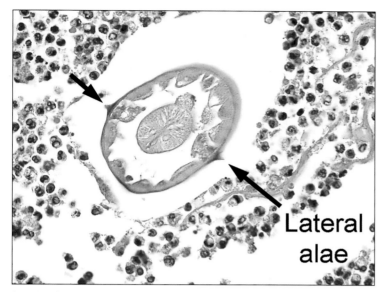

f3.28 *Enterobius vermicularis* in cross section

Enterobius vermicularis	Trichuris trichiura	Ascaris lumbricoides		Hookworm
		fertile	infertile	

scale: ⊢⊣ = 10 µm

f3.29 Nematode eggs

hyperbilirubinemia (raised indirect bilirubin), elevated lactate dehydrogenase, and reticulocytosis. Elevated liver function tests and thrombocytopenia are sometimes observed. The definitive diagnosis is based upon identification of the organism on Wright or Giemsa stained blood smears. Antibabesial antibodies may be misleading, particularly in places with high prevalence, where most infections are thought to be asymptomatic; nonetheless, antibabesial antibody titer, by IFA, of ≥1:1,024 is thought to indicate active infection. Patients who have had remote infection typically have a titer of ≤1:64. Molecular methods, such as PCR, have been developed to detect and differentiate *Babesia* species.

Metazoa

The metazoa belong to the phylum helminth (helmins = worms) and are further divided into 2 subphyla, nemathelminths (nema = thread) and the platyhelminths (platys = flat). The nemathelminths includes the nematodes (roundworms) and the platyhelminths include the trematodes (flukes) and the cestodes (tapeworms).

Nematodes, intestinal

Intestinal nematodes spend most of their time in the intestinal tract and are typically diagnosed by finding characteristic eggs (or larvae) in stool. With the exception of pinworm, all eggs require a soil incubation stage before becoming infectious; therefore, infection with these parasites can be prevented by adequate sanitary measures, including provision of clean water and proper treatment of human feces. Although mortality due to infection is rare, intestinal nematodes can cause significant morbidity, with severity usually correlated to worm burden. Up to a third of the world's population is infected.

Enterobius vermicularis (pinworm, oxyuriasis)

The adult female worm has a slightly bent & pointed (pin-like) tail. In cross sections, such as may be seen in histologic sections of bowel and appendix, the adult worm has characteristic lateral alae f3.28. The egg is characterized as a thin-walled 30-50 µm oval with one side flattened. Unlike the other intestinal nematodes, the egg is not routinely found in stool specimens, necessitating a cellophane tape test; Clear (not frosted) tape is applied to the perianal skin in the early morning before the patient (usually a child) rises and is then applied to a slide and examined microscopically.

Pinworm is the most common helminthic infection in American children. Eggs are infectious shortly after being laid and autoinfection is common. Infection is acquired from ingestion of eggs which hatch in the small intestine to release larvae which mature and inhabit the large intestine (cecum). After mating, the gravid female undergoes nocturnal migration to lay eggs in the perianal region. Common symptoms are nocturnal anal pruritus, vaginitis, and/or enuresis. Appendicitis is an occasional complication. Eggs become lodged under the infected patient's fingernails and contaminate the environment, thus facilitating infection.

Trichuris trichiura (whipworm)

The adult worm measures up to 5 cm and has a whip-like anterior end. The male has a coiled posterior end, whereas females have a straight thickened posterior end containing the uterus with eggs. The characteristic eggs are found in stool; they measure 50 × 25 µm, have brownish thick-shells, and are barrel shaped with bilateral polar plugs.

Infection results from ingestion of embryonated eggs in contaminated food and water and causes large intestinal infection which may be asymptomatic. Heavy infections present with dysentery-like manifestations. Significant bowel edema and resultant tenesmus may produce rectal prolapse in young children. Eggs are passed into the soil where they mature and can contaminate food and water sources.

Ascaris lumbricoides (roundworm)

This is the largest nematode parasitizing the human intestine where adult females measure 20-35 cm and adult males measure 15-30 cm. The male has a terminal curvature which the female lacks. In feces, the fertilized egg is ~60 µm, bile-stained, and its thick hyaline shell has a rough, mammillated, exterior) f3.29. Larger, unfertilized forms are also commonly seen. Eggs that have lost the external mammillated shell (decorticate eggs) may resemble hookworm eggs, but have a much thicker shell.

ISBN 978-089189-5985

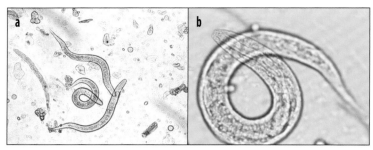

f3.30 a Rhabditiform larvae of *Strongyloides stercoralis*
b The short buccal cavity allows it to be differentiated from hookworm rhabditiform larvae

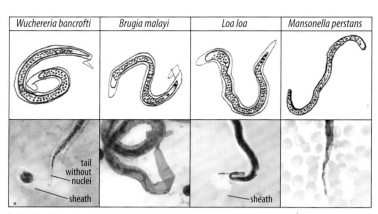

f3.31 Microfilariae found in peripheral blood

Infection results from ingestion of eggs which hatch in the small intestine, giving rise to larvae that penetrate the mucosa and enter the bloodstream to be carried to the lungs. There, they mature, are expectorated and swallowed, eventually to infect the duodenum. During migration through the lung, the larvae may provoke a Löeffler syndrome (transient pulmonary infiltrates with eosinophilia). Duodenal infection may be asymptomatic or result in abdominal discomfort, obstruction, cholangitis, or appendicitis. Worms live for ~1 year.

Necator americanus & Ancylostoma duodenale (hookworms)

Adult hookworms measure ~1 cm in length. The mouth parts of the 2 hookworms differ: *N americanus* has cutting plates; *A duodenale* has "teeth." In feces, the eggs of these 2 hookworms are indistinguishable from one another. They have a thin translucent wall that encloses a morula-like cluster of several spherical embryos. When stool is left at room temperature for several days, the eggs may hatch and release larvae, which must then be distinguished from the larvae of *Strongyloides stercoralis*, by their longer buccal cavity and indistinct genital primordium.

The largest number of infections worldwide are found in Asia and sub-Saharan Africa. Coastal regions are the preferred location for this organism, since larvae enjoy the sandy soil. *N americanus* (but not *A duodenale*) is found in some parts of the southeastern United States (eg, Appalachia). Infection results from penetration of skin by larvae rather than ingestion of eggs. Often this takes place in the feet, resulting in a localized pruritic lesion (ground itch). The larvae enter the circulation, trespass the lungs (sometimes associated with a Löeffler-like syndrome), are expectorated and swallowed. Intestinal (small bowel) infection may persist for years, often leading to iron deficiency anemia. *Ancylostoma braziliense* is a zoonotic hookworm that, rather than proceeding through the skin into the circulation, results in a cutaneous infection called *cutaneous larva migrans*.

Strongyloides stercoralis (thread worm)

Adult females measure ~3 mm and can be found burrowed into the intestinal crypts. The egg is identical to the hookworm egg but is not usually found in stool; instead, eggs hatch in the bowel and the organism appears in feces as rhabditoid larvae f3.30. The larvae are very similar to hookworm larvae but have a short buccal groove and prominent genital primordium. Duodenal aspirates or string test specimens may be helpful when stool examination is negative. Alternatively, microscopic examination of multiple stool specimens (7 or more) may be required. Most sensitive methods are the Baermann apparatus or agar culture.

In addition to being found in many tropical and subtropical regions throughout the world, *S stercoralis* is found in parts of the southeastern US. Infection results from penetration of skin, often the feet, by larvae. Like hookworm, these circulate to and migrate through the lungs, a trespass often associated with a Löeffler like syndrome. The larvae are then expectorated and swallowed, resulting in intestinal (duodenal) infection. Larvae mature into adults, and the females burrow into the intestinal crypts and begin to produce eggs. The eggs hatch within the small intestine, and mature into rhabditoid larvae which are passed into stool. Rhabditoid larvae mature in the environment into filariform larvae capable of penetrating skin. In some instances, particularly in a weakened (eg, malnourished) host, larvae mature into infective forms while still within the bowel; these are capable of penetrating the bowel wall, circulating through the lungs and reinfecting the duodenum in large numbers, a condition called autoinfection. Autoinfection results in long-term carriage, a state that is often asymptomatic or characterized by persistent eosinophilia, and sometimes by the formation of linear urticaria (larva currens). However, in immunocompromised hosts, autoinfection can lead to hyperinfection, a potentially deadly complication in which larvae penetrate the bowel wall and disseminate widely via the bloodstream. Hyperinfection often presents gastroenteritis, pneumonia, sepsis, and/or recurrent Gram– meningitis due to damage caused by the invasive larvae and the gut bacteria they carry with them.

Nematodes, filarial

These nematodes are transmitted to humans through the bite of an infected arthropod. Microfilaria are the diagnostic forms, while the adults often cause significant morbidity. The presence or absence of a sheath and the pattern of nuclei in the tail are the main features which allow distinction of the various microfilariae t3.21, f3.31.

t3.21 Microfilariae in blood

Organism	Sheath	Tail nuclei	Periodicity of microfilariae in blood	Adult found in
Wuchereria bancrofti	+	None	Nocturnal	Lymphatics
Brugia malayi	+	2 discontinuous	Nocturnal	Lymphatics
Loa loa	+	Continuous row	Diurnal	Migrating through subcutis
Mansonella perstans	–	Continuous row	None	Body cavities or subcutis

Microfilaria found in blood

W bancrofti and *B malayi* are acquired through the bite of various mosquitoes. Both *W bancrofti* and *B malayi adults* infect the lymphatics, leading to lymphadenitis and lymphedema (elephantiasis). They are shed into the blood primarily at night (nocturnal periodicity), and therefore the highest likelihood of detection is between 10 PM and 2 AM.

Loa loa is acquired from the mango (*Chrysops*) fly. *Loa loa* adults inhabit and migrate through subcutaneous and conjunctival locations, causing transient migratory edema (calabar swellings). Microfilariae have diurnal periodicity.

Mansonella perstans are acquired from the biting midge (*Culicoides*) and inhabit body cavities. Infections usually are asymptomatic or associated with mild disease.

Microfilaria not found in blood

O volvulus is acquired from the bite of the *Simulium* black fly. The adults ball up in a subcutaneous nodule (onchocercoma), where the female releases microfilariae into the surrounding skin. Unlike the other microfilariae, *disease is caused by the microfilariae and not the adults*. Microfilariae, rather than circulating in the blood, migrate continuously through the skin and eye, resulting in dermatitis, keratitis, and corneal opacity. It is a leading cause of blindness (aka river blindness) in central Africa and parts of Central America. Diagnosis is by identifying characteristic larvae in skin snips.

Dirofilaria immitis (dog heart worm) is a zoonotic infection acquired from a mosquito. Humans are a dead-end host, and infection typically presents as a subcutaneous or pulmonary granulomatous nodule (depending on the species) surrounding a degenerating worm. Infections in the US are most common in the southeast.

Nematodes, zoonotic

These are primarily parasites of animals and humans are often a dead-end host.

Trichinosis

Trichinella spiralis is acquired by consumption of undercooked meat, especially pork and wild game. This results in infection of the skeletal muscle by encysted larvae, producing myositis and weakness. Encysted larvae can be seen on histologic sections of infected skeletal muscle within host muscle ("nurse") cells. More commonly, diagnosis is made by serology, in combination with the clinical presentation and associated risk factors.

Toxocara canis (dog roundworm) & *cati* (cat roundworm)

T canis and, to a lesser extent, *T cati* are the principal causes of visceral larva migrans (VLM) and ocular larva migrans (OLM). These typically affect children who ingest soil contaminated with cat or dog feces. The organism, incapable of completing its life cycle in humans, wanders throughout various organs. This produces a syndrome of hypereosinophilia, hepatosplenomegaly, and pneumonitis.

The organism is rarely identified in tissue sections. Diagnosis is usually clinical with or without serology.

Anisakiasis

Anisakiasis is acquired from ingestion of raw or undercooked fish, especially cod, containing the larvae of *Anisakis simplex* or *Pseudoterranova decipiens*. Within hours after ingestion of infected

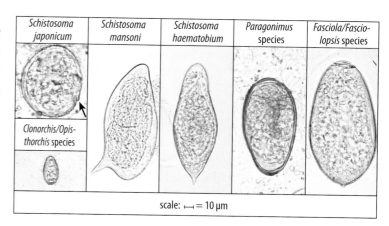

f3.32 Trematode ova; arrow denotes small lateral spine

larvae, the larvae may be coughed up or the patient may present with extreme gastric pain as the larvae burrow into the stomach wall. Less commonly, the worm may lodge in the bowel wall or even penetrate the wall and enter the peritoneal cavity. Diagnosis can be made by gastroscopic examination during which the 2 cm larva is visualized and removed, or by histopathologic examination of tissue removed at biopsy or during surgery. Biopsy may disclose an eosinophil-rich granuloma containing the nematode. Serology may aid in the diagnosis.

Trematodes (flukes) t3.22, f3.32

Trematodes have a flat, leaf-like, bilaterally symmetrical body. They are all hermaphroditic except for *Schistosoma* species which have separate sexes. Their life cycle is complex usually involving 3 hosts where the first asexual stage takes place in snails. The adult worms are rarely encountered and are usually seen after antihelminthic purging (for intestinal or biliary forms) or at autopsy. Diagnosis is usually made by direct observation of excreted eggs in stool, urine, or sputum, depending on the infecting species.

t3.22 Operculated eggs

Organism	Shoulder	Size (µm)	Abopercular knob
Clonorchis sinensis	+	30	+
Diphyllobothrium latum (only operculated tapeworm egg)	–	60	+
Paragonimus westermani	+	90	– (abopercular thickening)
Fasciola hepatica/ Fasciolopsis buski	–	120	+

Fasciolopsis buski (intestinal fluke)

The adult is a flattened worm with a pointed, but not conical, cephalad. The egg, at 100-150 µm, is one of the largest seen in human parasitology. It is oval with a thin shell and an unshouldered operculum (which resembles a hatch door). There is a small abopercular knob at the end opposite the operculum. The egg is identical to *F hepatica*. Diagnosis is usually by microscopic identification of eggs in stool. Less commonly, adults are seen on colonoscopy.

ISBN 978-089189-5985

F buski is acquired by ingestion of freshwater plants (eg, water chestnuts). It is found in Asia and the Indian subcontinent primarily and results in infection of duodenum.

Fasciola hepatica (liver fluke)

The adult is a flattened worm with a cephalic cone that distinguishes it from *F buski*. The egg is identical to that of *F buski*. Diagnosis is usually by microscopic identification of eggs in stool.

Fasciola is acquired by ingestion of freshwater plants (eg, watercress). It is found in parts of Asia and the Middle East and results in infection of the bile ducts. The fluke reaches the bile ducts by migrating through the liver, causing hepatic damage and fibrosis/cirrhosis.

Clonorchis sinensis/Opisthorchis species (liver fluke)

Adults are much smaller than *F hepatica* and have a snout-like cephalad. Eggs are oval and tiny, measuring ~30 µm, and are characterized by a shouldered operculum with a small abopercular knob. The eggs of *Clonorchis* and *Opisthorchis* are morphologically indistinguishable. Diagnosis is usually by microscopic identification of eggs in stool.

Both flukes are acquired through ingestion of undercooked freshwater fish. It is found in parts of Asia. Infection results in chronic biliary tract infection within the liver, leading to biliary fibrosis. Chronic infection is a risk factor for cholangiocarcinoma. Unlike *F hepatica* infection, the flukes do not enter the liver parenchyma and remain in the bile ducts.

Paragonimus westermani (oriental lung fluke)

The egg is oval, ~90 µm, and has a shouldered operculum at the thickened end. Diagnosis is based on the presence of excreted eggs in sputum or alternatively they are swallowed and passed in the stool.

Paragonimiasis is acquired by ingestion of undercooked crustaceans (eg, crab and crayfish), resulting in lung infection with pulmonitis. Infection in North America is associated with a different species of *Paragonimus* (*P kellicotti*).

Schistosomiasis (bilharziasis, blood flukes)

Schistosome eggs may be detected in stool, urine (*S haematobium*), or tissue (where they are usually surrounded by a granulomatous and fibrous reaction). They are oval, 75-150 µm, and have a single spine whose size and placement allows identification as follows: *S haematobium* has a terminal spine, *S mansoni* has a lateral spine, and *S japonicum* has a small, knob-like, spine. The small size and blunt spine of *S japonicum* allows it to sometimes disseminate within the host. Paired adult schistosomes have been likened to a hot dog in a bun; that is, the longer, more slender female (hot dog) resides within an anterior groove (gynecophoric canal) of the shorter, broader male (bun).

Schistosomes are acquired through penetration of the skin (swimmer's itch) by free-swimming, fork-tailed, cercariae found in snail-infested water. Cercariae migrate through the blood stream and mature to eventually make their way as adults into the mesenteric and pelvic blood vessels. The adults mate and the female releases numerous eggs into the blood stream; some of these eggs make their way through the bowel or bladder wall to be excreted in stool or urine.

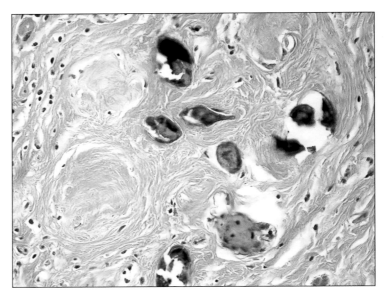

f3.33 Partially calcified *Schistosoma* species eggs lodged in the intestinal wall

During the acute stage of disease (weeks to months after infection), circulating immune complexes cause a systemic febrile illness called Katayama fever, with fever, fatigue, myalgia, urticaria, nonproductive cough, and eosinophilia. Patchy infiltrates may be observed on chest x-ray. Abdominal pain may be a prominent feature. The manifestations of Katayama fever are most pronounced in nonimmune individuals, ie, travelers to endemic regions, and are uncommon in indigenous populations.

The chronic stage of disease is caused by the host tissue reaction to retained eggs. Although some eggs are excreted from the human host, many remain lodged in tissue. Over time, the tissue reaction to eggs can lead to visceral dysfunction.

S mansoni is found in parts of South America and the Caribbean, Africa, and the Middle East. The adult worms infect the hepatic portal vasculature and the inferior mesenteric vessels. Eggs are passed into the intestine and excreted in the stool but are also deposited in the periportal hepatic parenchyma. Reaction to deposited eggs in the liver can lead to so-called pipestem portal fibrosis and eventual cirrhosis. In the intestine, retained eggs can result in colitis and fibrosis. Rectal biopsies reveal the characteristic eggs.

S japonicum is found in the Far East. Like *S mansoni*, it infects the liver, leading to cirrhosis. *S japonicum* may also, less commonly, disseminate to the brain and spinal cord. *S mekongi*, in many respects similar to *S japonicum*, is found focally in Southeast Asia.

S haematobium is found in Africa and the Middle East. The adult worms infect the venous plexus of the bladder and deposit eggs into the bladder wall, leading to hematuria and irritative bladder symptoms. Long term infection may result in squamous cell carcinoma of the bladder. A terminal urine specimen (the last 10-20 mL passed) is ideal for detection of *S haematobium*. The specimen is best collected around midday (greatest shedding) or following exercise. Eggs may also be seen in bladder biopsies. The eggs of *S intercalatum* closely resemble those of *S haematobium*; however, *S intercalatum* produces intestinal schistosomiasis f3.33, and the eggs are seen in feces instead of urine. *S intercalatum* is found focally in central West Africa.

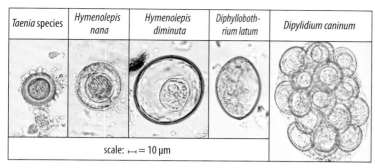

| *Taenia* species | *Hymenolepis nana* | *Hymenolepis diminuta* | *Diphyllobothrium latum* | *Dipylidium caninum* |

scale: ⊢⊣ = 10 μm

f3.34 Cestode eggs

Cestodes (tapeworms) f3.34

Adult cestodes have a flattened body composed of a scolex (head with attachment structures), a neck and a strobila (body) made up of numerous segments called proglottids. They resemble a strip of tape hence the common name tapeworm. Adult cestodes infect the human intestinal tract and are usually diagnosed by identification of characteristic eggs and/or proglottids in stool. 2 cestodes, *Taenia solium* and *Echinococcus* species, can infect humans as a larval form, in which case diagnosis is by clinical and radiologic features, macroscopic and/or microscopic morphology, and serology.

Taenia saginata (beef tapeworm)

The diagnosis is usually made by finding eggs in stool. The egg, which is identical to that of *T solium*, is 30-40 μm, spherical, has a thick radially striated wall, and contains 3 pairs of hooks. The finding of such eggs is reportable as "*Taenia* species" only. Further characterization relies upon examination of the scolex or proglottids. The scolex has 4 suckers and a smooth surface (unarmed rostellum). Each proglottid is longer than it is wide and has >13-15 lateral uterine branches. The uterine branches are classically visualized through India ink injection into the genital pore, a technique which requires considerable expertise to perform.

While common in South and Central America, *T saginata* is rare in North America. It is acquired by ingestion of encysted organisms (cysticerci) in beef. This results in intestinal (small bowel) infection by the adult worm. The eggs of *T saginata* are not infectious to humans unlike those of *T solium,* and thus cysticercosis (larval form of disease in humans) due to *T saginata* does not occur.

Taenia solium (pork tapeworm)

The egg is identical to that of *T saginata*. The scolex has 4 suckers and many tiny hooklets on its surface (armed rostellum). Each proglottid is longer than it is wide, and has <13 lateral uterine branches. The encysted larval form (as seen in cysticercosis) consists of a spherical cyst measuring ~1 cm. The wall of the cyst measures up to 200 μm in thickness. An invaginated scolex with a double row of hooklets (which are acid-fast and birefringent) is the key finding.

T solium is occasionally encountered in the US, most commonly in recent immigrants. Intestinal infection results from ingestion of encysted organisms (cysticerci) in "measly" pork. This situation is very similar to infection with *T saginata*.

Cysticercosis, a condition in which cysts, containing larvae, are found in the brain (neurocysticercosis) and elsewhere, results from ingestion of eggs shed in the feces of a human tapeworm carrier. Note that a person does not need to ingest meat to get cysticercosis.

Diphyllobothrium latum (broad fish tapeworm)

The diagnosis is usually made by finding eggs in stool. The egg is a 60 μm oval structure with a smooth shell and an unshouldered operculum (like a hatch door) at one end. A small abopercular (located on the other end from the operculum) knob is seen. This egg must be distinguished from the similarly appearing egg of *P westermani* which is larger and has a shouldered operculum (small swellings rise up on either side of the operculum). The scolex looks like an elongated almond with 2 longitudinal sucking grooves that are used for attachment. Each proglottid is characteristically much wider than it is long (hence the appellation "broad fish tapeworm") and contains a coiled uterus in the shape of a rosette. These features allow the proglottids to be easily differentiated from *Taenia* species proglottids.

D latum is somewhat unusual in that it is found in temperate zones—Scandinavia, Russia, Canada, northern US, and Alaska. It is acquired through ingestion of poorly-cooked freshwater fish, resulting in intestinal infection. In some cases, infection is complicated by vitamin B_{12} deficiency.

Hymenolepis nana (dwarf tapeworm)

The egg has thin inner and outer shells with a wide space in between containing 2 pairs of polar filaments that arise from the inner shell containing an embryo with hooklets. The egg of *H diminuta* is similar but lacks the polar filaments. The adult worm is very small (2-4 cm).

H nana is one of the most common cestodes recovered in the US. Intestinal infection typically follows accidental ingestion of infected arthropods (beetles). Person to person spread may occur through ingestion of eggs shed in feces.

Dipylidium caninum (double-pored dog tapeworm)

Eggs look somewhat like the eggs of *H diminuta*, except that they tend to occur in globular packets of 5-15 eggs enclosed by a thin membrane. The proglottid has a double genital pore, one exiting out of each side, and macroscopically resembles a rice grain.

D caninum commonly infects cats and dogs, but occasionally infects humans, especially children following accidental ingestion of infected fleas.

Echinococcus species

Protoscoleces (larval tapeworms) and free hooklets can be found in fluid from an echinococcal (hydatid) cyst; the aspirated material is referred to as hydatid sand. Care must be taken when aspirating a hydatid cyst due to the risk of anaphylaxis and dissemination of infection. Aspiration can be both diagnostic and curative when combined with antihelminth medication. In some settings, cysts are resected. Histopathology of *E granulosus* shows characteristic cysts with thick laminated membranes (laminations accentuated with GMS) containing protoscoleces and hooklets. In *E multilocularis*, cysts are separated by fibrous stroma rather than laminated material. Clinical and radiologic features, microscopic and macroscopic morphology and serology are commonly combined for definitive diagnosis.

Echinococcosis is acquired when ingesting food contaminated with eggs from the stool of an infected dog, the definitive host. Sheep, cattle, and other herbivores are intermediate hosts; thus, the infection is commonest in sheep and cattle-raising areas (pastoral infections). There is also a wild (sylvatic) life cycle that occurs between foxes and wolves and their herbivore prey. *Echinococcus* infection results in the formation of cysts in various organs, particularly the liver. A single hydatid cyst, sometimes containing daughter cysts, is seen in *E granulosis* infection, while multilocular cysts are seen with *E multilocularis*. Polycystic hydatid cyst disease is seen with *E vogeli*. Hepatic cysts may rupture through the diaphragm, giving rise to pulmonary cysts.

Additional pearls of parasitology t3.23-t3.26

t3.23 Dual infections involving parasites

Ascaris lumbricoides & *Trichuris trichiura*
Pinworm & *Dientamoeba fragilis*
Babesia, Lyme disease & *Anaplasma phagocytophilum*
Lepromatous leprosy or HTLV-1 & *Strongyloides stercoralis* hyperinfection

t3.24 Parasitic oculocutaneous infections

Loa loa—disease is caused by the adult worm
Onchocerca volvulus—disease is caused by the larvae

t3.25 Parasitic infections capable of person to person spread

Enterobius vermicularis
Hymenolepis nana

t3.26 Parasitic infections in immunodeficient patients

Type of immunodeficiency	Susceptibility
T cell (cellular) immunodeficiency	Many, eg, *Toxoplasmosis*, *Cryptosporidium*, *Cystoisospora*, *Cyclospora*, microsporidia, are more common Others, eg, *Strongyloides*, are more severe
B cell (humoral) immunodeficiency	*Giardia* more common
Splenectomy	Babesiosis more severe

Mycology
Laboratory methods
Direct examination

For examination of primary specimens, wet preparations are typically made using a stain for fungi, such as the calcofluor white stain. Calcofluor white is a fluorochrome that selectively binds to the cellulose and chitin in fungal cell walls. Human cells, which lack these targets, remain unstained. The slide is then examined using fluorescence microscopy. Fungal elements, whether yeasts or hyphae, appear bright white, blue or apple green, depending on the microscope's UV filter f3.35. The calcoflour white stain will highlight all fungi, including *Pneumocystis*, plus a few nonfungal organisms, including Prototheca and the cysts of *Acanthamoeba*.

The microscopic morphology of fungi in direct wet preparations can help with initial classification. *Yeasts* are unicellular organisms, most of which display budding, and many of which form pseudohyphae. Molds are multicellular organisms which form true hyphae. Hyphal structures may be further classified as septate, aseptate or pauciseptate.

India ink is used for the presumptive identification of *Cryptococcus neoformans*, particularly in CSF. A small amount of India ink is added to a drop of CSF on a slide. The slide is examined for the presence of encapsulated yeasts, which appear round, with wide variation in size, and narrow-based budding. A clear halo around the yeast cells indicates the presence of a capsule, which strongly suggests Cryptococcus as few other yeast species are encapsulated.

In tissue sections, fungi are difficult to detect by examining routine H&E-stained sections. The exception are the intrinsically pigmented (dematiaceous) molds. For sensitive detection of most fungi, special stains are needed. Commonly, either a Gormori methenamine silver (GMS) or periodic acid schiff (PAS) stain is used.

Fungal culture

For general purpose cultures, several media are typically inoculated and incubated simultaneously, including brain heart infusion (BHI) agar, Sabouraud dextrose agar, and inhibitory mold agar t3.27. Cultures are incubated at 25-30°C for 4-6 weeks. Special culture techniques may be applied either for initial isolation or for differentiation, in some circumstances t3.28

t3.27 Fungal media

Fungal medium	Principle	Purpose
Sabouraud dextrose agar (SDA)	Acid pH & high dextrose concentration inhibits bacterial growth but permits growth of fungi; some formulations also contain antibiotics	General-purpose medium for cultivation/isolation of many fungi
Inhibitory mold agar (IMA)	Nutrient-rich medium containing chloramphenicol & sometimes gentamicin or ciprofloxacin; chloramphenicol suppresses the growth of many bacteria	Selective isolation of fungi from specimens that may contain commensal bacterial flora
Brain heart infusion agar (BHI)	Nutrient-rich medium containing brain/meat infusion, peptone & dextrose Chloramphenicol & gentamicin can be added for selectivity	The nonselective formulation is a general purpose medium used in the cultivation/isolation of bacteria, yeasts & molds When supplemented with chloramphenicol & gentamicin, it is used for selective isolation of fungi from specimens that may contain commensal bacterial flora
Cycloheximide-containing media	Cycloheximide inhibits the growth of many saprophytic fungi, while permitting growth of most (but not all) pathogenic fungi Chloramphenicol & gentamicin can be added to inhibit bacteria	Selective isolation of slow growing pathogenic fungi that may be overgrown by rapidly growing saprophytic fungi Notably, cycloheximide also inhibits the growth of certain pathogenic fungi, including *C neoformans*, many *Candida* species, *Aspergillus* species & the zygomycetes, among others It is frequently used to target dermatophytes or thermally dimorphic fungi

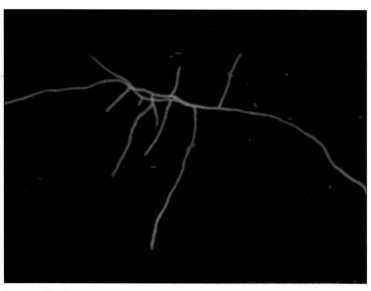

f3.35 Fungal hyphae stained with calcofluor white, viewed under UV light

Initial examination of a fungal isolate t3.29

The first clue is the colony morphology: yeast form creamy or mucoid colonies; molds make fuzzy colonies. Thermally dimorphic fungi grow as yeast when incubated at 37°C, but grow as molds when incubated at 25°C or 30°C.

A fuzzy colony usually indicates the presence of a mold. The major considerations in the differential diagnosis are the hyaline septate molds (also called hyaline hyphomycetes), the dematiaceous molds, the zygomycetes, and the thermally dimorphic fungi. In order to differentiate among these, 3 major characteristics are considered—rate of growth, hyphal septations, and pigmentation.

- The hyaline septate molds tend to grow moderately to rapidly, and have hyphae with frequent septations. The surface of the colonies may be white or colored, due to various (nonmelanin) pigments in their reproductive structures, but the reverse side of the plate is usually light, as the hyphae do not contain dark melanin pigment.

- The dematiaceous molds grow moderately to slowly, and have hyphae with frequent septations. Typically, these molds have melanin pigment in both their hyphae and their reproductive structures, and so the surface and reverse side of the plate are both dark.

- The zygomycetes are extremely rapidly growing molds that may cover the surface of the dish after overnight incubation (lid lifters). They are aseptate or, more commonly, pauciseptate. Like the hyaline molds, they do not contain melanin pigment and the reverse side of the plate is light.

- Thermally dimorphic fungi are slow growing, sometimes requiring several weeks for colonies to develop. When incubated at 30°C, the usual incubation temperature for fungal culture, young colonies tend to be white, and hyphae are septated. In order to confirm that the fungus is thermally dimorphic, it can be converted from the mold form to the yeast form by reincubating the colonies at 37°C. DNA-based testing is commercially available for some of the more common dimorphic fungi (eg, *H capsulatum*, *B dermatitidis* and *C immitis*). These tests employ labeled oligonucleotide probes complementary to segments of species-specific ribosomal RNA (rRNA).

t3.28 Specialized fungal culture media

Medium	Purpose
Cornmeal or potato dextrose agar	Promotion of characteristic reproductive structures & pigmentation useful for morphologic identification of mold isolates, when general-purpose media prove inadequate for a particular isolate
Cornmeal or rice agar with Tween 80	Promotion of characteristic structures (eg, chlamydospores, arthroconidia) useful for morphologic identification of yeast isolates, when more routine identification methods prove inadequate
Sabouraud dextrose agar, Dixon medium, or Leeming-Notman medium overlaid with sterile olive oil	Isolation/cultivation of *Malassezia species*, all of which (except *M pachydermatis*) require lipid supplementation for growth
Trichophyton agars	Differentiation between species of *Trichophyton*, which can be difficult to speciate based on morphology alone
Bird seed (niger seed) agar	Demonstration of phenol oxidase activity in *Cryptococcus neoformans* isolates

t3.29 Classification of fungi based on morphology

	Yeast			Mold			Thermally dimorphic
				Septate hyphae		**Pauciseptate hyphae**	
Morphology	Blastoconidia only	Blastoconidia with pseudohyphae	Arthroconidia	Hyaline molds (hyphae & other structures are non-melanized)	Dematiaceous molds (hyphae and/or conidia are darkly pigmented with melanin)		
Important examples	Cryptococcus Candida glabrata Rhodotorula Malassezia	Candida species (except C glabrata) Saccharomyces cerevisiae	Trichosporon Geotrichum	Aspergillus Penicillium Fusarium Dermatophytes (Epidermophyton, Microsporum, Trichophyton)	Alternaria P boydii/S boydii Scedosporium prolificans Curvularia	Zygomycetes (eg, Rhizopus, Mucor, Cunninghamella, Rhizomucor)	Histoplasma capsulatum Blastomyces dermatitidis Coccidioides immitis/posadasii* Paracoccidioides brasiliensis Sporothrix schenkii Penicillium marnefii

*In routine culture, Coccidioides produces the same structures (septate hyphae & arthroconidia) whether grown at 25°C or 37°C; it can technically be considered thermally dimorphic, though, because the structures it produces in tissue (spherules) can be induced in culture at 37°C using special media

ISBN 978-089189-5985

- Once a fungus has been placed into one of these broad categories, examination of its reproductive structures (conidia or spores) often provides the basis for a genus- or species-level identification.

A smooth, creamy or pasty colony usually indicates the presence of a yeast. *Cryptococcus* species may produce mucoid colonies, because they are encapsulated. *Candida albicans* may form "feet" or starlike projections, because of its ability to form true hyphae in addition to pseudohyphae and blastoconidia. The presence of yeast colonies can be confirmed by making a simple wet preparation, which will demonstrate budding yeast (blastoconidia) and may also demonstrate pseudohyphae and occasionally, true hyphae as well. A few yeast also produce arthroconidia. Once a yeast has been detected, it can be fully identified using several methods including biochemical testing, MALDI-TOF mass spectrometry or morphologic classification after growth on special yeast morphology medium.

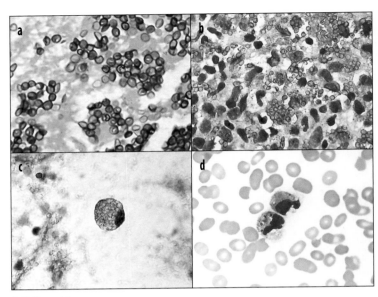

f3.36 *H capsulatum*
a GMS stained, b PAS stained tissue sections demonstrate small yeasts with narrow based budding; c H&E stained, d Wright stained smears demonstrate intracellular yeast forms

Fungal isolate growing as a mold in 25-30°C culture: thermally dimorphic fungi & thermally monomorphic molds

Thermally dimorphic fungi (also called endemic fungi) t3.30

t3.30 Summary of dimorphic fungi

Species	Yeast form characteristics	Mold form characteristics	Route of infection	Common sites of disseminated infection
H capsulatum var capsulatum	2-4 μm, narrow-based budding	Septate hyphae with tear shaped microconidia & thick-walled, tuberculate macroconidia	Inhalation	Reticuloendothelial system, mediastinum
B dermatitidis	8-15 μm thick-walled, broad-based budding	Septate hyphae with lollipop-like conidia atop unbranched conidiophores	Inhalation	Skin, mucous membranes
C immitis	10-100 μm spherules containing 2-5 μm (nonbudding) endospores	Barrel shaped arthroconidia alternating with empty cells	Inhalation	Skin, bone, joints
P brasiliensis	10-50 μm mariner's wheel (circumferential budding)	Septate hyphae with intercalary & terminal chlamydospores	Inhalation or traumatic inoculation	Skin, mucous membranes, bone marrow, lymphatics
S schenckii	4-6 μm elongated (cigars) with narrow-based budding	Rosettes of microconidia at the apex of swollen, delicate conidiophores	Traumatic inoculation	Regional lymphatics
P marneffei	3-5 μm ovoid, divide by fission	Colonies producing diffusible red pigment	Inhalation	Bone marrow, skin

Histoplasma capsulatum

In tissue sections f3.36 or primary wet preparations *H capsulatum var capsulatum* yeast cells typically are found within histiocytes or reticuloendothelial cells, where they are seen as 2-4 μm ovoid yeast with narrow-based budding. A retraction artifact in tissue sections may mimic encapsulation. *H capsulatum var duboisii* is contrasted with *H capsulatum var* capsulatum in t3.31.

In cultures incubated at 25-30°C, *H capsulatum* is a very slow growing, powdery or cottony white mold f3.37 that forms septated, hyaline hyphae with intermittent small (2-5 μm),

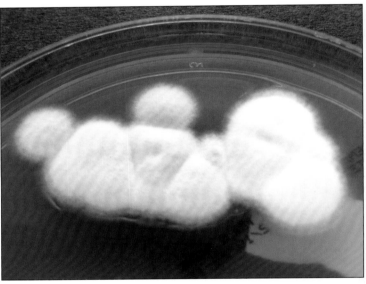

f3.37 *H capsulatum* cultured at 25-30°C colony morphology—powdery or cottony white mold

smooth, microconidia and large (7-15 μm), thick walled, spiny macroconidia f3.38. The latter are extremely helpful for morphology-based identification, but may be absent in immature cultures. This makes yeast conversion, exoantigen tests, or molecular confirmatory tests very important.

Histoplasmosis caused by *H capsulatum var capsulatum* is endemic in the eastern regions of the United States, and especially the Ohio and Mississippi River valleys. It is also found throughout Latin America. In the environment, the fungus favors soil contaminated by droppings from chickens, other birds, and bats, because of its high nitrogen content. *H capsulatum var duboisii* is found in Central and western Africa.

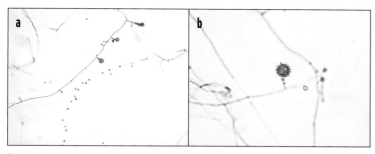

f3.38 *H capsulatum*; in mold form, demonstrates a septated, hyaline hyphae with intermittent small (2 μm), smooth, microconidia & b large (7-15 μm), thick walled, spiny macroconidia

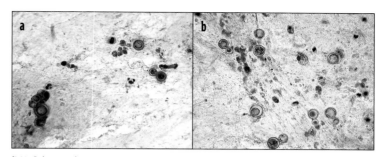

f3.39 *B dermatitidis*
a & b Smears demonstrate uniform, large (8-15 μm) yeasts with broad based budding; the yeast cell walls are thick & double contoured

t3.31 *Histoplasma capsulatum*

	var capsulatum	var duboisii
Geography	Worldwide, but most common in North and Central (Latin) America; eastern US represents the area of highest endemicity	Central and western Africa, especially Nigeria, Senegal, the Congo and Angola
Disease	Pulmonary, with or without dissemination to the reticuloendothelial system	May be localized or disseminated; most frequently involves skin, subcutaneous tissue & bone
Culture	Slowly growing, white cottony colonies; microscopic examination reveals hyaline, septate mold with smooth microconidia and thick-walled, tuberculate (spiked) macroconidia	Colony and microscopic morphology is indistinguishable from *var capsulatum*
Tissue	Often intracellular within histiocytes or reticuloendothelial cells; oval, small (2-4 μm) yeast bud on a narrow base	Often intracellular within giant cells or macrophages Round to oval, thick-walled yeast measuring 7-15 μm Bud on a narrow base, unlike *B dermatitidis*, the yeast of which are similar in size

Histoplasmosis caused by *H capsulatum var capsulatum* may be asymptomatic, or may cause acute or chronic pulmonary infection. Disseminated histoplasmosis may follow pulmonary infection, particularly in HIV/AIDS patients and other immunocompromised hosts. Disseminated infection may lead to oropharyngeal ulcers, hepatic and/or splenic involvement, or infection of the bone marrow, central nervous system, major arteries or cardiac valves. Histoplasmosis caused by *H capsulatum var duboisii* may be acquired by inhalation or by direct inoculation of the skin. It most often presents with skin (chronic ulcers), subcutaneous tissue involvement (nodules), or bone involvement (osteolytic lesions), and pulmonary infection is not a typical feature.

In addition to culture, the diagnosis of histoplasmosis can be made with an antigen test performed on urine or serum.

Blastomyces dermatitidis

In tissue sections, touch imprints f3.39, primary wet preparations, or culture at 37°C, *B dermatitidis* appears as fairly uniform, large (8-15 μm) yeasts with broad-based budding. The yeast cell walls are thick and double-contoured.

When cultured at 25-30°C, *B dermatitidis* is a slow growing mold, with a cottony, white surface that darkens to tan with age f3.40. Microscopic examination of the mold colonies reveals septate, hyaline hyphae with short, unbranched conidiophores producing single, pyriform to round, smooth conidia that measure 2-10 μm. The conidiophores together with their solitary conidia are sometimes referred to as "lollipops." Because this morphology is similar to that of certain nondimorphic molds

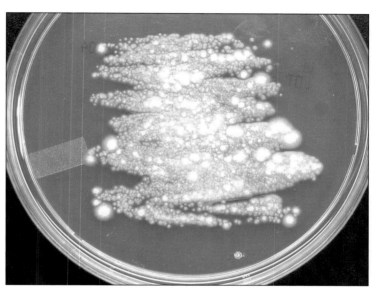

f3.40 *B dermatitidis*; the mold form has a cottony white surface that darkens to tan with age

(eg, *Chrysosporium*), definitive identification of *B dermatitidis* rests either on conversion to its yeast form at 37°C, or exoantigen tests or molecular confirmatory tests.

Blastomycosis has a geographic distribution that partly overlaps with that of Histoplasmosis, being endemic in the Mississippi and Ohio River valleys. It is also endemic in the Southeastern US and in areas bordering the Great Lakes (several states and Canadian provinces), and the St Lawrence Seaway (parts of New York and Canada). It is thought to thrive in the soil of wooded areas.

B dermatitidis initially infects the lung, where it can produce acute and/or chronic infection, although many infections are asymptomatic. Severe pulmonary disease and disseminated infection occur more frequently in immunocompromised hosts. Disseminated infection most often involves the skin or mucous membranes of the nasopharynx and mouth. Other common sites of disseminated infection include the bones, prostate, and central nervous system. Rare primary cutaneous blastomycosis may arise as a result of direct inoculation following trauma or dog bite. In addition to culture, the diagnosis can also be made with an antigen test performed on urine or serum.

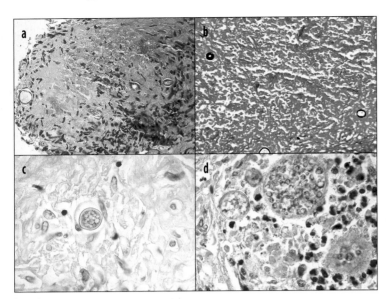

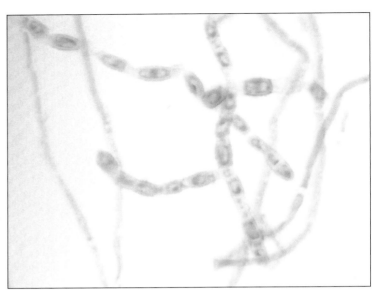

f3.41 *C immitis*
a, c-d In tissue sections stained with H&E, it appears as large (10-100 μm) spherules with thick, hyaline walls that enclose numerous tiny (2-5 μm) endospores, which do not bud
b The spherules are highlighted by GMS stain

f3.42 *C immitis*; in culture, mature arthroconidia are barrel shaped & alternate with empty cells

Coccidioides immitis/posadasii

In tissue sections f3.41 or primary wet preparations, *Coccidioides* is seen as large (10-100 μm) spherules with thick, hyaline walls that enclose numerous tiny (2-5 μm) endospores. The spherules may be confused with the sporangia of *Rhinosporidium seeberi* or *Prototheca* species. Sometimes the endospores are seen spilling from the spherules, and individual endospores may be confused with small yeasts such as those produced by *H capsulatum*. However, in contrast to yeast, the endospores of *Coccidioides* do not bud. Septated hyphae may also be seen in tissue, particularly in association with foreign material.

In routine culture, whether incubated at 25-30°C or 37°C, *C immitis* grows moderately to rapidly in its mold form, initially forming glabrous, moist, gray colonies that become white and cottony when mature. Microscopic examination reveals thin, hyaline, septate hyphae and arthroconidia. Mature arthroconidia are barrel shaped, and alternate with empty cells f3.42. However, immature arthroconidia are not barrel shaped and may resemble the arthroconidia of *Malbranchea* species. If special media are used, incubation at 37°C can produce the same morphology seen in tissue sections, including spherules.

Coccidioides has recently been divided into 2 separate species: *C immitis*, which is found mostly in the San Joaquin Valley of California, and *C posadasii*, which is found outside of California in the Southwestern United States (Arizona and New Mexico) as well as parts of Mexico and Central America. The 2 species are morphologically indistinguishable and produce the same clinical syndrome. The infectious arthroconidia are present in soil, and soil disruption or soil exposure are risk factors.

Coccidioides is acquired through inhalation of environmental arthroconidia, causing pulmonary infection. It may also disseminate, most commonly to skin but also to bone, joints, the meninges or other organs. Compromise of the immune system predisposes infected persons to dissemination (eg, HIV/AIDS, corticosteroid use), and for some reason those in certain ethnic groups (Filipino and African American) are at greater risk for dissemination. Pregnancy in the third trimester is another risk

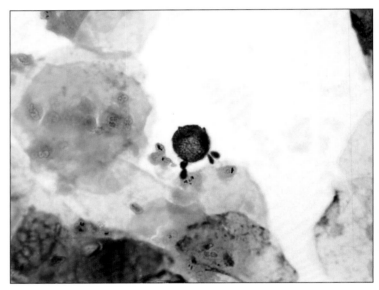

f3.43 *P brasiliensis* yeast form with circumferential budding

factor for severe disease. In addition to culture, the diagnosis can also be made with an antigen test performed on urine or serum, or with antibody testing.

Coccidioides is a risk to laboratory personnel and can be contracted from laboratory cultures.

Paracoccidioides brasiliensis

In tissue sections or primary wet preparations, the diagnostic form is a round, large (10-50 μm) yeast cell with circumferential budding, giving the appearance of a mariner's wheel f3.43. The daughter cells bud on a narrow base from the mother cell.

When cultured at 25-30°C, *P brasiliensis* is a slow growing mold with a white to tan surface and a variable texture that may be leathery, velvety or glabrous. Microscopic examination of the

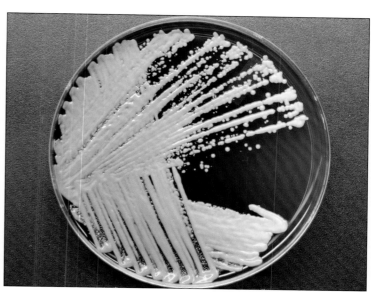

f3.44 *S schenckii* mold colonies cultured at 25-30°C

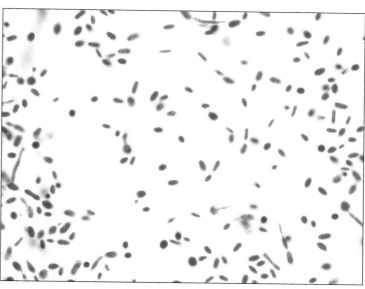

f3.46 *S schenckii*; yeast form cultured at 37°C

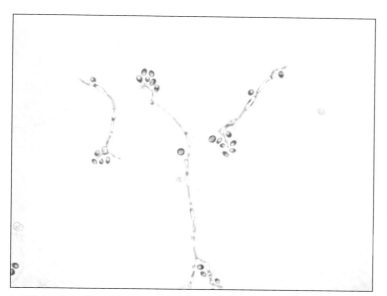

f3.45 *S schenckii* mold form; conidiophores topped by clusters of microconidia ("rosettes")

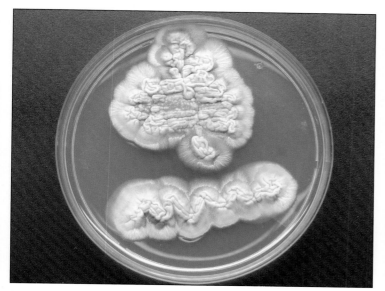

f3.47 *S schenckii* yeast form; "cigar bodies"

cultured mold reveals septate, hyaline hyphae with terminal and intercalary chlamydospores, and infrequent, pear shaped microconidia arranged along the hyphae. Definitive identification requires conversion of the mold form to the yeast form.

Paracoccidioidomycosis is encountered in the rainforests of Central and South America. It can be acquired either by inhalation or by direct inoculation during penetrating injury. In adults, pulmonary infection is chronic and indolent, and untreated infection often leads to dissemination involving the skin, oral mucosa, lymphatics, viscera or central nervous system. In children and immunocompromised hosts, the infection progresses more rapidly and frequently disseminates to involve bone marrow, lymphatics and the abdominal organs.

Sporothrix schenckii

In tissue sections or primary wet preparations, *S schenckii* appears as 4-6 µm elongated ("cigar shaped") yeasts with narrow based budding, usually seen in a background of purulent inflammation.

When cultured at 25-30°C, the mold form grows moderately to rapidly. Colonies are moist and white to pale orange initially, turning brown with age f3.44. Microscopic examination of the cultured mold reveals very delicate, hyaline, septate hyphae producing conidiophores topped by clusters of microconidia ("rosettes") f3.45. Definitive identification requires conversion of the mold form to the yeast form, which exists as tan to brown, creamy colonies f3.46. Yeast cells are oval or long and thin ("cigar bodies"), and bud on a narrow base f3.47.

Sporotrichosis is seen worldwide, although the majority of cases occur in North and South America. Infection is usually acquired by penetrating injury from contaminated plant material ("rose gardener's disease") or soil, although infection via the respiratory route occurs rarely. The most common clinical manifestation is lymphocutaneous infection, with nodular, ulcerative skin lesions following lymphatics.

Penicillium marneffei

In tissue sections or primary wet preparations, *P marneffei* appears as elongated, ovoid, small (3-5 µm) yeast that divide by fission rather than by budding. They are frequently found within histiocytes.

When cultured at 25-30°C, *P marneffei* forms rapidly growing, tan mold colonies that are initially powdery or velvety on the surface, and become colored with maturity (typically blue/green centrally, but other colors are also seen). A red pigment diffuses into the agar around and underneath the mold colonies; this is an important feature for correct identification. Microscopic examination of the mold colonies reveals features indistinguishable from other *Penicillium* species, including hyaline, septate hyphae with conidiophores and metulae producing brushlike clusters of phialides. Chains of small, oval conidia form at the terminal ends of the phialides. For concrete identification, thermal dimorphism should be demonstrated by converting the mold form to the yeast form at 37°C. Yeast colonies are off-white to pink, and consist of small (3-5 µm), oval yeastlike cells that reproduce by fission rather than by budding. Although they are yeastlike in appearance, they are actually single celled arthroconidia.

Penicilliosis marneffei is endemic in Southeast Asia, and is not found elsewhere. At particular risk are HIV/AIDS patients, among whom the infection is most prevalent. The usual portal of entry is the respiratory route, but pulmonary infection is not always a prominent clinical feature. Most cases lead to involving the bone marrow, skin, lymphatics, liver and spleen.

Thermally monomorphic molds
Hyaline septate molds (hyaline hyphomycetes)
Aspergillus species

Aspergillus species are ubiquitous in soil and on decaying vegetable matter. Hundreds of species have been described, but only a few are pathogenic for humans.

In tissue sections, *Aspergillus* species produce narrow (3-6 µm), uniform, hyaline, septate hyphae with characteristic acute-angle (45°) dichotomous, evenly-spaced (arboreal) branching f3.48. However, this appearance is not specific for aspergillosis and can represent other fungal species. The histologic differential diagnosis should also include *Fusarium*, *Scedosporium apiospermum* (*P boydii*), and many others. The exception is the rare circumstance in which the diagnostic fruiting heads of *Aspergillus* are seen in tissue sections. Normally, fruiting heads of *Aspergillus* are produced only in culture, and are not seen in vivo. However, if *Aspergillus* grows in an air-filled tissue pocket (as is sometimes the case in aspergilloma), its reproductive structures are produced and a definitive identification can be made by histology f3.49.

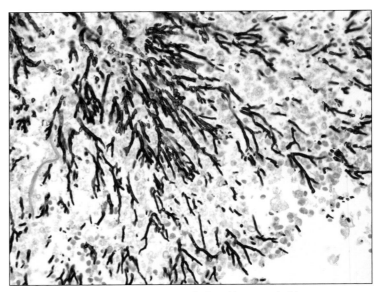

f3.48 *Aspergillus* species in tissue—narrow septate hyphae with acute-angle dichotomous evenly spaced branching is characteristic but not genus-specific

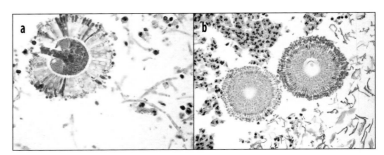

f3.49 *Aspergillus* species, when growing in an air-filled space (in this case a paranasal sinus) may demonstrate the formation of fruiting heads; in this case, *A niger*

On routine fungal media, *Aspergillus* is rapidly growing. Microscopically, all cultured *Aspergillus* species have in common that they produce a swollen vesicle ("aspergillum") at the end of each conidiophore. This feature is distinct to the genus. Identification to the species level is based on characteristic colony and microscopic morphology.

- *A fumigatus* colonies are blue-green with a distinct white apron f3.50a and a light reverse f3.50b. Microscopically, the species is notable for conidiophores that terminate in a swollen vesicle having a single row of phialides (uniseriate) that cover only the top 2/3 of the vesicle. Each phialide gives rise to a chain of small (2-4 µm), round conidia f3.51.

- *A flavus* produces yellow-green to olive colonies f3.52a with a light reverse f3.52b. Microscopic examination demonstrates circumferential phialides f3.53. Some strains are uniseriate, while others are biseriate. Importantly, when *A flavus* contaminates grains and other foodstuffs, it may produce aflatoxins, which are carcinogenic. Chronic exposure to aflatoxins by ingestion can lead to hepatocellular carcinoma.

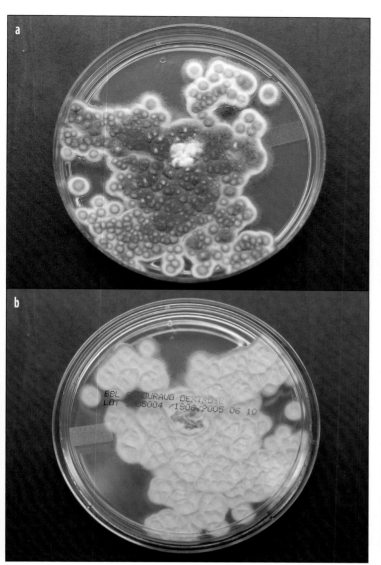

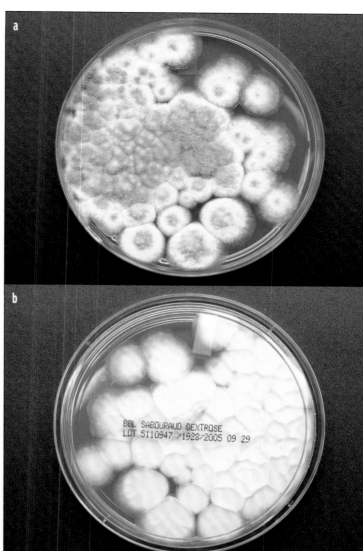

f3.50 *A fumigatus* colonies a are blue-green with a distinct white apron & b a light reverse

f3.52 *A flavus* colonies a are yellow-green to olive with b a light reverse

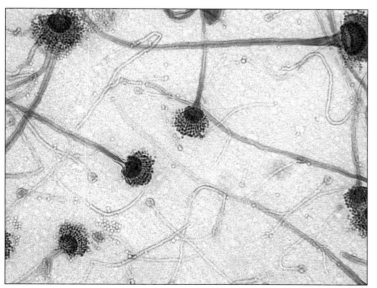

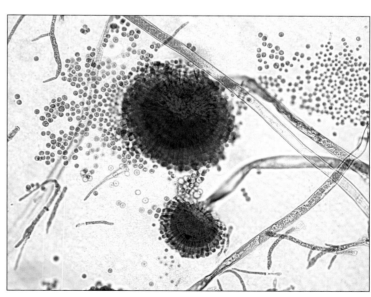

f3.51 *A fumigatus*: swollen vesicles with single row of phialides (uniseriate) that cover only the top 2/3 of the vesicle

f3.53 *A flavus*: circumferential phialides

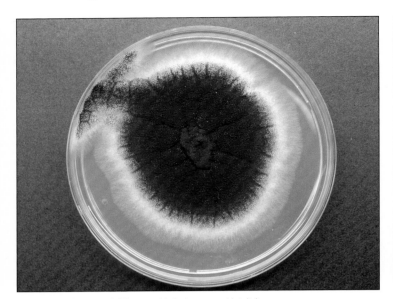

f3.54 *A niger* colonies are dark brown to black; the reverse side is light

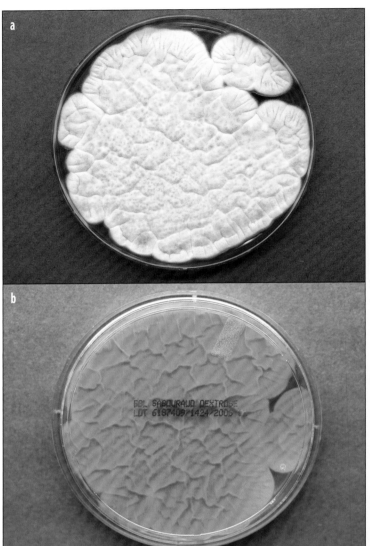

f3.56 *A terreus* colonies a are cinnamon brown on the surface with b a yellow or orange reverse

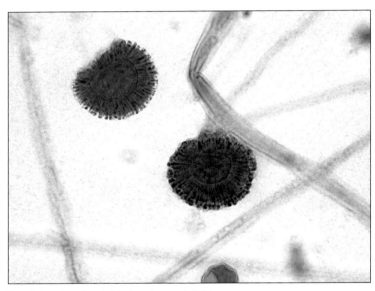

f3.55 *A niger*: circumferential biseriate pigmented phialides

- *A niger* cultures have a dark brown to black surface f3.54, due to the dark (non-melanin) pigmentation of the conidia, but the reverse side is light. This contrasts with cultures of dematiaceous molds, which tend to be darkly pigmented front and back, and contain melanin. Microscopic examination reveals vesicles with 2 rows of phialides (biseriate) covering the entire surface of the vesicle f3.55. Phialides produce chains of rough, round, dark conidia. Of note, *A niger* pulmonary infection is associated with oxalosis (calcium oxalate tissue deposition).

- *A terreus* colonies are cinnamon brown on the surface f3.56a, with a yellow or orange reverse f3.56b. Microscopically, *A terreus* looks superficially like *A fumigatus*, in that its phialides cover only the top 2/3 of the vesicle. In contrast to *A fumigatus*, though, *A terreus* is biseriate and typically has longer chains of conidia. *A terreus* is intrinsically resistant to amphotericin B, unlike *A fumigatus*, *A flavus* or *A niger*.

Aspergillosis most commonly affects the respiratory tract. The type of respiratory disease caused by *Aspergillus* depends on host factors. An immunocompetent individual with cavitary lung disease, such as from bronchiectasis or old tuberculosis, is prone to develop the saprophytic form of aspergillosis: an aspergilloma (fungus ball), which is a noninvasive colonization. Allergic bronchopulmonary aspergillosis (ABPA) is a condition in which *Aspergillus* colonizes the airway, without invasion, and elicits a marked allergic response characterized by mucus impaction, peripheral eosinophilia, and reactive airways. The inflammatory response can be sufficiently severe

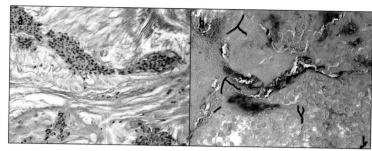

f3.57 Allergic fungal sinusitis
a A clue is eosinophil-permeated mucin containing b fungal hyphae on GMS stained sections

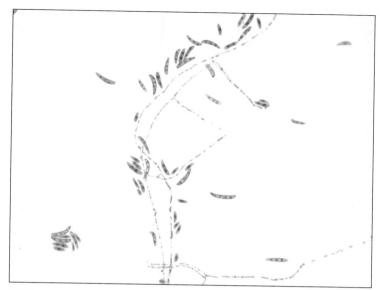

f3.58 *Fusarium* species

to cause hemoptysis and eventual bronchiectasis. This form of aspergillosis is often seen in patients with an atopic history; there is also an increased incidence of the cystic fibrosis transmembrane regulator (CFTR) gene mutations in patients with this condition. The diagnosis can be supported with tests for serum anti-*Aspergillus* IgE, elevated total serum IgE, *Aspergillus* skin tests, and peripheral eosinophilia. Allergic sinonasal aspergillosis (allergic fungal sinusitis) is a related condition which can be diagnosed on the basis of sinus curetting histology: inflamed sinonasal mucosa and eosinophil-permeated mucin containing fungal hyphae f3.57. An individual with emphysema or other structural lung disease, who is receiving steroid therapy, is prone to develop semi-invasive pulmonary aspergillosis, also called chronic necrotizing pulmonary aspergillosis. Here, the mold colonizes cavitary regions of the emphysematous lung parenchyma, and invades superficially into the surrounding lung tissue. Finally, profoundly immunosuppressed hosts are susceptible to invasive bronchopulmonary aspergillosis (IBPA) or invasive fungal sinusitis, very serious conditions in which the mold invades tissue and blood vessels, and may disseminate. *Aspergillus* species and the zygomycetes have a propensity to invade vessel walls (angioinvasion) and give rise to tissue infarction. Confirming the diagnosis of IBPA is difficult and may require lung biopsy. Therefore, there has been growing use of an ELISA assay for the serum marker galactomannan, a cell wall constituent released during tissue invasion by *Aspergillus*. The assay is best used as a screening tool for early detection in asymptomatic, immunosuppressed patients. Another fungal antigen assay can detect serum 1-3-β-D-glucan, a marker for invasive fungal infection by a wide range of agents, including *Aspergillus* species. A positive serum 1-3-β-D-glucan test can complement a positive serum galactomannan test, increasing the positive predictive value.

Other hyaline hyphomycetes

This group of organisms is known for causing such infections as mycotic keratitis, onychomycosis, and eumycotic mycetoma, and some genera are associated with more serious invasive infections. *Fusarium* species cause a spectrum of infections overlapping with those caused by *Aspergillus* species, including invasive pulmonary and sinus infections, and disseminated infection, in immunocompromised hosts, and fungus ball or allergic bronchopulmonary disease in immunocompetent hosts. *Fusarium* species also cause fungal keratitis, particularly in contact lens wearers, as well as onychomycosis.

In addition, *Fusarium* has recently emerged as an important opportunistic pathogen in burn wounds. *Pseudallescheria boydii/Scedosporium boydii* causes eumycotic mycetoma after penetrating trauma, fungal keratitis, and pneumonia after near-drowning accidents. In immunocompromised hosts, *P boydii/S boydii* causes invasive pulmonary or sinus infections, and disseminated infection. It is intrinsically resistant to amphotericin B.

The hyaline hyphomycetes can be distinguished based on their colony and microscopic morphology. One key aspect of their microscopic morphology is the arrangement of their conidia. Useful information can be acquired simply by observing whether the conidia occur singly, in clusters, or in branching chains.

Conidia arranged in clusters: *Fusarium, Acremonium, Gliocladium. Fusarium* species form canoe shaped, multicellular macroconidia with 3-6 cells each, often clumping together f3.58. Some strains may also produce smaller, 1-2 celled microconidia in clusters at the apex of unbranched conidiophores. *Acremonium* species are characterized by long, threadlike, unbranched phialides bearing clusters of single celled microconidia. *Gliocladium* species have branching conidiophores bearing flask shaped phialides, resembling *Penicillium*. However, microconidia do not chain but rather cluster in a ball, resembling a golf ball held at the end of outstretched fingertips.

Conidia arranged in chains: *Penicillium, Paecilomyces, Scopulariopsis. Penicillium* species are characterized by a brush-like arrangement of flask shaped phialides that give rise to unbranching chains of microconidia. The phialides are present on metulae (secondary branches of conidiophores). *Paecilomyces* species have branching conidiophores with elongated, flask shaped phialides arranged in pairs or brush-like groups. Long chains of oval or spindle shaped microconidia emanate from the phialides. *Scopulariopsis species* have single or branched conidiophores that give rise to annellides (similar to phialides). Annellides are often clustered in a brush-like

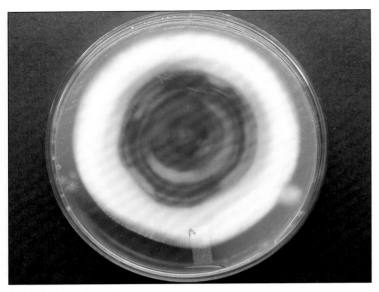

f3.59 *Trichophyton rubrum*; red reverse

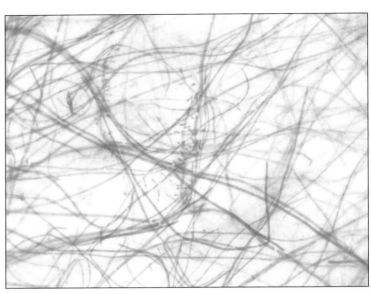

f3.60 *Trichophyton rubrum*; birds on a wire

arrangement. Each annellide bears a chain of rough-walled, round or truncated microconidia.

Conidia arranged singly: *Chrysosporium* species, *Sepedonium* species, and *Beuveria* species. *Chrysosporium* species form single, cutoff microconidia directly on hyphae or on the tips of simple conidiophores. They sometimes also produce intercalary, cylindrical conidia resembling arthroconidia. *Sepedonium* species have single-borne, hyaline conidia at the ends of branched or unbranched conidiophores. The conidia are large, thick walled and echinulate, resembling the macroconidia of the mold form of *H capsulatum*. *Beuveria* species are characterized by single, small, round or oval microconidia emerging from each inflection point in a zigzagging (geniculate), flask shaped conidiophore. Although the conidia appear singly, the conidiophores themselves typically cluster together.

Dermatophytes

Dermatophytes are considered separately from other hyaline septate molds because they share certain unique features. They are keratinophilic, meaning that they are able to digest keratin as nutrient source using keratinases. This special ability informs their pathogenicity, which is mostly limited to infection of superficial, keratinized structures such as hair, nails, and the stratum corneum of skin. In addition, they are uniformly resistant to cycloheximide, a feature that is leveraged in culture strategies by including a cycloheximide-containing medium when culturing for dermatophytes.

Rapid diagnosis of dermatophytosis can be made with a bedside KOH prep or calcofluor white prep of skin scrapings. This does not permit species identification, which is not always necessary to guide therapy.

Dermatophytes are speciated based upon characteristic colony and microscopic morphology after culture. *Trichophyton rubrum* has a particularly distinctive colony morphology, because it produces a red pigment that causes the reverse side of the plate to appear red f3.59. Microscopically, the dermatophytes appear as hyaline, septate hyphae that produce

microconidia, macroconidia, or both. These reproductive structures are often the key to a species-level identification.

- *Trichophyton rubrum*: tear shaped microconidia are arranged along the hyphae, producing a "birds on a telephone wire" appearance f3.60.

- *Trichophyton mentagrophytes*: microconidia are arranged in clusters, and occasional spiral hyphae may be seen. Club shaped macroconidia are sometimes present, containing 1-6 cells each. *T mentagrophytes* has the ability to penetrate hair shafts, unlike *T rubrum*, which can appear morphologically similar to some strains of *T mentagrophytes*.

- *Trichophyton tonsurans* is distinctive for the marked size and shape variability of its microconidia. Microconidia may be round, tear shaped, cigar shaped, or swollen and enlarged. Intercalary chlamydospores are common, particularly in mature cultures.

- *Microsporum canis*: macroconidia are spindle shaped and rough (echinulate), and taper to a knob-like end. Each macroconidium contains >6 cells, separated by transverse septae.

- *Microsporum gypseum*: macroconidia are oval shaped structures with rounded ends and transverse septae. Each macroconidium contains 3-6 cells.

- *Epidermophyton floccosum*: macroconidia are smooth, club shaped structures with rounded ends, which may be found singly or in characteristic clusters. Each macroconidium contains 2-6 cells, separated by transverse septae. Microconidia are never produced.

Dermatophyte infection may take many forms, including tinea capitis (scalp ringworm), tinea corporis (ringworm), tinea cruris (jock itch), tinea pedis (athlete's foot), and tinea unguium (onychomycosis). Multiple dermatophyte species can cause the same clinical manifestation.

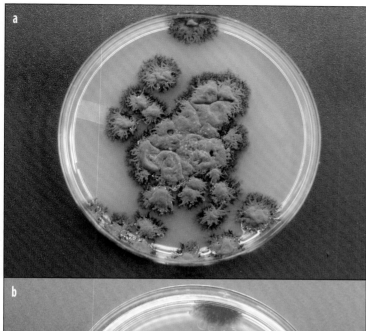

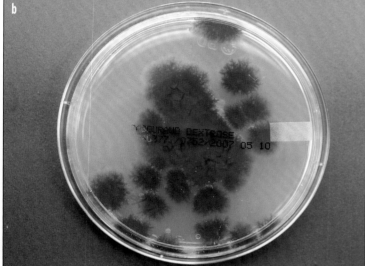

f3.61 Dematiaceous molds are typically pigmented a on the surface & b reverse side of the plate

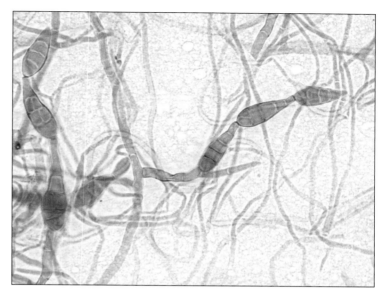

f3.62 *Alternaria* species form chains of conidia with transverse & longitudinal (muriform) septations; one end of each conidium is blunt & the other pointed

Dermatophytes may be classified according to their natural habitat, which informs the mode of transmission. Anthropophilic dermatophytes principally infect humans, and are transmitted between individuals either directly or via fomites. Major examples include *T rubrum*, *T tonsurans* and *Epidermophyton floccosum*. Zoophilic dermatophytes infect animals, and can be transmitted to humans by animal contact. Important examples include *T mentagrophytes* (rodents), *M canis* (cats and dogs), *T verrucosum* (cattle), and *T equinum* (horses). Geophilic dermatophytes are soil inhabitants that rarely infect humans, with the exception of *M gypseum*.

Dematiaceous molds

The unifying feature among dematiaceous molds is production of melanin pigment, conferring dark pigmentation. Dematiaceous molds typically are darkly pigmented on the surface and reverse side of the plate, because both their hyphae and conidia are melanized f3.61. However, some species are melanized only in their conidia, resulting in a dark surface

with a lighter reverse side, and other species do the opposite. The first 2 groups below (conidia with internal septae) grow relatively rapidly, while the last group is a short list of disparate slow growers. In tissue, there are no features that permit distinction to the genus level, but intrinsic dark pigmentation is a clue to the presence of a dematiaceous mold.

Conidia with transverse septae: *Bipolaris*, *Drechslera*, *Exserohilum*, *Helminthosporum*, *Curvularia*.

- *Bipolaris* is characterized by oval, transversely septated conidia that arise from bent (geniculate) conidiophores. *Bipolaris* gets its name from the production of germ tubes from both ends of the conidia in saline mounts incubated for 12-24 hours. Each conidium contains 3-5 septations.

- The genus *Drechslera* produces similar conidia but is distinguished from *Bipolaris* by its lack of production of bipolar germ tubes in saline incubation; instead, it produces germ tubes along the sides of the conidia.

- *Exserohilum* also resembles *Bipolaris*, except that its conidia are longer and thinner, and have more septations (5-12).

- *Helminthosporium* has a highly characteristic bottle brush-like microscopic appearance, with side by side conidia arranged in whorls along the conidiophores.

- *Curvularia* is easy to recognize, since its transversely septated conidia curve distinctly when mature.

Conidia with transverse & longitudinal septae: *Alternaria*, *Ulocladium*, *Stemphilium*.

- *Alternaria* species produce chains of transverse and longitudinally septated (muriform—resembling a brick wall) conidia that have alternating blunt and pointed ends f3.62.

- *Ulocladium* is characterized by oval muriform conidia borne singly on bent (geniculate) conidiophores. The conidiophores bend in a zigzag fashion.

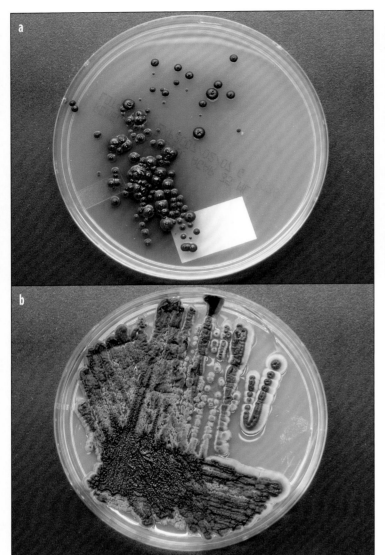

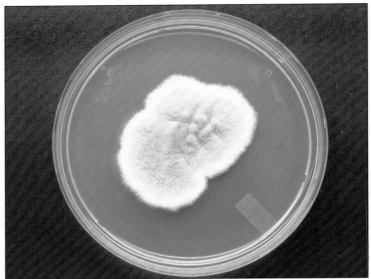

f3.64 *Pseudallescheria boydii/Scedosporium boydii* complex forms a mold colony with a light brown melanized surface

f3.63 A slow growing dematiaceous mold whose **a** early colony morphology is smooth & moist (yeastlike) & whose **b** late colony morphology is fuzzy (moldlike); this would be typical of *Exophiala, Wangiella* & *Hortaea*

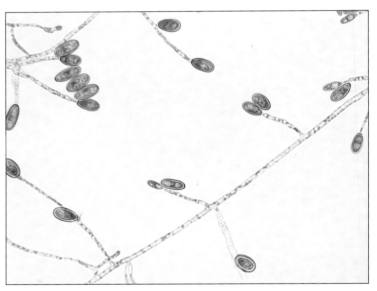

f3.65 *Pseudallescheria boydii/Scedosporium boydii* complex: oval, truncated, melanized microconidia with non-melanized hyphae

- *Stemphilium* conidia resemble those of ulocladium but are borne upon straight conidiophores, and frequently the conidiophores will each produce only a single, terminal conidium.

Slow growing dematiaceous molds may be grouped into 2 categories: those whose early growth is yeastlike (becoming moldlike with age), and those whose early and late growth is moldlike. Those with yeastlike early growth produce smooth, moist colonies in early culture f3.63a, composed of budding yeastlike cells. With age, the colonies become fuzzy f3.63b and the microscopic morphology converts to septate hyphae with conidia formation. Examples include *Exophiala, Wangiella,* and *Hortaea.* Those with moldlike early growth produce fuzzy colonies from the beginning. Examples include *Pseudallescheria boydii/Scedosporium boydii* complex and *Scedosporium prolificans.*

The name "*P boydii*" refers to the sexual state of the mold, whereas *S boydii* refers to its asexual state. In either state, the mold has a light gray or brown surface f3.64, owing to melanization of its oval, truncated microconidia f3.65. Its septate hyphae are hyaline (non-melanized), resulting in a light reverse, which can darken with age. In its sexual state, the mold produces large (50-200 μm), dark cleistothecia f3.66, whereas the asexual form lacks this feature but is otherwise indistinguishable. An alternative asexual form of the same mold, called *Graphium,* is also sometimes seen. Its colony morphology is indistinguishable from *P boydii* or *S boydii,* but microscopically it is characterized by thick mats of long conidiophores stuck together side by side, resembling the bristles of a broom f3.67. *P boydii/S boydii* complex molds are intrinsically resistant to amphotericin B, but are usually susceptible to triazoles such as voriconazole and posaconazole. A closely related species, *Scedosporium apiospermum* was thought until recently to be an

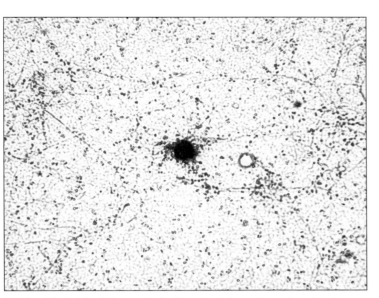

f3.66 *Pseudallescheria boydii/Scedosporium boydii* complex: in the sexual state, the mold produces large dark cleistothecia

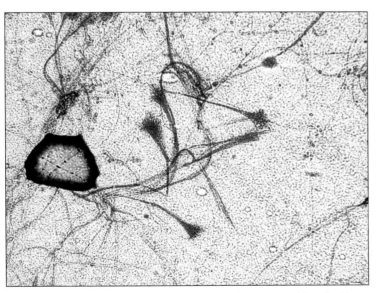

f3.67 *Pseudallescheria boydii/Scedosporium boydii* complex: the alternative asexual form, *Graphium*, characterized by thick mats of long conidiophores stuck together side by side, resembling the bristles of a broom

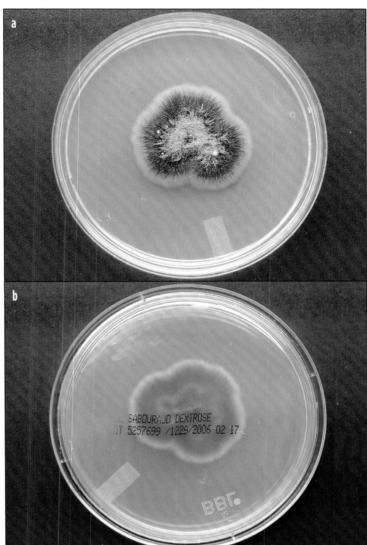

f3.68 *Scedosporium prolificans* has a gray or black a surface & b reverse

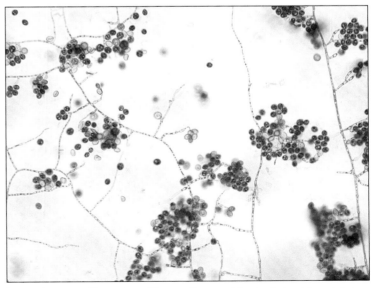

f3.69 *Scedosporium prolificans* microconidia are oval & truncated, forming clusters at the end of annellides, which have swollen bases & thin necks

asexual form of *P boydii*, but is newly recognized as a separate species. It is morphologically identical to *S boydii*, and is best distinguished using molecular methods.

Scedosporium prolificans has a gray or black surface and reverse f3.68. Unlike *P boydii/S boydii*, its growth is inhibited by cycloheximide, and it has no sexual state. Microconidia are oval and truncated, forming clusters at the end of annellides (conidiogenous cells) f3.69. The annellides have swollen bases and thin necks. *S prolificans* is intrinsically resistant not only to amphotericin B, but also to the azoles and echinocandins, making antifungal therapy ineffective.

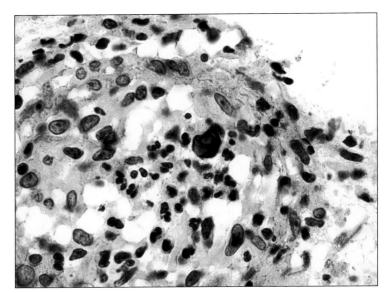

f3.70 Chromoblastomycosis, demonstrating muriform bodies (sclerotic bodies having internal septations in more than one plane)

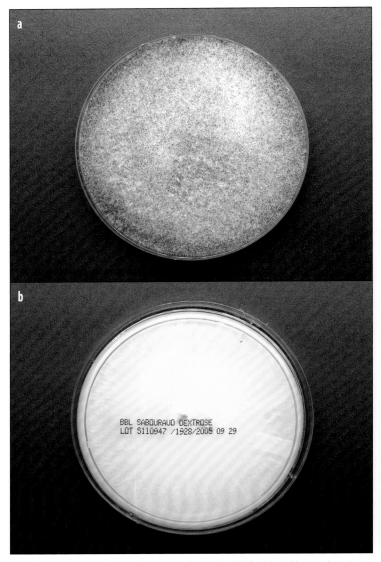

f3.71 *Rhizopus* species in culture: colonies are rapidly growing (lid lifters) & quickly cover the entire agar surface; they are initially cottony & white, turning light brown with sporulation

Infections caused by dematiaceous molds can be classified as chromoblastomycosis, mycetoma, or phaeohyphomycosis, based on the appearance of the fungus in tissue and the associated clinical manifestations.

Chromoblastomycosis is a subcutaneous mycosis associated with prominent pseudoepitheliomatous hyperplasia of the overlying skin (cauliflower-like or warty lesions). In tissue, one sees pigmented hyphae and sclerotic bodies. The latter are small (5-12 μm) round, dark structures with internal septations in more than 1 plane (muriform) f3.70. *Fonsecaea pedrosoi*, *Phialophora verrucosa*, and *Cladophialophora carrionii* are the principal agents of chromoblastomycosis, which is found in tropical and subtropical areas, particularly where shoes are not regularly worn. The organisms gain entrance through puncture wounds, so infections tend to be found on the lower extremities. Lesions are usually solitary and may take the form of verrucous lesions, nodules, or massive tumors.

Mycetoma (also known as Madura foot or Maduromycosis) is another form of subcutaneous infection, in which a slowly-developing subcutaneous nodule is formed, often with draining sinus tracts to the skin. Mycetoma can be caused by filamentous bacteria (actinomycotic mycetoma) or by molds (eumycotic mycetoma). Eumycotic mycetoma is frequently caused by dematiaceous molds, although it can also be caused by certain hyaline molds. Within the subcutaneous nodule are granules composed of clusters of the infectious agent within a proteinaceous matrix. Like chromoblastomycosis, mycetoma is usually the result of a puncture wound. The causes of eumycotic mycetoma include *Madurella, Exophiala, Wangiella*, and *P boydii/S boydii*. Actinomycotic mycetomas are caused by aerobic actinomycetes, such as *Nocardia* species

Phaeohyphomycosis is a catch-all term for infections caused by dematiaceous molds that do not fit into the chromoblastomycosis or eumycotic mycetoma categories. Infections may involve any organ system. In tissue, agents of phaeohyphomycosis form dark, septate hyphae, as well as yeastlike forms and forms that resemble pseudohyphae.

Zygomycetes (pauciseptate molds)

The zygomycetes grow extremely rapidly both in vivo and in culture. The hyphae are broad and have few septations, making them floppy and ribbonlike. Branching is infrequent, haphazard, and nondichotomous. Care must be taken not to grind specimens prior to culture if zygomycosis is a clinical consideration, as the grinding process can easily disrupt all the viable hyphae. Tissue specimens should be minced instead.

The zygomycetes can be distinguished from one another based on certain microscopic features. It is important to note the presence or absence of rootlike structures called rhizoids, and their location, and to determine whether the sporangiophores are branched or unbranched (simple). The presence or absence of an apophysis at the sporangiophore's apex should also be noted. Distinguishing features of some commonly isolated zygomycetes are described below.

- *Rhizopus* species f3.71, f3.72 produce rhizoids and unbranched sporangiophores that arise directly over the rhizoids. Their sporangia (sack-like structures that

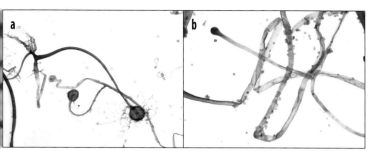

f3.72 *Rhizopus* species produce rhizoids & unbranched sporangiophores that arise directly over the rhizoids; their sporangia are prominent spherical structures that tend to collapse when mature, resembling a collapsed umbrella; their sporangiophores lack an apophysis

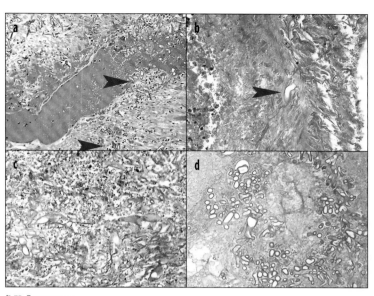

f3.75 Zygomycetes
a A necrotic vessel containing angioinvasive ribbonlike hyphae seen better b at high magnification in H&E stained sections
c The trichrome stained section highlights the residual vessel wall
d A residual thrombosed vessel in cross section, with numerous mural hyphae

contain spores) are prominent spherical structures full of tiny spores which tend to collapse when mature, resembling a collapsed umbrella. Sporangiophores lack an apophysis.

- *Mucor* species f3.73, f3.74 do not produce rhizoids. Sporangiophores can be branched or unbranched, but lack an apophysis. Their sporangia are large spherical structures that tend to fall apart, releasing their numerous spores.

- *Lichtheimia* (formerly *Absidia*) produces rhizoids but its sporangiophores arise at points between rhizoids, rather than over the rhizoids. Sporangiophores are branched and form a conical apophysis at the top.

- *Cunninghamella* species differ from most zygomycetes in that their branched sporangiophores are topped by large vesicles. The vesicles are covered with spines (denticles), each of which supports a single spore contained within a round sporangiolum.

Zygomycetes may produce several forms of invasive infection: rhinocerebral, pulmonary, gastrointestinal, and cutaneous. Hosts are typically immunocompromised, and important risk factors include uncontrolled diabetes (especially ketoacidosis), stem cell or solid organ transplantation, neutropenia, corticosteroid therapy or severe burns. Like *Aspergillus* species, the zygomycetes characteristically invade vessel walls and thereby produce parenchymal infarction and sometimes disseminated infection. They can be seen in routine H&E-stained sections f3.75.

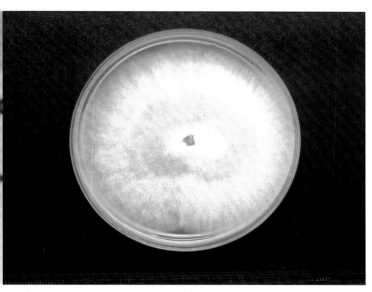

f3.73 *Mucor* species: colonies are rapidly growing (lid lifters), fluffy & become pigmented with the development of sporangia

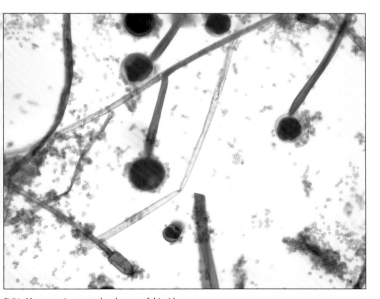

f3.74 *Mucor* species: note the absence of rhizoids
Sporangiophores can be branched or unbranched, but lack an apophysis
Their sporangia are large spherical structures that tend to fall apart, releasing their numerous spores

Fungal isolate growing in culture at 25-30°C as yeast: yeast & yeastlike fungi

Approach to identification

Presumptive identification methods

Chromogenic agar plates (Chromagar) are available that are selective for yeast, while inhibiting the growth of bacteria, and allowing for differentiation between some common *Candida* species on the basis of colony color after incubation. Chromogenic compounds within the medium are used to demonstrate enzyme activity that is species specific. If primary specimens are directly cultured on this medium, a presumptive identification of *C albicans*, *C tropicalis*, or *C krusei* can be made after 24-48 hour incubation at 35-37°C. This method is particularly useful in fungal culture of specimens from the vagina, oropharynx, stool or urine, where *Candida* species are frequently encountered along with resident bacterial flora.

Germ tube test

This assay can be performed on yeast isolates (after initial culture) to rapidly identify *C albicans* presumptively. The test relies on 2 principles

1. Yeast cells of *C albicans* begin to produce hyphal elements (pseudohyphae and true hyphae) more rapidly than most other species

2. *C albicans* yeast cells are able to produce true hyphae without a constriction between the mother cell and the hyphal element, whereas most yeast species can produce only pseudohyphae, which do have a constriction

Briefly, yeast are suspended in serum and incubated at 37°C for up to 3 hours (no more). A wet mount is prepared and examined for the formation of germ tubes—yeast cells producing hyphae with no constriction at the juncture with the yeast cell. Sensitivity is good but not 100%, and the absence of germ tubes does not rule out *C albicans*. Specificity is also high, but *C dubliniensis* also produces germ tubes within 3 hours.

Rapid trehalose assimilation

This test can presumptively identify *C glabrata*, using yeast isolates after initial culture. Unlike most other yeast, *C glabrata* has the ability to ferment trehalose rapidly at 42°C. To perform the test, a yeast isolate is inoculated into broth containing trehalose and a pH indicator. After a short (3 hour) incubation at 42°C, fermentation of the substrate causes a color change, indicating a positive result. The test is very sensitive, and specificity is high, particularly if one only tests isolates with appropriate microscopic morphology (small budding yeast producing no pseudohyphae, and germ tube negative).

Urease test

Detection of urease enzyme activity can distinguish ascomycetous yeasts, which do not have urease activity, from basidiomycetous yeasts, which do. It is most commonly used to presumptively identify *Cryptococcus* species isolates after initial culture. Urea disks are available for rapid testing and can detect urease activity by a color change within a few hours. An alternative method involves the use of urea agar slants, but this requires a longer incubation. A positive urease test can aid in the presumptive identification of *Cryptococcus* species, when accompanied by appropriate colony morphology and microscopic morphology. Importantly, other commonly isolated basidiomycetous yeasts are also urease+, including *Rhodotorula* species and *Trichosporon* species, so a positive urease test alone cannot be relied upon to presumptively identify *Cryptococcus* species

Phenol oxidase test

Demonstration of phenol oxidase enzyme activity can differentiate *Cryptococcus neoformans* from nonneoformans *Cryptococcus* species and from other yeast genera. *C neoformans* is uniquely able to oxidize diphenolic compounds such as caffeic acid, dopamine, and dopa to produce darkly pigmented melanin or melanin precursors. The classic phenol oxidase test involves culturing a yeast isolate on bird seed agar, a natural source of caffeic acid. Growth of brown-pigmented yeast colonies after overnight incubation supports the presumptive identification of *C neoformans*, whereas white or nonpigmented colonies indicate a negative result. A more rapid method involves the use of caffeic acid disks, which are inoculated with a yeast isolate and can demonstrate brown pigment production within a few hours.

Definitive identification methods

Assimilation tests

These tests assess the ability of an isolate to use a particular carbohydrate as its sole carbon source, or its ability to use nitrate as its sole source of nitrogen. Several commercially-available, biochemical identification systems are available that combine a battery of assimilation tests for yeast identification. Because these systems rely on yeast metabolism, a prolonged incubation period (18-48 hours) is required to obtain results. However, they are accurate and provide a species-level identification along with a confidence score, to help interpret the results.

MALDI-TOF mass spectrometry

This method allows for the analysis of yeast isolates without the need for growth and metabolism, and therefore can provide a full identification in a matter of minutes. In this method, an isolate taken from an agar plate is transferred to a target slide. The sample on the target slide is then overlaid with a matrix solution, and loaded into the ionization chamber of a matrix-assisted laser desorption/ionization time of flight (MALDI-TOF) mass spectrometer. The sample is irradiated by a laser, causing the sample/matrix mixture to vaporize. During this process, proteins in the sample acquire an electrical charge. Electric fields in the instrument then push the charged proteins into a vacuum tube. The time of flight through the vacuum tube is measured, and used to determine the mass of each protein within a certain size range. From these data, a mass spectrum is compiled, which serves as a type of fingerprint that can be used to identify the organism. The mass spectrum generated from the sample is compared to a database of spectra generated from known yeast species, to provide a species-level identification and an associated confidence score. The same methodology can be used to identify bacteria, mycobacteria, and molds.

Demonstration of specific morphology using specialized media: Certain media, especially rice or cornmeal agar supplemented with Tween 80, will reliably induce formation of characteristic yeast structures such as blastoconidia, pseudohyphae, true hyphae, arthroconidia or chlamydospores (chlamydoconidia). Microscopic examination can be performed by dropping

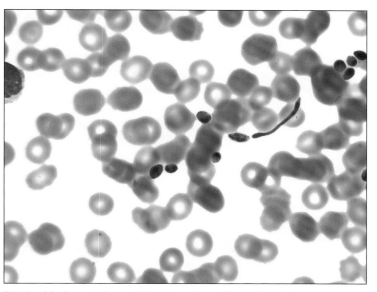

f3.76 Pseudohyphae: note the constriction between the yeast & the hyphal structure

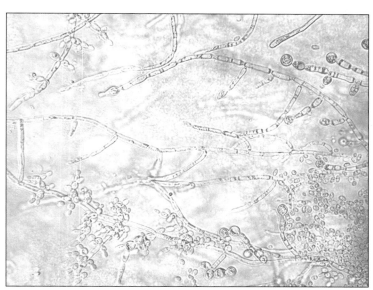

f3.78 *C albicans* on yeast morphology medium: pseudohyphae with clusters of blastoconidia at septations & single terminal chlamydospores

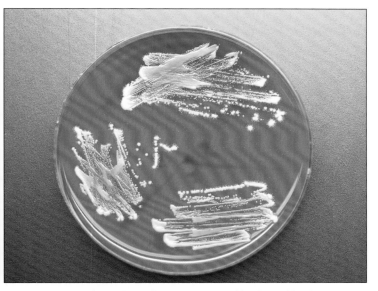

f3.77 *C albicans* colonies frequently form filamentous extensions ("feet") around the edges

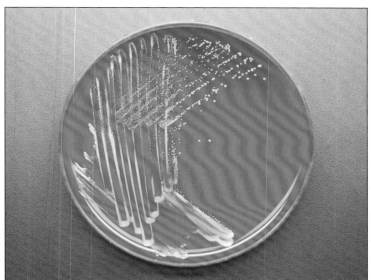

f3.79 *C glabrata*: slow growing smooth creamy colonies lacking "feet"

a coverslip directly on the agar and examining the yeast structures through the coverslip. This method can be used alone to identify yeast, but is more often used as a supplemental test when more convenient identification methods prove inadequate for definitive identification of a particular isolate.

Notes on specific yeasts
Candida species

C albicans is by far the most common *Candida* species isolated from humans, regardless of specimen type or host. On direct examination, *C albicans* appears as 3-5 µm budding yeast with accompanying pseudohyphae f3.76, and occasionally true hyphae as well. Colonies grown on solid medium frequently form filamentous extensions ("feet") around the edges f3.77—a characteristic that helps to differentiate *C albicans* from nonalbicans species. When cultured on yeast morphology medium (cornmeal or rice agar with Tween), *C albicans* forms pseudohyphae with clusters of blastoconidia present at the septations. In addition, single, terminal chlamydospores are seen f3.78. *C albicans* is positive by the germ tube test and forms green colonies on chromogenic agar. Most clinical isolates are susceptible to azole agents, echinocandins, and amphotericin B.

C glabrata is frequently isolated from blood and urine. Direct examination reveals small (2-4 µm) budding yeast (blastoconidia), without pseudohyphae or other structures. In culture, isolates are relatively slow growing in comparison to other *Candida* species, and may take an extra day of incubation for

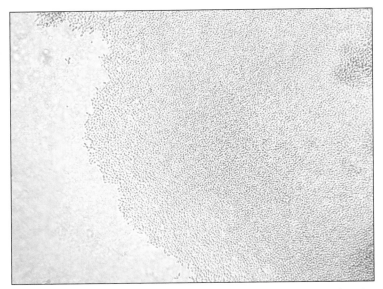

f3.80 *C glabrata* on yeast morphology medium: budding yeast with no additional structures formed

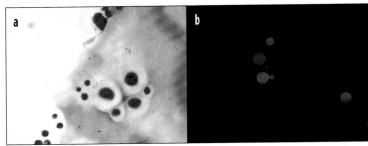

f3.81 *C neoformans*: a Wright stain & b calcofluor white show spherical, narrow-budding yeasts that vary greatly in size

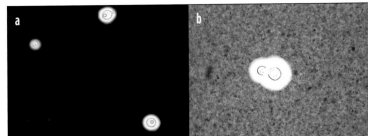

f3.82 *C neoformans*: India ink preparation at a low & b high magnification show spherical, narrow-budding yeasts with thick capsule

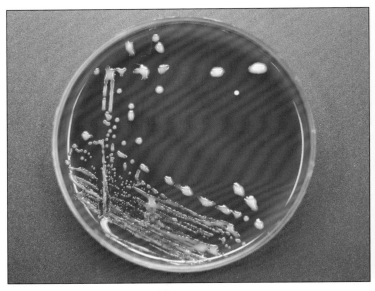

f3.83 *C neoformans*: mucoid colonies on solid agar

mature colony formation f3.79. Yeast morphology medium does not induce structures other than budding yeast f3.80. *C glabrata* is positive by the rapid trehalose assimilation test. A significant proportion of clinical isolates has reduced susceptibility or frank resistance to azole agents (both imidazoles and triazoles), but most isolates are susceptible to echinocandins and amphotericin B.

Certain other *Candida* species are predictably resistant to antifungal agents. *C krusei* is intrinsically resistant to fluconazole, but isolates are generally susceptible to the triazoles, echinocandins and amphotericin B. *C lusitaniae* is considered resistant to amphotericin B, despite low MICs in many cases by in vitro testing. *C parapsilosis*, *C krusei*, *C guilliermondii* and *C lusitaniae* sometimes exhibit relatively high MICs for echinocandins, but frank resistance is unusual.

Cryptococcus neoformans

Although there are numerous species within the genus, the main human pathogens are *C neoformans* and *C gattii*. Previously, *C gattii* was considered a variety of *C neoformans*, but these have now been classified as separate species. *C neoformans* is the cause of most infections in the US. *C gattii*, previously confined to tropical zones, has now been reported as an emerging infection in the Pacific northwest region of the United States.

In histologic sections or direct wet mounts, cryptococci present as spherical, narrow-budding yeasts that vary in size from 3-15 μm f3.81. The yeast are encapsulated (although rare capsule-deficient strains exist), a feature that can be highlighted in tissue using a mucicarmine stain, or in wet mounts using india ink f3.82. The yeast cell walls contain melanin, which makes them positive by the Fontana-Masson stain in tissue sections. Colonies grown on solid agar are frequently mucoid f3.83, owing to the capsular material. Whether visualized directly in primary specimens or after culture, *Cryptococcus* forms only budding yeast, and never forms other structures like pseudohyphae.

The cryptococcal capsular polysaccharide antigen can be detected in either serum or body fluids (usually CSF). Latex particles coated with antibodies against cryptococcal capsular antigen form the basis for this simple agglutination test.

C neoformans is acquired by inhalation during exposure to contaminated soil, particularly soil containing bird excreta (eg, pigeon, chicken). *C gattii* appears to be associated with trees, especially eucalyptus trees. *C gattii* has become increasingly relevant in the US for 2 reasons: it is an emerging infection in the Pacific northwest, and seems capable of causing infection in immunocompetent hosts.

Infected patients typically present with respiratory symptoms, especially tachypnea, bilateral interstitial infiltrates, and hypoxemia. Serum LD is usually very high. Serologic testing is not helpful. Respiratory samples such as bronchoalveolar lavage (BAL) are ideal, but induced sputum may provide sufficient sensitivity in severely immunocompromised hosts. The organisms, within typical exudate f3.84, are easily seen on Pap-stained, Giemsa-stained, and GMS-stained preparations. Immunofluorescent staining with anti-*Pneumocystis* monoclonal antibodies can provide greater specificity.

Bacteriology
Laboratory methods
Specimens

Routine aerobic and anaerobic cultures can be performed on a wide variety of specimens. Specimens for anaerobic culture should be transported to the lab immediately, or in anaerobic transport containers. Specimens transported anaerobically can be used for aerobic cultures as well. The following sites normally harbor indigenous anaerobic flora and should not be cultured for anaerobes: stool, skin, oropharynx, vagina, and urethra. Anaerobic culture is best reserved for specimens obtained from normally-sterile sites.

Blood culture bottles are ideally inoculated with 10 mL of blood per bottle (in adults), and typically a 2- bottle set (consisting of 1 aerobic and 1 anaerobic bottle) is collected from a given anatomic site (20 mL per set). Inoculation of <10 mL per bottle in adults reduces yield; likewise, collecting only a single set of bottles per episode is discouraged, because the total volume cultured is inadequate and interpretation of results is more difficult. The optimal number of blood cultures per episode is 3 sets, but the minimum should be 2 sets (40 mL total) drawn from separate sites. Bacteremic children tend to have a higher concentration of organisms in their blood than adults, and so collection of smaller quantities of blood for culture in children is acceptable. In children, the volume collected should not exceed 1% of total blood volume.

Direct examination

Gram staining is routinely performed on certain specimen types, especially those collected from normally-sterile sites. Blood and urine specimens are not examined directly, because Gram staining is too insensitive to be practical. For CSF, the specimen must be concentrated by cytocentrifugation prior to staining and examination. t3.32, t3.33

Gram stain procedure

- Heat-fix a smeared slide
- Apply crystal violet for 20 seconds, then wash with water
- Add iodine for 20 seconds, then wash with water
- Decolorize with acetone-alcohol, then wash with water
- Apply safranin for 20 seconds, then wash with water
- Blot dry and examine at 1,000× magnification (oil immersion light microscopy)

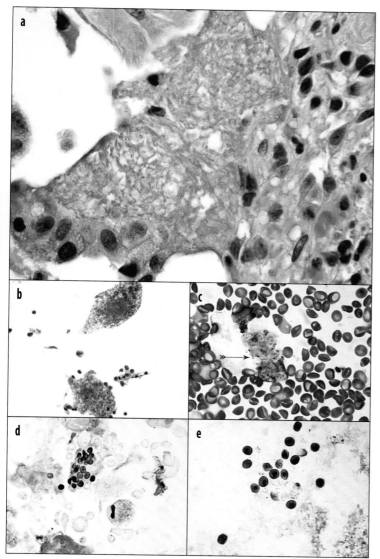

f3.84 *Pneumocystis*: characteristic exudative material is seen within alveolar airspaces on a an H&E stained lung section & b on Pap stained & c Wright stained sputum smears; note the central dot visible within the empty spaces on the Wright stained preparation
In GMS stained preparations at d low & e high magnification, the organisms are approximately the size of yeast but do not bud; they tend to cluster & have a central dark staining dot when stained with silver stains; cyst forms are round or cup shaped & have been likened to crushed ping pong balls

Pneumocystis jiroveci

Pneumocystis jiroveci (formerly known as *P carinii*) is an atypical fungus that cannot be cultured in vitro. Laboratory diagnosis depends upon direct examination of clinical specimens.

The organism was first recognized as a cause of human disease a century ago, at which time it mainly affected the severely malnourished. In this population it was generally associated with interstitial plasma cell pneumonitis or granulomatous pneumonitis. In the late 20th century, *P jiroveci* emerged as a major pathogen in HIV-infected patients. In HIV infected patients, the strongest risk factor is a CD4 count <200 cells/mL. In addition to the HIV infected, populations at risk include those with primary immunodeficiency, particularly severe combined immunodeficiency (SCID), patients undergoing chemotherapy, especially for lymphoma, and patients receiving immunosuppression for transplant or collagen vascular disease.

t3.32 Gram stain morphology of selected organisms

Organism	Gram stain morphology
Gram+ cocci	
Staphylococci	Gram+ cocci in grapelike clusters
Pyogenic streptococci	Gram+ cocci in pairs & short chains
Nonpyogenic streptococci	Gram+ cocci in long chains
Streptococcus pneumoniae	Gram+ lancet shaped diplococci
Enterococcus species	Gram+ diplococci
Gram– cocci	
Neisseria species	Gram– coffee-bean shaped diplococci
Gram+ rods	See t3.33
Gram– rods	
Vibrio species	Gram– curved, comma shaped short rods
Campylobacter species	Gram– curved, thin, rods (S-shaped, seagull shaped or corkscrew shaped)
Yersinia pestis	Gram– rods with bipolar staining ("closed safety pin")
Legionella species	Gram-invisible in primary smear

t3.33 Gram stain morphology: Gram+ rods

	Short, irregularly shaped, pleomorphic	Regularly shaped, monomorphic		Branching, filamentous
		Small to medium	**Large**	
Aerobic or facultatively anaerobic	*Corynebacterium* species Other coryneforms* Non-*Nocardia* aerobic actinomycetes†	*Listeria* species *Erysipelothrix* species	*Bacillus* species	*Nocardia* species
Aerotolerant	*Actinomyces* species‡ *Bifidobacterium* species	Aerotolerant *Lactobacillus* strains		
Anaerobic, nonspore-forming	*Propionibacterium* species	*Eubacterium* species *Lactobacillus* species	*Clostridium perfringens*	*Actinomyces israelii*
Anaerobic, spore-forming		*Clostridium ramosum*	Other *Clostridium* species§	

Examples include Arcanobacterium species, Rothia species & Arthrobacter species
†*Examples include Rhodococcus species, Gordonia species & Tsukamurella species*
‡*Examples include Actinomyces neuii, A odontolyticus, A viscosus*
§*Examples include C septicum, C difficile, C sordellii, C sporogenes, & C bifermentans*

Gram+ organisms have a thick peptidoglycan cell wall without a surrounding outer membrane. Bacteria with this structure will retain the purple crystal violet/iodine stain during the decolorization step. Gram– organisms have a much thinner peptidoglycan cell wall layer, surrounded by an outer membrane. Bacterial with this structure lose the crystal violet/iodine stain during decolorization, and are visualized using the red safranin counterstain.

The nuclei of human cells, such as neutrophils or squamous cells, stain red (Gram–). If present, these cells can be used to detect under-decolorization of the smear, in which case their nuclei will appear purple (Gram+).

Acid-fast stains

Mycobacteria have the cell-wall structure of Gram+ bacteria, but are usually Gram-invisible. Their cell walls contain mycolic acids, which create a hydrophobic barrier that prevents the crystal violet/iodine stain from reaching the peptidoglycan cell wall. Such organisms can be visualized using various acid-fast staining techniques. Acid-fast staining relies on heat and/or phenol to allow a fuchsin dye to penetrate the hydrophobic barrier and stain the mycolic acids in the cell wall. Once stained, the organisms resist decolorization, even with harsh decolorizers like hydrochloric acid. This is why they are termed "acid-fast."

In the classic Ziehl-Neelsen technique, a red carbol fuchsin dye containing phenol is heated during application, to aid penetration and staining of the bacterial cell wall. A strong acid, 3% HCl, is used for decolorization. A methylene blue counterstain is then added to provide contrast with the background. The slide must be examined at 1,000× magnification using oil-immersion light microscopy.

The Kinyoun (cold) acid-fast staining technique is a modification of the Ziehl-Neelsen method. Use of a higher concentration of phenol in the carbol fuchsin dye obviates the need for heating the stain, making the technique more convenient. The decolorization and counterstaining steps are identical to the Ziehl-Neelsen method.

An excellent alternative to fuchsin-based acid-fast stains for mycobacteria is the fluorescent auramine-rhodamine stain. Auramine and rhodamine stain mycolic acids, and fluoresce when exposed to ultraviolet light. The staining technique involves application of an auramine-rhodamine stain containing phenol, followed by an HCl decolorization step and sometimes a potassium permanganate counterstain. The slide is examined using fluorescence microscopy, with mycobacteria appearing bright yellow-green on a black background. The contrast is so great that the slide may be examined at relatively low magnification (200×), allowing more rapid slide review than traditional fuchsin based staining methods.

Modified acid-fast staining techniques are useful for direct visualization of weakly acid-fast bacteria, particularly *Nocardia* species and related aerobic actinomycetes. The cell wall of such organisms contains fewer mycolic acids than *Mycobacteria*, and strong decolorization with HCl washes away the fuchsin stain, making them invisible by traditional acid-fast staining techniques. Modified acid-fast staining methods employ a weaker decolorizing agent, such as 1% H_2SO_4, allowing these bacteria to retain the fuchsin stain. Modified acid-fast staining is also used to visualize the intestinal coccidia (*Cryptosporidium*, *Isospora*, *Cyclospora* and *Sarcocystis*) in smears prepared from concentrated stool specimens. *Legionella micdadei* is also modified acid-fast, unlike other *Legionella* species and other Gram– organisms in general.

Culture media t3.34, t3.35, t3.36

Media may be liquid or solid. Liquid media are especially helpful for isolating organisms present in rare amount, whereas solid media (in general) are less sensitive in this regard. However, solid media allow for separation of mixed organisms into pure-cultured isolates.

Nonselective media are designed to allow the growth of many organism types, limited only by the nutritional growth factors present in the medium's formulation. Selective media are intended to inhibit the growth of nontarget organisms, while allowing the growth of target organisms. Many nonselective media are also available with antimicrobial additives, making them selective. Differential media are designed to help differentiate among organisms whose growth is supported by the medium, by eliciting a phenotypic feature present in some but not others.

t3.34 Commonly used nonselective media

Medium	Type	Purpose
Sheep blood agar	Solid	General bacteriology; supports the growth of most bacteria, with important exceptions (eg, *N gonorrhea*, *H influenzae* & *Legionella*).
Chocolate agar	Solid	Cultivation/isolation of fastidious bacteria like *Neisseria* species & *Haemophilus* species, but not *Legionella* species
Buffered charcoal-yeast extract (BCYE) agar	Solid	Recovery of *Legionella* species; contains cysteine & iron supplementation, necessary to support growth of *Legionella* Activated charcoal helps bind & sequester growth inhibitors that may be present in the specimen
Mueller-Hinton agar	Solid	Antimicrobial susceptibility testing of many common bacteria
Thioglycolate broth	Liquid	Cultivation of bacteria, including microaerophilic & obligately anaerobic bacteria; oxygen tension decreases toward bottom of tube, permitting growth of obligate anaerobes & microaerophilic bacteria without incubation in an anaerobic atmosphere

t3.35 Commonly used selective media

Medium	Type	Basis for selectivity	Purpose
MacConkey agar (MAC)	Solid	Bile salts & crystal violet inhibit growth of Gram+ bacteria & delicate Gram− bacteria	Cultivation/isolation of hardy enteric Gram− rods
Eosin methylene blue (EMB)	Solid	Aniline dyes inhibit growth of Gram+ bacteria	Cultivation/isolation of hardy enteric Gram− rods
Campylobacter blood agar (Campy-BAP)	Solid	Antimicrobials to which *Campylobacter* species are resistant (cephalothin, vancomycin, trimethoprim, amphotericin B, polymyxin B)	Recovery of *Campylobacter* species
Hektoen enteric (HE) agar	Solid	Bile salts & the dyes bromthymol blue & acid fuchsin inhibit the growth of Gram+ organisms & some Gram− strains	Enhanced recovery of *Salmonella* & *Shigella*, compared with MAC or EMB
Salmonella-Shigella (SS) agar	Solid	Bile salts, sodium citrate & brilliant green dye inhibit Gram+ bacteria & many enterics other than *Salmonella*	Recovery of *Salmonella* & *Shigella*, although *Shigella* strains may be inhibited Not recommended for primary isolation of *Shigella*
Selenite broth	Liquid	Sodium selenite inhibits growth of Gram+ bacteria & many enterics other than *Salmonella*	Recovery & enrichment of *Salmonella*
Thiosulfate-citrate-bile salts-sucrose (TCBS) agar	Solid	Bile salts inhibit Gram+ bacteria Alkaline pH inhibits most enterics & enhances growth of *Vibrio* species	Recovery of *Vibrio* species
Cefsulodin-Irgasan-novobiocin (CIN) agar	Solid	Antimicrobials (cefsulodin, Irgasan, novobiocin) & crystal violet inhibit most Gram− & Gram+ bacteria other than *Yersinia* species	Recovery of *Yersinia* species
Anaerobic colistin-nalidixic acid (CNA) agar	Solid	Antimicrobials (colistin, nalidixic acid) inhibit Gram− bacteria	Recovery of anaerobic streptococci; blood in the agar allows differentiation based on hemolytic reactions
Lim broth	Liquid	Antimicrobials (colistin, nalidixic acid) inhibit Gram− bacteria	Recovery of Group B streptococci (*S agalactiae*)
Regan-Lowe medium	Solid	Antimicrobials to which *Bordetella* species are resistant (cephalexin)	Recovery of *Bordetella pertussis* & *Bordetella parapertussis*
Thayer-Martin medium	Solid	Antimicrobials to which *Neisseria* species are resistant (vancomycin, colistin, nystatin, & SXT)	Recovery of *Neisseria* species from nonsterile sites

t3.36 Commonly used differential media

Medium	Type	Basis for differentiation	Purpose
MacConkey (MAC) agar	Solid	Lactose fermentation results in pink or red coloration of colonies Lactose nonfermenters form translucent colonies	Differentiating between lactose fermenting & nonlactose fermenting enterics
Eosin methylene blue (EMB)	Solid	Lactose fermentation results in purple-black colonies or colonies with a green metallic sheen Lactose nonfermenters form translucent colonies	Differentiating between lactose fermenting & nonlactose fermenting enterics
Hektoen enteric (HE) agar	Solid	Lactose and/or sucrose fermentation results in yellow or orange coloration of colonies Lactose & sucrose nonfermenters form translucent colonies H_2S production results in black coloration of colonies	Differentiating between lactose and/or sucrose fermenting enterics & nonlactose or nonsucrose fermenting enterics Differentiating between H_2S-producing & non-H_2S-producing enterics
Salmonella-Shigella (SS) agar	Solid	Lactose fermentation results in pink or red colonies Lactose nonfermenters form translucent colonies H_2S production results in black coloration of colonies	Differentiating between lactose fermenting enterics & nonlactose fermenting enterics Differentiating between H_2S-producing & non-H_2S-producing enterics
Thiosulfate-citrate-bile salts-sucrose (TCBS) agar	Solid	Sucrose fermentation results in yellow colonies Sucrose nonfermenters form translucent colonies	Differentiating between sucrose fermenting *Vibrios* (eg, *Vibrio cholerae*) & sucrose nonfermenting *Vibrios*
Cefsulodin-Irgasan-Novobiocin (CIN) agar	Solid	Mannitol fermentation results in characteristic "bull's eye" colonies (colorless with red center) Mannitol nonfermenters form translucent colonies	Differentiating between mannitol fermenting *Yersinia* species (eg, *Yersinia enterocolitica*) & mannitol nonfermenting *Yersinia* species
Motility test agar	Semi-solid	Motile organisms show growth spreading away from the line or inoculation (stab), clouding the agar Nonmotile organisms stay within the stab, leaving the remaining agar clear	Differentiating between motile & nonmotile bacteria

Culture temperature

The optimal temperature for initial incubation is usually 37°C. *Yersinia enterocolitica* and certain *Pseudomonas* species (eg, *Pseudomonas fluorescens, Pseudomonas putida*) grow optimally at 25°C to 30°C, while the *Campylobacter* species most commonly associated with diarrheal illness (*C jejuni* and *C coli*) grow optimally at 42°C. *Listeria monocytogenes* grows optimally at 37°C, but displays its characteristic motility only at 25°C, and is notoriously able to multiply at refrigeration temperature (4°C).

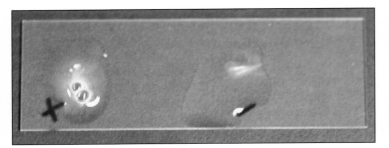

f3.85 Catalase test
Rapid & sustained effervescence (note bubbles on left) after addition of hydrogen peroxide to an isolate indicates the presence of catalase; staphylococci are catalase positive

Key biochemical tests

Catalase test f3.85

Catalase is a peroxidase enzyme that converts hydrogen peroxide (H_2O_2) to water and oxygen. To perform the catalase test, a colony is transferred to a glass slide, and a few drops of 3% hydrogen peroxide are added. Rapid and sustained effervescence indicates the presence of catalase. Care must be taken to avoid contaminating the colony with blood agar, as red blood cells produce catalase and can cause a false positive result. The catalase test is often the first test used to initially categorize Gram+ cocci. It differentiates staphylococci (catalase +) from streptococci and enterococci (catalase negative). Catalase activity is also characteristic of several other important bacterial pathogens, including *Campylobacter* species, Listeria species, and Bacillus species

Coagulase test

The coagulase test is used to distinguish *S aureus* (coagulase+) from other staphylococci (coagulase–). 2 test formats are used:

The tube coagulase test f3.86a detects free (secreted) coagulase and is the definitive coagulase test. To perform the test, a bacterial isolate is mixed with plasma in a tube. Free coagulase from *S aureus* complexes with coagulase reacting factor (CRF) in plasma, which then converts fibrinogen into fibrin, forming a clot. Examination of the tube after both 4 and 24 hours of 37°C incubation is necessary, since certain strains of *S aureus* produce a fibrinolysin, which will dissolve any coagulum (clot) that forms, giving a false negative result if only examined at 24 hours. Others produce a delayed reaction that will give false negative results if examined only at 4 hours.

The slide coagulase test f3.86b detects cell-bound coagulase, known as clumping factor. A bacterial isolate is mixed with plasma on the surface of a slide; clumping factor on the surface of *S aureus* crosslinks fibrinogen to create visible clumps. The reaction is immediate, making this a convenient, rapid test for *S aureus* identification. However, false negative results occur with a small proportion of *S aureus* that make free coagulase but not cell-bound coagulase. In addition, false positive results occur with certain nonaureus *Staphylococcus* species, especially *S lugdunensis* and *S schleiferi*, which produce clumping factor (but not free coagulase). For these reasons, the tube test is more accurate, and results obtained by the slide test should always be confirmed using the tube test.

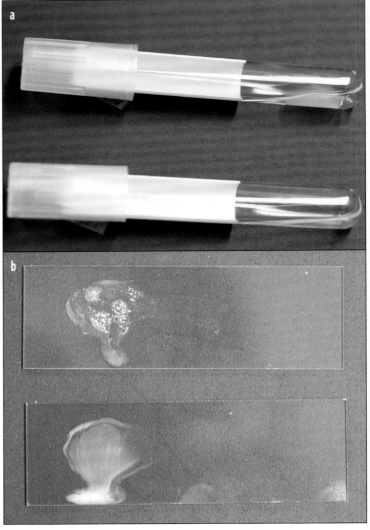

f3.86 The coagulase test is used to presumptively identify *S aureus*
a The tube coagulase test detects free coagulase, producing a coagulum in the presence of plasma (top tube); to avoid false negative reactions, it is necessary to examine the tube at both 4 & 24 hours
b The slide coagulase test detects bound coagulase, producing clumping in the presence of plasma (top slide); the slide test is faster but the tube test is required for confirmation

Novobiocin susceptibility

The novobiocin susceptibility test is used to distinguish *S saprophyticus*, a common uropathogen, from other coagulase– staphylococci. *S saprophyticus* is novobiocin resistant, while *S epidermidis* and other coagulase– staphylococci are susceptible.

Optochin susceptibility

The optochin susceptibility test (P-disk) f3.87 differentiates *S pneumoniae* from other α-hemolytic (viridans) streptococci. *S pneumoniae* is susceptible to optochin, whereas viridans streptococci are resistant.

CAMP test

The CAMP test is used to identify group B pyogenic streptococci (*Streptococcus agalactiae*) or *Listeria monocytogenes*, both of which produce CAMP factor. CAMP factor has a synergistic effect on staphylococcal β-hemolysin, producing enhanced

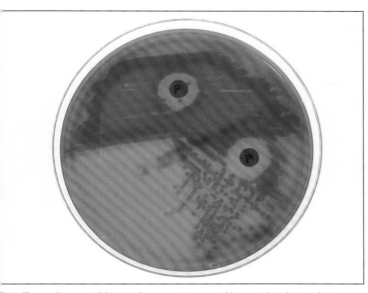

f3.87 The optochin susceptibility test: *S pneumoniae* is susceptible to optochin, showing clearing around P-disc, whereas viridans streptococci are resistant

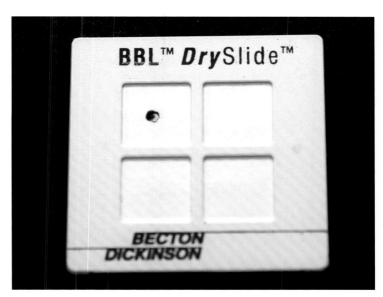

f3.89 Cytochrome oxidase test; oxidase positive organisms include *Neisseria, Moraxella, Pseudomonas, Legionella* & the curved Gram– rods (*Campylobacter, Vibrio* & *Helicobacter*); all Enterobacteriaceae are oxidase negative

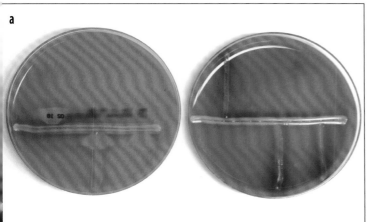

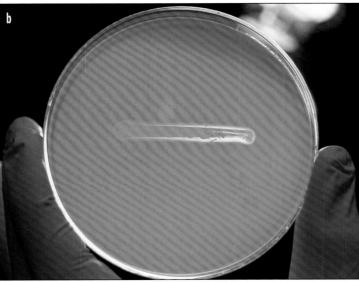

f3.88 CAMP test
a Arrowhead shaped enhancement of β hemolysis at the junction of the 2 streaks is characteristic of *S agalactiae* (left plate)
b Rectangular enhancement is characteristic of *Listeria* species

hemolysis of erythrocytes. To perform the test, a test isolate is streaked at a perpendicular angle to a *S aureus* streak. Arrowhead shaped enhancement of β-hemolysis at the junction of the 2 streaks is characteristic of *S agalactiae* f3.88a; rectangular enhancement is characteristic of *Listeria* species f3.88b.

PYR test

The PYR test is used to identify group A pyogenic streptococci and *Enterococcus* species. These bacteria enzymatically hydrolyze PYR substrate (L-pyrrolidonyl-β-naphthylamide) yielding β-naphthylamide which, in the presence of a detection reagent, yields a red color change.

Bile-esculin test

Enterococci and group D streptococci (*S bovis*) are able to hydrolyze esculin in the presence of bile. To perform the test, a bile-esculin agar slant is inoculated and incubated for 24 hours. Diffuse blackening of the medium indicates esculin hydrolysis. Rapid spot-test versions of this assay are also available.

Oxidase test

Cytochrome oxidase enzyme activity is characteristic of certain bacterial genera, including *Neisseria*, Moraxella, *Pseudomonas*, *Legionella*, and the curved Gram– rods (*Campylobacter*, *Vibrio*, and *Helicobacter*). In contrast, all Enterobacteriaceae are oxidase negative. The immediate development of a blue color after a colony is smeared on a reagent-impregnated strip, or after reagent is added to a colony, indicates oxidase activity. The reagent, p-phenylenediamine, is oxidized by cytochrome oxidase, forming iodophenol blue f3.89.

Indole test

The indole test determines an organism's ability to produce indole via deamination of tryptophan. There are many variations of this test, but a common version involves a test-strip

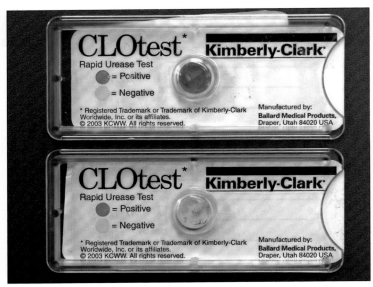

f3.90 Urease test, showing positive (top) & negative (bottom) results; rapid (within 4 hours) urease positive organisms include *Proteus* species & *H pylori*

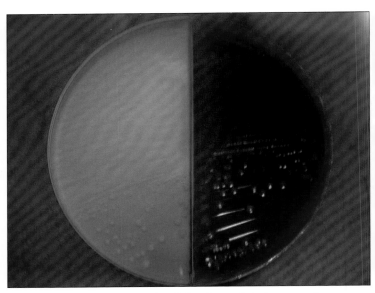

f3.91 A fluorometric substrate (MUG) can be added to culture media; in the presence of β-glucuronidase enzyme activity a fluorescent product can be seen under UV light; this is a key test in the presumptive identification of *E coli*

impregnated with Kovac reagent. Indole produced by the cultured organism combines with the reagent in the strip to produce a pink complex. Numerous bacteria produce indole, but the test is perhaps best known as a way to help identify *E coli*, which is characteristically indole+.

Rapid urease test

Organisms that produce urease can split (hydrolyze) urea present in the test medium, producing ammonia and thereby alkalinizing the medium, leading to pH-based color change (red or pink coloration). Many bacteria have urease activity, but only a few can degrade it quickly (within 4 hours) and are designated "rapid urease+" organisms. Notable examples include *Proteus* species and *H pylori* f3.90.

β-glucuronidase

β-glucuronidase enzyme activity is a key test in the presumptive identification of *E coli*, and also members of the anginosus group streptococci. It is detected using a colorimetric enzyme substrate (p-nitrophenyl-β-D-glucopyranoside or PNPG), which produces a yellow compound (p-nitrophenol) when hydrolyzed. Alternatively, a fluorometric substrate (4-methylumbelliferyl-β-D-glucuronide) can be employed, which produces a compound (4-methylumbelliferone) that fluoresces under UV light. MUG can be added to culture media like MacConkey, making the medium differential for β-glucuronidase activity f3.91.

Hippurate hydrolysis test

This rapid assay relies on ninhydrin reagent to detect glycine produced by hydrolysis of the hippurate substrate. Development of a blue-purple color indicates a positive result. It is a key test in the presumptive identification of *Campylobacter jejuni*, which is characteristically positive. It can also be helpful in the presumptive identification of *Listeria monocytogenes*,

Streptococcus agalactiae, *Gardnerella vaginalis*, and *Legionella pneumophila*.

Lysozyme test

This test determines an organism's ability to grow in the presence of lysozyme. Most bacteria are inhibited by lysozyme, but *Nocardia* species are resistant. To perform the test, growth of the test organism in lysozyme-containing broth medium is compared with growth in control medium that doesn't contain lysozyme.

Specific bacteria: key characteristics
Gram+ cocci

Once the obligate anaerobes have been excluded, the remaining pathogenic organisms, for practical purposes, include staphylococci, streptococci and enterococci.

Anaerobic Gram+ cocci

Until recently, most organisms in this group were classified as various *Peptostreptococcus* species. However, taxonomy is changing and expanding, and clinical isolates now fall within numerous genera in addition to *Peptostreptococcus*, including *Finegoldia*, *Peptococcus*, *Parvimonas*, *Anaerococcus* and others. Anaerobic Gram+ cocci are commensal flora of the oropharynx, GI tract, vagina and skin. They are associated with endogenous, usually polymicrobial infections, such as abscesses involving the skin, soft tissues, lung or brain; aspiration pneumonia, necrotizing pneumonia, or empyema; diabetic foot infections, crepitant cellulitis, synergistic gangrene or necrotizing fasciitis; septic abortion or intraabdominal infections; and other serious infections including bacteremia, endocarditis, and meningitis.

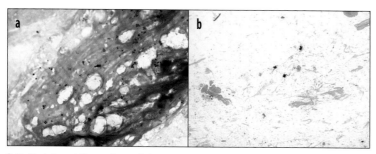

f3.92 Staphylococci: Gram stain morphology

Staphylococci (catalase+, Gram+ cocci)

Staphylococci appear as Gram+ cocci in grapelike clusters f3.92a and tetrads f3.92b in primary smears. In addition to Gram stain morphology, they are distinguished from streptococci and enterococci using the catalase test. Staphylococci are catalase+, whereas the other Gram+ cocci are catalase–. Plate morphology and Gram stain morphology are also useful, as staphylococci characteristically form creamy colonies on solid media, and grapelike clusters or tetrads in primary smears.

Staphylococci can be subdivided on the basis of the coagulase test. *S aureus* isolates are coagulase+, while other staphylococcal species are coagulase–.

Drug resistance among *S aureus* strains is a major problem. Most clinical isolates express a β-lactamase, conferring resistance to penicillin, ampicillin, and early generation cephalosporins. Consequently, antistaphylococcal penicillins such as nafcillin, dicloxacillin, or oxacillin, which are not inactivated by β-lactamases, are required to combat these strains. However, an increasing proportion of nosocomial and community acquired *S aureus* strains are also resistant to antistaphylococcal penicillins, via expression of altered penicillin-binding proteins. These so-called "methicillin-resistant *S aureus*" or MRSA strains carry the *mecA* gene, which allows them to express PBP2A, a penicillin target with little affinity for the drug. Clinical isolates can be identified as MRSA using routine phenotypic antimicrobial susceptibility testing methods (disk diffusion testing or MIC testing, using cefoxitin as the indicator drug), or with DNA hybridization probes to detect *mecA*, or by detection of PBP2A using latex agglutination. Patients may be screened for MRSA colonization t3.37 by analysis of a nasal swab either by culture on selective media or by PCR-based methods.

Coagulase negative staphylococci include *S epidermidis*, *S saprophyticus*, and *S lugdunensis*, among others. *S epidermidis* is a skin commensal and is relatively avirulent. It rarely causes infection in natural tissues, and its main pathogenic potential lies in its ability to colonize biomaterials. *S epidermidis* can cause bloodstream infections related to infected intravascular catheters, prosthetic vascular grafts, or prosthetic cardiac valves. It can also cause prosthetic joint infections or CNS infection related to ventricular shunts. *S saprophyticus* is a uropathogen and the only clinically significant coagulase negative *Staphylococcus* that is novobiocin resistant. It causes urinary tract infection in healthy, young, sexually-active, female outpatients. *S lugdunensis* (SLUG) is a skin commensal that is more virulent than other coagulase– staphylococci, and causes infections similar in severity to *S aureus*. It causes aggressive native valvular and prosthetic valvular endocarditis, skin infections, prosthetic joint infections, and osteomyelitis, among other clinical syndromes. When isolated from superficial skin infections, it is less likely than other coagulase– staphylococci to represent a contaminant, and should always be considered a potential pathogen. SLUG isolates are often positive by the slide coagulase test, but unlike *S aureus* are negative by the tube coagulase test. In addition, SLUG is PYR+ and ornithine decarboxylase positive.

Coagulase– Gram+ cocci

Catalase–, Gram+ cocci are streptococci or enterococci t3.38. One can begin to classify them based on their hemolytic properties when grown on blood agar plates: complete (β) hemolysis (clear zone surrounding colonies), incomplete (α) hemolysis (green pigment surrounding colonies), or no (γ) hemolysis.

t3.38 Catalase–, Gram+ cocci

Hemolysis	Organism	Properties
β	*S pyogenes*	PYR+, bacitracin susceptible, expresses Lancefield group A antigens
	S dysgalactiae	PYR–, bacitracin resistant (usually), expresses Lancefield group C or G antigens
	S agalactiae	PYR–, bacitracin resistant (usually), CAMP factor+, hippurate hydrolysis+, expresses Lancefield group B antigens
	Some strains of enterococci	PYR+, bile esculin+, bacitracin resistant, expresses Lancefield group D antigens
	Some strains of anginosus group streptococci	PYR–, bacitracin resistant, small colonies, butterscotch odor, may express Lancefield group A, C, F or G antigens
α	*S pneumoniae*	Optochin susceptible
	Most viridans streptococci	Optochin resistant, PYR–, bile esculin–
	Some strains of *S bovis*	Optochin resistant, PYR–, bile esculin+
	Some strains of enterococci (especially *E faecium* strains)	Optochin resistant, PYR+, bile esculin+
γ	Most strains of enterococci	PYR+, bile esculin+
	Most strains of *S bovis*	PYR–, bile esculin+
	Some strains of viridans streptococci	PYR–, bile esculin–

t3.37 Carriage rates for a variety of bacterial species

Organism		Carriage rate	Site
Staphylococcus aureus		50%	Nares
Streptococcus pneumoniae	Adults	5%	Oropharynx
	Children	50%	
Group B streptococci	Pregnant women	10-30%	Rectum/vagina
Clostridium difficile	Healthy infants	30%	Colon
	Healthy adults	<3%	
	Adults in long term care facilities	4-20%	
Neisseria meningitidis		10%	Oropharynx

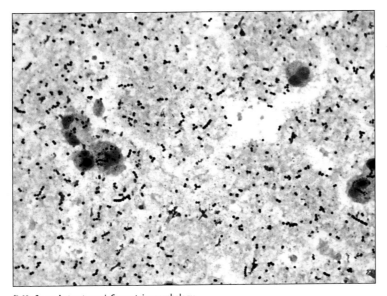

f3.93 Group A streptococci: Gram stain morphology

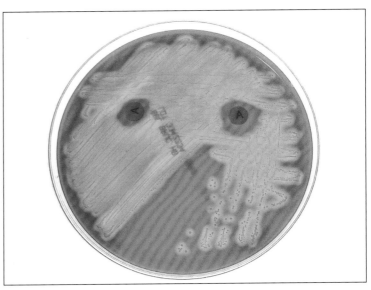

f3.95 Group A streptococci: characteristic bacitracin (A disc) susceptibility

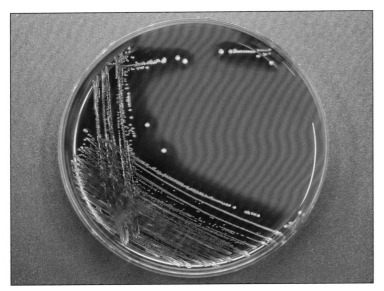

f3.94 Group A streptococci: colony morphology showing a wide zone of β hemolysis on blood agar

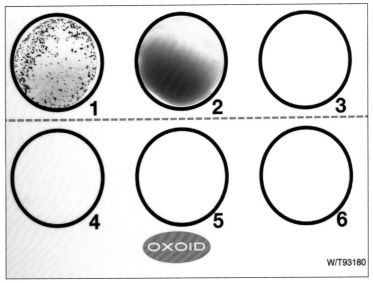

f3.96 A latex agglutination test for the identification of streptococcal groups A, B, C, D, F & G
In well 1, *S pyogenes* was agglutinated using Lancefield group A reagent
In well 2, *S pyogenes* did not agglutinate using Lancefield group B reagent

β hemolytic, catalase–, Gram+ cocci

Streptococcus pyogenes (group A streptococci)

Group A streptococci (GAS) appear as Gram+ cocci singly, in pairs, and in short chains in primary smears f3.93. On blood agar, colonies are large and are surrounded by a wide zone of β-hemolyis f3.94. GAS is characteristically susceptible to bacitracin (A disk) f3.95, positive for PYR hydrolysis, and expresses Lancefield group A antigens f3.96. In addition to culture-based methods, GAS can be detected directly using rapid antigen tests. The sensitivity of antigen detection is inferior to culture, however, so negative results cannot rule out infection and should be followed up with standard culture. Serologic testing is useful in the diagnosis of post-streptococcal disease, when antecedent infection was not documented. For increased sensitivity, the antistreptolysin O test should be combined with the anti-DNase B test. A fourfold rise in antibody titer defines antecedent infection.

Group A streptococci colonize the oropharynx and skin and cause a wide variety of infections including pharyngitis, retropharyngeal abscess, bacteremia, and several skin and soft tissue infections including impetigo, erysipelas, and necrotizing fasciitis. GAS also causes toxin-mediated illnesses, such as toxic shock syndrome and scarlet fever, as well as immune-mediated complications, including acute rheumatic fever (ARF), post-streptococcal glomerulonephritis, and pediatric autoimmune neuropsychiatric disorders. ARF

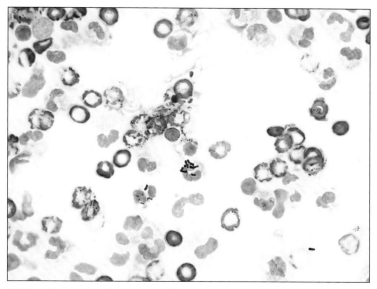

f3.97 Group B streptococci: Gram stain morphology

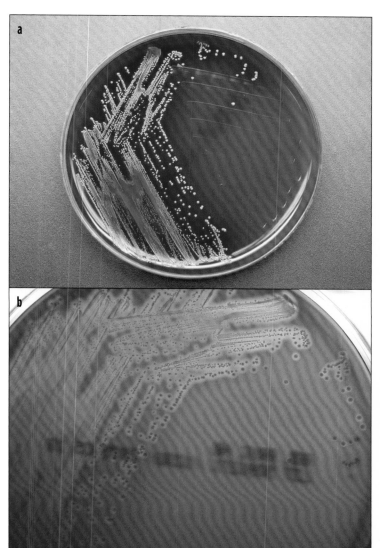

f3.98 Group B streptococci: colony morphology

is a potential complication of untreated streptococcal pharyngitis. The diagnosis of ARF depends upon fulfillment of the Jones criteria t3.39 or the somewhat less stringent WHO criteria. In contrast to ARF, post-streptococcal glomerulonephritis may be associated with both skin and pharyngeal infection. Furthermore, unlike ARF, the incidence of AGN is unaffected by antimicrobial treatment. Renal biopsy shows a proliferative and exudative lesion in a pattern that is difficult to distinguish from idiopathic membranoproliferative glomerulonephritis.

t3.39 Jones criteria*

Major criteria	Minor criteria
Carditis	Arthralgia
Polyarthritis	Fever
Chorea (Sydenham)	Elevated ESR or CRP
Erythema marginatum	Prolonged PR interval
Subcutaneous nodules	
Gram– cocci	

*2 major criteria or 1 major + 2 minor & evidence of antecedent group A streptococcal infection (+ throat culture, + rapid antigen test, or rising streptococcal antibody titer)

Streptococcus agalactiae (group B streptococci)

Group B streptococci (GBS) appear as Gram+ cocci in pairs and short chains f3.97. In culture, it forms gray-white colonies f3.98a, is β hemolytic with a narrow zone of hemolysis f3.98b, CAMP test +, and hippurate hydrolysis +. Pregnant females should be screened for GBS colonization at 35-37 weeks gestation. Screening can be accomplished by culture-based methods or by amplified molecular methods, although in either case an enrichment broth step must first be performed. Specimens should be obtained from the vagina and rectum, using a single swab. The enrichment step usually involves overnight incubation in a selective broth medium, such as Lim broth, containing antibiotics to inhibit the growth of other commensal organisms. PCR-based methods can then be applied to the enrichment broth, or the broth can be subcultured to selective or nonselective media. Several differential media are available with colorimetric indicators, which simplify detection of GBS in culture.

GBS can cause serious, invasive infection in neonates born to colonized women. Neonatal infection is acquired through an ascending route, often associated with placental funisitis and chorioamnionitis, or during passage through the birth canal at delivery. Neonates may have early onset (within 7 days of birth) or late-onset manifestations, including sepsis, pneumonia, or meningitis. Maternal risk factors correlating with early onset neonatal infection include preterm delivery, prolonged rupture of membranes, intrapartum fever, and prior affected infant. Efforts are directed at prevention through identification of colonized women.

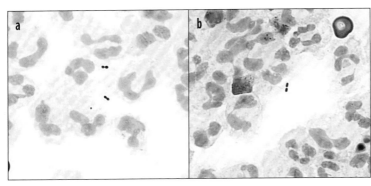

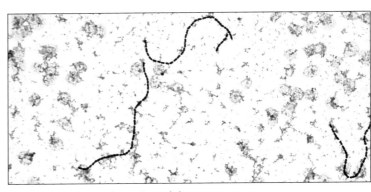

f3.99 *S pneumoniae*: Gram stain morphology

f3.101 Viridans streptococci: Gram stain morphology

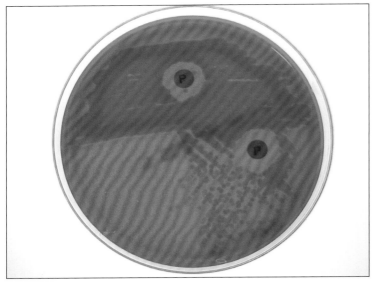

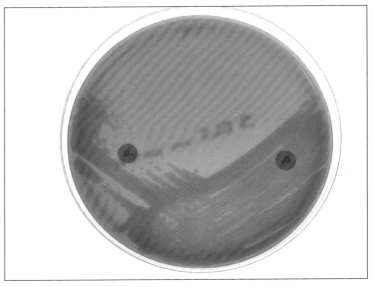

f3.100 *S pneumoniae*: colony morphology & characteristic optochin (P disk) susceptibility

f3.102 Viridans streptococci: colony morphology & characteristic optochin (P disc) resistance

α-hemolytic, catalase–, Gram+ cocci

Streptococcus pneumonia

S pneumoniae appears as lancet shaped, Gram+ diplococci in primary smears f3.99. It is α-hemolytic on blood agar, and susceptible to optochin (P disk) f3.100. Strains causing invasive disease have an antiphagocytic polysaccharide capsule that results in smooth colonies. In addition to culture-based methods, invasive infections in adults can sometimes be detected directly using a urine antigen test, although sensitivity is inferior to culture. The urine antigen test is especially useful as a rapid diagnostic tool, or when antibiotic therapy has been initiated prior to specimen collection for culture. Oropharyngeal colonization can lead to false positive results, rendering the test inadequately specific in infants and children, where colonization rates are very high.

S *pneumoniae* is the leading cause of community acquired pneumonia. Invasive infection may also lead to bacteremia and meningitis. Noninvasive infection (eg, otitis media, sinusitis) is also common. Vaccination can prevent invasive disease; young children are offered a 7-valent conjugate vaccine, whereas adults over age 65 (or others with risk factors) are offered a 23-valent polysaccharide vaccine.

Viridans streptococci

Viridans streptococci tend to form long chains of Gram+ cocci f3.101, are α-hemolytic on blood agar, and are optochin resistant f3.102. They colonize the oral cavity and sometimes the GI tract or female genital tract. Viridans streptococci can be subclassified into 4 species groups: the *S mitis* group, the *S mutans* group, the *S salivarius* group, and the *S anginosus* group. *S mitis* group strains are a frequent cause of native-valve endocarditis and late-onset prosthetic valve endocarditis. *S mutans* group strains are the principal agent of dental caries and can cause endocarditis. S salivarius group strains are an occasional cause of bacteremia and endocarditis. Anginosus group streptococci cause abscesses at various sites. One species, *S intermedius*, is particularly associated with brain or liver abscesses. Anginosus group streptococci can be α-, β-, or nonhemolytic, and can express Lancefield group A, C, F and/or G antigens, or none at all. However, β-hemolytic strains form small colonies (<0.5 mm) after overnight incubation, distinguishing them from pyogenic streptococci.

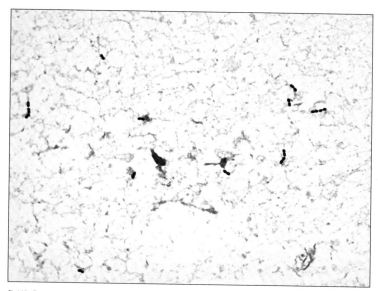

f3.103 Enterococci: Gram stain morphology

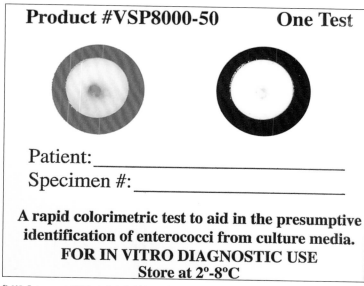

Product #VSP8000-50   **One Test**

Patient: _____

Specimen #: _____

A rapid colorimetric test to aid in the presumptive identification of enterococci from culture media. FOR IN VITRO DIAGNOSTIC USE
Store at 2°-8°C

f3.105 Enterococci: PYR hydrolysis (left) & esculin hydrolysis (right)

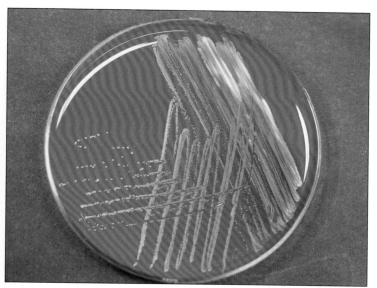

f3.104 Enterococci: colony morphology

Nonhemolytic, catalase–, Gram+ cocci

Enterococcus species

Enterococci grow as streptococcus-like diplococci and short chains f3.103, and form small, gray, usually nonhemolytic colonies on blood agar f3.104. They hydrolyze esculin in the presence of bile, hydrolyze PYR f3.105, and grow in the presence of 6.5% NaCl. They also express Lancefield group D antigens. Enterococci are normal inhabitants of the lower gastrointestinal tract, and cause urinary tract infection (usually nosocomial and related to indwelling catheters), bacteremia, endocarditis, and intraabdominal and pelvic infections. *E faecalis* and *E faecium* account for most clinical isolates.

Enterococci are intrinsically resistant to certain classes of antibiotics and can acquire resistance to several others. The cephalosporins (with a few exceptions), the antistaphylococcal penicillins (eg, methicillin), and the carboxypenicillins (eg, ticarcillin) have little activity against all species of *Enterococcus*. In addition, enterococci characteristically display low level resistance to penicillin and aminoglycosides. However, this intrinsic, low level resistance can be overcome by proper dosing. In contrast, most *E faecium* strains (but only rare *E faecalis* strains) express altered penicillin-binding proteins with little affinity for penicillins, and are frankly resistant to penicillin, the aminopenicillins (eg, ampicillin) and the carbapenems. All *Enterococcus* species can also acquire high level resistance to aminoglycosides. *E gallinarum* and *E casseliflavus* display intrinsic, low level vancomycin resistance, due to the presence of the chromosomal *vanC* gene, which encodes peptidoglycan precursors with moderately reduced affinity for vancomycin. More problematic is the acquisition of high level vancomycin resistance, because it usually occurs in *E faecium* strains that are also highly resistant to penicillins. High level vancomycin resistance is conferred by acquisition of the *vanA*, *vanB*, or *vanD* gene clusters, which are found on transferable genetic elements.

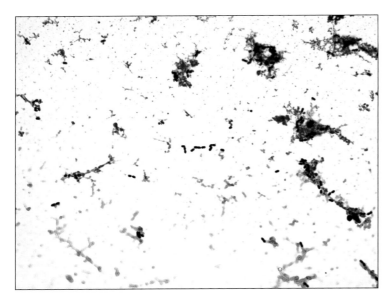

f3.106 *S bovis*: Gram stain morphology

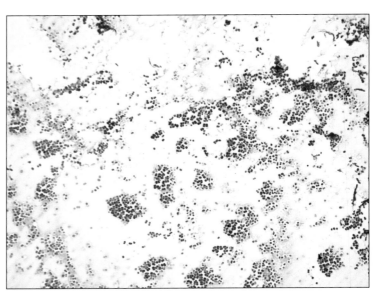

f3.108 *N gonorrhoeae*: Gram stain morphology

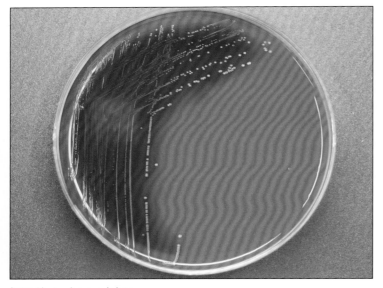

f3.107 *S bovis*: colony morphology

Streptococcus bovis group

S bovis appears as Gram+ cocci in pairs or short chains f3.106, and forms gray-white, nonhemolytic colonies on blood agar f3.107. Like *Enterococcus* species, *S bovis* group species express Lancefield group D antigens, and can hydrolyze esculin in the presence of bile, but *S bovis* group is PYR– and cannot grow in 6.5% NaCl. *S bovis* group colonizes the GI tract and causes bacteremia and endocarditis. Blood-borne infection by certain subspecies within the *S bovis* group, especially *S gallolyticus subspecies gallolyticus*, is associated with colonic malignancy.

Gram– cocci

Anaerobic Gram– cocci

Veillonella species and other anaerobic Gram– cocci are normal inhabitants of the oral cavity and GI, genitourinary and respiratory tracts. They are rare as pure isolates in human infection; instead, they are sometimes found as part of polymicrobial aerobic-anaerobic infections.

Neisseria species

Like Moraxella species (below), these organisms are fastidious and require prompt incubation in a CO_2-rich environment. *Neisseria* species are oxidase+, and appear as "coffee bean shaped" Gram– diplococci in smears. Chocolate agar with several antibiotics to inhibit indigenous flora (Thayer-Martin agar, Martin-Lewis, or New York City agar) is used to culture from nonsterile sites. In direct examination of clinical specimens (eg, urethral swabs), organisms often appear as intracellular Gram– diplococci.

N gonorrheae

There are numerous approaches to the identification of *N gonorrhoeae* in clinical samples. Presumptive diagnosis can be made by identifying intracellular, Gram– diplococci in specimens obtained from the urethra or cervix. For definitive diagnosis, culture or molecular techniques are most often employed. For culture, specimens are ideally plated onto chocolate-based agar at the point of care (the gonococcus will not grow on blood agar) and immediately incubated in 3-5% CO_2. Isolates can be confirmed as *N gonorrhoeae* by appropriate Gram stain morphology f3.108 and colony morphology f3.109, plus biochemical reactions or hybridization probe. Alternatively, a nucleic acid amplification test (NAAT) can be used for direct detection, without the need for culture. In addition

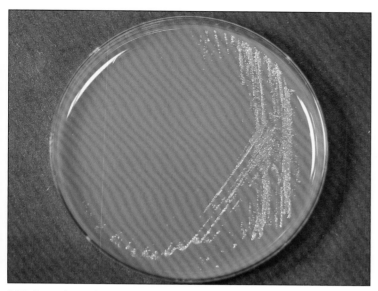

f3.109 *N gonorrhoeae*: colony morphology on chocolate agar

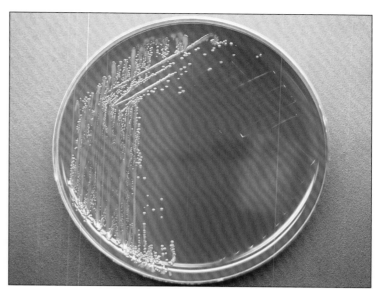

f3.110 *N meningitidis*: colony morphology on blood agar

to endocervical and urethral specimens, most commercial NAATs can be performed on urine due to their high sensitivity. This is a major advantage over culture, as is the shorter turnaround time associated with NAATs.

The clinical consequences of *N gonorrhoeae* infection range widely. Up to 10% of infected males are asymptomatic, and 50% of females with cervicitis are asymptomatic. Symptomatic males present with urethral discharge, and ascending infection may lead to acute epididymitis. In females, vaginal discharge, pruritus and/or urethritis are common symptoms. Ascending infection may lead to pelvic inflammatory disease (PID), which may be complicated by tubo-ovarian abscess or Fitz-Hugh Curtis syndrome, and can lead to infertility or ectopic pregnancy. Rectal and pharyngeal infections may also occur. Disseminated gonococcal infections arise in a small proportion of untreated patients, manifesting either as purulent arthritis or as a syndrome including tenosynovitis, dermatitis and polyarthralgias.

N meningitides

Culture is the usual approach to detecting the meningococcus. Like the gonococcus, meningococcus requires CO_2 supplementation and culture on chocolate agar (although it is capable of growth on blood agar as well) f3.110, f3.111. Multiple serogroups are defined by capsular polysaccharide antigens, with most human disease being related to serogroups A, B, C, Y, and W135. Serogroups B, C, and Y cause the majority of disease in the United States. Importantly, serogroup B is not represented in the tetravalent vaccines available.

Many people carry *N meningitidis* in their nasopharynx, and infection is transmitted via respiratory droplets. Invasive infection most often takes the form of bacterial meningitis.

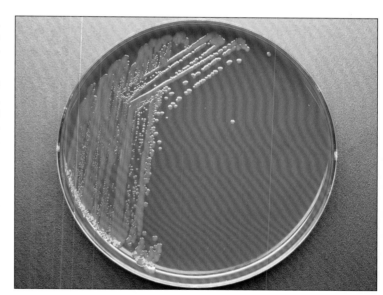

f3.111 *N meningitidis*: colony morphology on chocolate agar

Moraxella catarrhalis

In Gram stained smears, *M catarrhalis* can appear similar to *Neisseria* species, a Gram– diplococcus, or can be coccobacillary. Like *Neisseria*, *M catarrhalis* is oxidase+, but colonies grow well on blood agar and display the hockey puck sign (can be pushed intact along the surface of the agar). *M catarrhalis* is a common colonizer of the upper respiratory tract. It is a frequent cause of otitis media in children, and can cause COPD exacerbation in older adults. Species identification is usually achieved using biochemical tests.

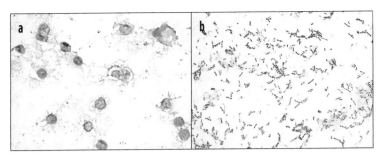

f3.112 *Kingella kingae*: Gram stain morphology

Kingella kingae

Kingella kingae is discussed here because of its taxonomic relationship to *Neisseria*. It is a β-hemolytic, Gram− coccobacillus that appears as pairs and short chains in Gram stained smears f3.112. *K kingae* is listed among the "HACEK" organisms and can cause endocarditis in adults. However, it is predominantly seen in young children, where invasive infection most commonly takes the form of septic arthritis, osteomyelitis, or occult bacteremia. Culture of synovial fluid or bone should be performed using an aerobic blood culture vial, rather than solid media, because the yield is significantly higher.

Gram+ bacilli

Gram+ bacilli can be classified according to Gram stain morphology, spore formation, and aerotolerance.

Anaerobic Gram+ bacilli

Spore formation indicates *Clostridium* species

C perfringens appears as large, somewhat short but wide "boxcar shaped" Gram+ rods, often in short chains. Although it is technically a spore-former, spores are rare and difficult to detect. Colonies produce a double zone of β-hemolysis on blood agar. Preliminary identification also involves demonstration of lecithinase activity, which is indicated by an opaque zone around colonies grown on egg yolk agar or on egg free agar containing purified lecithin. *C perfringens* causes several distinct clinical diseases, including trauma-related skin and soft tissue infections (clostridial myonecrosis [gas gangrene], anaerobic [crepitant] cellulitis), and food poisoning caused by ingestion of spores that germinate and produce enterotoxin. The organism is ubiquitous in soil and colonizes the GI tract.

C septicum is a large, long Gram+ rod that frequently forms chains. Subterminal spores may be seen. On nonselective agar medium, the organisms swarm rather than forming discrete colonies. Like *C perfringens*, *C septicum* causes gas gangrene, but the infection is usually "spontaneous" rather than related to trauma. *C septicum* is somewhat aerotolerant, which may explain why it can easily infect healthy (nontraumatized) tissue, unlike *C perfringens*. The underlying cause is bacteremia, which can be related to colonic carcinoma or other GI pathology that allows the bacteria to enter the bloodstream from the gut, such as diverticulitis or neutropenic enterocolitis. The organism may also cause bacteremia and sepsis, without associated tissue infection. Isolation of *C septicum* from blood or tissue should trigger an examination for GI malignancy.

C botulinum is ubiquitous in soil, dust and fresh water. It is the principal agent of botulism, a neurotoxin-mediated illness. Botulism is primarily a clinical diagnosis, and laboratory testing usually does not involve direct observation or cultivation of the organism. Instead, adjunctive laboratory testing relies on detection of botulinum toxin in serum, stool, vomitus, or food. The gold standard method is the mouse bioassay. Filtrates of the specimen are injected into mice intraperitoneally, and the animal is observed for paralysis. In parallel, control mice are injected with filtrates that have been preincubated with specific antitoxins, to demonstrate that antibotulinum toxin antibodies can neutralize the paralytic effects. Alternatives to the mouse bioassay include ELISA, cell culture toxicity assays, and real time PCR assays, although none is as sensitive or specific as the mouse bioassay. There are several forms of clinical botulism. Infant botulism, the most frequent form in the US, occurs sporadically when *C botulinum* spores are ingested and develop into vegetative cells in the gut, producing botulinum toxin. The exotoxin is absorbed into the bloodstream and is carried to nerve endings, where it blocks neurotransmitter release. Raw honey is a common source. More rarely, adults can be colonized with *C botulinum*, which can lead to a similar syndrome. Risk factors include GI surgery, recent antibiotic treatment, and/or inflammatory bowel disease or other chronic GI illness. Other forms of botulism include foodborne botulism, in which the preformed toxin is ingested in contaminated food such as fermented meat or canned goods, and wound botulism, in which the organism infects and grows within a wound, producing toxin that is absorbed into the blood stream.

C tetani is ubiquitous in soil, surviving in spore form, and colonizes the GI tract of many animals. During infection, it elaborates a neurotoxin, called tetanospasmin, which causes tetanus (lockjaw). Tetanus is a clinical diagnosis; useful laboratory tests for the toxin are unavailable. *C tetani* is very difficult to recover from clinical specimens, and culture is usually not attempted. Tetanus is always caused by entry of *C tetani* spores into wounds, especially deep puncture wounds. In this environment of low oxygen tension, the spores germinate to vegetative forms and elaborate exotoxin, which enters the bloodstream and affects neurons in the brain stem and spinal cord. Tetanospasmin blocks inhibitory neurotransmitters, leading to unchecked activation of motor neurons and muscle spasms. Tetanus can be prevented by vaccination, although booster immunization at 10-year intervals is needed for full immunity.

C difficile can be recovered in culture using a special selective medium, cycloserine-cefoxitin-egg yolk-fructose agar (CCFA), under strict anaerobic conditions. Colonies on CCFA are yellow, with a ground-glass appearance, and fluoresce when exposed to UV light. Cultured *C difficile* produces a characteristic "horse manure" odor. Gram stained smears of isolates show thin, regularly shaped Gram+ or Gram-variable rods, sometimes with subterminal and free spores. Because there are toxin-producing and nontoxigenic *C difficile* strains, "cytotoxic culture" (as opposed to culture alone) was traditionally performed to support the diagnosis of *C difficile*-associated diarrhea (CDAD). Cytotoxic culture involves culture isolation of *C difficile* from stool, as described above, after which isolates are assayed for toxin production by the cell cytotoxicity test. The cell cytotoxicity test is performed by exposing cell culture to an extract derived from the specimen, and observing for cytopathic effect

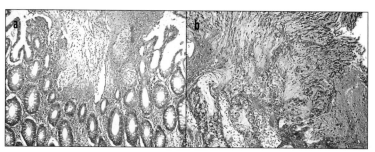

f3.113 Pseudomembranous colitis, demonstrating volcanolike fibrinopurulent exudate

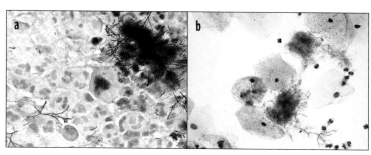

f3.114 *Actinomyces* species
a Gram stain morphology
b Pap stain morphology

caused by toxin. To demonstrate that the observed cytopathic effect is caused specifically by *C difficile* toxin, a parallel neutralization step is performed by preincubating the specimen extract with antitoxin B antibodies. The cell cytotoxicity test is now outdated, as it is labor intensive and turnaround time is slow. Most clinical laboratories now employ an alternative toxin-detection assay. Until recently, enzyme immunoassays for direct detection of toxins A and B in stool were popular, but sensitivity is poor. A much more sensitive alternative is real time PCR for toxin genes (*tcdA* for toxin A, *tcdB* for toxin B, and/or *cdt* for binary toxin). Often, DNA PCR assays are designed only to detect the gene for toxin B. Pathogenic strains are toxin A+B+ or toxin A–B+. To date, no pathogenic A+B– strains have not been reported. Another alternative is to screen stool specimens for glutamate dehydrogenase (GDH), an antigen produced by *C difficile* that can be detected using enzyme immunoassays or rapid immunochromatographic assays. This method is slightly less sensitive than PCR-based methods, but significantly more sensitive than enzyme immunoassays for toxins A and B. The major disadvantage is specificity, as GDH is produced both by toxigenic strains and nontoxigenic strains. Therefore, GDH tests are best used as a screening test in a multistep testing algorithm. Specimens that are GDH– can be reported as negative, whereas GDH+ specimens are evaluated by PCR or other means for toxigenic *C difficile*.

C difficile infection causes a range of clinical manifestations, from mild diarrhea to severe, bloody diarrhea or even pseudomembranous colitis f3.113. The latter can result in colonic perforation or toxic megacolon, requiring surgical intervention. Numerous antibiotic classes have been associated with *C difficile* infection, including clindamycin, fluoroquinolones, carbapenems, and cephalosporins.

The past decade was notable for a worldwide increase in severe cases of *C difficile* colitis, those complicated by fulminant colitis, colectomy, or death. This has been attributed to the emergence of a hypervirulent strain of *C difficile* that is commonly referred to as BI/NAP1/027. It is estimated that 30-50% of new cases are presently caused by the 027 strain. The BI/NAP1/027 causes severe disease, and antibiotic selection may be impacted. The newest PCR assays can detect, in addition to toxin-producing strains of *C difficile*, 027 strains. These assays detect the toxin gene(s) and the mutated form of the *tcdC* gene that typifies the 027 strain. It is not recommended that stool be tested in patients who have completed medical therapy and are symptom-free, because DNA detection may persist for weeks following successful treatment.

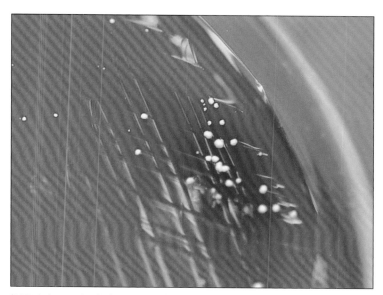

f3.115 *Actinomyces israelii*: slow growing, white colonies

Nonspore formers

Actinomyces species are branching, filamentous Gram+ rods f3.114 and can be difficult or impossible to distinguish from *Nocardia* species by Gram stain morphology. Both genera can also form macroscopic "granules" in vivo, although the term "sulfur granule" is reserved for granules composed of *Actinomyces* filaments. Unlike *Nocardia* species, *Actinomyces* species are anaerobes (or aerotolerant) and are not positive by acid-fast staining techniques. They grow slowly on routine media (eg, blood agar) under anaerobic conditions. One commonly-isolated species, *Actinomyces israelii*, forms white, cerebriform ("molar tooth") colonies on solid media f3.115. Actinomyces is a commensal organism in the oropharynx, lower GI tract, and vagina; infection usually results from a breech of the mucosal barrier or from aspiration. For this reason, infections are typically polymicrobial; they also tend to be indolent, as the organism grows slowly. Cervicofacial actinomycosis is usually the result of trauma (or surgery), and thoracic infection is usually the result of aspiration, although direct invasion into the thoracic cavity from cervicofacial infection can also occur. Infection of the female genital tract (endometritis, tubo-ovarian abscess) is associated with intrauterine devices (IUDs). Intraabdominal actinomycosis is often related

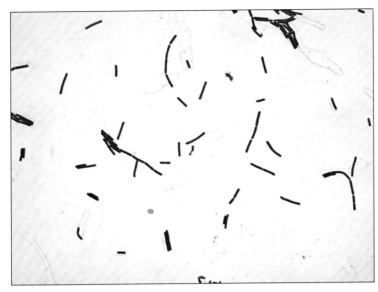

f3.116 *Bacillus* species: Gram stain morphology

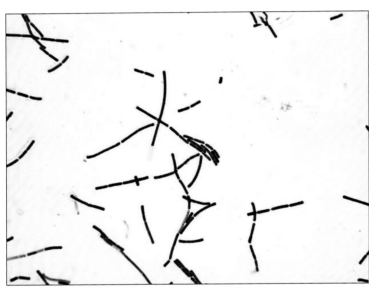

f3.117 *Bacillus anthracis*: Gram stain morphology

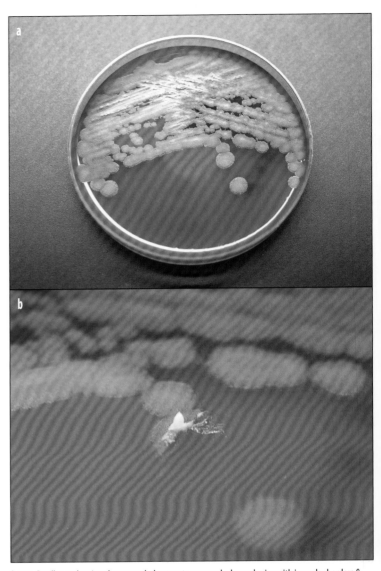

f3.118 *Bacillus anthracis*: colony morphology; note a ground-glass colonies with irregular borders & b tenaciousness

to appendicitis, diverticulitis, or surgery. Infections may be associated with significant local invasion, even traversing tissues (including bone) without respect for anatomic barriers.

Propionibacterium is notable for diphtheroid Gram stain morphology and propionic acid production. It grows slowly in culture and can require extended incubation (up to 14 days) for recovery. *P acnes* is a skin commensal that can cause significant infection of prosthetic joints and other foreign bodies, as well as endocarditis. *P propionicum* is a commensal in the oral cavity and causes indolent infections similar to *Actinomyces*.

Aerobic Gram+ bacilli

Spore-formers

Bacillus species are large, rectangular, Gram+ rods that form endospores and may form chains f3.116. They sometimes appear Gram-variable or even Gram−. Many are motile (*B anthracis* is an important exception) and most are catalase+.

B anthracis forms chains f3.117 and subterminal or central endospores, although the spores may be difficult to appreciate without performing a spore stain. On blood agar, colonies are nonhemolytic, with a ground-glass quality and irregular borders ("Medusa head" colonies) f3.118a. Colonies are tenacious and stand up when teased with a loop f3.118b. *B anthracis* is catalase+ and nonmotile. Nonmotility is best demonstrated using semi-solid agar (rather than a wet preparation) for safety reasons f3.119. Isolates with these features should be forwarded to a public health laboratory, where definitive identification is

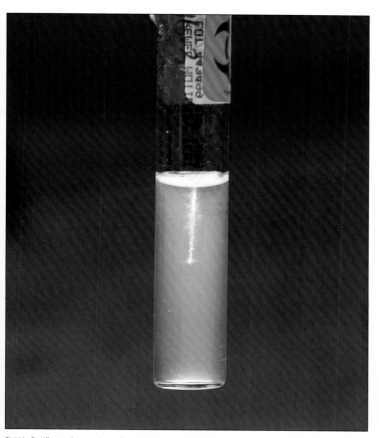

f3.119 *Bacillus anthracis*: the stab mark is clearly visible & the medium is nonturbid, indicative of nonmotility

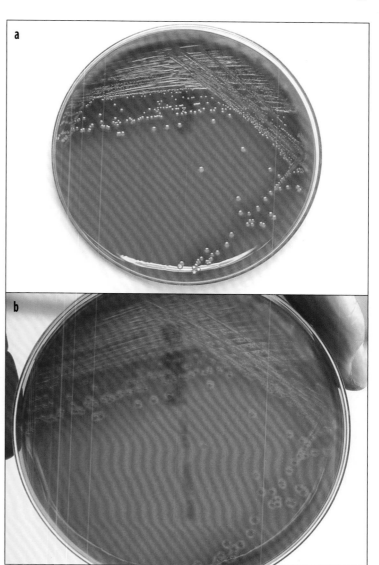

f3.120 *Listeria monocytogenes*: colony morphology

usually performed by PCR. Anthrax can take several forms, including cutaneous, gastrointestinal (ingestion), and inhalational anthrax. Cutaneous anthrax is the most common and least fatal form, and is typically acquired by inoculation of spores into a skin wound while handling animals or hides. A blackened eschar at the site of infection is the characteristic lesion. Gastrointestinal anthrax causes ulcerative lesions anywhere from mouth to colon, often with poor outcomes. Inhalational anthrax is classically associated with the processing of contaminated animal hides ("woolsorter's disease") but is also the form most commonly caused by the intentional release of purified spores as a terrorist act. The characteristic finding is a widened mediastinum, noted on anterior-posterior plain films of the thorax, caused by hemorrhagic mediastinitis.

B cereus forms chains and demonstrates subterminal spores. It is facultatively anaerobic, unlike many other *Bacillus* species which are strict aerobes. Colonies are large, β-hemolytic and nontenacious, and the organism is motile. Lecithinase activity can be demonstrated using egg yolk agar, and the catalase test is positive. *B cereus* causes food poisoning, leading either to a diarrheal syndrome or an emetic syndrome. Many foods have been associated with *B cereus* foodborne illness (Asian rice dishes are often associated with the emetic form), but the common feature is improper food storage (lack of

refrigeration) after cooking. *B cereus* can also cause a range of infections, including endophthalmitis, keratitis, bacteremia, meningitis, and many others. Typically, the host is immunocompromised, has an underlying illness (eg, malignancy, diabetes, alcoholism), and/or a catheter or shunt is involved.

Nonspore formers

Listeria monocytogenes grows somewhat slowly, forming small colonies in primary culture after 1-2 days of incubation f3.120a. Colonies are β-hemolytic, with a soft, narrow zone of hemolysis resembling the colonies of group B streptococci f3.120b. Gram stain reveals short, nonbranching, regularly shaped Gram+ rods, singly or in short chains. Isolates are catalase positive and demonstrate temperature-dependent tumbling motility in wet mounts (best seen at room temperature; not well demonstrated at 37°C.) The semi-solid agar motility

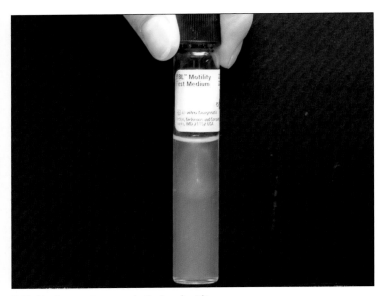

f3.121 *Listeria monocytogenes*: umbrella-shaped motility

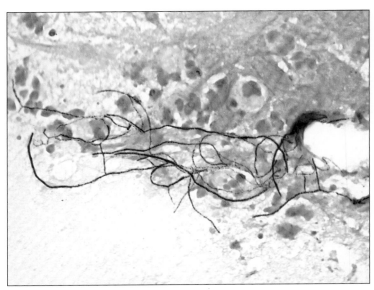

f3.123 *Nocardia*: Gram stain morphology

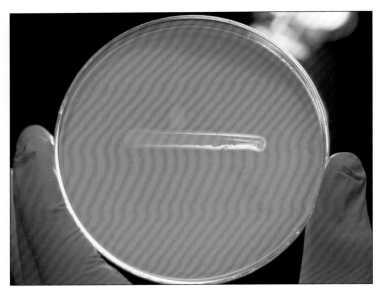

f3.122 *Listeria monocytogenes* : CAMP test with rectangular zone of hemolysis

test reveals umbrella shaped motility f3.121, and the CAMP test demonstrates a rectangular zone of enhanced hemolysis f3.122. A special feature of *Listeria* is its ability to grow at 4°C, which allows it to contaminate refrigerated foods in substantial quantity. Ingestion of contaminated foods, such as refrigerated deli meats, hot dogs or unpasteurized dairy products is the usual means of exposure. *Listeria* can cause a mild, flulike illness in pregnant women, but associated bacteremia can seed the placenta causing chorioamnionitis and/or intrauterine infection of the fetus. Live-born neonates who have acquired the infection in utero may have granulomatosis infantiseptica (widely distributed tissue abscesses), and neonates acquiring the infection during delivery may develop sepsis and meningitis. Other at-risk hosts include patients with compromised cell-mediated immunity and the elderly, in whom *Listeria* causes bacteremia, meningitis and/or encephalitis. Despite its name, *Listeria monocytogenes* rarely provokes monocytosis in humans.

Erysipelothrix rhusiopathiae is a regular, nonbranching, nonspore-forming Gram+ rod that can be short (even coccobacillary) and occur singly and in short chains, or can be long, thin and filamentous. Gram staining can be uneven, and sometime the cells will decolorize and appear Gram−. It is nonmotile and catalase negative, but characteristically produces H_2S on TSI slants, causing a blackened butt, which helps set it apart from Gram+ rods with similar microscopic morphology such as *Listeria* and *Lactobacillus*. *E rhusiopathiae* is intrinsically resistant to vancomycin. *E rhusiopathiae* causes erysipeloid, a cellulitis acquired when a skin wound comes in contact with a fish or other animal carrying the organism. It is an occupational hazard among anglers, butchers, farmers and others who handle fish, shellfish, birds or raw meat.

Nocardia are long, thin, filamentous, branching, beaded Gram+ rods f3.123 that are modified-acid fast positive f3.124. When causing indolent soft-tissue infection (mycetoma), they can form macroscopic granules similar to the sulfur granules of actinomycosis. They are aerobic and slow growing; cultures for *Nocardia* are best handled like fungal cultures (albeit with different media), because fungal cultures are incubated at 30°C and regularly examined over a long period of time. However, parallel bacterial culture at 37°C is also important, as some strains grow faster at higher temperature. Although many routine media will support its growth (eg, blood agar, brain heart infusion agar), BCYE is ideal for primary culture. Selective BCYE can be used for specimens obtained from nonsterile sites, such as sputum specimens. *Nocardia* typically produce chalky, white colonies, which become salmon orange-pink as colonies mature. They produce a characteristic

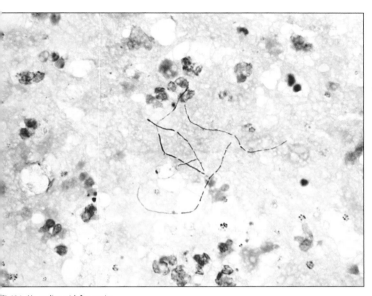

f3.124 *Nocardia*: acid-fast stain

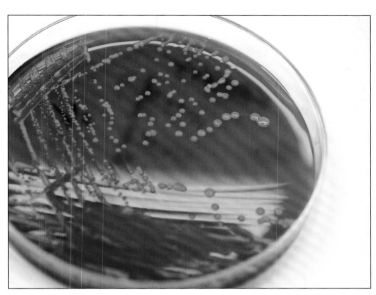

f3.125 *Rhodococcus equi*: colony morphology

"musty basement" odor. A presumptive identification can be made to the genus level by observing appropriate microscopic (Gram stain, modified acid-fast stain) and colony morphology, the presence of aerial hyphae, and lysozyme resistance. Species-level identification can be achieved by genetic methods (eg, PCR amplification of portions of the 16S rRNA gene, followed by sequence analysis of the amplicons) or by a combination of biochemical tests and susceptibility testing to look for species-specific susceptibility profiles.

Nocardia is ubiquitous in the environment, and infections are acquired from environmental sources. *N asteroides* complex species (*N asteroides sensu stricto, N nova, N farcinica, N abscessus*) and *N pseudobrasiliensis* cause invasive pulmonary infection and disseminated infection, often involving the central nervous system, in immunocompromised hosts. In such cases, the infection is acquired by inhalation. In contrast, *N brasiliensis* causes cutaneous and subcutaneous infections, such as mycetoma, in normal hosts who acquire the infection by penetrating injury.

Rhodococcus equi appears as Gram+ cocci, coccobacilli, or short, coryneform rods on direct examination of specimens by Gram stained smear. It is often found within phagocytes. When cultured on solid media, Gram stain morphology cycles between bacillary and coccoid, as the culture ages. In liquid culture, such as blood culture, it may even appear as minimally branching rods. An important microscopic feature is that the organisms are positive by the modified acid-fast stain procedure, like *Nocardia* and certain other aerobic actinomycetes (*Gordonia* and *Tsukamurella*). Growth of *Rhodococcus equi* is supported by routine media such as blood agar, and mature colonies are typically salmon colored and slimy f3.125. *R equi* does not produce aerial hyphae, and growth in lysozyme-containing medium is variable. Infection with *R equi* is rare, and usually affects immunocompromised patients. The most common presentation is a subacute pulmonary infection, eventually giving rise to cavitation in many cases. Histologic

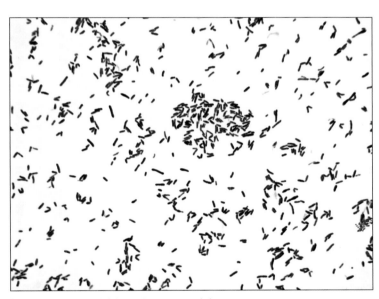

f3.126 *Corynebacterium diphtheriae*: Gram stain morphology

findings similar to malakoplakia have been described in patients with AIDS. Pulmonary infection can be complicated by dissemination to the brain or subcutaneous tissue, among other sites, causing abscess formation. Extrapulmonary infection without associated pulmonary disease can also occur. Examples include wound infection related to puncture wounds or other traumatic injury, bacteremia related to central venous catheters or severe immunosuppression, or peritonitis associated with peritoneal dialysis.

Corynebacterium diphtheriae appears as "coryneform" or "diphtheroid" pleomorphic, club shaped, irregular, short Gram+ rods that tend to palisade and cluster together f3.126. Although it grows well on routine media, such as blood agar

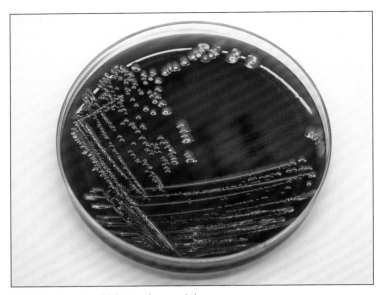

f3.127 *Corynebacterium diphtheriae*: colony morphology

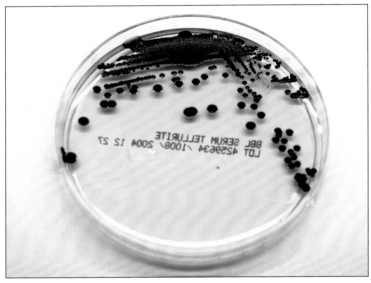

f3.128 *Corynebacterium diphtheriae* on agar containing tellurite

f3.127, isolation is improved by using selective media, such as Tinsdale agar. Potassium tellurite in tinsdale agar is a selective agent that inhibits upper respiratory tract commensals, and is also a differential agent. Presumptive identification of *C diphtheriae* involves demonstration of the organism's ability to reduce potassium tellurite to metallic tellurite f3.128, which distinguishes *C diphtheriae* from other diphtheroids in the upper respiratory tract. The appearance of brown-black colored colonies surrounded by brown-black halos on Tinsdale agar is presumptive evidence for *C diphtheriae*. Full identification is usually accomplished using biochemical tests. Diphtheria can be prevented by vaccination, making the disease a rare event in the United States. The most common site of infection is the oropharynx. Infection produces fever, sore

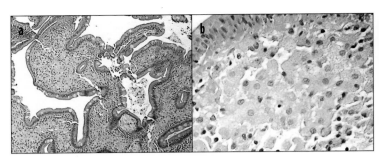

f3.129 Whipple disease: duodenal biopsy

throat, and development of a white, glossy pseudomembrane (turning gray-brown over time) covering the tonsils and other structures in the oro- and nasopharynx. This results from elaboration of a potent exotoxin. Aspiration of the membrane can lead to death in both children and adults.

Tropheryma whipplei

T whipplei is a Gram+ bacillus and the causative agent of Whipple disease.

Until recently, *T whipplei* could not be cultured. Cell culture on human fibroblasts has allowed further characterization of the organism by genome sequencing. Phylogenetic analysis has classified the bacterium as being closely related to *Actinomyces* species

T whipplei is ubiquitous in the environment; nevertheless, Whipple disease seems to develop only in individuals with selective immune deficiency. Most affected individuals are older males, with male to female ratio of 8-10:1. The most commonly affected structures are the gastrointestinal tract, joints, central nervous system, and heart valves.

In affected tissues, aggregates of foamy histiocytes are seen f3.129. Bacillary organisms can be highlighted by PAS stain; they are negative for AFB. PCR can be used to confirm the diagnosis.

Gram– bacilli

Once obligate anaerobes have been excluded, the Gram– bacilli can be initially classified by their growth characteristics on MacConkey agar. The Enterobacteriaceae and the nonfermenters are organisms that grow robustly on MacConkey. The so-called fastidious organisms that do not grow well on MacConkey are a large group of disparate species that must be grown on special media.

Anaerobic Gram– bacilli

Bacteroides, especially *B fragilis*, is the most common isolate but, like the others in this group, is usually a part of a polymicrobial infection. It is important to identify *Bacteroides* because of its potential for β-lactamase production (nearly all strains are resistant to penicillin) and association with high mortality. It grows readily on blood agar, where it forms small, shiny colonies whose Gram stain morphology is pleomorphic, ranging from bacillary to coccobacillary. In Gram stains from liquid media, *Bacteroides* appear as bacilli with bipolar vacuoles, described as having a "safety pin" appearance.

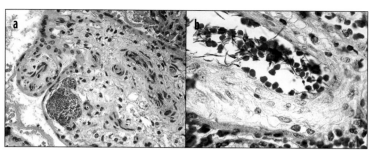

f3.130 *Fusobacterium necrophorum* in placenta on a H&E stained sections & b Gram stained sections

Porphyromonas/Prevotella are distinctive for production of a brick-red fluorescence when exposed to UV light; after several days of growth, the colonies appear brown-black in natural light.

Fusobacterium may appear as fusiform (spindle shaped) Gram– rods in Gram stained smears, although many strains have rounded ends rather than pointed ends. *F necrophorum*, an agent that may colonize or infect the tonsils, is associated with Lemierre syndrome (tonsillitis complicated by septic thrombophlebitis of the internal jugular vein). It has also been associated with placental infection complicated by preterm labor and/or stillbirth f3.130.

Growth on MacConkey glucose fermentation+, oxidase–: Enterobacteriaceae

Characteristics

Also known as "enterics" or "enteric Gram– rods," many of the Enterobacteriaceae are natural inhabitants of the colon. Nasopharyngeal carriage may occur in hospitalized patients, patients with uncontrolled diabetes mellitus, and chronic alcoholics. Enterobacteriaceae are commonly isolated from urine, blood, wounds, abscesses, and from the respiratory tract. Certain species, especially *Salmonella*, *Shigella*, Shiga-toxin producing *E coli* (STEC) and *Yersinia enterocolitica*, are GI pathogens. Lipopolysaccharide (LPS), a component of the outer membrane, is a major virulence factor. Lipid A, a component of LPS, is also called endotoxin. O antigen, a second LPS component, forms the basis for serogrouping.

Antimicrobial resistance among Enterobacteriaceae is a growing problem. For example, the emergence of extended-spectrum β-lactamase (ESBL)-producing Enterobacteriaceae and carbapenemase-producing Enterobacteriaceae is a major concern. All strains of *Klebsiella pneumoniae*, and many *E coli* strains, produce a serine β-lactamase (penicillinase) enzyme that inactivates penicillins and first-generation (narrow-spectrum) cephalosporins. This plasmid-mediated enzyme activity is typically susceptible to inactivation by β-lactamase inhibitors, making β-lactamase/β-lactamase inhibitor combinations an effective tool against these strains. In addition, oxyimino-cephalosporins (extended spectrum cephalosporins), monobactams and carbapenems are active against these strains. However, mutations in the parent β-lactamase genes can render the enzymes able to inactivate extended-spectrum cephalosporins and monobactams, in addition to penicillins and narrow-spectrum cephalosporins. These enzymes, termed ESBLs, are not very active against cephamycins (eg,

cefoxitin, cefotetan) or carbapenems, and remain susceptible to inactivation by β-lactamase inhibitors. Besides *K pneumoniae* and *E coli*, other Enterobacteriaceae may also harbor ESBLs, including *Klebsiella oxytoca*, *Proteus mirabilis*, *Salmonella*, and *Enterobacter* species. An even more ominous trend is the emergence of Enterobacteriaceae (primarily *Klebsiella pneumoniae*) that produce β-lactamase enzymes capable of inactivating carbapenems. These enzymes, termed carbapenemases, also inactivate penicillins, cephalosporins and in some cases aztreonam, leaving few good treatment options.

The Enterobacteriaceae are a large group of organisms t3.40 that can be difficult to sort out. Hallmark characteristics are reviewed in t3.41. With regard to Kligler iron agar & triple sugar iron (KIA/TSI) slants, recall that these are agar slants that contain proteins, sugars, and a phenol red indicator. The sugars are present in a 10:1 ratio of lactose to glucose for KIA, or 10:1 of lactose and sucrose to glucose for TSI. The phenol red indicator is yellow when the pH is below 6.8 and red when above 6.8. The organism is inoculated by stabbing all the way to the bottom (butt) of the tube then streaking the surface (slant). An organism's ability to ferment the sugars is evidenced by lowering the pH (yellowing of the indicator). The tubes are interpreted at 24 hours. After a short incubation (eg, 8 hours), a bacterium that ferments glucose but not lactose will produce an acidic (yellow) slant and acidic (yellow). However, after the limited quantity of glucose is consumed, the organism will begin oxidative metabolism of proteins, which can only take place in the oxygen rich environment of the slant; this will turn the slant back to alkaline (red) by 24 hours, while the butt will remain yellow. Organisms that ferment lactose, which is present in the agar at much higher concentration, will continue to ferment throughout the incubation period, maintaining a yellow slant and butt even after 24 hours. An H_2S indicator is also present in these slants; H_2S production will result in a black color. After 24-hour incubation, results are interpreted t3.42.

t3.40 Taxonomy of the Enterobacteriaceae

Family (tribe)	Genus & species
Escherichieae	Escherichia: E coli; Shigella: S sonnei, S flexneri, S dysenteriae, S boydii
Edwardsielleae	Edwardsiella tarda
Salmonelleae	Salmonella: S enteritidis, S typhi, S paratyphi, S choleraesuis
Citrobactereae	Citrobacter freundii
Klebsielleae	Klebsiella: K pneumoniae; Enterobacter: E aerogenes, E cloacae; Hafnia: H alvei Pantoea: P agglomerans; Serratia: S marcescens
Proteae	Proteus: P vulgaris, P mirabilis; Morganella: M morganii; Providencia: P stuartii
Yersinieae	Yersinia enterocolitica

t3.41 Enterobacteriaceae: key characteristics

Reduce nitrate to nitrite	All Enterobacteriaceae
Strong lactose fermenters (pink or red on MacConkey)	E coli, Klebsiella, Enterobacter
Hydrogen sulfide (H_2S) positive	Salmonella, Edwardsiella, Citrobacter freundii, Proteus
Strongly urease+	Proteus, Morganella, Providencia rettgeri
Nonmotile	Shigella, Klebsiella
Yersinia are non motile at 37°C, but motile at 22°C
Voges-Proskauer (VP) positive	Klebsiella, Enterobacter, Hafnia, Serratia, Pantoea
Phenylalanine deaminase (PAD) positive	Proteus, Morganella, Providencia
Kligler iron agar & triple sugar iron (KIA/TSI) slants	See t3.42

t3.42 KIA/TSI slant characteristics

Alkaline slant/alkaline butt (K/K, red over red)	Enterobacteriaceae excluded, as all are glucose fermenters
	Possibilities include nonfermentative bacteria such as *Pseudomonas*
Alkaline slant/acid butt (K/A, red over yellow)	Glucose fermented, lactose not fermented
	Possibilities include *Shigella, Serratia, Morganella, Providencia, Yersinia*
Alkaline slant/acid butt with H$_2$S production (K/A/H2S+)	Glucose fermented, lactose not fermented, H$_2$S produced
	Possibilities include *Salmonella, Edwardsiella, Citrobacter, Proteus*
Acid slant/acid deep (A/A, yellow over yellow)	Glucose & lactose fermenters
	Possibilities include *E coli, Klebsiella, Enterobacter*

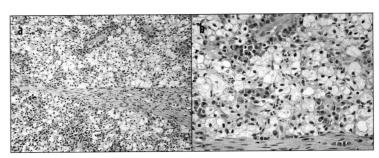

f3.131 Rhinoscleroma in H&E stained sections at a low & b high magnification

Escherichia coli

This species is presumptively identified when an Enterobacteriaceae isolate is lactose fermenting, indole+, and positive for β-glucuronidase activity. Although *E coli* is part of the normal gut flora, certain strains are diarrheagenic.

EHEC (enterohemorrhagic *E coli*) is capable of producing Shiga toxin (verotoxin) and is sometimes called STEC (Shiga toxin-producing *E coli*). The toxin inhibits protein synthesis, causing damage to enterocytes. Once released into the blood stream, the Shiga toxin causes damage to endothelial cells. EHEC has gained notoriety for its association with hemolytic uremic syndrome (HUS), in addition to production of a hemorrhagic colitis. HUS develops in ~10% of infected children, ~5-12 days after the onset of diarrhea. In North America, EHEC serotype O157:H7 is most commonly implicated in this syndrome. The major reservoir for EHEC is cattle, with ingestion of contaminated foods being the most common route of infection. Sorbitol-MacConkey plates can be used to detect EHEC O157:H7 in culture, as this strain (unlike routine *E coli* strains) does not ferment sorbitol. However, this method cannot be used to identify other non-O157 STEC strains, as these will ferment sorbitol. STEC (both O157 and non-O157) can be detected in stool using an ELISA or similar assay that detects Shiga toxins, or a PCR assay that detects the genes for these toxins.

ETEC (enterotoxigenic *E coli*) causes infection of the small intestine resulting in secretory (watery) diarrhea with clinical manifestations indistinguishable from cholera. It is the main cause of "traveler's diarrhea" and a major cause of childhood diarrhea worldwide. ETEC produces toxins similar to the cholera toxin, the so-called heat-stable and heat labile enterotoxins which stimulate guanylate and adenylate cyclase, respectively. Infection results from ingestion of contaminated water. The diagnosis of ETEC infection is usually clinical, but can be confirmed by PCR detection of the genes that encode its enterotoxins.

EIEC (enteroinvasive *E coli*) causes invasion of the colonic mucosa and clinical dysentery similar to that caused by *Shigella*. It is closely related to *Shigella*; it produces a Shiga-like toxin (T3SS) and, like *Shigella*, is nonmotile and lactose nonfermenting.

EPEC (enteropathogenic *E coli*) causes dysenteric illness without the production of a Shiga-like toxin. Clinically, it causes infant gastroenteritis in underdeveloped countries. Person to person spread is an important feature of EPEC outbreaks. The confirmation of EPEC infection depends upon PCR for detection of genes that encode strain-specific toxins.

EAggEC (enteroaggregative *E coli*) causes infant diarrhea in underdeveloped countries, traveler's diarrhea (particularly in children), and chronic refractory diarrhea in HIV infected patients. EAggEC is defined in vitro by an aggregative adherence to tissue culture cells.

Salmonella

Salmonellosis is most commonly manifested as enteritis. Certain *Salmonella* species have the potential to produce bacteremia, including *S choleraesuis, S paratyphi,* and *S typhi*. *Salmonella* sepsis is particularly a problem in children, and children with sickle cell disease are prone to develop salmonella osteomyelitis. Typhoid fever, caused by *S typhi* or *S paratyphi*, is yet another possible consequence of *Salmonella* infection. In this syndrome, bacteria traverse the bowel wall and entrench themselves within reticuloendothelial cells of the liver, spleen, and gallbladder. From these organs, repeated bouts of bacteremia are launched. The gallbladder may act as a reservoir, continually reinfecting the bowel, leading to long-term shedding of the bacterium.

Shigella

The most common cause of shigellosis in the United States is *S sonnei*. In underdeveloped countries, the most common isolate is *S flexneri*. *Shigella* infection requires the smallest inoculum of any form of bacterial gastroenteritis—only ~100-200 bacteria. Infection may be foodborne, waterborne, or can be transmitted by sexual contact. *Shigella dysenteriae*, like EHEC, can cause hemolytic uremic syndrome (HUS). *S flexneri* infection can lead to postinfectious arthritis, especially in individuals with the genetic marker HLA-B27.

Klebsiella

The most common manifestation of *K pneumoniae* infection is pneumonia, which tends to be necrotizing and productive of "currant jelly" sputum. Older debilitated patients are most susceptible, particularly older male alcoholics. *K oxytoca* may cause neonatal sepsis. Rhinoscleroma is a chronic granulomatous disease f3.131 of the upper airways, particularly the nasal cavity, which is endemic in tropical and subtropical areas. *Klebsiella rhinoscleromatis* is the causative agent.

Yersinia

Isolation of *Yersinia* relies on culture at room temperature, rather than body temperature, and is improved by the use of selective media (CIN agar). Cold enrichment, in which a specimen is stored at 4°C for 2 weeks prior to culturing, may also improve culture sensitivity. Most *Yersinia* infections are zoonotic. Humans are accidental hosts.

Y enterocolitica causes enterocolitis in places with cold climates. It characteristically targets the terminal ileum and can cause the misdiagnosis of appendicitis. *Y enterocolitica* is an important cause of transfusion related sepsis.

Y pseudotuberculosis is an uncommon cause of disease, but is noteworthy because it produces necrotizing granulomata resembling those caused by tuberculosis. Often these are found in the ileocecal region of the abdomen, including the appendix.

Y pestis causes plague. Sylvatic plague is the variety found in nonurban settings, and is transmitted by fleas that parasitize squirrels, field rats, domestic cats and other animals. Urban plague is found in densely populated areas and is carried by rats.

Growth on MacConkey, oxidase+, glucose fermentation+: nonenteric fermenters
Vibrio cholerae

Vibrio cholerae is sucrose-positive on selective TCBS agar (yellow colonies) and string test-positive. The El Tor biotype is distinctive for β-hemolysis, weak string test, & ability to agglutinate chicken erythrocytes. *V cholera* is traditionally classified by somatic O antigens (>150 O types currently recognized), by biotype (classic and El Tor), or by serotype (Ogawa, Inaba, and Hikojima). Based upon O antigens, isolates are broadly characterized as *V cholerae* O1 (etiologic agents of most cases of cholera) and non-O1 *V cholerae*. Serogroup O139 has emerged as an additional significant cause of cholera in the Indian subcontinent.

V parahaemolyticus

Sucrose– on TCBS (green colonies). Ingestion of contaminated seafood causes mainly gastroenteritis, sometimes with blood diarrhea.

V vulnificus

V vulnificus is found in warm, low-salinity marine environments, especially along the Gulf of Mexico, where contaminated oysters and crabs can be found. *V vulnificus* infection may present as gastroenteritis or skin/soft tissue infection, either of which may be complicated by severe sepsis. The gastroenteritis of *V vulnificus* features both vomiting and bloody diarrhea. Skin infection may follow trauma, or it may be caused by exposure of already open skin to infected water. The skin lesions initially resemble cellulitis, often with bullae, but may progress to necrotizing fasciitis. Patients with chronic liver disease, diabetes mellitus, or immunosuppression are at greatest risk of severe sepsis.

Aeromonas & Plesiomonas

Aeromonas and *Plesiomonas* are inhabitants of fresh and brackish water and may be found in hospital or household water, including fish tanks. Both are occasional causes of gastroenteritis and soft tissue (wound) infections. Several species of *Aeromonas* have been associated with infection, including *A hydrophila*, *A caviae*, *A schubertii* and *A veronii*; *P shigelloides* is the only pathogenic *Plesiomonas* species. Importantly, not all strains of potentially pathogenic species are capable of causing gastrointestinal illness, and the presence of *Aeromonas* or *Plesiomonas* in stool culture does not necessarily indicate infection.

Growth on MacConkey, glucose nonfermenters: nonenterics
Pseudomonas

Pseudomonas aeruginosa is an oxidase+, Gram– bacillus that is motile by means of polar monotrichous flagella. In culture, colonies are often β-hemolytic and produce a grapelike odor. Strains typically produce a green diffusible pigment (a combination of blue pyocyanin and yellow pyoverdin) which is best appreciated with growth on clear agars (eg, BHI, Mueller-Hinton). A few strains instead produce red (pyorubicin) or black (pyomelanin) pigments. Isolates are able to grow well at 42°C, both in culture and in the environment. Clinically, *P aeruginosa* is most important as a complication of cystic fibrosis and as a nosocomial pathogen. In the hospital, *P aeruginosa* is found in water wherever it collects, including sinks, showers, toilets, and water-containing equipment. Community acquired *P aeruginosa* infection, likewise, is associated with watery sources, including hot tubs and swimming pools. *P aeruginosa* endocarditis is encountered in intravenous drug abusers.

Stenotrophomonas

Stenotrophomonas maltophilia, previously *Xanthomonas maltophilia*, shares with *Pseudomonas* a preference for watery environments, including those found in hospitals, and frequent multidrug antimicrobial resistance. Unlike *Pseudomonas*, it is oxidase–. It is an opportunistic pathogen that most often causes nosocomial pneumonia or bacteremia.

Acinetobacter species

Oxidase–, nonmotile, Gram– coccobacilli that can appear sufficiently coccoid as to resemble *Neisseria*. Strains can be multiply drug resistant, and cause nosocomial pulmonary infections, bloodstream infections, wound infections and UTIs.

No growth on MacConkey, slow growth of pinpoint colonies on enriched media: fastidious Gram– rods
Tularemia

Francisella tularensis, the agent of tularemia, is a slow growing, Gram– coccobacillus. For in vitro growth, it requires supplementation with sulfhydryl compounds (eg, cysteine and cystine). Although it cannot grow on sheep blood agar, it will grow on BCYE, Thayer-Martin agar and in thioglycolate broth or routine blood culture bottles (with extended incubation). Some strains will also grow on chocolate agar. Isolates are oxidase– and urease–, and β-lactamase+.

Tularemia is usually acquired from arthropods or exposure to infected animals, but some infections are the result of inhalation of contaminated material. Also known as rabbit fever and deer fly fever, tularemia has a high fatality rate. Clinical presentations are variously described as ulceroglandular, oculoglandular, pneumonic, or typhoidal.

Although the organism can be cultured, the diagnosis is most often made by serologic testing. The agglutination method (either tube agglutination or microagglutination) remains the standard for serodiagnosis. PCR assays have also recently become available for direct detection in clinical specimens.

F tularensis is considered a potential agent of bioterrorism, and is on the select agent list.

Brucella

Brucella is a slow growing, Gram– coccobacillus that is urease+ and oxidase+. The organism is fastidious but can be isolated using routine blood culture bottles (sometimes requiring extended incubation) or chocolate agar with CO_2 supplementation. *Brucella* species can be isolated from blood, bone marrow, bone, and other tissues.

The major source of infection is livestock, particularly cattle (*Brucella abortus*), goats and sheep (*Brucella melitensis*), and swine (*Brucella suis*). Rare cases are due to *Brucella canis*, acquired by exposure to dogs. The epidemiology of brucellosis in the United States has undergone a change from occupational disease among livestock handlers and abattoir workers to foodborne illness acquired by consumption of unpasteurized goat and cow dairy products. Airborne transmission is possible, raising the possibility of use as an agent of bioterrorism.

The clinical manifestations are largely nonspecific, but fever is invariable. Lymphadenopathy, hepatosplenomegaly and inflammatory arthritis are common, and malodorous perspiration is considered nearly pathognomonic. Arthritis may affect the appendicular joints as well as the sacroiliac joint and spine. Other manifestations include spontaneous abortion, hepatitis (with granulomas in biopsies), and endocarditis (a principal source of mortality).

Serologic testing is the mainstay of diagnosis. Numerous methods can be employed, including agglutination tests, indirect fluorescent antibody tests, and ELISAs. PCR-based assays have also been developed for direct detection of the organism in primary specimens.

Bordetella

Bordetella is an aerobic small coccobacillus that requires nicotinic acid, cysteine, and methionine for growth. It does not require X or V factor. *Bordetella* characteristically grows in 2-4 days on Bordet-Gengou or Regan-Lowe media; incubation should be at 35°C with supplemental CO_2. Colonies are small, smooth and shiny and have been likened to a drop of mercury. *B pertussis* is the etiologic agent of whooping cough. *Bordetella parapertussis* rarely produces a pertussis-like illness. Laboratory isolation depends upon an adequate nasopharyngeal swab, with prompt inoculation of transport medium. Though a rapid DFA is available, its low sensitivity mandates culture, PCR or serologic testing in suspected cases.

Pasteurella

Gram– rod frequently associated with wound infection from animal bites. *P multocida*, which causes the majority of *Pasteurella* infections, is oxidase+, catalase+, and strongly indole+.

Legionella

Legionella is a Gram-invisible bacillus in primary Gram stained smears. Isolates require L-cysteine supplementation for in vitro culture, and thus will not grow on MacConkey, SBA or chocolate agar. *Legionella* forms whitish colonies in 2-5 days on BCYE medium, identification can be confirmed by direct fluorescent-antibody or latex agglutination methods. Infection with *L pneumophila* serogroup 1 (the most prevalent serogroup) can be detected using a urinary antigen test.

Campylobacter

The *Campylobacter* are tiny, thin, curved (seagull shaped) Gram– rods, which grow on selective media (Campy-BAP) at 42°C. Isolates are oxidase+, catalase+, and positive for hippurate hydrolysis. The hippurate hydrolysis test is key to distinguishing *C jejuni* from other *Campylobacter* species

Capnocytophaga

Capnocytophaga canimorsus is a spindle shaped, thin Gram– rod. Isolation requires CO_2 supplementation and may require enriched media such as chocolate agar. Isolation from blood is not always possible using routine blood culture media; blind subculture onto chocolate agar (or other enriched media) may be necessary. Isolates are catalase- and oxidase+. *C canimorsus* causes soft tissue infections after dog or cat bites, and leads to bacteremia and sepsis in susceptible hosts (asplenia, chronic liver disease).

Streptobacillus

Streptobacillus moniliformis forms puffball or cottonball-like colonies in serum-supplemented thioglycolate broth. Reliable isolation on solid medium also requires 15-20% serum or blood enrichment and CO_2 supplementation, with several days of incubation. Classically, the Gram stain shows tangles of Gram-variable, filamentous rods with moniliform swellings. *S moniliformis* is the causative agent of rat-bite fever.

Haemophilus species

Haemophilus species show no growth on MacConkey or SBA, but they form small colonies on chocolate agar. The species are classified according to hemolysis and growth requirements t3.43.

t3.43 Hemolysis & growth factor characteristics of *Haemophilus* species

Species	Requires X-factor	Requires V-factor	Hemolysis
H influenzae	+	+	–
H parainfluenza	–	+	–
H haemolyticus	+	+	+
H parahaemolyticus	–	+	+
H aegyptius	+	+	+
H ducreyi	+	–	

HACEK group

Acronym for a group of fastidious Gram– organisms causing endocarditis, including *Aggregatibacter* (formerly *Haemophilus*) *aphrophilus*, *Aggregatibacter* (formerly *Actinobacillus*) *actinomycetemcomitans*, *Cardiobacterium hominis*, *Eikenella corrodens*, and *Kingella* species. All are slowly growing, fastidious organisms that require 48-72 hours to grow in an enriched CO_2 environment on chocolate agar. Although in the past these organisms were considered common agents of "culture-negative endocarditis," modern blood culture techniques reliably detect them.

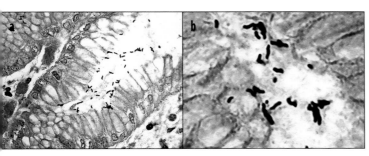

f3.132 *Helicobacter pylori* in Warthin-Starry-stained sections at **a** low & **b** high magnification

Helicobacter pylori

Helicobacter pylori is a Gram–, spiral bacillus that is the cause of the vast majority of cases of chronic gastritis and is the ultimate cause of gastritis complications—peptic ulcer disease, gastric adenocarcinoma (predominantly the intestinal type), and gastric MALT lymphoma. *H pylori* prevalence varies with patient age, socioeconomic status, and ethnic group. Typically, incidence increases with age. Infection has lowest prevalence in upper socioeconomic groups. In the US, prevalence is ~50% in African Americans, 60% in Mexican Americans, and 26% in caucasians. *H pylori* infection is a chronic condition. There tends to be a long latency period before manifestations develop. Eradication is recommended for all patients with the infection, regardless of symptoms, in order to reduce the risk of malignancy. Interestingly, treatment of *H pylori* may result in enhanced gastric acid production (due to reversal of atrophic gastritis), leading to unmasking of gastroesophageal reflux disease (GERD). The diagnosis may be made by a variety of methods. Anti–*H pylori* IgG antibodies typically become detectable by serologic testing after 4 weeks of infection. Since most patients who present for testing have been infected for many years, the sensitivity of this test is quite good. However, serology can remain positive for many years after eradication. Thus, serology cannot be used to confirm eradication. Urea breath testing can be used both to diagnose *H pylori* infection and to confirm eradication. The patient ingests radiolabeled urea which, if *H pylori* is present, is converted by bacterial urease into radiolabeled CO_2. Stool antigen testing and stool culture are available; stool antigen testing has become a useful way to confirm eradication. Histologic examination has the advantage of permitting not only detection of *H pylori* f3.132 but examination of the biopsy for premalignant changes (intestinal metaplasia, dysplasia). Additional tissue can be subjected to rapid urease testing or culture. Following treatment for *H pylori,* which has a high failure rate, confirmation of eradication is often undertaken. At least 4 weeks should elapse between cessation of treatment and confirmatory testing, to permit regrowth of residual *H pylori* bacteria; otherwise the false negative rate is unacceptably high. If a stool-based test is used for confirmation, 6-12 weeks should elapse.

Coxiella

Coxiella burnetii is the causative agent of Q fever, a zoonotic disease that is endemic worldwide. There are a large number of possible hosts, including livestock, pets, birds, fish, and ticks, and these hosts shed organisms in milk, feces, and birthing fluids. Human infection is usually the result of inhalation of the organisms during slaughter or while attending a birth. Thus, it is an occupational hazard for veterinarians, farmers, and abattoir workers. The organism can also be aerosolized and dispersed in the wind, leading to infection among patients without animal contact.

C burnetii is an obligate intracellular pathogen, and because of this was initially classified among the Rickettsiaceae. It is distinct from them genetically, however, and is now classified amongst the γ-Proteobacteria, with *Francisella* and *Legionella*. *C burnetii* is a pleomorphic Gram– coccobacillus with small-cell variants (SCV) and large cell variants (LCV) distinguishable by electron microscopy. The SCV survives well in the environment and is passively ingested by host monocytes, whereas the LCV cannot survive in the environment but is capable of multiplying within the phagolysosomes of monocytes.

Clinically, about half of infected persons remain asymptomatic. The other half have manifestations of acute Q fever, and ~1-2% of those develop chronic Q fever. While men and women are infected with equal frequency, men are much more commonly symptomatic. Children have a high rate of asymptomatic infection. Acute Q fever presents as a nonspecific flulike illness with pneumonitis and/or hepatitis. Thrombocytopenia is present in 25% of cases, hepatic enzymes are often elevated, and autoantibodies are frequent (including anti-mitochondrial and anti-smooth muscle antibodies). The fatality rate is 1-2%, often related to myocarditis. Granulomata can be found in the liver and bone marrow and have a classic fibrin-ring appearance. Chronic Q fever, which is associated with high mortality, most often takes the form of endocarditis, endovasculitis, or infection of the bone and joint. Q fever endocarditis usually forms no detectable vegetations, blood cultures are negative, and there is usually underlying valve disease. Immunosuppression is a major risk factor. Likewise, Q fever osteoarthritis develops in the immunocompromised or in those with prostheses. Endovasculitis may be complicated by arterial aneurysm. Histologically, Q fever endocarditis is characterized by inflammatory cells admixed with foamy histiocytes (containing organisms)—fibrin-ring granulomas are not seen. Recrudescence of Q fever may occur during pregnancy and often leads to premature birth, abortion, or neonatal death.

The diagnosis is based largely on serology, but this is not a simple matter. First, a significant proportion of people throughout the world have antibodies against *C burnetii* as a result of prior exposure. On the other hand, the use of recommended titer cutoffs may be associated with a high false negative rate. Furthermore, *C burnetii* has 2 significant antigenic states: bacteria obtained directly from infected humans or animals are in phase I, while those obtained after several passes through embryonated eggs are in phase II. The antibody response in acute human disease is primarily to phase II antigens, while antibodies to both the phase I and II organisms are elevated in chronic disease. For acute Q fever, a 4-fold rise in paired sera gives the highest specificity, but sufficiently elevated single titers may also provide the diagnosis. While there is controversy over diagnostic cutoffs, an IgM titer ≥1:50 by indirect immunofluorescence antibody testing (IFA) against phase II antigens is considered diagnostic of acute Q fever, as is an IgG titer ≥1:200. An IgG titer >1:800 against phase I antigens is usually found in chronic infection. Serology must

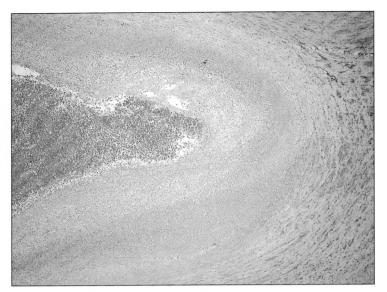

f3.133 *Treponema pallidum* associated necrotizing funisitis

be repeated 6 months after Q fever is diagnosed, to exclude chronic infection. Once chronic Q fever is diagnosed, antibody titers can be used to monitor treatment. PCR is highly sensitive when applied to tissue samples, such as heart valves, but is not useful for testing blood. Histological findings are generally nonspecific.

Spirochetes

A common feature of spirochetal infections is a triphasic clinical course. Initial manifestations are at the site of inoculation (primary phase). The secondary phase is marked by systemic manifestations of dissemination. Tertiary manifestations (latent phase) reflect sites of organism harbor. Diagnosis is usually serologic; however, direct visualization is sometimes possible.

Treponemes

Treponema are tightly coiled Gram– microaerophilic organisms with a characteristic flexing and bending motility.

T pallidum subspecies *pallidum* is distributed worldwide and causes venereal syphilis. The clinical types and stages of syphilis are distinctive t3.44. The laboratory diagnosis can be made by direct visualization or with various serologic strategies. In direct material from clinical lesions, one may visualize the organism using darkfield microscopy, direct fluorescent antibodies, immunohistochemistry, or silver stains.

Serologic tests are categorized as "treponemal-specific" or "nontreponemal." Early-generation treponemal-specific tests include the fluorescent treponemal antibody-absorption (FTA-ABS) test, the *Treponema pallidum* passive particle agglutination (TP-PA) test or the microhemagglutination assay for antibodies to *Treponema pallidum* (MHA-TP), among others. Recently, treponemal-specific enzyme immunoassays (syphilis IgG) using recombinant *T pallidum* target antigens have been developed, which are easier to perform, are objectively interpreted and are somewhat more sensitive. Nontreponemal tests include the rapid plasma regain (RPR) test and the venereal disease research laboratory (VDRL) test. The CDC

now recommends syphilis IgG as the primary screening test for syphilis, instead of RPR. Nontreponemal tests detect antibodies that bind such things as lecithin and cardiolipin, rather than components of the spirochete itself. One of the peculiarities of nontreponemal antibodies is their tendency to wane with treatment, whereas treponemal-specific antibodies remain positive indefinitely. Thus, treatment can be monitored with serial nontreponemal antibody titers.

Screening for syphilis can be performed using either a nontreponemal test, usually the RPR, or with a treponemal-specific enzyme immunoassay. False positive nontreponemal tests are a common occurrence, especially in patients with infectious mononucleosis, pregnancy, systemic lupus erythematosus and other collagen vascular diseases, and chronic infection. Thus, positive nontreponemal screening tests must be confirmed with a treponemal assay. Screening with a treponemal-specific test (currently recommended by the CDC) results in fewer false positive results, but positive tests should still be confirmed using a nontreponemal test.

T pallidum subspecies *pertenue* is found in Africa, Asia, and South America; it causes yaws.

T pallidum subspecies *endemicum* is found in Africa, Asia, and the Middle East; it causes endemic, nonvenereal syphilis (Bejel).

T carateum causes Pinta in South America.

t3.44 Clinical stages of syphilis

Stage	Definition	Possible complications	Pathology
Incubation	Period between exposure & symptoms is usually 3 weeks (range, 3-90 days)	None	None
Primary	Chancre, lasting 1-8 weeks	Regional lymphadenopathy, Jarisch-Herxheimer reaction	Obliterative endarteritis & plasmacytic infiltrate typify all phases
Secondary	Dissemination	Skin rash, condyloma lata, aseptic meningitis, hepatitis, arthritis, Jarisch-Herxheimer reaction, immune complex glomerulonephritis	
Early latent	Asymptomatic phase <4 years	Relapse	
Late latent	Asymptomatic phase >4 years		
Tertiary	Any of 3 complications:	Neurosyphilis: meningovascular, parenchymatous, tabes dorsalis, general paresis, otitis, optic neuritis Cardiovascular: aortic insufficiency and/or coronary artery stenosis Gummatous: bones and/or skin	
Congenital	Transplacentally acquired syphilis	Chorioamnionitis f3.133, hepatosplenomegaly, skin rash, rhinitis, periostitis, cytopenias, Clutton joints, saddle nose, sabre shins, Hutchinson teeth	

Borrelia

Borrelia are microaerophilic, loosely coiled bacteria with corkscrew motility.

Lyme disease is caused by *Borrelia* species within the *B burgdorferi sensu lato* complex, primarily *B burgdorferi sensu stricto* in North America, and other species (principally *B afzelii* and *B garinii*) in Europe. In the United States, Lyme disease is found in 3 distinct pockets, paralleling the distribution of its tick vectors, *Ixodes scapularis* and *Ixodes pacificus*: Northeastern states (New York, Pennsylvania, New Jersey, Massachusetts, Connecticut, Maryland, and Delaware), upper Midwestern states (Wisconsin and Minnesota), and West coast states (northern California and Oregon). The natural reservoir is the white-footed mouse, but in endemic areas, deer are an important reservoir. Coinfection with *Babesia* and/or *Anaplasma* is not uncommon.

Lyme disease, like syphilis, proceeds through distinct stages. The early stage of infection is characterized by a distinctive skin eruption at the inoculation site, termed erythema migrans (EM). EM is an annular, expanding lesion that appears within 2 weeks of inoculation and, if untreated, spontaneously fades by 4 weeks. Some patients develop satellite lesions that are smaller but otherwise resemble EM. The skin manifestation is the only really distinctive feature of Lyme disease; after it fades, or if it doesn't develop, the diagnosis becomes a significant challenge. EM is often accompanied by flulike constitutional symptoms. In the weeks to months that follow, untreated Lyme disease can progress to the second stage, which is characterized by neurologic or cardiac involvement. Neurologic involvement (neuroborreliosis) most commonly manifests as a facial nerve palsy, which may be bilateral. Less common are aseptic meningitis, with CSF lymphocytic pleocytosis and elevated protein, radiculopathy, or mononeuritis multiplex. A syndrome of recurring aseptic meningitis with simultaneous cranial nerve palsy is highly suggestive of Lyme disease. Cardiac involvement typically presents with atrioventricular (A-V) block, a manifestation of myocarditis. In third stage Lyme disease the joints are most commonly involved, with intermittent episodes of oligo- or polyarticular swelling and pain, especially involving the knee. In fact, American Lyme disease was first described in a group of children thought to be suffering from juvenile rheumatoid arthritis. Joint fluid is notable for leukocytosis, in the range of 500-100,000 WBC/mm^3, with a predominance of neutrophils. Other late stage manifestations may include acrodermatitis chronica atrophicans (a skin lesion) or late neurologic disease, including transverse myelitis and demyelinating disease or cognitive impairment.

The diagnosis of Lyme disease usually depends on recognition of its clinical features and serologic testing. The utility of direct detection using darkfield microscopy, fluorescence microscopy or silver stains is very limited, as organisms are very rare in primary specimens. Culture is possible using special media, but recovery from most specimen types is poor. Similarly, nucleic acid testing by polymerase chain reaction is possible, but sensitivity is poor except when applied to synovial tissue or fluid or skin biopsy of EM lesions. The most commonly used serologic methods are ELISA and western blot, performed upon serum or CSF. The CDC recommends a 2-tiered testing strategy, wherein serum testing positive by ELISA is then subjected to western blot. Specific criteria are applied to the interpretation of western blot, similar to HIV confirmatory testing. The sensitivity of this approach depends upon the stage of disease, with higher sensitivity in the later stages. More recently, enzyme immunoassays have been developed that detect antibodies directed against the variable-major protein-like sequence expressed (VlsE) lipoprotein of *B burgdorferi* or against a 26-mer peptide from the 6th invariable region of the protein (the C6 peptide). These assays are more sensitive than standard 2-tiered testing in early infection, and are gaining traction as a replacement for conventional ELISAs in the first tier of the 2-tiered testing algorithm.

Leptospirosis

Leptospira interrogans is a microaerophilic, tightly coiled, motile bacteria with hooked ends.

L interrogans is the causative organism of leptospirosis, a multisystem zoonotic disease sometimes characterized by the triad of meningitis, hepatitis, and nephritis (Weil disease). Presentations may be icteric or nonicteric. Nonicteric disease characterizes mild infections with a very low mortality. Icteric leptospirosis is a severe disease with up to 15% mortality. In this syndrome, one may see acute renal failure, pancreatitis, thrombocytopenia, and pulmonary involvement. In the latter circumstance, intraalveolar hemorrhage is a common pathologic finding. The occurrence of myocarditis is rare but carries a high mortality. Conjunctival suffusion is seen in the majority of patients, and in the presence of scleral icterus it is said to be pathognomonic of Weil disease.

Histopathologically, leptospirosis is characterized by vasculitis, endothelial damage, and inflammatory infiltrates. The histopathology is most marked in the liver, kidneys, heart, and lungs. In the liver, there may be intrahepatic cholestasis, hypertrophy of Küpffer cells, and erythrophagocytosis. The kidneys display interstitial nephritis. The heart may show lymphocytic myocarditis. In the lungs, pulmonary congestion and hemorrhage are common.

Humans are infected through contact with the urine of an infected animal, the usual portal of entry being the conjunctiva or abrasions or cuts in the skin. Within the US, the highest incidence is found in Hawaii. Rats are the usual hosts for the species that affect humans (*L interrogans* serogroup *icterohaemorrhagiae*). Domestic animals, like humans, often act as accidental hosts, and direct contact with them is the most common source of occupational infections (farmers, veterinarians, abattoir workers, meat inspectors). Indirect contact with rats is an important source for sewer workers. In tropical regions, infection may be acquired from walking in bare feet.

Laboratory findings in severe leptospirosis include a peripheral leukocytosis, thrombocytopenia, elevated creatinine, hyperbilirubinemia (with lesser increases in transaminases and alkaline phosphatase). The organisms may be visualized in tissue by dark-field microscopy, immunofluorescence microscopy, or immunohistochemical staining.

The mainstay of diagnosis is serology. However, *Leptospira* can also be grown on artificial growth media. Fletcher medium or Ellinghausen-McCullough-Johnson-Harris (EMJH) medium are primarily used. Growth in culture is possible but extremely slow, and cultures are retained for up to 13 weeks. Since organisms circulate only during the first stage of the disease, blood cultures should be taken as soon as possible after the patient's presentation. Other samples that may be cultured include CSF and urine (especially after the second week).

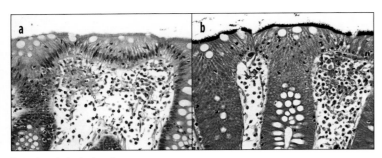

f3.134 Intestinal spirochetosis
a H&E stained section
b Steiner stained section

Brachyspira aalborgi

Though still a controversial clinical entity, this organism has been associated with intestinal spirochetosis.

In colorectal biopsy specimens f3.134, the organisms are visible as a "purple haze" of organisms lining the luminal surface of enterocytes. Closer inspection, especially on Steiner-stained slides, shows that the organisms stand on end on the surface of enterocytes (but not goblet cells).

The clinical significance of intestinal spirochetosis is controversial, and whether it is the cause of disease or an incidental finding remains unclear. *Brachyspira aalborgi* and another organism, *Brachyspira pilosicoli,* both anaerobic spirochetes, appear to be associated with most cases. Infections are seen in both asymptomatic and symptomatic individuals, and a significant minority of these occur in the setting of HIV infection. Spirochetosis may be found in any part of the colon and does not tend to elicit significant inflammation.

Chlamydiae

The *Chlamydiae* are obligate intracellular bacteria that cannot replicate outside cells or synthesize ATP. *Chlamydiae* exist in 2 forms: the elementary body is a 0.2-0.4 μm dense spherical structure that can briefly survive in the extracellular environment and is the infective form; the reticulate body measures 0.6-1.0 μm and is the intracellular form. The outer membrane of the bacterium contains the antigen known as major outer membrane protein (MOMP) which is exploited for clinical diagnosis.

C trachomatis infection is the most common sexually-transmitted disease in the United States; moreover, in the form of trachoma it is considered the most common preventable cause of blindness worldwide. It causes several clinical syndromes, including trachoma, lymphogranuloma venereum (LGV), urethritis, epididymitis, prostatitis, proctitis, cervicitis, and neonatal infections (inclusion body conjunctivitis, pneumonitis, and otitis). Serotypes A, B, & C are responsible for trachoma. Serotype L is responsible for LGV, which produces stellate microabscesses in lymph nodes that are histologically indistinguishable from the lesion of cat scratch disease. Serotypes D-K cause the remaining infections.

Presumptive diagnosis of trachoma has traditionally been based upon Wright-stained conjunctival smears/scrapings in which one sees cytoplasmic (reticulate body) inclusions in exfoliated cells. With regard to diagnosis of sexually transmitted *C trachomatis*, cell culture (McCoy cells) remains the gold standard; however, the sensitivity of culture is thought to

be low in comparison to molecular methods, while its specificity approaches 100%. Direct fluorescence antibody (DFA) tests may be applied to primary specimens, but sensitivity is suboptimal. Lastly, *C trachomatis* can be detected by nucleic acid amplification tests (NAATs). Suitable specimens include, for females, urine and endocervical swabs, and, for males, urine and urethral swabs; the suitability of urine for these assays is a tremendous advantage, particularly when applied to large-scale screening. Sensitivity using the commercially-available platforms is high, but varies slightly depending upon specimen type and format used.

C psittaci (now called *Chlamydophila psittaci*), the causative agent of psittacosis, infects individuals in contact with birds. The organism enters the body via the respiratory tract and then multiplies in the liver and spleen. It manifests primarily as pneumonitis. Diagnosis is usually based upon serology, the preferred method being microimmunofluorescence. Culture is also possible using special techniques.

C pneumoniae (TWAR bacillus, now called *Chlamydophila pneumoniae*) causes so-called walking or atypical pneumonia. Diagnosis can be established by applying PCR-based techniques to respiratory specimens, or by culture using special techniques.

Rickettsiae t3.45

t3.45 Rickettsial diseases

Disease	Organism	Vector
Rocky mountain spotted fever	*Rickettsia rickettsii*	Dog tick
Epidemic typhus	*Rickettsia prowazekii*	Louse
Scrub typhus	*Orientia* (previously *Rickettsia*) *tsutsugamushi*	Chigger
Murine typhus	*Rickettsia typhi*	Flea
Cat scratch disease	*Bartonella henselae*	Kitten
Bacillary angiomatosis	*Bartonella henselae*	Kitten
Boutonneuse fever	*Rickettsia conorii*	Tick
Rickettsialpox	*Rickettsia akari*	Mite
Human monocytic ehrlichiosis	*Ehrlichia chaffeensis*	Lone star tick (*Amblyomma americanum*)
Anaplasmosis	*Anaplasma* (previously *Ehrlichia*) *phagocytophilium*	Deer tick
Oroya fever bartonellosis	*Bartonella bacilliformis*	Sandfly
Verruga peruana	*Bartonella bacilliformis*	Sandfly
Trench fever	*Bartonella quintana*	Louse
Brill-Zinsser disease	*Rickettsia prowazekii*	None (Recrudescence of epidemic typhus)

Several genera now comprise this family: *Rickettsia, Ehrlichia, Bartonella, Orientia, Anaplasma,* and *Neorickettsia.* They prefer to replicate intracellularly, but unlike *Chlamydiae*, these organisms can survive for extended periods in the extracellular environment. All infections caused by these agents are transmitted by an arthropod vector.

Rocky mountain spotted fever (RMSF) is a disease of the western hemisphere that has been reported in the United States, Canada, Mexico, Panama, and several South American countries. It has occurred in nearly every state, but is most common in the Southeast where the American dog tick, *Dermacentor variabilis*, is the vector. In the Rocky Mountains, where it was first described, the vector is *Dermacentor andersoni*. The infection is caused by *R rickettsii*. Symptoms arise 2-14 days after exposure. The classic clinical triad of early infection includes fever, rash, and severe headache. Unfortunately, many patients experience a nonspecific flulike presentation that eludes specific diagnosis. The rash begins at the wrists and ankles. Early lesions are small erythematous macules, progressing to focally confluent maculopapular lesions with central petechiae. Eventually, the rash involves the palms, soles, arms, legs, and trunk. Renal failure, disseminated intravascular coagulation, and central nervous system involvement ensue in severe cases. A fulminant form, seen in African American males with glucose-6-phosphatase deficiency, is rapidly fatal. Serology does not typically become positive until the second week of infection and is generally useful only to confirm the diagnosis in retrospect. The traditional Weil-Felix test, a serological assay for RMSF, is no longer widely used. Currently, the serologic gold standard is the indirect fluorescent antibody (IFA) test. Skin biopsies may be taken when RMSF is suspected; this procedure may help when, instead of showing the lymphocytic vasculitis typical of RMSF, they show features of viral exanthema. In unclear cases, immunohistochemical (IHC) staining for rickettsial antigens may be useful. Sensitivity of IHC in this setting has been reported to be 70%.

Ehrlichiosis and anaplasmosis are found mainly in North America. The causative organisms can be seen on Wright-stained blood films within intracellular vacuoles, where they appear as mulberries or morulae. Both human monocytic ehrlichiosis (HME), caused by *E chaffeensis*, and human granulocytic anaplasmosis (HGA), caused by *Anaplasma phagocytophilum*, present as acute febrile illnesses with thrombocytopenia, leukopenia, and elevated transaminases. The agent of HME has a tropism for monocytes, whereas the agent of anaplasmosis has a tropism for granulocytes.

Bartonella species are numerous, but those most commonly associated with human disease are *B henselae*, *B bacilliformis*, and *B quintana*. Clinical syndromes classically associated with *Bartonella* include trench fever (*B quintana*), Oroya fever and Verruga peruana (*B bacilliformis*), cat-scratch disease and bacillary angiomatosis (*B henselae*).

Trench fever was a major cause of sickness and death in World War I, and has recently been noted in homeless alcoholics. It is transmitted by the human body louse (*Pediculus humanus corporis*).

Infection with *B bacilliformis* results in a bacteremia associated with hemolysis and spiking fevers (Oroya fever). Infection is seen predominantly in the Andean regions of South American countries, where the bloodsucking *Lutzomyia phlebotomine* sandfly is found. Some infected individuals develop a cutaneous manifestation (resembling bacillary angiomatosis) known as Verruga peruana. Unlike in bacillary angiomatosis, these patients are not typically immunocompromised. The Oroya fever—Verruga peruana spectrum has been called Carrion disease.

Cat scratch disease f3.135, caused by infection with *B henselae*, is characterized by lymphadenitis, usually at epitrochlear and/or axillary sites and is unilateral, with or without an inflamed inoculation site. *B henselae* has its natural reservoir in cats and is transmitted to humans through a scratch or bite. Human to human transmission has not been documented. Usually a single lymph node site is involved, but in 10% of cases more than 1 site is affected. The eye is the most common nonlymphoid site of *B henselae* infection. More recently,

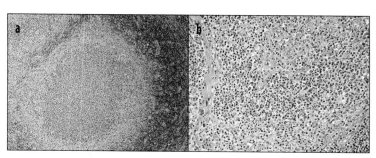

f3.135 Cat scratch disease
a H&E stained sections at low magnification showing necrotizing granuloma
b At high magnification a suppurative center is seen

Bartonella species have been associated with culture-negative endocarditis. In those with HIV, disseminated bartonellosis may occur. Alternatively, or in association with disseminated disease, HIV+ patients may develop bacillary angiomatosis (BA), within skin, lymph nodes, or viscera (sometimes called peliosis). Most cases are due to *B henselae*, but bone lesions are most often due to *B quintana*.

The laboratory diagnosis of *Bartonella* species is established principally by serology. It is useful to remember that many individuals, especially those with frequent contact with cats, have an IgG antibody titer of >1:64; thus, a high titer of IgG (>1:512) or an increasing titer (4 dilution change) must be shown to document infection. A positive IgM antibody is also suggestive of acute infection. Several IFA and EIA tests have been developed for serodiagnosis of *Bartonella* infection. However, there is tremendous crossreactivity among *Bartonella* species, and some crossreactivity with non-*Bartonella* species (*Coxiella burnetii*, *Chlamydia*, *Francisella tularensis*). Culture is not very practical for this organism, although it is sometimes possible in a CO_2-enriched environment, on enriched media, after prolonged periods of incubation. Molecular methods are also available, and can be especially useful when applied to fresh tissue.

Mycoplasma

Mycoplasma lack cell walls and are thereby distinct from bacteria. Their ability to replicate in cell-free media distinguishes them from viruses. Unlike both bacteria and viruses, they have cell membranes containing sterols. The lack of cell wall makes them insensitive to β-lactam antibiotics and invisible by Gram stain.

M pneumoniae causes atypical pneumonia (walking pneumonia), sometimes associated with autoimmune hemolytic anemia due to cold agglutinins (IgM anti-I antibodies). Cold agglutinins appear by the end of the first week in ~50% of infected persons, and this can serve as a nonspecific diagnostic test. Serology is the usual means of diagnosis, preferably using an enzyme immunoassay or indirect immunofluorescence assay applied to paired (acute and convalescent) sera. PCR is also available, and can be applied to respiratory specimens. Culture is possible but is challenging and is not superior to PCR or serology.

Ureaplasma urealyticum and *Mycoplasma hominis* cause nongonococcal urethritis. Infection can be detected by culture or PCR. *M hominis* classically produces "fried-egg" colonies in culture.

Mycobacteria
Laboratory methods
Direct examination of clinical specimens

On routine Gram stain, mycobacteria are typically Gram-invisible, although they are classified among the Gram+ rods based on their ultrastructure. Occasionally, isolates are visible as weakly Gram+ bacilli f3.136; this is most commonly observed with the rapidly-growing mycobacteria.

Mycobacteria are directly detectable either by traditional acid-fast staining methods (Ziehl-Neelsen, Kinyoun) f3.137 or by auramine-rhodamine fluorochrome staining techniques f3.138. The latter are excellent for initial screening of primary specimens, because acid-fast bacilli are detectable with high sensitivity at relatively low magnification (200×). Specimens must be concentrated by centrifugation prior to examination to enhance sensitivity.

Culture

Culture remains the gold standard for detection of mycobacteria in clinical specimens. It is more sensitive than the commercially-available NAATs, and cultured isolates are required for antimicrobial susceptibility testing.

Primary specimens should be cultured using both a liquid (broth) medium and a solid medium (plate or slant). Broth testing offers the advantage of speed, as most mycobacterial isolates will grow faster in liquid media than on solid media. In addition, modern broth systems offer automated growth detection and continuous culture monitoring. Depending on the platform, growth in liquid medium is detected by radiometric, colorimetric, barometric, or metabolic monitoring. Typically, a liquid Middlebrook broth is employed, with the addition of an antimicrobial cocktail designed to inhibit routine bacteria. The solid medium may either be egg based (eg, Lowenstein-Jensen) or agar based (eg, Middlebrook). Specimens from nonsterile sites, such as sputum, must be "decontaminated" prior to culture, using a strong alkaline solution to which mycobacteria (but not routine bacteria) are relatively resistant. Specimens must also be concentrated into a sediment by centrifugation to enhance culture detection.

Although liquid media generally provide more rapid mycobacterial growth detection than solid media, the use of solid media remains important. One reason is that a minority of mycobacterial strains prefer solid medium to broth medium, and can only be isolated on solid medium. In addition, the use of solid medium helps to detect mixed mycobacterial infections, which may be more difficult to detect in the broth medium component. Finally, if the broth medium becomes overgrown by contaminating commensal bacteria, the solid medium component serves as a backup.

When present, mycobacterial growth can usually be detected within 2-3 weeks, but cultures are generally held for ≥6 weeks. Any growth is first evaluated by examination of an acid-fast smear, to confirm that the organisms are mycobacteria. In addition, organisms growing in liquid broth can be assessed for cording, which is a characteristic feature of *M tuberculosis* complex species. The presence of cording acid-fast bacilli allows a preliminary identification of MTB complex, subject to confirmation by full identification. Noncording AFB are presumptively identified as nontuberculous mycobacteria.

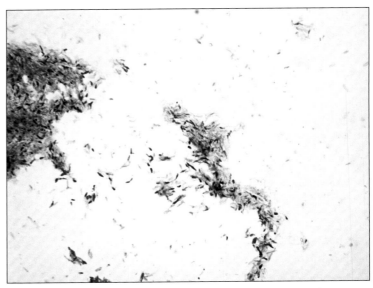

f3.136 Mycobacteria; occasionally, the organisms are visible by Gram stain as Gram+ rods

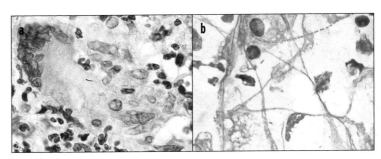

f3.137 Mycobacteria
a AFB stained tissue section
b AFB stained BAL specimen

f3.138 Mycobacteria: auramine-rhodamine fluorochrome stain

Full identification of mycobacteria isolated in culture can be approached in several ways. A popular molecular technique involves the application of nucleic acid hybridization probes for certain common species, namely MTB complex, *M avium* complex, *M kansasii* and *M gordonae*. When this method is unavailable, or if the hybridization probe tests are negative, alternative identification methods must be employed. One approach involves PCR directed against certain nucleic acid targets, such as the 65 kDa heat shock protein gene, or a short region within the gene encoding 16S rRNA, followed by analysis of the PCR amplicons either by DNA sequencing or RFLP analysis. Another involves elucidation of the isolate's growth characteristics and biochemistry. In this approach, the isolate is first classified either as a rapid grower or a slow grower based on measurement of time to mature colony formation on solid medium. The isolate is further subclassified based on its temperature preference and its pigmentation (nonchromogen, scotochromogen or photochromogen). Species-level identification is then achieved based on the outcome of a series of biochemical tests, which may take days to weeks. A third approach is analysis by MALDI-TOF mass spectrometry, which is a promising solution because of its speed and simplicity.

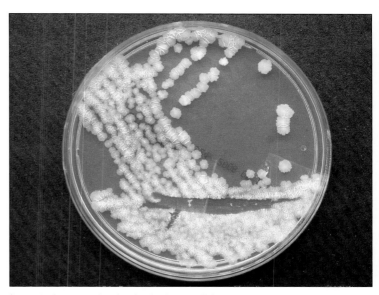
f3.139 *Mycobacterium tuberculosis* (MTB): colony morphology

Nucleic acid amplification tests (NAATs)

Several NAATs for the detection of MTB in primary specimens are commercially available, although at present only one is FDA-cleared. These tests are rapid, in comparison to culture, and are highly sensitive when the specimen is AFB smear-positive. However, sensitivity is relatively poor (compared with culture) when the primary AFB smear is negative, and the assays do not detect nontuberculous mycobacteria. Nevertheless, these assays are extremely useful, because a positive result (MTB detected) is highly reliable due to the assays' high specificity, and the predictive value of a negative result (MTB not detected) is high when the specimen is AFB-smear positive. A negative result cannot be relied upon to "rule out" tuberculosis when the specimen is AFB-smear negative.

Important species t3.46

t3.46 Important mycobacterial species

Site	Most common *Mycobacterium* species
Lung	MAC, M tuberculosis, M kansasii, M xenopi, M abscessus
Lymph node	MAC, M tuberculosis, M scrofulaceum, M haemophilum
Skin & soft tissue	M fortuitum, M chelonae, M abscessus, M marinum, M ulcerans, M haemophilum
GI	M tuberculosis, MAC

Mycobacterium tuberculosis (MTB)

Key characteristics include: slow growth, preference for incubation temperature of 37°C, cording in liquid media, lack of pigmentation (nonchromogenic), formation of flat, dry, white, wrinkled colonies on solid media f3.139.

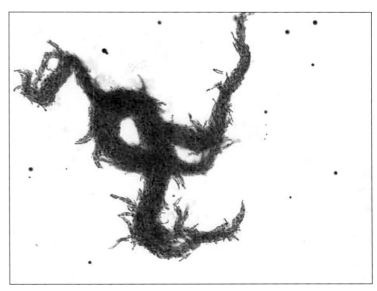
f3.140 *Mycobacterium tuberculosis* (MTB): cording

Cord factor is believed to be a virulence factor and is responsible for "cording" of organisms grown in broth, a morphological feature seen when the AFB line up end to end and side to side to form serpentine arrangements resembling stacked cord wood f3.140.

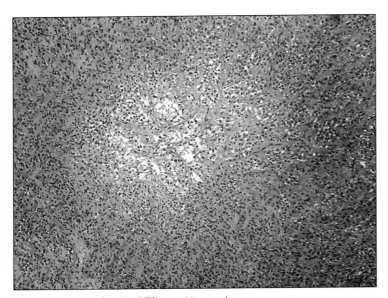

f3.141 *Mycobacterium tuberculosis* (MTB): necrotizing granuloma

Clinical features

Tuberculosis is a clinical disease with protean manifestations that may be caused by any of the *Mycobacterium tuberculosis* complex species. These include the most common agent, *M tuberculosis*, in addition to *M microti*, *M bovis*, *M africanum*, and *M canetti*. Tuberculosis is spread from person to person by respiratory droplets or aerosols. Primary infection is pulmonary and may have several outcomes, including spontaneous eradication, resolution without eradication (latency), and active disease. Most primary cases are asymptomatic and result in latency; cell-mediated immunity controls the infection by localizing it into caseating granulomas (tubercles), most often in the upper lobes f3.141. Latent foci eventually reactivate in 5-10% of immunocompetent individuals and a larger number of immunocompromised individuals.

Active tuberculosis may therefore be a feature of acute infection or reactivation infection. Active TB is usually pulmonary but may be extrapulmonary or involve multiple organs. Active pulmonary TB may manifest as pneumonia or miliary disease. Infants and immunocompromised individuals are most susceptible to miliary TB in the setting of acute infection, but any patient may be so affected. The most common extrapulmonary sites of involvement are the kidneys, bone, GI tract, and meninges. Tuberculous meningitis is characteristically a "basilar" meningitis, in which meningismus may be subtle and cranial nerve palsies are common. About half of patients with tuberculous meningitis are HIV+. Abdominal TB may present as nonspecific abdominal complaints or as an acute abdomen, due to perforation or obstruction. The manifestations of abdominal TB are caused by infection of the Peyer patches, especially in the terminal ileum. In the preantibiotic era, laryngeal tuberculosis was seen in about a third of patients with active pulmonary tuberculosis; it is now rare. TB secondarily involves the larynx because of repeated expectoration, and it presents with upper airway symptoms caused by ulcerated nodular masses that may clinically resemble squamous cell carcinoma.

Establishing the diagnosis of active tuberculosis is of paramount importance, since the disease is often fatal if untreated and is easily spread from person to person. The diagnosis depends upon direct smear examination, culture, and/or NAATs. None of these tests is adequate in isolation, so the CDC recommends that they be used in combination. In particular, the CDC recommends the availability of

1. rapid microscopic examination for acid-fast bacilli

2. nucleic acid amplification testing (PCR)

3. culture, with the capacity to both detect and subsequently identify an isolate within 3 weeks (ie, use of automated broth culture methods)

4. drug susceptibility testing; susceptibility testing is often carried out in state epidemiology laboratories

In a case of suspected pulmonary tuberculosis, an initial effort is made to support the diagnosis by direct examination of expectorated sputum. 3 first-morning samples on 3 separate days are submitted for AFB smear and culture. Ideally, one sputum specimen should also be analyzed by NAAT. Pleural effusion fluid, if present, should be obtained and studied by smear, culture, and NAAT. Adenosine deaminase (ADA) testing of effusion fluid should also be considered. In patients incapable of producing an adequate sputum sample, sputum induction may be attempted. In patients with repeatedly negative sputa, invasive sampling may be undertaken, in the form of bronchoscopy or gastric lavage. In patients with suspected extrapulmonary TB, the testing recommended for suspected pulmonary tuberculosis is carried out, in addition to multimodality testing of tissue from suspected extrapulmonary sites.

The tuberculin skin test (TST) has limited value in the diagnosis of active tuberculosis. Tuberculin is a filtrate of *M tuberculosis* broth culture, whose manufacture has been refined over time to become the presently-used purified protein derivative (PPD). PPD, a precipitate of tuberculosis culture supernatant, contains a large number of antigens, some of which are shared with other, nontuberculous mycobacteria. Thus, a positive tuberculin skin test (PPD) may signify active tuberculosis, but could also indicate latent MTB infection, active or past infection with nontuberculous mycobacteria, or vaccination with BCG (Bacille Calmette-Guérin, a vaccine prepared from an attenuated strain of *M bovis*, which is closely related to MTB). Anergy, for example due to HIV infection, is a common cause of false negative results in latent infection, and false negative results are also seen in a substantial proportion of patients with active tuberculosis (~20%). Poor standardization of test application and interpretation further compound these problems.

Recently discovered unique sequences in the *M tuberculosis* genome, sequences absent in *M bovis*, BCG and in most nontuberculous mycobacteria, have provided a basis for more useful tests based on the host's immunological response. One is the Region of Differentiation (RD)-1, found only in *M tuberculosis*, *M szulgai*, *M marinum*, and *M kansasii*, where the genes for ESAT-6 (early secretory antigen target-6) and CFP-10 (culture filtrate protein-10) are located. The proteins encoded by these genes can be used to stimulate host T cells in vitro. Thus stimulated, T cells that have been previously exposed to these unique proteins, ie, the T cells of persons infected with *M tuberculosis*, release interferon-γ (IFN-γ) in large quantities. Detection of interferon-γ after T cell stimulation with ESAT-6 and CFP-10 forms the basis of several commercially available interferon-γ release assays (IGRAs). One major advantage of IGRAs, in comparison to TSTs, is their high specificity for *M tuberculosis* infection. For this reason, IGRAs are very useful in determining the cause of a positive or intermediate PPD reaction in patients with a history of BCG vaccination or nontuberculous mycobacterial infection.

Serology (antibody testing) remains a poor test for TB infection, because of inadequate sensitivity and specificity.

Nontuberculous mycobacteria

Nontuberculous mycobacteria are ubiquitous in the environment, and unlike *M tuberculosis* complex agents, their isolation does not necessarily indicate clinical infection. Instead, isolation may sometimes reflect environmental contaminants or patient colonization.

The route of transmission is unclear for nontuberculous mycobacteria. There is not definitive evidence for person to person transmission, no known vector, and no evidence of transmission from animals. It is thought that bodies of water, such as swimming pools and holding tanks, are the environmental reservoirs for these agents. Still, the ubiquity of these agents in the environment and the relative rarity of clinical infection point towards crucial host factors in pathogenesis. In fact, these infections are more common in patients with compromised immunity; in immunocompetent hosts, underlying pulmonary disease appears to be an important factor.

The American Thoracic Society recommends the following criteria for the diagnosis of pulmonary disease caused by nontuberculous mycobacteria. First, pulmonary symptoms and cavitary or noncavitary lung disease must be present, and other potential causes excluded. Second, there must be microbiologic confirmation in the form of one of the following:

1. positive culture from ≥2 separate sputum samples

2. positive culture from at least 1 bronchial washing or BAL specimen

3. transbronchial or lung biopsy showing mycobacterial histopathological features (granulomata and/or acid-fast bacilli) and positive culture for nontuberculous mycobacteria

Mycobacterium avium complex (MAC) organisms, including *M avium* and *M intracellulare*, are now more common clinical isolates in the United States than *M tuberculosis*. Clinical infection may be seen in immunocompromised and immunocompetent individuals. Amongst the immunocompetent, there are 3 predominant forms of pulmonary disease. The first is seen in heavy smokers, often males, with upper lobe cavitary disease. This form of disease resembles classic tuberculosis. The second has been called "Lady Windermere syndrome" and is seen commonly in elderly women with weak cough,

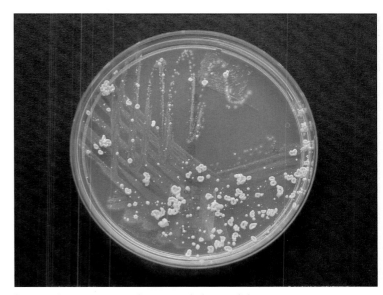

f3.142 *Mycobacterium avium* complex: pigmented colony morphology

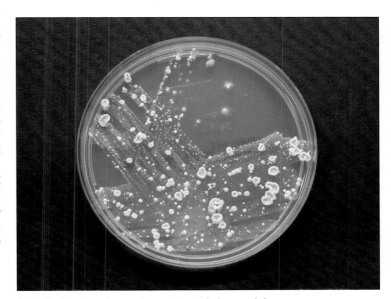

f3.143 *Mycobacterium avium* complex: nonpigmented colony morphology

either for structural reasons or because of voluntary cough suppression. This form of disease is mild and akin to colonization. Lastly, lung disease may be caused by a hypersensitivity reaction to MAC after exposure to hot tub water contaminated with the organisms. MAC is also the most common cause of scrofula (cervical lymphadenitis due to mycobacteria) in developed countries like the US. In culture, MAC organisms are slow growing and may be pigmented or nonpigmented f3.142 & f3.143.

M kansasii causes chronic pulmonary infection, often resembling tuberculosis. Extrapulmonary involvement and dissemination are rare. Risk factors for infection include underlying

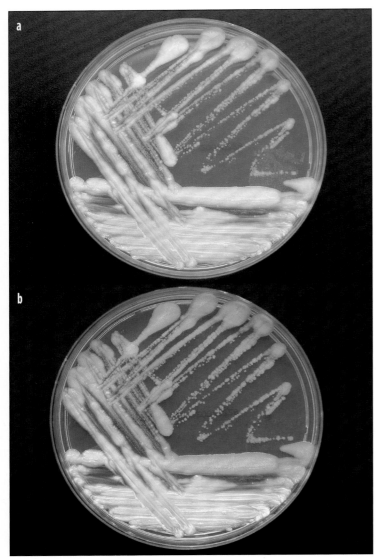

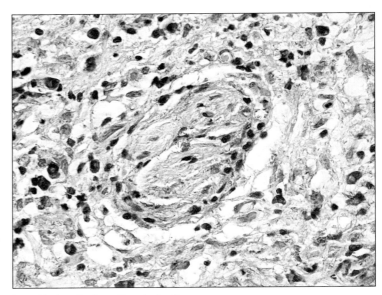

f3.145 *Mycobacterium leprae*: Fite stained section

f3.144 *Mycobacterium kansasii*: colonies are nonpigmented when incubated in the dark, but produce pigment after light exposure (photochromogenic)

pulmonary diseases such as COPD or pneumoconiosis, immunosuppression from HIV infection or drug therapy, malignancy, and alcoholism. *M kansasii* is a slow growing photochromogen f3.144.

The mycobacterial species that are typically associated with skin and soft tissue infections include the rapidly growing mycobacteria (especially *M fortuitum* group, *M chelonae*, and *M abscessus*), *M marinum*, *M ulcerans* and *M haemophilum*. Infection often follows trauma to the skin. In addition to post-traumatic skin infections, *M abscessus* causes chronic pulmonary infection, particularly in patients with cystic fibrosis. The most clinically important rapidly growing mycobacteria are nonpigmented, and grow optimally at lower temperatures (25-30°C). *M marinum* is associated with wound exposure to

freshwater fish tanks or saltwater, and causes localized cutaneous infection ("fishtank granuloma"). In some cases, secondary lymphadenitis resembling sporotrichosis is also seen. *M marinum* is photochromogenic and grows best at 25-30°C. *M ulcerans* causes indolent, necrotizing, ulcerating cutaneous lesions (Buruli ulcer). It is heat sensitive and requires low-temperature incubation (25-30°C). *M haemophilum* typically causes skin nodules in immunocompromised patients. It must be cultured at 25-30°C in media containing hemin (eg, chocolate agar).

M leprae is the cause of leprosy (Hansen disease). Leprosy, in addition to causing disfigurement, is a leading cause of blindness worldwide. In the United States, *M leprae* is found in Hawaii, Texas, and Louisiana (where it is harbored by armadillos). The cardinal clinical signs include hypoesthetic skin lesions and prominent thickening of peripheral nerves. Lepromatous and tuberculoid leprosy are polar clinicopathologic forms of leprosy, between which there is a range of indeterminate forms which can undergo progression in either direction. The anergic (lepromatous) form of leprosy, characterized by widespread skin involvement mostly on cool skin surfaces, is notable for larger numbers of acid-fast bacilli and sheets of foamy histiocytes identifiable within lesions. The tuberculoid form is characterized by one to several localized lesions containing noncaseating granulomata having few to no identifiable acid-fast organisms. *M leprae* cannot be cultured on artificial media. In tissue biopsy, it is best visualized using the Fite stain f3.145.

References

Agan BK, Dolan MJ [2002] Laboratory diagnosis of *Bartonella* infections. *Clin Lab Med* 22:937-962.

Aguero-Rosenfeld ME, Wang G, Schwartz I, Wormser GP [2005] Diagnosis of lyme borreliosis. *Clin Microbiol Rev* 18(3):484-509.

Aguero-Rosenfeld ME [2008] Lyme disease: laboratory issues. *Infect Dis Clin N Am* 22:301-313.

Albrich WC, Kraft C, Fisk T, Albrecht H [2004] A mechanic with a bad valve: blood-culture negative endocarditis. *Lancet Infect Dis* 4:777-784.

Alkalay AL, Pomerance JJ, Rimoin DL [1987] Fetal varicella syndrome. *J Pediatr* 111:320-323. PMID:12489289.

Allander T [2008] Human bocavirus. *J Clin Virol* 41:29-33. PMID:18055252.

Amchentsev A, Kurugundla N, Saleh AG [2008] *Aspergillus* related lung disease. *Respir Med* 1:205-215.

American Thoracic Society [2007] Diagnosis, treatment, and prevention of nontuberculous mycobacterial disease. *Am J Respir Crit Care Med* 175:367-416. PMID:17277290.

Anaissie EJ, McGinnis MR, Pfaller MA, eds [2009] *Clinical Mycology, 2nd Edition.* Philadelphia: Churchill Livingstone. ISBN:978-1416056805.

Archibald LK, Banerjee SN, Jarvis WR [2004] Secular trends in hospital acquired *Clostridium difficile* disease in the United States, 1987-2001. *J Infect Dis* 189:1585-1589. PMID:15116293.

Atkins BL, Athanasou N, Deeks JJ, Crook DWM, Simpson H, Peto TEA, McLardy-Smith P, Berendt AR [1998] Prospective evaluation of criteria for microbiological diagnosis of prosthetic-joint infection at revision arthroplasty. *J Clin Microbiol* 36:2932-2939. PMID:9738046.

Avidor B, Varon M, Marmor S, et al [2001] DNA amplification for the diagnosis of cat-scratch disease in small-quantity clinical specimens. *Am J Clin Pathol* 115:900-909. PMID:11392888.

Babel BS, Decker CF [2008] Microbiology and laboratory diagnosis of MRSA. *Dis Mon* 54:769-773. PMID:18996278.

Bacon RM, Biggerstaff BJ, Schriefer ME, et al [2003] Serodiagnosis of Lyme disease by kinetic enzyme linked immunosorbent assay using recombinant VlsE1 or peptide antigens of *Borrelia burgdorferi* compared with 2-tiered testing using whole-cell lysates. *J Infect Dis* 187:1187-1199. PMID:12695997.

Bangham CRM [2000] HTLV-1 infections. *J Clin Pathol* 53:581-586. PMID:11002759.

Barenfanger J, Drake CA [2001] Interpretation of Gram stains for the nonmicrobiologist. *Lab Med* 7:368-375.

Barlow GB, Dickson JAS [1978] Purple urine bags. *Lancet* 28:220-221.

Barlow K, Tosswill J, Clewley J [1995] Analysis and genotyping of PCR products of the amplicor HIV-1 kit. *J Virol Methods* 52:65-74. PMID:7769040.

Bartlett JG, Dowell SF, Mandell LA, File TM, Jr, Musher DM, Fine MJ [2000] Practice guidelines for the management of community acquired pneumonia in adults. *Clin Infect Dis* 31:347-382. PMID:10987697.

Beigel JH, Farrar J, Han AM, et al [2005] Avian influenza A (H5N1) infection in humans. *N Engl J Med* 353(13):1374-1385. PMID:16192482.

Blum JA, Zellweger MJ, Burri C, Hatz C [2008] Cardiac involvement in African and American trypanosomiasis. *Lancet Infect Dis* 8:631-641. PMID:18922485.

Bori G, Soriano A, Garcia S, et al [2006] Low sensitivity of histology to predict the presence of microorganisms in suspected loosening of a joint prosthesis. *Mod Pathol* 19:874-877. PMID:16607374.

Branson BM, Handsfield HH, Lampe MA, et al [2006] Revised recommendations for HIV testing of adults, adolescents, and pregnant women in health-care settings. *MMWR* 55 PMID:16988643.

Breman JG, Henderson DA [2002] Diagnosis and management of smallpox. *N Engl J Med* 346(17):1300-1308. PMID:11923491.

Brett-Major DM, Walsh TE [2006] Laboratory diagnosis of tuberculosis in primary care. *Dis Mon* 52:450-458. PMID:17157619.

Bush LM, Abrams BH, Beall A, Johnson CC [2001] Index case of fatal inhalational anthrax due to bioterrorism in the United States. *New Engl J Med* 345(22):1607-1610. PMID:11704685.

Carapetis JR, McDonald M, Wilson NJ [2005] Acute rheumatic fever. *Lancet* 366:155-168. PMID:16005340.

Carrigan CD, Scott G, Tabrizian M [2004] Toward resolving the challenges of sepsis diagnosis. *Clin Chem* 50(8):1301-1314. PMID:15166107.

Caserta MT, Mcdermott MP, Dewhurst S, Schnabel K, Carnahan JA, Gilbert L, Lathan G, Lofthus GK, Hall CB [2004] Human herpesvirus 6 (HHV6) DNA persistence and reactivation in healthy children. *J Pediatr* 145:478-484. PMID:15480370.

Centers for Disease Control and Prevention [2005] Controlling tuberculosis in the United States: recommendations from the American Thoracic Society, CDC, and the Infectious Diseases Society of America. *MMWR* 54(No. RR-12):1-81. PMID:16267499.

Centers for Disease Control and Prevention [2006] Hantavirus pulmonary syndrome—5 states, 2006. *MMWR* 55:627-629. PMID:16760891.

Centers for Disease Control and Prevention [2010] Prevention of perinatal group B streptococcal disease. *MMWR* 59(RR-10):1-32. PMID:21088663.

Chavez-Bueno S, McCracken, GH, Jr [2005] Bacterial meningitis in children. *Pediatr Clin N Am* 52:795-810. PMID:15925663.

Chen X-M, Keithly JS, Paya CV, LaRusso NF [2002] Cryptosporidiosis. *N Engl J Med* 346(22):1723-1731. PMID:12037153.

Chevaliez S, Pawlotsky J-M [2005] Use of virologic assays in the diagnosis and management of hepatitis C virus infection. *Clin Liver Dis* 9:37-382. PMID:16023971.

Chiesa C, Panero A, Osborn JF, et al [2004] Diagnosis of neonatal sepsis: a clinical and laboratory challenge. *Clin Chem* 50(2):279-287. PMID:14752012.

Chng WJ, Lai HC, Earnest A, Kuperan P [2005] Haematological parameters in severe acute respiratory syndrome. *Clin Lab Haem* 27:15-20. PMID:15686503.

Cleghorn FR, Manns A, Falk R, et al [1995] Effect of human T-lymphotropic virus type I infection on non-Hodgkin's lymphoma incidence. *J Natl Cancer Inst* 87:1009-1014. PMID:7629870.

Cohen A, Wolf DG, Guttman-Yassky E, Sarid R [2005] Kaposi's sarcoma-associated herpesviruses: clinical, diagnostic, and epidemiological aspects. *Crit Rev Clin Lab Sci* 42(2):101-153. PMID:15941082.

Connor DH, Chandler FW, Schwartz DA, Manz HJ, and Lack EE, eds [1997] *Pathology of Infectious Diseases.* Stamford CT: Appleton & Lange. ISBN:978-0838516010.

Cutler SJ, Bouzid M, Cutler RR [2007] Q fever. *J Infect* 54:313-318. PMID:17147957.

Daar E, Little S, Pitt J [2001] Diagnosis of primary HIV-1 infection. *Ann Intern Med* 134:25-29. PMID:11187417.

Dalton HR, Bendall R, Ijaz S, Banks M [2008] Hepatitis E: an emerging infection in developed countries. *Lancet Infect Dis* 8:698-709. PMID:18992406.

Dantas-Torres F [2007] Rocky Mountain spotted fever. *Lancet Infect Dis* 7:724-732. PMID:17961858.

De Silva T, Chapman A, Kudesia G, McKendrick M [2006] Ongoing queries: interpretation of serology in asymptomatic or atypical chronic Q fever. *J Infect* 52:e113-e116 PMID:16126277.

Dealler SF, Hawkey PM, Millar MR [1988] Enzymatic degradation of urinary indoxyl sulfate by *Providencia stuartii* and *Klebsiella pneumoniae* causes the purple urine bag syndrome. *J Clin Microbiol* 26(10):2152-2156. PMID:2846640.

Del Pozo JL, Patel R [2009] Clinical practice: infection associated with prosthetic joints. *New Engl J Med* 361(8):787-794. PMID:19692690.

Drosten C, Gunther S, Preiser W, et al [2003] Identification of a novel *Coronavirus* in patients with severe acute respiratory syndrome. *N Engl J Med* 348(20):1967-1976. PMID:12690091.

Duchin JS, Koster FT, Peters CJ, et al [1994] Hantavirus pulmonary syndrome: a clinical description of 17 patients with a newly recognized disease. *N Engl J Med* 330:949-955. PMID:8121458.

Dylewski J, Luterman L [2010] Septic arthritis and *Clostridium septicum*: a clue to colon cancer. *CMAJ* 182(13):1446-1447. PMID:20855487.

Enders G, Miller E, Cradock-Watson J, et al [1994] Consequences of *Varicella* and *Herpes zoster* in pregnancy: prospective study of 1739 cases. *Lancet* 343:1548-1551. PMID:7802767.

Enright AM, Prober CG [2004] Herpesviridae infections in newborns: varicella zoster virus, herpes simplex virus, and cytomegalovirus. *Pediatr Clin N Am* 51:889-908. PMID:15275980.

Feng H, Shuda M, Chang Y, et al [2008] Clonal integration of a polyomavirus in human Merkel cell carcinoma. *Science* 319:1096-1100. PMID:18202256.

Fenner L, Widmer AF, Goy G, et al [2008] Rapid and reliable diagnostic algorithm for detection of *Clostridium difficile*. *J Clin Microbiol* 46:328-30. PMID:18032627.

Fernández-Valencia JA, Garcia S, Prat S [2008] *Pasteurella multocida* septic shock after a cat scratch in an elderly otherwise healthy woman: A case report. *Am J Emerg Med* 26:380.e1-380.e3 PMID:18358966.

Fihn SD [2003] Clinical practice. Acute uncomplicated urinary tract infection in women. *N Engl J Med* 349:259-266. PMID:12867610.

Fine MJ, Smith MA, Carson CA, et al [1996] Prognosis and outcomes of patients with community acquired pneumonia. *JAMA* 275:134-141. PMID:8531309.

Fox JD [2007] Nucleic acid amplification tests for detection of respiratory viruses. *J Clin Virol* 40Suppl1:S15-S23 PMID:18162249.

Franks TJ, Chong PY, Chui P, et al [2003] Lung pathology of severe acute respiratory syndrome (SARS): a study of 8 autopsy cases from Singapore. *Hum Pathol* 34(8):743-748. PMID:14506633.

Garcia LS [2010] Malaria. *Clin Lab Med* 30:93-129. PMID:20513543.

Gaydos CA [2005] Nucleic acid amplification tests for gonorrhea and *Chlamydia*: practice and applications. *Infect Dis Clin N Am* 19:367-386. PMID:15963877.

Ginocchio CC [2007] Detection of respiratory viruses using nonmolecular based methods. *J Clin Virol* 40Suppl1:S11-S14 PMID:18162248.

Goede MR, Coopersmith CM [2009] Catheter-related bloodstream infection. *Surg Clin N Am* 89:463-474. PMID:19281894.

Goodgame R [2006] A Bayesian approach to acute infectious diarrhea in adults. *Gastroenterol Clin N Am* 35:249-273. PMID:16880065.

Goodgame RW [2003] Emerging causes of travelers diarrhea: *Cryptosporidium, Cyclospora, Isospora,* and *Microsporidia*. *Curr Infect Dis Rep* 5:66-73. PMID:12525293.

Gopal R, Ozerek A, Jeanes A [2001] Rational protocols for testing faeces in the investigation of sporadic hospital acquired diarrhoea. *J Hosp Infect* 47:79-83. PMID:11170768.

Graham JC, Galloway A [2001] The laboratory diagnosis of urinary tract infection. *J Clin Pathol* 54:911-919. PMID:11729209.

Granville L, Chirala M, Cernoch P, Ostrowski M, Truong LD [2004] Fungal sinusitis: histologic spectrum and correlation with culture. *Hum Pathol* 35(4):474-481. PMID:15116329.

Gratz NG [1999] Emerging and resurging vector-borne diseases. *Annu Rev Entomol.* 44:51-75. PMID:9990716.

Guerrant RL, Gilder TV, Steiner TS, et al [2001] Practice guidelines for the management of infectious diarrhea. *Clin Infect Dis* 32:3431 350 PMID:11170940.

Guleria R, Nisar N, Chawla TC, Biswas NR [2005] *Mycoplasma pneumoniae* and central nervous system complications: a review. *J Lab Clin Med* 146(2):55-63. PMID:16099235.

Gutierrez Y, Bhatia P, Garbadawala ST, Dobson JR, Wallace T, Carey TE [1996] *Strongyloides stercoralis* eosinophilic granulomatous enterocolitis. *Am J Surg Pathol* 20(5):603-612. PMID:8619425.

Habib G, Thuny F, Avierinos JF [2008] Prosthetic valve endocarditis: current approach and therapeutic options. *Progress in Cardiovascular Diseases* 50(4):274-281. PMID:18156006.

Hall CB [2001] Respiratory syncytial virus and parainfluenza virus. *N Engl J Med* 344(25):1917-1928. PMID:11419430.

Haque R, Huston CD, Hughes M, Houpt E, Petri WA [2003] Amebiasis. *N Engl J Med* 348:1565-1573. PMID:12700377.

Harris KR, Dighe AS [2002] Laboratory testing for viral hepatitis. *Am J Clin Pathol* 118:S18-25. PMID:14569810.

Hoagland RJ [1975] Infectious mononucleosis. *Prim Care* 2:295-307. PMID:1046252.

Hogenauer C, Langner C, Beubler E, et al [2006] *Klebsiella oxytoca* as a causative organism of antibiotic-associated hemorrhagic colitis. *N Engl J Med* 355:2418-2426. PMID:17151365.

Hotez PJ, Brooker S, Bethony JM, Bottazzi ME, Loukas A, Xiao S [2004] Hookworm Infection. *N Engl J Med* 351(8):799-807. PMID:15317893.

Houpikian P, Raoult D [2005] Blood culture-negative endocarditis in a reference center: etiologic diagnosis of 348 cases. *Medicine* 84(3):162-173. PMID:15879906.

Hovelius B, Mardh PA [1984] *Staphylococcus saprophyticus* as a common cause of urinary tract infections. *Rev Infect Dis* 6:328-337. PMID:6377440.

Hughes RA, Cornblath DR [2005] Guillain-Barré syndrome. *Lancet* 366:1653-1666. PMID:16271648.

Hurlbut TA III, Littenberg B [1991] The diagnostic accuracy of rapid dipstick tests to predict urinary tract infection. *Am J Clin Pathol* 96:582-588. PMID:1951183.

Hurt C, Tammaro D [2007] Diagnostic evaluation of mononucleosis-like illnesses. *Am J Med* 120:911.e1-911.e8 PMID:17904463.

Hviid A, Rubin S, Mühlemann K [2008] Mumps. *Lancet* 371:932-944. PMID:18342688.

Jackson AC [2008] Rabies. *Neurol Clin* 26:717-726. PMID:18657723.

Jacob JT, Mehta AK, Leonard MK [2009] Acute forms of tuberculosis in adults. *Am J Med* 122:12-17. PMID:19114163.

Jensen JU, Heslet TH, Espersen K, et al [2006] Procalcitonin increase in early identification of critically ill patients at high risk of mortality. *Crit Care Med* 34:2687-2688. PMID:16915118.

Jiang M, Abend JR, Johnson SF, Imperiale MJ [2009] The role of polyomaviruses in human disease. *Virology* 384:266-273. PMID:18995875.

Jones TD [1944] The diagnosis of acute rheumatic fever. *JAMA* 126:481-484.

Kanner WA, Saleh KJ, Frierson HF [2008] Reassessment of the usefulness of frozen section analysis for hip and knee joint revisions. *Am J Clin Pathol* 130:363-368. PMID:18701408.

Karch H, Tarr PI, Bielaszewska M [2005] Enterohaemorrhagic *Escherichia coli* in human medicine. *Int J of Medical Microbiology* 295:405-418. PMID:16238016.

Kass EH [1957] Bacteriuria and the diagnosis of infections of the urinary tract. *Arch Intern Med* 100:709-714. PMID:13468815.

Kessler HH, Sanker B, Rabenau H, et al [1997] Rapid diagnosis of *Enterovirus* infection by a new one-step reverse transcription-PCR assay. *J Clin Microbiol* 35:976 PMID:9157166.

Koneman EW [2005] *Color Atlas and Textbook of Diagnostic Microbiology, 5th ed.* Lippincott Williams & Wilkins. ISBN:978-0781730143.

Kostman JR [1996] Laboratory diagnosis of rickettsial diseases. *Clin Dermatol* 14:301-306. PMID:8727134.

Koteish A, Kannangai R, Abraham SC, Torbenson M [2003] Colonic spirochetosis in children and adults. *Am J Clin Pathol* 120:828-832. PMID:14671970.

Kravetz JD, Federman DG [2005] Toxoplasmosis in pregnancy. *Am J Med* 118:212-216. PMID:15745715.

Kunst H [2006] Diagnosis of latent tuberculosis infection: the potential role of new technologies. *Resp Med* 100:2098-2106. PMID:16650976.

Lamps LW, Havens JM, Sjostedt A, Page DL, Scott MA [2004] Histologic and molecular diagnosis of tularemia: a potential bioterrorism agent endemic to North America. *Mod Pathol* 17:489-495. PMID:15001997.

Larsen SA, Steiner BM, Rudolph AH [1995] Laboratory diagnosis and interpretation of tests for syphilis. *Clin Microbiol Rev* 8:1-21. PMID:7704889.

Larsen JW, Sever JL [2008] Group B *Streptococcus* and pregnancy: a review. *Am J Ob Gyn* 440-448. PMID:18201679.

Lemee L, Dhalluin A, Testelin S, et al [2004] Multiplex PCR targeting *tpi* (triose phosphate isomerase), *tcdA* (toxin A), and *tcdB* (toxin B) genes for toxigenic culture of *Clostridium difficile*. *J Clin Microbiol* 42:5710-14. PMID:15583303.

Levett PN [2001] Leptospirosis. *Clin Microbiol Rev* 14(2):296-326. PMID:11292640.

Liang FT, Steere AC, Marques AR, et al [1999] Sensitive and specific serodiagnosis of Lyme disease by enzyme linked immunosorbent assay with a peptide based on an immunodominant conserved region of *Borrelia burgdorferi* vlsE. *J Clin Microbiol* 37:3990-3996. PMID:10565920.

Loeffelholz MJ [2010] Avian influenza A H5N1 virus. *Clin Lab Med* 30:1-20. PMID:20513539.

Looney WJ, Narita M, Mühlemann K [2009] *Stenotrophomonas maltophilia*: an emerging opportunist human pathogen. *Lancet Infect Dis* 9:312-323. PMID:19393961.

Magill AJ, Grogl M, Gasser RA, et al [1992] Visceral infection caused by *Leishmania tropica* in veterans of Operation Desert Storm. *N Engl J Med* 328:1384 PMID:8292114.

Maguina C, Garcia PJ, Gotuzzo E, et al [2001] Bartonellosis (Carrion's disease) in the modern era. *Clin Infect Dis* 33:772-779. PMID:11512081.

Mandell GL, Bennett JE, Dolin R, eds [2010] *Principles and Practice of Infectious Diseases, 7th edition.* Philadelphia: Churchill Livingstone. ISBN:978-0-443-06839-3.

Mandell LA, Wunderink RG, Anzueto A, et al [2007] Infectious Diseases Society of America/American Thoracic Society consensus guidelines on the management of community acquired pneumonia in adults. *Clin Infect Dis* 44Suppl2:S27-72. PMID:17278083.

Marchand E, Verellen-Dumoulin C, Mairesse M, et al [2001] Frequency Of cystic fibrosis transmembrane conductance regulator gene mutations and 5T allele in patients with allergic bronchopulmonary aspergillosis. *Chest* 119(3):762-767. PMID:11243954.

Marik PE [2001] Aspiration pneumonitis and aspiration pneumonia. *New Engl J Med* 34(9):665-671. PMID:11228282.

Marr KA, Carter RA, Boeckh M, et al [2002] Invasive aspergillosis in allogeneic stem cell transplant recipients: changes in epidemiology and risk factors. *Blood* 100(13):4358-4366. PMID:12393425.

Martin GS, Mannino DM, Eaton S, Moss M [2003] The epidemiology of sepsis in the United States from 1979 through 2000. *N Engl J Med* 348:1546-1554. PMID:12700374.

Massei F, Gori L, Macchia P, Maggiore G [2005] The expanded spectrum of bartonellosis in children. *Infect Dis Clin N Am* 19:691-711. PMID:16102656.

McDonald JR, Olaison L, Anderson DJ, Hoen BM, Miro JM, Eykyn S, Abrutyn E, Fowler VG, Habib G, Selton-Suty C, Pappas PA, Cabell CH, Corey GR, Marco F, Sexton DJ [2005] Enterococcal endocarditis: 107 cases from the International Collaboration on Endocarditis merged database. *Am J Med* 118:759-766. PMID:15989910.

McDonald LC, Killgore GE, Thompson A, et al [2005] An epidemic toxin gene variant strain of *Clostridium difficile. N Engl J Med* 353:2433-41. PMID:16322603.

Mead PS, Slutsker L, Dietz V, McCaig LF, Bresee JS, Shapiro C, et al [1999] Food-related illness and death in the United States. *Emerg Infect Dis* 5(5):607-625. PMID:10511517.

Mendelson CL [1946] The aspiration of stomach contents into the lungs during obstetric anesthesia. *Am J Obstet Gynecol* 52:191-205. PMID:20993766.

Milei J, Guerri-Guttenberg R, Grana D, Storino R [2009] Prognostic impact of Chagas disease in the United States. *Am Heart J* 157:22-29. PMID:19081392.

Mirza NN [2009] *Clostridium septicum* sepsis and colorectal cancer—a reminder. *World J Surg Oncol* 7:73 PMID:19807912.

Molyneux EM, Walsh AL, Phiri AJ, et al [1999] Does the use of urinary reagent strip tests improve the bedside diagnosis of meningitis? *Trans R Soc Trop Med Hyg* 93:409-410. PMID:10674090.

Moosa AA, Quortum HA, Ibrahim MD [1995] Rapid diagnosis of bacterial meningitis with reagent strips. *Lancet* 345:1290-1291. PMID:7746063.

Moran GJ, Talan DA, Abrahamian FM [2008] Diagnosis and management of pneumonia in the emergency department. *Infect Dis Clin N Am* 22:53-72. PMID:18295683.

Moscona A [2005] Neuraminidase inhibitors for influenza. *N Engl J Med* 353(13):1363-1373. PMID:16192481.

Mungai M, Tegtmeier G, Chamberland M, Parise M [2001] Transfusion transmitted malaria in the United States from 1963 through 1999. *N Engl J Med* 344:1973-1978. PMID:11430326.

Nafziger SD [2005] Smallpox. *Crit Care Clin* 21:739-746. PMID:16168312.

Nagai M, Usuku K, Matsumoto W [1998] Analysis of HTLV-I proviral load in 202 HAM/TSP patients and 243 asymptomatic HTLV-I carriers: high proviral load strongly predisposes to HAM/TSP. *J Neurovirol* 4:586-593. PMID:10065900.

Nguyen HB, Rivers EP, Abrahamian FM, et al [2006] Severe sepsis and septic shock: review of the literature and emergency department management guidelines. *Ann Emerg Med* 48:28-54. PMID:16781920.

Ochola LB, Vounatsou P, Smith T, et al [2006]The reliability of diagnostic techniques in the diagnosis and management of malaria in the absence of a gold standard. *Lancet Infect Dis* 6:582-588. PMID:16931409.

Orth G, Favre M, Majewski S, et al [2001] *Epidermodysplasia verruciformis* defines a subset of cutaneous human papillomaviruses. *J Virol* 75:4952-4953. PMID:11336049.

Pachner AR, Steiner I [2007] Lyme neuroborreliosis: Infection, immunity, and infl ammation. *Lancet Neurol* 6:544-552. PMID:17509489.

Pantulu ND, Pallasch CP, Kurz AK, et al [2010] Detection of a novel truncating Merkel cell polyomavirus large T antigen deletion in chronic lymphocytic leukemia cells. *Blood* 116:5280-5284. PMID:20817850.

Pappas G, Akritidis N, Bosilkovski M, Tsianos E [2005] Brucellosis. *N Engl J Med* 352:2325-2336. PMID:15930423.

Parvizi J, Jacovides C, Antoci V, Ghanem E [2011] Diagnosis of periprosthetic joint infection: the utility of a simple yet unappreciated enzyme. *J Bone Joint Surg Am* 21;93(24):2242-2248. PMID:22258769.

Pasvol G [2005] Management of severe malaria: interventions and controversies. *Infect Dis Clin N Am* 19:211-240. PMID:15701555.

Patel MM, Hall AJ, Vinjé J, Parashar UD [2009] Noroviruses: a comprehensive review. *J of Clin Virol* 44:1-8. PMID:19084472.

Pawlotsky JM [2002] Use and interpretation of virological tests for hepatitis C. *Hepatology* 36(Suppl 1):S65-S73 PMID:12407578.

Peiris JS, Yuen KY, Osterhaus AD, et al [2003] The severe acute respiratory syndrome. *N Engl J Med* 349(25):2431-2441. PMID:14681510.

Pialoux G, Gaüzère B, Jauréguiberry S, Strobel M [2007] Chikungunya, an epidemic arbovirosis. *Lancet Infect Dis* 7:319-327. PMID:17448935.

Piersimoni C, Scarparo C [2008] Pulmonary infections associated with nontuberculous mycobacteria in immunocompetent patients. *Lancet Infect Dis* 8:323-834. PMID:18471777.

Pillai BP, Chong VH, Yong AML [2009] Purple urine bag syndrome. *Singapore Med J* 50(5):e193 PMID:19455508.

Pitout JDD, Laupland KB [2008] Extended-spectrum beta-lactamase-producing Enterobacteriaceae: an emerging public-health concern. *Lancet Infect Dis* 8:159-166. PMID:18291338.

Pizon AF, Bonner MR, Wang HE, et al [2006] Ten years of clinical experience with adult meningitis at an urban academic medical center. *J Emerg Med* 30(4):367-370. PMID:16740443.

Planche T, Aghaizu A, Holliman R, et al [2008] Diagnosis of *Clostridium difficile* infection by toxin detection kits: a systematic review. *Lancet Infect Dis* 8:777-784. PMID:18977696.

Podzorski RP [2002] Molecular testing in the diagnosis and management of hepatitis C virus infection. *Arch Pathol Lab Med* 126:285-290. PMID:11860301.

Poutanen SM, Simor AE [2004] *Clostridium difficile*-associated diarrhea in adults. *CMAJ* 171:51-58. PMID:15238498.

Powderly WG, Stanley Jr SL, Medoff G [1986] Pneumococcal endocarditis: report of a series and review of the literature. *Rev Infect Dis* 8:786-791. PMID:3538318.

Procop GW, Burchette JL Jr, Howell DN, Sexton DJ [1997] Immunoperoxidase and immunofluorescent staining of *Rickettsia rickettsii* in skin biopsies. A comparative study. *Arch Pathol Lab Med* 121:894-899. PMID:9278621.

Queiroz-Telles F, McGinnis MR [2003] Subcutaneous mycoses. *Infect Dis Clin N Am* 17:59-85. PMID:12751261.

Raad I, Hanna H, Maki D [2007] Intravascular catheter related infections: advances in diagnosis, prevention, and management. *Lancet Infect Dis* 7:645-657. PMID:17897607.

Ramoz N, Rueda LA, Bouadjar B, et al [2002] Mutations in 2 adjacent novel genes are associated with *Epidermodysplasia verruciformis. Nat Genet* 32:579-581. PMID:12426567.

Ramzan NN [2001] Traveler's diarrhea. *Gastroenterol Clin North Am* 30:665-678. PMID:11586551.

Raoult D, Birg ML, LaScola B, et al [2000] Cultivation of the bacillus of Whipple's disease. *New Engl J Med* 342:620-625. PMID:10699161.

Ray P, Badarou-Acossi G, Viallon A [2007] Accuracy of the cerebrospinal fluid results to differentiate bacterial from non-bacterial meningitis, in case of negative Gram-stained smear. *Am J Emerg Med* 25:179-184. PMID:17276808.

Rebucci C, Cerino A, Cividini A, et al [2003] Monitoring response to antiviral therapy for patients with chronic hepatitis C virus infection by a core-antigen assay. *J Clin Microbiol* 41:3881-3884. PMID:12904409.

Regev-Yochay G, Raz Meir, Dagan R, et al [2004] Nasopharyngeal carriage of *Streptococcus pneumoniae* by adults and children in community and family settings. *Clin Infect Dis* 38: 632-9. PMID:14986245.

Reithinger R, Dujardin J, Louzir H, et al [2007] Cutaneous leishmaniasis. *Lancet Infect Dis* 7:581-596. PMID:17714672.

Roberts AR, Hilburg LE [1958] Sickle cell disease with salmonella osteomyelitis. *J Pediatr* 53:170-175. PMID:13502825.

Rogers KL, Fey PD, Rupp ME [2009] Coagulase-negative staphylococcal infections. *Infect Dis Clin N Am* 23:73-98. PMID:19135917.

Ronald A [2002] The etiology of urinary tract infection: traditional and emerging pathogens. *Am J Med* 113(Suppl 1A):14S-19S PMID:12113867.

Ross AGP, Bartley PB, Sleigh AC, et al [2002] Schisotosomiasis. *N Engl J Med* 346(16):1212-1220. PMID:11961151.

Ross AG, Vickers D, Olds GR, et al [2007] Katayama syndrome. *Lancet Infect Dis* 7:218-224. PMID:17317603.

Rothberg MB, Haessler SD, Brown RB [2008] Complications of viral influenza. *Am J Med* 121:258-264. PMID:18374680.

Salkin I, Graybill JR [2000] Nucleic acid amplification tests for tuberculosis. *MMWR* 49(26):593-594. PMID:10921499.

Saltini, C [2006] Chemotherapy and diagnosis of tuberculosis. *Resp Med* 100:2085-2097. PMID:17113007.

Sander A, Berner R, Ruess M [2001] Serodiagnosis of cat scratch disease: response to *Bartonella henselae* in children and a review of diagnostic methods. *Eur J Clin Microbiol Infect Dis* 20:392-401. PMID:11476439.

Scarborough M, Thwaites GE [2008] The diagnosis and management of acute bacterial meningitis in resource-poor settings. *Lancet Neurol* 7:637-648. PMID:18565457.

Schneider T, Moos V, Loddenkemper C, et al [2008] Whipple's disease: new aspects of pathogenesis and treatment. *Lancet Infect Dis* 8:179-90. PMID:18291339.

Schuachat A, Robinson K, Wenger JD, Harrison LH, Farley M, Reingold AL, et al [1997] Bacterial meningitis in the United States in 1995. *N Engl J Med* 337:970-976. PMID:9395430.

Shlim DR [2002] Cyclospora cayetanensis. *Clin Lab Med* 22:927-936. PMID:12489288.

Shuda M, Feng H, Kwun HJ, et al [2008] T antigen mutations are a human tumor-specific signature for Merkel cell polyomavirus. *Proc Natl Acad Sci USA* 105:16272-16277. PMID:18812503.

Sigurdardottir B, Bjornsson OM, Jonsdottir KE, et al [1997] Acute bacterial meningitis in adults: a 20-year overview. *Arch Intern Med* 157:425-430. PMID:9046894.

Singh B, Kim Sung L, Matusop A, et al [2004] A large focus of naturally acquired *Plasmodium knowlesi* infections in human beings. *Lancet* 363(9414):1017-1024. PMID:15051281.

Sloots TP, Whiley DM, Lambert SB, Nissen MD [2008] Emerging respiratory agents: New viruses for old diseases? *J Clin Virol* 42:233-243. PMID:18406664.

Spangehl MJ, Masri BA, O'Connell JX, Duncan CP [1999] Prospective analysis of preoperative and intraoperative investigations for the diagnosis of infection at the sites of 2 hundred and 2 revision total hip arthroplasties. *J Bone Joint Surg Am* 81:672-683. PMID:10360695.

Steingart KR, Henry M, Ng V, Hopewell PC, Ramsay A, Cunningham J, Urbanczik R, Perkins M, Aziz MA, Pai M [2006] Fluorescence versus conventional sputum smear microscopy for tuberculosis: a systematic review. *Lancet Infect Dis* 6:570-581. PMID:16931408.

Steketee RW, Abrams EJ, Thea DM, et al [1997] Early detection of perinatal human immunodeficiency virus type 1 infection using HIV RNA amplification and detection. *J Infect Dis* 175:707-711. PMID:9041350.

Stoll BJ, Hansen N, Fanaroff AA, et al [2002] Changes in pathogens causing early onset sepsis in very-low birthweight infants. *N Engl J Med* 347:240-7. PMID:12140299.

Sunenshine RH, McDonald LC [2006] *Clostridicum difficile*-assoacited disease: New challenges from an established pathogen. *Cleve Clin J Med* 73(2): 187-197. PMID:16478043.

Svenungsson B, Lagergren A, Ekwall E, et al [2000] Enteropathogens in adult patients with diarrhea and healthy control subjects: a 1-year prospective study in a Swedish clinic for infectious diseases. *Clin Infect Dis* 30:770-778. PMID:10816147.

Swarz MN [2001] Recognition and management of anthrax—an update. *N Engl J Med* 345(22):1621-1626. PMID:11704686.

Syed FF, Millar BC, Prendergast BD [2007] Molecular technology in context: a current review of diagnosis and management of infective endocarditis. *Progress in Cardiovascular Diseases* 50(3):181-197. PMID:17976503.

Taylor GP, Tosswill JHC, Matutes E [2000] A prospective study of HTLV-I infection in an initially asymptomatic cohort. *J Acquir Immune Defic Syndr* 22:92-100. PMID:10534152.

Tigges S, Stiles RG, Roberson JR [1994] Appearance of septic hip prostheses on plain radiographs. *Am J Roentgenol* 163:377-380. PMID:8037035.

Tissot-Dupont H, Raoult D [2008] Q fever. *Infect Dis Clin N Am* 22:505-514. PMID:18755387.

Trampuz A, Steckelberg JM, Osmon DR, Cockerill FR, Hanssen AD, Patel R [2003] Advances in the laboratory diagnosis of prosthetic joint infection. *Rev Med Microbiol* 14:1-14.

Trampuz A, Hanssen AD, Osmon DR, Mandrekar J, Steckelberg JM, Patel R [2004] Synovial fluid leukocyte count and differential for the diagnosis of prosthetic knee infection. *Am J Med* 117:556-562. PMID:15465503.

Trampuz A, Piper KE, Jacobson MJ, et al [2007] Sonication of removed hip and knee prostheses for diagnosis of infection. *N Engl J Med* 357:654-663. PMID:17699815.

Troy SB, Rickman LS, Davis CE [2005] Brucellosis in San Diego: epidemiology and species-related differences in acute clinical presentations. *Medicine* 84(3):174-187. PMID:15879907.

US Preventive Services Task Force [2007] Screening for *Chlamydia*l infection: US Preventive Services Task Force recommendation statement. *Ann Intern Med* 147:128-133. PMID:17576996.

Ugolini V, Pacifico A, Smitherman TC, et al [1986] Pneumococcal endocarditis update: analysis of 10 cases diagnosed between 1974 and 1984. *Am Heart J* 112:813-819. PMID:3766382.

Vannier E, Gewurz BE, Krause PJ [2008] Human babesiosis. *Infect Dis Clin N Am* 22:469-488. PMID:18755385.

Versalovic J, Carroll KC, Funke G, Jorgensen JH, Landry ML, Warnock DW, eds [2011] *Manual of Clinical Microbiology*, 10th ed. ASM Press (Washington DC). ISBN:978-1555814632.

Venneti S [2010] Prion diseases. *Clin Lab Med* 30:293-309. PMID:20513552.

Ventetuolo CE, Levy MM [2008] Biomarkers: diagnosis and risk assessment in sepsis. *Clin Chest Med* 29:591-603. PMID:18954695.

Vincent JL, Korkut HA [2008] Defining sepsis. *Clin Chest Med* 29:585-590. PMID:18954694.

Von Eiff C, Becker K, Machka K [2001] Nasal carriage as a source of *Staphylococcus aureus* bacteremia. *N Engl J Med* 344:11-16. PMID:11136954.

Wang TS, Byrne PJ, Jacobs LK, Taube JM [2011] Merkel cell carcinoma: update and review. *Semin Cutan Med Surg* 30:48-56. PMID:21540020.

Warny M, Pepin J, Fang A, et al [2005] Toxin production by an emerging strain of *Clostridium difficile* associated with outbreaks of severe disease in North America and Europe. *Lancet* 366:1079-84. PMID:16182895.

Weber DJ, Wolfson JS, Swartz MN, et al [1984] *Pasteurella multocida* infections. Report of 34 cases and review of the literature. *Medicine* 63(3):133-54. PMID:6371440.

Weisfelt M, van de Beek D, Spanjaard L, Reitsma JB, de Gans J [2006] Clinical features, complications, and outcome in adults with pneumococcal meningitis: a prospective case series. *Lancet Neurol* 5:123-129. PMID:16426988.

Whipple GH [1907] A hitherto undescribed disease characterized anatomically by deposits of fat and fatty acids in the intestinal and mesenteric lymphatic tissues. *Bull Johns Hopkins Hosp* 18:382-93.

Winn HN [2007] Group B *Streptococcus* infection in pregnancy. *Clin Perinatol* 34:387-392. PMID:17765489.

Wiwanitkit V [2006] Hematologic manifestations of bird flu, H5N1. *Infection Infect Dis Clin Pract* 14:9-11.

Workowski KA, Levine WC [2002] Sexually Transmitted Diseases Treatment Guidelines 2002. *MMWR* 51RR-7:18-30.

Yagupsy P [2004] *Kingella kingae*: From medical rarity to an emerging paediatric pathogen. *Lancet Infect Dis* 4:358-367. PMID:15172344.

Zerr DM, Frenkel LM, Huang H-L, Rhoads M, Nguy L, Del Beccaro MA, Corey L [2006] Polymerase chain reaction diagnosis of primary human herpesvirus-6 infection in the acute care setting. *J Pediatr* 149:480-485. PMID:17011318.

Zimmerli W, Trampuz A, Ochsner PE [2004] Prosthetic-joint infections. *N Engl J Med* 351(16):1645-1654. PMID:15483283.

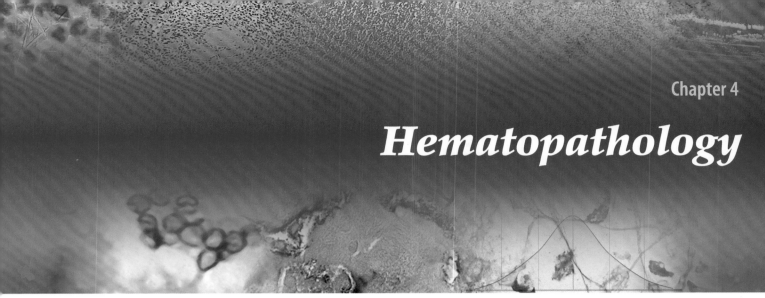

Hematopathology

Diseases of red blood cells

The most common red cell abnormality we confront is a decrement in their number (anemia). One approach to discovering the cause of anemia is discussed on p 233. Erythrocytosis is discussed on p 236. Our inability to produce a synthetic red cell capable of supplanting transfused blood is a testament to the complexity of this seemingly rudimentary structure, one with neither nucleus nor organelles. It is far more than a membrane-bound sack of hemoglobin. The litany of disorders discussed immediately below reflect defects in the complex systems that permit the red cell to survive the intemperate climates through which it must repeatedly pass during its average 120-day life span.

The key red cell systems include its membrane and embedded transmembrane proteins, its flexible cytoskeleton immediately beneath, and enzymes. A simple lipid bilayer would not permit the exchange of fluid and electrolytes needed to keep the red cell inflated; needed for this are the transmembrane proteins that are involved in sodium/potassium exchange. Furthermore, a simple bilayer might quickly emulsify in the blood; preventing this is a hexagonal array of spectrin, which outwardly attaches to the inner lipid layer and to the transmembrane proteins band 3 and glycophorin and inwardly to a meshwork of actin filaments. Hinged protein-protein linkages are formed by a variety of small proteins, including ankyrin and protein 4.1. In addition to keeping the lipid bilayer together, the cytoskeleton is designed to fold, bend, and return to its original biconcave discoid shape that is optimized for gas exchange.

Red cell enzymes include those involved in energy production, enzymes important in preventing hemoglobin oxidation, and enzymes involved in keeping the hemoglobin molecule soluble. There are 3 main metabolic cascades occurring in the red cell. The first is the Embden-Meyerhof pathway that anaerobically metabolizes glucose to form ATP; this is the only source of ATP, which is needed to drive sodium/potassium pumps. A byproduct of the Embden-Meyerhof pathway, produced via the hexose monophosphate shunt, is reduced nicotinamide adenine dinucleotide (NADH), which is important in preventing oxidation. A second by-product, produced via the Rapoport-Luebering shunt, is 2,3-diphosphoglycerate (2,3-DPG), which has the effect of reducing the affinity of hemoglobin for oxygen.

Cytoskeletal disorders

Hereditary spherocytosis (HS)

A plurality of underlying molecular defects contributes to the marked clinical heterogeneity noted in HS, with phenotypes ranging from mild to severe. Some cases present at birth as neonatal jaundice, while others are concealed well into adulthood. Most cases, in fact, are mild and well-compensated. Severely affected patients may require splenectomy, which usually results in clinical remission. Mildly affected patients may be notable only for mild reticulocytosis, reflecting low grade chronic hemolysis. Jaundice, gallstones, and splenomegaly may be noted in more severely affected patients.

In the United States, the incidence of HS is ~1 in 5,000; in parts of northern Europe the incidence approaches 1 in 1,000. HS is the most common red cell disorder in persons of northern European descent. Most affected families display autosomal dominant inheritance, but ~1 in 4 have an autosomal recessive pattern. The variable inheritance patterns derive from the fact that the HS phenotype can be caused by any one of several cytoskeletal protein defects. The most commonly affected gene is the *ANK1* (ankyrin) gene located on 8p (~60% of cases), followed by the band 3 (AE1) and spectrin β chain genes.

The most characteristic CBC abnormality is an increased MCHC. The MCV and MCH are usually normal. The peripheral blood film shows numerous spherocytes f4.1, lacking in central pallor. There is usually an elevated reticulocyte count.

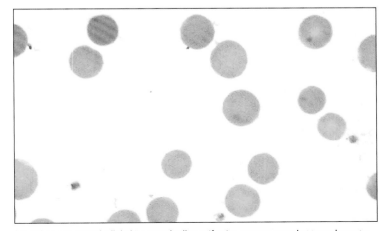

f4.1 Spherocytes are red cells lacking central pallor; artifact is a common cause, but true spherocytes are most often seen in autoimmune hemolytic anemia & hereditary spherocytosis

215

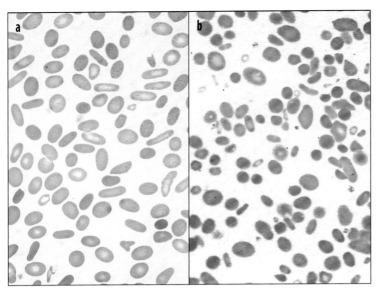

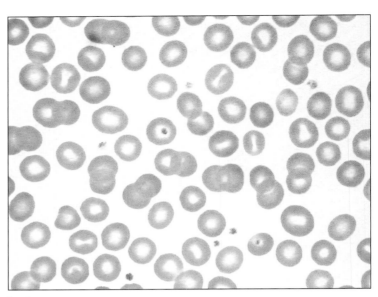

f4.2 Elliptocytes are red cells that are twice as long as they are wide
a While they are the hallmark of hereditary elliptocytosis, they are usually seen (in small numbers) in iron deficiency anemia & myelodysplasia
b Hereditary pyropoikilocytosis

f4.3 Stomatocytes

Typical of extravascular hemolysis, the lactate dehydrogenase (LD) and bilirubin are elevated. Either the osmotic fragility or autohemolysis test may be used for screening. The osmotic fragility test is performed by incubating the red cells in incrementally hypotonic NaCl solutions and measuring the degree of hemolysis. Spherocytic cells hemolyze more readily in hypotonic saline than normal cells; however, this test merely serves to identify the presence of spherocytes from any cause. The autohemolysis test is performed by incubating the red cells at 37°C for 48 hours and measuring hemolysis. HS cells autohemolyze more readily than normal, but this can be ameliorated by incubating with excess glucose as an energy source.

When spherocytes are noted in a peripheral smear, the differential diagnosis includes immune-mediated hemolysis and HS. The direct antiglobulin test (DAT) is negative in HS and usually positive in immune-mediated hemolysis. In the face of spherocytosis, negative DAT, and elevated reticulocytes, the diagnosis is most likely HS.

Hereditary elliptocytosis (HE)/hereditary ovalocytosis

HE is, like HS, a phenotype that can result from several genotypes. HE is usually inherited as an autosomal dominant disorder and most commonly caused by mutations in the spectrin α chain, resulting in defective formation of spectrin tetramers. However, many cases have been described in association with mutations in band 3 protein and protein 4.1.

By definition, HE is diagnosed when >25% of circulating red cells are elliptocytes f4.2, defined as cells twice as long as they are wide. Elliptocytes in lower proportion are seen quite commonly in patients with iron deficiency, B$_{12}$ deficiency, folate deficiency, or myelophthisis.

The incidence of HE, like that of G6PD deficiency (see p 217), appears to vary with the historical incidence of malaria; presumably, these anomalies confer some survival advantage in malaria-ridden areas. The incidence varies from 1 in 2,500 (United States) to 1 in 100 (parts of Africa).

There are 3 types of HE. The common type is found mostly in African Americans; the heterozygotes have mild or no hemolysis, while the homozygotes have moderate to severe anemia. A variant of common HE is hereditary pyropoikilocytosis (HPP), which is characterized by unusual sensitivity of red cells to heat. It is most common to see HPP as a transient finding in neonates having common HE; HPP as a permanent aberration is rare. The spherocytic type of HE results from double heterozygosity for HS and HE. Lastly, the stomatocytic type, also known as Southeast Asian ovalocytosis (SAO), is a common finding in Malaysia. It is caused by a specific band 3 protein defect (a 27 base pair gene deletion resulting in a 9 amino acid deletion resulting in a 9 amino acid deletion) and confers protection against *P vivax* malaria.

Hereditary stomatocytosis (HSt)

HSt is a group of autosomal dominant disorders in which red cells have an elongated, mouthlike, central pallor f4.3, in association with abnormal sodium/potassium permeability. There are 2 main types, including the severe hydrocytotic (overhydrated) type, in which red cells take on extra water, and a less severe xerocytotic type, in which they lose water. Stomatocytosis is also a feature of the Rh null red cell phenotype. Stomatocytosis, macrocytosis, moderate to severe hemolysis, and a low MCHC characterize the hydrocytosis syndromes. Affected red cells have decreased production of the membrane protein stomatin. The xerocytosis syndromes have normocytic red cells characterized morphologically as spiculated dessicocytes, accompanied by mild stomatocytosis and target cells. The gene for xerocytic HSt has been mapped to 16q23-q24. HSt syndromes have a marked tendency towards thrombosis following splenectomy, so therapeutic splenectomy is generally avoided (and usually unnecessary).

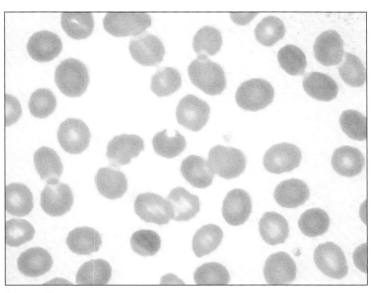

f4.4 Bite cells

Enzyme disorders

Red blood cell (RBC) enzyme defects may cause chronic (eg, pyruvate kinase deficiency) or episodic (glucose-6-phosphate deficiency) hemolysis. Since spherocytes are not found in these disorders, they are sometimes called chronic nonspherocytic hemolytic anemias (CNSHA).

Glucose-6-phosphate dehydrogenase (G6PD) deficiency

Even in normal circumstances G6PD deteriorates over the life of the blood cell, such that reticulocytes have significantly more G6PD activity than older RBCs. The most common forms of G6PD deficiency are associated with an accentuation of this pattern, in which RBC G6PD is exceptionally fragile and short-lived. G6PD is involved in the production of NADPH (through the hexose monophosphate shunt), which maintains glutathione, and consequently other proteins, in the reduced state when erythrocytes are subjected to an oxidant stress. When hemoglobin becomes oxidized, it precipitates as Heinz bodies. When RBCs bearing Heinz bodies pass through the spleen, they are targeted by sinusoidal macrophages, which ingest a portion of the RBC membrane, producing bite cells f4.4.

G6PD deficient RBCs are therefore hypersensitive to sources of oxidant stress, such as certain medications (methylene blue, sulfa-containing drugs, nitrofurantoin, and primaquine), fava beans (hemolysis associated with ingestion of fava beans is called favism), and infection. Following oxidant exposure, the peripheral smear shows poikilocytosis, Heinz bodies (with supravital dyes such as methyl violet, crystal violet, or brilliant cresyl blue), bite cells, and blister cells.

The most common clinical manifestations are neonatal jaundice and episodic hemolytic anemia, which in most patients is triggered by an exogenous oxidant. Geographically, the prevalence of G6PD deficiency parallels that of *Plasmodium falciparum* malaria, and G6PD deficiency is thought to have persisted in the population because of a protective effect. There is a high prevalence of G6PD deficiency in Africa, southern Europe, the Middle East, Southeast Asia, and Oceania. Because G6PD deficiency is an X-linked disorder, the clinical manifestations are seen primarily in males. In areas where G6PD deficiency is prevalent, females will occasionally be affected. The 3 mechanisms by which X-linked recessive traits affect females are homozygosity, asymmetric lyonization, or Turner syndrome.

The gene for G6PD is found on the X chromosome. There are >300 G6PD alleles, grouped into 3 categories. The most common category encompasses variants with acute intermittent hemolysis. The second and third categories are relatively rare, including variants with chronic hemolysis and variants with no hemolysis (polymorphisms). G6PD deficiency affects 12% of African Americans, most of whom have the G6PD A– allele. In G6PD A–, young RBCs (including reticulocytes) have adequate G6PD levels; however, G6PD is exceptionally fragile and short-lived, accentuating the discrepancy between young and old RBCs. A rise in enzyme activity caused by reticulocytosis may cause G6PD activity to appear to be within the normal range if the G6PD A– patient is tested immediately after a hemolytic episode. The ability to produce young RBCs imposes a limitation on the extent of hemolysis in G6PD A–, a limitation not available to those with the G6PD-Mediterranean allele. The G6PD-Mediterranean allele is found in Italy, Greece, Spain, Arabia, and among Sephardic Jews. The G6PD-Mediterranean mutation causes severe G6PD deficiency, because even very young RBCs are depleted of G6PD. Hemolytic episodes may be quite fulminant, resulting in extreme anemia. Lastly, Asian variants such as G6PD Mahidol Thailand, G6PD Chinese-1 through 3, and G6PD Canton resemble African variants clinically. Several polymorphic alleles, which produce no hemolysis, are prevalent within the population. These include the functionally normal alleles G6PDB (the wild type) and G6PDA (a normal variant common in African Americans).

Other inherited enzyme deficiencies involving the hexose monophosphate shunt are rare, including glutathione synthetase deficiency, glutathione reductase deficiency, and γ-glutamyl cysteine synthetase deficiency. These cause syndromes similar to G6PD deficiency.

The fluorescent spot test is performed by incubating RBCs with NADP and G6P and measuring the production of NADPH (which fluoresces). Note that in most forms of the disease, G6PD is abundant in younger RBCs, and older cells are selectively destroyed during acute hemolytic episodes. In the days following a hemolytic crisis, the surviving RBCs have normal G6PD activity; therefore, testing during this time may yield falsely negative (normal) results. Repeat testing in >3 months should confirm the diagnosis in these individuals.

Pyruvate kinase (PK) deficiency

Pyruvate kinase deficiency is inherited as an autosomal recessive trait. Rarely, myelodysplastic syndrome or acute myelogenous leukemia may result in acquired PK deficiency. PK deficiency is distributed worldwide, with a relatively high frequency in northern Europe and Pennsylvania Amish.

PK catalyzes the rate-limiting step in the Embden-Meyerhof (glycolysis) pathway, which is the main source of RBC ATP. PK deficiency is not the only known inherited glycolytic pathway enzyme defect, but it is the most common. Others, such as aldolase deficiency, hexokinase (glucokinase) deficiency, and glucose-6-isomerase deficiency have autosomal

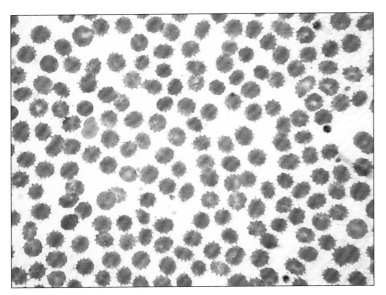
f4.5 Burr cells

Unmetabolized pyrimidines precipitate within the cell, recognizable as basophilic stippling, and cause hemolysis. Incidentally, lead inhibition of pyrimidine 5′ nucleotidase is the source of the basophilic stippling observed in lead poisoning.

Structurally abnormal hemoglobin variants (hemoglobinopathies)

A variety of normal hemoglobin molecules is synthesized throughout life t4.1. Hemoglobin A is a tetramer composed of 2 α chains and 2 β chains. The α genes are located on chromosome 16, and β genes are located on chromosome 11p15.5. There is 1 copy of the β (*HBB*) gene on each chromosome 11, for a total of 2 productive genes in normal cells. In adult life, the capacity to produce β chain substitutes (δ and γ) is preserved; thus, diminished production of β can be partially compensated by increased production of HbA2 and HbF. There are 2 copies of the α genes on each chromosome 16, for a total of 4 α chain-producing gene loci in each normal cell. Even at birth, the capacity to produce α chain substitutes is lost; thus, there is no transcriptional way to compensate for α chain defects.

t4.1 Normal hemoglobins

Hemoglobin	Chains	Role
HbA	$\alpha_2\beta_2$	Major adult hemoglobin
HbA2	$\alpha_2\delta_2$	Minor adult hemoglobin
HbF	$\alpha_2\gamma_2$	Major late fetal hemoglobin
Hb Gower1	$\zeta_2\varepsilon_2$	Major early fetal hemoglobin
Hb Gower2	$\alpha_2\varepsilon_2$	Minor early fetal hemoglobin

Hemoglobinopathy refers to the production of a structurally abnormal globin chain t4.2. Structurally abnormal hemoglobins are most often the results of genetic alterations in the coding sequence of α or β genes, but in some cases result from anomalies in posttranslational modification of normal hemoglobin. Thalassemia refers to a quantitative abnormality of structurally normal globin chain synthesis. Thalassemia, discussed below, usually results from genetic alterations in a noncoding sequence, such that the quantity of normal chain production is affected.

t4.2 β chain variants

Variant	Amino acid	Alteration
S	6	Glu→Val
C	6	Glu→Lys
C$_{Harlem}$	6 & 73	Glu→Val & Asp→Asn
E	26	Glu→Lys
D (D-Los Angeles, D-Punjab)	121	Glu→Gln
O$_{Arab}$	121	Glu→Lys

recessive patterns of inheritance; phosphofructokinase deficiency is X-linked recessive. ATP depletion causes impaired ion pumps, RBC dehydration, and finally hemolysis. A byproduct of the glycolytic pathway, which is exploited for diagnostic purposes, is the conversion of NADH to NAD. PK deficiency causes chronic hemolysis at a relatively constant rate, with the usual manifestations of chronic hemolysis—gallstones, jaundice, and splenomegaly. Severity differs from one patient to the next. Echinocytes (dessicocytes) are the classic peripheral smear finding f4.5, but these appear in large numbers only after splenectomy. The benefit of splenectomy is well established.

The autohemolysis test is positive, as in HS, but unlike HS autohemolysis does not correct with the addition of glucose. It does normalize with the addition of ATP. A fluorescent spot test may be used for screening. RBCs are incubated with NADH (which fluoresces under UV light at 340 nm) to check for conversion to NAD (which does not). The quantitative PK assay, which measures the rate of decrease of absorbance at 340 nm, is used for confirmation.

2 separate genes, *PKLR* (expressed in liver and RBCs) on 1q21 and *PKM* (expressed in muscle and leukocytes) on 15q22, encode pyruvate kinase. *PKLR* transcription is under the control of 2 separate promoters, each resulting in a distinct transcript. One leads to translation of the R isoenzyme (present in mature RBCs), and the other leads to the L isoenzyme (liver). Mutation of the *PKLR* gene results in a labile form of PK, leading to PK deficiency (unlike the anucleate RBC, the liver can compensate by making more PK).

Pyrimidine 5′ nucleotidase deficiency

There are groups of pyrimidine 5′ nucleotidases, one of which is unique to RBCs. RBC pyrimidine 5′ nucleotidase is responsible for the degradation of RNA that is present within reticulocyte (this degradation changes the tinctorial features of reticulocytes to resemble those of a mature erythrocyte).

Hemoglobin S (β$_6$ glu→val)

The allele that encodes hemoglobin S (the sickle cell gene) is found in parts of the world where *P falciparum* is prevalent. In the United States, it is mainly found in African Americans, in whom the prevalence of sickle cell trait (genotype SA) is ~10%. The S allele has valine in place of glutamate at position 6 of the hemoglobin β chain (β6 glu→val).

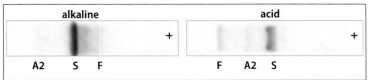

f4.6 Sickle cell disease as seen on alkaline gel in hemoglobin electrophoresis (left) & acid gel (right)

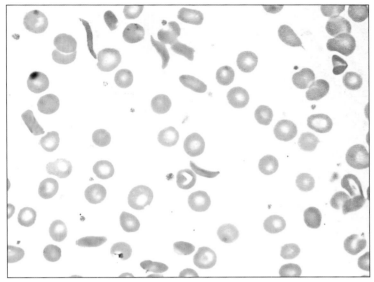

f4.7 Sickle cells

Sickle cell disease is a severe hemolytic disease. Hemoglobin S demonstrates abnormal polymerization when deoxygenated, but only when conditions are right; first among these conditions is reaching a threshold concentration of hemoglobin S, generally >50%, within the RBC. Clinical manifestations are thus not limited to those with the homozygous SS genotype, being more or less similar in sickle cell-β^0-thalassemia, sickle cell-β^+-thalassemia, and SC disease (genotype SC). Patients with sickle cell trait (genotype SA) who usually have around 40% HbS and 60% HbA, are generally asymptomatic.

The erythrocytes in sickle cell disease (homozygous SS) have shortened survival, with an average lifespan of 17 days (normal is 120 days). The electrophoresis shows >80% HbS, 1-20% HbF, 1-4% HbA2, and 0% HbA f4.6. At birth, HbF is much higher and exerts an inhibitory effect on HbS polymerization. The manifestations of sickle cell disease are not apparent until HbS levels increase beyond 50%, usually at ~6 months of age. In patients with combined sickle cell disease-hereditary persistence of fetal hemoglobin (SS-HPFH) clinical manifestations are mild. Treatment (hydroxyurea) to raise HbF lessens the severity of SS. The lower intraerythrocyte concentrations of HbS associated with α-thalassemia also lessen the hematologic and clinical manifestations of disease.

Theoretically, sickled cells should return to their normal shape upon exposure to atmospheric oxygen. Sickled cells seen on the peripheral smear of patients with sickle cell disease f4.7 are cells that have remained sickled despite reoxygenation, so-called irreversibly sickled cells (ISCs). The ISC percent is more or less constant in an individual and does not appear to predict or reflect episodic crises; however, it does seem to be correlated inversely with that patient's RBC survival. Sickled cells may also be seen in S-β thalassemia, S-C, S-D, and C_{Harlem}.

Clinically, sickle cell disease is characterized by chronic hemolytic anemia and recurrent crises. Thrombosis is thought to contribute significantly to the clinical manifestations. Aplastic crises are caused by transient arrests of erythropoiesis and are characterized by an abrupt drop in hemoglobin, reticulocytes, and RBC precursors in the marrow. Although these episodes typically last only a few days, the level of anemia may be severe. Parvovirus B19 accounts for nearly 70% of aplastic crises in children. Splenic sequestration crisis presents as worsening of anemia in association with an enlarged, tender spleen. These episodes often occur during a viral illness. Children (whose spleens have not yet undergone fibrosis) and adults with SC disease or sickle cell-β^+ are most susceptible. Worsening of anemia in a more slowly progressive fashion may be due to progressive renal insufficiency (with decreasing erythropoietin) or supervening iron/folate/B_{12} deficiency. Hyperhemolytic crisis presents as a sudden exacerbation of anemia in association with profound reticulocytosis and hyperbilirubinemia. This complication may be caused by concomitant G6PD deficiency. Acute pain crisis (acute painful episode) is thought to be due to a vaso-occlusive event within bone. These episodes often follow exposure to cold, dehydration, infection, or alcohol consumption. The acute chest syndrome presents with dyspnea, cough, chest pain, and fever. One may find tachypnea, leukocytosis, a pulmonary infiltrate on chest x-ray, and progressive hypoxia. This syndrome is thought to be related to either vaso-occlusive events or bacterial pneumonia. Priapism has been reported in up to 40% of males with sickle cell disease. Ocular complications (proliferative retinopathy) occurs with greater frequency in SC disease and sickle cell-β^+-thalassemia than in SS. Osteonecrosis is a common complication and may affect the vertebrae, hands, feet, and femoral and humeral heads.

There are 7 so-called sickle cell nephropathies, including gross hematuria, papillary necrosis, nephrotic syndrome, renal infarction, isosthenuria, pyelonephritis, and renal medullary carcinoma. The risk of the latter is also increased in sickle cell trait and SC.

Infections are a major source of morbidity and mortality, made worse by the functional asplenia that is so common in sickle cell disease. *S pneumoniae* infections, including pneumococcal sepsis, pneumonia, meningitis, and arthritis, are the most common overall. Other common infections include salmonellae, *Haemophilus influenza* type B, and *M pneumoniae*. The association of SS with salmonella infections, particularly of the bone, was first recognized >70 years ago. The condition can be difficult to distinguish from a pain crisis.

Neurologic complications are frequent and may manifest as transient ischemic attacks (TIAs), cerebral infarcts, cerebral hemorrhage, cord infarction, and meningitis. In sickle cell patients under the age of 20, the incidence of stroke is nearly 10%. Such a devastating complication as this has received much attention, and in clinical trials, aggressive transfusion strategies and the use of hydroxyurea have demonstrated the ability to prevent stroke. Approximately 1 in 3 patients with sickle cell disease will

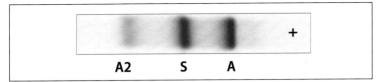

f4.8 Sickle cell trait as seen on alkaline gel

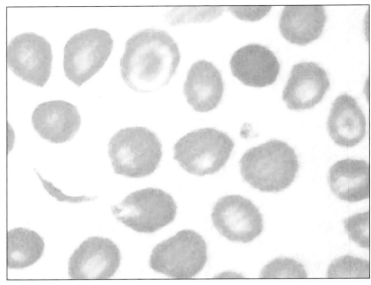

f4.9 Compound heterozygote for hemoglobin S & hemoglobin C (hemoglobin SC disease), showing sickle cell & numerous target cells

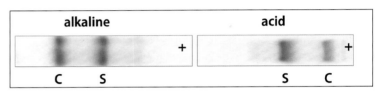

f4.10 Hemoglobin SC disease as seen in hemoglobin electrophoresis on alkaline gel (left) & acid gel (right)

have an angiographic appearance of moyamoya disease (segmental arterial stenoses with "puff of smoke" collaterals).

Acute hepatic cell crisis (right upper quadrant syndrome) manifests as progressive jaundice, elevated LFTs, and a tender, enlarged liver. This usually resolves within 2 weeks, it may progress to liver failure. Chronic nonspecific hepatomegaly and liver dysfunction are also common in sickle cell disease, thought to be related to centrilobular congestion. Gallstones (pigmented type) are ubiquitous in sickle cell disease, and may be present in patients as young as 3 years.

Pregnancy is a unique problem in sickle cell disease, with an increased rate of both maternal and fetal deaths. There is certainly an increased risk of pregnancy induced hypertension (preeclampsia), but there is also an increased incidence of intrauterine growth retardation, intrauterine fetal demise, and prematurity.

Patients with sickle cell disease, as a result of numerous transfusions, are prone to develop alloantibodies, with associated immediate and delayed hemolytic transfusion reactions. A paradoxical worsening of anemia following transfusion is sometimes observed. The mechanism for this is unclear, but it has been theorized that it results from "innocent bystander" destruction of host RBCs in the presence of a minor antigen incompatibility.

Sickle cell trait (genotype SA) is usually asymptomatic and associated with a normal CBC and peripheral smear. The peripheral blood smear shows no sickle cells. The electrophoresis shows 35-45% HbS, <1% HbF, 1-3% HbA2, and 50-55% HbA f4.8. The ~60:40 ratio of A:S is due to a greater affinity of α chains for β^A chains over β^S chains. As with all individuals with HbS, the metabisulfite and dithionate tests are positive. Sickle trait is generally thought of as a benign condition that renders a degree of protection against *P falciparum* malaria. In fact, several disorders have greater frequency in sickle cell trait than in the general population, including hematuria, isosthenuria, renal papillary necrosis, splenic infarction, exercise induced rhabdomyolysis, exercise induced sudden cardiac death, and renal medullary carcinoma. Renal medullary cancer is a rare aggressive tumor that arises almost exclusively in patients with sickle cell trait. In the original reported series of 34 cases, 33 had sickle cell trait. Nearly all patients present before the age of 40 years, many in their 20s, and most (2:1) are male. For unknown reasons, the right kidney is disproportionately affected (3:1). The tumor usually presents at an advanced stage, with median survival of <6 months. Splenic infarcts in sickle cell trait are usually restricted to patients experiencing hypoxic environmental conditions, such as exposure to high altitudes. If splenectomy occurs in such cases, sickled RBCs can be seen within the red pulp. Hematuria is extremely common in sickle cell trait and may be caused by renal papillary necrosis. The renal papillae are particularly susceptible to infarctions, because the arterial blood in this region, having traversed the loops of Henle, is acidotic, hypoxemic, and hypertonic;

thus promoting polymerization of even a low proportion of hemoglobin S. A variety of conditions predispose to renal papillary necrosis, including sickle hemoglobins, diabetes mellitus, pyelonephritis, renal outflow obstruction, and analgesic abuse. Isosthenuria refers to a loss of renal concentrating ability and is thought to be the result of numerous small papillary microinfarcts. The result may be hypertonicity of the blood.

When α-thalassemia is coinherited with sickle cell trait (S-α thalassemia), there is a decreased percentage of hemoglobin S. The degree to which HbS is decreased is relative to the number of α-globin genes deleted. In single gene α gene deletion (−α/$\alpha\alpha$), there is ~30-35% HbS. In 2 α gene deletions (−−/$\alpha\alpha$ or −α/−α) there is 25-30% HbS. When β thalassemia is coinherited with HbS (S-β thalassemia), there is an increased proportion of HbS (S usually above 50%). Disease manifestations can be quite severe, depending upon the type of β thalassemia defect.

SC disease, the result of double heterozygosity for HbS and HbC, results in ~50% HbS and clinical manifestations intermediate in severity between SS and SA. SC RBCs have an average lifespan of 27 days (compared with 17 days for SS and 120 days for normal RBCs). The various SS associated complications are about half as frequent in SC, but avascular necrosis of bone and proliferative retinopathy are equally common or more common in SC. The peripheral smear is remarkable for mild sickling and abundant target cells f4.9, f4.10. In patients initially diagnosed as SC who manifest an unexpectedly complicated clinical course, consider S-O$_{Arab}$ or S-C$_{Harlem}$, both of which run with C on the alkaline gel but can be resolved by other techniques.

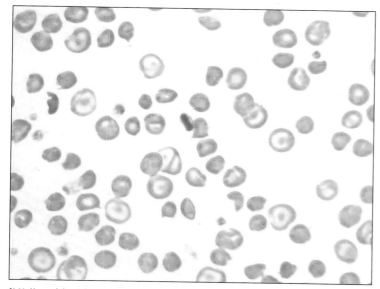

f4.11 Hemoglobin C disease (homozygous CC) peripheral blood smear, showing hemoglobin C crystals & numerous target cells

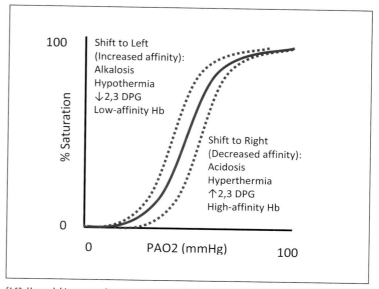

f4.12 Hemoglobin-oxygen dissociation (oxygen affinity) curves

Hemoglobin C (β_6 glu→lys)

Hemoglobin C trait (heterozygous AC) is characterized by an electrophoretic pattern showing 40-50% of hemoglobin within the C band (the C band contains both HbA2 and HbC). It is generally asymptomatic, though the peripheral smear has scattered target cells.

Hemoglobin C disease (homozygous CC) has an electrophoretic pattern showing 90% HbC, 7% HbF, 3% HbA2, 0% HbA. It is characterized by mild hemolytic anemia, splenomegaly, and numerous target cells. Hexagonal or rod shaped crystals f4.11 may be found in the RBCs, especially after splenectomy.

Hemoglobin E ($\beta_2$6 glu→lys)

Hemoglobin E is common in Southeast Asia and is the second most common abnormal hemoglobin worldwide (after hemoglobin S). The CBC shows thalassemic indices and the peripheral smear numerous target cells. The electrophoresis demonstrates an abnormal band in the C band (with A2). By itself, hemoglobin E is typically benign; however, its co-inheritance with β thalassemia may be clinically severe. In this regard, it can be helpful to know whether the hemoglobin A2 is elevated, but A2 runs with E on conventional gel electrophoresis and on HPLC. Capillary electrophoresis (CE) is capable of distinguishing HbE from HbA2. In one study, mean HbA2 in patients with HbE trait was 3.4%, and the mean HbA2 of HbE homozygotes was 4.4%.

Hemoglobins D & G

Patients with HbD and HbG are clinically normal. Usually, these variants are of significance only because they run with HbS on alkaline gel. The absence of HbS can be rapidly determined by a sickle screen study or by the fact that HbD and HbG run with HbA on citrate gels. Often D & G can be distinguished from one another, because HbD is a β chain defect, while HbG is an α chain defect; thus, HbG may produce 2 HbA2 bands (one normal, the other abnormal) separated by a distance equal to that separating HbA from HbG.

Hemoglobin Lepore

Hb Lepore is a common variant in geographic regions around the Mediterranean, especially Italy. Hb Lepore runs with HbS on alkaline gel, but is typically present in low proportions; thus, one may suspect Hb Lepore whenever around 15% of "hemoglobin S" is present on the electrophoresis. Actual HbS is rarely present in this quantity, unless aggressively transfused. Hb Lepore is the result of a fusion between δ and β genes.

Hemoglobin constant spring (HbCS)

HbCS causes thalassemic-type RBC indices. It results from a mutation in the α-globin gene stop codon, producing an abnormally long transcript that is unstable. The termination codon TAA is mutated to CAA which, instead of indicating the cessation of transcription, encodes the amino acid glutamine. The αcs allele is thus inefficient, producing thalassemia. This mutation is common in Southeast Asia. If the αcs allele arises in association with α-globin gene deletion (on the homologous chromosome), hemoglobin H disease can result.

In the heterozygote, the hemoglobins produced are: α-β (HbA), αcs-β (HbCS), α-δ (HbA2), αcs-δ (4 bands are seen in the adult on cellulose acetate electrophoresis). In the newborn, α-γ (HbF), and αcs-γ are also seen.

Altered oxygen affinity hemoglobins

This is a group of hemoglobins with shifted oxygen dissociation curves f4.12, the result of mutations that affect conformation-sensitive amino acids in the globin chains. High oxygen affinity hemoglobins result in a leftward shift in the curve and erythrocytosis. Examples include Hb Chesapeake, J-Capetown, Malmo, Yakima, Ypsilanti, Rainier and Hb Denver. Low oxygen affinity hemoglobins result in a rightward shift in the curve, anemia, and cyanosis. Examples include Hb Beth Israel, Kansas, and Providence. Most altered oxygen affinity hemoglobins cannot be resolved on either gel electrophoresis or HPLC, but the HbO_2 dissociation curve (P50) is diagnostic.

Unstable hemoglobins

This group of hemoglobin variants is associated with Heinz bodies and bite cells, a presentation that can mimic glucose 6 phosphate deficiency. This is the result of hemoglobin variants with unusual sensitivity to oxidative stress. Thus, exposure to oxidative stresses may precipitate hemolytic crisis. Screening for unstable hemoglobins is carried out by incubating lysed RBCs with 17% isopropanol which causes precipitation of unstable hemoglobins. Examples include Hb Hasharon, Koln, Seattle, Tacoma, Ann Arbor, & Zurich. There is variable clinical severity, ranging from severe (Hb Hammersmith, Ann Arbor, Koln) to mild (most others). Note that Hb Barts and HbH (severe α thalassemia) are also associated with Heinz body anemia.

Methemoglobin (Hi, hemiglobin)

Methemoglobin (Hi) is hemoglobin in which iron is in the oxidized ferric (Fe^{+++}) state instead of the usual ferrous (Fe^{++}). Hi is incapable of combining with oxygen. Under normal circumstances, up to 1.5% of total Hb is Hi; Hi is maintained at this relatively low level by the action of the NADH-dependent methemoglobin reductase system.

Elevated Hi may be the result of hereditary and acquired states. Hereditary methemoglobinemia can result from deficiency in the methemoglobin reductase system or abnormal hemoglobins (HbM) upon which this enzyme cannot act. HbM is actually a group of hemoglobins that, because of various amino acid substitutions, prefer the ferric (methemoglobin) state. Cyanosis appears at 6 months of age, unless there is M fetal hemoglobin in which case cyanosis abates at ~6 months. Most M hemoglobins run with HbA on routine gels. Examples include HbM-Iwate, HbM-Boston, HbM-Saskatoon, and HbM-Hyde Park. Acquired methemoglobinemia may result from exposure to drugs or chemicals that increase the formation of Hi, common examples being nitrites, quinones, phenacetin, and sulfonamides. The most common cause of a defective methemoglobin reductase system is inherited cytochrome b5R deficiency. This is inherited in an autosomal recessive manner and is particularly common in Navajo Indians and the Yakutsk of Siberia. There is a type I deficiency (mild, cyanosis only) and a type II deficiency (severe, causing neurologic deficits).

Clinically, elevated Hi presents with cyanosis and poor tissue oxygenation. Cyanosis results when Hi reaches 10% of total Hb or around 1.5 g/dL. The blood is grossly chocolate-brown. The cooximeter is capable of measuring methemoglobin directly. Both pulse oximetry and arterial blood gas analyzers estimate oxygen saturation by emitting a red light (wavelength of 660 nm) absorbed mainly by reduced hemoglobin and an infrared light (wavelength of 940 nm) absorbed by oxyhemoglobin. Since methemoglobin absorbs equally at both of these wavelengths, it is essentially undetectable by these modalities; in fact, increasing levels of methemoglobin result in regression of the measured oxygen saturation towards 85%. This is a form of oxygen saturation gap.

Hi has a very high affinity for cyanide, so part of the treatment for cyanide toxicity involves administration of nitrites to generate Hi which will chelate cyanide. Treatment for methemoglobinemia is methylene blue, which reduces Hi to Hb.

Sulfhemoglobin (SHb)

SHb is formed when hemoglobin is oxidized in the presence of sulfur. If further oxidized, SHb precipitates to form Heinz bodies. SHb cannot transport oxygen. Normally, SHb is <1% of total Hb. SHb may increase after exposure to sulfonamides and in the presence of C perfringens bacteremia (enterogenous cyanosis). Unlike, Hi, SHb cannot be reduced to Hb. Cyanosis manifests at around 3-4% or 0.5 g/dL.

Carboxyhemoglobin (HbCO)

CO binds tightly (with 200× the affinity of oxygen) to hemoglobin forming carboxyhemoglobin (HbCO), thus reducing the available binding sites for oxygen. CO has even greater avidity for fetal hemoglobin, placing infants (and fetuses) at great risk. Furthermore, CO is directly toxic to intracellular oxidative mechanisms and appears to enhance production of nitric oxide (NO), causing vasodilation. The clinical effects of carbon monoxide intoxication vary with the proportion of HbCO t4.3.

t4.3 Clinical effects of carbon monoxide poisoning

Level of HbCO	Clinical findings
0.4-2%	Normal nonsmoker
2-6%	Normal smoker
10-20%	Mild symptoms: dyspnea on exertion
20-50%	Severe symptoms: intoxication, with headache, lethargy, loss of consciousness
>50%	Coma & death

CO is produced when there is partial combustion of carbon-containing fossil fuels (complete oxidation leads to CO_2 production). It is normally produced endogenously from only one source: the breakdown heme, resulting in HbCO levels ≤1%. Carbon monoxide may also be generated in the hepatic metabolism of dichloromethane (methylene chloride), found in paint and varnish removers. Accidental poisoning results most often from house fires, engine exhaust, indoor heaters, and stoves. In fact, unventilated burning of charcoal or gas is a common source of poisoning during power outages in the winter. Intentional poisoning is a common means of suicide.

HbCO can be measured by the cooximeter, and venous blood is as good as arterial for this determination. Blood gas analyzers, in contrast to cooximeters, do not measure hemoglobin variants and determine oxyhemoglobin by calculation. Pulse oximetry may give falsely reassuring oxygen saturation. The oxygen gap (difference between pulse oximetry cooximetry) reflects the level of HbCO. HbCO levels correlate well with clinical effects; however, there is some variability in the clinical effects of the 20-60% range. Additional laboratory testing in support of the patient with CO poisoning may include measurement of lactate, calculation of the anion gap, myocardial markers, and cyanide levels (smoke inhalation also poses a risk of cyanide inhalation, depending upon the materials present in the fire).

CO is eliminated by slowly being replaced by oxygen on hemoglobin molecules. The half life of CO depends on the oxygen tension. The t½ on room air is ~6 hours, while the t½ on 100% O_2 is 1 hour.

Thalassemia

General features

Thalassemia refers to a quantitative abnormality of structurally normal globin chain synthesis. This is distinguished from hemoglobinopathy, which refers to the production of a structurally abnormal globin chain. Thalassemia is prevalent in the Mediterranean, Africa and Southeast Asia, paralleling the prevalence of malaria.

There is one copy of the β gene (*HBB*) on each chromosome 11, for a total of 2 productive β genes in normal cells. The *HBB* gene is regulated by an upstream (5′) promoter sequence and an upstream regulatory gene known as the locus control region (LCR). Nearby (within the *HBB* gene cluster) are the genes for the δ globin chain, γ globin chains, and a pseudo-*HBB* gene. There are a large number of possible abnormal alleles at the *HBB* gene locus (>200). The vast majority of these result from point mutations. Large deletions, such as those that underlie α-thalassemia, are rarely seen in the *HBB* gene. Based upon their impact on β globin chain production, these alleles can be categorized as β^0 or β^+. β^0 alleles are those that result in complete absence of β chain production. Usually these are caused by nonsense or frameshift mutations. β^+ alleles result in diminished β chain production, usually from mutations in the promoter sequence, LCR, or 5′ untranslated region. The β^+ alleles are variable in their severity; β^+ Mediterranean is more severe than β^+American, the latter found in American blacks. Lastly, silent alleles exist that have almost no impact on chain production. Such mutations affect the promoter's CACCC box or the 5′ untranslated region. With regard to genetic testing, the large number of possible disease associated alleles requires targeted mutation analysis. That is, within any given ethnic group, particular molecular defects will be more or less common. Using the appropriate primers for amplification or dot-blot analysis, one can screen for the most commonly expected alleles. Failing this, direct sequence analysis must be undertaken.

There are 2 copies of the α genes on each chromosome 16, for a total of 4 α chain-producing gene loci in each normal cell. α thalassemia alleles usually result from a large structural deletion within the translated portion of the gene, but occasionally result from a point mutation in the untranslated region (eg, Hb constant spring). One potential genotype, α thalassemia 2 (α+ thalassemia) refers to a genotype in which chromosome 16 has one normal and one deleted α gene (−α/). This is the most common genotype in African Americans. Another genotype, α thalassemia 1 (α^0 thalassemia) refers to a genotype in which chromosome 16 has 2 deleted α genes (−−/). α thalassemia 1 genotype is prevalent in Asians. Deletion testing by PCR is clinically available and can help to predict the carrier status. Deletion types common in certain populations are likely to be present on a single chromosome (α thalassemia 1), while others are likely to be present on complementary chromosomes.

Reduced synthesis of either α or β chains results in decreased total hemoglobin production, leading to hypochromasia and microcytosis. Continued synthesis of normal

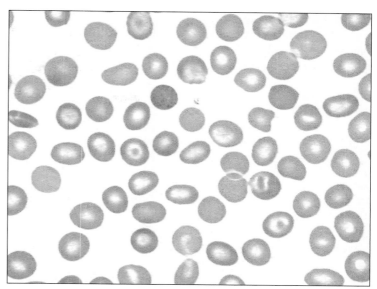

f4.13 Thalassemia blood smear; red cells are microcytic & there are numerous target cells

amounts of the unaffected chain leads to its relative abundance and precipitation of these chains in the RBC, reducing the cell's lifespan. In α thalassemia, β_4 and γ_4 tetramers form. In β thalassemia, α_4 tetramers form.

CBC findings typical of thalassemia ("thalassemic indices") include elevated RBC count (>5.5 × 10^{12} in men, >5.0 × 10^{12} in women), reduced MCV (65-75 fL in α thalassemia, 55-65 fL in β thalassemia), and low hematocrit t4.4. The RDW is typically normal to slightly increased, in contrast to the markedly increased RDW of iron deficiency. An MCV/RBC count ratio <13 favors thalassemia, while a ratio >15 favors iron deficiency. Peripheral smear findings include microcytic hypochromic cells, occasional target cells (more in β thalassemia than α thalassemia), and basophilic stippling f4.13.

t4.4 Typical CBC parameters in thalassemia trait & iron deficiency

Parameter	Thalassemia trait	Iron deficiency	Note
RBC (×10^6/μL)	5.50	3.90	Elevated in uncomplicated thalassemia
Hgb (g/dL)	12	8.2	May be decreased in both
Hct (%)	40	26.3	May be decreased in both
MCV (fL)	69.2	74.3	Decreased in both
RDW (%)	14.1	19.0	Much higher in IDA
Plt (×10^3/μL)	162	480	Usually higher in IDA

Double heterozygosity for β thalassemia and an abnormal β chain results in an increased percentage of the abnormal β chain; eg, in S-β thalassemia, there is >50% HbS with 1-15% HbF.

α thalassemia leads to decreased percentage of abnormal β chains; eg, in S-α thalassemia there is 30-35% HbS with 1 α gene deletion, and 25-30% HbS with 2 α gene deletions.

α thalassemia syndromes

α thalassemia is most common in those of sub-Saharan African and southeast Asian descent. The α thalassemia 1 gene is prevalent in Asians, and it is they who are at risk for the very severe kinds of α thalassemia (hemoglobin Barts and hemoglobin H diseases). The α thalassemia 2 gene is most prevalent in African Americans.

A single gene deletion is entirely asymptomatic, with normal CBC, and normal electrophoresis t4.5. Though it is of interest clinically for genetic counseling, the hematology lab is of little use in identifying these individuals. α thalassemia trait, the condition of having 2 mutated α genes, manifests as thalassemic indices and an electrophoresis with normal percentage of A2. In the absence of iron deficiency, this can be interpreted as consistent with α thalassemia trait. Unlike β thalassemia, the manifestations of α thalassemia are present at birth.

t4.5 α thalassemia syndromes

Syndrome	Genotype	CBC	Electrophoresis
Normal adult	αα/αα	Normal	Normal
Silent carrier	−α/αα	Normal	Normal
α thalassemia trait	−α/−α or −−/αα	Thalassemic	Normal
HbH disease	−−/−α or −−/αCSα	Thalassemic Heinz bodies	Fast-migrating HbH HbH = β4 tetramers
Hb Barts disease (hydrops fetalis)	−−/−−	Hypochromia nRBCs	Fast-migrating Hb Barts Hb Barts = γ4 tetramers

Hemoglobin H disease results from 3 mutated α genes. Hemoglobin H disease is usually of intermediate severity, with only a minority of patients having symptomatic anemia. Although many require transfusion at one time or another, very few are transfusion-dependent. More prevalent are late manifestations, including gallstones and iron overload.

β thalassemia syndromes

β thalassemia is most common in Mediterranean populations. Manifestations do not become fully evident until 6-9 months of age. β thalassemia minor typically results from inheritance of one abnormal β gene, either $β^+$ or $β^0$. On hemoglobin electrophoresis, one of several patterns emerges. In the most common situation, one sees high HbA2 (>2.5%, usually 4-8%) and normal HbF. In the second most common situation, the electrophoresis may show normal A2, because the patient is also iron deficient. This pattern may be erroneously interpreted as consistent with α thalassemia. When the electrophoresis is done for a CBC with thalassemic indices, many labs perform parallel iron studies to exclude this possibility. If the results of these indicate iron deficiency and the percent A2 is normal, electrophoresis should be repeated following iron repletion.

In δ-β thalassemia (deletion of both the δ and β genes) there is a normal quantity of HbA2 and elevated HbF (5-20%). In heterozygous Hb Lepore (fusion of δ and β) there is a normal quantity of HbA2, slightly elevated HbF, and a band in the S region comprising 6-15% (Hb Lepore).

β thalassemia major results from inheritance of 2 abnormal β genes such as $β^0β^0$, $β^{+med}β^{+med}$, or $β^0β^{+med}$. Severe anemia develops by 1 year of age. The hemoglobin electrophoresis shows increased HbF (50-95%), normal to elevated HbA2, and little to no HbA. β thalassemia intermedia and major (Cooley anemia) are distinguished by the dependence of the latter on transfusions. The HbF in this condition, as in most things other than HPFH (below) is present in a heterocellular distribution (some cells with and some cells without on the Kleihauer-Betke stain).

Hemoglobin A2 prime (HbA2′)

HbA2′ is a clinically insignificant δ-chain variant that occurs in 1-2% of African Americans. It is significant mainly because it may affect the interpretation of hemoglobin electrophoresis. Recall that the δ-chain combines with an α chain to make HbA2. When heterozygotes A2′ undergo gel electrophoresis, the HbA2′ chains are barely detectable, leading to underestimation of the A2 and therefore underdiagnosis of β thalassemia trait. In looking for an elevated A2 as part of excluding β thalassemia trait HbA2 and HbA2′ levels must be added. A2′ is easily detectable by HPLC, in which it produces a minor peak in the S area.

Hereditary persistence of fetal hemoglobin (HPFH)

During fetal life, γ chain production is high, resulting in a predominance of HbF. Production of β chains begins in late gestation, such that HbA represents ~30-40% of total hemoglobin at term. Production of HbF progressively diminishes, such that by 6 months of age HbF is usually <10%, and by 1 year of age it is usually <5%. By the age of 2 years and thereafter, HbF is normally <2%. HPFH results from a delayed switch from γ to β or δ chains. This can result from deletion of the β and δ genes; in contrast to most other conditions in which HbF is elevated, HPFH is characterized by HbF in a pancellular distribution.

These other causes of elevated HbF generally are pathologic conditions, in which HbF is present in only some cells (heterocellular). These so-called F cells (HbF-bearing cells) may be observed in normal pregnancy but are more numerous in molar pregnancy. F cells may be seen in bone marrow failure syndromes, particularly megaloblastic anemia, myelofibrosis, aplastic anemia, paroxysmal nocturnal hemoglobinuria, and some leukemias. High levels of HbF and of F cells are found in Fanconi anemia, juvenile myelomonocytic leukemia, and erythroleukemia (FAB M6).

Combined sickle cell-HPFH is found in ~1 in 100 of those with homozygous HbSS. These individuals have a pancellular distribution of ~25% HbF and suffer from neither anemia nor vaso-occlusive episodes. Note that an adult hemoglobin electrophoresis with HbS, FHb, and HbA2 has 2 possible causes. First is combined sickle cell-HPFH. Second is combined sickle cell-β-thalassemia. These can be distinguished by the pancellular distribution in the former and heterocellular in the latter; moreover the SS-HPFH patient is clinically much healthier than the SS-β.

Immune hemolytic disorders

Warm autoimmune hemolytic anemia (WAIHA)

WAIHA is mediated by a warm reacting IgG antibody t4.6. The pathogenic antibody usually has broad reactivity with RBC antigens, especially Rh antigens. Uncommonly, the antibody has a narrow specificity; eg, for a specific Rh antigen, Kell, Kidd.

t4.6 Warm autoimmune hemolytic anemia (WAIHA), cold agglutinin disease (CAD), paroxysmal cold hemoglobinuria (PCH)

Syndrome	WAIHA	CAD	PCH
Ig	IgG Anti-broad Rh	IgM anti-I, i	IgG anti-P
DAT	IgG only (2/3); IgG/C3 (1/4)	C3	C3
Serum	All cells in panel react (AHG phase)	Most cells in panel react (IS/AHG phases)	Antibody panel negative Biphasic hemolysin
Setting	Lymphoma, medications	*M pneumoniae* (anti-I), infectious mono (anti-i), lymphoma	Young children—viral Syphilis

Cold autoagglutinins

The DAT (direct antiglobulin test, Coombs test) is the crucial test in diagnosis. It is positive in nearly all cases of WAIHA, and is usually reactive with polyspecific and anti-IgG reagents. Uncommonly, reactions are observed only with anti-C3 reagent. Infrequently, the DAT may be falsely negative, because of very rapid intravascular destruction of erythrocytes or low titer antibody. Furthermore, a small percentage of healthy people have a positive DAT.

Antibody bound to the RBC acts as an opsonin that provokes RBC destruction by splenic macrophages (extravascular hemolysis). Some partially degraded RBCs are seen in the peripheral smear as spherocytes. In some cases, the antibody activates complement, and depending upon a range of factors may either produce intravascular hemolysis (through the completion of the cascade through the formation of C5-9 membrane attack complex) or cause opsonization (cascade arrested at C3b) and extravascular hemolysis. Lastly, in some cases, the antibody is incapable of producing RBC destruction and only coats the RBC. In fact, 5-10% of hospitalized patients develop such a nonhemolytic RBC antibody; most are due to a medication, and most inconsequential. The particular consequences of antibody binding depend upon several factors, including the density of the target antigen on the RBC surface, the avidity of the antibody, the titer of the antibody, the thermal amplitude of the antibody, and the isotype (complement can be activated by IgA, IgM, IgG1, and IgG3; IgG tends to produce extravascular hemolysis in the spleen; IgM tends to produce extravascular hemolysis in the liver).

Patients present with variable severity. Some have an abrupt onset and severe symptomatic anemia, while others have a chronic low grade hemolysis perhaps detected only incidentally. While these patients have less severe manifestations, the bad news is that they are much more likely to have a serious underlying disease. WAIHA may be primary (idiopathic) or secondary (~70% of cases). Secondary WAIHA occurs in hematolymphoid neoplasms (especially CLL/SLL), inherited autoimmunity (especially antibody deficiency—common variable immunodeficiency, IgA deficiency, Bruton agammaglobulinemia), collagen vascular disease, and thymoma. Stem cell transplantation has also been associated with AIHA.

Cold agglutinins are IgM antibodies with specificity that is most commonly anti-I. Others include anti-i, anti-H, anti-Pr, and anti-IH t4.7. Cold agglutinins may be pathologic or nonpathologic. The most important laboratory features in predicting pathogenicity are titer and thermal range (thermal amplitude). Nonpathologic (benign) cold agglutinins react most strongly at

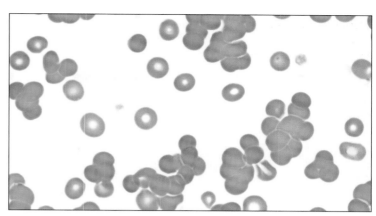

f4.14 Cold agglutinin disease; red cell clumps are the morphologic hallmark

4°C, but some have wide thermal amplitudes and may react up to 22°C. They may react at or near room temperature, making such things as automated CBCs unreliable. The only reliable CBC index in the presence of cold agglutinins is the hemoglobin. The titer of benign cold agglutinins is usually <64 at 4°C. Most are IgM and can activate complement, thus reactions may be seen at the antiglobulin phase using polyspecific antisera. If monospecific reagents are used, the cells are agglutinated by anti-C3d but not anti-IgG. Pathologic cold agglutinins are reactive over a broad thermal range, up to 37°C. They cause spontaneous autoagglutination in anticoagulated blood at room temperature f4.14. As with benign cold agglutinins, automated CBCs may be unreliable. The titer is often >1,000 when tested at 4°C.

t4.7 Antibody specificities in cold agglutinin disease

O cord	O adult	A1 adult	A2 adult	Specificity	Notes
–	+++	+++	+++	I	While often benign, anti-I is the most common cause of CAIHA; sometimes associated with *M pneumoniae*; enzymes enhance
+++	–	–	–	i	Sometimes associated with EBV infectious mono
+++	+++	–/+	+	H	Neutralized by saliva; almost always benign
±	+++	±	+++	IH	Neutralized by saliva; almost always benign
+++	+++	+++	+++	Pr	Rare; destroyed by enzymes; do not confuse with anti-P (see below)

There are 2 etiologic types: idiopathic and secondary. Idiopathic cold autoimmune hemolytic anemia (CAIHA) or cold agglutinin syndrome (CAS) is a chronic condition found predominantly in older individuals complaining of acrocyanosis and Reynaud phenomenon with a moderate hemolytic anemia. The responsible antibody is usually an IgM that is monoclonal. It may have anti-I, anti-i, anti-H, anti-IH or anti-Pr specificity t4.6, t4.7. The antibody causes agglutination in the extremities and fixing of complement, leading to eventual intravascular lysis. Secondary CAIHA is a transient condition often associated with infection. *M pneumonia* infection is associated with an anti-I, and EBV associated infectious mononucleosis is associated with anti-i.

As with warm autoantibodies, the task is to look beyond the cold reacting antibody for masked alloantibodies. Options include a prewarmed screen or crossmatch, using serum from a cold autoadsorption or adsorption with rabbit erythrocyte

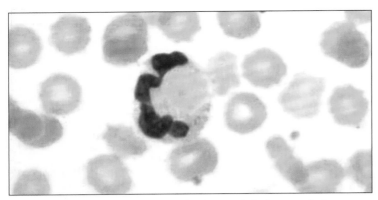

f4.15 Paroxysmal cold hemoglobinuria; neutrophils with ingested red cells are a rare finding

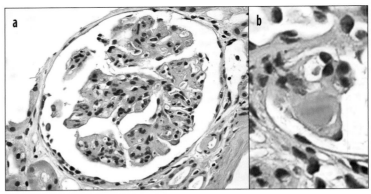

f4.16 Cryoglobulinemia
a The characteristic glomerular lesion has a resemblance to membranoproliferative glomerulonephritis
b At high power, characteristic bland intracapillary thrombi are seen

stroma (REST), or serum pretreated with DTT or 2-ME (disrupt IgM sulfhydryl bonds).

PCH is most often seen in children with viral illnesses such as measles, mumps, chickenpox, and infectious mono. The original description was in the setting of syphilis. PCH presents with paroxysmal episodes of hemoglobinuria associated with cold exposure. Sudden fever, chills, abdominal and back pain, hemoglobinuria, and jaundice characterize acute attacks. The resultant anemia is usually severe (eg, Hgb <5). Occasionally the peripheral blood smear shows unique intraneutrophilic hemophagocytosis f4.15. Treatment consists of keeping the patient warm and transfusing prewarmed blood as necessary.

The responsible antibody is an IgG biphasic hemolysin with anti-P specificity (Donath-Landsteiner antibody). It is called a biphasic hemolysin because of its capacity to produce hemolysis only when incubated at 2 different temperatures in vitro t4.8. To confirm the diagnosis, the Donath-Landsteiner test is performed on 2 vials of blood at 2 different temperatures: 4°C and 37°C. A positive test is obtained if only incubation of the patient's RBCs at 4°C then 37°C leads to hemolysis. Like CAIHA, the DAT is positive with polyspecific AHG, negative with anti-IgG, and positive with anti-C3.

t4.8 Example positive Donath-Landsteiner test

Procedure	Vial 1	Vial 2
30 minutes	37°C	4°C
30 minutes	37°C	37°C
Results	No hemolysis	Hemolysis

Cryoglobulinemia

Cryoglobulins are immunoglobulins that precipitate reversibly at low temperatures. To detect cryoglobulins, blood is drawn and kept at 37°C until clotted. It is centrifuged at 37°C, and the remaining serum is stored at 4°C for ≥3 days. It is then centrifuged at 4°C. Any precipitate that forms is a cryoprecipitate which can be subjected to electrophoresis for characterization. Note that cryoglobulins are found in temperature-manipulated serum (as opposed to plasma, where cryofibrinogen can be found).

3 types of cryoglobulins are recognized: type I and the mixed types, II & III. Type I cryoglobulins are monoclonal immunoglobulins found in association with multiple myeloma or Waldenström macroglobulinemia. Type II cryoglobulins are a mixture of a monoclonal IgM and a polyclonal IgG. The IgM has rheumatoid factor activity (anti-IgG). Type II is the most common type of cryoglobulin. Type III is a mixture of 2 polyclonal immunoglobulins. Mixed cryoglobulinemia (types II & III) affects individuals with a variety of clinical conditions, including lymphoproliferative disorders, chronic infections, chronic liver diseases, and autoimmune diseases (especially SLE). It is most common in women in the 4th and 5th decades. In the past, ~30-50% were associated with no underlying disorder (essential mixed cryoglobulinemia). With the advent of testing for hepatitis C virus, it was found that most of these had underlying hepatitis C virus infection. HCV is the most common cause of mixed cryoglobulinemia.

Clinically, cryoglobulinemia is a systemic immune complex disease characterized by a distinctive clinical syndrome of palpable purpura (leukocytoclastic vasculitis), arthralgia, hepatosplenomegaly, lymphadenopathy, anemia, sensorineural deficits, and glomerulonephritis. Most patients are variably hypocomplementemic, reflecting the immune complex nature of the disease. Renal involvement trails the onset of disease by 4-5 years, manifests as either nephrotic or nephritic syndrome, and is associated with severe hypocomplementemia. In renal biopsies, the most common finding is membranoproliferative glomerulonephritis (MPGN) type II f4.16. In some cases, usually when acute, the deposits produce the appearance of thrombotic microangiopathy f4.16. In all tissues, as in the kidney, the basic pathologic lesion is vasculitis. Electron microscopy demonstrates subendothelial immune complex deposits with a fibrillary or tubular structure in a fingerprint-like pattern. In blood, smears, pale purple cloudy aggregates of protein are observed.

Cryofibrinogens are composed of a mixture of fibrin, fibrinogen, factor VII, and fibronectin that precipitate out of plasma stored at 4°C. Cold induced precipitation of proteins from plasma, but not serum, forms the distinction between cryofibrinogens and cryoglobulins. Like cryoglobulins, cryofibrinogens can be classified as primary (essential) and secondary. Essential cryofibrinogenemia is extremely rare, and most cases are secondary to such things as collagen vascular disease, infection, and malignancy. In a recent report of several hundred patients with cryofibrinogens, only ~10% had persistent cryofibrinogenemia without cryoglobulinemia. Associated conditions in isolated cryofibrinogenemia included connective tissue diseases or vasculitis (~70%), malignancy (20%), and infection (10%). Complications associated with cryofibrinogenemia included

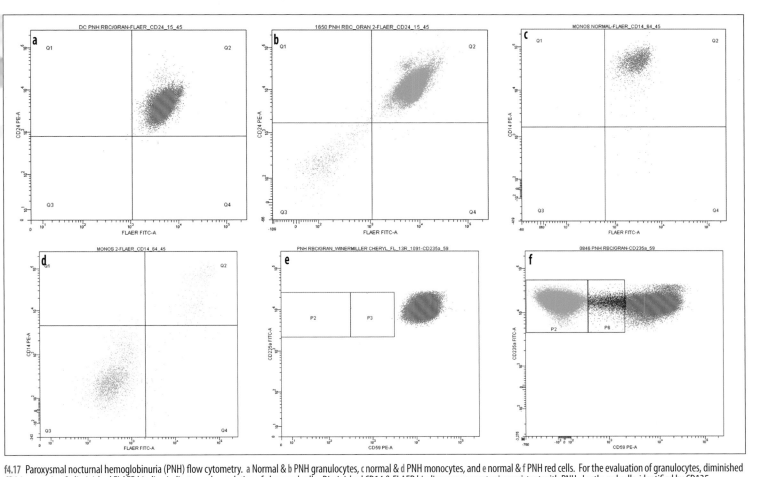

f4.17 Paroxysmal nocturnal hemoglobinuria (PNH) flow cytometry. **a** Normal & **b** PNH granulocytes, **c** normal & **d** PNH monocytes, and **e** normal & **f** PNH red cells. For the evaluation of granulocytes, diminished CD24 expression & diminished FLAER binding indicate a subpopulation of abnormal cells. Diminished CD14 & FLAER binding on monocytes is consistent with PNH. Lastly, red cells, identified by CD135 (glycophorin) expression show diminished CD59 in PNH cells. Red cells with normal CD59 expression (red population in f) are classified as type I cells. Red cells with complete CD59 deficiency (green population in f) are classified as type III cells, and cells with partial CD59 deficiency (blue) are classified as type II cells.

purpura, skin necrosis, sepsis and thrombosis. Biopsies of the skin were notable for bland intravascular thrombi as would be seen in TTP, coumarin skin necrosis, or cryoglobulinemia.

Paroxysmal nocturnal hemoglobinuria (PNH)

PNH is an acquired clonal RBC disorder. The defect is acquired at the level of a hematopoietic stem cell, and the affected clone has a set of intrinsic defects. Over time, this clone expands to ultimately dominate the RBC population and variable proportions of the white cell and platelet populations. All anomalies intrinsic to this clone appear to spring from a single molecular defect—decreased glycosyl phosphatidyl inositol (GPI) anchors. The GPI anchor is a protein whose function is to attach an array of proteins to the cell surface. Many of the GPI-anchored proteins function to deflect complement-mediated destruction by the immune system. The initial step in GPI synthesis is encoded by the phosphatidyl inositol glycan class A (PIG-A) gene located on the X chromosome. PNH is the result of various PIG-A mutations. The affected RBCs display a set of characteristic abnormalities, including diminished cell surface decay-accelerating factor (DAF, CD55), decreased membrane inhibitor of reactive lysis (MIRL, CD59), decreased acetylcholinesterase (AchE), decreased CD16, and decreased CD48. They are hypersensitive to complement-mediated lysis.

Clinically, patients are classically described as having episodic hemolysis, characterized by abdominal pain, back pain, and headaches, especially at night. More commonly, affected individuals slowly develop a chronic normocytic, normochromic hemolytic anemia. The DAT is negative, and there is hemoglobinuria (indicative of intravascular hemolysis). At this stage in the illness, the bone marrow is mildly hypercellular, with erythroid hyperplasia, depleted iron stores, and possibly mild dyserythropoiesis. Over time, transient thrombopenias and leukopenias develop. Eventually, there may be evolution to aplastic anemia and/or acute myelogenous leukemia. Furthermore, PNH may evolve out of aplastic anemia; thus, all patients with newly diagnosed aplastic anemia should be tested for PNH, and all patients recovering from aplastic anemia should be monitored for the development of PNH. Lastly, PNH may present with thrombosis, and exclusion of PNH should be considered in all patients with unexplained thrombophilia. Note also that the leukocyte alkaline phosphatase (LAP) score is decreased in PNH.

The traditional screening tests—Ham test and the sucrose hemolysis test—suffer from low sensitivity. The sucrose hemolysis test is performed by incubating the patient's RBCs in serum and isotonic sucrose (which promotes complement binding). Enhanced hemolysis in comparison with control RBCs is consistent with PNH. The acidified serum (Ham) test is performed by incubating the RBCs in heterologous and homologous serum that has been acidified (activating complement). Enhanced hemolysis in both types of sera is consistent with PNH.

Flow cytometry f4.17 is significantly more sensitive. Affected individuals demonstrate diminished expression of GPI-anchored proteins on the surfaces of neutrophils, monocytes, and RBCs. For definitive diagnosis, it is considered essential that deficiency of ≥2 GPI-anchored antigens be demonstrated on 2 cell lines. RBCs, granulocytes, and/or monocytes are most often studied. Lymphocytes are thought to give lower sensitivity because of their prolonged lifespan. Peripheral blood is the specimen of choice. For RBC analysis, CD55 and CD59 are most frequently studied. In patients who have not been transfused PNH, RBCs are classified as type I (normal antigen expression), type II (partial antigen deficiency) and type III (complete deficiency). Patients with >20% type III cells are usually clinically affected. Recent transfusion or recent hemolysis can falsely reduce the percentage of type III cells. In the study of granulocytes, patients with myelodysplasia and hypogranular neutrophils can present a difficulty if traditional cell gating is employed; a lineage marker (eg, CD15 vs side scatter) is recommended in initial gating of such specimens. The choice of GPI-anchored antigens in analysis of granulocytes and/or monocytes is highly variable from one laboratory to the next. Typical examples include CD14, CD15, CD16, and CD33. Aerolysin is a bacterial toxin obtained from *Aeromonas hydrophila* that binds specifically to GPI; fluorescent aerolysin (FLAER) can be used instead of antibodies against GPI-anchored antigens, providing greater sensitivity.

Patients with a diagnosis of PNH may be monitored over time with serial flow cytometry. Patients with type III erythrocytes exceeding 20% or abnormal granulocytes exceeding 50% have been noted to be at high risk for thrombosis and hemolysis. When patients are studied serially by flow cytometry, the abnormal cell population may initially be small in proportion. It expands with successive studies as the disease progresses.

Disorders of marrow production

Disorders of marrow production may result from inherited (germline) genomic abnormalities, acquired (somatic) genomic abnormalities, toxin, or nutritional deficiency. Production defects may concern a single cell line (eg, congenital neutropenia) or all cell lines (aplastic anemia). Lastly, a disorder that affects one cell line may progress to involve all lines (eg, Fanconi anemia, B_{12} deficiency).

It is common for the inherited disorders to come to clinical attention at a young age, but some (eg, Fanconi anemia) may present initially in an adult. Subtle physical anomalies, a family history, or a tendency to develop solid tumors may be the only clues at this point.

Iron deficiency

Iron deficiency anemia (IDA) is slowly acquired and progresses through a series of physiologic derangements. The earliest finding is a decrease in serum ferritin, making this one of the most sensitive tests. Next, there is a decrease in the percent saturation of transferrin, followed by decreased serum iron, and increased zinc protoporphyrin (ZPP). Lastly, there is decreased hemoglobin. Anemia is initially normocytic and becomes progressively hypochromic and microcytic t4.9, f4.18, f4.19.

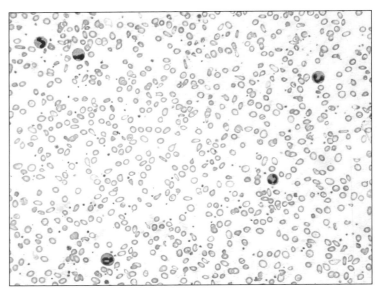

f4.18 Iron deficiency anemia; note hypochromic red cells & frequent thin elliptocytes (pencil cells)

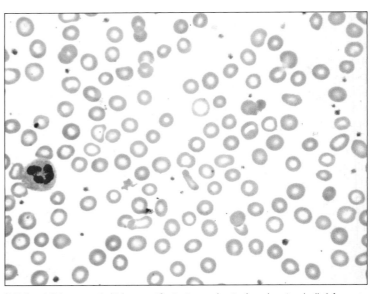

f4.19 Iron deficiency anemia; higher magnification image, showing hypochromic red cells & frequent thin elliptocytes (pencil cells)

t4.9 **Manifestations of iron deficiency**	
Blood	Microcytosis (↓ MCV)
	Hypochromia (↓ MCH)
	Anemia
	Anisocytosis (↑ RDW)
	Poikilocytosis (pencil cells)
	Thrombocytosis
Marrow	↓ iron stores
	Mild erythroid hyperplasia
Chemistries	↑ zinc protoporphyrin (ZPP)
	↓ iron
	↑ total iron binding capacity (TIBC)
	↓ iron saturation
	↓ ferritin
	Iron deficiency anemia

The morphology of IDA overlaps with that of thalassemia and anemia of chronic disease (ACD). IDA and thalassemia are more likely to be microcytic and demonstrate target cells than ACD. IDA demonstrates higher RDW (often >17) than either thalassemia or ACD. Pencil cells and prekeratocytes are typical of IDA and are not a common finding in either thalassemia or ACD.

Serum ferritin, usually <10 µg/L in established iron deficiency, is the best single test to make this diagnosis. However, ferritin is an acute phase reactant and may be elevated in hepatic insufficiency (impaired clearance), so adjunctive tests are sometimes required. Adjunctive tests include serum iron (low), total iron binding capacity (normal to high), percent transferrin saturation (low), and the serum soluble transferrin receptor (SSTR). The percent saturation of transferrin is calculated from the serum iron and the total iron binding capacity:

$$\% \text{ saturation} = [\text{serum iron}]/\text{TIBC} \times 100$$

In health, ~33% of the circulating iron binding sites are occupied (range: 20-50%). In iron deficiency, the percent saturation is generally <15%. SSTR is elevated whenever there is a relative lack of iron (iron deficiency and in erythroid hyperplasia such as hemolytic anemia, hemorrhage, or polycythemia). Zinc protoporphyrin (ZPP) and free erythrocyte protoporphyrin (FEP) are both elevated in iron deficiency but also elevated in lead poisoning and anemia of chronic disease. Lastly, direct microscopic examination of marrow for iron stores remains one of the most accurate tests of iron status, assuming enough bone spicules are obtained.

Iron metabolism begins with ingestion t4.10. Iron is ingested and absorbed predominantly in the duodenum, transported in bloodstream by transferrin, and eventually stored. Most of the body's iron is found in heme (hemoglobin, myoglobin, oxidative enzymes) and in storage (ferritin, hemosiderin). One mL of whole blood contains 0.5 mg of iron (1 mL of RBCs contains 1 mg of iron).

In children, there appears to be a relationship between iron and lead levels. Children with elevated lead levels are more likely to have iron deficiency, even after controlling for socioeconomic status. It appears that lead ingestion inhibits the intestinal absorption of iron. Furthermore, iron deficiency may enhance intestinal absorption of any ingested lead.

t4.10 Causes of iron deficiency

Infants & children	Decreased intake; increased use with inadequate intake (growth spurts)
Adult	Blood loss (eg, colon cancer, menses); decreased intake (strict vegetarianism); decreased absorption (celiac sprue, small bowel resection); increased use with poor intake (pregnancy, lactation)

Folate & vitamin B$_{12}$ t4.11, t4.12

The active form of folate, tetrahydrofolate (THF), acts as a cofactor in methyl transfer reactions. An important methyl transfer reaction is the conversion of dUMP to dTMP for use in DNA synthesis. Folate deficiency leads to impaired DNA synthesis which leads to impaired nuclear maturation. Folate is ingested in green vegetables (mostly), absorbed in jejunum, and released from enterocytes as N5-methyl folate. After transport in blood stream, it is converted in target cells to THF by a B$_{12}$-dependent methyltransferase.

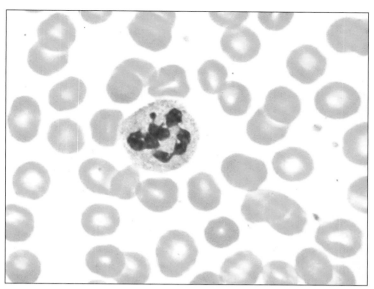

f4.20 Megaloblastic anemia; note hypersegmented neutrophil & numerous oval macrocytes

t4.11 Causes of folate & vitamin B$_{12}$ deficiency

	Folate deficiency	B$_{12}$ deficiency
Diet	Common (alcoholics)	Rare (strict vegetarians)
Malabsorption	Sprue	Pernicious anemia
		Post-gastrectomy
		Pancreatic insufficiency
		Crohn disease
		Diphyllobothrium latum infestation
Increased demand	Pregnancy	Pregnancy
	Hemolysis	Hemolysis
Drugs	Methotrexate (MTX)	Dilantin
Inherited	none	Transcobalamin II deficiency

t4.12 Manifestations of folate & vitamin B$_{12}$ deficiency

Peripheral blood		Oval macrocytosis
		Hypersegmented neutrophils
		Pancytopenia (when severe)
		Anisopoikilocytosis (variable)
Bone marrow		Hypercellularity
		Megaloblastic changes
		Erythroid hyperplasia with left shift
Chemistry	Folate deficiency	↑ LD & indirect bilirubin
		↓ serum & RBC folate
		↑ urinary FIGLU (formiminoglutamic acid)
	B$_{12}$ deficiency	↑ LD & indirect bilirubin
		↓ serum B$_{12}$
		↑ urinary methylmalonic acid
		↓ RBC folate (2/3 of cases)

B$_{12}$ is a cofactor for methyltransferase enzymes necessary for the conversion of the circulating form of folate (N5-methyl folate) to the active form (THF). In B$_{12}$ deficiency, methyl folate accumulates (the "methyl folate trap"). B$_{12}$ is also a cofactor for methylmalonyl CoA mutase which converts methylmalonyl CoA to succinyl CoA. In B$_{12}$ deficiency, methylmalonyl CoA accumulates. B$_{12}$ is ingested in animal products (mostly), bound to R factor in the stomach, released from R factor in the duodenum by pancreatic enzymes, and bound to gastric derived intrinsic factor (IF). IF-bound B$_{12}$ is absorbed in the ileum, bound to transcobalamin I & II (TC-I and TC-II) in enterocytes, and exported to the bloodstream.

The findings in B_{12} and folate deficiency are similar. The blood smear shows the classic features of megaloblastic anemia, which include oval macrocytosis, hypersegmented neutrophils, and large platelets f4.20. Erythropoiesis is ineffective, resulting in a hypercellular marrow. Nuclear maturation arrest associated with essentially normal cytoplasmic maturation leads to nuclear:cytoplasmic dyssynchrony. Many erythroblasts perish while still in the marrow. Thus megaloblastic anemia is in part a hemolytic anemia, and is commonly associated with a very high LD and a mild to moderate elevation in serum bilirubin. The RBCs that do proceed to maturity are macrocytic, with the MCV in fully developed megaloblastic anemia exceeding 115 fL.

Folate deficiency does not cause the neurologic defect that vitamin B_{12} deficiency causes. However, supplementation of folate in early pregnancy is known to reduce the incidence of neural tube defects. No clear mechanism for this effect has been established, but there appears to be an increased incidence of antifolate antibodies in women whose pregnancy has this complication.

The diagnosis of folate deficiency can be confirmed by measuring the serum or RBC folate. However, there are several confounding factors. One to several balanced meals can quickly normalize the serum folate, but the RBC folate is more stable over time. On the other hand, B_{12} deficiency can produce a falsely low RBC folate but does not affect the serum folate.

The diagnosis of B_{12} deficiency is a 2-step process, beginning with documentation of B_{12} deficiency and proceeding to identification of its cause. Serum vitamin B_{12} level can be measured directly by immunoassay. Serum B_{12} levels are often low in patients with HIV infection, but true B_{12} deficiency is very uncommon in this situation. The mechanism for this is unclear. B_{12} deficiency may be difficult to diagnose in patients with leukocytosis, especially in myeloproliferative diseases, since these conditions produce a falsely elevated B_{12} level through increased levels of TC-I and TC-II. A similar mechanism creates falsely elevated B_{12} in hepatic and renal disease. In such scenarios, and when B_{12} levels are borderline, serum methylmalonic acid (MMA) and/or plasma total homocysteine may be useful tests. Both are metabolites that become elevated even in mild B_{12} deficiency (and are unaffected by folate deficiency).

If B_{12} deficiency is diagnosed, identifying its cause is the next step. The Schilling test, while no longer commonly performed, was designed elegantly for this purpose. The patient was given a parenteral dose of unlabeled B_{12} followed by an oral dose of radiolabeled vitamin B_{12}. The purpose of the unlabeled dose is to fully saturate the body with B_{12} so that the radiolabeled dose will be quickly excreted in the urine. A 24-hour urine sample is then collected. A low level of urinary radioactivity confirms B_{12} malabsorption, but it does not identify the specific gastrointestinal defect. The second part of the Schilling test is then undertaken. The patient is given another oral dose of radiolabeled B_{12} in addition to oral intrinsic factor. Patients with pernicious anemia will demonstrate enhanced absorption (increased urinary radioactivity) in this second part of the test. Simpler adjunctive tests are available today, including the test for anti-intrinsic factor (anti-IF) antibody, a sensitive and specific marker of pernicious anemia.

Anemia of chronic disease (ACD)

Systemic inflammation alters marrow iron utilization and suppresses erythropoietin secretion and RBC sensitivity to erythropoietin. This combination of factors leads to a mild, refractory,

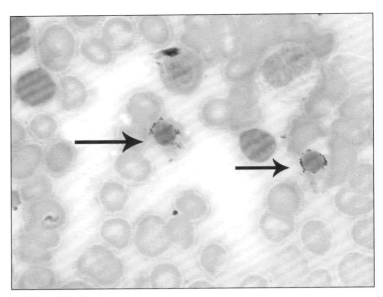

f4.21 Ringed sideroblasts

hypo-regenerative anemia that is usually normocytic and normochromic, but is microcytic in up to a third of cases. ACD is the most common cause of anemia in hospitalized patients in the United States. Most cases are associated with rheumatoid arthritis, collagen vascular disease (eg, lupus), chronic infection (eg, osteomyelitis, bronchiectasis), or malignancy.

The challenge in laboratory diagnosis consists in distinguishing ACD from iron deficiency t4.13. ACD typically presents as normocytic or microcytic anemia with low reticulocyte count and characteristic iron studies that reflect diminished RBC iron in the face of adequate to increased iron stores. Increased iron stores are identified as normal to high serum ferritin or increased stainable iron in a bone marrow biopsy. Note again that ferritin must be interpreted in light of its positive acute phase response; thus, a low ferritin is essentially diagnostic of iron deficiency, but normal ferritin does not exclude it. In confusing situations, the soluble serum transferrin receptor assay may be helpful. This analyte is increased in iron deficiency anemia and usually normal in ACD.

t4.13 Anemia of chronic disease (ACD) vs iron deficiency anemia (IDA)					
	Serum iron	TIBC	% transferrin saturation	SSTR	Ferritin
IDA	↓	↑	<10%	↑	↓
ACD	Normal to ↓	Normal to ↓	>15%	Normal	Normal to ↑

Sideroblastic anemia

The term sideroblastic anemia refers to a group of disorders unified by the presence of anemia and ringed sideroblasts f4.21 in the marrow. The peripheral blood contains hypochromic RBCs that may be microcytic, normocytic, or macrocytic. Microcytic presentations are more common in inherited sideroblastic anemia, while macrocytosis is more often a feature of acquired forms. The classic finding of a bimodal RBC volume distribution is also more commonly a feature of inherited sideroblastic anemia. Basophilic stippling may be noted and is attributable to iron-containing Pappenheimer bodies.

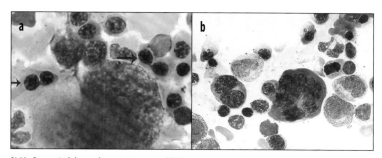

f4.22 Congenital dyserythropoietic anemia (CDA)
a Type I demonstrating internuclear bridges
b Type II demonstrating multinucleated erythroid precursors

The bone marrow shows, in addition to ringed sideroblasts, increased iron stores and erythroid hyperplasia. There may be a mild degree of dyserythropoiesis. Laboratory studies show elevation of the serum iron concentration, with high transferrin percent saturation, and high ferritin. Sideroblastic anemia, particularly hereditary forms, must be distinguished from hereditary hemochromatosis, since both produce a clinical picture of iron overload. Often, because of ineffective erythropoiesis and intramedullary hemolysis, there is hyperbilirubinemia, high LD, and a drop in the serum haptoglobin.

Sideroblastic anemia may be acquired or inherited. Acquired forms include a clonal stem cell defect (a form of myelodysplasia called refractory anemia with ringed sideroblasts), medications (isoniazid, chloramphenicol, chemotherapy), irradiation, copper deficiency, and alcohol abuse. The vast majority of acquired cases are in fact associated with a clonal stem cell defect (myelodysplasia). This typically presents in older adults with macrocytic, hypochromic anemia. The bone marrow aspirate shows >15% ringed sideroblasts. Cytogenetic studies find a chromosomal anomaly in 25-50% of cases. Inherited forms are rare and usually display X-linked recessive inheritance. Some inherited sideroblastic anemia can be overcome with large doses of pyridoxine (B6). The responsible gene is most often *ALAS2*, found on the X chromosome, in which a large number of different mutations have been found. Inherited sideroblastic anemia usually manifests initially in childhood, and organ dysfunction due to iron overload may occur. The MCV is usually low, and the RDW is usually high, with a distribution that may be bimodal. A rare inherited form of sideroblastic anemia is Pearson syndrome (sideroblastic anemia with pancreatic insufficiency). The marrow shows sideroblastic anemia with vacuolization of precursors, and the pancreas shows fibrosis typical of chronic pancreatitis. The molecular defect is a microdeletion within the mitochondrial DNA.

Congenital dyserythropoietic anemia (CDA)

CDA type II is by far the most common in this uncommon group of RBC disorders. CDA II is recessively inherited and characterized by multinucleate erythroid precursors **f4.22** with abnormal mitoses and increased karyorrhexis, and a positive acidified serum test. This constellation of findings underlies the alternative term, HEMPAS (hereditary erythrocyte multinuclearity with positive acidified serum). CDA I is characterized by dysplastic erythroid precursors with frequent internuclear bridges **f4.22**.

There is an important distinction between the positive acidified serum (Ham) test in CDA type II and that seen in paroxysmal nocturnal hemoglobinuria (PNH). Enhanced lysis in CDA type II is observed in heterologous serum only, whereas that in PNH is seen in autologous and heterologous serum. The positive Ham test in CDA II is due to an abnormal RBC antigen to which 1/3 of normal individuals have a naturally occurring IgM antibody. Unlike PNH, the sucrose hemolysis test is negative in HEMPAS.

The erythrocytes manifest a high density of the I antigen and the i antigen. Electron microscopy shows abnormally abundant endoplasmic reticulum located adjacent and parallel to the cell membrane (resembling a double cell membrane).

Fanconi anemia (FA)

Fanconi anemia is an inherited (autosomal recessive) chromosomal breakage syndrome that is complicated by aplastic anemia, usually by the age of 10 years. Often macrocytic anemia (or thrombocytopenia) exists in isolation for a period of time before pancytopenia emerges. In those who do not succumb to marrow failure, clonal hematopoietic defects may develop, including myelodysplasia (MDS) and acute myelogenous leukemia (AML). The predominant type of AML has monocytic differentiation (M4 or M5). There is increased incidence of epithelial malignancies as well, including cutaneous malignancies (squamous cell carcinoma), hepatocellular carcinoma, gastric carcinoma, and others. Associated findings are variable and may include absent thumbs or radii, microcephaly, renal anomalies, short stature, café au lait spots, and elevated HbF.

There are several genes in which mutations have been identified in association with FA. Mutations in *FANCA*, *FANCC*, and *FANCG* account for the great majority of cases. Additional genes—*FANCB*, *FANCD1*, *FANCD2*, *FANCE*, *FANCF*, and *BRCA2*—have been reported, each accounting for ~1% of cases. If all genes are included, it is estimated that 1 in 300 Americans are carriers. The overall incidence is ~1 in 100,000, and particularly high incidence has been noted in descendants of white South Africans.

The screening test is based upon the known hypersensitivity of FA cells to DNA crosslinking agents (mitomycin C, diepoxy butane, cisplatin). Cells grown in culture are exposed to one of these agents and their metaphase spreads examined. Increased chromosomal breaks, gaps, radials, and rearrangements are consistent with a diagnosis of FA.

Dyskeratosis congenita (Zinsser-Engman-Cole syndrome)

Dyskeratosis congenita may initially present with leukopenia, anemia, or thrombocytopenia, but isolated cytopenias progress to pancytopenia. Other findings include reticulated skin hyperpigmentation, nail dystrophy, oral leukoplakia, lacrimal duct atresia (causing overflow lacrimation), and testicular atrophy. The most common causes of death are fatal opportunistic infections, hemorrhage, and malignancy.

Dyskeratosis congenita has X-linked forms (most common) and autosomal forms (recessive and dominant) and results from a variety of genetic defects. The common thread is telomere maintenance. *DKC1* (Xq28) encodes the protein dyskerin and is responsible for X-linked cases, while a majority of autosomal cases is related to mutations in the *TERC* gene.

Telomeres function in the stabilization of chromosome during DNA replication. They are composed of hexanucleotide repeats (TTAGGG) that are associated with a set of proteins (including telomerase) and nucleic acids whose function is to maintain the telomere. Paucity or impaired function of telomerase leads to progressive shortening of telomeres with each round of cell division. At a critical length, the cell is signaled to stop dividing. Telomere shortening has been noted in patients with dyskeratosis congenita. Telomerase expression in tissue is proportional to the rate of proliferation. The more rapidly a tissue type proliferates, the more sensitive it is to telomerase anomalies; thus, bone marrow is very sensitive.

Anticipation, the finding of increased severity or younger age at onset in successive generations, usually thought of as a feature of trinucleotide repeat disorders, is found in many families with dyskeratosis congenita. This is believed to be due to inheritance of progressively shorter telomeres (in addition to inheritance of the mutant allele).

Pure red cell aplasia (PRCA)

PRCA may be acquired (eg, in thymoma and infection with parvovirus B19) or congenital. Congenital PRCA (Diamond-Blackfan syndrome) is rare, with an incidence of ~1 in 200,000. Median age at diagnosis is 3 months, with nearly all cases becoming evident by 5 years of age. Leukocytes and platelets typically are unaffected. Marrow erythroid precursors are sparse or absent. The i antigen is overexpressed on RBCs, erythrocyte adenosine deaminase (ADA) is increased, and the HbF is increased. About 75% of patients respond to corticosteroids. Mutations in the *RPS19* gene (19q1.32) are found in ~25% of cases. Another locus, at 8p23.2, appears to harbor a second disease associated gene.

Acquired PRCA, in over half of cases, is associated with a thymoma (especially the spindle cell/medullary/type A variant). Other cases are associated with collagen vascular disease, lymphoproliferative disorders of large granular lymphocytes, or medications. Pure RBC aplasia has been increasingly seen as a complication of erythropoietin therapy. Antierythropoietin antibodies are detected in many of these cases.

Parvovirus B19 may cause transient arrests of RBC production in healthy children and adults without serious consequences. Infection usually lasts ~2 weeks, and in those with a normal RBC life span of 120 days, this may be barely noticed. However, in those with chronic hemolytic anemia, a transient arrest of erythropoiesis may be catastrophic. The virus infects erythroid progenitor cells, causing a maturation arrest at the pronormoblast stage. Marrow examination finds numerous giant pronormoblasts, a reduction of the more mature forms, and viral nuclear inclusions. Parvovirus gains access to erythroids via the P antigen.

Transient erythrocytopenia of childhood (TEC) is a self-limiting disorder arising in previously healthy children, 1-4 years of age. The peripheral blood shows reticulocytopenia and a normochromic, normocytic anemia. Often, there is thrombocytosis. The marrow is hypocellular due to erythroid hypoplasia. The etiology in at least some of the cases appears to be parvovirus B19.

Congenital amegakaryocytic thrombocytopenia (CAMT)

CAMT is an autosomal recessive disorder presenting in neonates with severe thrombocytopenia and the absence of megakaryocytes in the marrow. Progressive thrombocytopenia proceeds to pancytopenia by the second decade of life. Mutations of the thrombopoietin receptor (MPL) gene are the cause of CAMT.

Thrombocytopenia with absent radii (TAR) syndrome

In the TAR syndrome, there is defective development of the bilateral radii and thrombocytopenia that is most profound at birth and becomes less severe during the first year of life. TAR does not proceed to aplastic anemia.

Congenital neutropenia (Kostmann syndrome) & cyclic neutropenia

Neutropenia syndromes t4.14 usually present with recurrent fever, cervical lymphadenopathy, oral ulcers, gingivitis, sinusitis, and pharyngitis. The more severe form of congenital neutropenia (Kostmann syndrome), may present in the neonatal period with omphalitis, followed in infancy by infectious complications such as pneumonia, intractable diarrhea, and abscesses, complicated by the later development of acute myelogenous leukemia (AML) in some. The milder form (cyclic neutropenia) is marked by intervals of fever, often accompanied by one or more foci of inflammation—such as oral ulcers, pharyngitis, sinusitis, perianal ulceration, or colonic ulceration—during which neutropenia can be found. The neutrophil count varies from normal to essentially none in a ~21-day cycle; the period of neutropenia lasts several days during which the patient is at risk for severe infections. Lastly, there are autosomal recessive and autosomal dominant forms of less severe congenital neutropenia, collectively termed benign familial neutropenia.

t4.14 Inherited causes of isolated neutropenia

Kostmann syndrome
Cyclic neutropenia
Myelokathexis (WHIM syndrome)
Chédiak-Higashi syndrome
Reticular dysgenesis
Shwachman-Diamond syndrome
Glycogen storage disease type 1b
Barth syndrome
Dyskeratosis congenita
Common variable immunodeficiency
Hyper-IgM syndrome
Hyper-IgE syndrome

Examination of the bone marrow finds a maturation arrest at the promyelocyte stage. Maturation arrest is intermittent in cyclic neutropenia, but even in intercritical periods, the neutrophil count rarely exceeds 2,000/μL.

Mutations in the *ELA2* (neutrophil elastase) gene, located at 19p13, are responsible for both Kostmann syndrome and cyclic neutropenia. Mutations in *GFI1*, a gene whose expression exerts control over that of *ELA2*, can also cause these syndromes.

Shwachman-Diamond syndrome

Shwachman-Diamond syndrome is an autosomal recessive disease characterized by neutropenia or pancytopenia, pancreatic dysfunction with fatty replacement of pancreatic parenchyma, and skeletal anomalies (metaphyseal dysostosis). Note that this is distinct from Diamond-Blackfan syndrome (pure RBC aplasia, no pancreatic or bone disease). Hematologic findings include neutropenia, eventually leading to aplastic anemia, myelodysplasia, and possibly acute leukemia. The bone marrow is hypocellular, usually with paucity of granulocytic precursors, and these may appear dysplastic. Neutropenia leads to recurrent infections, particularly skin infections. Shwachman-Diamond syndrome is caused by mutations in a gene known as *SBDS* (Shwachman-Bodian-Diamond syndrome) on chromosome 7.

Myelokathexis (& WHIM syndrome)

Myelokathexis is an autosomal dominant disorder, with neutropenia and recurrent bacterial infections. Circulating neutrophils have characteristic morphology, appearing degenerative, with pyknotic nuclei, fine chromatin filaments, and hypersegmentation. Neutrophils with similar morphology may be seen in patients treated with mycophenolate mofetil. The marrow discloses only hypercellularity with myelocytic hyperplasia. WHIM is an acronym that refers to a subset of myelokathexis cases, in which there are warts, hypogammaglobulinemia, infections, and myelokathexis. Both WHIM and myelokathexis in general are related to defective release of mature granulocytes from the marrow, reduced expression of bcl-x in granulocytic precursors, and for some reason, enhanced apoptosis in circulating granulocytes. Mutations in the *CXCR4* (chemokine receptor) gene have been identified as the cause of WHIM syndrome.

Barth syndrome

Barth syndrome is an inherited X-linked recessive syndrome of dilated cardiomyopathy, skeletal myopathy, aminoaciduria of 3-methylglutaconic acid, cardiolipin deficiency, and neutropenia. Marrow examination reveals maturation arrest at the myelocytic stage. Barth syndrome is caused by mutations in the *TAZ* gene, which encodes taffazin proteins involved in phospholipid biosynthesis.

Autoimmune neutropenia

Autoimmune neutropenia usually occurs as part of a systemic autoimmune condition, particularly rheumatoid arthritis (Felty syndrome). Most affected patients are positive for HLA-DR4. The presence of HLA-DR4 is also a feature of large granular lymphocyte leukemia, a disorder often associated with neutropenia.

Aplastic anemia

The term aplastic anemia refers to pancytopenia associated with a hypoproliferative marrow. The marrow is hypocellular and replaced with fat. The causes of aplastic anemia are numerous and include many of the inherited causes of isolated cytopenia t4.15. Most cases (60-70%) are idiopathic. Another 10% are due to medication or toxin exposure, and another 5% are related to viral hepatitis (especially hepatitis C). Before making a diagnosis of aplastic anemia, a careful search for its mimics must be conducted t4.16.

t4.15 Germline causes of aplastic anemia

Syndrome	Gene	Comment
Fanconi anemia	FANCA (16q24)	Autosomal recessive chromosomal breakage syndrome
	FANCC (9q22)	Initially anemia or thrombocytopenia
	FANCG (9p13)	Café au lait spots
		Thumb & radial anomalies
		Short stature
		Microcephaly
Diamond-Blackfan syndrome	DBA1/RPS19 (19q13.2)	Autosomal dominant
		Initially anemia
		Thumb & radial anomalies
		Short stature
		Cardiac septal defects
Dyskeratosis congenita	DKC1 (Xq28)	X-linked recessive
	TERC	Nail dystrophy
		Reticulated skin pigmentation
		Oral leukoplakia
		Lacrimal duct atresia
		Testicular atrophy
Kostmann syndrome	ELA2 (19p)	Autosomal dominant
		Initially neutropenia, uncommonly progresses to aplastic anemia
Congenital amegakaryocytic thrombocytopenia (CAMT)	CMPL (1p34)	Autosomal recessive
		Initially thrombocytopenia
		Thumb & radial anomalies
Shwachman-Diamond syndrome	SBDS (7q11)	Autosomal recessive
		Pancreatic exocrine insufficiency
		Short stature
		Reticular dysgenesis
		AR form of SCID
Down syndrome	Trisomy 21	

t4.16 Mimickers of aplastic anemia

Paroxysmal nocturnal hemoglobinuria
Hairy cell leukemia
T-cytotoxic large granular lymphocytic leukemia
Hypoplastic myelodysplastic syndrome
Hypoplastic acute myelogenous leukemia

Approach to the diagnosis of quantitative abnormalities

Anemia

There is no universally accepted definition of anemia. Perhaps the most influential definition is that published by the WHO, in which anemia is defined as a hemoglobin level <13 g/dL for adult men and 12 g/dL for adult women (11 for pregnant women), 12 g/dL for children aged 6-14 years, and 11 g/dL for children aged 6 months to 6 years. However, the WHO definitions are considered inadequate by many, and other definitions have been offered t4.17.

t4.17 Definitions of anemia

Author	Adult men (g/dL)	Adult women (g/dL)
WHO	13	12 (11 if pregnant)
Wintrobe	13.2	11.6
Williams	14	12.3

The evaluation of anemia should be guided by the morphologic findings t4.18 and the reticulocyte count. The reticulocyte count is pivotal in distinguishing production defects from consumptive processes. Anemia caused by a production defect is associated with a low or normal reticulocyte count (hyporegenerative anemia). Anemia with reticulocytosis (hyperregenerative anemia) suggests either hemolysis or hemorrhage. Several caveats should be noted. First, partially treated iron, folate, or B_{12} deficiency may be associated with reticulocytosis.

Uncommonly, immune hemolysis targets not only mature erythrocytes but also maturing marrow erythroid precursors, resulting in reticulocytopenia. Both hemolytic and blood-loss anemia may eventually lead to depletion of iron, folate, or B_{12} and present with reticulocytopenia. Lastly, while hemorrhage is usually apparent, significant blood loss into the retroperitoneum or pelvis may go unnoticed. In neonates, intracranial hemorrhage of sufficient quantity to cause anemia may occur.

t4.18 Morphologic findings in RBCs

Finding	Definition	Associated conditions
Acanthocytes (spur cells)	RBCs that have unevenly distributed, blunt & spiny projections with bulbous tips f4.23	Liver disease Abetalipoproteinemia McLeod (Kell-null) phenotype
Basophilic stippling	Small blue dots in RBCs, caused by clusters of ribosomes (RNA) Do not stain for iron f4.24	Hemolytic anemias Lead poisoning Arsenic poisoning Thalassemia Megaloblastic anemia Alcoholism Pyrimidine 5′ nucleotidase deficiency
Dacrocytes (teardrop cells)	Teardrop or pear shaped erythrocytes f4.25	Can be seen in relatively benign conditions (thalassemia, megaloblastic anemia) Often seen in myelophthisis
Echinocytes (burr cells)	RBCs that have circumferential undulations or spiny projections with pointed tips	Uremia Gastric cancer Pyruvate kinase deficiency Postsplenectomy Often artifact
Elliptocytes	RBCs twice as long as they are wide	Iron deficiency B_{12} & folate deficiency Myelodysplasia Hereditary elliptocytosis
Heinz bodies Bite cells	Heinz bodies: gray-black round inclusions, seen only with supravital stains (crystal violet) Bite cells: sharp bitelike defects in RBCs where a Heinz body has been removed in the spleen Both are due to denatured hemoglobin	Oxidative injury: G6PD deficiency or unstable hemoglobins
Howell-Jolly bodies Cabot rings	Howell-Jolly body: dot-like dark purple inclusion f4.26 Cabot ring: ring shaped dark purple inclusion Both represent a residual nuclear fragment	Asplenia Myelodysplasia
Macrocytosis	Enlarged RBCs (confirm with MCV, with age appropriate reference range)	Reticulocytosis Oval macrocytes: megaloblastic (folate or B_{12} deficiency) Round macrocytes: chronic liver failure, hypothyroidism, myelodysplasia
Microcytosis	Small RBCs (confirm with MCV)	Iron deficiency Thalassemia Anemia of chronic disease (usually normocytic) Immune hemolysis Lead poisoning Sideroblastic anemia
Pappenheimer bodies	Larger, more irregular & grayer than basophilic stippling, caused by iron-containing mitochondria f4.27	Asplenia Sideroblastic anemia
Rouleaux	Adherent RBCs laying side by side, usually caused by abnormal plasma proteins (immunoglobulin or fibrinogen) Unlike RBC aggregates caused by immune phenomena, rouleaux are reversible with dilution & do not affect automated CBC parameters f4.28	Monoclonal immunoglobulin Marked hyperfibrinogenemia
Schistocytes	Fragmented RBCs, taking shapes such as helmet shaped cells, due to mechanical RBC fragmentation f4.29	Microangiopathic hemolytic anemias (MHA): DIC, TTP, HUS, HELLP Mechanical heart valves 58% of normal adults have schistocytes, with mean of 0.05% of RBCs, range 0-0.27%
Spherocytes	RBCs without central pallor, due to decreased RBC membrane, often with high MCHC	Immune hemolytic anemia Hereditary spherocytosis
Stomatocytes	RBCs whose area of central pallor is elongated in a mouthlike shape	Alcohol Dilantin Rh null phenotype (absence of Rh antigens) Hereditary stomatocytosis Often artifact
Target cells	RBCs with a dark circle within the central area of pallor, reflecting redundant membrane f4.30	Thalassemia Hemoglobin C Liver disease

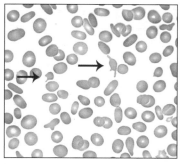

f4.23 Acanthocytes

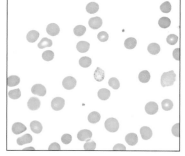

f4.24 Basophilic stippling

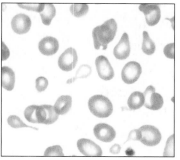

f4.25 Teardrop cells (dacrocytes)

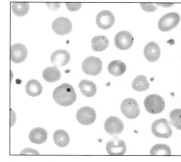

f4.26 Howell-Jolly body

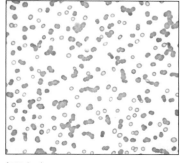

f4.27 Rouleaux

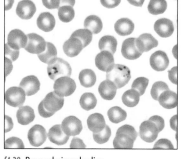

f4.28 Pappenheimer bodies

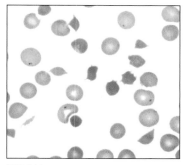

f4.29 Schistocytes

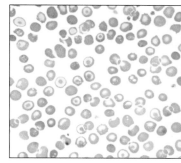

f4.30 Target cells

Neonatal anemia brings up several unique etiological possibilities. Loss of blood volume in the neonate can occur before, during, or after delivery. While fetomaternal hemorrhage is usually of low volume, significant fetomaternal hemorrhage (exceeding 30 cc) is estimated to occur in up to 0.25% of all pregnancies. Twin-twin transfusion occurs in 1/3 of monochorionic twin gestations. The donor twin in this scenario may become anemic. Intrapartum injuries to the umbilical cord are another cause of significant fetal hemorrhage; velamentous cord insertion and vasa previa are major predisposing factors. Lastly, rare inherited forms of marrow failure may present in the neonate, including Fanconi syndrome and Diamond-Blackfan syndrome.

Hyperregenerative anemia may be caused by hemolysis or blood loss. Blood loss is usually clinically apparent and most often results from surgery, trauma, or gastrointestinal pathology. Occasionally, hemorrhage is occult, as in the case of large retroperitoneal or pelvic hemorrhages, or occurs in the prehospital setting, where its volume cannot be estimated. While acute blood loss is usually associated with symptoms, chronic slow blood loss is generally well-tolerated and usually presents late, as iron deficiency anemia. Note also that acute blood loss is not the only form of anemia that can present abruptly t4.19. Causes other than hemorrhage that may present as rapid-onset severe anemia include intravascular hemolysis and acute exacerbations of a chronic compensated hemolytic anemia such as sickle cell disease.

t4.19 Nonhemorrhagic causes of acute severe anemia

Acute intravascular hemolysis	Acute exacerbation of chronic hemolysis
Microangiopathic hemolytic anemia	Aplastic crisis (parvovirus B19)
Mechanical hemolysis (eg, heart valve)	Splenic sequestration crisis
Toxins (eg, venoms)	Hyperhemolytic crisis
Infections (eg, malaria, *Clostridium*)	
Oxidant stress (especially G6PD deficiency)	
Hemolytic transfusion reaction (usually ABO)	
Paroxysmal nocturnal hemoglobinuria	
Paroxysmal cold hemoglobinuria	

Good screening tests for hemolysis are the serum lactate dehydrogenase (LD) (elevated), haptoglobin (decreased), and bilirubin (elevated). Note that most of these tests, particularly bilirubin and LD, will be abnormal in conditions associated with intramedullary hemolysis, such as vitamin B_{12} deficiency. Hemolysis may occur within the blood stream (intravascular hemolysis) or within the reticuloendothelial system (extravascular hemolysis). The differential diagnosis hinges first on whether the hemolysis is intra- or extravascular t4.20. Intravascular hemolysis is caused by microangiopathic hemolytic anemia (DIC, HUS, TTP, HELLP), complement fixation on the RBC surface (eg, ABO incompatibility, PNH, PCH), mechanical heart valves, snake envenomation, and infection (malaria, babesiosis, *Clostridium*). Most other forms of hemolysis are extravascular.

t4.20 Intravascular vs extravascular hemolysis

Intravascular hemolysis	Extravascular hemolysis
Schistocytes	Microspherocytes
↑ LD	↑ LD
↓ haptoglobin	Normal to ↓ haptoglobin
↑ free Hb, ↑ urine Hb	↑ indirect bilirubin
Hemosiderinuria	↑ urine & fecal urobilinogen

The peripheral blood smear can be examined for specific morphologic clues. The automated MCV is the best determinant of RBC size, and blood film cell size is subjective and artifact-prone. In thicker regions of the smear, erythrocytes appear smaller than they are, and in thinner regions appear larger. If the hematocrit is either too high or too low, there may be no "good" part of the smear in which to estimate size. Note also that the MCV is a volume and that the blood film provides only a sense of cell diameter; thus the 2 may not agree. Spherocytes, for example, may have normal MCV but appear small on the blood film. Variability in RBC size and shape are termed anisocytosis and poikilocytosis, respectively. RBC shape changes t4.18 may be artifactual, and many are nonspecific. RDW can act as a quantitative assessment of anisocytosis, but there is no such parameter for quantifying poikilocytosis. Hypochromia, the observation of increased central pallor, is reflected in the MCHC.

RBC size (MCV) is most often used to guide further diagnostic considerations f4.31.

t4.21 Polycythemia vera (PV) vs secondary erythrocytosis

Parameter	PV	Secondary
RBC mass	↑	↑
PaO$_2$	Normal	Normal to ↓
Leukocytes & basophils	↑	Normal
LAP score	↑	Normal
Serum B$_{12}$	↑	Normal
EPO	↓	↑
Serum iron/stainable iron	↓	Normal
Platelet aggregation studies	Abnormal	Normal

Erythrocytosis t4.21

The differential diagnosis for erythrocytosis includes myeloproliferative neoplasm, reactive erythrocytosis, and spurious erythrocytosis of dehydration (Gaisböck syndrome). If the latter 2 can be excluded through history and erythropoietin (EPO) measurements, then a myeloproliferative neoplasm should be suspected. The causes of reactive erythrocytosis are hypoxia (lung disease, smoking, high altitude), high oxygen-affinity hemoglobins, and certain EPO-secreting neoplasms (renal cell carcinoma, cerebellar hemangioblastoma, uterine leiomyoma, and hepatocellular carcinoma). Transient neonatal polycythemia may be seen in infants of diabetic mothers and Down syndrome.

Neutrophilia

Reactive neutrophilia usually does not exceed $30 \times 10^3/\mu L$, and is often accompanied by toxic granulation f4.32, Döhle bodies, and cytoplasmic vacuoles. Immature cells may be present (left shift), but mainly in the form of bands and some metamyelocytes. Myelocytes and promyelocytes are very uncommon, and there should be no blasts. Most importantly, reactive neutrophilia resolves either spontaneously or following treatment. The most common cause of reactive neutrophilia is infection. Other causes include medications (epinephrine, corticosteroids), trauma, burns, systemic inflammation (collagen vascular diseases, gout), seizure, exercise, postsplenectomy, leukocyte adhesion defect, and pregnancy. In children, juvenile rheumatoid arthritis (JRA) is a consideration.

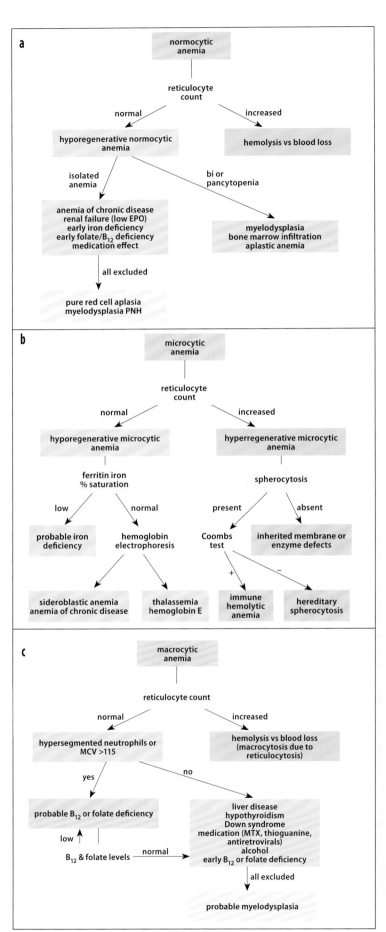

f4.31 Algorithms for anemia: a normocytic, b microcytic, c macrocytic

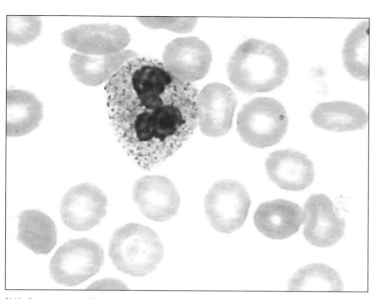

f4.32 Reactive neutrophil with toxic granulation

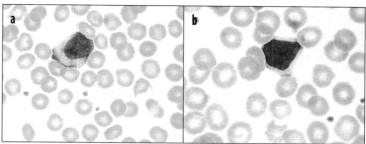

f4.33 Atypical (reactive) lymphocytes having abundant cytoplasm with 'burnt' cytoplasmic edges

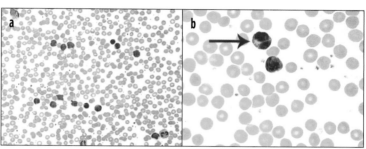

f4.34 Marked lymphocytosis in pertussis a composed of cells with irregular nuclear contours, b some of which are clefted, typical of Reider cells

GM-CSF causes leukocytosis with prominent toxic granulation, nRBCs, and abnormal nuclear segmentation. Lastly, a type of reactive neutrophilia in which toxic changes are regularly absent is that associated with the hantavirus pulmonary syndrome (HPS). During the HPS prodrome, thrombocytopenia is the only dependable finding. Once pulmonary edema is established, however, there is a highly reproducible pentad of findings—thrombocytopenia, left-shifted neutrophilia, lack of significant toxic granulation, increased hemoglobin concentration (hemoconcentration), and >10% of lymphocytes having immunoblastic morphology. In fact, having 4 of these 5 has a high sensitivity and specificity for HPS.

Myeloproliferative neoplasms should be suspected if neutrophilia is unexplained and prolonged. Clues include basophilia, lack of "toxic" morphology, and a "myelocyte bulge" (myelocytes outnumbering metamyelocytes). The leukocyte alkaline phosphatase (LAP) score is decreased in chronic myelogenous leukemia, while it is increased in reactive neutrophilia.

Lymphocytosis

Reactive lymphocytosis may be caused by medication or infection. Viral infection (EBV, CMV, acute HIV) and toxoplasmosis are the most common causes of the infectious mononucleosis syndrome, in which the peripheral blood "mononucleosis" is caused by a proliferation of reactive T lymphocytes. Often, these have a spectrum of morphologic appearance. The most common cell type takes the form of so-called atypical lymphocytes (ATLs f4.33) which are enlarged lymphocytes with moderate to abundant cytoplasm (Downey II cells). Often, there is cytoplasmic granulation, and the cytoplasmic borders have characteristic "burnt" edges that may be indented by adjacent erythrocytes.

Transient stress lymphocytosis is characterized by a proliferation of reactive T cells, B cells, and NK cells, often with no change in proportions. Morphologically these present a spectrum of morphology. The predominant cell type has a small, indented, eccentric nucleus, and there may be cytoplasmic granulation. Transient stress lymphocytosis is seen in acutely ill or traumatized patients and generally resolves within days.

The syndrome of persistent polyclonal B lymphocytosis usually affects young adult females who smoke. It presents as a mild absolute increase in small lymphocytes with indented to bilobed nuclei and abundant pale staining cytoplasm. There is a polyclonal IgM hypergammaglobulinemia, and there are no cytopenias. The vast majority of patients are HLA-DR7+.

Reactive lymphocytosis in children can sometimes take the form of small mature lymphocytes with clefted nuclei (Reider cells). Reider cells are classically associated with pertussis f4.34, in which the lymphocyte count can be quite high.

Absolute lymphocytosis in adults over the age of 40 years must be considered suspicious. Mild absolute lymphocytosis composed of reactive T cells (ATLs) may be occasionally observed in this age group, but follow-up to ensure resolution is always indicated. The likelihood of neoplasm is relative to the degree of lymphocytosis. Other clues to neoplasm include irregular nuclear contours, clumped nuclear chromatin, cytopenias, persistent lymphadenopathy, and increasing age. Chronic lymphocytic leukemia (CLL) is the most common neoplastic consideration.

Monocytosis

Monocytosis is a frequent reactive finding, but persistent monocytosis, if not otherwise explained, may represent chronic myelomonocytic leukemia (CMML). Causes of reactive monocytosis include collagen vascular diseases, chronic infection (classically *Listeria* or tuberculosis), malignancy, and neutropenia (a compensatory response). A neoplasm is suggested by the presence of promonocytes and/or splenomegaly. Serum lysozyme is usually elevated in monocytic proliferations, but it is not useful to distinguish reactive from neoplastic conditions. It is useful to clarify that a neoplastic process has monocytic differentiation. An additional caveat is that some automated counters may misclassify hairy cells, blasts, or immature hypogranular neutrophils as monocytes.

Eosinophilia

Eosinophilia is almost always a reactive change, most commonly related to allergy. Worldwide, the most common cause is helminthic infections. Other causes of reactive eosinophilia include collagen vascular disease, malignancy (T cell neoplasm, Hodgkin lymphoma, and colonic carcinoma), inflammatory bowel disease, and GM-CSF therapy. Of the cytokines, interleukin-5 (IL-5) is the most specific for the eosinophil lineage and is responsible for selective differentiation of eosinophils and release of eosinophils from bone marrow. Several named syndromes are associated with eosinophilia and eosinophilic infiltration of specific organs: eosinophilic cellulitis (Well syndrome), eosinophilic pneumonia (Löeffler syndrome), eosinophilic fasciitis (Shulman syndrome), and eosinophilic vasculitis (Churg-Strauss syndrome).

After excluding the enormous list of causes of reactive eosinophilia, one may consider a myeloproliferative neoplasm or hypereosinophilic syndrome (HES). There are very few morphologic clues to help distinguish reactive from neoplastic eosinophilia, but if eosinophils are morphologically abnormal (trilobate, monolobate) and/or there is splenomegaly, the likelihood of a neoplastic eosinophilic proliferation is increased.

Neutropenia (agranulocytosis)

The most common cause of neutropenia is medication. Medication related neutropenia may be pathophysiologically related to increased destruction or decreased production. Antithyroid agents (methimazole, propylthiouracil, carbimazole) are a common culprit. Agranulocytosis is not dose dependent, and its incidence is somewhere between 0.05 and 0.5% of all antithyroid drug users. Neutropenia usually occurs within the first 3 months of treatment, often presenting with pharyngitis, and patients are specifically instructed to seek attention if they develop sore throat, fever, an oral ulcer, or other symptoms of infection. Other medications commonly associated with neutropenia include antibiotics (penicillins, chloramphenicol, sulfasalazine), anticonvulsants (valproate, carbamazepine), and procainamide.

Causes of increased neutrophil destruction include autoimmunity, splenomegaly, medications, or infection. Infections that cause neutropenia include typhoid fever, brucellosis, tularemia, rickettsial infection, and, particularly in neonates and the elderly, overwhelming sepsis of any bacterial cause. Autoimmune neutropenia takes 2 forms. In adults, it is usually associated with lupus or rheumatoid arthritis (the triad of RA, splenomegaly and neutropenia is Felty syndrome). In infants and children, it is often idiopathic, with no identifiable underlying disease.

Decreased production, when isolated to neutrophils, may be caused by medications, large granular lymphocytic leukemia, and the constitutional neutropenias. The constitutional neutropenias include cyclic neutropenia, Kostmann syndrome, Shwachman-Diamond syndrome (not to be confused with Diamond-Blackfan syndrome which is similar but affects erythrocytes), Chédiak-Higashi, Fanconi anemia, dyskeratosis congenita, benign familial neutropenias, glycogen storage disease type Ib, WHIM syndrome (myelokathexis), reticular dysgenesis, and Wiskott-Aldrich syndrome.

Lymphopenia

Isolated lymphopenia is uncommon but may be seen in systemic lupus erythematosus, HIV infection, severe acute respiratory syndrome (SARS), anti-CD20 (rituxan) therapy, steroid therapy, and congenital immunodeficiency (Bruton, severe combined immunodeficiency, DiGeorge, common variable immunodeficiency). Since T cells are normally more numerous than B cells, T cell deficiency is more likely to be noticed in the lymphocyte count. Flow cytometry for lymphocyte subsets can be helpful.

Monocytopenia

Consider hairy cell leukemia or steroid therapy. In patients undergoing chemotherapy, monocytopenia heralds the onset of neutropenia.

Thrombocytopenia

An algorithmic approach to thrombocytopenia is offered in f4.35. The first question to be asked concerns the age of the patient, since the likelihood of the various possibilities differs with age at onset. In neonates, the common causes are infection induced bone marrow suppression (toxoplasmosis, rubella, CMV), neonatal alloimmune thrombocytopenia (NAIT), maternal immune thrombocytopenic purpura (passive transfer of antibodies), inherited thrombocytopenia syndromes, and chromosomal anomalies (trisomy 18, trisomy 13, trisomy 21, Turner). Inherited thrombocytopenia usually presents in the first year of life and is chronic or recurrent, but mild disorders may be noted only much later, either at the time of menarche, trauma, or surgery, or on a routine CBC. Since many of the inherited syndromes have recognizable changes in platelet morphology, examination of the peripheral blood smear should be carried out in all cases of newly recognized thrombocytopenia, particularly in search of giant platelets (megathrombocytes), very small platelets (microthrombocytes), abnormal platelet granules, and Döhle bodies. In children, immune thrombocytopenic purpura (ITP) is the most common cause. A rapid response to steroids is consistent with a diagnosis of ITP. A poor response to steroids but good response to transfused platelets is consistent with an inherited syndrome. In adults, thrombocytopenia is caused most commonly by ITP, a drug, or hypersplenism. The most common drugs implicated include antibiotics, alcohol, antiarrhythmics, thiazides, abciximab, quinidine, and heparin. Hypersplenism

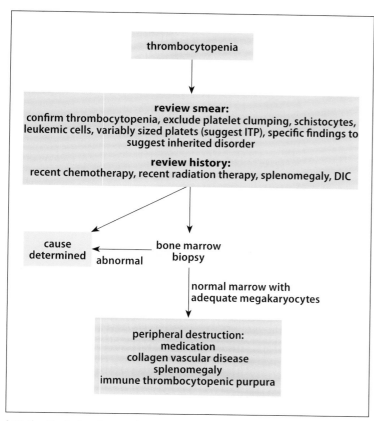

f4.35 Algorithm for thrombocytopenia

t4.22 Inherited thrombocytopenias classified by size

Small platelets	Giant platelets (megathrombocytes)
Wiskott-Aldrich syndrome	*MYH9* syndromes (May-Hegglin, Sebastian, Fechtner, Epstein)
CAMT syndrome	Bernard-Soulier syndrome
TAR syndrome	Grey platelet syndrome
	DiGeorge syndrome
	X-linked macrothrombocytopenia
	Mediterranean macrothrombocytopenia

A marrow biopsy may disclose underlying marrow pathology responsible for decreased platelet production (eg, myelodysplasia). A marrow showing numerous and focally clustered morphologically normal megakaryocytes would support peripheral destruction (eg, ITP).

Immune thrombocytopenia (ITP) is an autoimmune disorder that results in the splenic destruction and sequestration of platelets. The antigenic target in ITP varies, and may be GPIIb, GPIIIa, GPIb, or GPV. Definitive diagnosis, though not usually pursued, can be made by flow cytometry or ELISA to demonstrate increased platelet surface immunoglobulin. Most often, ITP is a clinical diagnosis of exclusion that, in the most straightforward cases, is made in an otherwise healthy individual who presents with isolated thrombocytopenia, a peripheral smear that is unremarkable aside from enlarged platelets, and no other obvious causes of thrombocytopenia. A substantial response to immunomodulatory treatment is the best diagnostic test for ITP, and >80% of ITP patients will respond to initial therapy, usually consisting of methylprednisolone with or without intravenous immunoglobulin (IVIG). Failure to respond suggests either an incorrect diagnosis or refractory ITP. Approximately 10% of patients with ITP have refractory disease, meaning that a platelet count of 30,000 cannot be achieved with initial therapy. Another 5% or so can be maintained ~30K only with chronic treatment. Splenectomy is considered for those who are refractory to medical treatment. Splenectomy is often an effective treatment for ITP, with 2/3 of patients achieving a sustained complete response. Some patients either fail to respond to splenectomy or suffer relapses after an initial response. No preoperative factor has been found to correlate with the likelihood of response, although younger age has been associated with response in some studies. In postsplenectomy patients who still require treatment, anti-CD20 antibodies may be used. The mortality rate for open splenectomy is around 1%, with 0.2% mortality from laparoscopic splenectomy. Alternatives to splenectomy, including corticosteroids and other immunosuppressants, also carry significant risks.

Neonatal alloimmune thrombocytopenia (NATP or NAIT) is caused by anti-PLA1 (HPA-1a) antibodies in ~80% of cases. Approximately 98% of the US population has platelets that are PLA1 positive. The remaining 20% of cases are most commonly related to Bra (HPA-5b), PLA2 (HPA-1b), or Baka (HPA-3a). The antibodies are of maternal origin and directed at fetal/neonatal platelet antigens. Sensitization ordinarily occurs during pregnancy of a PLA1 negative mother by PLA1 positive fetal platelets. In some cases, sensitization is from prior transfusion or other event. Nearly half of cases affect the first pregnancy, unlike hemolytic disease of the newborn in which the first pregnancy is usually spared. Affected neonates should be transfused with maternal platelets.

resulting in significant thrombocytopenia is most often secondary to liver disease. ITP is usually a diagnosis of exclusion. Uncommon causes include systemic lupus or other autoimmune disease (secondary ITP), antiphospholipid syndrome, B cell neoplasm, HIV infection, HCV infection, and *H pylori* infection. Particularly in older individuals or those who do not respond to treatment, a bone marrow biopsy may be undertaken to exclude MDS. Thrombotic thrombocytopenic purpura (TTP) is an uncommon cause of thrombocytopenia but one always worth considering, particularly because platelet transfusion is absolutely contraindicated. Lastly, heparin induced thrombocytopenia (HIT) syndrome must always be considered in new-onset thrombocytopenia.

It is important to review the peripheral smear, especially to exclude platelet satellitosis and platelet clumping. Platelet clumping is an EDTA-related artifact that occurs in up to 1% of hospitalized patients. This can be ameliorated by re-collection in citrate or acid-citrate-dextrose (ACD). Second, observe the size of the platelets. Large and variably sized platelets are seen in Bernard-Soulier syndrome and May-Hegglin anomaly t4.22, but more commonly indicate increased marrow production (ITP). Platelets with small size are seen in production defects and Glanzmann thrombasthenia. Third, look for schistocytes. Thrombocytopenia associated with schistocytes suggests a microangiopathic hemolytic anemia (DIC, TTP, HUS, HELLP). The number of schistocytes is usually high in TTP (>3/hpf), and lower in the other conditions. Clotting times are normal in TTP/HUS and prolonged in DIC/HELLP.

Posttransfusion purpura (PTP), like NAIT, is related to the PLA1 antigen. Thus, the 2% of blood recipients who are PLA1 negative are at risk. PTP classically presents as severe thrombocytopenia in a female recipient of cellular blood products, ~7-10 days following transfusion. Often there is a history of prior pregnancy or transfusion. For unknown reasons, the recipient's own platelets are destroyed in addition to the antigen-positive platelets, such that thrombocytopenia is profound. Usually platelet counts recover within several weeks.

Quinidine is associated with an immune-mediated thrombocytopenia in which the responsible antigen is the GPIX component of the GPIb/V/IX complex.

May-Hegglin anomaly f4.36 is an autosomal dominant disorder expressing a triad of giant platelets, thrombocytopenia, and Döhle-like leukocyte inclusions. Several similar disorders are known to be closely related to May-Hegglin, including Fechtner, Sebastian, and Epstein syndromes. Some of these have associated Alport syndrome-like nephritis and sensorineural hearing loss. All are autosomal dominant giant platelet disorders, and all are linked to anomalies on chromosome 22q12-13, where the *MYH9* gene, encoding a nonmuscle type of myosin heavy chain, is found. Aggregates of this heavy chain appear to comprise the Döhle-like bodies found in neutrophils. Mutations of *MYH9* have also been identified in an autosomal dominant form of sensorineural hearing loss without hematologic anomalies. Different disease-causing alleles at this locus appear to result in slightly different clinical expressions.

Mediterranean macrothrombocytopenia is a relatively common cause of mild thrombocytopenia in southern Europe. A mutation on chromosome 17 results in decreased expression of the GPIb/IX/V complex (the vWF receptor). Thus, the syndrome is essentially the same as the BSS carrier state.

Congenital amegakaryocytic thrombocytopenia (CAMT) is an autosomal recessive disorder that should be considered in a neonate with severe thrombocytopenia and the absence of megakaryocytes in the marrow. Patients with CAMT develop progressive thrombocytopenia and eventual pancytopenia by the second decade of life. Thus, they may be mistaken for other marrow failure syndromes (Fanconi anemia, dyskeratosis congenita). Mutations of the thrombopoietin receptor (MPL) gene are the cause of CAMT.

The thrombocytopenia with absent radii (TAR) syndrome includes defective development of the bilateral radii and severe thrombocytopenia. Thrombocytopenia is most profound at birth, and becomes less severe during the first year of life. The molecular basis of TAR remains unknown.

Thrombotic thrombocytopenia purpura (TTP) is a syndrome resulting from the widespread formation of microvascular platelet thrombi. It presents with the classic pentad of thrombocytopenia, microangiopathic hemolytic anemia, neurologic abnormalities, renal dysfunction, and fever. Platelets usually number <20,000/μL, and schistocytes are numerous in the peripheral smear f4.29. See chapter 5.

Alloimmune thrombocytopenia (platelet refractoriness) may develop in repeatedly transfused patients. The classic scenario is a patient receiving chemotherapy who needs repeated prophylactic platelet transfusions who attains progressively

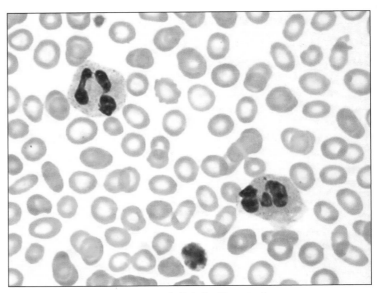

f4.36 May-Hegglin anomaly; note numerous Döhle bodies & large platelet

smaller platelet count increments following transfusion. The most common mechanism is the development of anti-HLA antibodies directed against class I HLA antigens, especially HLA-A and B.

Thrombocytosis

Reactive thrombocytosis must be distinguished from a myeloproliferative neoplasm. Evaluation is initially centered upon identifying clues to a secondary thrombocytosis. Elevated C-reactive protein, erythrocyte sedimentation rate, and iron studies may point to an unrecognized inflammatory condition or iron deficiency.

Nearly all cases of childhood thrombocytosis are reactive, benign, and self limited. In young infants, the likelihood of finding an underlying cause is low. In older children, thrombocytosis is often an acute phase reaction to an identifiable condition. In a study of Japanese children, the most common underlying condition was infection, followed by Kawasaki disease and iron deficiency. In a European study, infection was also the most common cause, followed by iron deficiency and malignancy (most commonly lymphoblastic leukemia). In adults, the causes of reactive thrombocytosis include systemic inflammation, malignancy, and splenectomy. Postsplenectomy thrombocytosis does not often exceed 600×10^9/L. Neither thrombosis nor hemorrhage is usually a risk in reactive thrombocytosis, even at very high counts.

Myeloproliferative thrombocytosis is suspected when the platelet count is very high. It is difficult to give a particular number at which thrombocytosis definitely represents a myeloproliferative neoplasm (MPN), but is found in >95% of patients with 2 million platelets/dL, >80% at 1 million, and >70% at 600,000. Thrombocytosis caused by myeloproliferative neoplasm does place the patient at significant risk for thrombosis and bleeding.

Neoplastic hematopathology
B cell neoplasms
General clinical considerations

Nearly 90% of lymphoid neoplasms are composed of mature B cells. The remaining are Hodgkin lymphoma and T cell neoplasms. Most B cell neoplasms initially present with lymphadenopathy. The remaining cases present as peripheral blood lymphocytosis, extranodal tumors, or other manifestations (eg, cytopenia, M protein, B symptoms). B symptoms consist of fever, drenching night sweats, and weight loss of >10% of body weight. The most common sites of extranodal B cell lymphoma are, in decreasing order, the gastrointestinal tract, skin, bone, and central nervous system. The most common site in the GI tract is the stomach.

Some B cell neoplasms tend to be tissue-based (lymphomas), while others tend to present as leukemia, involving primarily the peripheral blood and marrow. B cell neoplasms usually presenting as leukemia include chronic lymphocytic leukemia, prolymphocytic leukemia, hairy cell leukemia, and B-acute lymphoblastic. The remaining B cell neoplasms tend to present as lymphomas, with variable rates of marrow/peripheral blood involvement t4.23. Low grade B cell lymphomas are often disseminated at presentation, often involving the marrow at initial staging. High grade lymphomas are often localized, usually not involving the marrow at presentation. About 40% of patients have marrow involvement overall. Bilateral bone marrow sampling increases sensitivity, as compared to unilateral biopsy, by ~15%.

t4.23 Frequency of bone marrow & peripheral blood involvement by B cell neoplasms

Lymphoma type	Frequency of marrow involvement (predominant pattern)	Peripheral blood involvement	Notes
Follicular lymphoma	30-40% (paratrabecular)	15-20%	Discordance in ~1/3
Diffuse large B cell lymphoma	15% (diffuse)	20-30%	Discordance in ~1/3
Mantle cell lymphoma	10-20% (nodular)	40-50%	
Lymphoplasmacytic lymphoma	10% (interstitial)	5-10%	
Marginal zone lymphoma	5% (nodular)	70-80%	
Burkitt lymphoma	2-5% (diffuse)	30-40%	

Low grade B cell lymphomas largely afflict older adults. High grade lymphomas (especially Burkitt lymphoma and diffuse large B cell lymphoma) typically affect young adults and children. Most B cell lymphomas display slight male predominance, with mantle cell lymphoma (MCL) and hairy cell leukemia (HCL) having marked male predominance (3-5:1). But both follicular lymphoma (FL) and MALT lymphomas have a slight female predominance, and primary mediastinal (thymic) large B cell lymphoma has a marked female predominance (2:1).

The only significant risk factors are immunodeficiency and autoimmunity. Patients born with primary immunodeficiency and patients with long term autoimmunity states such as Sjögren syndrome are at particularly high risk.

Rituximab is widely used in the treatment of B cell neoplasms, either alone or in combination with other chemotherapy. It is increasingly being used in nonneoplastic B cell disorders, such as autoimmune disease. The effect of rituximab is depletion of even nonneoplastic circulating and tissue-based B cells. This effect may be rapid and profound and may take up to a year to replete after cessation of therapy. Furthermore, large lymphoid aggregates, composed predominantly of reactive T cells, may be seen in the marrow during or after rituximab therapy. At the same time, the neoplastic B cells often demonstrate diminished or absent CD20 expression by both flow cytometry and immunohistochemistry, necessitating the use of other B cell markers to detect recurrent/residual disease.

The most common types of B cell neoplasms, in decreasing order, are diffuse large B cell lymphoma (DLBCL), follicular lymphoma (FL), chronic lymphocytic leukemia/small lymphocytic lymphoma (CLL/SLL), and mantle cell lymphoma. FL is relatively common in the West (United States and western Europe) but uncommon in the East (eastern Europe, Africa and Asia). Burkitt lymphoma is endemic in equatorial Africa. T cell neoplasms are significantly more common in the Far East, while CLL/SLL is very uncommon there.

Small lymphocytic lymphoma/chronic lymphocytic leukemia (SLL/CLL)

CLL is the most common B cell leukemia in adults residing in the western hemisphere. SLL, its lymphomatous counterpart, is the third most common B cell lymphoma. SLL/CLL is uncommon in far eastern populations. These differences appear to arise from genetic rather than environmental influences. SLL/CLL displays the strongest genetic influence of all the B cell neoplasms, with familial clustering in 5% of cases. The risk of CLL in first-degree relatives is around 5× baseline. The incidence increases with age, with a median age of 65 years.

Clinically, SLL/CLL presents in a generalized fashion—generalized adenopathy, splenomegaly, peripheral blood and bone marrow involvement. Paraneoplastic autoimmunity and immunodeficiency are common. Cytopenias are unusual in SLL/CLL and are more likely to be caused by autoimmunity than by marrow replacement. A positive DAT is identified in >30% of cases, with fully developed autoimmune hemolytic anemia in 15-20%. Hypogammaglobulinemia is common, arising in about half of cases. A small minority display hypergammaglobulinemia. An M protein is occasionally present.

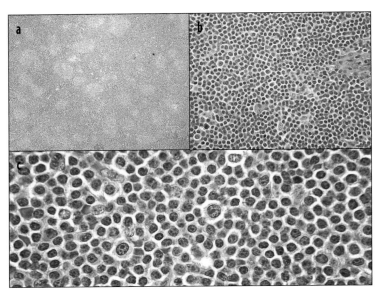

f4.37 Small lymphocytic lymphoma (SLL)
a At low magnification, proliferation centers (pale areas) can be seen
b & c At high magnification, a nearly monomorphous population composed largely of small round lymphocytes with occasional prolymphocytes (large cells with nucleoli)

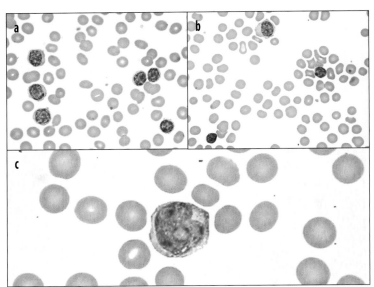

f4.38 Chronic lymphocytic leukemia (CLL)
a Usual cytologic features, consisting of small lymphocytes (nuclei not much bigger than a red cell) with scant cytoplasm & characteristic clumpy (checkerboard or cracked-earth) chromatin
b 2 typical CLL cells in addition to a single prolymphocyte, with a moderate quantity of eccentric cytoplasm & a prominent nucleolus
c shows a single prolymphocyte

Morphologically, SLL f4.37 presents as diffuse nodal efface-ment by predominantly small, mature-appearing lymphocytes with rounded nuclear contour, coarsely clumped chromatin, and scant cytoplasm. Occasionally, the nuclear contours are irregular or clefted (resembling mantle cell or follicular lymphoma), and some cases have plasmacytoid features (dis-tinguished from lymphoplasmacytic lymphoma by the expres-sion of CD5 and CD23). Mitoses are low in number, higher numbers suggesting mantle cell lymphoma. The diffuse pat-tern is interrupted in places by so-called proliferation centers (pseudofollicular growth centers) notable at low magnification as pale nodules and at high magnification for a large propor-tion of prolymphocytes and paraimmunoblasts. The presence, size, and number of proliferation centers—in fact all facets of lymph node histology in SLL—have no proven impact upon prognosis.

CLL f4.38 presents with lymphocytosis, composed of small, mature-appearing lymphocytes with scant cytoplasm, rounded nuclear contours, and a coarsely clumped chromatin (block-like, checkerboard-like, cracked earth-like), with numerous smudged cells (an EDTA artifact not seen on heparin smears). Absolute lymphocyte count is high (>6,000/μL) but usually not extremely high (usually <30,000/μL). By WHO definition, the count must exceed 5×10^9/L (5,000/μL) to serve as the sole cri-terion for diagnosis (ie, in the absence of tissue involvement). Cases falling short of this threshold, in which there is a mono-clonal B cell population immunophenotypically identical to CLL, are classified as monoclonal B cell (MBL) lymphocytosis;

MBL can be found in 3.5% of the population over the age of 40 years. Prolymphocytes, characterized by an increased volume of cytoplasm, open chromatin, and central prominent nucleoli, comprise 10% or less of the population. When 11-55% prolym-phocytes are identified, the condition is defined as chronic lymphocytic leukemia/prolymphocytic leukemia (CLL/PLL).

Atypical CLL is a term that has been inconsistently applied to neoplasms with most but not all the typical features of CLL. The most common variations ascribed to "atypical CLL" are irregular nuclear contour and immunophenotypic changes (eg, bright CD20, bright sIg, and/or +CD38). Atypical CLL is more often seen in association with trisomy 12.

The bone marrow is commonly involved at presentation. 1 of 3 patterns is observed: nodular, interstitial, or diffuse. The diffuse pattern is associated with a worse prognosis.

The immunophenotype f4.39 is highly characteristic. The neoplastic cells are positive for CD19, CD20 (dim), CD22, CD5, CD23, sIg (dim), CD43, CD79a, and CD11c (dim and variable). Dim expression of CD20 and surface immunoglobulin are nearly constant observations. The cells are negative for FMC-7, a particular epitope on CD20 that is consistently expressed in other B cell neoplasms. The cells are negative for CD10 and bcl-6 (in contrast to most cases of follicular lymphoma) and negative for bcl-1 (in contrast to mantle cell lymphoma). As in most B cell lymphomas, bcl-2 is overexpressed. CD38 and/or ZAP-70 expression is present in about half of cases and implies an unmutated IgVH status and an unfavorable prog-nosis. ZAP-70, the ζ (zeta) chain associated protein (ZAP), is a

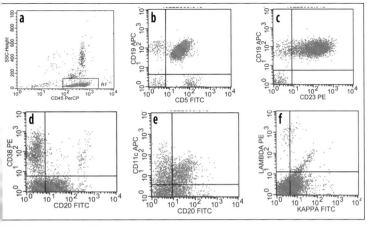

t4.24 **CLL staging**

Original Rai	Modified Rai	Survival (years)	Binet	Survival (years)
0. lymphocytosis (>5,000/mL)	Low risk	>13	A. <3 lymphoid areas	15
I. lymphadenopathy II. hepatosplenomegaly	Intermediate risk	8	B. >3 lymphoid areas	5
III. anemia (<11 g/dL) IV. thrombocytopenia (<100,000/mL)	High risk	2	C. Anemia (<11 g/dL) or thrombocytopenia (<100,000/mL)	3

4.39 Flow cytometry in CLL
a Gating around cells with bright CD45 & low side scatter (SSC), typical of the lymphocyte gate
b Plot of CD5 vs CD19, in which the neoplastic cells have characteristic coexpression, a feature shared with mantle cell lymphoma (MCL)
c Bright expression of CD23, typical of CLL but not seen in MCL
d No expression of CD38 in this case, indicating an indolent variety of CLL, with the typically dim CD20 expression
e Dim CD11c expression, expected in CLL but rare in MCL
f κ restriction, with dim expression typical of CLL

tyrosine kinase normally associated with the T cell receptor (TCR) ζ chain. Note that coexpression of CD5 and CD19 is a normal feature of a very small B cell subset. An increase in polyclonal lymphocytes coexpressing CD5/19 is sometimes seen in autoimmune disorders, especially rheumatoid arthritis (RA), in chronic hepatitis C, and post-bone marrow transplant.

With regard to molecular findings, older texts state that fewer than half of cases have chromosomal aberrations and that the most common of these is trisomy 12, biased by the fact that a trisomy is relatively easy to observe in karyotypic analyses. With more sensitive techniques, in fact, only 20% of cases have a normal karyotype. The most common chromosomal anomaly is deletion of 13q14 (>50%); other frequent findings are trisomy 12 (15-20%), del(11q), del(14q), and del(17p). About 30% of cases have complex abnormalities.

The most common form of transformation is prolymphocytic, heralded immunophenotypically by stronger expression of CD22, sIg, and CD20, weaker CD5 and CD23. CLL/PLL is present when prolymphocytes comprise 11-55% of the neoplastic cells. True PLL, defined as having >55% prolymphocytes, rarely evolves from CLL and more often arises de novo. Richter syndrome, the transformation to large cell lymphoma, occurs in 3-15% of cases. Rarely, histologic transformation to classic Hodgkin lymphoma has been reported.

Multiple factors relate to prognosis, stage among them **t4.24**. The Rai staging system was initially proposed as a 5-tiered system and subsequently revised to 3 tiers: low-risk (original Rai stage 0), intermediate-risk (stages I and II), and high risk (stages III and IV). The Binet staging system classifies noncytopenic patients as stage A or B, depending upon the number of lymph node areas involved, and patients with anemia or thrombocytopenia as stage C.

The "lymph node areas" include cervical nodes, axillary nodes, inguinal nodes (each side counting as one), liver, and spleen. B symptoms (fever, weight loss, and night sweats) are thought to correlate with shortened survival. Peripheral lymphocyte doubling time of ≤1 year and higher initial lymphocyte count (especially >30,000) correlate with worsened survival. The nodular pattern of marrow infiltration is correlated with a better prognosis, while the diffuse pattern implies worse prognosis. ZAP-70 and CD38 expression have been correlated with atypical morphology, an unmutated IgVH gene, and a worsened prognosis. With regard to chromosomal abnormalities, a relatively stable clinical course is seen with a normal karyotype or with del(13q) as the sole abnormality. The shortest survival has been noted in those with 11q and 17p deletions. The impact of isolated trisomy 12 is unclear but generally considered adverse. The t(14;19)(q32;q13) translocation results in juxtaposition of the *BCL3* gene and the immunoglobulin heavy chain gene, leading to enhanced expression of bcl-3 protein. This genetic change is present in 5% of cases of CLL and is rare in other types of B cell leukemia/lymphoma (bcl-3 protein overexpression is significantly more common than the t(14;19) rearrangement, being found in ~10% of B cell lymphomas overall, 20% of B-CLL and T cell lymphomas, and 40% of Hodgkin lymphomas). The t(14;19) translocation has been associated with atypical morphology, trisomy 12, and aggressive disease.

The mutation status of immunoglobulin heavy chain gene variable region (IgVH) is the single most powerful prognostic factor. CLL cells with somatic hypermutation of IgVH resemble post-germinal center B cells ("memory" B cells) and are observed in about half of CLL cases. Such cases have a stable course, good prognosis, and may be managed conservatively. CLL cells with unmutated IgVH resemble pregerminal center B cells. Such cases are likely to progress, have poor prognosis, and are candidates for treatment. Mutation analysis consists of RNA extraction and reverse transcriptase amplification with VH leader and JH primers. The amplified products are then sequenced, and the clonal VH sequence is then searched against a database of all known VH germline sequences. The closest matching germline VH sequence is compared, and the percent homology determined. If >98% homology is observed, then the case is considered nonmutated. If there is <98% homology, then it is considered mutated. Mutation analysis is obviously labor intensive and not widely available. CD38 and/or ZAP-70 (both tending to be expressed in nonmutated cases) may serve as surrogate markers. For a designation of CD38+, ≥30% of neoplastic cells should express CD38.

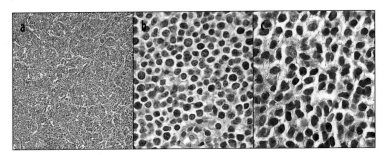

f4.40 Mantle cell lymphoma (MCL)
a At low magnification, note an effaced lymph node with vaguely nodular architecture
b & c Typical slightly irregular nuclear contours & small distinct nucleoli; prolymphocytes are absent

It is difficult to decide when or if to start treatment in patients diagnosed with CLL. Most patients are discovered incidentally, because of an abnormal CBC. Many cases do not progress. Therefore, most cases are approached initially with a period of watchful waiting, monitoring the patient for the development of symptoms, tumor growth, or cytopenias. At present, the prognostic markers noted above are not codified into national guidelines. If treatment is undertaken, the purine analogue fludarabine, alone or in combination with chemotherapy and rituximab, is commonly used.

Mantle cell lymphoma (MCL)

MCL occurs mainly in adults, affecting males disproportionately. It is often generalized at the time of diagnosis and has a tendency to involve the Waldeyer ring and the gastrointestinal tract. Endoscopic evidence of gastrointestinal involvement is found in nearly 60% of patients, most commonly presenting in upper endoscopy as "gastritis" and in lower endoscopy as polyps (lymphomatous polyposis). MCL follows an aggressive clinical course, with median survival of 3-4 years.

Morphologically f4.40, MCL presents as diffuse or "vaguely nodular" lymph node effacement. The neoplastic cell is a small to medium-sized lymphocyte with an irregular nuclear contour and a small subtle nucleolus. Mitoses are frequent. Typically there are admixed histiocytes, in sheets and aggregates, and hyalinized small vessels. There are no proliferation centers, and no "transformed" cells such as immunoblasts, paraimmunoblasts, and centroblasts. MCL may present as lymphomatous polyposis, in which 1 to several polyps are found in the colon. Biopsy f4.41a discloses a polyp whose core is composed of an expansile proliferation of monomorphic lymphocytes. MCL variants include blastoid, pleomorphic, small-cell, marginal zone-like, and peripheralized MCL. The blastoid variant f4.41b-d is composed of large cells with open chromatin and a high mitotic rate. It must be distinguished from several varieties of high grade lymphoma, especially lymphoblastic lymphoma/leukemia which lacks bcl-1 and CD5 but expresses CD99 and Tdt. The pleomorphic variant

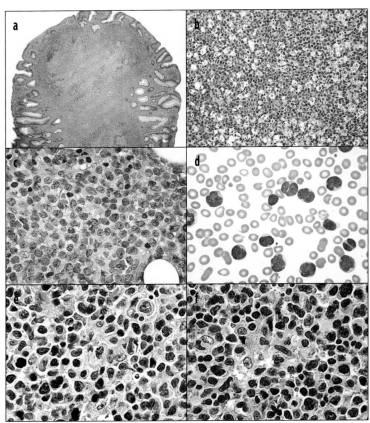

f4.41 a A low magnification image of lymphomatous polyposis, a variant of MCL
MCL blastoid variant
b-d MCL blastoid variant; b At low magnification, there is a diffuse proliferation of cells with numerous tingible body macrophages, reminiscent of the starry sky pattern of Burkitt lymphoma
c At high magnification, there are large lymphocytes with prominent nucleoli & irregular nuclear contours
d In the peripheral blood, one can again see the irregular nuclear contours in large lymphocytes with prominent nucleoli
e & f Pleomorphic MCL demonstrates a variety of cell sizes exhibiting many large cells with nucleoli

has a mixture of cell sizes and many large cells with nucleoli f4.41b-c. Blastoid and pleomorphic variants are considered more aggressive. The small cell variant is significant mainly for its resemblance to SLL; likewise, the marginal zone-like variant resembles MZL. While most cases of MCL have circulating cells detectable by flow cytometry, there is a subset of cases with a penchant for significant peripheral blood involvement, tending to have cytogenetic aberrations involving 17, 21, and 8 (in addition to the requisite t(11;14)). Peripheralized MCL happens often enough that the leukemic phase of MCL must be excluded whenever a diagnosis of CLL is entertained.

Immunophenotypically f4.42, the neoplastic cells are positive for CD19, CD20 (bright), CD22, FMC-7, CD5, sIg (bright), CD43, and bcl-1 (cyclin D1/prad1). They are negative for CD23, CD11c, and CD10. Particularly when studied by flow cytometry, some cases may express CD23, usually dimly. For this reason, it is

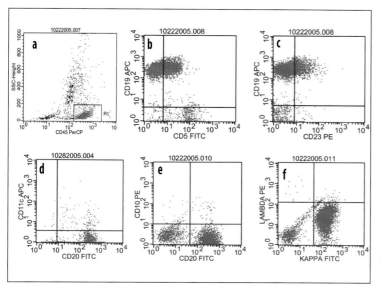

f4.42 MCL flow cytometry
a Gating around cells with bright CD45 & low side scatter (SSC), typical of the lymphocyte gate
b Plot of CD5 vs CD19, in which the neoplastic cells have characteristic coexpression, a feature shared with CLL
c Dim to absent CD23, typical of MCL
d No expression of CD11c, with bright expression of CD20, in contrast to the dim expression of both in CLL
e Absence of CD10
f κ restriction, with the bright expression typical of MCL, in contrast to the dim expression seen in CLL

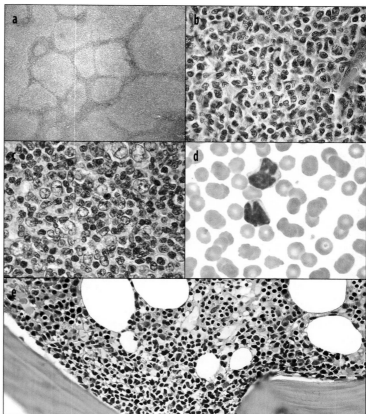

f4.43 Follicular lymphoma (FL)
a low magnification; note distinctly follicular proliferation in which follicles are confluent & geographic
b high magnification; low grade FL, composed predominantly of small lymphocytes with twisted nuclei (centrocytes) & few large lymphocytes with nucleoli (centroblasts)
c high magnification; high grade FL, with numerous large lymphocytes with nucleoli (centroblasts)
d FL involving the peripheral blood
e FL in marrow, which usually takes the form of paratrabecular lymphoid aggregates

important to pay attention to the other immunophenotypic features, such as the brightness of expression of CD20 and surface immunoglobulin. Unlike lymphoblastic lymphoma, the blastoid variant is negative for CD99 and Tdt. MCL is slightly more likely to be λ-restricted than κ-restricted. Note that up to 1/3 of primary splenic MCL and blastoid MCL may be CD5–.

The characteristic cytogenetic finding is t(11;14), resulting in translocation of JH region of the IgH (14q32) gene to the CCND1 (11q13) gene, resulting in cyclin D1 (bcl-1) amplification. Cyclin D1 (prad1, bcl-1), the product of the CCND1 gene, is a protein that appears to stimulate entrance into the G1-phase of the cell cycle. Note that the sensitivity for detection of t(11;14)/BCL1 rearrangements in MCL varies with the methodology employed. ~50% of rearrangements affect a single breakpoint area, referred to as the major translocation cluster (MTC) region. Thus, Southern blot (SBA) using a single MTC region probe, or PCR, using flanking primers to this region, will detect only about half of rearrangements. The use of multiple probes or multiplex primers can raise this detection rate to ~70%. Fluorescence in situ hybridization (FISH) assays, however, can detect nearly 100% of rearrangements and are therefore the clear choice for finding t(11;14)/BCL1–IgH fusions in MCL. Most cases display more than just this molecular anomaly, with second anomalies most commonly affecting chromosome 13, and ~25% of cases demonstrating trisomy 12. As in CLL, hypermutation of the Ig heavy chain has been found in a subset of MCL, but unlike CLL there is no clinical significance of this finding in MCL.

The single most important prognostic factor is the mitotic rate. While studies have shown prognostic significance for other factors (histologic variants, peripheral blood involvement, molecular parameters), none appear to be independent of the rate of mitoses. Specifically, >10 mitoses/hpf is considered adverse. Ki-67 immunostaining may be used as an adjunct, with staining in >40% of nuclei correlating with an adverse mitotic rate.

Follicular lymphoma (FL)

Clinically, FL presents with isolated lymphadenopathy without constitutional symptoms. The bone marrow is involved in over half of cases at presentation.

FL presents morphologically f4.43 as a nodular lymphoid proliferation that often overruns the lymph node capsule, consisting of back to back or fused follicles with attenuated mantles, lost polarity, absence of tingible body macrophages, and diminished mitoses. Within the follicles are 2 cell types in varying proportions, small cleaved cells (centrocytes) and large noncleaved cells (centroblasts). Grading t4.25 is based upon the proportion of large noncleaved cells (centroblasts) found in 40× fields of 10 randomly selected different neoplastic follicles (random, not worst areas). The 2008 WHO classification does not require stringent distinction of grades 1 and 2, encouraging the designation "grade 1-2" in low grade cases.

t4.25 FL Grade

Grade	Centroblast number
Grade 1	0-5/40× field
Grade 2	6-15/40× field
Grade 3	>15 per 40× field
3A	Some residual centrocytes
3B	No residual centrocytes

Diffuse growth is defined as an area in which follicular architecture is lost and that lacks follicular dendritic cells by CD21 and/or CD23 immunohistochemistry. Diffuse growth, when composed largely of grade 1-2 cells, is of unclear clinical significance, but it is recommended that the architecture be noted in the report according to the traditional classification. When diffuse areas are grade 3, then a diagnosis of DLBCL should be rendered (with background FL also noted).

FL variants include intrafollicular, isolated cutaneous, isolated gastrointestinal, and pediatric FL. Intrafollicular FL (FL in situ) may be overlooked at low magnification, because of intact interfollicular zones and open sinuses. Furthermore, there may be a mixture of reactive and neoplastic follicles. Upon close inspection, at least a portion of the follicles contain a "pure" population of centrocytes and centroblasts that coexpress bcl-2. The prognosis is not well understood. Isolated cutaneous FL has a low rate of lymph node involvement and an excellent overall prognosis. It is notable for a lack of CD10 and bcl-2 expression (bcl-6 is positive) and lack of *BCL2* rearrangement. Any FL in skin with expression of CD10 and/or bcl-2 should be suspected of having disseminated from a primary node-based FL. Isolated gastrointestinal FL also has a low rate of lymph node dissemination and an excellent prognosis. It typically involves the duodenum. Pediatric FL often presents with localized cervical lymph node involvement. They lack bcl-2 expression, lack *BCL2* rearrangement, and are usually grade 3.

In the marrow, FL typically presents as focal paratrabecular aggregates f4.43e. Only FL and T cell rich B cell lymphoma (TCRBCL) are commonly found in this form. Bone marrow discordant morphology is a common finding, usually in the form of high grade lymph node with low grade in the marrow. This form of discordance implies a slightly better prognosis as compared to patients with concordant (high grade/high grade) findings.

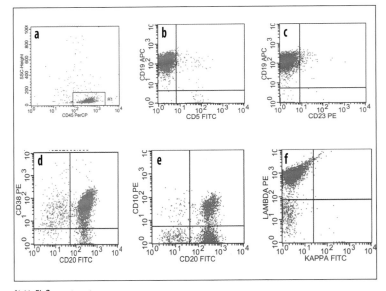

f4.44 FL flow cytometry
a Gating around cells with bright CD45 & low side scatter (SSC), typical of the lymphocyte gate
b Plot of CD5 vs CD19, in which the neoplastic cells strongly express CD19 but lack CD5; occasionally, FL has diminished or absent CD19
c CD23 is absent, but some cases of FL express dim or variable CD23
d Expression of CD38 (typical of FL) & bright CD20
e Distinct CD10 expression by a subset of cells; some FL does not express CD10, and expression is progressively lost with higher grade
f Bright λ expression

Immunophenotypically f4.44, f4.45, the neoplastic cells are usually positive for CD19, CD20, FMC-7, CD22, CD23, CD10, sIg (bright), bcl-2, and bcl-6. They are negative for CD5, CD43, and CD11c, with variable expression of CD23, CD19, CD10, bcl-6, and bcl-2. Many cases are dim or variable for CD19, and many, particularly with ascending grade, are negative for CD10 and/or bcl-2. Ki-67 expression increases with grade and may be used as an adjunct in grading (<20% in grade 1-2, >20% in grade 3). CD21 and CD23 can be used to highlight the background of follicular dendritic cells (FDC) in follicular areas, and absence of CD21 and CD23 can be used to support an impression of diffuse growth.

bcl-6 and bcl-2 must be interpreted with care. bcl-6 expression is common in reactive germinal centers, whereas bcl-2 is not expressed by B cells in benign germinal centers. However, bcl-2 is expressed by germinal center T cells, B cells in primary follicles, and mantle B cells; so it is important to pay careful attention to the morphology of the staining cells. bcl-6 is relatively specific for follicular derived lymphomas but is also expressed by Burkitt lymphoma and a subset of diffuse large B cell lymphomas (DLBCLs). Likewise, bcl-2 is also expressed in most B and T cell neoplasms. If interpreted appropriately, bcl-2 is a marker that can support a diagnosis of neoplasia in follicular proliferations, and bcl-6 can support follicular differentiation in a known neoplasm.

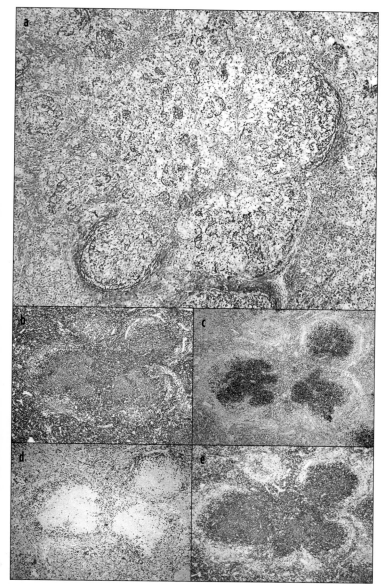

f4.45 FL immunohistochemistry
a CD21 reaction, highlighting the residual follicular dendritic cell meshwork; this stain can be used in unclear cases to distinguish diffuse from follicular growth
b CD20, highlighting several confluent follicles
c BCL2, which is positive in neoplastic follicles but would be negative in reactive follicles
d CD3, which highlights a few residual T cells around the follicle
e CD10 expression

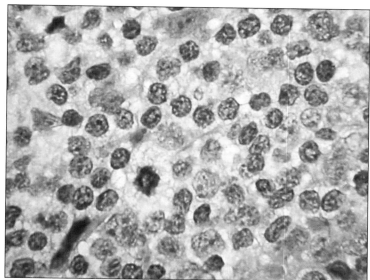

f4.46 Marginal zone lymphoma (MZL) usually consists of small lymphocytes with an abundance of clear cytoplasm ("fried eggs"), many of which have bilobed or indented nuclei ("monocytoid")

CD10 is expressed in early B cell maturation and then again in reactive germinal centers. Most FLs display cytoplasmic CD10 as do Burkitt lymphomas and a subset of DLBCL. CD10 expression in the follicle does not help to diagnose malignancy; however, increased expression of CD10 in the interfollicular zones (indicative of permeation of the sinuses by lymphoma) does.

The t(14;18)(p32;q21) translocation forms the basis for FL. This is best determined by FISH (the sensitivity of PCR ranges from 40-90%). The translocation juxtaposes the *BCL2* gene on chromosome 18 with the J region of the immunoglobulin heavy chain gene (JH) on chromosome 14 with a resulting overexpression of the bcl-2 protein. The gene product of *BCL2*, bcl-2 protein, is an antiapoptotic molecule capable of aborting the normal process of programmed cell death. Most t(14;18) translocations occur within a 150 base pair region (the major breakpoint region—MBR). The translocation is not unique to FL; t(14;18) is the most common translocation encountered in B-lineage lymphoma of all stripes. A 5' region of *BCL2*, the variant cluster region (VCR) may be rearranged in CLL/SLL. In DLBCL, the presence of the t(14;18) rearrangement has been associated with a "germinal center" phenotype and a relatively favorable prognosis. *BCL2* gene rearrangement is nearly always associated with overexpression of bcl-2 protein. The converse is not true—bcl-2 overexpression is often not associated with *BCL2* gene rearrangement. Many B cell neoplasms overexpress bcl-2, and most of these do not have structural *BCL2* gene rearrangements; instead having deregulated *BCL2* for other reasons. Lastly, a small number of benign cells harboring a *BCL2/IGH* rearrangement can be found in ≥25% of healthy adults.

Prognostically, FL has a median survival of 8-10 years. Most eventually progress (transform) to high grade FL or DLBCL. Factors known to correlate with progression include age, stage, bone marrow involvement, B symptoms, performance status, serum lactate dehydrogenase levels, and anemia. It appears that bcl-6 and CD10 expression favorably impact prognosis.

Marginal zone lymphoma (MZL)

MZL is a neoplasm of marginal zone B cells with several distinct clinicopathologic presentations. Nodal marginal zone B cell lymphoma presents as a proliferation of small round lymphocytes with abundant pale cytoplasm and indented nuclei (monocytoid B cells) **f4.46**. The pattern may be diffuse, sinusoidal, or interfollicular. Often, the neoplastic cells proliferate around residual follicles and demonstrate follicular permeation (colonization). Clonal plasma cells are often present, and rare intranuclear Dutcher bodies can be found within them. Extranodal marginal zone B cell lymphoma of mucosa associated lymphoid tissue (MALT lymphoma) presents as a variably destructive and/or tumefactive proliferation of monocytoid B cells and plasma cells (some with Dutcher bodies). The cells may permeate background epithelium, forming lymphoepithelial lesions f4.47. The plasma cells are monoclonal. Reactive (polyclonal) lymphoid follicles with germinal centers may be present. The WHO does not recognize a high grade variety of MALT; such tumors should be regarded as DLBCL. MALT lymphomas are associated with chronic antigenic stimulation t4.26, usually from infectious agents. The most common site is the GI tract, especially the stomach. Lastly, splenic marginal zone lymphoma involves the spleen (mainly white pulp), splenic hilar lymph nodes (but not other nodal sites), liver (sinusoids) and peripheral blood (usually at very low levels).

t4.26 MZL: associated antigenic stimulation

Gastric MALT	H pylori
Ocular MALT	C psittaci
IPSID (α chain disease)	C jejuni
Cutaneous MALT	B burgdorferi
Salivary MALT	Sjögren syndrome
Thyroid MALT	Hashimoto
Splenic MZL	HCV

The leukemic phase of splenic MZL is synonymous with splenic lymphoma with villous lymphocytes (SLVL) f4.47c-e, in which the leukemic cells morphologically resemble hairy cell leukemia (HCL). The leukemic cells have small nuclei, abundant pale cytoplasm, irregular cytoplasmic borders, and polar villous projections f4.47. Characteristic differences with HCL include a distinct nucleolus (usually absent in HCL), polar villi (usually circumferential in HCL), and a nodular pattern of bone marrow involvement (interstitial or diffuse in HCL). Blood lakes and reticulin fibrosis, common in marrows involved by HCL, are not seen in SLVL. In the spleen, HCL diffusely involves the red pulp, while SLVL is found in the white pulp. Lastly, hairy cells are diffusely and strongly positive for tartrate-resistant acid phosphatase (TRAP), while SLVL is weakly positive at best. With regard to mantle cell lymphoma (MCL), it should be noted that a significant minority of primary splenic MCL is CD5–; attention to irregular nuclear contour and other clinical features (lymphadenopathy) should prompt a bcl-1 study. Splenic MZL is associated with hepatitis C virus (HCV) infection in >30% of cases. Remission can often be achieved by splenectomy.

Immunophenotypically, MZL is positive for CD19, CD20, CD79a, FMC-7, bcl-2, and sIg (IgM). It is negative for CD5, CD23, CD10, CD103, Annexin A1, and CD11c. Plasma cells contain monoclonal cytoplasmic light chains. CD43 is negative in all except MALT lymphoma (<30% of cases positive).

Extranodal marginal zone (MALT) lymphomas often demonstrate cytogenetic abnormalities which are loosely site-specific. The t(11;18) translocation, a rearrangement of the *API2* and *MALT1* genes, is common in tumors of the stomach and lung. The t(14;18) translocation results in a *MALT1*-IgH gene

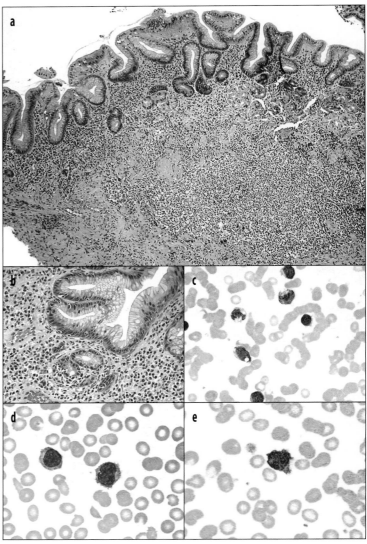

f4.47 Extranodal MZL
a Gastric extranodal marginal zone lymphoma (MALT lymphoma), low magnification view, showing an expansile lymphoid proliferation in the deep mucosa & mucosal gastritislike infiltrate in the superficial mucosa
b High magnification image of the superficial mucosa of a showing many plasma cells in this region, also depicted is a lymphoepithelial lesion
c Peripheral blood involvement by splenic lymphoma with villous lymphocytes, in which lymphocytes with distinct nucleoli are associated with voluminous cytoplasm that is bipolar & has polar villi

fusion. *MALT1*–IgH translocation tumors are found largely in ocular, parotid, and cutaneous sites. The t(3;14) translocation (*FOXP1-MALT1*) is associated with ocular, thyroid, and cutaneous sites. Translocation t(1;14) is seen in lung and small bowel. Lastly, +3 and +18 are seen nonspecifically in all sites.

A monoclonal gammopathy is present in 30-50% of cases.

Hairy cell leukemia (HCL)

HCL is an easily overlooked cause of new onset neutropenia, monocytopenia, or aplastic anemia. When it presents with splenomegaly, clinical suspicion is higher and the diagnosis therefore easier. In the literature that has accumulated since its first description as "leukemic reticuloendotheliosis,"

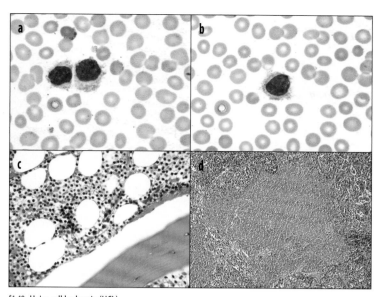

f4.48 Hairy cell leukemia (HCL)
a & b Peripheral blood involvement by cells with large nuclei, approximately twice the size of a red cell, no nucleoli & an abundance of cytoplasm with frayed edges (hairy projections)
c Marrow involvement by cells with abundant clear cytoplasm ("fried eggs")
d Blood lake in the spleen

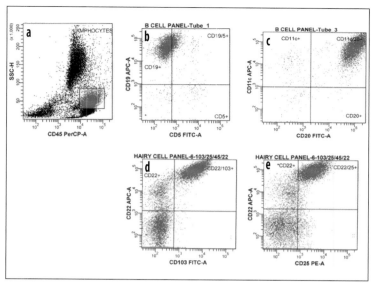

f4.49 HCL flow cytometry
a Gating around cells with bright CD45 & moderate side scatter (SSC), somewhat removed from the typical lymphocyte gate
b Plot of CD5 vs CD19, in which the neoplastic cells have characteristically very bright CD19 expression, lacking CD5
c Very bright CD20 & CD11c expression, in contrast to the dim 11c expression seen in CLL
d & e Expression, again very bright, of CD22, CD103 & CD25

a striking 4:1 male:female ratio has been consistent. At presentation, the most common symptoms are constitutional (fatigue), but there may be left upper quadrant pain referable to splenomegaly. Splenomegaly is present at presentation in nearly all patients and may be massive. Lymphadenopathy is uncommon. Cytopenias are common, including anemia, thrombocytopenia, and leukopenia. The presence of monocytopenia has been stressed in the literature of the HCL. In fact, the diagnosis of HCL is unlikely without monocytopenia. Note, however, that some automated analyzers will mistake hairy cells for monocytes. Infectious complications are common and remain a leading cause of death in HCL.

HCL morphology f4.48 in peripheral blood smears and cytologic preparations is highly characteristic. Hairy cells are large in comparison to mature lymphocytes, with a nucleus about twice the size. The nuclei vary in outline—they may be round, oval, reniform, or bilobed. The nuclear outline is sharp and smooth, and the chromatin is usually described as "ground glass" because of its even dispersal. Nucleoli are usually absent or indistinct. Hairy projections are in fact neither a consistent nor a unique feature. When present, however, hairy projections are circumferential. They are formed by a cytoplasmic margin that is indistinct and frayed. The cytoplasm of the cells is pale, textured, and flocculent.

In tissue, such as in bone marrow and spleen, hairy cells have "fried egg" morphology, with small dark nuclei and abundant pale cytoplasm. In marrow, these are easily identifiable when in sheets but often form subtle interstitial infiltrates. The marrow itself may be extremely hypocellular, mimicking aplastic anemia. Reticulin fibrosis is common, causing a typically inaspirable (dry tap) marrow. In whatever tissue it involves, there is frequent formation of "blood lakes." These are blood-filled spaces without endothelial lining. Mast cells are also frequent in HCL infiltrates. In the spleen, the cells infiltrate the red pulp. In the liver, the cells infiltrate the hepatic sinusoids. Angiomatoid foci have been described, which appear to represent the hepatic version of a blood lake. In lymph nodes, HCL tends to be sinusoidal.

There is a variety of HCL mimics. Splenic lymphoma with villous lymphocytes (SLVL), the leukemic phase of splenic marginal zone lymphoma (MZL), displays moderate to abundant cytoplasm and may have cytoplasmic projections; however, these tend to be polar, and the flocculent quality of HCL cytoplasm is lacking. The chromatin in SLVL lacks the dispersed ground-glass quality of HCL, being more clumped, and the nucleolus is typically more prominent in SLVL. Prolymphocytic lymphoma (PLL) is characterized by a significantly higher peripheral white count and much more prominent nucleoli. Mastocytosis may produce a cytologic and histologic appearance similar to HCL in many respects. The nuclei tend to be oval to reniform, there is dispersed chromatin, and there is abundant cytoplasm. Both may be associated with fibrosis, and an infiltrate of mast cells is common to both. The finding of granular cytoplasm and numerous admixed eosinophils are important clues to mastocytosis. In some cases, even AML (particularly M3 and M5) may enter the differential diagnosis.

Ultrastructurally, ribosome-lamellar complexes have been described as the most distinctive feature of HCL. These are annular structures with a central empty zone surrounded by concentric tubules and ribosomes. These may be large enough to see with light microscopy, appearing as Döhle-like inclusions.

The cells contain tartrate-resistant acid phosphatase (TRAP) in cytologic preparations. TRAP is not unique to HCL and weak staining may be seen in prolymphocytic leukemia (PLL), Waldenström macroglobulinemia, mast cell disease, and the histiocytes of Gaucher disease. However, strong TRAP staining is relatively specific.

Immunophenotypically f4.49, HCL is positive for CD19, CD20, CD22, sIg, CD11c (bright), CD25 (bright), CD103, DBA.44, Annexin A1, and cyclin D1 (dim, nuclear). It is negative for CD5, CD43, CD23, and CD10 t4.27. In the plot of CD45 vs side-scatter, there is often a dual lymphoid population, HCL having strong CD45 and moderate side-angle light scatter, such that it may be found in the monocyte region. About 10% are CD10+, and these cases do not appear to differ clinically. While CD11c is commonly expressed in CLL and SLVL, expression is typically brighter in HCL. CD25 is also commonly expressed in MZL, but again expression is much brighter in HCL. Annexin A1 is the most specific of the hairy cell antigens; CD103 is sometimes expressed in SLVL and so-called variant HCL (HCLv), both of which may not respond favorably to HCL-directed therapy. It has been suggested that CD103+ neoplasms that coexpress neither CD25 nor Annexin A1 should be treated differently. Note that Annexin A1 is expressed in some T cells and myeloid cells. DBA.44 is also expressed in a majority of SLVL and a significant minority of follicular lymphoma, mantle cell lymphoma, and diffuse large B cell lymphoma.

There are no signature molecular findings. Noted abnormalities include duplications of a region in 14q, t(14;18), and abnormalities of a region of chromosome 5. The finding of bcl-1 overexpression, in many cases of HCL, does not appear to be associated with structural rearrangements of the *BCL1* locus (11q13).

Prolymphocytic leukemia (PLL)

PLL is an uncommon neoplasm that presents abruptly with a very high white count >100,000/µL, B symptoms, cytopenias, and splenomegaly. By WHO criteria, there are >55% prolymphocytes, defined as lymphoid cells with prominent nucleoli and a moderate quantity of slightly eccentric cytoplasm. Morphologically, PLL is similar to and must be distinguished from MZL, HCL, and blastoid MCL. The immunophenotype differs from SLL/CLL with >80% of cases negative for CD5 and CD23, most cases expressing bright CD11c, bright sIg, bright CD20, CD22, and FMC-7 t4.27. There are no consistent molecular findings, but molecular and cytogenetic studies are useful to exclude MCL.

t4.27 Immunophenotype of mature B cell neoplasms composed of small lymphocytes

	CD19	CD20	CD79a	CD5	CD23	FMC-7	CD11c	CD25	CD10	sIg
CLL	+++	+	–/+	+	+	–	±	–	–	±
PLL	+++	+++	+	–	–	+	–	–	–	+++
MCL	+++	+++	+	+	–	+	–	–	–	++
FL	++/±	+++	+	–	+	+	–	–	+	+++
MZL/SLVL	+++	+++	+	–	–	+	+	–/+	–	+++
HCL	+++	+++	+	–	–	+	+++	++	–	+++

CLL = chronic lymphocytic leukemia, PLL = prolymphocytic leukemia, MCL = mantle cell lymphoma, FL = follicular lymphoma, MZL/SLVL = marginal zone lymphoma/splenic lymphoma with villous lymphocytes, HCL = hairy cell leukemia

Lymphoplasmacytic lymphoma (LPL)/Waldenström macroglobulinemia

LPL must be distinguished from other B cell neoplasms that have plasmacytoid differentiation or a bona fide plasmacytic component, including SLL/CLL, MCL, and marginal zone cell lymphoma. Essentially, the term LPL should be applied only to cases lacking features of these other lymphomas. LPL displays a spectrum of cellular morphology, from small lymphoid cells to fully developed plasma cells. Individual cases may be dominated by cells anywhere in this spectrum. Dutcher bodies can be found in the plasmacytic component (a monoclonal protein is usually present). Lymph node architecture may be preserved (LPL present in interfollicular spaces and sinuses) or effaced. PAS+ material may be found in sinuses (and Dutcher bodies are PAS+). Proliferation centers (SLL) and monocytoid B cells (MZL) are absent. In the marrow, an infiltrate of mast cells often accompanies LPL (similar finding in HCL). Waldenström macroglobulinemia is LPL with an IgM monoclonal gammopathy and marrow involvement. Some cases are found in association with hepatitis C and cryoglobulinemia; these respond to antiviral therapy. Immunophenotypically, the neoplastic cells are positive for CD19, CD20, CD38, Sig (bright), and cIg (plasma cells). CD5, CD23, CD43, and CD10 are negative or dim.

A recently described t(9;14)(p13;q32), involving the *PAX5* gene, appears to be a reproducible finding in LPL. *PAX5* encodes a B cell-specific transcription factor that is involved in the control of B cell differentiation (eg, into plasma cells). While the chromosome 14 breakpoint involved in *BCL1* and *BCL2* rearrangement is usually within the JH sequence, the *PAX5* rearrangement involves the C region of the IgH gene. Southern blot analysis, PCR, or FISH may be used to detect *PAX5* rearrangements.

Heavy chain disease

Heavy chain disease is a rare lymphoproliferative disorder productive of immunoglobulin heavy (H) chains only. The most common form is α H chain disease. α H chain disease is seen in association with immunoproliferative small intestine disease (IPSID), also known as Mediterranean lymphoma, a type of MALT lymphoma that is thought to be stimulated by infection with *Campylobacter jejuni*. Less common are γ heavy chain disease, found in some cases of lymphoplasmacytic lymphoma (LPL), and μ heavy chain disease found in some cases of CLL. In 1/3 of patients with γ heavy chain disease, also called Franklin H chain disease, there is a history of rheumatoid arthritis.

Diffuse large B cell lymphoma (DLBCL)

DLBCL, NOS is the term applied to large B cell lymphomas that do not conform to any of the several well defined clinicopathologic entities discussed below. DLBCL, NOS accounts for around 30% of all non-Hodgkin lymphomas. Clinically, it presents as a rapidly enlarging lymph node or extranodal (most often gastrointestinal) site. DLBCL tends to be localized at the time of presentation, with bone marrow involvement at the time of diagnosis being uncommon (10%). About a third of patients have "B" symptoms, and about half have an elevated LD at presentation.

Morphologically f4.50, DLBCL presents with diffuse nodal effacement by predominantly large cells (larger than a macrophage nucleus). The large cells are often "centroblastic," with vesicular nuclei having one or more nucleoli and basophilic cytoplasm. Some cases have immunoblastic cytology, with prominent single nucleoli. Others resemble anaplastic large cell lymphoma. Some DLBCL closely resembles Burkitt

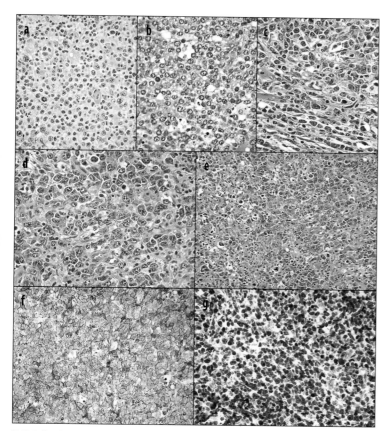

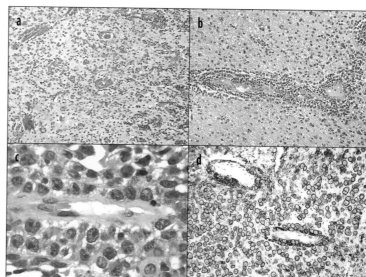

f4.51 Primary CNS lymphoma
a & b Note the tight perivascular nature of the proliferation
c At high magnification, note that the cells are large lymphocytes, in contrast to encephalitis, in which predominantly small lymphocytes are seen
d Strong CD20 expression

f4.50 Diffuse large B cell lymphoma (DLBCL)
a-e A variety of morphologic expressions of DLBCL
f Typical CD20 reaction
g Nuclear expression of Ki67; typically 30-95% of the cells express Ki67, in contrast to lower rates of expression in indolent lymphomas & higher rates of expression in Burkitt lymphoma

lymphoma and has features intermediate between the 2 (discussed below under the heading of "Burkitt lymphoma").

Immunophenotypically, the neoplastic cells are positive for CD19, CD20, CD22, and CD45. They are usually positive for bcl-2, with variable expression of CD10, CD5, and bcl-6. CD5–expressing cases must be distinguished from blastoid MCL by evaluating for bcl-1 overexpression or CCND1 rearrangement.

At the molecular level, BCL2 or BCL6 rearrangements are present in 20-30% of cases. The BCL6 gene is located on chromosome 3(q27), and it rearranges with a wide variety of partners, a common example being t(3;14)(q27;q32), joining BCL6 with the IgH locus. bcl-6 protein is overexpressed in FL, a large number of DLBCL, and Burkitt lymphoma/leukemia, but structural BCL6 rearrangements are found in only 10% of FL and 30% of DLBCL.

The prognosis is difficult to predict. Overall, DLBCL responds well to chemotherapy, with complete response in around 80% of patients and long term disease-free survival nearly 50%. However, there is great variability in clinical course, and morphologic findings correlate poorly with prognosis. The distinction of germinal center B cell-like (GCB) and activated B cell-like (ABC) phenotypes has shown initial promise in prognostication, with GCB-like DLBCL having better response to treatment. The GCB vs ABC distinction arose out of gene expression profiling (GEP) studies in which it was found that most large B cell lymphomas had resemblance

to either GCB cells or cells mitogenically activated in vitro (ABC). GEP is not widely available, however, and more widely available surrogate markers have been used to assist in making this distinction t4.28. Generally speaking, expression of CD10 and BCL6 correlates with the more favorable GCB phenotype, while expression of MUM1 and CD138 correlates with the ABC phenotype. Morphologically, GCB DLBCL is more likely to have centroblast-predominant morphology, while ABC often has immunoblast-predominant morphology. The BCL2, t(14;18), rearrangement is common in the GCB type, while rearrangement of BCL6, t(3;X), is more common in the ABC type.

t4.28 Stepwise evaluation of DLBCL subtypes by immunohistochemistry (Hans method)

Step	Marker(s)	Interpretation
1	CD10	If CD10+ in >30% of cells, then GCB
		If CD10–, proceed to step 2
2	BCL6	If BCL6–, then non-GC (ABC)
		If BCL6+, proceed to step 3
3	MUM1	If MUM1+, then non-GC (ABC)
		If MUM1–, then GCB

DLBCL subtypes by immunohistochemistry

CD10	BCL6	MUM1	Phenotype
+	+	–	GCB
+	–	–	GCB
–	+	–	GCB
–	+	+	Non-GC (ABC)
–	–	+	Non-GC (ABC)

Distinct clinicopathologic types of DLBCL

Primary DLBCL of the CNS f4.51 is defined by the 2008 WHO to specifically exclude those associated with HIV infection. With HIV associated cases excluded, the median age is ~60

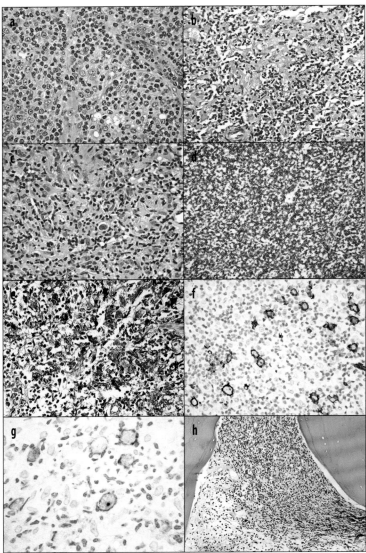

f4.52 T/histiocyte rich B cell lymphoma (TCRBCL)
a proliferation consisting of small lymphocytes (T cells) & large lymphocytes with prominent nucleoli
(B cells)
b & c Prominent eosinophilia in the background is due to histiocytes
d Reaction with CD3 highlighting background cells
e CD68, also highlighting background cells
f & g CD20 & CD10 reactions, respectively, in the large cells
h Marrow involvement with TCRBCL, typically paratrabecular as seen also in FL

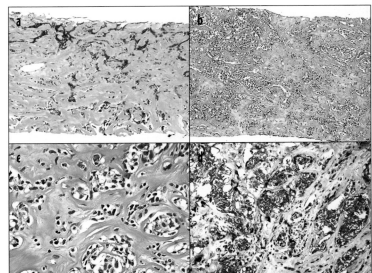

f4.53 Primary mediastinal lymphoma
a-c Densely sclerotic stroma surrounds compressed groups of large B cells
d CD20 reaction

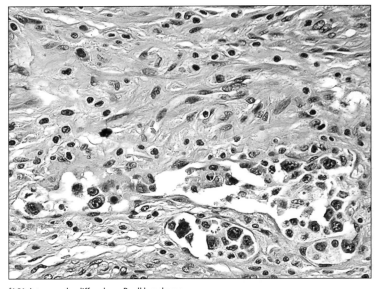

f4.54 Intravascular diffuse large B cell lymphoma

years. Primary DLBCL of the CNS presents as a supratentorial mass, within the frontal, temporal, or parietal lobes. Usually it produces a solitary lesion with radiographic features that mimic glioblastoma multiforme (GBM), including a tendency to spread along white matter tracts and cross the midline. Primary DLBCL of the CNS may present or recur as intraocular lymphoma. Histologically, the neoplastic cells are typically found in perivascular cuffs and express pan-B cell antigens. A large number of cases demonstrate a *BCL6* rearrangement and overexpress bcl-6, but *BCL2* rearrangement is rare.

T cell/histiocyte rich large B cell lymphoma (TCRBCL) presents at a mean age 40 years, but age at presentation ranges from childhood to old age. Morphologically, TCRBCL has a distinct appearance, consisting of a diffuse proliferation of small lymphocytes and clusters of pink histiocytes within which scattered large (neoplastic) B cells can be found f4.52. The pattern

may be mistaken for Hodgkin lymphoma (HL), especially the lymphocyte rich variant or classic HL or nodular lymphocyte predominant HL. The small lymphocytes are a mixture of CD4+ and CD8+ T cells. In contrast to the similar HL variants, CD57+ T cells are absent, T cell rosettes are absent, small B cells are essentially absent, and there is no CD21+/CD23+ follicular dendritic cell meshwork. The large B cells express pan-B markers in addition to bcl-6; some express bcl-2 and EMA, but they are negative for CD15, CD30, and EBV. Like follicular lymphoma, TCRBCL involves the marrow as paratrabecular lymphoid aggregates f4.53.

Primary mediastinal (thymic) large B cell lymphoma most commonly affects young adult females, with a male:female ratio of 1:2. It is a sclerosing process that may diffusely infiltrate the mediastinum and usually remains confined to the mediastinum. Morphologically, large centroblast-like B cells are entrapped within bands of sclerosis f4.54. Sclerosis may cause the cells to resemble small lymphocytes, appear epithelial, or become obscured entirely. The histologic differential diagnosis includes sclerosing mediastinitis, thymoma, carcinoma, and Hodgkin lymphoma. The neoplastic cells are positive for CD45, CD19, CD20, CD79a, and CD30. They are negative for surface immunoglobulin, CD10 and CD5. Primary mediastinal large B cell lymphoma harbors alterations in the *MAL* gene, gains in 9p (the location of *JAK2*), and lacks rearrangement of *BCL2* and *BCL6*.

ALK+ large B cell lymphoma is a rare tumor composed of immunoblastic/plasmablastic cells that express ALK. CD30 is negative t4.29.

Plasmablastic lymphoma is a rare tumor composed of large B cells that may have immunoblastic or plasmablastic t4.29 morphology and have the immunophenotype of plasma cells. The neoplastic cells are CD38+, CD138+, IRF4/MUM1+, cIg+, CD45−, CD20−, and EBV+. CD56 is usually negative, in contrast to plasmacytoma. Plasmablastic lymphoma is seen in HIV+ adults and arises mostly in extranodal sites such as the mucosa of the oral cavity.

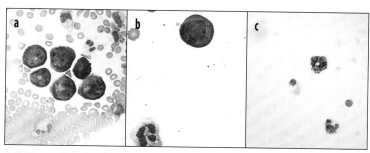

f4.55 Primary effusion lymphoma (PEL)
a & b Markedly atypical lymphoid cells with somewhat plasmacytoid morphology
c Nuclear expression of HHV-8

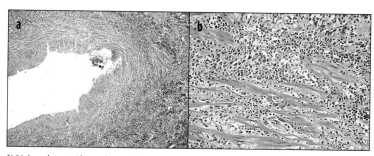

f4.56 Lymphomatoid granulomatosis
a At low magnification, the process resembles vasculitis
b At high magnification, the infiltrate is composed of large atypical B lymphocytes

t4.29 B cell neoplasms with plasmablastic morphology

Neoplasm	Notes
Plasmablastic lymphoma	Extranodal, especially oral cavity
	HIV+, EBV+
	If arising from multicentric Castleman disease, HHV8+
Primary effusion lymphoma	Extranodal, pleural cavity
	HIV+, EBV+, HHV8+
ALK+ DLBCL	Nodal
	Not associated with HIV or EBV
PTLD	Polymorphous PTLD
	EBV+
Plasmacytoma, anaplastic	Medullary
	Not associated with HIV or EBV

Intravascular large B cell lymphoma f4.55 has over the years been called "angioendotheliomatosis," "angiotropic lymphoma," and "intravascular lymphomatosis." Its symptoms are related to small-vessel obstruction by large B cells. Lymph node involvement is rare, and the tumor is often diagnosed in skin biopsies.

Primary effusion lymphoma (PEL) is strongly associated with HHV-8 (the same virus that has been implicated in Kaposi sarcoma and multicentric Castleman disease) and was initially recognized in patients with advanced AIDS. PEL presents with effusions (pleural, pericardial, peritoneal) containing large atypical B lymphocytes with immunoblastic, plasmablastic, or anaplastic morphology and cytoplasmic vacuolization f4.56. Cases of PEL have now been reported with primary soft tissue and lymph node presentations. PEL has an unusual immunophenotype, lacking expression of typical B cell, T cell, and myeloid antigens (CD20, CD79, CD19, CD10, CD3, CD5, CD13, CD14, CD33) and positive for CD45, CD30, CD38, CD138, and EMA. HHV-8 can be displayed in all cases by immunohistochemistry or molecular studies.

Leg-type primary cutaneous DLBCL affects predominantly elderly women, 90% of cases being found on the lower extremity. Morphologically, it presents a deep seated (nonepidermotropic) infiltrate of large B cells which express pan-B markers in addition to bcl-2 (note that primary cutaneous FL is bcl-2−) and bcl-6; CD10 is negative.

EBV+ DLBCL of the elderly is a neoplasm that affects elderly adults, usually in extranodal sites, that is most common in Asian populations. By definition, patients are over the age of 50, and this neoplasm is thought to be related to immune system senescence. EBV+ large B cell neoplasms are listed in t4.30.

t4.30 EBV+ large B cell neoplasms

Neoplasm	Notes
Plasmablastic lymphoma	Often seen in HIV infection; usually extranodal
Primary effusion lymphoma	Co-infection with HHV-8; usually seen in immunodeficiency
Lymphomatoid granulomatosis	Usually extranodal (lung, skin, brain)
DLBCL associated with chronic inflammation	Classically arising in longstanding pyothorax
EBV+ DLBCL of the elderly	Usually extranodal; by definition >50 years old
EBV+ DLBCL, NOS	Usually arises in immunodeficiency; if no immunodeficiency, by definition under age of 50 years

Lymphomatoid granulomatosis (LG) is a neoplasm composed of cells that destructively invade vessel walls in a pattern resembling primary vasculitis f4.56. The neoplastic B cells are often obscured by large numbers of reactive T cells, in addition to plasma cells and histiocytes. Granulomas are actually very uncommon. LG most commonly affects the lungs, where it presents as one or several tumors, but may involve the upper aerodigestive tract, brain, kidneys, and liver. It is associated with both EBV and immunodeficiency. It must be distinguished from nasal-type T/NK cell angiocentric lymphoma.

DLBCL associated with chronic inflammation is a high grade B cell lymphoma that arises at sites of longstanding inflammation. The prototype is lymphoma arising within a longstanding pyothorax. The neoplastic cells express EBV.

Immunodeficiency associated lymphoproliferative disorders

Lymphoproliferative disorders (LPD) arising in primary immunodeficiency (PID) are treated as a distinct group in the 2008 WHO classification. The PIDs manifest an increased risk of malignancy, especially lymphoma, and diagnosis of lymphoma in PID is often made with great difficulty, since many of them are associated with impressive benign lymphoid proliferation; furthermore, in most of these there is an anomalous response to EBV infection that may either mimic neoplasm or actually become neoplastic. The most common PIDs in which LPD develops are ataxia-telangiectasia (AT), Wiskott-Aldrich syndrome (WAS), common variable immunodeficiency (CVI), X-linked lymphoproliferative disorder (Duncan disease), and Nijmegen chromosomal breakage syndrome. The most common lymphoproliferative disorders to arise in PID are DLBCL, LG, and T cell neoplasms.

The most common lymphomas in HIV infection are Burkitt lymphoma, DLBCL (especially in the CNS), primary effusion lymphoma (PEL), plasmablastic lymphoma, and HL.

Posttransplant lymphoproliferative disorder (PTLD) is an abnormal lymphoid proliferation that arises following transplantation, usually within the first posttransplant year. EBV has been implicated in most cases of PTLD, especially in early posttransplant cases. Several studies suggest that an elevated EBV-DNA viral load is predictive of an emerging PTLD. Late (>5 years) posttransplant lymphomas tend to be EBV negative and more aggressive. The likelihood of PTLD depends partly upon the type of allograft, with renal and bone marrow transplant recipients having the lowest incidence and heart-lung and liver-bowel recipients have the highest incidence. Risk further depends upon recipient age (children are most at risk), recipient pretransplant EBV status (EBV negative at higher risk), and degree of immunosuppression (most suppressed at greatest risk). Most PTLD clones are of recipient origin; <10% are of donor origin. PTLD often involves the allograft itself. There is a spectrum of B lymphoproliferative lesions, including reactive plasmacytosis, infectious mononucleosis-like proliferations, polymorphous (lymphocytes, immunoblasts, plasma cells) proliferations, and monomorphous PTLD. Most monomorphous PTLDs take the form of a conventional high grade B cell lymphoma. A smaller number of T cell lymphomas and Hodgkin lymphomas occur in this setting.

Burkitt lymphoma/leukemia (BL)

Highly aggressive treatment regimens are usually restricted to patients with highly aggressive lymphomas, including BL and T or B lymphoblastic lymphoma/leukemia. Treatment involves highly intensive combination chemotherapy regimens, which can be curative. Some treat so-called Burkitt-like lymphoma similarly. 3 clinicopathologic types of Burkitt lymphoma are recognized. African (endemic) BL often presents as a jaw mass in childhood and is strongly associated with EBV. Western (sporadic) BL presents in nodal or extranodal sites, often intraabdominal, and is not strongly associated with EBV.

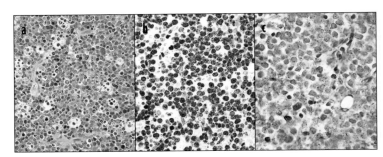

f4.57 Burkitt lymphoma (BL)
a Lymph node is diffusely effaced by a proliferation of large lymphoid cells with numerous tingible body macrophages & a high rate of both mitosis & apoptosis
b Neoplastic cells express Ki67 in nearly 100% of nuclei
c Neoplastic cells are BCL2−

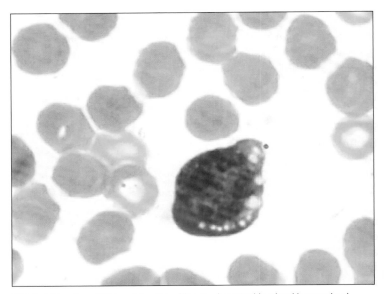

f4.58 Burkit lymphoma (BL) in peripheral blood (& in touch imprints) has deep blue vacuolated cytoplasm

It affects children and young adults. Lastly, Burkitt-like lymphoma most often presents nodally; many cases of Burkitt-like lymphoma arise in immunocompromised hosts, and these are classified under "immunodeficiency associated lymphoproliferative disorders."

In tissue, BL presents as a diffuse proliferation of monomorphic cells with a distinct rim of basophilic cytoplasm and medium-sized (about the size of a tissue macrophage nucleus) round nuclei having 2-5 nucleoli. Numerous tingible-body macrophages are scattered throughout, and there is a high rate of both mitosis and apoptosis, imparting the classic starry sky appearance f4.57. In peripheral blood or cytologic preparations, the cells are notable for deep blue cytoplasm (Wright stains) with lipid-containing vacuoles f4.58. This characteristic morphology is not specific for BL, however, and may be found in DLBCL, plasmablastic lymphoma, and lymphoblastic lymphoma. Thus, a combination of morphology and immunophenotyping is required to make the diagnosis, and in difficult cases molecular testing is required.

Immunophenotypically, the cells of BL are positive for CD19, CD20, CD22, CD10, bcl-6, sIg (light chain restricted), and c-myc. They are negative for CD5, CD23, Tdt, and CD34. PCNA

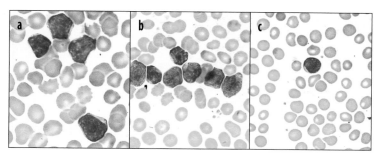

f4.59 Acute lymphoblastic leukemia (ALL)
a & b Large B lymphoblasts with relatively sparse agranular cytoplasm
c T lymphoblasts which are morphologically identical to B lymphoblasts

(Ki67) is positive in >99% of cells by immunohistochemistry. In contrast to DLBCL, BL is positive for c-myc, negative for bcl-2, and has a Ki-67 score of >99%. On the contrary, BL is extremely unlikely if CD10–, bcl-6–, bcl-2+, or if either the *BCL2* or *BCL6* rearrangement is present. In contrast to lymphoblastic lymphoma/leukemia, BL is TdT negative and sIg positive. There are exceptions; the classic BL phenotype was observed in only 89% of 34 cases recently studied. In the variant cases, findings included the absence of sIg by flow cytometry and, in some cases, absence of CD20. These findings would make the distinction from B-lymphoblastic lymphoma/leukemia very difficult and require molecular confirmation.

At the molecular level, BL is characterized by rearrangements involving the *CMYC* gene on chromosome 8. Most commonly, the *CMYC* gene is translocated to the IgH locus as a result of t(8;14); however, in many cases it is rearranged with Igκ (2p12) or Igλ (22q11). The result of these rearrangements is c-myc protein overexpression. c-myc and its partner protein—Max—combine to activate a number of genes involved in driving the cell into the cell cycle.

Lymphoblastic leukemia & lymphoma (ALL/LBL)

General features

The 2008 WHO classification recognizes these 3 categories: B acute lymphoblastic leukemia/lymphoblastic lymphoma not otherwise specified, B acute lymphoblastic leukemia/lymphoblastic lymphoma with recurrent cytogenetic abnormalities, and T-ALL/LBL. By convention, lesions involving tissue and sparing the peripheral blood and bone marrow are termed lymphoblastic lymphoma (LBL); lesions heavily involving the marrow (>25% blasts) and peripheral blood (>20%), regardless of tissue involvement, are considered acute lymphoblastic leukemia (ALL).

B lineage neoplasms represent ~80% of ALL, but only 20% of LBL. Conversely, T lineage neoplasms represent ~20% of ALL, and 80% of LBL. ALL is the most common malignancy of children, in whom ALL is significantly more common than AML; in adulthood the converse is true. ALL peaks in incidence at ~3 years of age. Risk factors include Down syndrome, Fanconi anemia, Li-Fraumeni syndrome, Ataxia-telangiectasia, Bloom syndrome, and other chromosomal breakage syndromes.

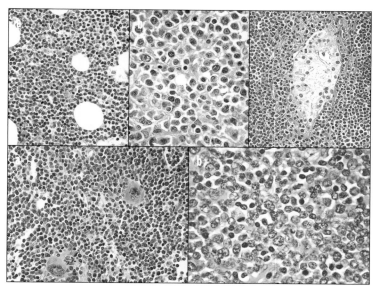

f4.60 Lymphoblastic lymphoma (LBL); B-LBL in a-b lymph nodes, presenting as a diffuse proliferation of large lymphoid cells; lymphoblastic neoplasms may localize to the c testis, d bone marrow or brain. e T-LBL is morphologically similar

T-LBL typically presents as an anterior mediastinal mass and may be associated with hypercalcemia, while B-LBL involves lymph nodes, CNS, liver, spleen, and testes but is uncommon in the mediastinum. ALL usually presents with manifestations of cytopenias—fatigue, bleeding (petechiae), and infection. Hepatosplenomegaly is present in ~2/3 of patients. Bone pain (resulting from rapid intramedullary growth) is a common presenting complaint. Extramedullary sites—especially the central nervous system and testes—are a common source of disease relapse.

Morphologically, ALL/LBL presents as a monotonous proliferation of undifferentiated blasts f4.59-f4.60. Initially, the morphologic differential diagnosis includes undifferentiated varieties of AML (M0, M1, M2). In tissue, T-LBL is sometimes associated with an infiltrate of eosinophils. Cytochemically, lymphoblasts are negative for MPO and SBB. They have PAS positivity in a block-like or coarse granular pattern.

Precursor B-ALL/LBL, NOS

Immunophenotypically, the neoplastic cells are usually positive for CD19, CD10, *PAX5*, CD34, CD99, HLA-DR, and nuclear Tdt t4.31.

t4.31 Immunophenotypes in ALL/LBL & BL

	Tdt	HLA-DR	CD19	CD20	CD10	sIg	CD7
Precursor B	+	+	+	–/+	+/–	–	–
Burkitt	–	+	+	+	+	+	–
Precursor T	+	–	–	–	–	–	+

CD19 is the earliest B-lineage specific antigen; while CD19 may be dim, lack of CD19 essentially excludes B lineage ALL. CD19 expression is not uncommon in AML, however, where it is typically dimly expressed. CD20 is usually negative, as is sIg. CD45 may be dim and sometimes absent. CD10 is more often expressed in childhood ALL than adult ALL, and absence of CD10 suggests the possibility of an *MLL* gene anomaly. Immunophenotypic aberrancy is found in virtually all cases, a feature that is useful for diagnosis, for detection of minimal residual disease, and for distinction of residual ALL from hematogone rich populations. Between 30 and 50% of cases express at least one myeloid antigen, usually CD13 or CD33, usually dimly. Some cases express NK antigens. Amongst B cell antigens, anomalies are found in the form of underexpression (of CD45, for example) or dyssynchronous expression (coexpression of CD34 and CD20 or of CD10 and CD22, for example).

Without chemotherapy, B-ALL/LBL is uniformly fatal. With therapy, B-ALL/LBL has a good prognosis in children (CR in >95%) and fair prognosis in adults (CR in ~80%). Cure is achieved in 80% of children and 50% of adults. The major prognostic factors are initial white count, age, gender, and initial response to therapy. Initial leukocyte count is inversely related to prognosis. With regard to patient age, the best outcomes are observed in those diagnosed between the ages of 2 and 10 years. Infants have a high incidence of anomalies within band 11q23 [eg, t(4;11)] which may account for the adverse prognosis in this age group. Females have a better outcome than males. Lastly, failure to achieve complete remission (usually assessed in the day 14 marrow) following induction chemotherapy is an adverse prognostic sign. Hypodiploidy (<46 chromosomes) is associated with a relatively poor prognosis, and the prognosis worsens the fewer the chromosomes. Cases with 45 chromosomes comprise the largest share in this group. Cases having 33-44 chromosomes are rare but have a poorer overall outcome than those with 45, and cases with so-called near-haploidy (23-29 chromosomes) are rarer and gloomier still, with a median survival of <1 year.

Posttreatment marrows pose the difficulty of distinguishing hematogone rich recovering marrow from residual ALL. Even untreated marrows of pediatric patients can present this difficulty, particularly if they are undergoing recovery from aplastic anemia. A combination of flow cytometric and immunohistochemical immunophenotyping can aid in this distinction. In regard to flow cytometry, hematogone rich populations present a spectrum (noticeable spectrum of strength of CD10 expression, for example); whereas ALL is characterized by a distinct immature population (a tight cluster of cells expressing a uniform strength of CD10, for example). Hematogone rich populations consist of very immature (CD34+, TDT+), maturing (CD10+, CD19+), and mature (CD20+, sIg+) cells; importantly, mature cells represent a major component of the overall lymphoid population. ALL consists of an isolated population of immature cells, predominating over any mature cells in the sample. The authors of a study comparing the 2 types of marrows attempted to objectify these findings as follows: hematogone rich populations tend to have

1. >25% of CD20+ (mature) cells

2. >20% of sIg+ (mature) cells

3. <20% of TdT+ (immature) cells

4. CD20+ cells outnumber CD34+ cells

In regard to immunohistochemistry, hematogone rich populations are dispersed. That is, immunohistochemical stains for CD34 or TdT do not show clusters of >5 positive cells.

Common molecular findings include abnormalities of 6q, 9p, and 12p, all of which are unrelated to prognosis. By definition, none of the recurrent genetic abnormalities described below may be present in B-ALL/LBL, NOS.

B-ALL/LBL with recurrent genetic abnormalities t4.32

The most common structural abnormality in B-ALL/LBL is t(9;22)(q34;q11), the BCR/ABL translocation, a distinctly unfavorable finding. At the cytogenetic level, the t(9;22) of ALL appears identical to that of CML; however, the translocations differ. The major breakpoint (M-bcr) rearrangement, resulting in a chimeric protein of 210 kD, is common in CML. The minor breakpoint (m-bcr) rearrangement results in a chimeric protein of 190 kD and is common in ALL. PCR and FISH are capable of distinguishing these rearrangements.

t4.32 B-ALL/LBL with recurrent genetic abnormalities

Abnormality	Genetics	Age group	Prognosis	Morphology	Immuno-phenotype
t(9;22) (q34;q11.2)	BCR/ABL1	25% of adults 3% of children	Poor	Usual	CD19+, CD10+, Tdt+, CD34+ CD13/33+ (weak), CD25+
t(v;11q23), usually t(4;11)	MLL	Infants	Poor	Usual	CD19+, CD10−, CD15+ Overexpress FLT3
t(12;21) (p13;q22)	TEL-AML1 (ETV6-RUNX1)	25% of children	Good	Usual	CD19+, CD10+, CD9− CD13/33+ (weak)
Hyperdiploid	>50; extra copies esp of 21, 4, 14, X	25% of children	Good	Usual	CD19+, CD10+, Tdt+, CD34+
Hypodiploid	<46	<5% of children & adults	Poor	Usual	CD19+, CD10+, Tdt+, CD34+
t(1;19) (q23;p13.3)	E2A-PBX1 (TCF3-PBX1)	5% of children	Poor	Usual	CD19+, CD10+, CD34−
t(5;14) (q31;q32)	IL3-IGH	<1% of children & adults	Usual	Eosinophilia	CD19+, CD10+, Tdt+, CD34+

T-ALL

T-ALL most commonly presents in adolescence. Immunophenotypically, the neoplastic cells are positive for CD99, CD7, CD2, CD5, CD3 (cytoplasmic), and TdT (nuclear). CD34 is variable, and HLA-DR is usually negative. CD4 & CD8 are often both positive or both negative. Some cases express CD13 and/or CD33. TCR genes are rearranged in nearly all cases, and 10-20% have IgH rearrangements.

Difficulty may be encountered in anterior mediastinal tumors, where both T-ALL and thymoma commonly present. Thymic T cells are often quite numerous in thymoma, so much so that they often obscure the thymic epithelial nature of the tumor. Furthermore, thymic T cells may have distinctly unusual immunophenotypic features that can lead to misdiagnosis as T cell lymphoma. In particular, the majority of thymic T cells coexpress CD4 and CD8. The most important finding in this distinction is the finding of obscured epithelial cells in thymomas when stained by immunohistochemistry with epithelial markers such as EMA. When studied by flow cytometry, plots of CD4 vs CD8 show a dark cluster of CD4+/CD8+ thymic T cells, with thinner "tail" clusters of CD4+/CD8− and CD4−/CD8+ T cells. Likewise, CD45 vs CD3 shows a spectrum of immature to mature cells. In contrast, T-ALL that coexpresses CD4 and CD8 demonstrates a pure population of such cells, without tails on the plot of CD4 vs CD8, and without a spectrum on the plot of CD45 vs CD3.

A unique clinicopathologic form of T-ALL consists of coexistent chronic eosinophilic leukemia and T-lymphoblastic lymphoma (8p11-12 stem cell syndrome). While reactive hyper-eosinophilia is common in T cell malignancies, hyper-eosinophilia associated with the *FGFR1* (fibroblast growth factor receptor-1) gene at 8p11-12 is a distinct entity that presents as coexistent myeloid and lymphoid neoplasms. The latter most often take the form of a T-ALL. This disorder has been called the 8p11-12 stem cell syndrome and is a rare but aggressive neoplasm. The diagnosis requires demonstration of the same translocation breakpoint at 8p11-12 in both myeloid and lymphoid cells.

Acute leukemia with mixed lineage

It is common for unilineage acute leukemia to express a mixture of lymphoid and myeloid antigens. In such cases, classification may be somewhat challenging, and one must consider the lineage specificity of each positive marker as well as its strength of expression. For example, CD13 and CD33 are relatively nonspecific antigens and may be seen in many cases of B- or T-ALL. On the other hand, CD117 is nearly 100% specific for AML. CD4, CD5, and CD7 are nonspecific lymphoid antigens that are expressed in 20-40% of AML. CD2 and CD3 are nearly 100% specific for T-ALL. Likewise, CD19 is present in 10-20% of AML, but CD79a and CD10 are nearly 100% specific for B-ALL.

Taking these considerations into account (scoring systems have been devised), most acute leukemias can be classified as one of the following:

1. myeloid antigen positive ALL, which behaves like ALL

2. lymphoid antigen positive AML, which behaves like AML

Rare cases cannot be classified as either of these. Mixed lineage acute leukemia is diagnosed when there is noncommittal morphology (M0, L1, L2), negative cytochemistry, and a roughly equal expression of myeloid and lymphoid antigens, both in number and intensity. Lastly, rare cases are categorized as biphenotypic acute leukemia, in which 2 distinct populations are identified, 1 myeloid and 1 lymphoid.

Plasma cell neoplasms

Plasma cell myeloma/multiple myeloma (MM)

Myeloma is a disease of older adults, with median age at onset of 70 years. Blacks are affected significantly more often than whites, males more than females, and there is familial clustering (3-4× increased risk in first-degree relatives).

The WHO 2008 classification recognizes 2 forms of myeloma: symptomatic and asymptomatic (smoldering). The clinical manifestations that define symptomatic myeloma fall into 4 categories denoted by the acronym CRAB t4.33. "C" refers to hypercalcemia, which may be quite severe, often initially presenting with altered mental status. "R" is for renal insufficiency, which may come about through a variety of mechanisms. "A" refers to anemia. Lastly, "B" refers to bone lesions, which may take the form of distinct lytic lesions or generalized osteoporosis.

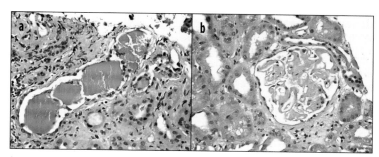

f4.61 a Myeloma cast nephropathy; b light chain deposition disease

t4.33 **Diagnostic criteria for multiple myeloma**

Symptomatic myeloma	Asymptomatic (smoldering) myeloma
M protein (any measurement)	M protein >3.0 g/dL (30 g/L)
&	or
Clonal plasma cells in marrow (any percentage) or plasmacytoma	Clonal plasma cells in marrow >10%
&	
Organ impairment (CRAB: high calcium, renal insufficiency, anemia, bone lesions)	

Renal manifestations are often found at presentation and are often in fact the presentation of myeloma. Both hypercalcemia and hyperuricemia can cause damage, which may be undetectable by light microscopy, to the proximal tubules. This may result in acquired renal Fanconi syndrome. The most common morphologic pattern of injury is AL amyloidosis, which is most commonly found in association with λ light chains. Amyloid is found in vessel walls and within glomeruli, predominantly within the mesangium. Once Congo Red or other stains confirm the presence of amyloid, immunohistochemistry for κ and λ light chains can confirm the diagnosis of AL amyloidosis. Light chain deposition disease, on the other hand, is more common with κ light chains. Most often, this presents morphologically in a pattern of nodular glomerulosclerosis, resembling diabetic glomerulosclerosis. κ and λ light chain immunohistochemistry can help to confirm the diagnosis. An easily overlooked pattern is that of myeloma cast nephropathy, the result of intratubular crystallization of M protein f4.61. Unlike the typical hyaline casts that one learns to overlook in renal biopsies, these are angulated and cracked, often found in association with adherent epithelioid histiocytes. Again, κ/λ immunohistochemistry can be confirmatory.

Several additional manifestations are not considered amongst the diagnostic criteria. Many patients suffer from a bleeding diathesis, caused by interference with coagulation factors and/or thrombocytopenia (amyloidosis, if present, may lower factor X). Hyperviscosity syndrome may arise, depending upon the immunoglobulin isotype (IgM, IgA, and IgG3 paraproteins are most often associated with hyperviscosity). Amyloidosis (AL type), with its widespread manifestations, develops in 10-30% of patients. Immunodeficiency, attributable to hypogammaglobulinemia, predisposes to infection with encapsulated organisms such as *S pneumoniae*.

A monoclonal immunoglobulin paraprotein is present in the vast majority of cases. The isotype (heavy chain) is most commonly IgG (55%), followed by IgA (22%), none—light chain only (18%), IgD (1-2%), biclonal (1-2%), and IgE (1-2%). IgM-producing myeloma is rare, and IgM paraproteinemia is much more commonly found in association with

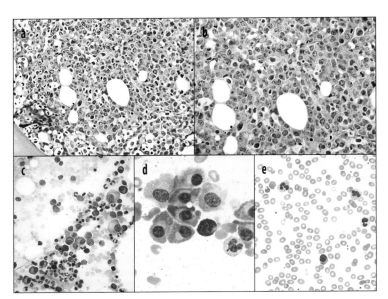

f4.62 Multiple myeloma in marrow; the tumor often forms sheets of cells ranging from a evidently plasmacytic to b poorly differentiated
c There is a spectrum from minimally atypical on the left to moderately atypical on the right
d Prominent paranuclear hoffs are evident
e A case of plasma cell leukemia in the peripheral blood

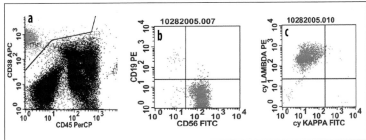

f4.63 Myeloma flow cytometry
a Gating around cells with bright CD38 & dim to absent CD45, typical of the plasma cell gate
b Plot of CD56 vs CD19, in which the neoplastic cells have characteristic dim to absent CD19 but express CD56
c Cytoplasmic λ light chain restriction

lymphoid neoplasms, especially lymphoplasmacytic lymphoma (Waldenström), chronic lymphocytic leukemia/small lymphocytic lymphoma, and marginal zone lymphoma. The idiotype (light chain) is most commonly κ; interestingly, IgD myelomas are associated with λ in 90% of cases. Nonsecretory myeloma is found in ~5% of cases; the plasma cells often contain stainable immunoglobulin (85%); in others (15%) the plasma cells are truly nonproducing. There are no prognostic differences in nonsecretory myeloma. Many cases thought initially to be nonsecretory turn out to be light chain-only when urine is subjected to electrophoresis.

Initial laboratory detection of monoclonal proteins has traditionally required study of serum and urine, the latter to detect light chain-only producing myeloma. Often, urine is not provided for examination; thus, many advocate addition of a serum free light chain assay to conventional SPEP in the initial evaluation of patients suspected of having myeloma. The quantification of serum free light chains is more sensitive than SPEP for the detection of light chain-only disease, nonsecretory myeloma, and AL amyloidosis. It is actually somewhat less sensitive than SPEP in the detection of intact immunoglobulin-producing myeloma. Lastly, there is evidence for a significant role of serum free light chain measurement in the monitoring of myeloma.

Morphologically, the neoplastic cells range from typical to anaplastic f4.62. A variety of cytoplasmic changes have been described (Mott, flame, morula, Russell bodies, Gaucher-like), none of which are diagnostic of myeloma and all of which may be seen in reactive conditions. Rod shaped inclusions are rare but relatively specific for myeloma. Nuclear changes, including significant atypia, are also relatively specific for myeloma. In bone marrow biopsies, myeloma is often associated with clustering or sheeting of plasma cells; in the absence of these findings, there is often an alteration in the topography of plasma cells, with neoplastic cells being found away from arterioles, within the interstitium of the marrow.

Immunophenotypically f4.63, neoplastic plasma cells do not usually express CD45 or B cell antigens (CD19, CD20, CD21, CD22, sIg). Most neoplastic plasma cells express CD38, CD138, CD56, cytoplasmic κ or λ, and PCA-1. CD56 expression not only implies the neoplastic nature of a plasma cell population, but when present is suggestive of behavior that is more aggressive. Some cases are bcl-1+ (cyclin D1+), correlating with the presence of a t(11;14) translocation. 10-30% express myelomonocytic markers (CD117, CD13, CD33, CD11b, CD15). 10-50% express CALLA (CD10). Occasional cases express EMA and CD30. Notably, CD56 is often absent in plasmablastic lymphoma and plasma cell leukemia.

Mean survival is 3-5 years. Factors indicating a poorer prognosis include higher levels of β2 microglobulin, high plasma cell labeling index, which reflects the number of plasma cells in S-phase, and high stage. Chromosomal abnormalities are among the most important prognostic parameters. Plasma cells are difficult to culture for cytogenetics, so FISH studies are typically used. Over 80% of cases are found to have 4 or more chromosomal anomalies, the most common of which affect 14q32, 13q14, 19p, and 17p13.1. The most commonly abnormal locus in MM is 14q32 (IgH gene), and the most common rearrangement is t(11;14)(q13;q32) producing *CCND1*/IgH. Chromosome 14q32 translocations (IgH translocations) appear to be common early events and are found in >70% of myeloma and 50% of MGUS. Based upon FISH results, patients can be stratified into 3 distinct prognostic groups t4.34.

Complete remission in multiple myeloma has been defined as the disappearance of paraprotein from serum and urine (confirmed by immunofixation electrophoresis) and <5% plasma cells in the marrow. The status of the marrow has traditionally been assessed by morphology alone. This practice is somewhat complicated by the sometimes anomalous cytology of neoplastic plasma cells and the common presence of nonneoplastic plasma cells in the marrow. Furthermore, complete remission by these criteria is associated with almost universal recurrence of disease. Several additional modalities have been explored in regard to MRD testing for myeloma, the most sensitive of which appear to be immunohistochemistry or flow cytometry. Immunohistochemistry for CD138 (syndecan-1), when used in the appropriate context, is a specific marker for plasma cells (while expressed in a wide range of tissues and neoplasms, CD138 is not expressed by other hematopoietic cells). In one study, CD138 immunostaining combined with immunostains for κ and λ light chains provided the highest rate of MRD detection. However, the technique has certain limitations: not all biopsies are big enough to provide a useful immunohisto-chemical study, light chain immunohistochemistry is some-times of poor technical quality, and plasma cell quantitation is somewhat unreliable (the denominator is at most several hundred RBCs). Flow cytometry, using CD38 (bright) vs CD45 (dim to absent) expression gating, can be used to detect and quantify small populations of clonal plasma cells. Assessment of CD19, CD56 and cytoplasmic κ/λ expression can confirm the neoplastic nature of the gated plasma cells (benign reactive plasma cells are CD19+/CD56–/light chain unrestricted, while neoplastic plasma cells are usually CD19–/CD56+/light chain restricted). FISH can be applied to posttreatment marrow, espe-cially if a specific pretreatment anomaly is known. However, it appears to be less sensitive than immunohistochemistry and/or flow cytometry. PCR, for detection of IgH gene rearrangement, performs poorly in post-germinal center B cells (eg, follicular lymphomas, myelomas) due to somatic IgH hypermutation. A way around this is patient or clone-specific primers, but this is expensive and requires pretreatment PCR analysis. Lastly, it has been demonstrated that in patients with a previously char-acterized paraprotein, negative high-resolution serum or urine protein electrophoresis with immunofixation can obviate the need for bone marrow biopsy.

t4.34 Myeloma prognosis by FISH

Group	Findings
Shortest survival, median of 24 months	t(4;14), t(14;16), or 17p13.1 deletion
Intermediate survival, median 42 months	13q14 deletions alone
Longest survival, median of >50 months	No anomalies or only t(11;14)

Plasma cell leukemia (PCL)

PCL is defined as >20% or $>2.0 \times 10^9$/L plasma cells in the peripheral blood. Half of cases present de novo, and half develop in patients with established MM. PCL presents abruptly and follows an aggressive course, with mean survival <1 year. It is notable for a relatively high incidence of IgE, IgD, or light chain only paraprotein, high incidence of monosomy 13, and the plasma cells are often CD56–.

Solitary plasmacytoma (osseous & extraosseous)

Solitary osseous plasmacytoma (solitary plasmacytoma of bone) arises most commonly in the vertebrae, ribs, and pelvis. About half have a detectable M protein, and most (75%) develop MM within 10 years.

Solitary extraosseous (extramedullary) plasmacytoma arises most commonly in the nasal cavity, oropharynx or larynx. Most do not have a detectable M protein, and most do not develop MM.

Monoclonal gammopathy of unknown significance (MGUS)

MGUS t4.35 is a term applied to the very common scenario in which a patient is found to have a monoclonal gammopathy but lacks criteria for the other plasma cell neoplasms defined above (and lacks a B cell neoplasm capable of producing an M-spike). Patients with MGUS may have suppression of immunoglobulins, amyloidosis, and other complications. Chromosomal abnormalities are often detected with FISH.

t4.35 Diagnostic criteria for MGUS

Monoclonal gammopathy <3.0 g/dL (30 g/L)
<10% PCs in bone marrow
No CRAB (eg, normal Ca²⁺, normal renal function, no lytic bone lesions)
No B cell neoplasm

MGUS is found in 3% of adults over the age of 50 years and 5% of adults over the age of 70; 60% of patients with a known M protein are classified as MGUS. Several studies have asked the question: what is the significance of monoclonal gammopathy of unknown significance? Overall, these have demonstrated a ~0.5-1%/year risk of progression to multiple myeloma or another plasma cell neoplasm. In one study, ~1 in 3 patients had developed overt myeloma by 20 years after the detection of MGUS. In the most recent large study, that of the Dutch Comprehensive Cancer Centre, MGUS patients were found to have a higher rate of all-cause mortality than a matched control population, with albumin at presentation being strongly predictive of survival.

Osteosclerotic myeloma (POEMS syndrome)

POEMS is an acronym for a very rare syndrome consisting of polyneuropathy, organomegaly, endocrinopathy, M-protein, and skin changes. Affected individuals usually have a solitary intraosseous plasmacytoma with associated thickening of bony trabeculae (osteosclerotic myeloma). There appears to be a greater than chance association between POEMS syndrome, the plasma cell variant of Castleman disease, and HHV-8.

T cell neoplasms
General features

T cell neoplasms account for only ~5% of lymphoid neo-plasms overall. Incidence varies markedly with geography, being highest in Asia. This is attributed to the higher rate of HTLV-1 infection and a peculiar susceptibility to EBV asso-ciated lymphoid neoplasms in Asians. As an exception, enteropathy associated T cell lymphoma (EATCL) is strongly associated with Welsh and Irish ancestry. The most common T cell neoplasms, in decreasing order, are peripheral T cell lymphoma, not otherwise specified (PTCL, NOS), angioim-munoblastic T cell lymphoma (AITL), anaplastic large cell lymphoma (ALCL), and adult T cell lymphoma (ATCL).

The role of immunophenotyping in T cell neoplasms is 2-fold. First, if the proliferation is obviously neoplastic on morphologic grounds, then immunophenotyping is mainly performed to confirm T-lineage and further sub-classify the lymphoma, if possible. Second, if a reactive process is in the differential, then immunophenotyping may disclose antigenic aberrancies that help confirm a diagnosis of malignancy. Immunophenotypic aberrancies may include an unnaturally large preponderance of T cells over B cells, but this is among the softest of findings. A very large preponderance of CD4 over CD8 or CD8 over CD4 may further support the impres-sion of malignancy. Coexpression of CD4 and CD8 or lack of both CD4 and CD8 are very strong indicators of malignancy, as is the unequivocal loss of pan-T cell markers such as CD2, CD3, CD5 or CD7. T cell neoplasms positive for CD4 include cutaneous T cell lymphoma (CTCL)/Sézary syndrome, periph-eral T cell lymphoma (PTCL), adult T cell leukemia/lymphoma

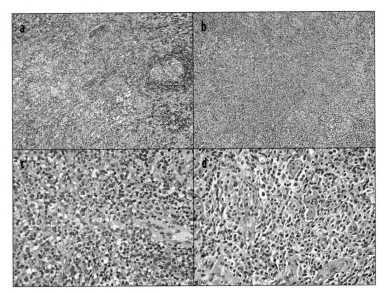

f4.64 Peripheral T cell lymphoma (PTCL)
a Low magnification image showing an interfollicular expansion, pushing atretic follicles apart; at this magnification, one can see prominence of high-endothelial venules & a distinctly mixed population, more evident in b
c & d At high magnification, there is a mixture of small & large lymphocytes, all of which are neoplastic; within the background, there is characteristically an admixture of histiocytes & eosinophils

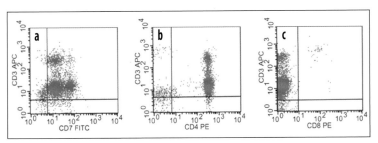

f4.65 PTCL flow cytometry
a Distinctly bimodal population of T cells, one with dim CD7 expression & a range of CD3 expression
b This population expresses purely CD4
c CD8 is not expressed

(ATCL), anaplastic large cell lymphoma (ALCL), angioimmunoblastic T cell lymphoma (AITCL), and CD4+,CD56+ hematodermic neoplasm. CD8+ T cell neoplasms include large granular lymphocytic leukemia (LGL), subcutaneous panniculitic T cell lymphoma, and hepatosplenic T cell lymphoma. Some PTCL and ATCL may be positive for both CD4 and CD8, and enteropathy associated T cell lymphoma (EATCL) is usually negative for both.

Peripheral T cell lymphoma (PTCL)

PTCL has the distinction of being the most common T cell lymphoma, largely because it is the designation given to T cell neoplasms that do not fit any of the defined clinicopathologic entities that follow. The PTCLs are predominantly nodal-based neoplasms, with wide-ranging morphology. In most cases, it appears as a diffuse proliferation of polymorphic small and large lymphoid cells, but either small cells or large cells may predominate. The neoplastic lymphocytes are distinctive for their multilobate (cloverleaf) nuclei. Admixed eosinophils, plasma cells, and/or histiocytes may be numerous, and post-capillary venules may be prominent, features that are common to many T cell neoplasms f4.64. Architectural variants include an interfollicular (T-zone) variant and a Lennert-like (lymphoepithelioid/lymphohistiocytic) variant. Immunophenotypically, PTCL is characteristically CD4+ and CD8– f4.65. It commonly demonstrates loss of one or several pan-T cell markers, and it is negative for CD25. There is no consistent structural chromosomal abnormality, but trisomy 3 is frequent in Lennert-like variants.

Adult T cell leukemia/lymphoma (ATCL)

ATCL is a peripheral T cell neoplasm caused by HTLV-1. HTLV-1 is endemic in southern Japan, parts of Oceania (Papua New Guinea, Solomon Islands, and Vanuatu), and parts of the Caribbean (Jamaica, Martinique, Guyana). HTLV-1 is rare in North America. In Southwest Japan, the incidence of HTLV-1 is nearly 10%. The lifetime risk of ATCL in HTLV-1+ persons is estimated to be around 5% (7% for infected males and 3% for females). There are several types of ATCL, including acute (55%), lymphomatous (20%), chronic (20%), and smoldering (5%). Regardless of type, most patients present with lymphadenopathy and hepatosplenomegaly, with or without visceral involvement (CNS, lungs, GI tract). Some patients manifest a skin rash, hypercalcemia (caused by elaboration of OAF [osteoclast activating factor]), and lytic bone lesions. The neoplastic lymphoid cells have pronounced nuclear irregularity, producing cloverleaf or flowerlike forms. Immunophenotypically, ATCL is positive for CD2, CD3, CD5, CD4, and CD25. It is usually CD7– and CD8–.

Angioimmunoblastic T cell lymphoma (AITL)

AITL is an EBV associated neoplasm that affects older adults. It presents abruptly with a unique syndrome that is dominated by constitutional symptoms including fever, night sweats, weight loss, and generalized lymphadenopathy. Pleural effusion is commonly present, and many patients manifest a Coombs+ autoimmune hemolytic anemia, pruritic skin rash, and cold agglutinins. Patients with AITL frequently develop anti-smooth muscle antibody, rheumatoid factor, and polyclonal hypergammaglobulinemia. The morphologic presentation consists of diffuse nodal effacement with a characteristic prominence of post-capillary venules, deposition of PAS+ extracellular material, and a mixed lymphoid infiltrate. Lymph nodes with early involvement may display hyperplastic follicles; later there is absence of apparent follicles. CD21 immunostaining displays hyperplastic follicular dendritic cells in areas infiltrated by neoplasm f4.66. The cytology presents a mixed population of immunoblasts, lymphocytes, plasma cells, and eosinophils. Aggregates of cells with clear cytoplasm are characteristic. Immunophenotypically, the neoplastic cells are positive for CD4 and most pan-T cell markers—CD2, CD3, CD5, CD7. They are negative for CD8, and display loss of 1 or several pan-T cell markers—CD2, CD3, CD5, CD7. They have the immunophenotypic features of follicular helper T cells—CD10+, bcl-6+, CXCL-13+. Despite the association with EBV, the neoplastic T cells are EBV– (EBV is present in B cells). At the molecular level, TCR is clonally rearranged in most cases. The most common karyotypic abnormalities are trisomy 3, trisomy 5, and duplication of the X chromosome.

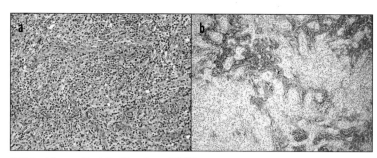

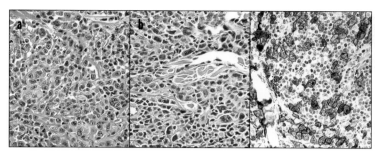

f4.66 Angioimmunoblastic T cell lymphoma (AILTCL)
a Low magnification image showing a diffuse proliferation amidst prominent high endothelial veins, of a mixed hematolymphoid population
b CD21 stain highlights the residual follicular dendritic cell meshwork

f4.67 Anaplastic large cell lymphoma (ALCL)
a & b Typical cytologic features, consisting of large lymphoid cells, some appearing epithelioid, with admixed "hallmark" cells
c ALK is expressed

Anaplastic large cell lymphoma (ALCL)

ALCL is most frequent in children and young adults. It is responsible for half of childhood high grade lymphomas and ~5% of adult high grade lymphomas. In the 2008 WHO classification, ALCL is formally divided into those that are Alk+ and those that are negative for Alk.

Most ALCLs have 4 things in common: nodal disease, anaplastic cytology, expression of CD30, and expression of Alk. There are many variations on this theme, however, including Alk– cases, leukemic presentations, extranodal presentations, and small cell variants that resemble PTCL. The bone marrow is involved in 10-30% of cases. The typical ALCL f4.67 presents with a diffuse nodal proliferation of lymphocytes, many having pleomorphic nuclei containing one or more nucleoli, and a variable number of anaplastic cells (multinucleated, horseshoe shaped, and Reed-Sternberg-like cells). When low in number, anaplastic cells can be found near blood vessels where they tend to cluster. They often grow in a cohesive-appearing manner and often involve lymph node sinuses; as such, they may be mistaken for a carcinoma or melanoma. The small cell variant is composed of large, but not anaplastic, lymphoid cells and may be mistaken for PTCL. In the leukemic cases, small cell cytology predominates. The vast majority of leukemic cases occur in children, and despite expressing Alk have a poor prognosis.

Prognosis depends heavily upon the expression of Alk. Cases that are Alk+ and arise in children have the best prognosis overall (so long as there is not a leukemic presentation). Alk– ALCL is a more aggressive disease (48% 5-year survival as contrasted to 80% in Alk+) and occurs mainly in adults. Alk– ALCL should be distinguished from PTCL, NOS, which carries a worse prognosis still. Widespread and uniform expression of CD30 is the most useful finding in this distinction. Clusterin and EMA expression also favor Alk– ALCL.

Immunophenotypically, nearly all cases are positive for CD30 (membranous and Golgi staining), Alk (nucleus, cytoplasm, or both), clusterin (Golgi pattern), EMA, CD45, at least one myeloid antigen (CD13 and/or CD33) and at least one T cell antigen. The most sensitive T cell antigens in ALCL are CD4, CD7, and CD2. CD3 is relatively insensitive and is more commonly expressed in Alk– ALCL. Overall, T antigen negative cases (null cell type) display no clinical differences with T cell type ALCL. Expression of Alk correlates with the presence of a t(2;5) rearrangement. In cases having the usual t(2;5)/NPM-ALK translocation, Alk expression is both cytoplasmic and nuclear; variant translocations result in various patterns of Alk expression. ALCL is negative for B cell antigens, CD15, and EBV antigens.

The t(2;5)(p23;q35) rearrangement is present in >95% of cases. The t(2;5) results in relocation of the ALK (anaplastic lymphoma kinase) gene on 2p23 to the NPM (nucleophosmin) gene on 5q35. Since the ALK-NPM rearrangement occurs regularly within the same intron, PCR has no difficulty detecting the fusion gene. Less common ALK rearrangements include t(1;2), t(2;3), and inv(2). Clonal TCR rearrangement is present in ~90% of cases

Large granular lymphocytic leukemia (LGL leukemia)

The LGLs that circulate in low numbers in healthy adults are a mixture of Tc cells (T-cytotoxic T cells) and NK cells. This population expands in response to viral infection, rheumatoid arthritis, other autoimmune disorders, and splenectomy. Following allogeneic bone marrow transplant, there is frequently an oligoclonal expansion in Tc LGLs; care should be taken in diagnosing LGL leukemia in this setting. Furthermore, oligoclonal but reactive LGL populations are often found in association with mature B cell neoplasms, another potential pitfall. LGL leukemia is a condition in which there is an unexplained sustained (>6 month) increase (>2 × 10⁹/L) in LGLs. This has previously been called large granular lymphocytosis, T-CLL, and T-γ lymphoproliferative disorder. Like benign LGLs, LGL leukemia is a neoplasm that may be composed of either Tc cells or NK cells.

T-cytotoxic LGL leukemia is associated with neutropenia, a helpful finding when present. Most patients are older males (median age 60) who present with either sustained lymphocytosis, unexplained infections (neutropenia), or splenomegaly. Anemia may also be seen, in addition to polyclonal hypergammaglobulinemia. Lymphadenopathy is rare. In the peripheral blood, the neoplastic cells appear as typical LGLs; ultrastructurally, the granules have been described as consisting of parallel tubular arrays. In the marrow, there may be left-shifted granulocytic maturation and reticulin fibrosis. The neoplastic cells are quite subtle in marrow, presenting as sparse interstitial or intrasinusoidal infiltrates. In the spleen, the cells are found expanding the red pulp. There apparently is an increased incidence of rheumatoid arthritis in patients with T-cytotoxic LGL leukemia; in fact, some cases of Felty syndrome may actually represent T-cytotoxic LGL. Clonality can be demonstrated by TCR gene rearrangement studies. There are no recurring karyotypic findings. T-cytotoxic LGL is largely an indolent disease; however, a small group experiences aggressive disease that is often linked to CD56 expression and blastlike morphology. The

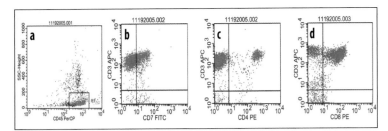

f4.68 Large granular lymphocytic (LGL) leukemia flow cytometry
a Gating around cells with bright CD45 & low side scatter (SSC), typical of the lymphocyte gate
b Plot of CD3 vs CD7, in which there is bright CD3 (indicating Tc rather than NK phenotype) & a subset with anomalously weak CD7 & somewhat weak CD3
c In this plot, the anomalous population is CD4−
d The anomalous population is CD8+

cells f4.68 are positive for CD2, CD3, CD8, and CD16. They are negative for CD4. In keeping with the T-cytotoxic phenotype, they are also positive for CD57, TIA, granzyme M, and granzyme B. TCR is predominantly of the αβ type. CD5 and/or CD7 may be diminished or absent; the distribution of CD5 in flow plots is characteristically bimodal.

NK cell LGL leukemia arises in a slightly younger population who present with fever, jaundice, and hepatosplenomegaly. Neutropenia and anemia are common. EBV is negative and the disease is indolent (to be distinguished from aggressive NK cell leukemia, which is EBV+). There are no recurring karyotypic anomalies, and TCR is germline. Demonstration of clonality is difficult. The cells are positive for CD2 but negative for surface CD3 (cytoplasmic ε chain of CD3 are present when studied immunohistochemically). They are positive for CD16 and CD56, and have variable expression of CD7, CD8, and CD57. They are usually CD4−.

Aggressive NK cell leukemia (ANKL)

ANKL has similarities to both NK-LGL (see above) and nasal-type NK cell lymphoma (see below), causing conceptual difficulties in this group of disorders. In contrast to NK-LGL, ANKL is strongly associated with EBV and follows an aggressive clinical course. In contrast to nasal-type NK cell lymphoma, ANKL is mainly leukemic (peripheral blood, bone marrow, and hepatosplenic involvement), affects younger patients, spares the skin, expresses CD16, and is uniformly fatal. ANKL is much more common among Asians, with a mean age of around 40 years. It presents with constitutional symptoms, hepatosplenomegaly, a leukemic blood picture, and markedly elevated serum LD. Some cases are complicated by hemophagocytosis. Morphologically, the neoplastic cells range from large atypical lymphocytes to LGL-like cells. The immunophenotype is that of typical NK cells; notably, CD16 is usually positive in contrast to nasal-type lymphoma.

Nasal type NK/T cell (NTNKT) lymphomas

NTNKT lymphomas arise both nasally and extranasally, but are essentially always extranodal. Morphologic findings that are highly characteristic include angioinvasion and extensive necrosis; cytologic findings are highly variable, neoplastic cells ranging from small to large. NTNKT lymphoma affects especially Asian and Native American groups of Central and South America. Nasal examples present clinically as so-called lethal midline granuloma and have previously been called angiocentric T cell lymphoma or polymorphic reticulosis. Immunophenotypically, the cells are EBV+ and most have a typical NK cell phenotype (positive for CD2 and CD56, negative for surface CD3) with CD16−. In this and other EBV associated neoplasms, in situ hybridization for EBV-encoded RNA (EBER) is the most reliable way to demonstrate the presence of EBV.

Blastic NK cell lymphoma

This is a neoplasm involving mainly the skin, with some cases also involving lymph nodes, peripheral blood, and bone marrow, consisting of a lymphoblastic appearing lymphoma with an NK immunophenotype. The cells express CD45, CD4, CD43, CD56, and the relatively unique antigen CD123 (shared only with so-called plasmacytoid dendritic cells). They are nearly always negative for CD2, CD3, CD5, CD7, CD8, CD30, CD138, B cell antigens, and myelomonocytic antigens. TCR and Ig genes are usually germline.

Enteropathy associated T cell lymphoma (EATCL)

EATCL is a high grade T cell lymphoma arising in patients with longstanding celiac sprue. The emergence of lymphoma is often preceded by refractory sprue with mucosal ulceration (ulcerative jejunoileitis). EATCL typically affects the jejunum and/or ileum. The incidence of EATCL parallels that of sprue, appearing most frequently in those of northern European descent, especially Welsh and Irish. Like sprue, the great majority of patients with EATCL have the HLADQA1*0501, DQB1*0201 genotype. The neoplastic cells are derived from intraepithelial T lymphocytes and are typically found within a mixed inflammatory background adjacent to flattened mucosa having the usual morphologic features of sprue. The neoplastic cells are CD3+ and usually CD4−/CD8− (some are CD8+); CD30 expression is usually present.

Hepatosplenic T cell lymphoma (HSTCL)

Splenic lymphomas account for ~1% of NHLs, most being B cell lymphomas. The γδ type of HSTCL occurs in young males who present with constitutional ("B") symptoms, hepatosplenomegaly, and cytopenias. Lymphomatous infiltrates are seen in the red pulp of the spleen and sinusoids of the liver, and they are composed of CD8+ cytotoxic T cells that express an γδ TCR, and isochrome 7q. These usually pursue an aggressive clinical course. The αβ T cell lymphomas are very similar, except for a female predominance and wider age distribution. In neither is peripheral blood or nodal involvement seen. A proportion of HSTCL arise in the setting of immunosuppression for transplant; these are regarded as a form of late-onset PTLD. Lastly, some cases arise in children treated for Crohn disease with azathioprine and infliximab.

Subcutaneous panniculitic T cell lymphoma

Subcutaneous panniculitic T cell lymphoma presents as a superficial soft tissue mass. Histologically, there is a proliferation of atypical lymphoid cells within the subcutaneous fat, often associated with extensive karyorrhexis. The neoplastic cells express CD3, CD8, and TCR αβ. A proportion of patients have associated systemic lupus erythematosus, and in this instance it must be distinguished from lupus profundus.

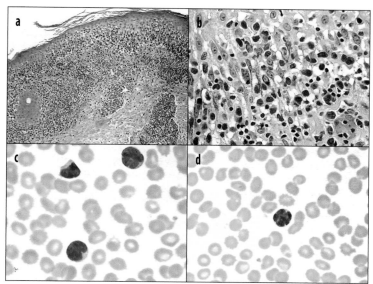

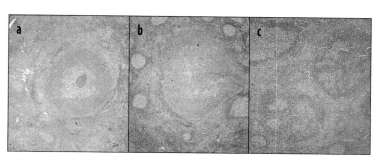

f4.71 Progressive transformation of germinal centers

f4.69 a-b Skin biopsy showing epidermotropic lymphoid infiltrate typical of mycosis fungoides
c-d Peripheral blood involvement by mycosis fungoides (Sézary syndrome) consisting of cells with markedly irregular (cerebriform) nuclear contours

represents peripheralized (circulating) mycosis fungoides, characterized by circulating cerebriform T lymphocytes. The incidence of circulating malignant cells is highest for the generalized erythroderma presentation (90%), while usual-type localized MF has a very low incidence of peripheralization. Marrow involvement, even when there is peripheral blood involvement, is rare. Lymph nodes are often enlarged in MF, but their histology is usually that of dermatopathic lymphadenopathy. Later, there may be colonization of nodes by malignant T cells. The immunophenotype of the neoplastic cells is characterized by expression of CD2, CD3, CD5, and CD4, usually with loss of CD7. The cells are negative for CD8 and CD25.

Hodgkin lymphoma (HL)

Nodular lymphocyte predominant Hodgkin lymphoma (NLPHL)

NLPHL must be distinguished from T cell/histiocyte rich B cell lymphoma (TCRBCL) and classic Hodgkin lymphoma (CHL). Morphologically, NLPHL presents as a lymph node effaced by a nodular or vaguely nodular proliferation f4.70a-c. Classic Reed-Sternberg cells are rare, and there is instead the characteristic L&H cell, a cell having abundant cytoplasm and a large vesicular convoluted (popcorn) nucleus f4.70d-f. Progressive transformation of germinal centers is thought to be a precursor lesion f4.71. The distinction with TCRBCL is mainly based upon the background, while the distinction with CHL rests upon the large neoplastic cells themselves t4.36.

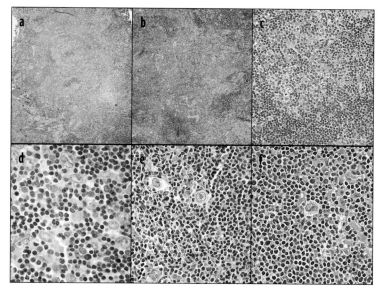

f4.70 Nodular lymphocyte predominant Hodgkin lymphoma (NLPHL)
a & b Low magnification vaguely nodular appearance
c Intermediate magnification shows a mixture of small & large cells
d-f The cytologic features of the large (L&H) cells of NLPHL; note the pronounced irregularity of the nuclear membrane

Cutaneous T cell lymphoma (CTCL), mycosis fungoides (MF) & Sézary syndrome

CTCL is an entity not specifically recognized in the WHO classification, but has been taken to refer to any primary cutaneous T cell malignancy, most often composed of CD4+ T lymphocytes. CTCL is an epidermotropic malignancy of small to large lymphoid cells having cerebriform nuclei f6.69. MF is CTCL which involves lymph nodes. Sézary syndrome

t4.36 TCRBCL vs NLPHL vs LRCHL

	TCRBCL	NLPHL	LRCHL
Architecture	Diffuse	Nodular	Nodular/diffuse
Classic R-S cells	−/+	−/+	+
CD45 (neoplastic cell)	+	+	−
CD30 (neoplastic cell)	−	−	+
CD15 (neoplastic cell)	−	−	±
CD20 (neoplastic cell)	+	+	−/+
CD79a (neoplastic cell)	+	±	−
EBV	−	−	±
Background lymphs	T >>> B	B >>> T	B > T
CD3+/CD57+ rosettes	−	+	−
CD21+ FDC	−	+	−
Bone marrow involved	±	−/+	−/+

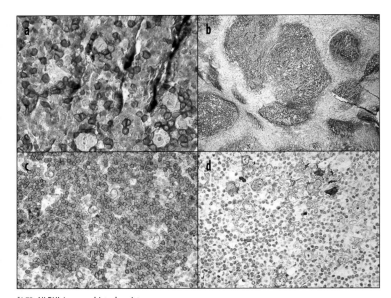

f4.72 NLPHL immunohistochemistry
a CD3 highlights rings of T cells encircling neoplastic cells
b CD21 highlights the residual follicular dendritic cell meshwork
c CD20 expression by the neoplastic cells
d EMA expression by the neoplastic cells

The background has 3 distinctive features f4.72. First, there is a meshwork of follicular dendritic cells that are responsible for the nodular architecture and which can be highlighted by CD21 or CD23 immunohistochemistry. Second, the predominant small infiltrating lymphocytes are CD20+ B cells. Last, a wreath of CD3+ (and CD57+) T cells can often be found around the neoplastic L&H cells. The neoplastic (L&H) cells express CD45, CD20, surface Ig, bcl-6, and EMA. They are negative for CD30, CD15, OCT2, BOB1, and EBV. L&H cells have clonally rearranged IGH genes and frequent *BCL6* rearrangement.

Classic Hodgkin lymphoma (CHL)

Common features to all subtypes of CHL include the presence of Reed-Sternberg cells or Reed-Sternberg variants f4.73 that represent neoplastic B cells with a typical immunophenotype. The cells express CD15, CD30, and fascin and often express IRF4/MUM1, PAX5, and EBV antigens (LMP-1+, EBER1/2+, EBNA2–). They are negative for CD45, CD20, bcl-6, ALK, and EMA. The CD15 is often dim and limited to the golgi zone. About 10-20% of cases express CD20; most such cases are CD79a negative. Background lymphocytes are a mixture of T and B cells.

A history of infectious mononucleosis raises the risk of CHL, but EBV is not found in all cases. EBV is found most commonly in MC and LD subtypes, and in tropical regions EBV is present in nearly all cases. The incidence of CHL is bimodal, showing a peak between the ages of 15-35 years (predominantly NS and NLPHL) and a second peak after age 50 (LD).

HL presents with localized lymphadenopathy in the vast majority of cases. The cervical lymph nodes are most often affected, followed by the mediastinum, and intraabdominal nodes. When presenting in the mediastinum, the NS subtype is usually identified. Intraabdominal CHL is more frequently MC. HL has a habit of spreading via contiguous lymphatic sites, but noncontiguous spread is often manifested by LD.

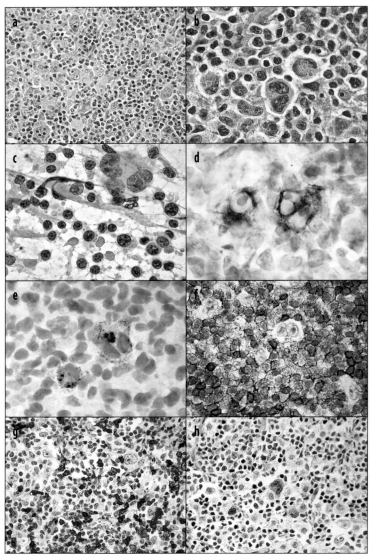

f4.73 Classic Hodgkin lymphoma (CHL)
a & b A mixed hematolymphoid background & several classic Reed-Sternberg cells
c Reed-Sternberg cell in H&E stained alcohol-fixed touch imprint
d CD30 stains Reed-Sternberg cells in membranous pattern with Golgi accentuation
e CD15 stains Reed-Sternberg cells primarily within the Golgi region
f CD20 is usually negative in Reed-Sternberg cells but may be positive in up to 20% of cases
g CD45 is nearly always negative in Reed-Sternberg cells
h PAX5 demonstrates dim nuclear expression in Reed-Sternberg cells

Disseminated disease is uncommon but may be seen in LD and HIV associated CHL. So-called "B" symptoms are present in some patients and include fever, night sweats, and weight loss. The bone marrow is not frequently involved. The incidence of marrow involvement is highest for LD (50%) and HIV associated (60%), lowest for LP (<1%) and ~10% overall. Marrow involvement f4.74 takes the form of focal collections of lymphocytes, histiocytes, plasma cells, and Reed-Sternberg cells, usually with a degree of fibrosis. WHO 2008 criteria for bone marrow (or other secondary site) involvement require an atypical mononuclear (CD30+) cell in the appropriate background; a classic Reed-Sternberg cell is not mandatory.

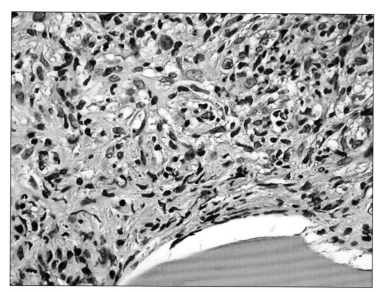

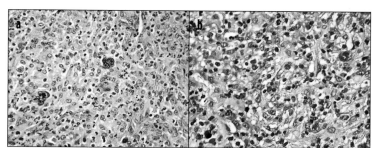

f4.76 Mixed cellularity variant of classic Hodgkin lymphoma

f4.74 CHL in marrow typically presents as fibrous lesions within which atypical CD30+ cells can be found

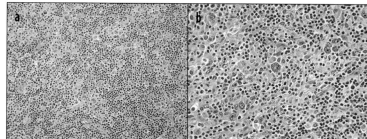

f4.77 Lymphocyte rich classic Hodgkin lymphoma

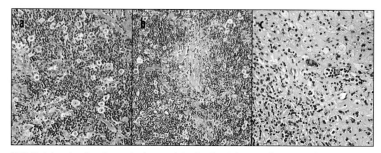

f4.75 Nodular sclerosis variant varies from a minimally sclerotic lesion with numerous lacunar cells to b moderately sclerotic lesions to c near complete sclerosis

t4.37 Subtypes of CHL

Subtype	Sites	Epidemiology	Hodgkin cell type	Background	EBV
NS	Mediastinum	70% of CHL 15-35 years	Lacunar	Mixed	25%
MC	Peripheral nodes	25% of CHL 25-45 years HIV associated Developing nations	Classic R-S	Mixed	75%
LR	Peripheral nodes	5% of CHL 35-55 years	Classic R-S Mononuclear Popcorn	Lymphs	50%
LD	Retroperitoneum	<1% of CHL 30-40 years HIV associated Developing nations	Classic R-S Pleomorphic	Mixed	50%

Nodular sclerosis (NS) subtype of CHL is the most common type in the western world, accounting for 70% of cases t4.37. It typically is found in young females and typically presents in the mediastinum. The morphology is characterized by a nodular proliferation carved out by bands of sclerosis. Classic Reed-Sternberg and Hodgkin cells are present, but the lacunar cell is the predominant R-S variant found f4.75. The lacunar cell resides within a lacune produced by a formalin fixation induced retraction artifact. Lacunes are not seen with other fixatives. It is the lacunar cell, not the sclerosis, which is the constant and defining feature of NS; prior to sclerosis and nodularity, lacunar cells are present in the cellular phase of NS. Also characteristic are so-called mummified cells, which resemble lacunar cells with shrunken and dark, structureless pyknotic nuclei. In the background is an abundance of small lymphocytes, plasma cells, and eosinophils. Histiocytes, including well formed epithelioid granulomas, are often present. Syncytial NS refers to an aggressive form of CHL that often presents at a high stage with bulky mediastinal disease. Confluent sheets of R-S cells and R-S variants proliferate and may undergo focal necrosis.

Mixed cellularity (MC) subtype of CHL accounts for ~25% of all cases. It is more common in underdeveloped parts of the world and in patients infected with HIV. The morphology is characterized by a diffuse proliferation of lymphocytes, eosinophils, histiocytes, and plasma cells, with varying numbers of classic R-S cells and mononuclear Hodgkin cells f4.76. The interfollicular variant is a form of partial nodal involvement by MC that may be subtle. R-S cells are present within the interfollicular compartment and around reactive-appearing follicles.

Lymphocyte rich (LR) subtype is responsible for ~5% of all cases of CHL. Morphologically, it is similar to NLPHL but has the typical immunophenotype of CHL f4.77.

The lymphocyte depleted (LD) subtype is infrequent overall but increases with age. It presents at a higher stage than other subtypes and is relatively aggressive. Classic R-S cells and variants usually number >15/hpf. The background cells are markedly decreased compared to MC.

ISBN 978-089189-5985

Myeloid neoplasms

Assessment

Manual 200-cell count of peripheral blood is recommended. Manual 500-cell count is recommended in marrow, conducted as close to particles as possible, enumerating blasts, promonocytes, promyelocytes, myelocytes, metamyelocytes, bands, segmented neutrophils, eosinophils, basophils, monocytes, lymphocytes, plasma cells, and erythroids. Note that megakaryocytes are not counted.

Normally, blasts are understood to include myeloblasts, monoblasts, and megakaryoblasts. In certain instances, other cells are considered "blast-equivalents." In considering the diagnosis of monocytic or myelomonocytic leukemia (FAB M4 or M5), promonocytes are considered "blast-equivalents." Promyelocytes are considered "blast-equivalents" for the diagnosis of acute promyelocytic leukemia (APML). Erythroblasts are not included in the blast count except in "pure erythroleukemia" variant of M6. Note that morphologic blast counts may be compared to flow cytometry, but in this comparison, flow cytometry usually underestimates blasts.

The bone marrow trephine biopsy should be assessed for overall cellularity, topography, and fibrosis. The WHO recommends, for an adequate exam, a biopsy that is ≥1.5 cm and contains ≥10 inter-trabecular areas.

Cytogenetic culture should be initiated in all cases, at initial diagnosis and at regular intervals thereafter. The morphologic differential diagnosis should guide the use of specific molecular assays t4.38. Depending on the abnormality found (eg, *BCR/ABL*) quantitative PCR should be ordered to determine a baseline for treatment.

t4.38 Tyrosine kinase anomalies in myeloproliferative neoplasms

Disorder	Associated abnormalities
CML	*BCR/ABL* translocation
PV	*JAK2* V617F, *JAK2* exon 12 mutation
PMF & ET	*JAK2* V617F, *MPL* W151L, *MPL* W151K
Eosinophilia related disorders	*PDGFRα, PDGFRβ, FGFR1* mutations
Mastocytosis	*KIT* D816V

Myelodysplastic syndromes (MDS)

Common features to this group of disorders include cytopenias, dyspoiesis, and a tendency to develop acute leukemia t4.39.

t4.39 General overview of myeloid neoplasm categories

Category	Peripheral blood	Marrow aspirate	Marrow biopsy	Splenomegaly
MDS	Cytopenia(s)	Dysplasia ± blasts (<20%)	Hypercellular	No
MD/MPN	Cytosis, usually leukocytosis	Dysplasia ± blasts (<20%)	Hypercellular	Yes
MPN	Cytosis, any	Orderly maturation ± blasts (<20%)	Hypercellular	Yes
AML	Cytopenia ± blasts	Blasts ± dysplasia	Hypercellular	No

The clinical presentation is reflective of cytopenias—fatigue, infection, bleeding. Splenomegaly is usually absent. Most cases of MDS present in older adults and are not associated with a known exposure (primary MDS). Secondary MDS follows such things as chemotherapy (usually with alkylating agents), radiation exposure, benzene exposure, or Fanconi anemia. Secondary MDS may present in young adults who were previously exposed to treatment for a childhood malignancy. The risk is highest following treatment with alkylating agents, and therapy related MDS caused by alkylating agents is often associated with anomalies in chromosome 5q or 7q.

The spleen is usually not enlarged in MDS, a clinical feature that supports distinction from myeloproliferative neoplasms (MPN). Radiographic criteria for splenomegaly, however, are fulfilled in up to 10% of patients with low grade MDS and in up to 20% of patients with RAEB or RAEB-T. It is present in >50% of patients with chronic myelomonocytic leukemia (CMML), a combined MDS/MPN.

Morphologically f4.78, the marrow biopsy is usually hypercellular. By definition, blasts are <20%, and dyspoiesis is present in one or more cell lines. Dyspoiesis in the erythroid cell line may be reflected in the peripheral blood as basophilic stippling, poikilocytosis, and macrocytosis. Erythroid precursors may be megaloblastoid (dyssynchrony of nuclear and cytoplasmic maturation) and may have nuclear lobation, internuclear bridging, multinuclearity, and karyorrhexis. Additional features may include ringed sideroblasts (defined by the WHO as an erythroid precursor with ≥5 siderosomes that surround at least a third of the nucleus), cytoplasmic PAS positivity, and cytoplasmic vacuolization. Functional changes are frequently noted in RBCs, including increased susceptibility to complement-mediated lysis (resulting in a positive Hams test), increased HbF, abnormal expression of RBC antigens, acquired enzyme defects (eg, pyruvate kinase deficiency), and acquired thalassemia. Granulocytic (myeloid) series dysplasia may appear in the peripheral blood as neutropenia, abnormal cytoplasmic granulation, or abnormal nuclear segmentation (including pseudo-Pelger-Huët anomaly). There is an increased rate of bacterial infection due to neutrophil dysfunction. In the marrow, there may be left-shifted maturation and megaloblastoid maturation. Megakaryocytic dysplasia may be reflected in peripheral thrombocytopenia. In the marrow, one may see hypogranulation, micromegakaryocytes, "pawn ball" (multinucleated) nuclei, and hypolobated nuclei. There may be a qualitative defect as well, reflected in abnormal platelet aggregometry. Clusters of very immature cells located away from bony trabeculae or vessels are known as abnormal localization of immature precursors (ALIP). This finding suggests an increased likelihood of leukemic evolution.

Note that the marrow of healthy subjects contains a few dyspoietic cells, ordinarily representing <5% of any cell line, and there is a tendency for these findings to increase if the specimen is not immediately processed. The current WHO classification requires that dyspoiesis be present in 10% or more of any cell line for that lineage to be declared dysplastic. Mild dyspoiesis and hypercellularity are particularly common in B_{12} and folate deficiencies. It is important to exclude these deficiencies as well as dyspoiesis related to alcohol consumption, HIV infection, lead poisoning, arsenic poisoning, copper deficiency/zinc intoxication (prominent erythroid vacuolization and iron-laden plasma cells are clues), or medications (isoniazid, chloramphenicol, chemotherapeutic agents).

At the molecular level, cytogenetic abnormalities are present in 30-40% of low grade cases (RA, RARS) and 70-80% of high grade cases. The most common karyotype, present in ~25% of cases, is one with complex abnormalities (2 or

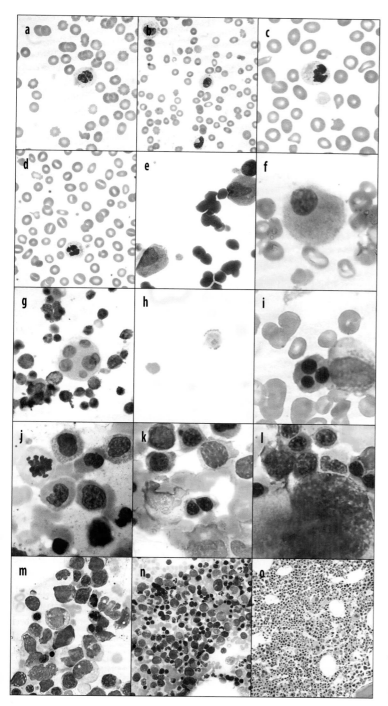

f4.78 Myelodysplastic syndrome (MDS)
a–d Peripheral blood in MDS showing a variety of findings, including neutrophils that are hypogranular & hyposegmented, enlarged hypogranular platelets, and erythroid anisopoikilocytosis
e–o Bone marrow aspirates in MDS showing a variety of finding, including **e** abnormal granulocyte granulation, **f** small mononuclear megakaryocytes, **g** multinucleated (pawn ball) megakaryocytes, **h** ringed sideroblasts, **i** multinucleate erythroid precursors, **j** irregular nuclear contours & karyorrhexis, **k & l** internuclear bridges & nuclear blebs, **m** karyorrhexis, **n** erythroid hyperplasia
o In most cases the marrow is hypercellular, as is the case with myeloid neoplasms generally, but some cases present as hypoplastic MDS

more clonal abnormalities), and this is associated with a poor prognosis. The second most common finding (15%) is isolated monosomy 7 or 7q–. Third most common (10%) is isolated 5q–, which is associated with a good prognosis.

Immunophenotyping has recently shown promise in evaluating the marrow for dysplasia. Certain reproducible patterns of abnormal antigenic maturation are found in dysplastic

marrow. Frequently reported abnormalities include altered (diminished) side-angle light scatter by maturing myeloid cells as well as altered expression of CD13 vs CD16 or CD11b vs CD16. Maturing neutrophils normally demonstrate increasing expression of CD16 simultaneous with decreasing expression of CD13 and/or CD11b. Furthermore, any expression of nonmyeloid antigens by a significant proportion of maturing myeloid or monocytic cells is supportive of MDS. Among experienced observers, the sensitivity and specificity of this modality may be >90%, greatly exceeding that of morphology or cytogenetics alone.

Prognosis depends on 4 main variables, including the type of MDS t4.40, percentage of blasts, cytogenetics t4.41, and the number of depressed cell lines. With regard to type, RA and RARS are the most stable. The overall rate of progression to acute leukemia is ~10% for RA and RARS, 45% for RAEB. Favorable cytogenetics include loss of Y, del(5q), and del(20q).

t4.40 Myelodysplastic syndromes

Type	Peripheral blood	Bone marrow
Refractory cytopenia with unilineage dysplasia	Anemia or thrombocytopenia or neutropenia No blasts (<1%) or Auer rods No monocytosis (<1,000/µL)	Unilineage dysplasia <5% blasts & no Auer rods ≤15% ringed sideroblasts
Refractory anemia with ringed sideroblasts (RARS)	Anemia ± dimorphic RBCs & Pappenheimer bodies No blasts (<1%) or Auer rods No monocytosis (<1,000/µL)	Dysplastic erythroids <5% blasts & no Auer rods >15% ringed sideroblasts
Refractory cytopenia with multilineage dysplasia (RCMLD)	Bi- or pancytopenia <1% blasts No Auer rods	<5% blasts & no Auer rods Dysplasia in >10% of >1 cell line ≤15% ringed sideroblasts
Refractory cytopenia with multilineage dysplasia with ringed sideroblasts (RCMLD-RS)	Bi- or pancytopenia <1% blasts No Auer rods	<5% blasts & no Auer rods Dysplasia in >10% of >1 cell line >15% ringed sideroblasts
Refractory anemia with excess blasts (RAEB)	Bi- or pancytopenia <5% blasts, no Auer rods—RAEB-1 5-19% blasts or Auer rods—RAEB-2	5-9% blasts, no Auer rods—RAEB-1 10-19% blasts or Auer rods—RAEB-2 Dysplasia
MDS with del(5q)	Anemia, normal to increased platelets <5% blasts No Auer rods	Hypolobated megakaryocytes <5% blasts & no Auer rods Isolated 5q– karyotype

t4.41 Cytogenetic risk categories for patients with myelodysplastic syndrome

Favorable prognosis	Normal karyotype or isolated loss of Y, 5q–, 20q–
Intermediate prognosis	Other findings
Unfavorable prognosis	3 or more anomalies (so-called complex karyotype) or anomalies of chromosome 7

The 5q– syndrome results from isolated loss of the long arm of chromosome 5. This presents in a reproducible syndrome that disproportionately affects elderly females and follows an indolent clinical course, progressing uncommonly to acute leukemia (~20%). 5q– syndrome manifests mainly with anemia; there is little or no neutropenia, and platelets are normal to elevated in number.

Hypocellular MDS is similar to other forms of MDS, aside from posing a more challenging diagnosis. Usually, MDS presents with hypercellular marrow, but ~10% of cases present instead with hypocellular marrow. This may be confused with aplastic anemia unless careful attention is paid to the findings in the touch imprints or aspirate material.

Rarely, reticulin fibrosis is found in MDS. This diagnosis is difficult to make and should only be entertained when there is significant dyspoiesis and no splenomegaly.

Myelodysplastic/myeloproliferative neoplasms (MD/MPN)

The MD/MPN category includes disparate entities united by the coexistence, at presentation, of dyspoiesis and increased production of mature cells. Thus, there are overlapping features of myelodysplasia and myeloproliferation.

Chronic myelomonocytic leukemia (CMML) is diagnosed when there is persistent absolute monocytosis ($>1 \times 10^9$/L or $>1,000$/μL), marrow dysplasia (usually dysgranulopoiesis), <20% blasts, and absence of a Philadelphia chromosome. The blast count should include blasts and promonocytes. CMML is further subdivided into CMML-1 (in which blasts and promonocytes are <5% in peripheral blood and <10% in marrow) and CMML-2 (5-19% in peripheral blood, 10-19% in marrow). There may be hepatosplenomegaly, and there is often anemia and thrombocytopenia. Enlarged spleens in patients with CMML have been found to fall into 3 broad categories when studied histologically: erythrophagocytosis-predominant, plasmacytosis-predominant, and extramedullary hematopoiesis (EMH)-predominant. Each represents about a third of the cases. Despite the requisite monocytosis, about half of cases present with a normal or low leukocyte count, because of neutropenia. The monocyte morphology varies from essentially normal to mildly atypical f4.79. When (rarely) lymph nodes are enlarged, they are found to have an infiltrate of so-called plasmacytoid monocytes having an unusual immunophenotype (CD14+, CD68+, CD56+, CD4+, CD2+, and CD5+). Some cases display clonal cytogenetic anomalies, but none that are specific for this entity. *JAK2* mutations are present in a small proportion of cases. If eosinophilia ($>1.5 \times 10^9$/L) is present, then rearrangement of *PDGFRα* and *PDGFRβ* should be excluded. CMML with eosinophilia can be diagnosed if no *PDGFRα* or *PDGFRβ* rearrangement is found.

Atypical chronic myelogenous leukemia (aCML) is diagnosed when there is neutrophilia, composed of a spectrum of mature neutrophils, metamyelocytes, myelocytes, and promyelocytes, in conjunction with marrow dysplasia, <20% blasts, and absence of a Philadelphia chromosome. Most cases have clonal cytogenetic anomalies, most commonly +8 or del(20q), but none are specific. Some cases have *JAK2* mutations.

Juvenile myelomonocytic leukemia (JMML) usually affects children, presenting with monocytosis and/or granulocytosis, hepatosplenomegaly, and constitutional symptoms. Findings may also include anemia, thrombocytopenia, increased HbF, and clonal chromosomal abnormalities (monosomy 7 in 25%). In vitro spontaneous formation of granulocyte-macrophage colonies that are hypersensitive to GM-CSF is confirmatory. Nearly 10% of patients have neurofibromatosis type 1 (NF-1).

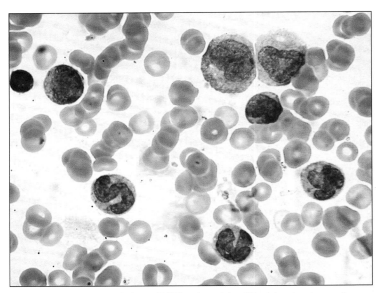

f4.79 Chronic myelomonocytic leukemia (CMML); in the peripheral blood, there is an increased absolute number of monocytes that are mildly atypical

Myeloproliferative neoplasms (MPN)

Myeloproliferative neoplasms are clonal nondysplastic proliferations of marrow elements, usually resulting in increased production of mature cells. An MPN is nearly always associated with splenomegaly at presentation. All have a tendency to progress to eventual marrow failure and/or acute leukemia.

Chronic myelogenous leukemia (CML)

CML is defined by the presence of the Philadelphia chromosome, consisting of a reciprocal translocation of chromosomes 9 and 22—t(9;22)(q34;q11). As a result of this rearrangement, the *ABL* locus at the 9q34 is translocated to the *BCR* locus at 22q11. The gene product is a chimeric Bcr-Abl protein with enhanced tyrosine kinase activity. The mutation occurs within an early marrow stem cell, such that it can be found in all marrow cell lines, including endothelial cells. Sometimes it is even found in lymphoid cells. Most commonly, the translocation occurs within the major breakpoint cluster (M-BCR), spanning exons 12-16, productive of a p210 fusion protein. The translocation may occur at other breakpoints, however. The μ-BCR breakpoint produces a p230 fusion protein; this is associated with marked thrombocytosis and relatively mature leukemic neutrophils. The m-BCR breakpoint (p190 fusion protein) is associated with marked monocytosis and is the breakpoint of Ph+ ALL. Mutation of *JAK2* is not seen in CML. Without treatment, CML progresses through an accelerated phase to an eventual blast phase, often within 2-3 years. Among the MPNs, CML has the highest rate of progression (95% compared to 10% in the others).

The initial chronic phase of CML presents f4.80 with leukocytosis attributable to increased neutrophils in all stages of maturation, basophilia, eosinophilia, and thrombocytosis. The leukocyte count is usually $>50 \times 10^9$/L and may exceed 300×10^9/L (median 100×10^9/L). Characteristically, the proportion of myelocytes and neutrophils exceeds that of the other stages (myelocyte "bulge"). This, especially when accompanied by basophilia, is highly specific for CML and is seen in neither

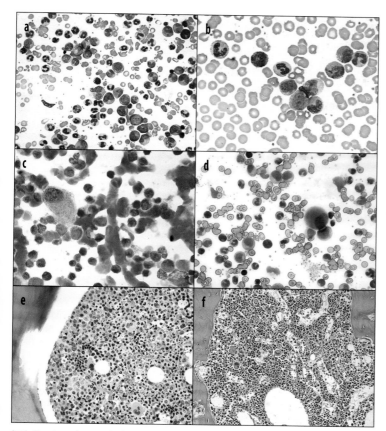

f4.80 Chronic myelogenous leukemia (CML)
a & b In the peripheral blood, there is leukocytosis composed of a range of myeloid progenitors, including a pronounced proportion of myelocytes; basophils & eosinophils are increased as well, and there is usually thrombocytosis
c & d In the marrow aspirate there are, in addition to a range of myeloid precursors, small mononuclear ("dwarf") megakaryocytes
e & f The marrow biopsy shows hypercellularity with a thickened regenerative zone

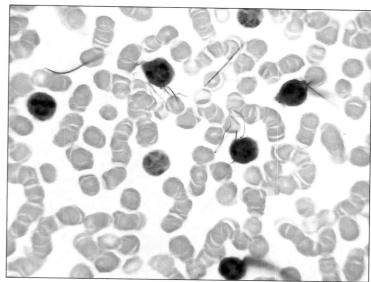

f4.81 Leukocyte alkaline phosphatase (LAP) test in normal peripheral blood

other MPNs nor in reactive conditions. Absolute monocytosis is also present in most cases, but the proportion of monocytes is usually <3%; even larger numbers of monocytes are seen in cases harboring the p190 *BCR-ABL* variant translocation, and this may cause confusion with CMML. Eosinophils are often elevated. Blasts are rare (usually <1%). At this stage there is the distinctively low leukocyte alkaline phosphatase (LAP) score **f4.81**. The marrow is frequently inaspirable, because of reticulin fibrosis. Examination of the marrow discloses hypercellularity, with an increased M:E ratio, and a myelocyte "bulge" similar to that seen in the peripheral blood. There is an increase in megakaryocytes, which are often small and hypolobated ("dwarf" megakaryocytes). The topography is altered, with migration of immature myeloids away from bony trabeculae and thickening of the paratrabecular cuff of immature cells. One can easily find scattered histiocytes—gray-green crystal containing, Gaucher-like, and sea-blue histiocytes—that are merely indicative of increased cell turnover and nonspecific. Dyspoiesis is unusual; dysgranulopoiesis in CML has a strong association with chromosome 17p abnormalities and may herald an accelerated phase. As with all MPNs, splenomegaly is common at presentation. There is a platelet aggregation defect characterized by impaired aggregation in response to epinephrine, and CML is a cause of markedly elevated B_{12} levels, thought to be due to increased transcobalamin I.

The accelerated phase is marked by the emergence of one or more of the following: progressive basophilia (>20%), thrombocytopenia (<100×10⁹/L), thrombocytosis (>1,000×10⁹/L) or leukocytosis, clonal cytogenetic progression (Philadelphia chromosome in addition to, eg, +8, i(17q), +19, another Ph), or increasing blasts >10% (but <20%). At this stage one can often find clusters of abnormal megakaryocytes. The LAP score tends to rise. The blast phase is marked by one of the following: >20% blasts in blood or marrow, a tissue infiltrate of blasts (chloroma), or a prominent focal accumulation of blasts in the marrow biopsy (filling an inter-trabecular space). In the blast phase, 70% are of the AML type, and 30% are ALL type (often coexpressing myeloid antigens). Most patients in blast crisis have additional cytogenetic abnormalities, most commonly duplication of the Philadelphia chromosome, +8, or i17q. Conventional chemotherapy prolongs progression to 3-5 years; however, tyrosine kinase inhibitor therapy (imatinib and second-line agents nilotinib and dasatinib) results in prolonged survival. The most powerful prognostic factor is the response to tyrosine kinase inhibitor therapy as measured by quantitative RT-PCR.

Imatinib functions through competitive inhibition of the ATP binding site of bcr-abl. It is active against not only bcr-abl, but also against PDGFR (platelet derived growth factor receptor) and c-kit. Imatinib resistance is present initially in 5% of cases and emerges during treatment in many more. Resistance is often the result of distinct mutations within the *BCR-ABL* gene, especially the tyrosine kinase domain and the so-called P loop. Within the tyrosine kinase domain, the substitution of isoleucine for threonine at position 315 (T315I) has been frequently associated with resistance. A variety of assays are available for detection of *BCR-ABL* resistance associated mutations. These include direct sequence analysis (limited to the kinase domain), denaturing high pressure liquid chromatography, allele-specific oligonucleotides, and others. Additional mechanisms of imatinib resistance include P-glycoprotein (MDR-1) overexpression, amplification of *BCR-ABL* leading to increased bcr-abl kinase, acquisition of additional non-*BCR-ABL* genetic anomalies (clonal evolution). It appears that early treatment with imatinib lessens the incidence of acquired resistance, as patients who begin therapy >2 years after diagnosis have a significantly higher incidence of resistance than those who begin treatment before 2 years; furthermore, those initially treated while in the accelerated or blast phase have a much higher incidence of imatinib resistance.

Minimal residual disease (MRD) in CML has had a shifting definition over the years, as newer technologies emerged. Broadly speaking, it refers to a level of leukemic cells too low to produce clinical manifestations or to be visible microscopically. Several concepts are worth noting. First, it is estimated that, at presentation, patients with CML have around 10^{12} leukemic cells; when clinical remission is reached, there are around 10^9-10^{10} leukemic cells (about a 2- to 3-log reduction). Thus, MRD generally refers to a number of leukemic cells $<10^9$-10^{10}. Second, there are several modalities for detecting MRD in CML, including conventional cytogenetics, FISH, PCR, and flow cytometry. Each has its unique lower limit of detection. A complete cytogenetic response (undetectable Philadelphia chromosome in 20 metaphases by conventional cytogenetics) generally is achieved when the number of leukemic cells is below 10^9 (a 3-log reduction). A true 3-log reduction at 12 months, as confirmed by quantitative PCR for the *BCR-ABL* transcript, predicts a nearly 0% likelihood of disease progression over the ensuing 2 years. There is a ~5% likelihood of progression when the reduction is <3 logs.

Conventional cytogenetics can be used

1. to initially detect CML, by identifying a Philadelphia chromosome, and additional anomalies, if any

2. to follow CML, by looking for cytogenetic progression

Cytogenetic remission (the lack of cyogenetically detectable Philadelphia chromosomes in 20 metaphases) is too insensitive an index of remission for clinical utility. The major advantage of cytogenetics is its ability to find additional chromosomal abnormalities (indicative of progressive disease). PCR is also of value initially for 2 reasons:

1. to characterize the *BCR-ABL* fusion gene for later detection of molecular remission

2. to provide greater sensitivity in the initial detection of *BCR-ABL* than cytogenetics can provide

Thus, it is reasonable to obtain both cytogenetics and qualitative PCR whenever bone marrow tissue is obtained in patients with known or suspected CML. The *BCR-ABL* translocation can be studied by either qualitative or quantitative assays. When testing a patient for the first time, the qualitative assay should be ordered and, if positive, a quantitative assay performed on the same sample. The *BCR-ABL* quantitative assay is used to establish a baseline for future MRD monitoring but should be ordered after the qualitative assay because it does not distinguish the different types of *BCR-ABL* breakpoints. FISH, using a fusion probe for *BCR* and *ABL*, can detect the Philadelphia chromosome. Normal cells would be expected to show 2 red and 2 green nuclear signals. In CML, cells have 3 signals—1 red, 1 green, and 1 yellow (the fusion signal). FISH is more sensitive for the Philadelphia chromosome than cytogenetics, but it cannot detect additional chromosomal aberrations. Furthermore, while FISH

has a level of sensitivity that is generally considered sufficient for detecting MRD, a high rate of false positive and false negative results preclude its routine use. Thus, FISH has a limited role overall in CML diagnosis and management. Quantitative PCR (reverse transcriptase real time polymerase chain reaction [RT-PCR]) is considered the method of choice for MRD detection in patients who have achieved a complete cytogenetic remission. RT-PCR monitoring can be performed with equivalent efficacy on either peripheral blood or bone marrow. Nested RT-PCR is the amplification of an initial amplicon (by performing an amplification within the initial amplicon using consecutive primer sets). While capable of increased sensitivity (1 in 10^6 as compared to 1 in 10^4-10^5 cells) as compared to routine PCR, it is unclear that this degree of sensitivity offers any advantage, and nested PCR is prone to contamination. At this time it is not recommended.

Flow cytometric immunophenotyping has traditionally not had a role in the diagnosis of CML. Like MDS, however, it has now been demonstrated that there are characteristic immunophenotypic abnormalities in CML, having to do with the aberrations in the normal temporal acquisition of myeloid antigens or the anomalous expression of nonmyeloid antigens.

Non-CML myeloproliferative neoplasms

Polycythemia vera (PV) presents at a median age of 60 years with manifestations of polycythemia—hypertension, thrombosis, pruritus, plethora, erythromelalgia, or headache. The spleen is typically enlarged at presentation. PV must be distinguished from relative polycythemia, secondary polycythemia, and CML t4.42.

t4.42 Criteria for PV: both major criteria + 1 minor criterion or 1st major criterion + 2 minor criteria		
Major criteria	1. Hgb>18.5 g/dL (men), >16.5 g/dL (women), or increased RBC mass	
	2. *JAK2* V617F or other functionally similar *JAK2* mutation	
Minor criteria	1. Bone marrow panmyelosis (megakaryocytes, granulocytes, erythroids)	
	2. Endogenous erythroid colony formation in vitro	
	3. Normal serum EPO	

Relative polycythemia is seen in the setting of stress or dehydration and has been called Gaisböch syndrome. Secondary polycythemia is associated with low PaO_2 states (such as smoking and living at high altitudes), high oxygen affinity hemoglobin variants, and certain neoplasms (renal cell carcinoma, cerebellar hemangioblastoma) that produce excess erythropoietin.

The initial proliferative phase is marked by erythrocytosis. The erythrocytes are usually normocytic, but may become microcytic and hypochromic. Neutrophilia is common, and sometimes there is basophilia and/or thrombocytosis. The marrow is hypercellular, usually with a low M:E ratio. Megakaryocytic hyperplasia is often quite prominent and may distract from the erythroid hyperplasia. Stainable iron is characteristically decreased or absent. The spent phase (post-polycythemic myelofibrosis with myeloid metaplasia—PPMM) is heralded by a peripheral myelophthisic pattern, marrow reticulin fibrosis, and extramedullary hematopoiesis. The cause of death is most commonly thrombosis (31%), followed by acute leukemia (19%). MPNs, particularly PV, are the most common cause of the Budd-Chiari syndrome. PV alone accounts for 10-40% of cases. Endogenous erythroid colony formation may be seen in >80% of patients thought to have idiopathic Budd-Chiari syndrome. RBC mass is measured using isotope dilution, in which a sample of patient RBCs is labeled with a radioactive isotope and reinfused. The RBC mass can then be calculated from the degree of dilution of the labeled RBCs. This direct measurement of the RBC mass distinguishes reduced plasma volume from a true absolute erythrocytosis. Endogenous erythroid colony formation is assessed in a culture of patient marrow. In PV, one can observe the spontaneous formation of erythroid colonies (without addition of erythropoietin). In healthy patients or those with secondary erythrocytosis, erythroid colony formation requires exogenous erythropoietin.

The *JAK2* (Janus kinase 2) mutation is identified in the majority of cases of non-CML myeloproliferative neoplasms, including in >90% of cases classified as PV and >50% of ET and PMF. Notably, the *JAK2* mutation can be found in the peripheral blood of many patients presenting with idiopathic venous thrombosis, including nearly 9% of patients with Budd-Chiari syndrome. The Jak2 protein is a tyrosine kinase involved in the pathway that stimulates so-called signal transducers and activators of transcription (STAT) proteins. Jak2 is a member of the Janus kinase family. These are tyrosine kinases that are activated by cell surface growth factor receptors and, when activated, phosphorylate other proteins in the pathway (the STATs). Phosphorylated STATs enter the nucleus where they act as transcription factors for a number of genes. The common *JAK2* mutation is a guanine to thymine substitution at nucleotide 1849, resulting in a valine to phenylalanine substitution at codon 617 (Val617Phe). The mutation affects the protein's JH2 domain, a normally inhibitory domain. Alteration in JH2 has a net gain of function effect that leads to constitutive *JAK2* activation, with the effect of cytokine-independent growth. A second activating mutation—within *JAK2* exon 12—produces a small proportion of PV cases. Mutations in *MPL*—the *MPL* W515L or *MPL* W515K mutations—produce a small subset of PMF and ET but are not seen in PV. Unlike *BCR/ABL*, a *JAK2* mutation is not required for the diagnosis of these MPNs; nor is it specific for these neoplasms, with *JAK2* mutations found in some types of MD/MPN. The major practical question at this time concerns the best diagnostic assay for detection of the *JAK2* mutation. The physicochemical significance of a G to T mutation (with a 3-2 hydrogen bond change) has been evaluated; indeed, there appears to be somewhere between 6°C to 10°C difference between the melting points of the wild-type and mutant alleles, as well as, eg, differences in denaturing gradient gel electrophoretic velocity, single strand conformation. Sequence-based testing, such as allele-specific oligonucleotide (ASO) PCR and quantitative real time PCR, remain the most sensitive assays.

Essential thrombocythemia (ET) is the least common MPN, in part because the diagnosis is made only after all the others have been excluded t4.43. It demonstrates a bimodal age distribution, with peaks at age 30 and 60, and female preponderance. Patients with ET have the longest survival of the MPNs, with the lowest likelihood (5%) of transformation to acute leukemia. <1/2 of patients have splenomegaly.

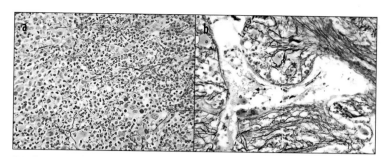

f4.82 Bone marrow reticulin fibrosis in myeloproliferative neoplasms, ranging from a mild to b severe, in which one can see gaping sinuses, pulled open by the fibrosis

ET presents as isolated thrombocytosis, with some patients presenting with thrombosis or mucosal hemorrhages. Aside from variable size, the platelets are not morphologically noteworthy. The bone marrow shows an increase in mature-appearing, large, hyperlobated megakaryocytes which are paratrabecular and may display marked emperipolesis. Unlike PV and PMF, the megakaryocyte topography is not extensively altered, and megakaryocyte clustering is not significant. Proliferation of other elements (erythroid, granulocytic) is not a feature of ET (consider PV, PMF, or CML). Megakaryocytes with very atypical or bizarre nuclei are not a feature of ET (consider PV or PMF). Stainable iron is usually present (helpful to exclude iron deficiency). Lastly, significant reticulin fibrosis at presentation is not a feature of ET. ET must be distinguished from reactive thrombocytopenia that occurs in iron deficiency, chronic inflammation, asplenia, and other hematolymphoid malignancies (such as CML).

Primary myelofibrosis (PMF) has been given a variety of names over the years, including myelofibrosis with myeloid metaplasia (MMM), agnogenic myeloid metaplasia (AMM), and chronic idiopathic myelofibrosis (CIMF). About 30-40% of cases present with unexplained splenomegaly or hepatosplenomegaly. The cellular (prefibrotic) phase presents with anemia, mild leukocytosis, and thrombocytosis. The marrow at this stage shows hypercellularity due to increased granulocytic precursors and megakaryocytes. Erythroid precursors are relatively diminished and may demonstrate maturation arrest. The granulocytes have a normal distribution and lack a myelocyte bulge. The megakaryocytes are both morphologically abnormal—aberrantly lobulated with clumped, hyperchromatic, and inky chromatin—and topographically abnormal—in clusters found adjacent to sinuses and trabeculae. As mentioned, this phase is often characterized by thrombocytosis; attention paid to the megakaryocyte morphology generally permits appropriate diagnosis of PMF instead of ET, the significance being the very high likelihood of progression to fibrotic-phase myelofibrosis. The fibrotic phase, in which most patients present, has a leukoerythroblastic pattern in the peripheral blood, with dacrocytosis and anisocytosis. The bone marrow is inaspirable. Characteristic bone marrow findings include reticulin and/or collagen fibrosis f4.82, intrasinusoidal hematopoiesis, and morphologically abnormal, clustered megakaryocytes.

t4.43 Criteria for ET

Sustained thrombocytosis >450 × 10⁶/μL (>450 × 10⁹/L)
Bone marrow shows megakaryocytic hyperplasia, without panmyelosis (no significant increase in granulocytic/erythroid precursors)
Fails to meet criteria for PV, PMF, CML, or MDS
JAK2 V617F mutation + or no evidence for reactive thrombocytosis

Chronic eosinophilic leukemia (CEL) is predominantly a disease of men, with a 9:1 male:female ratio. It usually presents in males between the ages of 25 and 45 years. CEL is characterized by peripheral blood eosinophilia ($>1.5 \times 10^9$/L), often with evidence of tissue infiltration and damage. The eosinophils may be hypogranular, in which case histochemical staining for cyanide-resistant myeloperoxidase (eosinophils are positive) can be helpful. Common sites of tissue infiltration include the heart, GI tract, lung, and CNS. In the heart, endomyocardial fibrosis may result. To diagnose CEL, there must be no identifiable cause of secondary eosinophilia. Common causes of secondary eosinophilia include allergic reactions, parasitic infestations, collagen vascular disease, mastocytosis, and other hematolymphoid neoplasms. Furthermore, there must be no evidence of one of the defined syndromes with eosinophilia (ie, no *PDGFRα* rearrangement, no *PDGFRβ* rearrangement, and no *FGFR1* rearrangement—see below). When evidence of clonality can be found, such as a cytogenetic abnormality or increased blasts (but not >20%), CEL is diagnosed. Lacking this, the diagnosis is hypereosinophilic syndrome (HES).

Myeloid & lymphoid neoplasms with eosinophilia with abnormalities of *PDGFRα, PDGFRβ,* or *FGFR1*

The 2008 WHO classification separates 3 gene rearrangement-defined entities that are associated with eosinophilia t4.44. Endomyocardial fibrosis may complicate all of these disorders.

t4.44 Myeloid & lymphoid neoplasms with eosinophilia with abnormalities of *PDGFRα, PDGFRβ,* or *FGFR1*

Gene	Usual presentation	Other presentations	Epidemiology	Abnormal karyotype	Usual rearrangement
PDGFRα	CEL-like	AML with eos T-ALL with eos	M:F=17:1 Median 40 years	No	NFIP1L1/PDGFRα— cryptic del(4q12)
PDGFRβ	CMML-like	AML with eos	M:F=2:1 Median 40 years	Yes	ETV6/PDGFRβ (TEL/ PDGFRβ)—t(5;12)
FGFR1	T-ALL with eos	CEL-like	M:F=1.5:1 Median 30 years	Yes	ZNF198/ FGFR1—t(8;13)

Unlike most fusion genes that result from a balanced translocation, the one responsible for the CEL-like myeloid neoplasm in this category results from a deletion of genetic material between genes. Specifically, an interstitial deletion in the long arm of chromosome 4, del(4)(q12;q12), results in the *FIP1L1-PDGFRα* fusion gene. The deletion cannot be seen in routine cytogenetic studies (cryptic interstitial deletion). The Fip1l1-pdgfr fusion protein is a tyrosine kinase that can often be inactivated by imatinib and similar tyrosine kinase inhibitors. The dose required for inhibition is much lower than that needed for bcr-abl inhibition.

PDGFRβ rearrangements usually result from the translocation t(5;12). Like *PDGFRα* rearrangements, such neoplasms are responsive to imatinib and similar tyrosine kinase inhibitors.

Acute myelogenous leukemia (AML)

General features

Most adult and infantile acute leukemia is myeloid. Only 10-15% of childhood acute leukemia is myeloid. The median age overall is 65 years. AML ordinarily presents with a very high WBC count attributable to abundant circulating blasts f4.83. It is not uncommon, however, to present with pancytopenia. Uncommonly, AML presents as a soft tissue mass (so-called

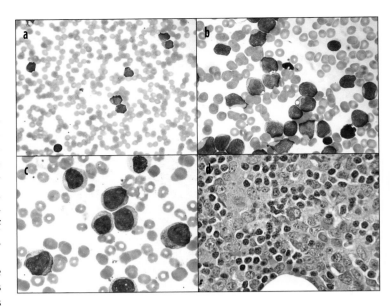

f4.83 Acute myelogenous leukemia (AML)
a–c In contrast to lymphoblasts, the cells tend to have more complex nuclei & cytoplasm, including granulation; the only specific finding, however, is the Auer rod
d In some cases, it presents as chloroma with eosinophilic myelocytes being a helpful clue

chloroma, extramedullary myeloid cell tumor, or myeloid sarcoma). The diagnosis of AML can be established in 2 ways:

1. blast percentage >20%
2. <20% blasts if there is pure erythroleukemia, myeloid sarcoma, or certain genetic abnormalities (eg, t(8;21) and other recurrent genetic abnormalities)

Blast percentages should be based upon a 500 cell count of marrow and 200 cell count of blood, noting that in acute promyelocytic leukemia (APML) promyelocytes are included in the blast percentage, and in acute monocytic leukemia, promonocytes are included.

Immunophenotypically f4.84, the general features of AML include the expression of CD13, CD33, HLA-DR, and CD45. APML is usually negative for HLA-DR, however. CD34 is often present, but in subtypes with maturation may be absent. AML is usually negative for lymphoid markers, but a significant minority expresses CD7 and/or CD19. Flow cytometry is a sensitive and widely available means of detecting minimal residual disease (MRD). MRD is that level of residual disease that is undetectable by light microscopic examination; it is estimated that visual examination of marrow is sensitive to ~1-5% leukemic blasts. Flow cytometry is sensitive to as little as 0.001% leukemic blasts, with enhanced sensitivity if there are previously defined immunophenotypic aberrations.

The 2008 WHO classification t4.45 recognizes 4 major categories of AML. The first category is AML with recurrent genetic abnormalities, a group of well characterized clinicopathologic entities. The second and third categories include AMLs arising secondary to therapy or myelodysplasia. The fourth category consists of all remaining cases (AML, NOS), which are further subclassified according to a system resembling the old French-American-British (FAB) categories. AML, NOS may have normal or abnormal cytogenetics and a variety of genetic anomalies, so long as none in the first category is present.

t4.45 **Classification of AML**

Group	Category	Morphology	Immunophenotype	Molecular	Age	Prognosis
AML with recurrent genetic abnormalities	t(8;21)	Abundant grey-blue cytoplasm, Auer rods, large granules (M2-like)	CD34+, HLA-DR+, CD13+, CD33+, CD19±,	*RUNX1/RUNX1T1* (*AML1/ETO*)	Young adult	Favorable
	inv(16) or t(16;16)	M4-like, increased/abnormal eosinophils	CD34+, HLA-DR+, CD13+, CD33+, CD11b+, CD14+, CD64+	*MYH11/CBFβ*	Young adult	Favorable
	t(15;17)	Promyelocytes	CD34–, HLA-DR–, CD13+, CD33+, CD15±, CD2±	*PML/RARα*	Middle age	Favorable
	t(9;11)	M5-like	CD34–, HLA-DR+, CD13+, CD33+, CD56±, CD14+, CD64+, CD11b+	*MLLT3/MLL*	Children	Intermediate
	t(6;9)	Any, especially M4, with basophilia	CD34+, HLA-DR+, CD13+, CD33+, Tdt±	*DEK/NUP214*	Children & adults	Poor
	t(1;22)	Megakaryocytic (M7-like)	CD34–, HLA-DR–, CD13+, CD33+, CD41+, CD61+	*RBM15/MKL1*	Infants	Intermediate
	inv(3) or t(3;3)	M0, M1, or M7-like. Thrombocytosis, giant agranular platelets		*RPN1/EVI1*	Adults	Poor
AML, therapy related		Multilineage dysplasia, RS, increased basophils	CD34+, HLA-DR+, CD13+, CD33+, CD56+	Topo II: 11q23 (*MLL*) or 21q22 (*RUNX1*)	T + 5 years	Poor
AML with myelodysplasia related changes		Variable	Variable	MDS-like	Elderly	Slowly progressive, unresponsive to treatment
AML, NOS	AML, NOS, M0	Undifferentiated blasts, <3% positive for SBB or MPO	CD34+, HLA-DR+, CD13+, CD33+, CD117+	No reproducible findings		Poor
	AML, NOS, M1	≥3% positive for SBB or MPO	CD34+, HLA-DR+, CD13+, CD33+, CD117+	No reproducible findings		Poor
	AML, NOS, M2	Abundant grey-blue cytoplasm, Auer rods, large granules	CD34+, HLA-DR+, CD13+, CD33+, CD117+	No reproducible findings		Variable
	AML, NOS, M4	Monocytic cells >20%, granulocytic cells >20%	CD34–/+, HLA-DR+, CD13+, CD33+, CD117+, CD14+, CD11b+, CD64+	No reproducible findings		Variable
	AML, NOS, M5	≥80% show monocytic differentiation	CD34–/+, HLA-DR+, CD13+, CD33+, CD117+, CD14+, CD11b+, CD64+	No reproducible findings		Poor
	AML, NOS, M6 (erythroleukemia)	≥50% erythroblasts & ≥20% myeloblasts in nonerythroid cells	CD34–/+, HLA-DR+, CD13+, CD33+, CD117+, CD235 (glycophorin)+	No reproducible findings		Poor
	AML, NOS, M7 (megakaryoblastic)	Blasts with blebbing	CD34–/+, HLA-DR–/+, CD13+, CD33+, CD117+, CD41+, CD61+	No reproducible findings		Poor

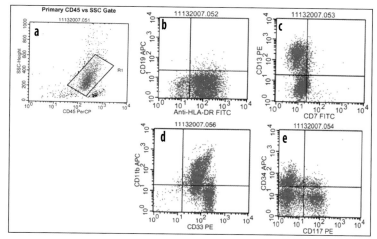

f4.84 AML flow cytometry in a case with monoblastic differentiation
a Gating around cells with dim CD45 & moderate side scatter (SSC); depending upon the morphology of the blasts, they may have minimal to moderate side scatter
b Plot of HLA-DR vs CD19, in which the neoplastic cells have expression of HLA-DR but no CD19 expression; most types of AML express HLA-DR, with the notable exception of acute promyelocytic leukemia; CD19 may be anomalously expressed, particularly in AML with t(8;21)
c Variable expression of CD13 & no expression of CD7; anomalous CD7 expression is not uncommon in AML
d Expression of CD33 & variable CD11b, typical of monoblasts
e Variable expression of CD34; CD34 is positive in most cases of AML but may be lost in more differentiated forms, such as acute promyelocytic leukemia & M5

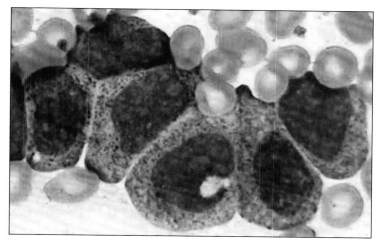

f4.85 AML with t(8;21)

AML with t(8;21)(q22;q22)

AML with t(8;21)(q22;q22) accounts for 8-10% of all de novo cases of AML. This translocation results in the transposition of the AML1 (*RUNX1*) and ETO (*RUNX1T1*) genes. The AML1 gene encodes the α chain of core binding factor (CBFα). This translocation may be found by conventional cytogenetics, or with greater sensitivity by FISH or PCR.

The blasts are characterized by pronounced azurophilic granularity **f4.85**, sometimes having large (pseudo Chédiak-Higashi) granules, and Auer rods. Such blasts would

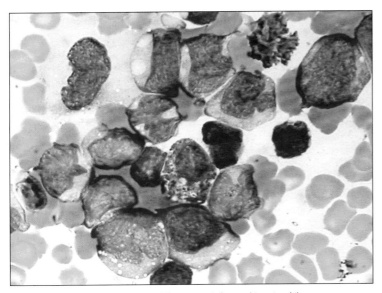

f4.86 AML with t(16;16); note monocytic differentiation & dysmorphic eosinophils

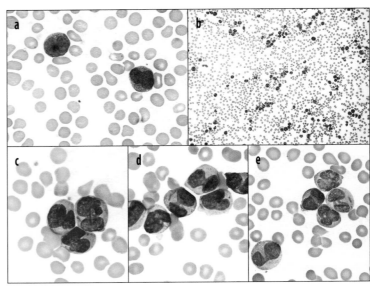

f4.87 Acute promyelocytic leukemia (APML)
a In the classic variant, there is usually a low blast count & cytoplasmic granules are prominent
b-e In the microgranular variant, there is usually a high blast count & granules are absent; the cells are notable for indented nuclei & occasional Auer rods

otherwise be characterized as AML with maturation (FAB M2). Dysplastic mature granulocytes are present in the blood and marrow, displaying pseudo-Pelger-Huët nuclei and homogeneous pink cytoplasm.

Immunophenotypically, the blasts express CD34, CD13, CD33, CD56, and HLA-DR. Many express CD15. In most cases, the blasts also express CD19, a significant clue to the possibility of t(8;21). In fact, one study found that 100% of AML cases expressing CD19, CD56, and CD34 had t(8;21). Lack or diminution of CD19 expression, with retention of CD56 expression, in a t(8;21)+ AML is correlated with the presence of coexisting *KIT* mutations (see below).

AML with t(8;21) tends to affect young adults and to be relatively chemosensitive, with overall 96% rate of remission and 70% 5-year survival. A subset of cases displays a tenacious tendency to relapse. In this subset of cases, there is a high rate of activating *KIT* mutations.

AML with inv(16)(p13q22) or t(16;16)(p13;q22)

AML with inv(16)(p13q22) or t(16;16)(p13;q22) harbors translocations that result in the apposition of the *MYH11* (myosin) and *CBFβ* genes. This may be found by conventional cytogenetics, or with greater sensitivity by FISH or PCR. The blasts demonstrate myelomonocytic differentiation and are found in association with abnormal eosinophils f4.86. The eosinophils have abnormally large granules, some of them basophilic, that stain positively with α naphthyl acetate esterase (negative in normal eosinophils). There is usually no eosinophilia in the peripheral blood. The designation acute myelomonocytic leukemia with eosinophilia (M4Eo) was given to this type of neoplasm in the FAB. Immunophenotypically, the blasts express CD13, CD33, CD14, CD64, CD11b, HLA-DR, lysozyme, and often express CD2. AML with inv(16)(p13q22) or t(16;16)(p13;q22) affects younger adults and is relatively chemosensitive.

AML with t(15;17)(q22;q21)—acute promyelocytic leukemia (APML)

AML with t(15;17)(q22;q21) is the FAB subtype AML M3, also called acute promyelocytic leukemia (APML). It is important to recognize because of its tendency to present in DIC and its responsiveness to all trans retinoic acid (ATRA). The age associated incidence of APML is as a plateau beginning in the late teen years and extending to the age of 60 years. This is in marked contrast to other subtypes of AML, whose incidence increases steadily with age.

APML f4.87 is a neoplasm of abnormal promyelocytes that have kidney shaped or bilobed nuclei, with cytoplasm varying from intensely granulated to agranular (microgranular variant). The microgranular variant may resemble acute monocytic leukemia. The MPO reaction is quite strong in both variants, sometimes obscuring nuclei, being weak or negative in monoblasts. The typical (hypergranular) variant often presents with very few leukemic cells in the peripheral blood, while the microgranular variant presents with a high blast count. The neoplastic cells express CD33 and CD13 strongly and express CD15 weakly (in contrast to normal promyelocytes that ar CD15 bright). They are negative for HLA-DR and CD34 f4.88. CD34 and HLA-DR expression may be features of so-called variant M3 (M3v), in addition to expression of CD2.

The defining chromosomal abnormality, t(15;17) results in juxtaposition of the retinoic acid receptor (RARα) gene and the PML gene. Several variant translocations involving RARα have been documented, usually resulting in morphologic APML that is relatively insensitive to ATRA; these include t(11;17) and t(5;17). In addition, there are 3 major RARα breakpoints—bcr1 (located within intron 6), bcr2 (exon 6), and bcr3 (intron 3)—that lead to the production of 3 different transcripts—long, variable, and short. This last transcript (short, bcr3) may have the features of variant M3 (M3v), with shorter survival and relative insensitivity to ATRA.

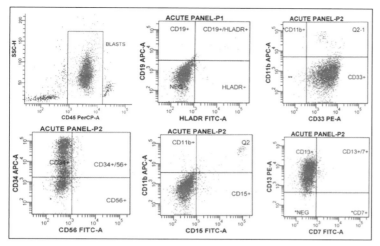

f4.88 APML flow cytometry
a Gating around cells with dim CD45 & moderate side scatter (SSC)
b Plot of HLA-DR vs CD19, in which the neoplastic cells do not express HLA-DR or CD19
c Homogeneous expression of CD33 with no expression of CD11b
d Variable expression of CD34, which is often entirely absent in APML
e CD15 expression is absent
f CD13 is expressed

Suspicion of APML requires urgent communication with the treating physician. Most oncologists prefer to await molecular confirmation before administering definitive treatment, but differentiation therapy (ATRA) and supportive therapy should commence immediately if clinicopathologic features support the diagnosis of APML. Molecular testing can be commenced on peripheral blood samples, to avoid waiting for bone marrow sampling. If bone marrow is subsequently obtained, it is wise to also order molecular testing on the marrow aspirate, in case the peripheral blood is insufficient. Conventional cytogenetics should be initiated, mostly to exclude other forms of AML, but is usually not sufficiently sensitive or timely to detect t(15;17). RT-PCR is capable of characterizing the specific breakpoint for future evaluation of MRD, but it takes days to get results and may miss cryptic rearrangements. FISH is both timely and sensitive.

Therapy is usually initiated without awaiting molecular confirmation, because hemorrhagic complications may otherwise occur. All-trans retinoic acid (ATRA; tretinoin) represents the earliest example of targeted therapy for cancer. It is usually employed in conjunction with anthracycline-based chemotherapy or arsenic trioxide (ATO). Before ATRA, survival rates with conventional chemotherapy were in the range of 35%; furthermore, conventional chemotherapy often had the effect of provoking or worsening coagulopathy. Survival rates now exceed 70%. Supportive care is aimed primarily at detecting and treating coagulopathy and preventing and treating differentiation syndrome (DS). DS, also called retinoic acid syndrome, is a potentially life threatening complication of treatment with ATRA. It presents with fever, weight gain, anasarca, effusions, hypotension, and renal failure. The overall incidence was as high as 20% before the recognition that dexamethasone treatment can prevent or ameliorate it; with dexamethasone, the incidence is around 1%. DS is bimodal, with peaks observed in the first and third weeks of treatment. Risk is correlated with initial WBC count $>5 \times 10^9$/L.

AML with t(9;11)(p22;q23)—AML with MLL gene anomalies

AML with t(9;11)(p22;q23) is common in children. The leukemic cells usually show monoblastic (FAB M4-M5) differentiation, with expression of CD4, CD14, CD64, CD11b, and lysozyme. CD34 is usually negative. The 11q23 locus contains the *MLL* gene. Most cases of AML that harbor *MLL* abnormalities have a poor prognosis, but AML with t(9;11)(p22;q23) has a better prognosis than other 11q23 aberrations, and an intermediate prognosis overall. Cytogenetics has limited sensitivity for 11q23 rearrangements; furthermore, cytogenetics cannot distinguish 11q23 rearrangements with and without *MLL* abnormalities. FISH is significantly more sensitive and is capable of making the *MLL* distinction. The most common rearrangements are t(9;11)(p21;q23), producing an *MLL/AF9* gene fusion, and t(4;11), producing the *MLL/AF4* gene fusion and common in infants.

AML with t(9;22)—Philadelphia chromosome positive AML

This is not yet a WHO-recognized subtype of AML but is notable for its uniquely bad behavior. Philadelphia chromosome positive AML here refers to de novo AML with t(9;22) rather than post-CML transformation into AML, but it is debatable whether such cases merely represent transformation of subclinical CML. Most such cases harbor a typical p210 *BCR-ABL* translocation.

AML with FLT3 mutation

The WHO classification does not recognize AML with *FLT3* internal tandem duplication (ITD) mutation as a distinct entity, but this anomaly is present in a sizable proportion of cytogenetically normal cases of AML. FLT3+ AML is notable for minimally differentiated to monoblastic morphology, poor outcome, and aberrant expression of CD7.

AML with myelodysplasia related changes

AML with myelodysplasia related changes t4.46 represents ~30% of AML. It affects mainly the elderly and often follows a period of antecedent MDS, but it may arise de novo. By definition, these cases of AML have one of 3 features: evolution from known MDS, certain MDS associated cytogenetic abnormalities, or dysplasia within >50% of the cells in ≥2 cell lines. They may present with any variety of immunophenotype, but are typically CD34, CD13, and CD33+. The genetics are typically quite complex, reflecting an evolving myelodysplastic substrate. The prognosis is relatively poor; these leukemias are unresponsive to treatment though slowly progressive.

t4.46 Criteria for AML with myelodysplasia related changes

1. At least	20% blasts
2. And one of	History of MDS
	MDS-related cytogenetic abnormality
	Multilineage dysplasia (>50% of 2 cell lines)
3. And absence of	Prior cytotoxic chemotherapy
	Any of the "AML with recurrent genetic abnormality" abnormalities

AML, *therapy related*

Therapy related AML and MDS may result from treatment with topoisomerase II inhibitors, alkylating agents, or ionizing radiation. There is an average latency of 5 years (1-5 for topo II inhibitors, 5-10 for alkylating agents and radiation) following treatment, and the incidence is dose dependent. The response to treatment is poor.

AML, NOS

AML, NOS, minimally differentiated (FAB M0) is an acute leukemia whose blasts have agranular cytoplasm which lacks cytochemical evidence of myeloid differentiation. That is, <3% of blasts stain positively with SBB, MPO, and NSE. Myeloid differentiation, therefore, is demonstrable only by immunophenotyping (or ultrastructural cytochemical reactions which are rarely available). The blasts typically express myeloid markers (CD13, CD33, CD117), CD34, and HLA-DR. Myeloid antigens indicative of greater degrees of maturation (CD14, CD15, CD11b) are negative. Lymphoid antigens are usually negative or of low intensity, and Tdt is positive in up to 30% of cases. The prognosis is poor.

AML, NOS, without maturation (FAB M1) is defined as acute leukemia in which >90% of blasts show no maturation (maturation in 10% or fewer blasts). The cells may display obvious granulation or Auer rods, but often do not. At least 3% of the blasts stain with MPO, CAE, or SBB. The cells usually express CD34, CD13, CD33, HLA-DR, and CD117. Prognosis is poor.

AML, NOS, with maturation (FAB M2) is acute leukemia with maturation in >10% of blasts; undifferentiated myeloblasts represent <89% of cells. Monocytic differentiation is present in <20% of nonerythroid cells (or else M4/M5 must be considered). Cytoplasmic granulation and Auer rods are frequent. Neoplasms with this type of morphology may turn out to have the t(8;21) translocation, requiring reclassification as such. M2 blasts may or may not express CD34, but they are usually positive for HLA-DR, CD13, CD33, CD117, and CD15. Abnormalities of chromosome 12p may be present and are associated with increased basophils. AML with maturation is frequently responsive to therapy.

Acute myelomonocytic leukemia (FAB M4) is diagnosed when, amongst nonerythroid cells, there are ≥20% with monocytic and ≥20% with neutrophilic maturation. The immunophenotype is typically myelomonocytic: CD13, CD33, CD4, CD14, CD64, CC11b positive. A smaller population of cells may be CD34+. M4 is frequently responsive to therapy.

Acute monocytic/monoblastic leukemia (FAB M5) demonstrates monocytic differentiation f4.89 in over >80% of nonerythroid cells (including monoblasts, promonocytes, and monocytes). Monoblast nuclei are round, contain lacy chromatin, and nucleoli. Monoblasts have abundant cytoplasm that is usually basophilic, and may show pseudopod formation. Promonocytes have infolded or lobated nuclei, with nucleoli. The cytoplasm is lighter blue-gray, and it may display granules and/or vacuoles. M5a (WHO acute monoblastic leukemia) exists when >80% of the monocytic cells are monoblasts, while M5b (WHO acute monocytic leukemia) has <80% monoblasts. Prominence of promonocytes, with their lobated nuclei, may lead to confusion with the microgranular variant of acute promyelocytic leukemia. The distinction is easily made with

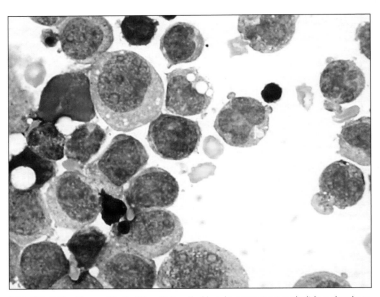

f4.89 AML, NOS, with monoblastic differentiation; the blasts have prominent nucleoli & an abundance of pale blue cytoplasm with occasional vacuoles

cytochemistry, flow, and/or cytogenetics. Flow cytometry shows expression of HLA-DR, monocytic markers (CD4, CD14, CD64, CD11b, lysozyme), variable myeloid markers (CD13, CD33, CD117), and a usually negative CD34. The translocation t(8;16) is sometimes present, and this is associated with the presence of hemophagocytosis by the neoplastic cells. M5 is apt to affect younger individuals and often manifests bleeding disorders and some degree of soft tissue infiltration, notably gingival enlargement and CNS infiltration. The course is variable but the prognosis is relatively poor.

Acute erythroid leukemia (FAB M6, diGuglielmo syndrome) is fairly rare. The WHO recognizes 2 subtypes. In the more common erythroleukemia subtype, >50% of all nucleated cells are erythroids f4.90 and >20% of nonerythroids are myeloblasts. In the extremely rare pure erythroid leukemia subtype (true erythroleukemia, acute erythremic myelosis), >80% of all nucleated cells are erythroid precursors; the neoplastic cells are immature erythroids without an excess of myeloblasts. Peripheral anemia, not erythrocytosis, is the rule, often with numerous circulating nRBCs. In the marrow, both the erythroid precursors and the myeloids are dysplastic and megaloblastoid. Erythroid cytoplasm may contain vacuoles and display globular PAS positivity (like ALL blasts are prone to do). The myeloblast population variably express CD34, HLA-DR, CD13, CD33, and CD117. The erythroid population expresses HLA-DR, CD34, glycophorin (CD235a), and CD71 (which may be aberrantly dim). M6 responds poorly to treatment and has a poor prognosis. The natural history is characterized by a progressive expansion in the myeloblast population, such that the marrow devolves into something resembling AML, NOS, M1-M2. The differential diagnosis includes other acute leukemias (particularly therapy related and myelodysplasia related) and myelodysplasia. B_{12} and folate deficiency must be excluded, particularly in the pure erythroid leukemia subtype; in B_{12} and folate deficiency, the dysplastic features are not quite as pronounced. Toxic exposures, such as

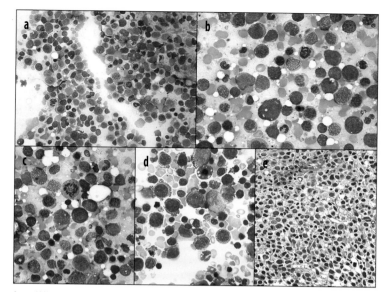

f4.90 AML, NOS, with erythroid maturation; note the predominance of erythroid precursors, many of which have dyspoietic morphology

arsenic and heavy metals, and erythropoietin therapy should be excluded. Note also that cases with >50% erythroids but <20% myeloblasts may be classified as MDS (RAEB), and cases with dysplasia in more than just the erythroid series may qualify as AML with myelodysplasia related changes. Lastly, therapy related AML often demonstrates a marked erythroid hyperplasia.

Also rare is acute megakaryoblastic leukemia (FAB M7). The criteria for M7 are that >50% of blasts are demonstrably megakaryocytic, either by the platelet peroxidase (PPO) technique (electron microscopy with staining for peroxidase), or by immunophenotyping (CD41 or CD61). There is an association with mediastinal germ cell tumors, with both neoplasms demonstrating i(12p). Note also that the AMLs and transient myeloproliferative disorders (TMD) that are associated with Down syndrome most often take the form of an M7 AML.

Acute basophilic leukemia is rare, if it exists at all as a distinct entity. Other AML types may demonstrate basophilic differentiation, notably AML with t(9;22) and AML with t(6;9). AML with inv(16) demonstrates abnormal basophil-like eosinophils.

Acute panmyelosis with myelofibrosis is defined as an acute neoplastic proliferation of pan-myeloid elements, in conjunction with marrow fibrosis. End-stage MPN, AML with myelodysplasia related changes, and M7 AML must be excluded.

Acute leukemia in Down syndrome (DS)

There is a many-fold increased risk of acute leukemia in DS, somewhat evenly divided between lymphoblastic (ALL) and myeloblastic (AML) phenotypes. In contrast to AML in non-DS children, DS associated AML shows increased chemosensitivity, particularly to methotrexate (MTX), a relatively favorable prognosis, and a peculiar tendency towards megakaryoblastic differentiation. This subtype is unusual overall and exceedingly rare in karyotypically normal children.

DS associated AML arises at an early age (1-5 years) in 1-2% of children with DS.

Transient myeloproliferative disorder (TMD), also called transient abnormal myelopoiesis (TAM), arises in ~10% of neonates with DS. TMD nearly always arises in the first week of life (ranging from 30 weeks' gestation to 6 months of age). It presents with a very high white cell count and hepatosplenomegaly. It is somewhat difficult to distinguish from congenital acute leukemia, but when the newborn has the obvious stigmata of DS, it is best to err on the side of TMD and withhold treatment. However, many cases arise in trisomy 21 mosaics or, in some cases, the trisomy 21 anomaly is confined to the clone itself. Thus, in children with apparent congenital acute leukemia, a crucial first step in the evaluation, regardless of the child's appearance, is cytogenetics. Some patients develop hepatic fibrosis, attributed to megakaryoblast infiltration of the liver; others may develop heart failure. But in most, there is complete clinicopathologic resolution without therapy. Nonetheless, ~30% of children with TMD go on to develop true DS associated AML during childhood.

Somatic (acquired, not germline) mutations in the *GATA-1* gene are present in the blasts of both TMD and DS associated AML. In both DS associated AML and TMD, the blasts type as megakaryoblastic or mixed megakaryoblasts-erythroblasts. TMD blasts are reported to be negative for CD11b and CD13, positive for CD34; in contrast to true DS associated AML which expresses CD11b and CD13 and is negative for CD34.

Congenital acute leukemia

Congenital acute leukemia is arbitrarily defined as an acute leukemia presenting before the age of 4 weeks and must be distinguished from a leukemoid reaction (sepsis, hemolytic disease of the newborn) and TMD. In contrast to other childhood acute leukemias, congenital acute leukemia is most commonly (~65%) myeloblastic (AML). About 25% is lymphoblastic (ALL), and most of the remaining cases have mixed lineage. While the vast majority of congenital AML falls into the M4/M5 category, TMD usually has an M7 phenotype and, of course, trisomy 21. A large proportion of newborns and infants with AML have associated leukemia cutis, often described as "blueberry muffin" babies. A significant minority (~10%) of congenital acute leukemias have abnormalities of 11q23 (*MLL* gene).

Mast cell neoplasms

Mastocytosis is a term that encompasses a group of disorders ranging from the solitary cutaneous mastocytoma to systemic mastocytosis. Types of cutaneous mastocytosis include solitary mastocytoma, diffuse erythrodermic mastocytosis, telangiectasia macularis eruptiva perstans (TMEP), and urticaria pigmentosa (UP). UP is the most common form and is characterized by oval or round red-brown macules. Urtication upon stroking is characteristic of these lesions and is called the Darier sign. Systemic mastocytosis is a multifocal disease that may involve the skin, spleen, bone marrow, and GI tract.

Useful laboratory tests include the serum tryptase level, urine N-methylhistamine (NMH), and urine prostaglandin D2 (PGD2). Histamine levels are elevated but nonspecific, as hypereosinophilic states can also raise histamine.

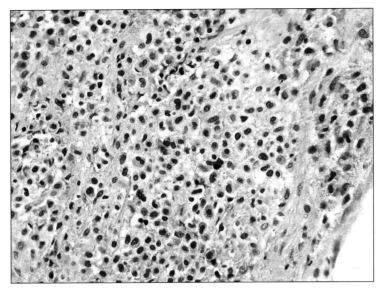

f4.91 Mastocytosis in marrow; sheets of cells with pale granular cytoplasm, in this case demonstrating predominantly round cell morphology; other cases have predominantly spindled morphology

Systemic mastocytosis appears in the marrow f4.91 as spindled or round cell infiltrates, usually accompanied by fibrosis and a smattering of eosinophils. Thus, the differential includes a wide range of entities—spindle cell infiltrates such as AILT; fibrotic processes such as MPD, HL, and HCL; round cell processes such as PLL and HCL.

Nonneoplastic mast cells are consistently positive for LCA, CD11c, CD33, CD43, CD117, and FcεRI. They are negative for CD25 and CD34, in addition to the plasma cell marker CD138, the monocyte markers CD14 and CD15, and the lymphoid markers CD2, CD3, CD5, CD19, and CD20. Neoplastic mast cells usually demonstrate an abnormal phenotype with aberrant expression of CD25 and CD2, often with diminished intensity of expression of CD117.

Expression of CD25 correlates with the presence of *CKIT* mutation and is indicative of malignancy. The most common *CKIT* mutation is the D816V mutation found in exon 816.

The diagnostic criteria for mastocytosis include a single major criterion and 4 minor criteria; the diagnosis is predicated upon fulfillment of the major criterion or 3 of the minor criteria. The major criterion is morphologic evidence of a mastocytoma (a discrete tissue infiltrate of essentially pure mast cells). The minor criteria are

1. prominent (>25%) spindling in the mast cells

2. expression of CD25

3. activating *CKIT* mutation in codon 816

4. chronic elevation (>20 ng/mL) of serum tryptase

Methods
RBC indices
Manual techniques

The manual hematocrit is performed by simply centrifuging a tube of whole blood. The ratio of the packed RBC column height to the total height is the hematocrit (Hct). Sometimes a capillary tube is used (internal bore of 1 mm); in this procedure, commonly called microhematocrit, blood is drawn up by capillary action, capped with wax, and centrifuged. The Hct is a unitless value (mm/mm) expressed as a percentage.

With the use of a hemocytometer, erythrocytes, leukocytes, and platelets can be counted manually. A hemocytometer (counting chamber) is an etched glass chamber with raised sides that holds a coverslip exactly 0.1 mm (0.01 cm) above the chamber floor. A pipette is used to dispense whole blood into the notched edge of the hemocytometer and allowed to fill the chamber by capillary action. The counting chamber is etched in a total surface area of 9 mm^2. The cell concentration is based upon the number of cells counted and the volume examined. One large square has a volume of 0.0001 mL (0.1 cm × 0.1 cm × 0.01 cm).

When Hct and RBC count are determined manually, the following calculations can be performed (note that mean corpuscular volume [MCV] is expressed in femtoliters (fL); 1 fL = 10^{-9} μL = 10^{-15} L; mean corpuscular hemoglobin concentration [MCHC] is expressed in g/dL)

$$MCV = Hct \times 10/RBC$$
(where Hct is expressed as a %, eg, 42%)

$$MCHC = (Hgb/Hct) \times 100$$
(where Hct is expressed as a % and Hgb in g/dL)

The manual differential is performed most commonly by examining 100 cells and categorizing them according to lineage. This results in a percentage of neutrophils (bands and segmented neutrophils are generally lumped together), lymphocytes, monocytes, basophils, eosinophils, and any unusual cells present (metamyelocytes, myelocytes, blasts). This technique provides at best a broad stroke reflection of the true distribution of cells and is prone to statistical error, by virtue of the relatively low number of events counted. There is also interobserver error; this error has profound impact on the band count (the separate enumeration of mature segmented neutrophils from bands), still considered crucial in some clinical circles. Interobserver agreement on the border between band and segmented neutrophil is dismal, and proficiency testing surveys have firmly established that this practice is too imprecise for clinical utility. Still, until recently there have been few alternatives; modern analyzers offer the ability to enumerate immature granulocytes with greater precision.

Automated techniques

Automated analyzers use a variety of methods, including impedance, optical, radio frequency, and conductivity, to detect and thereby count cells in a chamber. Overall, they provide excellent precision in most major parameters—the leukocyte count (WBC), RBC count (RBC), mean corpuscular volume (MCV), and hemoglobin (Hgb). There remains a high level of imprecision in platelet counts (Plt), particularly when counts are low. Automated analyzers are capable of producing a 5-part differential similar to that performed manually, only it does so based upon physic-optic analysis of thousands of cells, thereby reducing both statistical and interobserver error. 2 major hurdles have been the counting of bands, which has been impossible and generally relegated to a qualitative "flag," and the counting of basophils, which until recently has been inferior to manual counts.

Modern analyzers also offer qualitative information—generally called "flags"—that suggest the presence of abnormal cell types such as blasts, nucleated RBCs, and immature granulocytes. Such flags are generally calibrated to provide high sensitivity but low specificity; that is, many flags are false alarms. Many modern analyzers are capable of reporting new parameters that can be extremely helpful, including immature reticulocyte fraction, immature platelet fraction (reticulated platelets), immature granulocyte fraction (IG), schistocytes (FRBC), and reticulocyte hemoglobin concentration (CHr or Ret-He, depending upon the manufacturer). The immature reticulocyte fraction can be determined by automated analysis following incubation with dyes that bind RNA. The brighter the signal, the more immature the reticulocyte. This permits sensitive classification of anemia (hyper-regenerative vs hypo-regenerative) and early detection of marrow recovery or response to nutritional replenishment. Similarly, RNA-avid dyes can be used to provide an immature platelet fraction, useful for categorizing thrombocytopenic conditions as hyper-regenerative or hypo-regenerative. The mean platelet volume (MPV) has been a flawed surrogate for this, based upon the observation that there is an inverse relationship between platelet count and MPV in healthy subjects (the lower the platelet count, the higher the MPV, maintaining a steady overall platelet mass). Thus, barring the rare patient with congenital giant platelets, high MPV suggested a marrow response to peripheral platelet destruction/consumption. The immature granulocyte (IG) fraction is the sum of the metamyelocytes, myelocytes, and promyelocytes in the sample and has demonstrated utility in diagnosing sepsis, offering a superior alternative to the manual "band" count. Schistocytes can be enumerated using the platelet channel, with fragmented RBCs having size similar to, but refractive index different from, large platelets. The reticulocyte hemoglobin concentration (CHr or Ret-He) is a reflection of the availability of marrow iron (functional iron deficiency and actual iron deficiency).

In impedance counting, pioneered by Coulter, cells are suspended in a conductive diluent and passed one by one through an aperture across which a DC current flows. A cell within the aperture causes a momentary increase in electrical resistance (impedance). The instrument interprets a momentary increase in voltage as a single cell. The amount of voltage change is proportional to the size of the cell. Optical methods employ detectors to measure light scattered by the cell, including forward and side scatter; the degree of forward angle light scatter is proportional to the size of the cell, and side scatter is mainly affected by cell complexity. Conductivity, assessed with an AC current, provides a measure of the internal complexity of the cell (nuclear convolution and cytoplasmic granularity).

Hemoglobin (Hgb) is most commonly measured by the cyanohemoglobin, or hemiglobin cyanide (HiCN) method, in which lysed blood is dissolved in a solution of potassium ferricyanide and potassium cyanide which oxidizes Hb to hemiglobin cyanide (HiCN) whose concentration is measured by spectrophotometry. The absorbance at 540 nm reflects the amount of Hb. The HiCN method detects all forms of hemoglobin except sulfhemoglobin (SHb); that is, it detects unmodified Hb, hemiglobin (Hi), and carboxyhemoglobin (HbCO). Anything that raises the turbidity of blood, such as lipidemia and paraproteinemia, can falsely raise the hemoglobin measurement. Some instruments use a cyanide-free method, such as sodium lauryl sulfate (SLS), which still relies on absorbance.

Cell counts, such as the red blood cell count (RBC) and white blood cell count (WBC) are carried out by one of the particle detection methods mentioned above. As stated, impedance counting calibrates the amount of voltage change in proportional to cell size. If limits are set, the instrument can count all events within a range of sizes. Particles measuring between 36 and 360 fL are counted as RBCs. Note that leukocytes, which are within this size range, will be counted as erythrocytes, but (usually) their effect is negligible. Platelets are counted as particles <36 fL; note that falsely low platelet counts may result if platelets are abnormally large or if they are clumped.

The mean corpuscular volume (MCV) and RBC distribution width (RDW) are determined statistically. Once a large number of cells are analyzed, RBC size (volume) will be distributed in a roughly Gaussian fashion. The mean of this distribution is taken as the mean corpuscular volume (MCV); note that reticulocytes are larger than mature RBCs, such that pronounced reticulocytosis can raise the MCV. The coefficient of variation in the curve is the RBC distribution width (RDW). The RBC distribution width (RDW) is reflective of anisocytosis. RDW is useful in the differential diagnosis of microcytic anemia, for example, where RDW is higher in iron deficiency anemia than in thalassemia.

The rest of the RBC indices can be calculated

$$Hct = MCV \times RBC/10$$

$$MCHC = (Hgb/Hct) \times 100$$

The MCHC usually is in the range of 32-36%. High MCHC may indicate spherocytosis or cold agglutinin. This may also be seen in lipemic specimens.

When using automated hematology analyzers, it is important to have criteria for manual blood smear review. These include objective criteria for determining when a technologist must make and examine a smear and when such a smear should be submitted for pathologist review. The purpose of the blood smear review is to evaluate instrument "flags," to verify the automated indices prior to releasing the results, or to evaluate abnormal indices with a view towards making a specific diagnosis; after review, the automated indices may be altered or released unaltered, and an interpretive comment may be appended. In some cases, the instrument is incapable of providing an accurate differential for a variety of reasons, and a manual differential is undertaken; a manual differential is distinct from a blood smear review. Criteria for blood smear review may include such things as high and low cell counts, high and low differential counts, certain "flags," and significant changes from prior counts (deltas). One may choose to publish some criteria that apply only to first-time abnormalities.

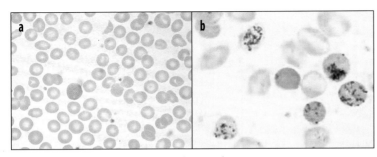

f4.92 Reticulocytes on a Wright stained smear & b supravital stain

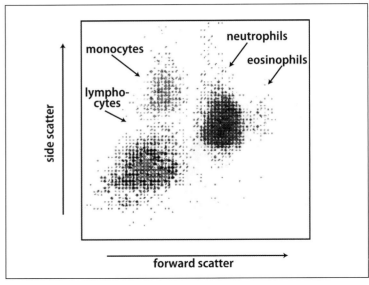

f4.93 Automated differential

Counting reticulocytes

Techniques for differentiation of reticulocytes from mature RBCs are based upon the abundance of ribosomal RNA in the reticulocyte f4.92. These techniques include manual counting by light microscopy, optical light scatter, and flow cytometry. In the first 2 methods, RBCs are stained with a supravital dye (eg, new methylene blue or azure B) which highlights residual cytoplasmic RNA. In flow cytometry, the cells are stained with an RNA-specific fluorochrome. Because of the large number of cells counted, automated techniques are much more precise than manual methods.

The reticulocyte count may be reported as a percentage of RBCs or as an absolute number/unit volume. The absolute number is calculated by multiplying the reticulocyte percentage by the RBC count. The reticulocyte percentage in normal adults is between 0.5-1.5%. In anemic patients, corrections must be made in order to properly interpret the reticulocyte percentage.

Absolute reticulocyte count = % reticulocytes × RBC count

Corrected reticulocyte count (CRC) = % reticulocytes × Hct/45

Reticulocyte production index (RPI) = CRC × 1/maturation index

The maturation index corrects for the longer life span of prematurely released reticulocytes in the blood, which is a phenomenon of increased RBC production t4.47.

t4.47 Maturation index

Maturation index	Hematocrit
1.0	36-45
1.5	26-35
2.0	16-25
2.5	≤15

Leukocyte indices

Total leukocyte count

RBCs are lysed, and the remaining cells are subjected to counting in a manner similar to that for RBCs. Particles larger than 36 fL are counted as leukocytes.

Leukocyte differential

Some instruments use light scatter to create a 5-part leukocyte differential f4.93. Others use light scatter combined with a peroxidase stain. Another approach is to assess differential resistance to lysis, particularly for enumerating eosinophils and basophils. For example, Coulter instruments create a 5-part differential by performing measurements of electrical impedance (varies with volume), electrical conductivity (cell complexity), and side-angle light scatter (cytoplasmic granularity). This "VCS" technology allows identification of neutrophils, lymphocytes, monocytes, eosinophils, and basophils.

All instruments are capable of "flagging" a specimen for various reasons. Often, this requires the preparation of a smear and manual review. For example, all can "flag" for immature granulocytes, requiring a manual review. Note that neither instruments nor humans can precisely count bands.

Platelet indices

Particles measuring between 2 fL and 20 fL are counted as platelets. In a manner analogous to the MCV, the mean platelet volume (MPV) is also determined. The platelet count is the least reliable of all the values generated by automated analyzers. This results from the wide range in platelet size, the tendency to overlap with RBCs at the high end of the range, and the overlap with debris at the low end. Furthermore, platelets may be consumed in an in vitro clot that forms as a result of inadequate anticoagulation. In some patients platelets tend to aggregate in either EDTA or citrate, resulting in a falsely low count. Platelet aggregates are not formed in samples collected in heparin. Platelet aggregates can be seen in the peripheral blood smear.

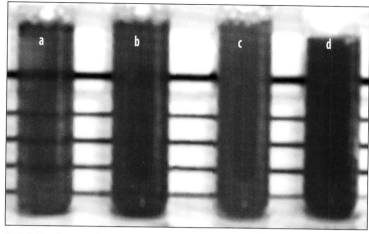

f4.94 Sickle cell screen; tubes **a** & **b** are negative (background lines can be seen throughout); tubes **c** (sickle trait) & **d** (sickle cell disease) are positive (lines obscured)

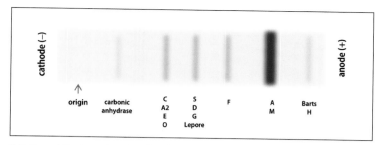

f4.96 Hemoglobin electrophoresis at pH 8.6 (alkaline electrophoresis), showing the positions of the various hemoglobin variants

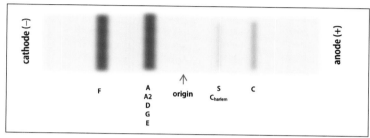

f4.97 Hemoglobin electrophoresis at pH 6.8 (acid electrophoresis), showing the positions of the various hemoglobins

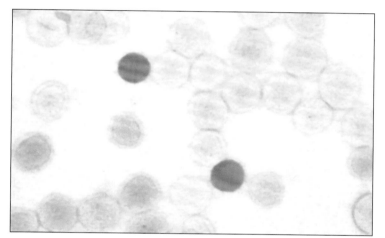

f4.95 Kleihauer-Betke preparation; the pale cells have no fetal hemoglobin, while the bright red cells have fetal hemoglobin

Detection of normal & variant hemoglobins

Rapid detection of hemoglobin S

The hemoglobin solubility (dithionate) test detects insoluble forms of hemoglobin within a lysate of blood. The development of marked turbidity is a positive screen f4.94. The test is sensitive to any hemoglobin with altered solubility; it may be positive in SS, SA, SC, SD, and C$_{Harlem}$. The dithionate test may be negative when the concentration of HbS is too small; eg, in neonates.

The sickling (metabisulfite) test detects cells that contain sickling hemoglobins. A smear is examined microscopically for sickling after metabisulfite is added. The metabisulfite test may be positive in SS, SA, SC, SD, and C$_{Harlem}$. The metabisulfite test requires ≥10% HbS to be positive; it may be falsely negative in neonates or the very aggressively transfused.

Detection of hemoglobin F

The acid elution technique (Kleihauer-Betke) may be used to detect RBCs containing HbF. In an acid buffer, HbA elutes from RBCs, but HbF does not. A smear is examined microscopically for cells with persistent eosinophilia following acid elution, to enumerate the cells containing HbF f4.95. 2 patterns may be observed in blood smears. The heterocellular pattern, in which some but not all cells contain HbF, is the most common pattern. This is typical of fetomaternal hemorrhage and thalassemia. The pancellular pattern, in which all cells contain HbF, is seen in hereditary persistence of fetal hemoglobin (HPFH).

The alkali denaturation technique may be used to quantify HbF. HbF is resistant to alkali denaturation (in 1.25 M NaOH). HbA is denatured and precipitated out; the optical density of the remaining supernatant reflects the quantity of HbF.

High pressure liquid chromatography (HPLC) provides a highly accurate method of HbF quantitation.

Hemoglobin electrophoresis

In routine hemoglobin electrophoresis f4.96, lysed blood on cellulose acetate at pH 8.6 (alkaline electrophoresis) is subjected to electromotive force, fixed, and stained. The normal adult has >97% HbA, <3% HbA2 (seen in the C band), and nothing else. The quantity of the Hb variants can be determined by densitometric reading of the gel. Densitometry is usually not sufficiently accurate for quantification of small quantities of HbA2 or HbF. A separate quantitative assay should be performed to obtain the exact amounts of HbA2 and HbF.

Hemoglobinopathies, caused by a structurally abnormal hemoglobin molecule, usually a distinct band on electrophoresis. The identity of many abnormal hemoglobins can be determined by routine electrophoresis, particularly when supplemented with some clinical information and CBC data. When there is uncertainty, electrophoresis on citrate agar f4.97 at pH 6.2 (acid electrophoresis) produces a different set of electrophoretic positions which, in combination with the alkaline gel, can help identify most, but not all, abnormal hemoglobins. Fast hemoglobins are those that migrate beyond HbA on the alkaline gel. Fast hemoglobins can be mimicked by hyperbilirubinemia, a common feature in neonates. The most commonly encountered fast hemoglobins are HbH and Hb Barts. When a band is present in the S region, its identity can be confirmed by the sickle screen. If the screen is negative, this may indicate D, G, or Lepore.

Thalassemia, being a quantitative defect in the production of entirely normal hemoglobins, does not produce abnormal bands on the electrophoresis. Instead, β thalassemia is diagnosed by the presence of "thalassemic indices" (low hematocrit, increased RBC count, low MCV) and a quantitatively increased HbA2. α thalassemia has "thalassemic indices" and normal HbA2.

Capillary electrophoresis is carried out using thin-bore capillary tubes within which there is a pH gradient. Hemoglobins migrate through the capillary tubes at differing rates, resulting in very good resolution of the hemoglobin variants present. In contrast to routine agar electrophoresis, the level of HbA2 can be accurately quantified even at low levels. Furthermore, HbE can be quantified separately from HbA2. HbC, if present still runs with HbA2, however.

High pressure liquid chromatography (HPLC)

Alkaline electrophoresis has limitations. For example, it is incapable of separating HbS from HbD, HbG, and Hb-Lepore. It does not resolve HbC, HbA2, HbO_{Arab}, and HbE. Acid electrophoresis is needed for clarifying these variants, but does not help to separate HbD from HbG and Hb-Lepore or HbE from HbO_{Arab}. Rare variants may be misinterpreted as a more common Hb variant. Lastly, electrophoresis does not permit accurate quantitation of A2 or F.

In HPLC, hemolysate is injected under high pressure into a column containing a negatively charged resin causing variable delay in elution of the positively charged hemoglobins. Individual molecules elute at different and characteristic rates, allowing identification of Hb variants f4.98. A light source produces a deflection on a spectrophotometer proportional to Hb variant concentration. The degree of separation is greater than electrophoresis permits, and A2 and F can be accurately quantified. One limitation with HPLC is that HbE and HbA2 have similar retention times, such that these hemoglobins cannot be easily separated. HbC and HbO_{Arab} also cannot easily separated for quantification. Note also that bilirubin elutes with Hb Barts on HPLC. Bilirubinemia should be excluded in HPLCs demonstrating Hb Barts; alternatively, confirmation by gel electrophoresis is an option.

Molecular methods for hemoglobin identification

~1-2% percent of variant hemoglobins detected by HPLC or gel electrophoresis cannot be definitively identified. Sequencing the hemoglobin gene by PCR can characterize the exact genotype for a given individual. This is especially useful in prenatal diagnosis, in which PCR can be used to sequence the hemoglobin gene from any sample of fetal tissue.

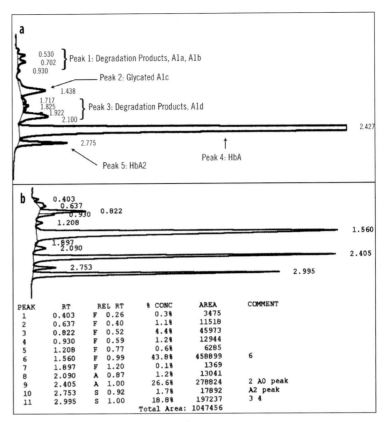

PEAK	RT	REL RT		% CONC	AREA	COMMENT
1	0.403	F	0.26	0.3%	3475	
2	0.637	F	0.40	1.1%	11518	
3	0.822	F	0.52	4.4%	45973	
4	0.930	F	0.59	1.2%	12944	
5	1.208	F	0.77	0.6%	6285	
6	1.560	F	0.99	43.8%	458899	6
7	1.897	F	1.20	0.1%	1369	
8	2.090	A	0.87	1.2%	13041	
9	2.405	A	1.00	26.6%	278824	2 A0 peak
10	2.753	S	0.92	1.7%	17892	A2 peak
11	2.995	S	1.00	18.8%	197237	3 4
					Total Area: 1047456	

f4.98 High pressure liquid chromatography (HPLC)
a HPLC in a patient with normal hemoglobin genotype; 5 major peak regions are present, including some caused by degradation products (peaks 1 & 3), the HbA$_{1c}$ peak (peak 2), the HbA peak (peak 4), and the HbA2 peak (peak 5)
b HPLC in a neonate with S trait, showing peaks for F, A & S

Hemoglobin oxygen saturation

Pulse oximetry is based upon 2 wavelengths of light-emitting diodes (LEDs), one that emits light at 660 nm (red) and another that emits at 940 nm (infrared). Deoxyhemoglobin has an absorption peak at 660 nm, while oxyhemoglobin has a peak at 940 nm. By simultaneously measuring at these wavelengths, the pulse oximeter can estimate arterial oxygen saturation (SaO_2). The pulse oximeter can identify only oxyhemoglobin and deoxyhemoglobin; it cannot measure carboxyhemoglobin, methemoglobin, or sulfhemoglobin and will therefore overestimate the oxygen saturation in these settings. Carboxyhemoglobin has an absorbance peak at approximately the same wavelength as oxyhemoglobin; therefore, the oxyhemoglobin saturation may be reported as quite artificially high. In contrast, while also overestimating the percent saturation, methemoglobin tends to produce a reading of ~85%. Arterial blood gas analyzers calculate the percent saturation after directly measuring the pH, PCO_2, and PO_2. The calculation assumes a normal Hb-O_2 saturation curve, normal 2,3-DPG, and an absence of abnormal hemoglobins. The cooximeter utilizes multiple wavelengths of light and can specifically measure carboxyhemoglobin and methemoglobin (in addition to oxyhemoglobin and deoxyhemoglobin).

Histochemistry & cytochemistry
Wright stain

The Wright stain is a Romanowsky type stain made by mixing methylene blue dye with eosin and alcohol. James Homer Wright did not invent the stain but refined it; it was first used by Romanowsky and first refined by Leishman. Credit goes to Dr Wright primarily for the many discoveries and careful descriptions he made using the stain, including the origin of blood platelets from marrow megakaryocytes and the derivation of multiple myeloma from plasma cells. In Wright stained smears, basic cellular components attract the acidic dye eosin; thus hemoglobin and the granules of eosinophils appear red. Acidic components of the cell, such as nucleic acids and ribosomes, take up the basic dye component, methylene blue. The term neutrophil derives from the fact that neutrophilic granules stain equally with the red and the blue and are thus "neutral." The pH must be carefully controlled through the use of a buffer. Too acidic and cells take on a pinkish tint and nuclear structures are obscure. Too alkaline and cytoplasmic structures turn blue-black and obscure.

Cytochemical stains for typing blasts t4.48

t4.48 Cytochemical stains for typing blasts						
Blast type	PAS	SBB	MPO	CAE	NSE	Auer rods
Undifferentiated (M0)	–	–	–	–	–	rare
Myeloblasts (M1, M2, M4)	–	+ black	+	+	–	50%
Promyelocytes (APML)	–	+ black	+	+	–	95%
Monoblasts (M4, M5)	–	–	–	–	+ Inhibited by NaF	0%
Erythroblasts	+ diffuse granular	–/+	–/+	–	–/+ Resists NaF	50%
Megakaryoblasts	+ diffuse granular	–	–	–	± Resists NaF	rare
Lymphoblasts	+ block, rosary bead	–/+ faint grey	–	–	–	–

Myeloperoxidase (MPO) stains the primary (azurophilic) granules of cells within the granulocytic line. Staining is coarse and Golgi-predominant. MPO is negative in lymphoblasts, erythroblasts, megakaryoblasts, most monoblasts (fine dusty positivity may be seen), and very early blasts. Note that MPO degrades quickly in wet specimens, but is stable in smears for up to a month. Because of rapid degradation, a negative MPO reaction should not by itself exclude AML. Sudan black B (SBB) stains lipid material, present in the granulocytic series, black. Reactivity parallels that of MPO, but some cases of ALL display faint light-grey granules. Chloroacetate esterase (CAE), also known as the Leder stain, is positive in granulocytic cells, including mast cells. It is frequently positive in abnormal (neoplastic) eosinophils but negative in normal eosinophils. Nonspecific esterases (NSE) comes in 2 varieties, α naphthyl acetate esterase and α naphthyl butyrate esterase. Both stain the monocytic series and, to lesser extents, megakaryocytic, lymphocytic, granulocytic, and erythroid series. The NSE activity of monocytes is inhibited by sodium fluoride (NaF). Periodic acid Schiff (PAS) is positive in most lymphoid and some myeloid blasts. ALL shows "block" positivity, often encircling the nucleus in a "rosary bead" fashion. AML may show diffuse, granular staining. The vacuoles of L3 blasts stain positively with the oil red O stain.

Leukocyte alkaline phosphatase (LAP) score

LAP hydrolyzes naphthol AS-biphosphate, a component of the neutrophil granule, to form a colored product. The LAP score is derived by visual examination of 100 bands and neutrophils, scoring each cell on the basis of the intensity of cytoplasmic staining from 0-4+. The sum of the 100 values is the LAP score. Normal adults have an LAP score between 40 and 120. In chronic myelogenous leukemia (CML), the score is typically low, between 0 and 15. Other conditions with low LAP score include paroxysmal nocturnal hemoglobinuria, some myelodysplastic syndromes, congenital hypophosphatasia, and neonatal septicemia (LAP paradoxically decreased). Elevated LAP score is seen in the leukemoid reaction (reactive neutrophilia), polycythemia vera, primary myelofibrosis, glucocorticoid administration, and third trimester of pregnancy.

Immunophenotyping
Flow cytometry

Flow cytometry is a technique that is capable of detecting cell surface expression of a large number of antigens. In some instances, it can be adapted to detecting intracytoplasmic expression, such as for expression of light chains in plasma cells. The specimen is distributed among several tubes into which are added various fluorochrome-labeled antibodies against cell surface antigens. The "stained" cells are run through the flow cytometer, and as a cell passes through the counting chamber multiple parameters are measured: size (forward light scatter [FLS]), nuclear complexity/cytoplasmic granularity (90° light scatter or side scatter [SSC]), and the intensity of fluorochrome on the cell surface.

Fluorochromes are substances that absorb light at a certain wavelength and emit it at a different wavelength. This difference in absorbed and emitted wavelength is essential so that one can simultaneously detect both the original wavelength (to determine size and complexity characteristics of the cell) and the fluorochrome-emitted wavelength (to determine antigen expression), and this difference is called the Stokes shift. Common fluorochromes include fluorescein isothiocyanate (FITC), allophycocyanin (APC), and phycoerythrin (PE), but there are many.

The simplest flow cytometers have the capacity to analyze 2 fluorochromes simultaneously (2-color flow cytometry). Recently, instruments that can simultaneously detect up to 10 fluorochromes simultaneously have become commercially available. This allows not only an increase in the number of queried antigens but also the ability to informatively evaluate smaller samples in a fewer number of tubes.

Gating, in which cells of interest are digitally selected for consideration, is the key first step in flow interpretation. For example, if one seeks to examine lymphocytes in a sample, one could "gate" around those cells which have low side scatter and strong CD45 expression on a graph of CD45 expression vs side scatter. Plasma cells can be selected out of a mixed population (eg, bone marrow) with CD45 vs CD38 gating, wherein the plasma cells have very low CD45 and very high CD38 expression.

Immunohistochemistry

Antibodies are tagged with an enzymatic chromagen to allow visualization of antibody binding to corresponding surface and cytoplasmic antigens. Many but not all antigens detectable by flow cytometry are also detectable by immunohistochemistry.

Antigens

Alk is expressed in anaplastic large cell lymphoma (ALCL) that is t(2;5)+. It is also commonly expressed in inflammatory myofibroblastic tumor from multiple sites.

bcl-1 (cyclin D1, prad1) is expressed in mantle cell lymphoma. Hairy cell leukemia and plasma cell myeloma are also sometimes bcl-1+. Numerous epithelia and epithelial neoplasms express bcl-1, including breast and colon.

bcl-2, in normal and reactive lymph nodes, is expressed by T cells, mantle B cells and the small number of mantle B cells that normally permeate the follicle center (this number is increased in follicular lysis). Expression by T cells makes it necessary to compare reactivity to concomitant expression of CD3 and CD20. bcl-2 is expressed by most low grade B cell lymphomas and many high grade B cell lymphomas. Expression in follicular lymphoma decreases with grade, varying from >95% in grade 1 to 75% in grade 3. Thus, bcl-2 is useful in distinguishing neoplastic from reactive germinal centers, but it is not useful to distinguish FL from other B cell lymphomas. In this latter regard, CD10 is preferable. bcl-2 is not expressed by Burkitt lymphoma, a fact that is helpful to separate Burkitt from Burkitt-like DLBCL. bcl-2 is expressed in a large proportion of breast carcinomas, and can be used to differentiate breast carcinoma from other sites of origin. Unfortunately, bcl-2 expression in breast cancer decreases with grade, such that ER negative tumors are likely to also be bcl-2 negative. Lastly, bcl-2 is expressed in a large proportion of solitary fibrous tumors and synovial sarcomas.

bcl-6 is strongly expressed in normal germinal center B cells. It is also expressed in some lymphomas, including Burkitt lymphoma, follicular lymphoma, nodular lymphocyte predominance Hodgkin lymphoma, anaplastic large cell lymphoma, and a subset of DLBCL. In DLBCL, bcl-6 overexpression has been associated with a translocation involving the bcl-6 gene on chromosome 3q and the IgH gene on 14q.

CD1a is expressed by Langerhans cells, dendritic reticulum cells, interdigitating reticulum cells, and cortical thymocytes. Langerhans cell histiocytosis is characterized by coexpression of S100 and CD1a.

CD2 is expressed by T lymphocytes and NK cells, even from a very early stage.

CD3 is expressed by T lymphocytes (mature nonneoplastic and neoplastic) in tight but noncovalent association with the TCR. The CD3 molecule is composed of 3 chains—γ, δ, and ϵ. Cytoplasmic expression precedes surface expression and may be detectable by immunohistochemistry (eg, in immature T cells and NK cells) when surface expression is not detected by flow cytometry. CD3 is not expressed on the surface of very immature T lymphocytes or NK cells.

CD4 is expressed by a subset of T lymphocytes, specifically, T-helper cells. It is also expressed by monocytes, histiocytes, and dendritic cells. The normal CD4:CD8 ratio in blood and tissue is 2-4:1. CD4+/CD8+ coexpressing T cells are normal only in the thymic cortex. Likewise CD4–/CD8– T cells are not normal and probably neoplastic. The vast majority of T cell neoplasms are CD4+.

CD5 is expressed by normal and neoplastic T cells and a small, normally inconspicuous, B cell subset. It is not expressed by NK cells. Occasional patients have increased (polyclonal, benign) circulating CD19+/CD20+/CD5+ B cells, particularly those with connective tissue diseases such as rheumatoid arthritis. CD5 coexpression in B cells is the hallmark of SLL/CLL and MCL. CD5 is sometimes lost in T cell neoplasms, a helpful clue if present. CD5 is expressed in most thymic carcinomas, a fact that can help distinguish them from lung and other primaries. CD5 expression in thymic carcinomas appears to be restricted to frank malignancies of the thymus; ie, the ones that would enter into the differential diagnosis of metastatic lesions. The so-called well differentiated thymic carcinomas in the Müller-Hermelink classification are typically CD5–.

CD7 is expressed by both T cells and NK cells. CD7 loss is a common form of aberrant phenotype in T cell neoplasms, particularly common in cutaneous T cell lymphoma/mycosis fungoides. CD7 is sometimes expressed in myeloblasts (~10% of cases—especially types M4 and M5).

CD8 is expressed by the CD4– subset of T lymphocytes and neoplastic NK, T cytotoxic and T suppressor cells.

CD10 (CALLA) is the antigen characteristic of follicle center lymphocytes, including follicle center B cells and T cells, and it is expressed by both normal and neoplastic follicle center cells. Thus it is expressed by follicular lymphoma, nodular lymphocyte predominant Hodgkin lymphoma, and angioimmunoblastic T cell lymphoma, neoplasms thought to be derived from follicle center lymphocytes. CD10 is also present on B cell acute lymphoblastic leukemia (B-ALL), normal granulocytes, and neoplastic plasma cells. Lastly, CD10 is expressed by a large number of nonhematolymphoid tumors, including renal cell carcinoma, tumors derived from endometrial stroma, hepatocellular carcinoma (in canalicular pattern), and a variable proportion of numerous other tumors.

CD11b (MAC-1) is normally expressed by monocytes & granulocytes. It is expressed by hairy cell leukemia.

CD11c (C3r) is normally expressed by monocytes & granulocytes. Amongst B cell neoplasms, CD11c expression is distinctive for CLL/SLL (weak and variable expression is characteristic) and hairy cell leukemia (bright expression).

CD13 is expressed by granulocytes and precursors. In acute leukemia, CD13 expression is characteristic of AML types M1, M2, M3 (APML), M4, M5, and M6 (not M7).

CD14 is a marker of monocytic differentiation and a variable marker of monocytic precursors. It is often (but not uniformly) expressed in AML types M4 and M5. It is also commonly expressed in B-CLL and FL.

CD15 (Leu-M1) is expressed in mature monocytes and granulocytes, Reed-Sternberg cells, and most adenocarcinomas. In practice, CD15 expression in Reed-Sternberg cells is somewhat unreliable, and positivity, when present, is often limited to faint Golgi zone staining. Its absence is a distinctive feature of anaplastic large cell lymphoma (ALCL). In the setting of AML, CD15 indicates a maturing phenotype; for example, it is strongly expressed in APML (M3).

CD16 is expressed by normal and neoplastic NK cells and granulocytes.

CD19 is expressed by B cells from the pre-B stage onward. It is expressed by normal plasma cells, but expression is typically lost in neoplastic plasma cells. CD19 is not expressed in classic Hodgkin lymphoma or T cell neoplasms. It is often dimly expressed in follicular lymphoma (FL). CD19 may be present on some myeloblasts, especially in AML with t(8;21) (q22;q22).

CD20 is expressed on the surface of mature B cells just after the appearance of CD19 and before CD22. It is not expressed by plasma cells. In classic Hodgkin lymphoma, Reed-Sternberg cells express CD20 in ~20% of cases (these are CD79a–). Nodular lymphocyte predominant Hodgkin lymphoma is uniformly CD20+. CD20 expression by CLL/SLL is distinctively dim. FMC-7 is an antibody that recognizes a particular epitope of CD20. Cells with weak CD20 (CLL/SLL) tend to be FMC-7–. Cells with bright CD20 (most other B-NHLs) tend to be FMC-7+.

CD23 (the IgE receptor) is useful in the distinction of CLL (CD23+) from MCL (CD23–).

CD25 (the IL-2 receptor) is expressed by activated lymphoid cells (T and B). It is characteristically expressed by hairy cell leukemia and adult T cell leukemia/lymphoma (ATCL). Furthermore, soluble IL-2 receptor is usually elevated in the serum of patients with ATCL. CD25 expression in mast cell proliferations is indicative of clonality.

CD30 (Ki-1; Ber-H2) is expressed by normal plasma cells, immunoblasts (such as in viral [EBV] lymphadenopathy) and NK cells. In neoplasms, it is expressed by Reed-Sternberg cells, anaplastic large cell lymphoma (ALCL), embryonal carcinoma, and mediastinal B cell lymphoma.

CD33 is expressed by normal and neoplastic myeloid and monocytic cells, usually positive in AML types M1-M5.

CD34 is a marker of immature mesenchymal cells. It is expressed by normal and neoplastic endothelial cells, immature hematolymphoid cells, gastrointestinal stromal tumor, dermatofibrosarcoma protuberans, and solitary fibrous tumor.

CD38 is normally expressed by activated T and B cells and plasma cells. It is commonly expressed in B cell, T cell, and plasma cell neoplasms. CD38 expression in CLL/SLL is, like ZAP-70, indicative of IgVH nonmutated status and a more aggressive clinical course.

CD41 and CD61 are expressed by normal and neoplastic megakaryocytes.

CD43 is expressed by normal and neoplastic T cells and is characteristically underexpressed in Wiskott-Aldrich syndrome. It is anomalously expressed on B cells in majority of cases of MCL, SLL, and some cases of MZL (especially MALT-type MZL). It is not expressed in FL.

CD45 (leukocyte common antigen, LCA) is found in nearly all normal and neoplastic leukocytes. As they differentiate CD45 expression by hematolymphoid cells changes, with mature lymphocytes and monocytes having bright expression, granulocytes with intermediate intensity, and erythrocytes with almost none. Dim to absent CD45 (usually with strong CD34) is the immunophenotypic signature of blasts, and dim to absent CD45 (with strong CD38) is typical of plasma cells. CD45 is not expressed by Reed-Sternberg cells.

CD45-RO (UCHL-1) is expressed by normal and neoplastic T cells.

CD56 is expressed by normal and neoplastic NK cells, plasma cells, and neuroepithelial cells (an excellent marker for small cell carcinoma).

CD57 (Leu-7) is expressed by a subset of normal and neoplastic NK cells and neuroepithelial cells.

CD59 is present on nearly all human cells. Decreased (along with CD55-DAF) cell surface expression is a feature of the affected clone in paroxysmal nocturnal hemoglobinuria (PNH).

CD68 is expressed by macrophages and histiocytes, but its specificity is poor.

CD71 is the transferrin receptor, which is highly expressed in highly metabolic cells. In general, higher levels of CD71 expression tend to correlate with tumor grade in a variety of hematolymphoid neoplasms.

CD79a is expressed by normal and neoplastic B cells and plasma cells. It is negative in Reed-Sternberg cells.

CD99 (p30/32, mic-2; O-13) is expressed in lymphoblastic lymphomas, PNET/Ewing, granulosa cell tumors, synovial sarcoma, rhabdomyosarcoma, solitary fibrous tumor, and others.

CD103 is a very sensitive and specific marker for hairy cell leukemia (HCL).

CD117 (c-kit) is a tyrosine kinase whose gene is found on chromosome 4q12, adjacent to *PDGFRα*. It is expressed by the so-called interstitial cell of Cajal (the precursors of GI stromal tumors), melanocytes (particularly junctional), seminomas, progenitor myeloid cells (AML, CML) and mast cells (mastocytomas).

CD138 is a marker of plasma cells. Among hematolymphoid proliferations, CD138 is a very specific marker of plasma cell differentiation; however, CD138 is positive in a wide range of epithelial and mesenchymal proliferations.

Clusterin expression in a discrete Golgi pattern appears to be unique to ALCL. Cytoplasmic staining may be seen in several epithelial neoplasms and occasional Reed-Sternberg cells. Strong cytoplasmic reactivity is noted in megakaryocytes.

Epithelial membrane antigen (EMA) is expressed by plasma cells, anaplastic large cell lymphoma, nodular lymphocyte predominant Hodgkin lymphoma, primary effusion lymphoma, and T cell rich B cell lymphoma.

Fascin is expressed by Reed-Sternberg cells and dendritic reticulum cells.

FMC-7: See CD20.

HLA-DR is normally expressed by monocytes, B cells, and activated T cells. It is expressed in most B-ALL but is negative in T-ALL. HLA-DR is positive in most myeloblasts but notably absent in APML.

PAX5 is positive in nearly all B cell neoplasms and most classic Hodgkin lymphoma. It is negative in T cell neoplasms and plasma cell neoplasms. All B cell lineage neoplasms, from those of precursor B cells to mature B cells, express PAX5, but expression is lost at the plasma cell stage. Some other small round blue cell tumors, such as Merkel cell carcinoma and small cell carcinoma of lung, may also express PAX5. PAX5 can differentiate classic Hodgkin lymphoma (PAX5+) from null cell anaplastic large cell lymphoma (PAX5–). It can also differentiate B cell neoplasms with plasmacytic differentiation, such as marginal zone lymphoma, lymphoplasmacytic lymphoma, and CLL (PAX5+) from plasma cell neoplasms (PAX5–).

S100 is a calcium binding protein that is expressed in both nuclear and cytoplasmic compartments. It is largely found in neural and neural crest tissues (glial cells, Schwann cells, melanocytes, sustentacular cells of the adrenal medulla), chondrocytes, adipocytes, myoepithelial cells (the cell of origin of most salivary and skin adnexal tumors). Of relevance to hematopathology, S100 is expressed by a subset of histiocytic cells; in particular, interdigitating reticulum cells, dendritic reticulum cells, and Langerhans cells.

ZAP-70 is a tyrosine kinase that in normal circumstances is expressed primarily by T and NK cells. ZAP-70 is expressed by some B cell neoplasms, notably a subset of CLL/SLL and B-ALL, and most T cell neoplasms. Expression can be assessed either by immunohistochemistry or flow cytometry, but many flow cytometry laboratories experience difficulties with it. Expression in CLL/SLL correlates with immunoglobulin heavy chain variable region gene mutational status; overexpression is correlated with nonmutated status and a more aggressive clinical course.

Immunophenotypic evolution in hematolymphoid cells

The lymphoid constituent of the immune system is divided into 2 parts: innate and adaptive. The innate immune system is a relatively primitive first-line immune defense that somewhat nonspecifically targets polysaccharide antigens. Cells of the innate immune system are situated mainly in mucosa and skin, and their antigenic response is MHC-independent. Innate immunity is mediated by NK cells, NK-like T cells (CD3+, CD56+), and γδ T cells. Lymphomas derived from cells of the innate immune system (aggressive NK cell lymphoma, systemic EBV+ T cell lymphoproliferative disease, hepatosplenic T cell lymphomas, and γδ T cell lymphomas) are relatively common in children and young adults and are largely extranodal, reflecting the physiologic location of these cells. The adaptive immune system is significantly more refined. Highly specific antibodies are formed through an MHC-dependent exposure to polypeptide antigens. The adaptive immune system displays memory. It is mediated by T cells and B cells.

The earliest precursors of B lymphocytes (progenitor B cells or B lymphoblasts) express CD34, Tdt, CD38, dim CD45, CD10, and CD19 t4.49. They undergo immunoglobulin gene rearrangement to become cytoplasmic μ heavy chain+ pre-B cells and subsequently develop into mature surface immunoglobulin-expressing (sIg+) B cells, expressing both IgM and IgD. At this stage B cells often coexpress CD5. CD5+ naïve B cells are found circulating in low number in the peripheral blood, within mantle zones, and within resting (unstimulated) follicles. By the time IgM is expressed on the surface of the B cell, all of the immature antigens are lost except CD19 and CD45, and the cell gains expression of CD20, CD22, CD79, and CD40 (CD38 is expressed again in activated B cells). When B cells are exposed to antigen, some of them mature into plasma cells, losing CD45 and most pan-B antigens (CD20, CD22, CD40, surface Ig), but expressing CD19, CD79a, CD38 and CD138. Others migrate into the center of the follicle and populate the germinal center as centroblasts, turning off expression of bcl-2 and gaining expression of CD10 and bcl-6. In the germinal center, somatic

hypermutation of the immunoglobulin heavy chain variable region (IgVH) occurs, leading to more or less avid Ig (cells expressing more avid Ig are permitted to re-express bcl-2 and thereby saved from apoptosis), and class switching may occur (to IgG, IgE, or IgA).

T cell precursors (prothymocytes) express CD34, Tdt, HLA-DR, CD38, dim CD45, CD2, CD7, and have cytoplasmic CD3 t4.49. As they mature, T cells begin to express CD5, CD1a, surface CD3 (expression coincides with the expression of surface TCR), CD4, and CD8. Simultaneously, there is progressive diminution of CD34, Tdt, CD1, and HLA-DR. T cells having TCR that reacts with self antigens are killed by apoptosis. Selection leads to loss of either CD4 or CD8, coincident with the loss of CD1a. Note that there is a stage of T cell maturation in which the cell is both CD4–, CD8–, followed by a period of both CD4+, CD8+, with eventual expression of one or the other. CD38 is re-expressed upon T cell activation. In the normally functioning immune system the CD4:CD8 cell ratio is 2:1, and the normal T:B cell ratio is 2:1. CD4+ T cells come in 4 types: Th1 (activating mainly other T cells and macrophages), Th2 (activating B cells), T-regulatory (Treg) cells (suppressor cells which express CD25), and follicular Th (FTH) cells (populate the germinal center and, in addition to normal T markers, express bcl-6 and CD10). Angioimmunoblastic T cell lymphoma (AITL) is composed of FTH cells (explaining its tendency to be associated with expansion of FDCs and polyclonal hypergammaglobulinemia). Adult T cell lymphoma (ATCL) is related to Treg cells (thus profound immunosuppression is a feature of ATCL). The vast majority of mature T cells have TCRs with αβ light chains (noncovalently associated with the antigen CD3). γδ T cells are functionally a part of the innate immune system. They normally represent a small (3-5%) population of overall T cells, but a large proportion of dermal, intestinal, and splenic T cells. Furthermore, there may be an expansion in the peripheral blood population of γδ T cells in certain reactive conditions and in postsplenectomy states. γδ T cells express neither CD4 nor CD8 and usually have weak or absent CD5; as such, an expansion in this population may raise suspicion for T cell neoplasm.

t4.49 B & T cell maturation

B cell stage	Features	T cell stage	Features
Lymphoid stem cell	CD34+, Tdt+, HLA-DR+ IgH gene germline, TCR gene germline	Lymphoid stem cell	CD34+, Tdt+, HLA-DR+ TCR gene germline, IgH gene germline
Pro-B cell	CD34+, Tdt+, HLA-DR+, CD19+, CD10+ Ig H chain rearranging	Prothymocyte	CD34+, Tdt+, CD2+, CD7+
Pre-B cell	CD34–, Tdt–, HLA-DR+, CD19+, CD10+, CD20+ Cytoplasmic μ heavy chains Ig L chain rearranging	Immature/ common thymocyte	CD34–, Tdt+, CD1+, CD2+ Cytoplasmic CD3+, CD5+, CD7+, CD4+ & CD8+ TCR rearranged
B cell	All of the above plus surface Ig, CD21+, CD22+	Mature thymocyte	All of the above, except Tdt– & CD1–, CD4+ or CD8+
Plasma cell	Loss of B cell markers (CD20–) Cytoplasmic (not surface) Ig+	Mature T cell	All of the above, plus surface CD3+

NK cells bear neither the TCR nor immunoglobulin. They lack surface CD3 (CD3– by flow cytometry), but contain cytoplasmic δ and ε chains of CD3 (CD3+ by immunohistochemistry). NK cells are positive for CD2, CD7, CD16, CD56, and CD57. CD16 is the receptor for the Fc portion of γ heavy chains (FcγR). Some NK cells express CD8. The TCR genes are germline (not rearranged). NK cells utilize antibody dependent cellular cytotoxicity (ADCC) to kill cells bearing foreign antigen; as part of this killing mechanism, they display killer inhibitory receptors (KIRs) and a group of cytolytic molecules including granzymes (eg, granzyme B and granzyme M).

Early granulocytes (myeloblasts) express CD34, HLA-DR, CD38, CD117, dim CD13, and CD33. Promyelocytes become negative for CD34 and HLA-DR, continue to express dim to moderate CD13 and CD33, and acquire bright CD15. Metamyelocytes acquire CD11b. As they mature into mature bands and segmented neutrophils, CD10 is expressed, along with bright CD13, CD15 and CD11b. In bone marrow specimens, plots of CD45 vs side scatter show myeloids with dimmer CD45 expression than lymphocytes and monocytes, and a broad range of side scatter. Immature myeloids have dim CD45 and low to intermediate side scatter. Mature myeloids have high side scatter and bright CD45.

The monocyte also derives from the myeloblast. In the promonocyte stage, there is loss of CD34 and expression of CD11b. With additional maturation, there is expression of CD64 and CD14. Throughout maturation, they are CD15– or dim.

Conventional cytogenetics & molecular techniques

Cytogenetics

Cytogenetics is the evaluation of chromosome structure and is used to detect structural chromosomal aberrations such as t(9;22). Cytogenetic studies require specimens that contain viable cells; eg, fresh lymph node tissue for lymphomas, fresh whole blood or fresh marrow specimens for leukemia or myelodysplasia. Administration of chemotherapy may decrease yield. Generally speaking, adequate examination (adequate exclusion of an abnormal clone) requires examination of ≥20 metaphases. If an abnormal metaphase is identified, the same abnormality must be found in at least 1 additional cell to confirm a clone. See chapter 7.

Molecular examination of lymphocytes

B and T cells undergo somatic gene rearrangements in order to produce the genes that will ultimately encode their respective immunoglobulin (Ig) and T cell receptor (TCR) proteins. A primitive B cell begins life with its genes in a germline (embryonic) configuration. In the germline configuration, the segments of DNA that will encode the Ig heavy (IgH) chain are all found on chromosome 14 but separated by considerable distances. These separate segments of DNA are called V, D, J and C (variable [V] segment, diversity [D] segment, joining [J] segment, and constant [C] segment). Analogously, the germline κ light chain gene segments, on chromosome 2, consist of separately located V, J and C segments (no D), and the germline λ light chain gene segments, on chromosome 22, also are V, J, and C. All these segments become linked closely enough together to produce a functional protein following gene rearrangement. In B cell maturation, the IgH genes rearrange first, followed by the kappa (κ) light chain genes. If the κ rearrangement is nonproductive, then lambda (λ) rearranges. Finally, with all the rearranging complete, the cell begins to make immunoglobulin in its cytoplasm (cIg+). Later, it will incorporate this immunoglobulin into its cell membrane (sIg+) and will be defined as a mature B cell. The process is similar for T cells.

A clonal rearrangement supports a diagnosis of neoplasia. The finding of only germline genes with no clonal rearrangements is indicative of

1. a benign lymphoid proliferation

2. a lymphoid neoplasm composed of very early lymphoid cells

3. nonlymphoid neoplasm

A couple of caveats are worth noting. First, a not insignificant number of B cell neoplasms will display, in addition to rearrangement of Ig genes, rearrangement of TCR genes (lineage infidelity). T cell neoplasms may do the same t4.50. Second, clonal populations can be detected where no neoplasm exists, particularly in immunocompromised individuals. In general, a clone representing >1-5% of cells is required for a confident diagnosis of malignancy. This threshold happens to be the lower limit of detection for Southern blot hybridization.

t4.50 Rate of detection of clonal receptor gene rearrangements in lymphoid neoplasms

Neoplasm	Clonal IgH rearrangement	Clonal TCR rearrangement
Mature B-NHL	>99%	5-7%
Mature T-NHL	4-6%	>90%
B-ALL	>99%	20-40%
T-ALL	10-15%	85-95%

The techniques in wide use for detection of clonal IgH gene rearrangements include Southern blot analysis (SBA) and polymerase chain reaction (PCR). In PCR for IgH, DNA is amplified using a number of consensus primers that are designed to amplify several members of the V gene class and several of the J gene class. The amplicon is then subjected to electrophoresis, and if there is a major population of lymphocytes having the same IgH gene rearrangement, it will appear as a distinct band. A mixture of polyclonal B cells will produce a ladderlike distribution of bands. Southern blot hybridization (SBH) with restriction fragment length polymorphisms (RFLP) consists of a process in which radiolabeled probes for the IgH gene, Igκ gene, and TCRβ gene, are applied to an agarose gel that contains DNA which has been

1. extracted from the cells of interest

2. cut with restriction enzymes (EcoRI, BamHI, HindIII)

3. electrophoresed

The resulting clonal band (restriction fragment), if any, is then displayed on an autoradiograph. A lymphoid neoplasm will show a strong clonal band. A polyclonal proliferation shows many individual rearranged genes, none hybridizing strongly enough to resolve into a distinct band. While Southern blot is still considered the gold standard, it requires high quality DNA and is labor intensive. As a result, it is being replaced by PCR which can be automated and performed on formalin fixed, paraffin embedded material. PCR is not perfect, however, as results are dependent upon a host of considerations, especially the choice of primers.

In PCR, the choice of primers is responsible for the specificity of this technique, as they anneal preferentially to the genomic areas of interest, usually sequences known to lie on either side of the target gene. At the end of this process, if the target gene is present, there will be a dark blot corresponding to the known size of the gene. PCR is preferred for detecting many, but not all, chromosomal translocations. In particular, the t(11;14) *BCL1* translocation of MCL is poorly suited for detection by PCR t4.51.

t4.51 Detection of *BCL1* rearrangement

Method	Sensitivity (%)
FISH	>95
Cytogenetics	80
Southern blot	70
PCR	40-50

FISH, or interphase FISH, is well suited for detecting most oncogene translocations. In particular, detection of the *BCL1*, *BCL2*, *BCL6*, and *CMYC* translocations is most sensitive by FISH.

A summary of important chromosomal and genetic associations is provided in t4.52.

t4.52 Selected molecular genetic associations

Disease	Rearrangement	Notes
Chronic myelogenous leukemia (CML)	t(9;22)(q34;q11.2)	*BCR/ABL*
	t(9;22) + Ph, +8, +19, i(17q), del(9q)	Indicates progression (clonal evolution)
Burkitt lymphoma	t(8;14), t(8;22), t(2;8)	cMyc/IgH; cMyc/Igλ; cMyc/Igκ
Chronic lymphocytic leukemia (CLL/SLL)	del(13q), del(11q), +12, del(17p), del(14q)	20% have a normal chromosomes 30% of cases have complex abnormalities
Follicular lymphoma (FL)	t(14;18)(q32;q21)	*BCL2/IgH*
Mantle cell lymphoma (MCL)	t(11;14)(q13;q32)	*BCL1/IgH*
MALT lymphoma	t(11;18)(q21;q21) & others	*MLT/API2*
Lymphoplasmacytic lymphoma (LPL)	t(9;14)(p13;q32)	PAX5/IgH
Anaplastic large cell lymphoma (ALCL)	t(2;5)(p23;q35)	ALK/NPM Good prognosis
Myelodysplasia	−5, −5q, −7, −7q, or −8	Most commonly seen are complex abnormalities involving one or more

Bone marrow biopsy

Sites of hematopoiesis

Hematopoiesis begins in the fetus during the first trimester, and by early in the second trimester, nucleated RBCs can be found within the vessels of the chorionic villi. By the end of the first trimester, hematopoiesis is taking place in multiple sites, including the liver, spleen, thymus, lymph nodes, and marrow. Extramedullary hematopoiesis (hematopoiesis taking place outside the marrow) ceases around the time of birth, and indicates a pathologic condition thereafter. At birth, medullary hematopoiesis is occurring in essentially all bones. Gradually this regresses such that in adults, medullary hematopoiesis is confined to a few of the flat bones, such as the ilium and sternum, and the epiphyses of long bones, such as the femur and clavicle.

Indications

The most common indications for bone marrow biopsy are

1. to evaluate quantitative cellular abnormalities that have been detected in the peripheral blood

2. staging of hematolymphoid neoplasms

3. a monoclonal protein detected by serum/urine protein electrophoresis

Bone marrow biopsy was once considered a standard part of evaluating fever of unknown origin (FUO), but this is not so common any more.

Peripheral blood

A rough estimate of the cell counts can be achieved through low power (10× or 20× objective) review of the smear. The automated count is much more reliable in most instances, but smear examination may disclose major discrepancies; for example, the automated platelet count may be falsely low when platelets are markedly enlarged or clumped (EDTA artifact). Likewise, the automated RBC count may be falsely low when RBCs are clumped (cold agglutinins). Automated basophil counts are often inaccurate. The low power scan is also useful to detect rare abnormal cells such as blasts or promyelocytes, and to appreciate a bimodal RBC population (sideroblastic anemia, recent transfusion, marked reticulocytosis) and rouleaux (M protein).

Detailed morphologic evaluation of the cellular constituents is conducted under oil immersion (50× or 100× objective). The laboratory should adopt a scoring system for RBC morphologic abnormalities, usually one that is numeric (1+ to 3+) or description (slight, occasional, moderate, many). RBCs should be described according to size (normocytic, microcytic, macrocytic) and hemoglobinization (normochromic, hypochromic). Anisocytosis describes an increase in RBC size variability, and poikilocytosis refers to the presence of shape changes.

Leukocytes should be evaluated for overall distribution, maturity, and the presence of abnormal cells. A 200 cell count should be undertaken, particularly if myelodysplasia is being considered. Neutrophils should be evaluated for left shift (presence of bands, metamyelocytes, myelocytes) and quality of nuclear segmentation (hypo-, hypersegmentation). Left shift usually indicates infection but may indicate leukemia (CML); a reactive left shift rarely includes promyelocytes or blasts and is often accompanied by "toxic" changes (prominence of primary—blue—granules, Döhle bodies, vacuolization). Hyposegmented neutrophils (<3 lobes) may be seen in myelodysplasia, left-shifted smears, and inherited Pelger-Huët anomaly. Pelger-Huët anomaly is an otherwise benign condition in which neutrophils have 2 lobes of even size; occasional cells with a single lobe may be seen (Stodtmeister cells). Pseudo-Pelger-Huët cells are any cells resembling Pelger-Huët cells in a patient without the inherited anomaly. Hypersegmentation (6 or more lobes) is seen in megaloblastic anemia (B$_{12}$ or folate deficiency). Circulating lymphocytes normally consist of small mature cells with rounded nuclei. Lymphocytes with clefted nuclei (Reider cells) are sometimes seen in children with viral infection or pertusis. So-called atypical lymphocytes (variant lymphocytes, reactive lymphocytes) refer to lymphocytes with enlarged nuclei, open chromatin, sometimes nucleoli; the cytoplasm is increased in quantity, deformable (RBCs often impinge upon it), sometimes finely granulated, and with edges that resemble the edges of a burned page.

Platelets should be evaluated for size, variation in size, clumping, and granulation. Platelets are described as "large" when they are larger than usual and as "giant" when they are larger than a RBC. Enlarged and variably sized platelets may be seen in thrombocytopenic patients (ITP, typically), in acute phase reactions, and in myeloproliferative neoplasms. Pale, hypogranular platelets are often seen in myeloproliferative neoplasms, myelodysplasia, and rare inherited conditions (gray platelet syndrome).

Bone marrow aspirate & touch imprints

The bone marrow aspirate is prepared from smears and/or particle crushes at the bedside, and touch imprints are performed from the core biopsy before formalin fixation. These yield cytologic information about the cells in the marrow, and form the basis for evaluation of myelodysplasia (dyspoiesis). A qualitative assessment of adequacy should be made, based upon overall cellularity and the number of spicules present. A 500 cell count should be undertaken, enumerating blasts, promyelocytes, myelocytes, metamyelocytes, mature neutrophils (segmented neutrophils and bands), monocyte lineage cells, lymphocytes, plasma cells, megakaryocytes, and erythroid precursors. Metastatic tumor may be identified in these preparations.

The assessment of iron stores (Prussian blue or Perls stain) is best performed on the aspirate, if it is spicular; alternatively, this may be done on the clot section, and as a last resort on the trephine biopsy (the decalcification procedure often diminishes the stainable iron). Ideally, ≥7 spicules are examined. Stainable iron is often graded as increased, adequate, decreased, or absent. The Prussian blue stain is also examined for the presence of ringed sideroblasts; if present, the percentage should be determined (ringed sideroblasts/100 erythroid precursors).

Note that a certain degree of dyspoietic maturation can be found in the marrow of normal subjects. It is for this reason that a cell line is considered dysplastic only if dyspoiesis is present in >10% of its constituents. Dyserythropoiesis increases with time to fixation (smear preparation).

Bone marrow biopsy & clot section

The bone marrow (trephine) biopsy is the core of tissue retrieved from the trephine needle. Often, there is a variable quantity of debris and clot, which contains a wealth of marrow fragments and can be processed as a cell block (clot section). H&E stained 4 μm sections are usually adequate; although, some routinely perform PAS stains, trichrome stains, and/or reticulin stains. The biopsy and clot section are most useful for assessing semiquantitative overall cellularity and for detecting tumor. The overall cellularity is based upon an overall impression of the fat:cell ratio and is usually given as a percent cellularity. Cellularity decreases with age; roughly speaking, cellularity varies from essentially 100% at birth to around 30% by age 70 and progressively diminishes thereafter. Total fatty replacement of the marrow is consistent with aplastic anemia at any age, with the caveat that if peripheral counts are normal, sampling error should be considered. Adults with cellularity >70% are considered to have hypercellular marrow.

The myeloid to erythroid (M:E) ratio may be assessed from the 500-cell count (with the myeloid component including granulocyte and monocyte lineage) or from the marrow biopsy sections. The normal adult M:E ratio is between 2-4:1. Outside of this range, it is likely that one of the cell lines is either hypoplastic or hyperplastic; generally speaking, a hypercellular marrow (>70%) suggests hyperplasia of one of the cell lines, and normocellular or hypocellular marrow suggests hypoplasia. Thus, in a marrow with overall cellularity of 80% and M:E ratio of 8:1, the myeloid line is likely hyperplastic (rather than the erythroid line being hypoplastic).

Additional information may be gleaned by topography. Usually, the generative zone, a rim of immature cells, is paratrabecular and just 1-2 cells thick; an increase in the girth of the generative zone may be seen in myeloproliferative neoplasms and myelodysplastic syndromes. Megakaryocytes are typically scattered and only rarely touch one another; increased and clumped megakaryocytes are seen in myeloproliferative neoplasms and marrow reacting to peripheral platelet consumption. Intrasinusoidal hematopoiesis is a feature of fibrotic marrow, again seen in myeloproliferative neoplasms. A reticulin stain should be performed in selected cases, to evaluate for reticulin fibrosis. Generally reticulin fibrosis is apparent from the H&E stained sections, seen as "streaming" of the marrow elements. The normal marrow has minimal reticulin fibers that are restricted to paratrabecular and perivascular sites. Any reticulin outside of this distribution is abnormal and may suggest a myeloproliferative neoplasm or an infiltrative process such as hairy cell leukemia.

The marrow biopsy and clot section should be evaluated for the presence of metastatic tumor, granulomas, vascular alterations, and lymphoid aggregates. Small benign lymphoid aggregates, located in nonparatrabecular locations, increase with age. If evaluated by immunohistochemistry, these are usually a mixture of T cells and B cells with normal T:B ratio. If composed solely of B cells, consider lymphoma. Paratrabecular lymphoid aggregates are typical of marrow involvement by follicular lymphoma and T cell rich B cell lymphoma. Granulomas may indicate infection, and microbial stains (AFB and GMS) should always be done when granulomas are seen. Particularly when making the diagnosis of plasmacytoma, the vasculature should be examined for amyloid.

References

Ahmed S [2003] Diagnostic yield of bone marrow examination in fever of unknown origin. *Am J Med* 115(7):591-592. PMID:14599649.

Al-Mawali A, Gillis D, Lewis I [2009] The role of multiparameter flow cytometry for detection of minimal residual disease in acute myeloid leukemia. *Am J Clin Pathol* 131:16-26. PMID:19095561.

Amin HM, Medeiros LJ, Manning JT, Jones D [2003] Dissolution of the Lymphoid Follicle Is a Feature of the HHV8+ Variant of Plasma Cell Castleman's Disease. *Am J Surg Pathol* 27(1):91-100. PMID:12502931.

Arber DA, George TI [2005] Bone marrow biopsy involvement by non-Hodgkin lymphoma. *Am J Surg Pathol* 29(12):1549-1557. PMID:16327427.

Ataga KI [2003] Hypercoagulability in sickle cell disease: a curious paradox. *Am J Med* 115(9):721-728. PMID:14693325.

Baens M, Maes B, Steyls A, et al [2000] The product of the t(11;18), an API2–MLT fusion, marks nearly half of gastric MALT type lymphomas without large cell proliferation. *Am J Pathol* 156:1433-1439. PMID:10751367.

Bain BJ [1996] The Bone Marrow Aspirate of Healthy Subjects. *Br J Haematol* 94:206-209. PMID:8757536.

Bajwa RPS, Skinner R, Windebank KP, Reid MM [2004] Demographic study of leukaemia presenting within the first 3 months of life in the northern health region of England. *J Clin Pathol* 57:186-188. PMID:14747447.

Banerjee R, Halil O, Bain BJ, et al [2000] Neutrophil dysplasia caused by mycophenolate mofetil. *Transplantation* 70:1608-1610. PMID:11152223.

Baxter EJ, Scott LM, Campbell PJ, et al [2005] Cancer Genome Project. Acquired mutation of the tyrosine kinase JAK2 in human myeloproliferative disorders. *Lancet* 365:1054-1061. PMID:15781101.

Berliner N, Horwitz M, Loughran TP [2004] Congenital and acquired neutropenia. *Hematology* 63-79. PMID:15561677.

Beutler E, Waalen J [2006] The definition of anemia: what is the lower limit of normal of the blood hemoglobin concentration? *Blood* 107:1747-1750. PMID:16189263.

Bilalovic N, Blystad AK, Golouh R, et al [2004] Expression of bcl-6 and CD10 protein is associated with longer overall survival and time to treatment failure in follicular lymphoma. *Am J Clin Pathol* 121:34-42. PMID:14750238.

Binet JL, Auguier A, Dighiero G, et al [1981] A new prognostic classification of CLL derived from a multivariate survival analysis. *Cancer* 48:198-206. PMID:7237385.

Bizzarro MJ, Colson E, Ehrenkranz RA [2004] Differential diagnosis and management of anemia in the newborn. *Pediatr Clin N Am* 51:1087-1107. PMID:15275990.

Bohm J [2000] Gelatinous transformation of the bone marrow: the spectrum of underlying diseases. *Am J Surg Pathol* 24(1):56-65. PMID:10632488.

Bouroncle B, Wiseman BK, Doan C [1958] Leukemic reticuloendotheliosis. *Blood* 13(7):609-30. PMID:13560561.

Bovio IM, Allan RW [2008] The expression of myeloid antigens CD13 and/or CD33 is a marker of ALK+ anaplastic large cell lymphomas. *Am J Clin Pathol* 130:628-634. PMID:18794057.

Bresters D, Reus ACW, Veerman AJP, et al [2002] Congenital leukaemia: the Dutch experience and review of the literature. *Brit J Haematol* 117:513-524. PMID:12028017.

Burns ER, Lou Y, Pathak A [2004] Morphologic diagnosis of thrombotic thrombocytopenic purpura. *Am J Hematol* 75:18-21. PMID:14695628.

Campo E [2003] Genetic and molecular genetic studies in the diagnosis of B-Cell lymphomas I: mantle cell lymphoma, follicular lymphoma, and Burkitt lymphoma. *Hum Path* 34(4):330-335. PMID:12733111.

Caraway NP, Stewart J [2006] Primary effusion lymphoma. *Pathol Case Rev* 11:78-84.

Carella M, Stewart G, Ajetunmobi JF, et al [1998] Genomewide search for dehydrated hereditary stomatocytosis (hereditary xerocytosis): mapping of locus to chromosome 16 (16q23-qter). *Am J Hum Genet* 63:810-816. PMID:9718354.

Cataldo KA, Jalal SM, Law ME, et al [1999] Detection of t(2;5) in anaplastic large cell lymphoma comparison of immunohistochemical studies, FISH, and RT-PCR in paraffin-embedded tissue. *Am J Surg Pathol* 23:1386-1392. PMID:10555007.

Chan WC, Hans CP, Kadin ME [2003] Genetic and molecular genetic studies in the diagnosis of T-cell malignancies. *Hum Pathol* 34(4):314-321. PMID:12733109.

Chen FE, Ooi C, Ha SY, et al [2000] Genetic and clinical features of hemoglobin H disease in Chinese patients. *N Engl J Med* 343:544-550. PMID:10954762.

Chen Y, Tallman MS, Goolsby C, Peterson L [2005] Immunophenotypic variations in hairy cell leukemia. *Am J Clin Pathol* 125:251-259. PMID:16393677.

Chng WJ, Lai HC, Earnest A, Kuperan P [2005] Haematological parameters in severe acute respiratory syndrome. *Clin Lab Haem* 27:15-20. PMID:15686503.

Cioc AM, Vanderwerf SM, Peterson BA, et al [2008] Rituximab induced changes in hematolymphoid tissues found at autopsy. *Am J Clin Pathol* 130:604-612. PMID:18794054.

Clark BE, Thein SL [2004] Molecular diagnosis of haemoglobin disorders. *Clin Lab Haem* 26:159-176. PMID:15163314.

Cook JR, Shekhter-Levin S, Swerdlow SH [2004] Utility of routine classical cytogenetic studies in the evaluation of suspected lymphomas: results of 279 consecutive lymph node/extranodal tissue biopsies. *Am J Clin Pathol* 121:826-835. PMID:15198354.

Cooper DS, Goldminz D, Levin AA, et al [1983] Agranulocytosis associated with antithyroid drug: effects of patient age and drug dose. *Ann Intern Med* 98:26-29. PMID:6687345.

Cournoyer D, Toffelmire EB, Wells GA, et al [2004] Anti erythropoietin antibody-mediated pure red cell aplasia after treatment with recombinant erythropoietin products: recommendations for minimization of risk. *J Am Soc Nephrol* 15:2728-2734. PMID:15466278.

Cox MC, Panetta P, Lo-Coco F, et al [2004] Chromosomal aberration of the 11q23 locus in acute leukemia and frequency of *MLL* gene translocation results in 378 adult patients. *Am J Clin Pathol* 122:298-306. PMID:15323147.

Crespo M, Bosch F, Villamor N, et al [2003] ZAP-70 expression as a surrogate for immunoglobulin-variable-region mutations in CLL. *N Engl J Med* 348:1764-1775. PMID:12724482.

Cushing T, Clericuzio CL, Wilson CS, et al [2006] Risk for leukemia in infants without down syndrome who have transient myeloproliferative disorder. *J Pediatr* 148:687-689. PMID:16737888.

Davoren A, Curtis BR, Aster RH, McFarland JG [2004] Human platelet antigen-specific alloantibodies implicated in 1162 cases of neonatal alloimmune thrombocytopenia. *Transfusion* 44:1220-1225. PMID:15265127.

De J, Zanjani R, Hibbard M, Davis BD [2007] Immunophenotypic profile predictive of KIT activating mutations in AML1-ETO leukemia. *Am J Clin Pathol* 128:550-557. PMID:17875504.

Delaunay J [2004] The hereditary stomatocytoses: genetic disorders of the red cell membrane permeability to monovalent cations. *Semin Hematol* 41:165-172. PMID:15071792.

Delgado J, Matutes E, Morilla AM, et al [2003] Diagnostic significance of CD20 and FMC7 expression in B-cell disorders. *Am J Clin Pathol* 120:754-759. PMID:14608903.

Dickinson JD, Smith LM, Sanger WG, et al [2005] Unique gene expression and clinical characteristics are associated with the 11q23 deletion in chronic lymphocytic leukaemia. *Brit J Haematol* 128:460-471. PMID:15686453.

Dighiero G, Hamblin TJ [2008] Chronic lymphocytic leukaemia. *Lancet* 371:1017-1029. PMID:18358929.

Dohner H, Stilgenbauer S, Benner A, et al [2000] Genomic aberrations and survival in CLL. *N Engl J Med* 343:1910-1916. PMID:11136261.

Dong HY, Weisberger J, Liu Z, Tugulea S [2009] Immunophenotypic analysis of CD103+ B-lymphoproliferative disorders: hairy cell leukemia and its mimics. *Am J Clin Pathol* 131:586-595. PMID:19289595.

Dorfman DM, Shahsafaei A, Chan JK, et al [1997] Thymic carcinomas, but not thymomas and carcinomas of other sites, show CD5 immunoreactivity. *Am J Surg Pathol* 21(8)August:936-940. PMID:9255257.

Douglas VK, Gordon LI, Goolsby CL, et al [1999] Lymphoid aggregates in bone marrow mimic residual lymphoma after rituximab therapy for non-Hodgkin lymphoma. *Am J Clin Pathol* 112:844-853. PMID:10587708.

Du MQ, Liu H, Diss TC, et al [2001] Kaposi sarcoma associated herpesvirus infects monotypic (IgM lambda) but polyclonal naive B cells in Castleman disease and associated lymphoproliferative disorders. *Blood* 97:2130-2136. PMID:11264181.

Einerson RR, Kurtin PJ, Dayharsh GA, et al [2005] FISH is superior to PCR in detecting t(14;18)(q32;q21)–IgH/bcl-2 in follicular lymphoma using paraffin-embedded tissue samples. *Am J Clin Pathol* 124:421-429. PMID:16191511.

Elliot MA, Tefferi A [2004] Thrombosis and haemorrhage in polycythemia vera and essential thrombocythaemia. *Brit J Haematol* 128:275-290. PMID:15667529.

Emile C, Danon F, Fermand JP, Clauvel JP [1993] Castleman disease in POEMS syndrome with elevated interleukin-6. *Cancer* 71(3):874 PMID:8499003.

Escribano L, Montero ACG, Nunez R, Orfao A [2006] Flow cytometric analysis of normal and neoplastic mast cells: role in diagnosis and follow-up of mast cell disease. *Immunol Allergy Clin N Am* 26:535-547. PMID:16931292.

Eshoa C, Perkins S, Kampalath B, et al [2001] Decreased CD10 expression in grade III and in interfollicular infiltrates of follicular lymphoma. *Am J Clin Pathol* 115:862-867. PMID:11392883.

Facon T, Avet-Loiseau H, Guillerm G, et al [2001] Intergroupe Francophone du Myélome. Chromosome 13 abnormalities identified by FISH analysis and serum beta2-microglobulin produce a powerful myeloma staging system for patients receiving high dose therapy. *Blood* 97:1566-1571. PMID:11238092.

Fais F, Ghiotto F, Hashimoto S, et al [1998] CLL B cells express restricted sets of mutated and unmutated antigen receptors. *J Clin Invest* 102:1515-1525. PMID:9788964.

Flanagan MB, Sathanoori M, Surti U, et al [2008] Cytogenetic abnormalities detected by fluorescence in situ hybridization on paraffin-embedded chronic lymphocytic leukemia/small lymphocytic lymphoma lymphoid tissue biopsy specimens. *Am J Clin Pathol* 130:620-627.

Fohlem-Walter A, Jacob C, Lecompte T, Lesesve JF [2002] Laboratory identification of cryoglobulinemia from automated blood cell counts, fresh blood samples, and blood films. *Am J Clin Pathol* 117:606-614. PMID:11939736.

Foucar K [2001] *Bone Marrow Pathology*, 2nd ed. Chicago: American Society of Clinical Pathology; Chapters 7-18.

Franco V, Florena AM, Iannitto E [2003] Splenic marginal zone lymphoma. *Blood* 101:2464-2472. PMID:12446449.

Franklin EC [1964] Structural studies of human 7S gamma globulin: further observations of a naturally-occurring protein related to the crystallizable (fast) fragment. *J Exp Med* 120:691-709. PMID:14247713.

Frost M, Newell J, Lones MA, et al [2004] Comparative immunohistochemical analysis of pediatric Burkitt lymphoma and diffuse large B-cell lymphoma. *Am J Clin Pathol* 121:1-9. PMID:15023043.

Garcia DP, Rooney MT, Ahmad E, Davis BH [2001] Diagnostic usefulness of CD23 and FMC-7 antigen expression patterns in B-cell lymphoma classification. *Am J Clin Pathol* 115:258-265. PMID:11211615.

Gascoyne RD, Aoun P, Wu D, et al [1999] Prognostic significance of anaplastic lymphoma kinase (ALK) protein expression in adults with anaplastic large cell lymphoma. *Blood* 93:3913-3921. PMID:10339500.

Hagland U, Juliusson G, Stellan B, et al [1994] Hairy cell leukemia is characterized by clonal chromosome abnormalities clustered to specific regions. *Blood* 83: 2637-2645. PMID:8167343.

Han X, Bueso-Ramos CE [2007] Precursor T cell acute lymphoblastic lymphoma and acute biphenotypic leukemias. *Am J Clin Pathol* 127:528-544. PMID:17369128.

Hans CP, Weisenburger DD, Greiner TC, et al [2004] Confirmation of the molecular classification of diffuse large B cell lymphoma by immunohistochemistry using a tissue microarray. *Blood* 103:275-282. PMID:14504078.

Harrington A, Ward PCJ, Kroft SH [2008] Iron deficiency anemia, β-thalassemia minor, and anemia of chronic disease: a morphologic reappraisal. *Am J Clin Pathol* 129:466-471. PMID:18285271.

Hasserman RP, Howard J, Wood A, Henry K, Bain B [2001] Acute erythremic myelosis (true erythroleukemia): a variant of AML FAB-M6. *J Clin Pathol* 54:205-209. PMID:11253132.

Herrera G [2009] Renal lesions associated with plasma cell dyscrasias: practical approach to diagnosis, new concepts, and challenges. *Arch Pathol Lab Med* 133:249-267. PMID:19195968.

Hill PG, Forsyth JM, Rai B, Mayne S [2006] Serum free light chains: an alternative to the urine Bence Jones proteins screening test for monoclonal gammopathies. *Clin Chem* 52(9):1743-1748. PMID:16858075.

Hoffman MA [2006] Clinical presentations and complications of hairy cell leukemia. *Hematol Oncol Clin N Am* 20:1065-1073. PMID:16990107.

Hohlfield P, Forestier F, Kaplan C, et al [1994] Fetal thrombocytopenia: a retrospective survey of 5194 fetal blood samplings. *Blood* 84(6):1851-1856. PMID:8080991.

Howanitz PJ, Kozarski TB, Howanitz JH, Chauhan YS [2006] Spurious hemoglobin barts caused by bilirubin: a common interference mimicking an uncommon hemoglobinopathy. *Am J Clin Pathol* 125:608-614. PMID:16627270.

Hoyer JD [1993] Leukocyte differential. *Mayo Clin Proc* 68:1027-1028. PMID:8412355.

Huang L, Abruzzo LV, Valbuena JR, et al [2006] Acute myeloid leukemia associated with variant t(8;21) detected by conventional cytogenetic and molecular studies: a report of 4 cases and review of the literature. *Am J Clin Pathol* 125:267-272. PMID:16393685.

Hughes DA, Stuart-Smith SE, Bain BJ [2004] How should stainable iron in bone marrow films be assessed? *J Clin Pathol* 57:1038-1040. PMID:15452156.

Ibrahim S, Keating M, Do KA, et al [2001] CD38 expression as an important prognostic factor in B-cell CLL. *Blood* 98:181-186. PMID:11418478.

International Agranulocytosis and Aplastic Anaemia Study [1998] Risk of agranulocytosis and aplastic anaemia in relation to use of antithyroid drugs. *BMJ* 297:2651-2665. PMID:2458161.

Ioachim, Ratech [2002] *Ioachim's Lymph Node Pathology*, 3rd ed. Philadelphia: Lipincott Williams & Wilkons.

Jaffe, Harris, Stein, Vardiman Eds [2001] *Tumours of Haematopoietic and Lymphoid Tissues*. Lyon: International Agency for Research on Cancer.

Jamal S, Picker LJ, Aquino DB, et al [2001] Immunophenotypic analysis of peripheral T-cell neoplasms. *Am J Clin Pathol* 116:512-526. PMID:11601136.

Jasionowski TM, Hartung L, Greenwood JH, et al [2003] Analysis of CD10+ hairy cell leukemia. *Am J Clin Pathol* 120:228-235. PMID:12931553.

Joutovsky A, Hadzi-Nesic J, Nardi MA [2004] HPLC retention time as a diagnostic tool for hemoglobin variants and hemoglobinopathies: a study of 60,000 samples in a clinical diagnostic laboratory. *Clin Chem* 50(10):1736-1747. PMID:15388656.

Kadin ME [2003] Genetic and molecular genetic studies in the diagnosis of T-cell malignancies. *Hum Pathol* 34(4):322-329. PMID:12733110.

Kantarjian H, Sawyers C, Hochhaus A, et al [2002] Hematologic and cytogenetic responses to imatinib mesylate in chronic myelogenous leukemia. *N Engl J Med* 346:645-52. PMID:11870241.

Kantarjian H, Schiffer C, Jones D, Cortes J [2008] Monitoring the response and course of chronic myeloid leukemia in the modern era of BCR-ABL tyrosine kinase inhibitors: practical advice on the use and interpretation of monitoring methods. *Blood* 111(4):1174-1180. PMID:18055868.

Karandikar NJ, Hotchkiss EC, McKenna RW, Kroft SH. [2002] Transient stress lymphocytosis. *Am J Clin Pathol* 117:819-825. PMID:12090434.

Kelemen K, Braziel RM, Gatter K, et al [2010] Immunophenotypic variations of Burkitt lymphoma. *Am J Clin Pathol* 134:127-138. PMID:20551277.

Kenney B, Stack G [2009] Drug induced thrombocytopenia. *Arch Pathol Lab Med* 133:309-314. PMID:19195976.

Keren DF, Hedstrom D, Gulbranson R, et al [2008] Comparison of Sebia CapillaryS capillary electrophoresis with the Primus high pressure liquid chromatography in the evaluation of hemoglobinopathies. *Am J Clin Pathol* 130:824-831. PMID:18854277.

Keren DF, McCoy JP, Carey JL, eds [2007] *Flow Cytometry in Clinical Diagnosis*, 4th ed. Chicago: ASCP Press; Chapters 2, 9, 10. ISBN:978-089189-5480.

Kiss TL, Ali MAM, Livine M, Lafferty JD [2000] An algorithm to aid in the investigation of thalassemia trait in multicultural populations. *Arch Pathol Lab Med* 124:1320-1323. PMID:10975930.

Kjeldsberg CR, Perkins SL [2010] *Practical Diagnosis of Hematologic Disorders*, 5th ed. Chicago, ASCP Press. ISBN:978-089189-5718.

Koster F, Foucar K, Hjelle B, et al [2001] Rapid presumptive diagnosis of hantavirus cardiopulmonary syndrome by peripheral blood smear review. *Am J Clin Pathol* 116(5):665-672. PMID:11710682.

Kralovics R, Passamonti F, Buser AS, et al [2005] A gain-of-function mutation of JAK2 in myeloproliferative disorders. *N Engl J Med* 352:1779-1790. PMID:15858187.

Kraus MD, Bartlett NL, Fleming MD, et al [1998] Splenic pathology in myelodysplasia: a report of 13 cases with clinical correlation. *Am J Surg Pathol* 22(10):1255-1266. PMID:9777988.

Kussick SJ, Wood BL [2003] 4-color flow cytometry identifies virtually all cytogenetically abnormal bone marrow samples in the workup of non-CML myeloproliferative disorders. *Am J Clin Pathol* 120:854-865. PMID:14671974.

Kussick SJ, Fromm JR, Rossini A, et al [2005] 4-color flow cytometry shows strong concordance with bone marrow morphology and cytogenetics in the evaluation for myelodysplasia. *Am J Clin Pathol* 2005;124:170-181. PMID:16040286.

Kyle RA [1993] "Benign" monoclonal gammopathy—after 20 35 years follow-up. *Mayo Clin Proc* 68:26-36. PMID:8417251.

Kyle RA, Therneau TM, Rajkumar SV, et al [2002] A long-term study of prognosis in monoclonal gammopathy of undetermined significance. *New Engl J Med* 246:564-569. PMID:8417251.

Kyle RA, Gertz MA, Witzig TE, et al [2003] Review of 1027 patients with newly diagnosed multiple myeloma. *Mayo Clin Proc* 78:21-33. PMID:12528874.

Kyle RA, Therneau TM, Rajkumar SV, et al [2006] Prevalence of monoclonal gammopathy of undetermined significance. *New Engl J Med* 354:1362-1369. PMID:16571879.

Laran MJ, McErlean M, Wilner G [2006] Massive hemolysis associated with *Clostridium perfringens* sepsis. *Am J Emerg Med* 3(2):881-882. PMID:17098117.

Lecuit M, Abachin E, Martin A, et al [2004] Immunoproliferative small intestinal disease associated with *Camplyobacter jejuni*. *New Engl J Med* 350:239-248. PMID:14724303.

Lesesve J, Salignac S, Alla F, et al [2004] Comparative evaluation of schistocyte counting by an automated method and by microscopic determination. *Am J Clin Pathol* 121:739-745. PMID:15151214.

Levine RL, Loriaux M, Huntly BJP, et al [2005] The JAK2V617F activating mutation occurs in chronic myelomonocytic leukemia and acute myeloid leukemia, but not in acute lymphoblastic leukemia or chronic lymphocytic leukemia. *Blood* 106(10):3377-3379. PMID:16081687.

Li S, Juco J, Mann KP, Holden JT [2004] Flow cytometry in the differential diagnosis of lymphocyte-rich thymoma from precursor T cell acute lymphoblastic leukemia/lymphoblastic lymphoma. *Am J Clin Pathol* 121:268-274. PMID:14983942.

Lin P, Hao S, Medeiros LJ, et al [2004a] Expression of CD2 in acute promyelocytic leukemia correlates with short form of PML-RARα transcripts and poorer prognosis. *Am J Clin Pathol* 121:1-9. PMID:15023045.

Lin P, Owens R, Tricot G, Wilson CS [2004b] Flow cytometric immunophenotypic analysis of 306 cases of multiple myeloma. *Am J Clin Pathol* 121:482-488. PMID:15080299.

Lin P, Hao S, Handy BC, et al [2005] Lymphoid neoplasms associated with IgM paraprotein. *Am J Clin Pathol* 123:200-205. PMID:15842043.

Liu H, Ye H, Ruskone-Fourmestraux A, et al [2002] t(11;18) is a marker for all stage gastric MALT lymphomas that will not respond to *H pylori* eradication. *Gastroenterology* 1286-1294. PMID:11984515.

Mackay IR, Rosen FS [2000] The immune system: first of 2 parts. *New Engl J Med* 343:37-49.

Mackay IR, Rosen FS [2000] The immune system: second of 2 parts. *New Engl J Med* 343:108-117.

Macon WR, Levy NB, Kurtin PJ, et al [2001] Hepatosplenic αβ T-cell lymphomas: a report of 14 cases and comparison with hepatosplenic γδ T-cell lymphomas. *Am J Surg Pathol* 25(3):285-296. PMID:11224598.

Matsubara K, Fukaya T, Nigami H, et al [2004] Age-dependent changes in the incidence and etiology of childhood thrombocytopenia. *Acta Haematol* 111:132-137. PMID:15034233.

Mauro FR, DeRossi G, Burgio VL, et al [1994] Prognostic value of bone marrow histology in CLL: a study of 335 untreated cases from a single institution. *Haematologica* 79:334-341. PMID:7806088.

Means RT Jr, Allen J, Sears DA, Schuster SJ [1999] Serum soluble transferrin receptor and the prediction of marrow aspirate iron results in a heterogeneous group of patients. *Clin Lab Haem* 21:161-167. PMID:10448597.

Miralles GD, O'Fallon JR, Talley NJ [1992] Plasma cell dyscrasia with polyneuropathy: the spectrum of POEMS syndrome. *N Engl J Med* 327:1919-1923. PMID:1333569.

Miranda RN, Briggs RC, Kinney MC, et al [2000] Immunohistochemical detection of cyclin D1 using optimized conditions is highly specific for mantle cell lymphoma and hairy cell leukemia. *Mod Pathol* 13:1308-1314. PMID:11144927.

Montesinos P, Bergua JM, Vellenga E [2009] Differentiation syndrome in patients with acute promyelocytic leukemia treated with all-*trans* retinoic acid and anthracycline chemotherapy: characteristics, outcome, and prognostic factors. *Blood* 113:775-783. PMID:18945964.s

Morris MW, Davey FR [1996] Basic examination of blood. *Clinical Diagnosis and Management by Laboratory Methods,* 19th ed. Philadelphia: WB Saunders Company.

Mosca A, Paleari R, Ivaldi G, et al [2009] The role of haemoglobin A2 testing in the diagnosis of thalassaemias and related haemoglobinopathies. *J Clin Pathol* 62:13-17. PMID:19103851.

Nascimento AF, Pinkus JL, Pinkus GS [2004] Clusterin, a marker for anaplastic large cell lymphoma: immunohistochemical profile in hematopoietic and nonhematopoietic malignant neoplasms. *Am J Clin Pathol* 121:709-717. PMID:15151211.

Natkunam Y, Rouse RV [2000] Utility of paraffin section immunohistochemistry for C-kit (CD117) in the differential diagnosis of systemic mast cell disease involving the bone marrow. *Am J Surg Pathol* 24(1):81-91. PMID:10632491.

Needleman H [2004] Lead poisoning. *Annu Rev Med* 55:209-222. PMID:14746518.

Ng A, Taylor GM, Wynn RF, Eden OB [2005] Effects of topoisomerase 2 inhibitors on the *MLL* gene in children receiving chemotherapy: a prospective study. *Leukemia* 19:253-259. PMID:15592432.

Ng SB, Lai KW, Murugaya S, et al [2004] Nasal-type Extranodal natural killer/T cell lymphomas: a clinicopathologic and genotypic study of 42 cases in Singapore. *Mod Pathol* 17:1097-1107. PMID:15195107.

O'Brien LA, James, Othman M, et al [2003] Founder von Willebrand factor haplotype associated with type 1 von Willebrand disease. *Blood* 102:549-557. PMID:12649144.

O'Connell FP, Pinkus JL, Pinkus GS [2004] CD138 (Syndecan-1), a plasma cell marker: immunohistochemical profile in hematopoietic and nonhematopoietic neoplasms. *Am J Clin Pathol* 121:254-263. PMID:14983940.

O'Keefe EK, Rhodes MM, Woodworth A [2009] A patient with previous diagnosis of hemoglobin S/C disease with an unusually severe disease course. *Clin Chem* 55(6):1228-1233. PMID:19478026.

O'Shea J, Sherlock M, Philip R [2005] Thrombocytosis in childhood. *Acta Haematol* 113:212 PMID:15870494.

Ogawa M [1993] Differentiation and proliferation of hematopoietic stem cells. *Blood* 81:2844-2853. PMID:8499622.

Onciu M, Schlette E, Medeiros LJ, et al [2001] Cytogenetic findings in mantle cell lymphoma: cases with a high level of peripheral blood involvement have a distinct pattern of abnormalities. *Am J Clin Pathol* 116:886-892. PMID:11764078.

Onciu M, Behm FG, Raimondi SC, et al [2003] Alk-positive anaplastic large cell lymphoma with leukemic peripheral blood involvement is a clinicopathologic entity with an unfavorable prognosis: report of 3 cases and review of the literature. *Am J Clin Pathol* 120:617-625. PMID:14560573.

Orchard JA, Ibbotson RE, Davis Z, et al [2004] ZAP-70 expression and prognosis in CLL. *Lancet* 363:105-111. PMID:14726163.

Pagliuca A, Mufti GJ, Janossa-Tahernia M, et al [1990] In vitro colony culture and chromosomal studies in hepatic and portal vein thrombosis: possible evidence of an occult myeloproliferative state. *Q J Med* 76(281):981-989. PMID:2236481.

Pai MKR, Bedritis I, Zipursky A [1975] Massive transplacental hemorrhage: clinical manifestations in the newborn. *CMAJ* 112(5):585-589. PMID:1116088.

Petrella T, Bagot M, Willemze R, et al [2005] Blastic NK-cell lymphomas (agranular CD4+, CD56+ hematodermic neoplasms). *Am J Clin Pathol* 123:662-675. PMID:15981806.

Prassouli A, Papadakis V, Tsakris A, et al [2005] Classic transient erythroblastopenia of childhood with human parvovirus B19 genome detection in the blood and bone marrow. *J Pediatr Hemaol Oncol* 27(6):333-336. PMID:15956889.

Rai KR, Sawitsky A, Cronkite EP, et al [1975] Clinical staging of chronic lymphocytic leukemia. *Blood* 46:219-234. PMID:1139039.

Rai KR, Wasil T, Iqbal U, et al [2004] Clinical staging and prognostic markers in chronic lymphocytic leukemia. *Hematol Oncol Clin N Am* 18:795-805. PMID:15325699.

Raimondi SC, Chang MN, Ravindranath Y, et al [1999] Chromosomal abnormalities in 478 children with acute myeloid leukemia: clinical characteristics and treatment outcome in a cooperative Pediatric Oncology Group study-POG 8821. *Blood* 94:3707-3716. PMID:10572083.

Rajkumar SV, Kyle RA, Therneau TM, et al [2005] Serum free light chain ratio is an independent risk factor for progression in monoclonal gammopathy of undetermined significance. *Blood* 106:812-817. PMID:15855274.

Rao SP, Miller ST, Cohen BJ [1992] Transient aplastic crisis in patients with sickle cell disease. *Am J Dis Child* 146:1328 PMID:1415073.

Rausei-Mills V, Chang KL, Gaal KK, et al [2008] Aberrant expression of CD7 in myeloblasts is highly associated with de novo acute myeloid leukemia with FLT3/ITD mutation. *Am J Clin Pathol* 139:624-629. PMID:18343790.

Ray S, Craig FE, Swerdlow SH [2005] Abnormal patterns of antigenic expression in follicular lymphoma: a flow cytometric study. *Am J Clin Pathol* 124:576-583. PMID:16146823.

Remstein ED, Dogan A, Einerson RR, et al [2006] The incidence and anatomic site specificity of chromosomal translocations in primary extranodal marginal zone B cell lymphoma of mucosa associated lymphoid tissue (MALT lymphoma) in North America. *Am J Surg Pathol* 30:1546-1553. PMID:17122510.

Richards SJ, Barnett D [2007] The role of flow cytometry in the diagnosis of paroxysmal nocturnal hemoglobinuria in the clinical laboratory. *Clin Lab Med* 27:577-590. PMID:17658408.

Rimsza LM, Larson RS, Winter SS, et al [2000] Benign hematogone-rich lymphoid proliferations can be distinguished from B-lineage acute lymphoblastic leukemia by integration of morphology, immunophenotype, adhesion molecule expression, and architectural features. *Am J Clin Pathol* 114:66-75. PMID:10884801.

Robbins BA, Ellison DJ, Spinosa JC, et al [1993] Diagnostic application of 2-color flow cytometry in 161 cases of hairy cell leukemia. *Blood* 82:1277-1287. PMID:7688993.

Roberts AR, Hilburg LE [1958] Sickle cell disease with salmonella osteomyelitis. *J Pediatr* 53:170-5. PMID:13502825.

Roden AC, Morice WG, Hanson CA [2008] Immunophenotypic attributes of benign peripheral blood γδ T cells and conditions associated with their increase. *Arch Pathol Lab Med* 132:1774-1780. PMID:18976014.

Ross JS, Ginsburg GS. [2003] The integration of molecular diagnostics with therapeutics. *Am J Clin Pathol* 119:26-36. PMID:12520694.

Rothenberg ME [1998] Eosinophilia. *N Engl J Med* 338:1592-1600. PMID:9603798.

Saadoun D, Suarez F, Lefrere F, et al [2005] Splenic lymphoma with villous lymphocytes, associated with type II cryoglobulinemia and HCV infection: A new entity? *Blood* 105:74-76. PMID:15353484.

Saadoun D, Elalamy I, Ghillani-Dalbin P, et al [2009] Cryofibrinogenemia: new insights into clinical and pathogenic features. *Am J Med* 122:1128-1135. PMID:19958891.

Salama M, Lossos IS, Warnke RA, Natkunam Y [2009] Immunoarchitectural patterns in nodal marginal zone B cell lymphoma: a study of 51 cases. *Am J Clin Pathol* 132:39-49. PMID:19864232.

Salar A, Juanpere N, Bellosillo B, et al [2006] Gastrointestinal involvement in mantle cell lymphoma: a prospective clinic, endoscopic, and pathologic study. *Am J Surg Pathol* 30:1274-1280. PMID:17001159.

Salles GA [2007] Clinical features, prognosis and treatment of follicular lymphoma. *Hematology Am Soc Hematol Educ Program* 216-225. PMID:18024633.

Sanz MA, Grimwade D, Tallman MS [2009] Management of acute promyelocytic leukemia: recommendations from an expert panel on behalf of the European Leukemia Net. *Blood* 113:1875-1891. PMID:18812465.

Schaar CG, LeCessie S, Snijder S, et al [2008] Long-term follow-up of a population based cohort with monoclonal porteinaemia. *Brit J Haem* 144:176-184. PMID:19036113.

Schlette E, Fu K, Medeiros LJ [2003] CD23 expression in mantle cell lymphoma: clinicopathologic features of 18 cases. *Am J Clin Pathol* 120:760-766. PMID:14608904.

Schraders M, Oeschger S, Kluin PM, et al [2009] Hypermutation in mantle cell lymphoma does not indicate a clinical or biological subentity. *Mod Path* 22:416-425. PMID:19136929.

Scott JR, Warenski JC [1982] Tests to detect and quantitate fetomaternal bleeding. *Clin Obstet Gynecol* 25(2):277-282. PMID:6179677.

Seegmiller AC, Kroft SH, Karandikar NJ, McKenna RW [2009] Characterization of immunophenotypic aberrancies in 200 cases of B acute lymphoblastic leukemia. *Am J Clin Pathol* 132:940-949. PMID:19926587.

Sen F, Lai R, Albitar M [2002] Chronic lymphocytic leukemia with t(14;18) and trisomy 12: report of 2 cases and review of the literature. *Arch Pathol Lab Med* 126:1543-1546. PMID:12456221.

Shastri KA, Logue GL [1993] Autoimmune neutropenia. *Blood* 81(8):1984-1995. PMID:8471760.

Shetty S, Kulkarni B, Pai N, et al [2010] JAK2 mutations across a spectrum of venous thrombosis cases. *Am J Clin Pathol* 134:82-85. PMID:20551270.

Slone SP, Fleming DR, Buchino JJ [2003] Sinus histiocytosis with massive lymphadenopathy and langerhans cell histiocytosis express the cellular adhesion molecule CD31. *Arch Pathol Lab Med* 127(3):341-344. PMID:12653580.

Sotlar K, Horny HP, Simonitsch I, et al [2004] CD25 indicates the neoplastic phenotype of mast cells. *Am J Surg Pathol* 28(10):1319-1326. PMID:15371947.

Soupir CP, Vergilio J, Cin PD, et al [2007] Philadelphia chromosome positive acute myeloid leukemia. *Am J Clin Pathol* 127:642-650. PMID:17369142.

Staudt LM [2003] Molecular diagnosis of the hematologic cancers. *New Engl J Med* 348:1777-1785. PMID:12724484.

Steensma DP, Gibbons RJ, Higgs DR [2005] Acquired alpha-thalassemia in association with myelodysplastic syndrome and other hematologic malignancies. *Blood* 105(2):443-452. PMID:15358626.

Sutherland DR, Kuek N, Azcona-Olivera J, et al [2009] Use of a FLAER-based WBC assay in the primary screening of PNH clones. *Am J Clin Pathol* 132:564-572. PMID:19762534.

Swerdlow SH, et al, Eds [2008] *Tumours of Haematopoietic and Lymphoid Tissues,* Lyon: International Agency for Research on Cancer.

Tajiri J, Noguchi S, Murakami T, Murakami N [1990] Antithyroid drug induced agranulocytosis: the usefulness of routine white blood cell count monitoring. *Arch Intern Med* 150:621-624. PMID:2310281.

Tate JR, Gill D, Cobcroft R, Hickman PE [2003] Practical considerations for the measurement of free light chains in serum. *Clin Chem* 49(8):1252-1257. PMID:12881439.

Tatsas AD, Jagasia MH, Chen H, McCurley TL [2010] Monitoring residual myeloma: high-resolution serum/urine electrophoresis or marrow biopsy with immunohistochemical analysis? *Am J Clin Pathol* 134:139-145. PMID:20551278.

Tefferi A [2003] Anemia in adults: a contemporary approach to diagnosis. *Mayo Clin Proc* 78:1274-1280. PMID:14531486.

Thalhammer-Scherrer R, Mitterbauer G, Simonitsch I, et al [2002] The immunophenotype of 325 adult acute leukemias. *Am J Clin Pathol* 117:380-389. PMID:11888077.

Thomas C, Thomas L [2002] Biochemical markers and hematologic indices in the diagnosis of functional iron deficiency. *Clin Chem* 48(7):1066-1076. PMID:12089176.

Timuragaoglua A, Erkan Ç, Erbasan F [2004] The importance of platelet indexes in discriminating between β-thalassemia trait and iron deficiency anemia. *Acta Haematol* 111:235-236. PMID:15153720.

Tischkowitz M, Dokal I [2004] Fanconi anemia and leukemia—clinical and molecular aspects. *Br J Haematol* 126:176-191. PMID:15238138.

Trueworthy R, Shuster J, Look T, et al [1992] Ploidy of lymphoblasts is the strongest predictor of treatment outcome in B progenitor cell ALL of childhood: a Pediatric Oncology Group study. *J Clin Oncol* 10:606-613. PMID:1548523.

Tsaras G, Owusu-Ansah A, Boateng FO, Amoateng-Adjepong Y [2009] Complications associated with sickle cell trait: a brief narrative review. *Am J Med* 122:507-512. PMID:19393983.

Tworek JA, Singleton TP, Schnitzer B, Hsi ED, Ross CW [1998] Flow cytometric and immunohistochemical analysis of small lymphocytic lymphoma, mantle cell lymphoma, and plasmacytoid small lymphocytic lymphoma. *Am J Clin Pathol* 110:582-589. PMID:9802342.

Valla D, Casadevall N, Lacombe C, et al [1985] Primary myeloproliferative disorder and hepatic vein thrombosis: a prospective study of erythroid colony formation in vitro in 20 patients with Budd-Chiari syndrome. *Ann Int Med* 103(3):329-334. PMID:4026081.

Van Kirk R, Sandhaus LM, Hoyer JD [2005] The detection and diagnosis of hemoglobin A2' by high-performance liquid chromatography. *Am J Clin Pathol* 123:657-661. PMID:15981805.

Verdonck K, González E, Van Dooren S, et al [2007] Human T-lymphotropic virus 1: Recent knowledge about an ancient infection. *Lancet Infect Dis* 7:266-281. PMID:17376384.

Vyasa P, Crispino JD [2007] Molecular insights into Down syndrome associated leukemia. *Curr Opin Pediatr* 19:9-14. PMID:17224656.

Wang LJ, Glasser L [2002] Spurious dyserythropoiesis. *Am J Clin Pathol* 117:57-59. PMID:11789731.

Ward PCJ [2002] Modern approaches to the investigation of vitamin B_{12} deficiency. *Clin Lab Med* 22:435-445. PMID:12134470.

Went PT, Zimpfer A, Pehrs AC, et al [2005] High specificity of combined TRAP and DBA.44 expression for hairy cell leukemia. *Am J Surg Pathol* 29:474-478. PMID:15767800.

Willis MS, McKenna RW, Peterson LC, Coad JE, Kroft SH [2005] Low blast count myeloid disorders with auer rods: a clinicopathologic analysis of 9 cases. *Am J Clin Pathol* 124:191-198. PMID:16040288.

Wolf AW, Jimenez E, Lozoff B [2003] Effects of iron therapy on infant blood lead levels. *J Pediatr* 143:789-795. PMID:14657829.

Wu JM, Borowitz MJ, Weir EG [2006] The usefulness of CD71 expression by flow cytometry for differentiating indolent from aggressive CD10+ B cell lymphomas. *Am J Clin Pathol* 126:39-46. PMID:16753591.

Xu Y, Dolan MM, Nguyen PL [2003] Diagnostic significance of detecting dysgranulopoiesis in chronic myeloid leukemia. *Am J Clin Pathol* 120:778-784. PMID:14608906.

Zakai NA, Katz R, Hirsch C, et al [2005] A prospective study of anemia status, hemoglobin concentration, and mortality in an elderly cohort: The Cardiovascular Health Study. *Arch Intern Med* 165:2214-2220. PMID:16246985.

Zuo Z, Polski JM, Kasyan A, Medeios J [2010] Acute erythroid leukemia. *Arch Pathol Lab Med* 134:1261-1270. PMID:20807044.

Chapter 5

Coagulation

Hemostasis
Normal hemostasis occurs in 3 steps

Vasoconstriction

Vasoconstriction is the initial reaction to a vascular injury. This is mediated by vascular smooth muscle in response to local cytokines. There are disorders that cause vascular fragility and can result in abnormal bleeding, such as hereditary hemorrhagic telangiectasia (Osler-Weber-Rendu). Clinically, vascular fragility resembles bleeding caused by platelet defects.

Platelet aggregation (primary hemostasis)

Platelet aggregation is the second step, mediated by platelets in response to circulating and fixed agonists. Platelet aggregation is triphasic, consisting of adhesion, degranulation, and aggregation. Adhesion (attachment to a surface) is mediated by GPIb, the receptor for von Willebrand factor, and GPIa-IIa, a receptor for collagen. vWF and collagen are exposed on the denuded subendothelial basement membrane. The receptor GPIb is activated by shear forces in vivo and by ristocetin in vitro. Degranulation (the release reaction) refers to the release of α and dense granules and the simultaneous synthesis and release of thromboxane A2 (TXA2). The degranulation process is stimulated by any one of the platelet agonists, including epinephrine, ADP, thrombin, platelet activating factor (PAF), collagen, or TXA2. Lastly, aggregation (attachment to other platelets) is mediated by GPIIb/IIIa and fibrinogen. The latter is free in the extracellular space and can crosslink 2 platelets via their respective GPIIb/IIIa receptors.

Platelets are anucleate cells consisting of cytoskeleton, cytoplasmic granules, and a cell membrane. Platelets are normally smaller than red blood cells; mean platelet volume (MPV) is usually around 10 fL and tends to vary inversely with the platelet count. There are 2 types of platelet granules. Platelet α granules contain fibrinogen, platelet derived growth factor (PDGF), von Willebrand factor (vWF), P-selectin, and platelet factor 4 (PF4)—all large proteins. Platelet dense granules contain adenosine diphosphate (ADP), adenosine triphosphate (ATP), serotonin (5-HT), and calcium—all small molecules. Platelets bear a limited number of cell surface proteins t5.1.

t5.1 Platelet cell surface antigens

Antigen	Notes
GPIb/V/IX complex (CD42)	Receptor for vWF
GPIIb/IIIa complex (CD41 & CD61)	Receptor for fibrinogen GPIIIa is the basis for platelet antigens PL^{A1} & PL^{A2} GPIIb is basis for antigens bak^a & bak^b
GPIa/IIa complex	Collagen receptor Br^a/ Br^b antigen
GPIc/IIa complex	Fibronectin receptor
Red cell antigens ABO, P, I, i & Le	No Rh antigens
Class I MHC antigens	No class II antigens
IgG & coagulation factors	Passively adsorbed onto platelet surface

Fibrin formation (coagulation)

Fibrin formation is the final step in hemostasis, and it is mediated by the coagulation cascade f5.1 t5.2. For purposes of in vitro testing of the coagulation cascade, it is convenient

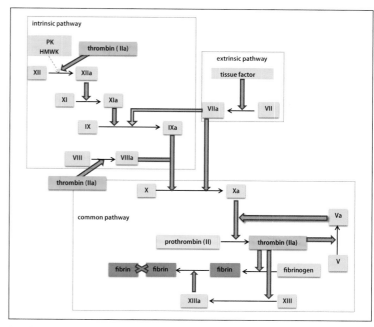

f5.1 The clotting cascades. The intrinsic cascade (left) is thought to have a minor in vivo significance. The extrinsic pathway (right) is initiated upon vascular injury, which leads to exposure of tissue factor (TF, factor III). There is thought to be a biologically significant interrelation of the extrinsic & intrinsic pathway, mediated by (1) factor VIIa crossing over & activating factor IX and (2) factor VIIa activating thrombin which in fact drives the intrinsic pathway. PK & HMWK were once thought to activate the intrinsic pathway, but their biologic significance is now unclear.

to distinguish 3 pathways: the extrinsic pathway, intrinsic pathway, and common pathway. These distinctions are not entirely valid in vivo.

t5.2 Coagulation factors

Factor	Other names	Vitamin K dependent	Where produced	Half life (hours)	% activity required for normal coagulation
I	Fibrinogen	–	Liver	100-150	30
II	Prothrombin	+	Liver	50-80	30
V		–	Liver	24	20
VII		+	Liver	6	20
VIII	Antihemophilic factor	–	Liver (Küpffer cells)	12	30
IX	Christmas factor	+	Liver	24	30
X	Stuart-Prower factor	+	Liver	25-60	20
XI		–	Liver	40-80	20
XII	Hagemann factor	–	Liver	50-70	<5
XIII	Fibrin stabilizing factor	–	Liver	150	<5
vWF	von Willebrand factor	–	Endothelial cells Megakaryocytes	24	30
Prekallikrein	Fletcher factor	–	Liver	35	<5
High molecular weight kininogen (HMWK)	Fitzgerald factor	–	Liver	150	<5

Others are factor IV (calcium) & factor III (tissue factor); activated factor V (Va) is sometimes called factor VI (accelerin)

The only factor unique to the extrinsic pathway is factor VII. The extrinsic pathway is initiated when tissue injury leads to the release of tissue factor (sometimes called factor III). Activated factor VII (VIIa), cleaves factor X to factor Xa; so VIIa is the "tenase" of the extrinsic pathway. Note that VIIa is capable of activating factor IX to IXa in vivo; so pathophysiologic activation of factor VII can drive the intrinsic pathway. This is thought to be a major mechanism by which the administration of factor VIIa exerts its therapeutic effect.

Intrinsic pathway factors include XII, XI, IX, VIII, prekallikrein, and high molecular weight kininogen (HMWK). Calcium (factor IV) and phospholipids are required in multiple steps. Like the extrinsic pathway, the endpoint is conversion of factor X to factor Xa. The intrinsic pathway is initiated by the proximity of prekallikrein, HMWK, factor XII and factor XI to one another and to a negatively charged surface (the contact phase). This results in conversion of prekallikrein to kallikrein, which in turn activates factor XII to factor XIIa. Factor XIIa can then activate more prekallikrein to kallikrein, establishing a cycle. The ultimate activation of factor X is carried out by the so-called tenase complex (calcium, VIIIa, IXa) on the surface of platelets. Platelets, when activated, express an abundance of phosphatidylserine (PS) and phosphatidylinositol (PI) on their surfaces, facilitating attachment of the tenase complex. Factor Xa is capable of activating VII to VIIa, thus providing another link with the extrinsic pathway.

The common pathway, while conceptually distinct, is required by the intrinsic and extrinsic pathways to produce a clot. Thus, while it is possible to separately test the pathways by mental subtraction, they are not truly isolatable in vivo. Common pathway constituents include X, prothrombin (II), and fibrinogen (I). It begins at the convergence of the intrinsic and extrinsic pathways, with the activation of factor X to factor Xa. Xa converts II to IIa (thrombin), and thrombin converts fibrinogen to fibrin (Ia). The so-called prothrombinase complex, like the tenase complex, forms on the surfaces of platelets, anchored by PS and PI, and consists of Va and Xa. Fibrinogen is composed of pairs of 3 polypeptides—α, β, and γ—thus it is a hexamer. Fibrinogen conversion to fibrin begins when thrombin cleaves the α and β chains, releasing their N-termini (fibrinopeptides A and B) and exposing the "sticky" ends of fibrin. The remaining fibrin molecules then polymerize, elongating into protofibrils; protofibrils associate side by side into fibrin fibers. Factor XIII is responsible for covalently crosslinking fibers.

Coagulation is under tight control normally. There is a delicate dynamic balance between the formation of thrombin on the one hand and fibrin degradation on the other. At nearly every step of the intrinsic and extrinsic pathways, there are feedback loops that are activated, usually leading to the rapid degradation of the step's product. A major mechanism in the extrinsic pathway is the inhibition of the tissue factor-VIIa-Xa complex by a protein known by several names: lipoprotein-associated coagulation inhibitor (LACI)/extrinsic pathway inhibitor (EPI)/tissue factor pathway inhibitor (TFPI)/anticonvertin. Furthermore, the activation of thrombin is directly controlled through the action of numerous factors: Antithrombin, α_2-macroglobulin, heparin cofactor II, and α1-antitrypsin. Antithrombin inactivates not only thrombin but also IXa, Xa, XIa and XIIa. Antithrombin can be further stimulated by heparin, forming the basis for heparin therapy. Lastly, thrombin combines with thrombomodulin on endothelial cell surfaces forming a thrombin-TM complex that converts protein C to activated protein C (APC). APC in turn inactivates Va and VIIIa, with protein S as its cofactor.

Plasmin is the primary agent of fibrin degradation, formed from plasminogen which is structurally incorporated into the fibrin clot. Tissue plasminogen activator (tPA) converts plasminogen to plasmin, and tPA is released from vascular endothelial cells following injury; thus the mechanisms for fibrin degradation and fibrin formation are set into motion simultaneously. Exposure to fibrin activates tPA. Plasmin itself is controlled by rapid degradation by α_2-antiplasmin as wells as inhibition by several agents: plasminogen activator inhibitors (PAI-1 and PAI-2).

Laboratory evaluation of hemostasis
Laboratory evaluation of platelets
The bleeding time (BT)

In the Ivy bleeding time, a blood pressure cuff is placed around the arm and inflated to 40 mm Hg. 2 standard incisions are made on the volar surface of the forearm. The cuts are blotted every 30 seconds until bleeding stops. The times for the 2 incisions are averaged. A normal adult bleeds for between

1½ and 13½ minutes. The Duke bleeding time is based upon an incision in the earlobe or fingertip. In the Mielke bleeding time, a template is used to standardize the incision depth and length. Despite extensive attempts at standardization, the bleeding time test has not achieved acceptable reproducibility. Mean interobserver variability is 135 seconds, and mean intraindividual variability (6 weeks apart) is 150 seconds. The coefficient of variation is estimated to be between 18 and 46%.

The bleeding time was proposed as an in vivo assessment of platelet function at a time when there were no other available tests of platelet function. It turns out to be a poor test of platelet function and is in particular not useful for predicting the risk of perioperative bleeding. It is currently the position of both the College of American Pathologists and the American Society for Clinical Pathology that the bleeding time is not effective as a screening test in patients without a history of excessive bleeding, including patients who have recently taken aspirin or NSAIDs. The only current indication for the bleeding time is to screen for qualitative platelet disorders and von Willebrand disease; even so, the PFA-100 assay (see below) is a more sensitive screening test for these disorders. The bleeding time is expected to be prolonged in von Willebrand disease, other inherited platelet disorders, uremia, aspirin ingestion, or low platelet counts (<100,000/µL).

PFA-100

PFA-100 is an instrument that may be used for platelet disorder screening. It utilizes an artificial vessel, and under standardized flow conditions measures the time required for anticoagulated whole blood to occlude a standard aperture (closure time). Shear forces arise at the aperture, simulating in vivo platelet plug formation. The aperture is covered by 1 of 2 types of thin membrane: one type is impregnated with collagen and epinephrine (Col/Epi), and the other with collagen and ADP (Col/ADP). Testing with the Col/Epi cartridge is sensitive to global platelet defects, and Col/ADP is sensitive to drug induced platelet defects (aspirin and aspirin-like agents). Trials comparing simultaneous PFA-100 and BT in identical patients show equivalent (normal vs abnormal) results in ~75% of cases. Discrepancies result from the low sensitivity of the BT to aspirin and von Willebrand disease. The closure time is dependent not only on platelet function but also on platelet number and hematocrit; a prolonged CT may be caused by anemia (hematocrit <25%) or thrombocytopenia (platelet count <100 × 10^9/L). The PFA-100 test is not useful for monitoring Plavix.

Platelet aggregometry

Standard preanalytic conditions must be maintained for reliable platelet aggregometry. Generally, the assay should be scheduled in advance so that there is not a significant delay in testing. Patients should not have taken aspirin or NSAIDs for >7 days. Tubes should be kept at room temperature (cold causes platelet activation), and the test should be performed within 2 hours.

Platelet aggregometry is performed on a sample of platelet rich plasma, which is prepared by slow-centrifugation of whole blood. The sample is stirred continuously within a cuvette while being exposed to various agonists, including ADP, epinephrine, arachidonate, collagen, and ristocetin. As

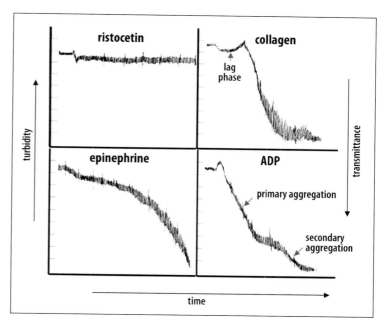

f5.2 Platelet aggregometry in a patient with von Willebrand disease

platelet aggregation takes place, the initially turbid mixture clears, light transmission through the cuvette increases, and turbidity increases. Normally there is no significant spontaneous aggregation. The normal adult displays >60% platelet aggregation in response to platelet agonists. Normal newborns tend to have decreased aggregation as compared to adults.

When transmittance is plotted against time, aggregation produces stereotypical curves. A biphasic curve is normally seen with low dose ADP and epinephrine, resulting from a primary and secondary wave of aggregation, the latter due to platelet degranulation. A monophasic curve (primary aggregation only) is seen with high dose ADP, collagen and ristocetin.

The response to ristocetin is normally seen with ristocetin concentration exceeding 1.2 mg/mL. There is normally little to no response to ristocetin <0.8 mg/mL. The response to collagen normally follows a short lag. The release of platelet dense granules, reflected in the secondary wave, can be monitored during aggregation by assaying secreted ATP using the firefly luminescence assay.

The most common cause of abnormal aggregometry is a medication. The typical result of aspirin and aspirin-like agents is decreased aggregation with arachidonate. Poor response to all agents (ADP, epinephrine, arachidonate, collagen) except ristocetin is typical of Glanzmann thombasthenia (rare). An absent secondary phase (with epinephrine and ADP) is seen in with storage pool defects and aspirin. A poor response to epinephrine is seen in myeloproliferative diseases. Response to everything but ristocetin f5.2 is the hallmark of von Willebrand disease. This pattern is also seen in Bernard-Soulier syndrome.

Platelet flow cytometry

Since flow cytometry is capable of detecting cell surface expression, it can be adapted to the diagnosis of most of the inherited platelet defects, particularly those in which a platelet surface receptor is quantitatively decreased. Furthermore, since platelet activation is associated with predictable changes in the expression of membrane constituents, functional defects can also be assessed. Currently, antibodies are available for a variety of platelet markers, including GPIIb/IIIa, CD62 (a component of the platelet α granule that is externalized if these are properly secreted), CD63 (lysosomal granule membrane protein), and the particular conformation of fibrinogen assumed only within the GPIIb/IIIa receptor.

Laboratory evaluation of coagulation

Activated clotting time (ACT)

The ACT is a point of care test that can be used to monitor high dose heparin therapy, particularly at ranges where the aPTT is immeasurable (>150 seconds). The ACT is performed on whole blood. Blood is collected into a tube that contains an intrinsic pathway activator (eg, kaolin, glass) and an analyzer measures the clotting time. This has utility in bypass surgery as well as in other instances when an immediate result is desired. If time permits, an anti-Xa assay is a favorable alternative to the ACT. In a normal adult, the ACT runs ~70-180 seconds. In high dose heparin therapy, a time of >400 seconds is often sought. The ACT is less precise than the aPTT, and, since it is performed on whole blood, a number of noncoagulation factors (eg, platelet count, hematocrit) influences it.

Activated partial thromboplastin time (aPTT)

Phospholipid, a contact activator of factor XII (eg, silica, kaolin), and excess calcium are added to citrated plasma. The time to clot formation is the aPTT. The aPTT can be used to screen for factor deficiency, but in the hospital setting its prolongation is often caused by inhibitors. Inhibitors come in 3 varieties: medications (heparin, argatroban), lupus anticoagulants, and, rarely, specific factor antibodies (anti-factor VIII antibody).

Prolongation of the aPTT may be caused by deficiencies of factors XII, XI, IX, VIII (intrinsic pathway constituents), X, V, II, or fibrinogen (common pathway) or by an inhibitor. Prolongation of both the PT and aPTT is caused by deficiencies of factors X, V, II, or fibrinogen (the common pathway) or an inhibitor. A factor generally must be below 30% to cause a prolonged aPTT. With multiple factor deficiencies, higher levels may shorten the aPTT. The aPTT is more sensitive to deficiencies in intrinsic pathway factors than common pathway factors. An elevated factor VIII level is capable of shortening the aPTT.

Determining the cause of a prolonged aPTT t5.3, t5.4, f5.3

- The first step is to exclude the effect of heparin through clinical inquiry or the use of a heparin neutralization procedure.

- If heparin neutralization does not correct the aPTT, then a mixing study (see below) is performed. If a mixing study fails to correct the aPTT, then an inhibitor is suspected (lupus anticoagulant, anti-factor VIII antibody). If a mixing study corrects the aPTT, then a factor deficiency is suspected. Specific assays for factor activities (XII, XI, IX, VIII) can be performed. If these are normal, consider common factor assays and/or a test for lupus anticoagulant (weak inhibitors sometimes correct in a 1:1 mix).

- Mixing studies may be performed to help determine the cause of prolonged clotting times (PT, PTT, or TT) and to screen for inhibitors. The patient's plasma is mixed with normal plasma, in 1:1 ratio, and the abnormal test (eg, PTT) is repeated, both immediately and after a 1-4 hour incubation. A 1:1 mix results in ≥50% activity of all clotting factors. Correction of the clotting time is the expected result if the prolongation is due to any factor deficiency. Anything less than complete correction to within the normal range (some use correction to within 10% of the upper limit of normal) suggests an inhibitor. Some inhibitors show a correction in the immediate aPTT, but prolongation of the incubated aPTT. This is particularly a feature of antibodies against specific factors (eg, anti-factor VIII antibody).

t5.3 Interpretation of screening coagulation tests

PT	aPTT	Likely factors involved	Clinical considerations
↑	Normal	Factor VII	Liver disease
			Vitamin K deficiency
			Warfarin
			Inherited factor deficiency
Normal	↑	Factor VIII	Acquired inhibitors
		Factor IX	Heparin
		Factor XI	Lupus anticoagulant
		Factor XII	Inherited factor deficiency
		Fitzgerald factor (HMWK)	
		Fletcher factor (prekallikrein)	
		LAC	
↑	↑	Factor V	Disseminated intravascular coagulation (DIC)
		Factor X	Heparin
		Fibrinogen	Amyloidosis (acquired factor X deficiency)
		LAC	Liver disease
			Prematurity (neonate)
			Polycythemia
			Inherited factor deficiency
Normal	Normal	XIII	Bleeding (with XIII)
		LAC	Normal or thrombophilic (with LAC)

t5.4 Causes of prolonged aPTT

Etiology	Protime	Additional tests
Deficiencies of factors XII, XI, IX, VIII, prekallikrein, HMWK	Normal	Specific factor assays
Deficiencies of factors X, V, II	Prolonged	Specific factor assays
Lupus anticoagulant	Normal or prolonged (PTT>PT)	LAC assay
Anti-factor VIII antibody	Normal	Anti-factor VIII antibody assay
Heparin	Usually normal (PTT>PT)	Heparin neutralization procedure
Hirudin	Prolonged	History
DIC	Prolonged (PT>PTT)	D-dimer
Liver disease	Prolonged (PT>PTT)	History, LFTs
Vitamin K deficiency/coumadin	Prolonged (PT>PTT)	Assays for II, VII, IX, X

- A 4:1 (4 parts patient plasma to 1 part normal plasma) mix has been advocated for the detection of weak inhibitors. Some inhibitors, especially weak ones, will correct with a 1:1 mix and may be missed. When a percent correction was calculated in one study, a percent correction cutoff of 50% in a 4:1 mix had a 100% sensitivity and 88% specificity for inhibitor. The sensitivity and specificity both approached 100% if a 10% cutoff is applied after incubation for 1 hour. For the 1:1 mix, the results were poor with any cutoff, with cutoffs of <58% indicating inhibitor, and >70% indicating deficiency.

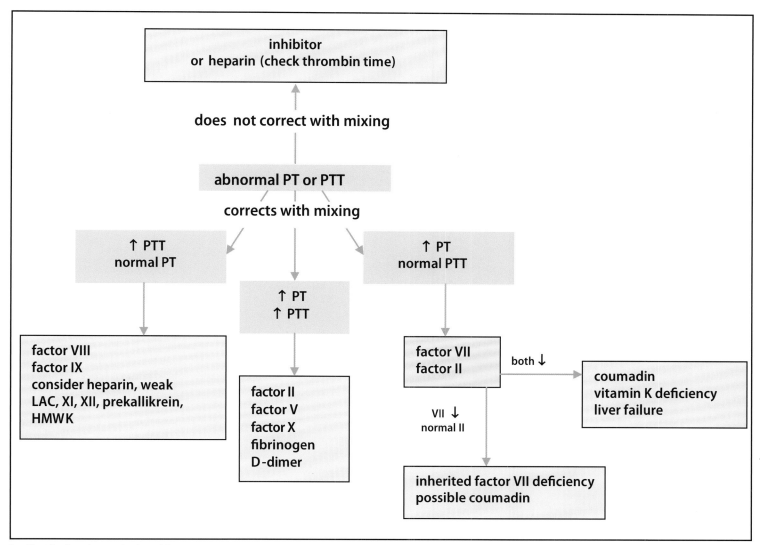

f5.3 Algorithm for evaluation of prolonged clotting times

$$\% \text{ correction} = \frac{\text{patient clotting time} - \text{mix clotting time}}{\text{patient clotting time} - \text{normal clotting time)}}$$

- Historically, mixing with various blood products was useful in determining the identity of a missing factor. For example, aged plasma lacks factors II, V, VIII, XIII. When a prolonged clotting test corrects with aged plasma, the prolongation cannot be due to any of these factors. Adsorbed plasma lacks factors II, VII, IX, X. Serum lacks fibrinogen and factors II, V, VIII, XIII.

Clinical utility of the aPTT

The PTT is used to monitor heparin therapy (unfractionated heparin). With very high doses of heparin, as used in cardiac bypass surgery, the aPTT is unmeasurable (often reported as >150 seconds). In this circumstance, the ACT is often used. The aPTT may also be used to monitor hirudin or argatroban. Xa assays are used to monitor therapy with low molecular weight heparin and to monitor unfractionated heparin in circumstances where the PTT is unreliable t5.5. The therapeutic PTT range for heparin is generally that which corresponds to

anti-Xa level of 0.3-0.7 U/mL. In some patients, heparin fails to prolong the PTT (heparin resistance). Often this is due to an acute phase response (combined effect of increased factor VIII and binding of heparin by acute phase reactants) or antithrombin deficiency t5.5.

t5.5 Sources of error in aPTT monitoring of anticoagulation	
aPTT may overestimate the degree of anticoagulation (be inappropriately prolonged)	aPTT may underestimate the degree of anticoagulation (be inappropriately shortened)
Antiphospholipid syndrome	Post-thrombosis acute phase reaction
Liver disease	Pregnancy
Inherited factor deficiencies	Antithrombin (AT) deficiency
Disseminated intravascular coagulation	Renal disease (acquired ATIII deficiency)
Low volume blood draw	Congenitally high factor VIII
Polycythemia	Marked anemia
Check	**Check**
Lupus anticoagulant factor levels	AT levels
D-dimer	Factor VIII levels

Pre-analytic aPTT considerations

Pretest variables can profoundly impact all in vitro clotting times. The anticoagulant (3.2% trisodium citrate) in coagulation collection tubes chelates calcium, preventing activation of the coagulation system until calcium is added back at the time of testing. The volume of anticoagulant in the collection tubes, ~0.5 mL, is intended to result in a final ratio of whole blood to anticoagulant of 9:1 and a ratio of plasma to anticoagulant of 5:1, assuming normal hematocrit (within the range of 35-55%). When the hematocrit is higher than this, the volume of plasma in a sample is proportionately reduced; thus in this instance the collected sample is over-anticoagulated, and the clotting time may be artifactually prolonged. The volume of anticoagulant may be manually adjusted for extreme hematocrits. Furthermore, if an inappropriate volume is drawn into the tube, this can affect results. Underfilling results in over-anticoagulation and inappropriately prolonged clotting times, and overfilling does the opposite. Numerous studies have confirmed that coagulation tests are reliable within 90-110% of the ideal volume, usually indicated by a marking on the tube. Modern instruments detect clot formation by photo-optical means, such that turbid, lipemic, icteric, or hemolyzed samples may suffer interferences. Traditional mechanical detection, still utilized on some instruments, is insensitive to these interferences. Plastic tubes differ slightly from glass tubes in many coagulation assays; a correlation study is required if making the switch to plastic tubes. Lastly, plasma should be separated from cells as soon as possible. This is particularly true when the PTT is being used for heparin monitoring, since platelets begin to release platelet factor 4 (PF4) which can artifactually shorten the PTT. The plasma should be kept cool until testing is completed (to minimize loss of coagulation factors). If testing will be delayed >4 hours, the specimen should be frozen. The normal neonate has a PTT up to 55 seconds. This shortens to the adult range by 6 months of age.

Activated protein C resistance (APCR) screening assay
See p 314

Anticardiolipin antibody (ACA)
See p 317

Anti-Xa assay (heparin antifactor Xa assay)

The anti-Xa assay can be used to monitor either unfractionated or low molecular weight heparin (LMWH). It is the test of choice for monitoring low molecular weight heparin and danaparoid. It is a useful alternative to the aPTT for monitoring unfractionated heparin, particularly in patients having abnormal baseline coagulation studies because of, eg, LAC or factor XII deficiency. Blood should be drawn 4 hours after a dose of LMWH; 6 hours after danaparoid.

In the chromogenic assay, the patient's plasma is added to a known amount of factor Xa with excess antithrombin. Heparin (or danaparoid) in the patient's plasma stimulates antithrombin to inhibit factor Xa. The quantity of residual factor Xa is measured with a chromogenic substrate which Xa cleaves to produce a colored compound that is detected by a spectrophotometer. The residual Xa is subtracted from the initial Xa to determine the anticoagulant concentration (expressed in antifactor Xa units/mL). Thus, when there has been no heparin administered, the antifactor Xa should be zero. The higher the heparin (or danaparoid), the higher the antifactor Xa.

Unlike unfractionated heparin, LMWH and danaparoid do not require strict monitoring in most patients. Monitoring may be required in renal failure, pregnancy, extremes of weight, and in children (particularly neonates).

Antithrombin (AT, previously antithrombin III)
See p 315

Bethesda assay (factor VIII inhibitor assay, anti-factor VIII antibody assay)

While factor VIII is the most common factor to which antibodies arise, this assay can be adapted to any factor (eg, anti-factor V, anti-factor IX). Anti-factor VIII antibodies (factor VIII inhibitors) have characteristic properties. First, they behave as inhibitors in coagulation screening assays; that is, they cause prolongation in the aPTT that fails to correct in a 1:1 mix. Second, while the immediate aPTT following a 1:1 mix may correct, the aPTT performed after 1-4-hour incubation is prolonged (time dependence). Third, if factor assays are performed, factor VIII will appear decreased. If serial dilutions are performed, each dilution will show progressively more factor VIII activity.

The Bethesda assay is performed by first making several dilutions of patient plasma with citrated saline. Each dilution is then mixed 1:1 with normal plasma and incubated for 1-2 hours. Factor VIII activity assays are then performed on each dilution. Control for expected factor VIII degradation is in the form of parallel incubation of either imidazole buffer with normal plasma (classic Bethesda assay) or factor VIII-deficient plasma with normal plasma (Nijmegen modification of the Bethesda assay). The dilution at which the factor VIII activity is 50% represents the inhibitor titer. The result is expressed in Bethesda units (if the 1:16 dilution results in 50% factor activity, then the result is 16 Bethesda units). Patients with low-titer antibodies (low responders) have <5 Bethesda units and can usually be successfully treated with DDAVP and higher doses of human factor VIII. In high responders, patients with >5 Bethesda units, the antibody cannot be overcome with high doses of human factor VIII. These patients require some combination of porcine factor VIII, activated prothrombin complex concentrate (APCC), or recombinant factor VII (NovoSeven).

Since one of the major therapeutic options in patients with anti-factor VIII antibodies is the use of porcine factor VIII, it can be helpful to know whether the patient's antibody will crossreact with the porcine product. Porcine factor VIII can be substituted for normal plasma in the above-described assay to make this determination.

Clot retraction test
See p 305

Clot stability test (urea solubility test, factor XIII deficiency screen)
See p 311

D-dimer & fibrin-degradation products (FDPs)

D-dimer is a type of fibrin-degradation product (FDP) or fibrin split product (FSP). At the end of the clotting cascade, fibrin monomers are generated through the action of thrombin on fibrinogen (fibrinopeptide removal from fibrinogen). Fibrin monomers spontaneously polymerize into fibrin strands which are later crosslinked by factor XIII. It is factor XIII that generates the D-dimer, by linking the D regions of fibrin molecules. Later, the fibrin clot is dis-assembled by plasmin, which is incapable of breaking up D-dimers. The plasmin-generated fibrin degradation products, including D-dimer, are released to the circulation. Note that D-dimer is not formed in the plasmin-mediated degradation of fibrinogen (which produces fibrinogen degradation products). Thus, the presence of D-dimer indicates that fibrin has been formed and then degraded. Assays for FDPs are a little less specific, because they detect fibrin degradation products, fibrinogen degradation products, and D-dimer.

D-dimers and FDP are most often increased in thrombosis and significant bleeding. They may also be elevated in atrial fibrillation and congestive heart failure. Cirrhotic patients, because of difficulty in clearing these products, may have persistent elevation of D-dimer and FDP in conjunction with low level chronic DIC. Patients with certain tumors, particularly mucin-secreting adenocarcinomas, may have elevated D-dimer and FDP. Lastly, D-dimer may be elevated in disseminated intravascular coagulation (DIC), infection, inflammation, and trauma (including surgery).

D-dimer has been widely applied to the diagnosis of venous thromboembolism (VTE) and pulmonary embolism (PE). In this setting, it is the negative predictive value of D-dimer that is most significant; a normal D-dimer measured by high-sensitivity assay largely excludes VTE and PE in selected patients. The usual D-dimer cutoff for quantitative assays is 500 ng/mL. D-dimer assays are most useful in patients with a low probability, based upon clinical parameters such as the Well prediction rules, of acute thromboembolic disease. In patients with clinical high probability, the D-dimer is not as useful. A positive D-dimer is relatively nonspecific in this setting. Patients with intermediate to high probability should undergo ultrasound of the lower extremities or other radiographic testing to exclude PE.

Assays for D-dimer and FDP include manual latex agglutination, enzyme linked immunosorbent (ELISA), turbidimetric, immunofiltration, and latex-enhanced photometric or immuno-chromatographic technologies. In latex agglutination, patient plasma is mixed with latex particles that are coated with anti-FDP or anti-D-dimer antibodies. If these are present, the latex particles will agglutinate as visible particles. Positive specimens can be serially diluted to provide a semiquantitative FDP or D-dimer titer. Automated versions of this assay are capable of providing quantitative or semiquantitative results. Not all of these assays have FDA approval for use in the exclusion of VTE or PE. When choosing a D-dimer assay, attention must be paid to the "intended use" statement in the package insert. D-dimer assays that have been approved for use in exclusion of VTE/PE will have an intended use statement to that effect and have been termed "high-sensitivity" D-dimer assays.

Factor assays (II, V, VII, VIII, IX, X, XI, XII)

Patient plasma is mixed with reagent plasma having a known factor deficiency. The resulting PT or PTT of this mixture can be compared to a standard curve, generated by plotting known factor levels against clotting times. Factor VIII, IX, XI, and XII assays are PTT-based. Factor II, VII, and X assays are PT-based. Factor V can be either. Serial dilutions are usually performed. An inhibitor is suggested if serial dilutions result in an apparent increase in factor activity. Chromogenic assays and antigenic assays are available for some factors (II, VII, VIII IX, X).

Factor assays are usually performed when a screening assay (PT, PTT, TT) is prolonged and mixing studies indicate a deficiency (full correction in a 1:1 mix). The specific factors assayed depend upon the screening test.

- Prolonged PTT, normal PT: factors XII, XI, IX, VIII.

- Normal PTT, prolonged PT: factor VII. In addition, consider common pathway constituents (I, II, X, V), since the PTT is insensitive to mild-moderate common factor deficiencies. Thus, these can sometimes produce a prolonged PT with normal PTT. Also, since coumadin is a common cause of a prolonged PT with normal PTT, it is often helpful to simultaneously assay other vitamin K-dependent factors (II, VII, IX, X).

- Prolonged PT and PTT: factors I, II, X, V (common pathway). Consider performing additional factors, as multiple factor deficiencies can produce this pattern. In clinical practice, isolated inherited factor deficiencies are less common than multiple acquired factor deficiencies (eg, DIC, liver disease, coumadin). Even when an apparent isolated factor deficiency is found, one must consider an acquired inhibitor (eg, anti-factor VIII antibody) t5.4.

The plasma should be separated as soon as possible, preferably within 2 hours. Plasma that cannot be tested within 4 hours should be frozen. Results are expressed as percent activity. Normal plasma, by definition, contains 100% activity (1 U/mL) for each factor; however, in actuality results for normal adults usually fall between 60-150%. With the exception of factor VIII, all factors are relatively low in neonates, reaching adult levels by 6 months of age.

Fibrinogen activity

The most common fibrinogen assays (the Clauss assay and the Ellis assay) are very similar to the thrombin time (see below). In the Clauss assay, the patient's plasma is diluted before the addition of excess thrombin. The lower the fibrinogen, the longer the clotting time, and when compared to a standard curve, the specific fibrinogen activity can be determined. In addition to specific fibrinogen assays, dys- and afibrinogenemia result in prolonged PT and PTT. The thrombin time and reptilase time are prolonged as well.

Lupus anticoagulant (LAC) assays

See p 317

Protein C activity

See p 316

Protein S activity

See p 316

Prothrombin variant (prothrombin 20210) test

See p 315

Prothrombin time (PT)

A source of tissue factor and phospholipid (thromboplastin) is added to citrated plasma with excess calcium. The time to clot formation is the PT. Many of the pretest variables that affect the aPTT (see above) apply as well to the PT.

Prolongation of the PT is caused by deficiencies of factors VII as well as common factor deficiencies (X, V, II, or fibrinogen) and inhibitors. While it seems intuitive that a common pathway factor deficiency should prolong the PT and PTT equally, in fact the effect is somewhat unpredictable. The PT is more sensitive to factor VII deficiency than it is to common pathway factor deficiencies. The PTT is much more sensitive to heparin, which acts largely upon the common pathway.

Shortened PT may cause confusion in automated analyzers. Many are set to begin assessing for clotting after a shortened PT has already clotted, leading to the inappropriate reporting of immeasurably long PT. It is important to look at the instrument graph if possible. Causes of shortened PT include traumatic blood draw, DIC, storage or transport at cool temperatures, or the therapeutic use of recombinant factor VIIa.

The PT is used to monitor warfarin (coumadin) therapy. Variations among thromboplastins result in differing sensitivity to coumadin and can result in differing PT results for the same level of anticoagulation. For this reason, the international sensitivity index (ISI) and international normalized ratio (INR) were invented. The manufacturer provides the ISI, based on comparisons between their thromboplastin and an international reference thromboplastin. A laboratory should calibrate/confirm the ISI locally through the use of a reference plasma and seek to use higher sensitivity reagents (low ISI reagents). In fact, most currently available reagents have an ISI very close to 1. Note that the INR is meant to reduce interlaboratory variation that results from differing thromboplastin sensitivities to coumadin. The INR is mainly valid as a standardizing calculation in coumadinized patients with PTs in the low range. In other clinical scenarios, the INR does not seek to nor does it succeed in reducing interlaboratory variation. The INR is calculated as follows:

$$INR = (PT \text{ measured} \div PT \text{ mean})^{ISI}$$

Chromogenic factor X assays are useful for monitoring warfarin in the presence of a lupus anticoagulant, hirudin, or argatroban. In these circumstances, the INR can overestimate the amount of coumadinization, leading to inappropriate dosing. The chromogenic assay for factor X is not affected by these agents. The laboratory must establish a curve that correlates factor X levels with INRs.

Thrombin time (TT)

Thrombin is added to patient plasma. The time to clot formation is the thrombin time. Prolongation of the TT is caused by deficiency of fibrinogen, defective fibrinogen (dysfibrinogenemia), or an inhibitor such as heparin, hirudin, argatroban, or fibrin degradation products (FDPs). In dysfibrinogenemia, both the thrombin time and reptilase time are prolonged (whereas inhibitors such as heparin do not affect the reptilase time). A prolongation of both the TT and reptilase time may also be caused by amyloidosis.

The thrombin time can be used to determine that heparin is present in a specimen, as a cause of a prolonged PTT. The TT is exquisitely sensitive to the presence of heparin, and the other main cause of prolongation, dysfibrinogenemia, is very rare. If the TT is prolonged, the presence of heparin can be confirmed by either the reptilase time or a mixing study. The reptilase time, a test of the same portion of the coagulation cascade that is unaffected by heparin, is normal in the presence of heparin. Alternatively the plasma can be mixed 1:1 with normal plasma. A 1:1 mix will fail to correct in the presence of heparin, but it will correct with dysfibrinogenemia. Note that these results can also be obtained with hirudin, argatroban, or FDPs. More commonly, a heparin neutralization procedure is used for this purpose.

Distinguishing dysfibrinogenemia from hypofibrinogenemia is difficult but of some clinical importance. In this regard, it is important to remember that an abnormal molecular form of fibrinogen (dysfibrinogenemia) is a bit of an inhibitor and will therefore show only partial correction in mixing studies; whereas hypofibrinogenemia will typically correct entirely.

von Willebrand factor assays

See p 306

Causes of excessive bleeding (hemophilia)
Laboratory evaluation f5.4
Clinical clues
Platelet-type bleeding, coagulation-type bleeding & nonbleeding patients with prolonged coagulation screening assays

Platelet-type bleeding manifests as easy bruising, petechiae, and purpura t5.6. It may be caused by thrombocytopenia, defective platelets, or von Willebrand disease. Manifestations similar to platelet-type bleeding may be produced by vascular disorders, including hereditary hemorrhagic telangiectasia (Osler-Weber-Rendu) and vasculitis. Congenital platelet disorders may present with a history of lifelong platelet-type bleeding despite normal coagulation assays. The most common congenital cause of platelet-type bleeding is von Willebrand disease, but one should also consider Wiskott-Aldrich syndrome, May-Hegglin anomaly, Bernard-Soulier syndrome, Glanzmann thrombasthenia, and platelet storage pool diseases. In clinical practice, acquired defects outnumber congenital ones and include idiopathic thrombocytopenic purpura (ITP), alcohol, aspirin, penicillin, uremia, disseminated intravascular coagulation (DIC), and myeloproliferative neoplasms.

Coagulation-type bleeding presents with deep-seated hemorrhages, such as hemarthrosis or intramuscular hematoma. Coagulation-type bleeding is usually the result of single or combined coagulation factor disorders; note that coagulation-type

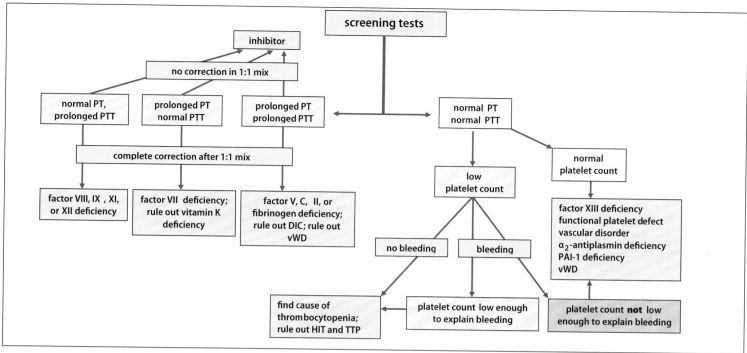

f5.4 Laboratory approach to the bleeding patient

bleeding may also be a feature of von Willebrand disease. Congenital forms of coagulation-type bleeding present with a lifelong history and, often, a family history. An acquired factor inhibitor presents with sudden-onset manifestations similar to hemophilia A or B. Disseminated intravascular coagulation usually arises in a typical clinical context and manifests as bleeding from multiple sites. Some patients simply are easily bruised, a condition called purpura simplex; a similar condition evolves in many elderly adults, a condition called senile purpura. Lastly, in children and elderly adults, one must consider abuse.

t5.6 Clinical manifestations of bleeding disorders

Findings	Coagulation-type bleeding disorders	Platelet-type bleeding disorders
Petechiae	Rare	Common
Hemarthroses	Common	Rare
Deep hematomas	Common	Rare
Delayed bleeding	Common	Rare
Mucosal bleeding	Rare	Common
Gender	Males>females	Females>males

The pathologist is often consulted in order to explain an unexpectedly abnormal screening test, perhaps performed as part of a preoperative evaluation, in a patient with no history of abnormal bleeding. Most commonly, an isolated abnormality in the platelet count, PT, or PTT has been reported. The first thing to do is repeat the test, taking care to control pre-analytic variables. If the assay remains abnormal, then further analysis may be indicated (see f5.3).

Family history

A pattern of X-linked inheritance is consistent with hemophilia A and hemophilia B. Autosomal inheritance is typical of von Willebrand disease. A negative family history does not exclude hemophilia, as ~30% are the result of new mutations.

Infants

In infants, the onset of bleeding after 1 to several weeks of life suggests the possibility of vitamin K deficiency. Prenatal exposure to phenytoin or phenobarbital may enhance vitamin K deficiency. Upper extremity defects may suggest the thrombocytopenia-absent radii (TAR) syndrome. Beyond these clues, the approach is as for adults. Laboratory testing must often be carried out on very small samples, raising the need for careful test selection. Laboratory testing must be interpreted in the light of an immature neonatal coagulation system, in which only factors VIII, fibrinogen, and vWF can be expected to have normal adult values. For all other values, repeat testing at around 6 months of age may be necessary.

Morphologic examination of platelets

One of the most unreliable tests in the clinical laboratory is the automated platelet count. This has a variety of causes. Platelets often form clumps or are present outside of their normal size range and are mistakenly counted along with the erythrocytes. It is for this reason that unexpectedly low platelet counts should always be confirmed by examination of a peripheral smear. Platelet aggregation (platelet-platelet binding) and/or satellitosis (platelet-neutrophil binding) are common causes of pseudo-thrombocytopenia. Markedly enlarged platelets are another. Platelet aggregation and satellitosis are EDTA induced artifacts. Patients on abciximab have been noted to be exceptionally prone to this artifact.

After excluding pseudo-thrombocytopenia, new-onset thrombocytopenia should prompt a search for schistocytes. These may be absent to numerous in disseminated intravascular coagulation (DIC). Schistocytes are typically numerous, however, in thrombotic thrombocytopenic purpura (TTP). Schistocytes point to microangiopathic hemolytic anemia (MHA), with a differential diagnosis of DIC, TTP, HELLP syndrome (hemolytic anemia, elevated liver enzymes, and low platelets), and mechanical trauma (heart valve).

Platelet size should be noted. In thrombocytopenic patients, platelet size is usually increased in immune thrombocytopenic purpura (ITP); release of large platelets into the circulation is analogous to reticulocytosis. Large platelets may also be seen in a variety of constitutional platelet anomalies t5.7. The mean platelet volume (MPV) is the automated measurement of platelet size. In general, consumptive platelet conditions (hyperproliferative thrombocytopenias) are associated with higher MPV, and hypoproliferative thrombocytopenias are associated with low MPV.

Lastly, look for clues to the uncommon constitutional platelet defects. In von Willebrand disease (vWD), platelets usually appear normal; however, large platelets have been described in type IIb. Bernard-Soulier syndrome is among the many settings in which one observes giant platelets t5.7. Agranular platelets are seen in gray platelet syndrome; in actual practice, agranular platelets are most commonly an artifact of in vitro platelet degranulation. Döhle bodies in leukocytes may point to May-Hegglin anomaly, Fechtner syndrome, or Epstein syndrome (see below). Wiskott-Aldrich syndrome is characterized by very small platelets.

t5.7 Giant platelet disorders

Bernard-Soulier syndrome (BSS)
Mediterranean macrothrombocytopenia (mild form of BSS)
May-Hegglin anomaly (giant platelets with Döhle bodies)
Fechtner syndrome (giant platelets with hearing loss, cataracts & nephritis)
Sebastian syndrome (giant platelets with leukocyte inclusions)
Gray platelet syndrome
Immune thrombocytopenic purpura
Montreal platelet syndrome

Platelet disorders t5.8

Bernard-Soulier syndrome (BSS)

BSS is an uncommon disorder caused by decreased or dysfunctional platelet GPIb/V/IX complex. This manifests with thrombocytopenia and giant platelets. GPIb is the von Willebrand factor (vWF) receptor, and the interaction of these 2 molecules is needed for platelet adhesion to denuded subendothelial tissue. In aggregometry studies, the platelets aggregate with all agonists except ristocetin (resembling the pattern of vWD). Unlike vWD, the peripheral smear contains large platelets. Failure to aggregate even in the presence of normal plasma distinguishes BSS from vWD.

BSS is inherited as an autosomal recessive trait. 2 genes—Ibα and Ibβ—encode the GPIb receptor. 2 additional genes—V and IX—encode the remaining components of the GPIb/V/IX complex. The Ibα and Ibβ genes are found on chromosomes 17 and 22, respectively, Ibα having a single exon, and Ibβ having 2. While most cases of BSS are due to mutations in the Ibα gene, the Ibβ gene may be affected in the DiGeorge (22q) microdeletion. Note that since the receptor is expressed as a complex, mutations in IX or V may also result in reduced expression of GPIb and a BSS phenotype.

t5.8 Summary of platelet disorders

Phase	Mediators	Inherited defects	Acquired defects
Adhesion	GPIb & vWF	Bernard-Soulier syndrome von Willebrand disease	Paraproteinemia
Release reaction	Granules & agonists	Platelet release defect Storage pool disease	Aspirin
Aggregation	GPIIb/IIIa & fibrinogen	Glanzmann thrombasthenia Dysfibrinogenemia	Dysfibrinogenemia

Mediterranean macrothrombocytopenia, a relatively common cause of mild thrombocytopenia in southern Europe, is caused by a mutation in Ibα (chromosome 17) that results in decreased expression of the GPIb/IX/V complex (the vWF receptor). Thus, this syndrome is essentially the same as the BSS carrier state.

Platelet storage pool disorders

Platelet-type (pseudo) vWD is caused by a gain of function mutation that enhances the avidity of GPIb for vWF. The high affinity leads to low plasma levels of vWF, mimicking vWD.

This group of disorders includes abnormalities of dense granules (Hermansky-Pudlak, Chédiak-Higashi, Wiskott-Aldrich) and abnormalities of α granules (grey platelet syndrome, white platelet syndrome, and Quebec platelet syndrome).

In the dense granule disorders, first wave aggregation is seen with all agents, but secondary aggregation is blunted or absent. Dense granule secretion, as quantified by ATP secretion using chemiluminescence, is markedly diminished. The absence of dense granules can be confirmed by electron microscopy. Recall that dense granules (essentially neurosecretory granules) store small molecules such as ADP, ATP, and serotonin and mediate the second wave of platelet aggregation.

Hermansky-Pudlak syndrome is particularly common in Puerto Rico and presents with epistaxis in childhood. Platelet counts are usually normal. Pulmonary fibrosis and granulomatous colitis complicated by bleeding have been reported in a significant minority of affected persons. Hermansky-Pudlak syndrome shares with Chédiak-Higashi syndrome the feature of oculocutaneous albinism, thought to reflect involvement of melanocytic dense granules (melanosomes). The macrophages in Hermansky-Pudlak syndrome contain ceroid-like inclusions. Biopsies in affected tissues show ceroid-like material within tissue macrophages (eg, alveolar macrophages). The genes associated with Hermansky-Pudlak syndrome include: *HPS1*(10q23), *HPS3*, *HPS4*, *HPS5*, *HPS6*, *AP3B1*, and *DTNBP1*. In Puerto Rican cases, nearly all patients are found to have a single duplication of 16 base pairs in exon 1 of the *HPS1* gene, and targeted mutation analysis is available for this defect. Among those of non-Puerto Rican descent, mutations are more variable or yet uncharacterized, and testing is not clinically available.

In Chédiak-Higashi syndrome, granulocytes, platelets, and melanocytes contain giant granules rather than ceroid bodies. A lymphoproliferative disorder ultimately arises in the vast majority of those affected by this syndrome. The responsible gene has been mapped to chromosome 13.

Wiskott-Aldrich syndrome in X-linked disorder that presents with the triad of thrombocytopenia, eczema, and immunodeficiency. The platelets are smaller than usual and demonstrate decreased aggregation with ADP, epinephrine, and collagen. A partial form of Wiskott-Aldrich syndrome manifests only with thrombocytopenia (X-linked thrombocytopenia). The basic defect appears to be a cytoskeletal anomaly that prevents movement of dense granules to the cell surface. Defects in the *WASP* gene are responsible for the Wiskott-Aldrich syndrome.

Platelet α granules store larger molecules than those found in the dense granules, including vWF, platelet derived growth factor, platelet factor 4, and fibrinogen, and give platelets their characteristic granular appearance.

Gray platelet syndrome is a recessively inherited mild bleeding disorder. Aggregation is blunted with all agents except ADP. The lack of platelet α granules imparts a uniform pale-grey tinctorial quality in Wright stained blood films, for which the disorder was named. Platelets fail to express CD62 following stimulation by high dose thrombin, and ELISA shows abnormally low PF4. Thrombocytopenia is common.

White platelet syndrome is named not for the microscopic appearance of the platelets but rather for the Minnesota family in whom this syndrome was described. It is characterized by a mild bleeding disorder with thrombocytopenia, mildly enlarged platelets, and impaired responses to all agonists. Ultrastructurally, the platelets have persistent Golgi complexes and poorly formed α granules.

Quebec platelet disorder is a mild bleeding disorder with autosomal dominant inheritance. Unlike gray platelet syndrome, the α granules form normally but fail to fully mature; thus, the tinctorial quality of platelets is unaltered. Platelet aggregation in response to epinephrine is abnormal.

Glanzmann thrombasthenia

First described in Switzerland by Glanzmann in 1918, Glanzmann thrombasthenia is an autosomal recessive disease caused by deficient GPIIb/IIIa complex. It is the function of GPIIb to bind fibrinogen, thus crosslinking platelets within a thrombus. The GPIIb/IIIa complex is responsible for the PLA1 antigen, so affected platelets are PLA1–. The peripheral smear shows a normal number of normally sized to small dispersed platelets.

In aggregometry studies, the platelets fail to aggregate with all agonists but ristocetin. There is a normal initial slope of ristocetin induced aggregation (mediated by the normal plasma vWF and normal GPIb/V/IX complex) but a blunted second wave of ristocetin induced aggregation (mediated by the diminished IIb/IIIa complex).

The in vitro clot retraction test was traditionally used to detect Glanzmann thrombasthenia, in which diminished clot retraction is observed. Clot retraction is a normal component of the physiologic formation of a thrombus and the beginning of wound healing. The normally functioning GPIIb/IIIa receptor is needed for proper clot retraction. In the performance of the clot retraction test, blood is kept at 37°C in a glass tube and observed at intervals for clot retraction. Normal adults should produce clot retraction within 4 hours. When the clot retracts, it pulls away from the walls of the tube, often resulting in the extrusion of a few red blood cells and a quantity of plasma.

The αIIb gene is large, consisting of 30 exons. The β₃ gene has 15 exons. Both are found at 17q. A large number of mutations in both genes can produce the Glanzmann phenotype. As such, molecular diagnosis is complicated, and flow cytometry for cell surface expression of GPIIb/IIIa is the preferred diagnostic modality.

von Willebrand disease (vWD)

vWD is notable for simultaneous impairment of the coagulation cascade and platelet function, since vWF participates in both. In coagulation, the function of vWF is to maintain high levels of circulating factor VIII. In platelet function, vWF is operant in the formation of platelet thrombi. vWD is the most common inherited bleeding diathesis overall (hemophilia A is considered the most common cause of severe hemophilia), with incidence varying from 1/100 in Italy to 1/100,000 in Great Britain.

Physiology of vWF begins with its synthesis in endothelial cells and megakaryocytes. After synthesis, it is stored in the Weibel-Palade bodies of endothelial cells and in the α granules of megakaryocytes. vWF is secreted by endothelial cells along the basolateral membrane, where it becomes an integral basement membrane protein, readily exposed in the case of endothelial injury. vWF is released into the circulation as a large multimer and broken down in serum by a protease. Thus, it circulates in variably sized multimers, most commonly dimers. vWF is sometimes called factor VIII-related antigen (factor VIIIR:Ag), because it complexes with and protects factor VIII from degradation within the bloodstream. The interaction of platelet glycoprotein Ib (GPIb) with ristocetin is stimulated by shear forces in vivo and by ristocetin in vitro; for this reason, another name for vWF is ristocetin cofactor.

There are 4 types of vWD and a type of pseudo-vWD t5.9.

t5.9 Types of vWD

Type	Ristocetin cofactor (vWF:Rco)	vWF antigen (vWF:Ag)	Ratio vWF Rco:Ag	Factor VIII activity	RIPA	Platelet count	Multimer pattern
1	↓	↓	Nl	↓-Nl	Nl	Nl-↓	Normal distribution, all diminished
2a	↓↓	↓	↓	↓-Nl	Nl-↓	Nl-↓	↓ HMW multimers
2b	↓	↓	Nl-↓	↓-Nl	↑ with low dose ↓	↓	↓ HMW multimers
Plt-type	↓	↓	Nl	Nl	Nl	↓	↓ HMW multimers
2N	↓-Nl	↓-Nl	Nl	↓	Nl	Nl-↓	Normal
2M	↓↓	↓	Nl-↓	↓-Nl	Nl-↓	Nl-↓	Normal
3	↓↓	↓↓	Nl	↓↓	↓	Nl-↓	Absent multimers

Type I vWD is a mild quantitative defect, type III is a severe quantitative defect, and the type II variants are qualitative (functional) defects. Type I vWD, the most common variant, is a quantitative defect that results in a mild bleeding disorder. There is usually a normal PT and platelet count, with prolonged PTT and bleeding time. There is decreased factor VIII, vWF antigen, and vWF activity. The decreases in these 3 analytes is "concordant," and the ratio of vWF activity to vWF antigen approaches 1 (nearly always >0.7). The multimer pattern shows a normal distribution, globally dim in comparison with normal adults. However, these parameters vary, and in fact the diagnosis of type I vWD can be challenging, requiring repeated testing over extended periods of time. Despite being responsible for 70-80% of vWD cases, there has been remarkably little progress in characterizing the underlying molecular defect in type I vWD. This may reflect the possibility that loci outside the *vWF* gene—perhaps those involved in biosynthesis or transport—are responsible in the majority of cases. A Canadian study found a single dominant *vWF* mutation—Tyr1584Cys—in ~15% of type I families.

Type IIa (10-15% of vWD cases) is a moderately severe bleeding disorder. It results largely from missense mutations in the *vWF* gene exon 28, a portion of the molecule that is involved in multimer stability. Multimer analysis shows absence of high weight multimers. The PT, fibrinogen, and TT are normal, while the PTT may be slightly prolonged. The factor VIII and vWF antigen are normal to decreased. The vWF activity (ristocetin cofactor) is decreased (<50%). Thus, there may be "discordance" between the markedly decreased ristocetin cofactor assay and normal to only mildly decreased factor VIII and vWF antigen. This discordance is the hallmark of the type II varieties of vWD, in which the ratio of vWF antigen to vWF activity is usually <0.7.

Type IIb, like IIa, has decreased high molecular weight multimers. Type IIb is unique in 2 important respects: there is enhanced ristocetin induced platelet aggregation, and there is profound thrombocytopenia and bleeding upon exposure to DDAVP. DDAVP should not be administered to patients with type IIb vWD. Type IIb results from spontaneous binding of vWF to platelets. Most cases are the result of a "gain of function" point mutation in the GP1b binding domain of vWF. Type IIb vWD must be distinguished from platelet-type vWD, which is caused by mutations in the gene that encodes the platelet GP1b receptor. In both cases, the enhanced binding is selective for high molecular weight multimers and results in clearance of both platelets and high molecular weight multimers from the blood. Thus, thrombocytopenia and decreased high molecular weight multimers are characteristic laboratory features in both disorders. In most other laboratory assays, it mimics type IIa.

Type IIM is extremely rare and caused by loss of function mutations in the GP1b binding domain. The basic defect prevents binding of vWF to GPIb. Multimer analysis appears entirely normal. Normal multimeric distribution distinguishes IIM from IIa and IIb.

Type II N (Normandy) is caused by a mutation in the domain that binds factor VIII, encoded in exons 18-20. This results in low levels of circulating factor VIII, mimicking hemophilia A. vWF quantity and function are otherwise unaffected. The resulting clinical disease resembles mild hemophilia A with the exception of an autosomal pattern of inheritance—ie, females are affected as commonly as males. 3 mutations (T791M, R816W, and R854Q) appear to account for most 2N cases. Multimer analysis is normal, RIPA is normal, and vWF antigen is normal.

Type III vWD is a severe disorder with virtually no vWF. factor VIII is low, vWF antigen and activity are low, and multimers are quite faint across the size spectrum. It results from frameshift mutations, nonsense mutations, and deletions in the *vWF* gene. Type III must be considered in kindreds in whom apparent hemophilia follows an autosomal recessive rather than X-linked inheritance.

Pseudo- or platelet-type vWD mimics some of the laboratory findings of type IIb. It is caused by an abnormality in platelet GP1b, leading to increased avidity for vWF. It can be distinguished by the observation that in pseudo-vWD, the platelets aggregate if exposed to cryoprecipitate, while in IIb they do not.

Type Vicenza vWD is believed to be caused by increased clearance of vWF from the blood. This variant is characterized by discrepant plasma (low) and platelet (normal) vWF and unusually large vWF multimers.

Acquired vWD occurs rarely. It has been reported in association with lymphoproliferative disorders, autoimmune disease, essential thrombocythemia, and aortic stenosis. The acquired defects of vWF observed in aortic stenosis is thought to be related to high shear stress. It mimics congenital type IIa vWD.

Laboratory diagnosis of vWD

The laboratory diagnosis of vWD is treacherous. Under ideal circumstances, low vWF antigen and low ristocetin cofactor activity make the diagnosis of the most common forms of vWD. However, several caveats are worth noting.

1. Both may be in the low end of the normal range in patients with vWD.

2. There are several genetic and environmental modifiers that affect measured levels of these analytes. The best known modifier is the ABO blood group. Normal individuals with blood group O have slightly lower vWF levels—~75% of normal. Thus, for a given genotype, affected individuals with the O blood group will be relatively more severely affected, and those with A, B, or AB will be less severely affected. However, the incidence of vWD is no different among the blood groups. A distinct vWF normal range for blood group O persons should be established by the laboratory. In one study, the mean vWF in each blood group were: O—75%, A—105%, B—117%, and AB—123%.

3. A variety of provocations, including vigorous exercise, inflammation, pregnancy, and estrogen therapy, may mask the diagnosis of mild vWD by increasing vWF levels. Estrogen-containing oral contraceptives have been demonstrated to increase vWF levels. Newborns tend to have high vWF activity, and the disease may not be detectable until 1 year of age.

4. vWF levels fluctuate. There is significant intraindividual day to day variation, and levels increase with age.
   As a result of all of these confounding factors, repeat interval testing is advised to both confirm or exclude the diagnosis.

The laboratory diagnosis of vWD begins with a panel of tests: ristocetin cofactor (vWF activity), vWF antigen, and factor VIII activity f5.5. It is often helpful to include an indicator of acute inflammation, such as the CRP or fibrinogen, and a blood group study. In some cases, a pregnancy test is important. Based upon the results of the initial panel, additional testing may include multimer analysis. Normal vWF activity, vWF antigen, and factor VIII results largely (though not entirely) exclude vWD. Patients with vWD may test as normal in the first year of life, in acute phase reactions, pregnancy, and exogenous estrogen use. Furthermore, if the diagnosis is

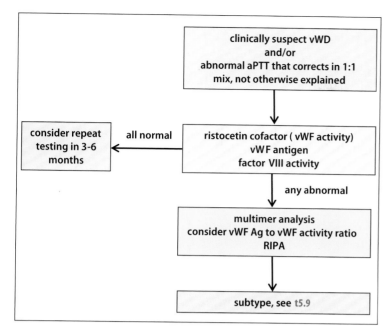

f5.5 Algorithm for suspected von Willebrand disease

strongly suspected, the tests should be repeated at a separate time. If all 3 tests are reduced mildly and proportionately, this is most consistent with type I vWD (if all tests are reduced profoundly, this is suggestive of type III vWD). When the vWD activity is reduced out of proportion to the vWF antigen and factor VIII, this is most consistent with a variant of type II vWD. Multimer analysis and low dose ristocetin aggregation are necessary to further elucidate these findings. When factor VIII is reduced out of proportion to vWF, consider hemophilia A, female hemophilia A carrier, specimen degradation (factor VIII is significantly more labile) or type IIN wVD.

The ristocetin cofactor assay (vWF activity assay) is a test in which patient plasma is added to formalin-fixed normal platelets in the presence of ristocetin, and aggregation is measured. Fixation precludes release of endogenous platelet vWF, so that only plasma vWF is operative in the reaction, but does not impair the function of platelet GPIb. (The routine platelet aggregation study using ristocetin and unfixed platelets is susceptible to spurious results). Under these circumstances, normal plasma will cause platelet agglutination, and plasma deficient in vWF does not fully aggregate. Current assays for vWF antigen (vWF:Ag) employ either ELISA or an immuno-turbidometric assay.

The factor VIII activity assay is an indirect test of vWF. Since factor VIII is bound to vWF in blood, adequate vWF must be present in order for factor VIII levels to be maintained. The PTT is often prolonged in vWD, but is often normal as well. In female carriers of the hemophilia A gene, ratio of factor VIII to vWF ratio is ~1:2 (0.5). The ratio in noncarriers and vWD is 1:1.

Platelet aggregometry can be used to detect vWD, but inherent limitations exist. These include the need for special handling to avoid pretest platelet activation and the precision-altering effects of inherent platelet vWF. Furthermore, even under ideal conditions the sensitivity of platelet aggregometry for vWD is low. The ristocetin cofactor test is therefore preferred. The low dose ristocetin induced platelet aggregation study may be needed, however, to detect type IIb vWD. Pronounced aggregation (hyperaggregation) of platelets in response to low dose ristocetin is consistent with type IIb. Platelet-type vWD also shows increased aggregation in this assay, due to a gain of function mutation on platelet GPIb. Like all forms of platelet aggregation, the low dose test is unreliable in the presence of thrombocytopenia, a common occurrence in IIB.

While the ristocetin cofactor assay measures vWF through its interaction with GPIb, a much more straightforward assay measures vWF through its interaction collagen. Measurement of collagen binding activity is possible with an ELISA-based assay that utilizes collagen-coated wells to capture vWF, which is then measured by labeled anti-vWF antibody. The value of this assay lies in the fact that high molecular weight multimers more readily bind collagen than do low molecular weight multimers; thus, the collagen binding assay has the potential to act as a surrogate for multimer analysis.

von Willebrand factor multimer analysis is performed by gel electrophoresis. Recall that vWF in blood exists in an array of sizes—monomers, dimers, and various multimers. When plasma is subjected to electrophoresis on a gel, vWF multimers separate according to size. Labeled anti-vWF antibody is added to permit visualization. The multimer patterns are the gold standard for classification of vWD (see below), but vWF electrophoresis is technically challenging and highly labor intensive, limiting its availability.

The bleeding time is often prolonged in vWD, but the PFA-100 assay is more sensitive. The PFA-100 has potential to become a screening assay for vWD, but additional study is needed.

It is still uncertain which laboratory test is best to follow the course of vWD severity and the efficacy of treatment. In surgical and acute bleed settings, factor VIII activity is considered the best monitoring test. Factor VIII levels should be monitored every 12 hours during these circumstances, both to ensure therapeutic effect and to prevent supranormal (>200%) factor VIII levels which may lead to thrombosis.

Type I vWD is treated with DDAVP or cryoprecipitate. DDAVP (desmopressin, 1-deamino-8-D-arginine vasopressin) is a synthetic derivative of antidiuretic hormone (ADH). Administration of desmopressin transiently increases factor VIII and vWF levels. Desmopressin must be given parenterally (usually by intravenous infusion in acute settings, but also available for subcutaneous injections and nasal inhalation). The effect of a single dose lasts for 8-10 hours. DDAVP is contraindicated in Type IIb. The adverse effects of desmopressin include, in addition to the generally mild tachycardia, headache, and facial flushing, and an important tachyphylaxis effect (the need for stronger dosing over time). While desmopressin is effective in patients with type I vWD, it is usually not useful in type II and III disease (type IIa patients experience an increase in the dysfunctional vWF they were already making, in IIb patients it is contraindicated, and type III patients cannot mount a significant secretory response). Thus, in most non-type I patients, administration of vWF is preferable. Fresh-frozen plasma contains both factor VIII and vWF, but large amounts are needed to attain hemostatic concentrations (20-25 mL/kg). 10 bags of cryoprecipitate, which also contains both factors, provide roughly equal clinical efficacy. Commercial concentrates (eg, Humate-P) contains vWF and factor VIII and have the advantage of being virus inactivated. Purified factor VIII products should not be used. Alloantibodies against vWF develop in 10-15% of patients with type III disease who undergo multiple transfusions.

Aspirin & NSAIDs

Aspirin and NSAIDs cause platelet impairment by inhibiting cyclooxygenase type 1 (COX-1), a key enzyme involved in the production of thromboxane A2 (TXA2). TXA2 exerts autocrine platelet stimulation, leading to dense granule release and the secondary wave of aggregation. The inhibitory effect of aspirin persists for the lifetime of the platelet (10 days), since it actually acetylates the enzyme; while the effect of other NSAIDs is reversible. COX-2, an enzyme present in endothelial cells, is involved in the production of prostacyclin, a platelet inhibitor. COX-2 is relatively resistant to the effect of aspirin, however. Furthermore, since endothelial cells have nuclei, they are able to replace COX-2, whereas platelets cannot replace COX-1; the balance, therefore, is shifted in favor of platelet inhibition.

The aspirin effect is detectable in the laboratory in the aggregometry responses of platelets to the so-called weak agonists: epinephrine, ADP, arachidonate, low dose collagen, and low dose thrombin. These are considered "weak agonists" because, by themselves, they are capable of producing only the first, reversible, wave of aggregation; they depend upon TXA2 to generate secondary-wave, irreversible, aggregation. The lag phase in collagen induced aggregation is often prolonged, and there is complete failure to aggregate in response to arachidonate. This combination of findings is collectively called the aspirin-like effect. The storage pool defect induced by aspirin can be distinguished from inherited storage pool defects by studying platelet secretion in response to high dose thrombin (normal in aspirin-like effect). High-dose thrombin (and high dose collagen) are capable of producing complete aggregation without TXA2.

Aspirin often, but inconsistently, prolongs the bleeding time. The PFA-100 is more sensitive to its effect. A relatively specific assay of aspirin effect is provided in the VerifyNow instrument.

Platelet defects in myeloproliferative neoplasms

Thrombosis is an extremely common cause of morbidity and mortality in the myeloproliferative neoplasms. Major thrombosis, such as hepatic vein thrombosis, is particularly common in polycythemia vera and essential thrombocythemia. These complications occur even with normal platelet counts, due presumably to clonal defects in megakaryocytes and platelets. The bleeding time is prolonged in only a small number of patients and predicts neither bleeding nor thrombosis. Very high platelet counts (>1.5 million) have been associated with an acquired vWD. The most common finding in platelet aggregometry is decreased aggregation and secretion in response to epinephrine, ADP, and/or collagen.

Uremia

Uremia impairs platelet function to a variable extent. It is capable of prolonging the bleeding time and altering platelet aggregation in vitro; however, the clinical effects appear to be milder than the in vitro effects. Dialysis seems to improve platelet function in this scenario, as does DDAVP and estrogen therapy.

Cardiopulmonary bypass

Cardiopulmonary bypass circuits cause both thrombocytopenia and platelet dysfunction. A prolonged bleeding time is a common finding in this circumstance, in addition to abnormal aggregometry (particularly with ristocetin). There appears to be depletion of dense granules and α granules.

Paraproteinemia

Paraproteinemia is a common cause of platelet dysfunction. This is particularly common in the immunoglobulin classes capable of forming multimers—IgA and IgM—but, due to its higher incidence, is seen commonly in IgG paraproteinemia. This is thought to be due to platelet "coating" with immunoglobulin, and the effect is noted to be proportional to the paraprotein concentration.

Thrombocytopenia

See p 320

Coagulation defects t5.10, t5.11

Hemophilia A

Hemophilia A is the most common form of inherited severe hemophilia, with an incidence of ~1 in 5000 live male births. Inheritance is X-linked recessive, implying that affected persons are male, and all mothers and daughters are obligate carriers. A female carrier has a 50% chance of passing the disease to a male offspring. A family history of hemophilia is present only ~60-70% of the time, however, since 30% of cases are due to a new spontaneous mutation.

Hemophilia is defined as severe when spontaneous bleeding occurs, and this develops when factor VIII is <1 U/dL (<1%). In moderate hemophilia, in the range of 1-5 U/dL of factor VIII, there is bleeding with minor trauma. With >5 U/dL of factor VIII, the patient is noted to have excessive bleeding following surgery or other significant trauma. The factor VIII activity must be <30% to prolong the PTT. The bleeding severity and factor VIII level is relatively constant within an individual patient and within a family, but there is variation among kindreds. Furthermore, rare patients with <1% factor VIII are found to have clinically mild disease, on the basis of co-inherited thrombophilic traits, eg, factor V Leiden or protein S deficiency.

t5.10 Inherited factor deficiencies

Deficiency	Prevalence	Chromosome	Inheritance	Bleeding
I (fibrinogen)	1 in 1 million	4	AR	Variable
II (prothrombin)	1 in 2 million	11	AR	Mild-moderate
V	1 in 1 million	1	AR	Mild-moderate
VII	1 in 500,000	13	AR	Mild-severe
VIII	1 in 10,000	X	XLR	Mild-severe
IX	1 in 30,000	X	XLR	Mild-severe
X	1 in 1 million	13	AR	Mild-severe
XI	1 in 1 million (higher in Ashkenazi Jews)	4	AR	Mild-severe
XII	1 in 1 million	5	AR	None
XIII	1 in 1 million	6 (XIIIA) 1 (XIIIB)	AR	Postoperative
Combined t5.12	1 in 1 million	18q & others	AR	Variable

AR = autosomal recessive; XLR = X-linked recessive

t5.11 Acquired factor deficiencies

VIII	Factor VIII inhibitors (autoantibodies) in hemophilia A patients on factor replacement therapy
	Factor VIII inhibitors (autoantibodies) in nonhemophilia patients
IX	Factor IX inhibitors (autoantibodies) in hemophilia B patients on factor replacement therapy
X	Acquired factor X deficiency associated with light chain amyloidosis (adsorption to amyloid)
Multiple	Disseminated intravascular coagulation (DIC)
	Extracorporeal membrane oxygenation (ECMO)
	Fibrinolytic drugs
	Liver disease
	Warfarin
	Neonatal or dietary vitamin K deficiency
	Nephrotic syndrome (usually most pronounced loss of AT, therefore prothrombotic)

The laboratory diagnosis is usually straightforward. The platelet count, PT and TT are normal, while the PTT is prolonged and corrects completely in the 1:1 mix. Factor levels demonstrate isolated deficiency in factor VIII. Note that there is often PTT prolongation in the cord blood of normal babies due to intrauterine vitamin K deficiency and a relative deficiency in contact factors (XI, XII). However, factor VIII activity can be reliably assayed in utero, from cord blood, and from neonatal and adult blood. In affected persons, the factor VIII level is <30%. There are several caveats. First, factor VIII is a labile factor, making expeditious measurement (or freezing for later measurement) important. Second, the effect of high hematocrit or inappropriately low volume draws into citrated tubes on functional clotting assays should be borne in mind. Lastly, the primary differential diagnostic consideration, once factor VIII deficiency is documented, is vWD. Especially difficult to exclude is vWD type N (Normandy).

Female carriers usually have >50% factor VIII activity and often fall within the normal range. They have a normal PTT and no history of abnormal bleeding (rare exceptions exist). The ratio of factor VIII to vWF, however, is usually ~1:2 (normal ratio is 1:1). Note that both factor VIII and vWF are positive acute phase reactants and may both be elevated in pregnancy. Note also that since factor VIII is labile, a decrease may be the result of delayed specimen processing. Clinically apparent hemophilia has arisen rarely in females, and 3 possible mechanisms may underlie this phenomenon:

very asymmetric lyonization, homozygosity (offspring of an affected male and carrier female), and hemizygosity (Turner syndrome). Confirmation of carrier status usually requires linkage analysis.

The factor VIII gene is found at Xq28. It is quite large, consisting of 26 exons, and it is transcribed mainly in hepatic endothelial cells. Upon entering circulation, factor VIII is bound to vWF, an association that prolongs its half life. Numerous disease-causing mutations have been identified, with a variety of mechanisms, including point mutations (missense, nonsense, and splicing error point mutations), frameshift mutations, small deletions, large deletions, small insertions, and inversions. A single inversion mutation of intron 22 has been shown to cause 40-45% of severe hemophilia A in Caucasians. This so-called common partial inversion can be found with Southern blot analysis, providing a useful assay for prenatal diagnosis and carrier detection. Certain mutations correlate with an increased likelihood of developing factor VIII antibodies. In particular, mutations that lead to production of no factor VIII or truncated factor VIII—inversions, gross deletions, and nonsense mutations—confer a higher risk of antibody development. Mutations associated with even minimal production of factor VIII have a low risk of antibody formation. The first step in the process of molecular diagnosis (eg, for prenatal or carrier detection) is to identify the causative mutation in an affected family member (a proband). If an affected family member is unavailable, testing can be performed on an obligate female carrier. For families with a history of severe hemophilia, the testing should be first performed for the intron 22 inversion, which can be detected by Southern blot analysis. This will be positive and thus provide a marker in ~45% of families with such a history. In the remaining families with severe hemophilia and the vast majority of families with mild to moderate hemophilia who do not have an intron 22 inversion, additional molecular testing is required. This can include direct sequence analysis and/or analysis for the intron 1 inversion (present in ~5% of families with severe hemophilia). Last, consideration should be given to testing for vWD, type IIN. If a specific mutation is identified, carrier or prenatal testing can be carried out either by inversion 22 testing (if this defect is present), direct DNA analysis, or RFLP-based linkage analysis. When attempting carrier detection or prenatal diagnosis in the face of an unidentified factor VIII mutation, RFLP linkage analysis can be applied if family members of the affected relative from 2 generations are available and willing to give blood samples.

Factor VIII is administered for treating spontaneous bleeds or for prophylaxis in surgery. Factor VIII is a high molecular weight compound that, when administered intravascularly, remains confined to the intravascular compartment (100% recovery of dose). The half life (t½) is 12 hours. The dose of factor VIII depends on the target activity desired and is repeated every 12 hours. Alternatively, DDAVP (desmopressin) can be used in mild hemophiliacs. Amicar (ε-aminocaproic acid) is an inhibitor of fibrinolysis that can be used as an adjunct.

Antibodies to factor VIII develop in up to 1/3 of patients who receive factor VIII replacement therapy. Most inhibitors develop during the first 50 treatment days, and the risk diminishes thereafter. The formation of anti-factor VIII antibodies (factor VIII inhibitors) is a dreaded consequence, because treatment is difficult, and there is a high rate of major morbidity and mortality. The strongest risk factor for development of factor VIII inhibitors is a genotype associated with zero production of factor VIII; such patients experience a high rate of exogenous factor VIII exposure, and lack of endogenous production precludes the development of immunologic tolerance to factor VIII. A factor VIII inhibitor is suspected when there is diminished response to factor VIII infusion, as measured by clinical response, half life of infused factor VIII, or factor VIII recovery (level of factor VIII after infusion). Suspected factor VIII inhibitory can be confirmed with a Bethesda inhibitor assay.

Rarely, factor VIII inhibitors arise in nonhemophiliacs. This scenario arises in 2 primary patient groups: elderly adults and young postpartum females. Thus, the incidence is bimodal but generally increases with age. While uncommon, this disorder must be thought of in patients with unexplained bleeding or unexpected aPTT prolongation, because it is associated with a high rate of morbidity and mortality. Severe bleeding occurs in up to 90% of affected patients. In about half of cases, there is no other associated illness, while the other half of patients has underlying autoimmunity, hematolymphoid neoplasm, or infection. Bleeding in patients with acquired factor VIII inhibitors presents as deep soft tissue hematoma or mucocutaneous bleeding (epistaxis, gastrointestinal bleed, cutaneous hematoma). Hemarthrosis is uncommon. Laboratory diagnosis of acquired factor VIII inhibitor is based upon isolated prolongation of the aPTT, which fails to correct in 2 hour incubation with a 1:1 mixture of reagent normal plasma (mixing study). Based upon this, in the appropriate clinical context, the diagnosis should be strongly suspected. Confirmation is based upon a low factor VIII level and subsequent measurement of factor VIII inhibitor activity (Bethesda assay). Characteristically, the inhibitor displays time dependence: the 1:1 mix must be incubated for 2 hours to bring out the inhibition. Most such anti-factor VIII antibodies are transient, disappearing within a few months. In the acute phase, treatment is directed at the acute bleed while efforts are made to reduce the titer of the inhibitor. For hemostasis, agents that bypass factor VIII are often required, such as recombinant activated factor VII (rFVIIa). For suppression of the inhibitor, immunosuppressive agents are required.

Hemophilia B (Christmas disease)

Hemophilia B is clinically indistinguishable from hemophilia A. It is an X-linked recessive congenital deficiency of fIX. The incidence is ~1 in 15,000 male births.

Like hemophilia A, the PT and TT are normal, while the PTT is usually prolonged. However, most commercially available PTT reagents are insensitive to mild factor IX deficiency, with the result that up to 30% of affected persons may show a normal PTT. Second, while not nearly as labile as factor VIII, factor IX is vitamin K-dependent, and vitamin K deficiency (as well as liver disease and coumadin ingestion) should be excluded. Third, unlike factor VIII, factor IX levels are low in neonates; actually, levels of factor IX increase progressively with age, even into old age. While up to 10% of carrier females manifest a bleeding diathesis, the majority have a normal PTT and factor IX level.

The factor IX gene is much smaller than the factor VIII gene, having 8 exons. It is found at Xq27, close to factor VIII, but far enough away to assort independently. Factor IX is synthesized in hepatocytes. Mild to moderate hemophilia B is most commonly caused by missense point mutations in the factor IX gene. Severe hemophilia B is usually caused by a nonsense mutation, microdeletion, gross deletion, or frameshift mutation. As is the case with hemophilia A, mutations resulting in essentially no production of antigenic factor IX (nonsense mutations and gross deletions) are associated with the greatest likelihood of developing anti-factor IX antibodies. The considerations for detecting carrier females and for prenatal diagnosis are similar to those for hemophilia A. The factor IX gene, being considerably smaller than the factor VIII gene, is more amenable to direct sequence analysis. By this method, a specific mutation in the factor IX gene can be detected in >99% of affected individuals. Like hemophilia A, molecular testing in hemophilia B is primarily applied to carrier detection and prenatal testing.

Factor IX Leiden is a particular type of hemophilia B characterized by spontaneous remission following puberty. A severe bleeding disorder is present during childhood, with <1% factor IX activity. With either puberty or the exogenous administration of androgens, factor IX levels rise to >30% and the bleeding disorder abates. Normal individuals experience a modest increase in factor IX activity at puberty as well. Interestingly, the genetic defect in factor IX Leiden appears to be located within the promoter region.

Factor IX replacement therapy differs from factor VIII in that there is only 30% dose recovery, and the half life is 8 hours.

Inherited deficiency of factors II, V, VII, X, or XI

Inherited deficiencies in factors II, V, VII, X, and XI have several features in common. They all display autosomal recessive inheritance, with heterozygotes having ~50% factor activity. Heterozygotes are usually asymptomatic and have normal PTT. Homozygotes have activity in the range of 1-5%, but tend to have somewhat milder disease than the X-linked recessive disorders, hemophilia A and B.

Factor V deficiency is rare and often associated with a consanguineous pedigree. The factor V gene is located at 1q21-25, and there is much homology with the factor VIII gene. Like factor VIII, the gene is quite large, and a variety of molecular defects have been described. (Of course, the most common mutation in the factor V gene is that leading to factor V Leiden.) Plasma factor V is synthesized in the liver. Platelet factor V is synthesized in megakaryocytes and found in platelet α granules. Severe factor V deficiency manifests as typical hemophilia. The PT and PTT are prolonged, and the thrombin time is normal. The bleeding time may be prolonged, due to a lack of platelet factor V. Isolated hereditary factor V deficiency is overall less common than the sum of the other causes of factor V deficiency—combined deficiency of factors V and VIII, acquired factor V deficiency (liver disease, amyloidosis), disseminated intravascular coagulation, and anti-factor V antibody inhibitors. The latter may develop spontaneously or after the administration of bovine thrombin preparations (which contain factor V).

Factor VII deficiency is the most common of the autosomal recessive coagulation factor deficiencies, but is quite rare, with an incidence of ~1 in 500,000. A unique feature of factor VII deficiency is poor association between factor VII levels and bleeding severity. In general, a complete absence of factor VII is incompatible with life, and a severe bleeding phenotype is mainly seen in those with factor VII activities <1-2%; however, many with activities in this range have only mild disease or no disease. Factor VII is a vitamin K-dependent factor synthesized in the liver. Circulating VII is activated by tissue factor to VIIa which can catalyze the formation of additional VIIa and activate factors X and IX. Thus, it is capable of driving both the extrinsic and intrinsic pathways. Factor VII deficiency is essentially the only inherited cause of an isolated prolongation of the PT. The PTT, TT, and bleeding times are normal. A factor VII assay will confirm the diagnosis. The factor VII gene is located on chromosome 13q, adjacent to the factor X gene. A wide variety of mutations have been reported with varying clinical phenotypes. Until recently, clinical severity could not be tied to genotype, suggesting other counterbalancing influences. It now appears that, at least in African Americans, the factor VII Padua genotype may account for many cases of asymptomatic factor VII deficiency (mild or no bleeding with factor VII<1%). The factor VII Padua mutation is a guanine to adenine substitution resulting in substitution of glutamine for arginine at amino acid 304. Molecular assays for factor VII gene mutations require direct DNA sequence analysis and are not widely available. Acquired factor VII deficiency can be caused by liver disease, warfarin, and vitamin K deficiency. These can be distinguished in the laboratory by the concomitant deficiency in other vitamin K-dependent factors.

Factor X deficiency is a rare autosomal recessive condition. Like factor VII, the factor X gene is located at 13q. It consists of 8 exons in which a large number of mutations have been described, the majority within exon 8. Nearly all of these have been missense mutations, and interestingly no nonsense mutations have been described. Factor X is synthesized in the liver as a vitamin K-dependent factor. In the circulation, it is activated either by the factor VIIa or the factor IXa-VIIIa complex. Russell viper venom (RVV) can activate factor X in vitro. The pivotal role of Xa is the conversion of prothrombin to thrombin. A multitude of gene mutations have been described in cases of factor X deficiency. The PT, PTT, and DRVVT are prolonged, with a normal TT and bleeding time. Amyloidosis is essentially the only cause of an acquired deficiency isolated to factor X. Interestingly, in this setting, transfused factor X does not effectively raise factor X levels. Acquired factor X deficiency in association with other factor deficiencies may be seen in liver disease, warfarin therapy, and vitamin K deficiency.

Factor XI deficiency, sometimes called hemophilia C, is an autosomal recessive condition that is unique in many respects when compared to other isolated coagulation factor deficiencies. While most of the conditions in this group are spread widely among geographic and ethnic groups, factor XI deficiency is found mainly in the Ashkenazim. In this population, the gene frequency may be as high as 5-10%. In addition, unlike the long list of unique mutations that give rise to other inherited factor deficiencies, 3 main mutations give rise to most cases of factor XI deficiency. Furthermore, genotype-phenotype correlations are not strong, and even very low factor XI levels may not result in a significant bleeding diathesis. In fact, most cases are mild; women may present with menorrhagia or prolonged puerperal hemorrhage, while males may present with epistaxis provoked by mild trauma. Interestingly, deficiency in factor XII, once thought to be the primary activator of factor XI, essentially never results in a bleeding diathesis. Factor XI deficiency is a common finding in Noonan syndrome.

Factor XIII deficiency

Factor XIII deficiency is rare. Inheritance is autosomal recessive, but while clinical abnormalities are most apparent in homozygotes, heterozygotes can have mild bleeding symptoms. The disorder in heterozygotes is characterized by delayed bleeding. Delayed bleeding is a reflection of the role of factor XIII: a normal fibrin clot can form in its absence but is weak because of an absence of factor XIII-mediated covalent crosslinking. Other symptoms include umbilical stump bleeding, frequent miscarriages, delayed wound healing and the formation of hypertrophic scars.

Homozygous factor XIII deficiency is associated with essentially normal PT, PTT, TT, and a severe bleeding diathesis. Unlike other AR deficiencies, deep hematomas and hemarthroses are unusual; instead, life threatening umbilical stump bleeding and intracranial bleeding are common.

Factor XIII consists of 2 catalytic A subunits and 2 noncatalytic B subunits, encoded on 2 separate chromosomes (6p and 1q). Most mutations causing factor XIII deficiency have so far been found in the A subunit. A factor XIII gene polymorphism (Val34Leu) is present in nearly half the population. It is believed to play a role in prevention of deep venous thrombosis. The polymorphism is found somewhat more commonly in patients with intracranial hemorrhage than in the general population.

Acquired factor XIII deficiency has been described in liver disease, DIC, inflammatory conditions (Crohn colitis, ulcerative colitis, Henoch-Schönlein purpura), and hematolymphoid neoplasms.

The assay traditionally used to detect factor XIII deficiency is the clot stability test. The clot stability test looks at the ability of an in vitro clot to withstand degradation by 5M urea. Clots formed in vitro by factor XIII-deficient patients disperse, usually within a few minutes, in these conditions. In the presence of >1-2% factor XIII activity, the clot should be stable for >24 hours. As such, this test is mainly for detecting homozyotes. The test is only valid if fibrinogen is qualitatively and quantitatively normal. Specific factor XIII assays can be used to confirm the diagnosis.

Contact factor deficiency (Factor XII, HMWK, prekallikrein)

Contact factor deficiency (factor XII, HMWK, or prekallikrein) cause marked prolongation of the aPTT without clinical bleeding (see p 314, causes of excessive thrombosis).

Inherited combined factor deficiency

While most single-factor deficiencies are the result of mutations within the gene that encodes the factor, there are mutations that affect genes involved in intracellular transport or posttranslational modification of multiple clotting factors. These can cause inherited combined deficiency states t5.12. The most common inherited combined deficiency is the combined factor V and factor VIII deficiency. This condition displays low levels of factors V and VIII coagulant activity and antigens. It appears that a gene on 18q—the *LMAN1* gene that encodes ERGIC-53—is responsible. ERGIC-53 is found within the rough endoplasmic reticulum and Golgi where it acts as a chaperone in the intracellular transport of factors V and VIII. Second most common is the combined deficiency of vitamin K–dependent factors. The syndrome of multiple deficiencies of vitamin K–dependent coagulation factors shows deficient factors II, VII, IX, X, and proteins C and S

t5.12 Familial combined factor deficiencies

Type	Deficiencies	Gene
I	V, VIII	*LMAN1* (ERGIC-53)
II	VII, IX	Unknown
III	II, VII, IX, X, C, S	Vitamin K Carboxylase
IV	VII, VIII	Unknown
V	VIII, IX, XI	Unknown

Fibrinogen defects: afibrinogenemia, hypofibrinogenemia & dysfibrinogenemia

Fibrinogen abnormalities may be congenital or acquired, and in both instances may be quantitative defects (afibrinogenemia, hypofibrinogenemia) or qualitative defects (dysfibrinogenemia). Furthermore, qualitative fibrinogen defects (dysfibrinogenemia) may cause either bleeding or thrombosis.

Inherited dysfibrinogenemia (autosomal dominant) is caused by various missense mutations. A cluster of 3 genes on chromosome 4q—fibrinogen α (FGA), fibrinogen β (FGB), and fibrinogen γ (FGG)—encode the protein fibrinogen. The fibrinogen molecule is a dimer, with each half composed of 3 polypeptide chains—Aα, Bβ, and γ. Deficiency-causing mutations are most often found in the Aα locus. Mutations in dysfibrinogenemia are more widespread throughout the several genes. Direct DNA sequence analysis is available through a small number of laboratories at this time.

Inherited afibrinogenemia and hypofibrinogenemia (autosomal recessive) are caused by mutations that severely truncate the protein. Umbilical cord hemorrhage is often the first manifestation of inherited hypo- or afibrinogenemia, followed by a life-long bleeding diathesis. Some patients, whose basic defect is the hepatocellular secretion of fibrinogen, succumb instead to cirrhosis (in a manner similar to that operative in α1-antitrypsin deficiency, in which abnormal protein accumulates in the endoplasmic reticulum of hepatocytes). Congenital afibrinogenemia is associated with an immeasurably prolonged PT and PTT and a clinical bleeding disorder similar to moderate to severe hemophilia A. Hypofibrinogenemia may be congenital or acquired (DIC, hepatic failure, and L-asparaginase therapy). Bleeding occurs when fibrinogen falls below 50 mg/dL.

Dysfibrinogenemia may be congenital or acquired (liver disease, biliary disease, hepatocellular carcinoma, and renal cell carcinoma). Clinically, it may be asymptomatic (50-60%), cause bleeding (30-40%) or cause thrombosis (10-20%), depending upon the particular mutation. Dysfibrinogenemia mutations associated with thrombosis tend to cluster in the γ gene. Recurrent miscarriages are a feature common to dysfibrinogenemia and factor XIII deficiency.

Acquired factor deficiencies

Factor X deficiency is sometimes found in patients with amyloidosis.

Liver disease causes a multitude of effects upon coagulation and thrombosis. First, there is decreased synthesis of most clotting factors, leading to clotting prolongation, particularly evident in the PT. Second, there is hypo- and dysfibrinogenemia, reflected in prolonged TT. Third, there is a poorly understood platelet functional abnormality. Lastly, there is chronic low grade DIC-like state caused by the impaired clearance of D-dimer.

Vitamin K deficiency leads to impaired production of the vitamin K-dependent factors II, VII, IX, X, protein C, and protein S. Vitamin K is necessary for γ-carboxylation of these factors within their so-called Gla domains. Note that, of these, factor VII has the shortest half life (2-5 hours). Protein C (6-8 hours) is a close second, and this, particularly in patients congenitally deficient in protein C, may lead to a transient thrombotic state often manifested by skin necrosis when treated with warfarin. Hemorrhagic disease of the newborn is a congenital form of vitamin K deficiency that typically presents at around 3 days of age. It is prevented by prophylactic vitamin K administration at birth. Vitamin K deficiency may result from the prolonged use of antibiotics, which diminish intestinal flora, the source of some of our vitamin K. Lastly, functional vitamin K deficiency may result from accidental or intentional ingestion of warfarin or warfarin-like compounds; warfarin-like compounds are present in the environment as a result of pesticide use. Such warfarin-like compounds are much more potent than pharmacologic warfarin, and are sometimes called "super-warfarins." One agent, brodifacoum, is widely used in pesticides in the United States; documented exposures have resulted from suicide attempts, occupational exposures, and from the smoking of marijuana or crack cocaine. Since it is highly lipophilic, skin exposure alone can lead to poisoning. Super-warfarin poisoning should be suspected when one encounters profound reduction in vitamin K-dependent factors that require significant replenishment (more than would be required for warfarin alone) for reversal.

Disseminated intravascular coagulation (DIC)

The formation of widespread microvascular thrombi is stimulated when there is a circulating substance capable of behaving like tissue factor. The fibrinolytic system responds by attempting to degrade the newly formed fibrin. The consumption of coagulation factors in numerous small clots leads to a bleeding diathesis, producing the seemingly paradoxical coexistence of excess bleeding and thrombosis. Causes of DIC include overwhelming infections (Gram–, usually), obstetric complications (abruption, amniotic fluid emboli), mucin-secreting adenocarcinomas, extensive trauma, prostatic surgery, and some venomous snake bites.

Laboratory tests useful to detect DIC are antithrombin (AT), fibrinopeptide A, D-dimer, and the platelet count. The PT and PTT are helpful if they are abnormal, but they are frequently normal. The fibrinogen measurement is fairly specific but insensitive (around 25-30%). It is best assessed serially, since many DIC-associated conditions create an acute phase elevation of the fibrinogen. If fibrinogen is low (<100), then DIC must be considered very likely. D-dimer is among the most sensitive tests for DIC (95% sensitive). AT and fibrinopeptide A are also reasonably sensitive (85%). Scoring systems have been developed, and that promulgated by the International Society of Thrombosis and Hemostasis (ISTH) has been validated in several studies t5.13.

t5.13 ISTH scoring system for DIC

Parameter	Scoring
Platelet count (×10⁹/L)	>100: score 0
	<100: score 1
	<50: score 2
D-dimer or FDP	Normal: score 0
	Elevated: score 2
	Marked (100× upper limit): score 3
PT prolongation	<3 seconds: score 0
	3-6 seconds: score 1
	>6 seconds: score 2
Fibrinogen	>100 mg/dL: score 0
	<100 mg/dL: score 1
Total score	5 or more: probable DIC
	<5: nonconfirmatory, follow serially

In patients who enter DIC when they harbor an anatomic bleeding source, such as obstetric patients and surgical patients, the likelihood of severe hemorrhage is high. In all other instances, however, bleeding is not the major problem in DIC; the prevalence of a major bleed in all patients with DIC is only ~10%. Patients with DIC and platelet counts below $50 \times 10^9/L$ are at greatest risk for major bleed. In the majority of instances it is thrombosis, at the microvascular level with attendant organ dysfunction, that produces morbidity and mortality.

The first principle of DIC treatment is to eliminate the underlying cause. Often the underlying cause is murky or untreatable, and the treating physician must attempt to control the clotting process. Treatment may target thrombosis, the process that most affects morbidity and mortality, bleeding, or both. There is, beyond these general statements, much controversy. Heparin administration is of empirically unclear value but there is a theoretical rationale—the mitigation of microvascular thrombosis—for its use; low dose subcutaneous heparin is the form usually administered. Antithrombin concentrates have been evaluated as a means to counteract microvascular thrombosis; studies show a small potential benefit. For the same reasons, administration of APC have been evaluated; these studies have shown a small but significant benefit. Further efforts may be directed at replenishing specific factor deficiencies and platelets, particularly in patients who are bleeding or who are at significant risk for bleeding. When fibrinogen is <100 mg/dL, FFP (15-20 mL/kg of body weight)

or cryoprecipitate (1 U/10 kg of body weight) should be considered. In the instances in which bleeding is severe, some would consider inhibition of the fibrinolytic system (δ-aminocaproic acid and tranexamic acid) or procoagulants (VIIa).

Nonhemostatic causes of excessive bleeding

Vascular & connective tissue disorders

Age related connective tissue fragility leads to easy rupture of superficial vessels, resulting in purpuric lesions, often seen beneath thin crepe-paper skin (actinic purpura). Solar damage and age related diminution in collagen and elastin conspire to cause these purpuric patches that are most often seen on the dorsum of the forearms and hands. A similar appearance may be seen in patients with glucocorticoid excess, from Cushing syndrome or glucocorticoid therapy.

Scurvy (vitamin C deficiency) is a disease of populations who lack access to dietary sources of vitamin C. Ascorbic acid (vitamin C) functions in a variety of biosynthetic pathways, chief among which is the biosynthesis of stable collagen. After 2-3 months of inadequate intake, the syndrome of scurvy develops. Characteristic findings include soft tissue swelling, joint pain, purpura, and follicular keratosis with entrapped corkscrew hairs. Humans cannot synthesize vitamin C, but it is plentiful in all but the most restrictive diets. In the 19th century, the British Royal Navy recognized that provision of citrus fruits could ward off the effects of scurvy; the practice resulted in the nickname "limey." Prior to this, navies were ravaged by deaths due to scurvy. Interestingly, the livers of rats, which ran in large numbers on most sailing vessels, are also a rich source of vitamin C. One perplexing feature of scurvy is that different individuals on ship were variably affected, some being spared entirely. Some ethnicities, moreover, were more susceptible than others, perhaps affecting seagoing migration. Recent studies have indicated that the genetic polymorphism in plasma haptoglobin may play a role. There are 2 major haptoglobin polymorphisms, Hp1 and Hp2, giving way to 3 major haptoglobin genotypes, Hp1-1, Hp2-1, and Hp2-2. Serum vitamin C is extremely labile because it is easily oxidized; haptoglobin, by binding up free hemoglobin, is prominent in protecting serum proteins such as vitamin C from oxidation. But polymorphic haptoglobins are variably effective in this regard, and serum vitamin C is lowest in Hp2-2 individuals.

Other acquired vasogenic sources of hemorrhage include amyloidosis, rickettsial infection, calciphylaxis, vasculitis, cirrhosis, atheroembolic disease, and fat emboli. Amyloid may cause small vessel hemorrhage by direct infiltration and weakening of vessel walls. A typical presentation is cortical hemorrhage in association with cerebral amyloid angiopathy. Rickettsiae are notable for a propensity to directly invade endothelial cells and cause vasculopathy. Calciphylaxis consists of dystrophic calcification and weakening of vessel walls in patients with altered calcium-phosphate product, such as patients with chronic renal failure. In cirrhosis, spider angiomata are typically found on the upper trunk and may rupture and hemorrhage. Both atheroembolic disease from cardiovascular sources and fat embolic disease from trauma may result in widespread petechiae and purpura.

Congenital considerations include constitutionally abnormal vascular connective tissue, such as in Ehlers-Danlos syndrome, hereditary hemorrhagic telangiectasia (Osler-Weber-Rendu), and ataxia-telangiectasia. In Fabry disease, numerous vascular lesions develop that are characterized histologically as angiokeratomas.

Causes of excessive thrombosis (thrombophilia)

Clinical considerations

When to suspect thrombophilia

All patients with a thromboembolic event under age 55 should be considered for further evaluation. One should not be deterred by the presence of a clinical "explanation" for the event (such as trauma or recent surgery), as more than half of individuals with an inherent thrombophilia experience their first event under such circumstances. Furthermore, elderly patients experiencing their first thrombotic event should be selectively considered for further evaluation as well. Hagemann himself, for whom factor XII is named, did not die of his massive PE until well into his golden years.

Clinical clues

The differential diagnosis of thrombophilia may be guided by the type of thrombosis—arterial or venous—but there is much overlap t5.14. In *venous thrombosis*, the most common sites are the deep veins of the lower extremities and iliofemoral veins. Other uncommon but characteristic sites include the mesenteric veins, renal veins, retinal veins, cerebral veins, and hepatic vein (Budd-Chiari syndrome). *Arterial thrombosis* generally takes the form of myocardial infarction in the young (<55, but often <35 year old) patient but can also manifest as thrombosis in carotid arteries, cerebral arteries, retinal arteries, subclavian or axillary artery, or mesenteric arteries.

Laboratory evaluation

The optimal laboratory evaluation takes place >2 months following the acute episode and >14 days following cessation of anticoagulant therapy. Alternatively, blood drawn immediately before the institution of anticoagulant therapy may be useful. Specifically, assays for protein C and protein S are unreliable when anticoagulant therapy is ongoing.

t5.14 Thrombophilia: differential diagnosis by type of thrombosis

Arterial thrombosis: eg, MI		Venous thrombosis: eg, DVT	
Common	Antiphospholipid syndrome (ACA) Prothrombin mutation (20210) HIT syndrome	Common	APCR Prothrombin mutation (20210) Antiphospholipid syndrome (ACA & LAC) Protein C deficiency Protein S deficiency ATIII deficiency
Uncommon	Elevated PAI-1 activity Hyperhomocysteinemia t-PA deficiency	Uncommon	Hyperhomocysteinemia Heparin cofactor II Factor XII deficiency
Also consider	Anomalous coronary arteries Vasculitis	Also consider	Immobilization Trauma Pregnancy

Management

Effective management, in addition to the specific measures discussed below, includes family studies to identify individuals at risk for thrombosis. Counseling for affected individuals is important, so that risk factors, such as obesity, oral contraceptive use, and immobility, can be managed, and prophylactic use of anticoagulants can be started in appropriate clinical situations, such as pregnancy, immobilization, and surgery.

Specific causes of thrombophilia

Activated protein C resistance (factor V Leiden)

In the normal course of events, APC degrades activated factors V and VIII (Va and VIIIa) by proteolytic cleavage, thus inhibiting coagulation. APC resistance (APCR) is an autosomal dominant inherited condition in which a mutant factor V is made (factor V Leiden) that is resistant to APC proteolysis. APCR is responsible for up to 50% of the cases of hereditary thrombophilia.

The factor V gene is found on chromosome 1q. APCR is caused by a G to A point mutation at nucleotide 1691 in the factor V gene that results in a glutamine for arginine substitution at position 506 (factor V R506Q) in the factor V protein. This change affects 1 of 3 APC cleavage domains. The result is a type of factor V (factor V Leiden) that is resistant to proteolytic cleavage by activated protein C (APC). Heterozygotes are affected by a 5- to 10- fold increased risk of thrombosis; thus the condition is considered autosomal dominant with variable penetrance. The risk of thrombosis increases dramatically for homozygotes and compound heterozygotes having factor V Leiden and protein C deficiency or antithrombin deficiency.

APCR heterozygosity is found in up to 5% of the Caucasian population. The factor V Leiden allele is quite infrequent in those of sub-Saharan African, Chinese, Japanese, or Native American descent.

Laboratory tests include a screening clot-based assay (phenotypic analysis) and confirmatory DNA-based assay (genotypic analysis). In the clot-based test, 2 aPTTs are performed, one with patient serum alone, and the other with patient serum in the presence of APC. The ratio of the clotting time with APC to the clotting time without APC (the resistance ratio) is normally >2. This test is unreliable in patients undergoing anticoagulation, in the presence of a lupus anticoagulant, and in normal neonates. Neonates have transient protein C resistance on the basis of low endogenous protein C levels. A modification of this technique, using an initial 1:11 dilution, has been recommended for neonates and infants <6 months. Discrepant results may be seen in compound heterozygotes having both the factor V Leiden mutation and a type I quantitative factor V deficiency, as well as in other rare scenarios. Otherwise, the APCR screen correlates very well with genotypic tests. The overall sensitivity and specificity of this assay are around 85% each. In a modification to this assay, plasma deficient only in factor V is added to the patient plasma (to control for any other factor deficiencies such as those due to warfarin therapy and to mitigate the effects of any lupus anticoagulants), and a heparin neutralizer is added (to control for any heparin). This modified APC resistance assay has sensitivity and specificity >95%. Clinically available molecular testing most often is in the form of RFLP analysis. The factor V Leiden mutation results in the loss of a restriction endonuclease recognition site, permitting discernment of the mutated allele from the normal allele. The sensitivity approaches 100%.

58% of APCR patients had an associated risk factor at their first thrombotic event, and one very important risk factor is estrogen: pregnancy and oral contraceptive use are associated with the first thrombotic episode in 35% and 30% of women, respectively. Furthermore, the factor V Leiden mutation is associated with a high risk of fetal loss and a high risk of intrapartum thrombosis.

Prothrombin variant (prothrombin G20210A mutation)

A single nucleotide substitution—G to A—at position 20210 in the 3'-untranslated region of the prothrombin gene results in *elevated* levels of prothrombin. This mutation is believed to enhance prothrombin gene transcription and translation. The abnormal allele is transmitted as an autosomal dominant trait.

The incidence of prothrombin 20210 approaches that of factor V Leiden—up to 4% of the general population and 20% of patients with thrombophilia. As such, the prothrombin variant is the second most common cause of inherited thrombophilia. The mutation is present in around 2% of those with European ancestry and ~0.5% of the black population. It is also interestingly present in up to 10% of those with the factor V Leiden mutation.

The mutation behaves as an autosomal dominant trait, substantially (~3×) increasing the risk of thrombosis (by comparison, the relative risk in factor V Leiden is ~6). Venous events outnumber arterial ones. In particular, there appears to be a risk for cerebral vein thrombosis. This risk is compounded greatly by the concomitant use of oral contraceptives. Both the factor V Leiden and the prothrombin variant are associated with pregnancy complications, including a high risk of fetal loss and a high risk of intrapartum thrombosis.

While those harboring the 20210 mutation tend to have high levels of prothrombin (usually >115% of normal), the prothrombin activity is a poor (insensitive) screening test for the mutation. Direct gene sequencing by PCR is clinically available to detect the prothrombin 20210 mutation. In fact, methods are now available to detect both the prothrombin G20210A mutation and factor V Leiden in the same reaction.

Antithrombin deficiency (antithrombin III deficiency)

Antithrombin (AT) inhibits factors II, IXa, Xa, XIa and XIIa and is a crucial part of physiologic anticoagulant mechanisms. When bound to heparin, the activity of AT is enhanced markedly, forming the basis for the anticoagulant effect of heparin. Inherited AT deficiency is an autosomal dominant disorder characterized by recurrent venous thrombosis. Heterozygotes have a 5-10× increased risk for venous thrombosis, and the homozygous state is considered incompatible with life. The age at onset of thrombosis is usually between 10-40 years. The prevalence of hereditary AT deficiency appears to be around 1 in 2,000. It is estimated to cause around 3% of unexplained venous thrombosis. Particular attention must be paid to AT-deficient individuals during pregnancy (the combined AT-lowering effect of pregnancy and the prothrombotic effect of pregnancy are a dangerous combination). AT deficiency may come to clinical attention by an apparent inability to achieve a therapeutic response to heparin therapy, as measured by the aPTT and Xa assay, and patients who are unresponsive to heparin should be tested for AT deficiency. For AT-deficient individuals, infusions of AT concentrate will permit therapeutic heparinization. Acquired AT deficiency may arise in nephrotic syndrome, L-asparaginase therapy, estrogen therapy, pregnancy, acute thrombosis, DIC, and colitis. AT levels may increase with coumadin therapy.

With regard to laboratory diagnosis, the normal range for AT is between 70 and 120%. Healthy newborns have levels in the range of 40-60%, achieving adult levels by 6 months of age. AT activity <60% is consistent with AT deficiency in an adult. Heterozygotes generally have AT levels between 40% and 70%. Note that recent DVT or PE causes decreased levels of AT, because of consumption of this factor. Estrogens may reduce AT levels by ~15%. Heparin therapy reduces the AT activity in normal adults, but never below 70%. Patients whose activity is tested below 60% should be considered AT deficient, even in the presence of heparin.

There are 2 varieties of AT assays: functional and antigenic. Of the 2, the functional assay yields more clinically useful information. If the result is abnormal, one may elect to perform an antigenic assay to distinguish types I and II inherited AT deficiency. Functional assays are usually chromogenic and based upon AT's ability to inhibit thrombin and Xa. These are performed by adding patient plasma to heparin, a known quantity of either thrombin or Xa, and a chromogenic substrate. Any uninhibited thrombin (or Xa) will convert the substrate to a colored product that can be measured spectrophotometrically. The quantity of product is inversely proportional to the AT activity.

Over 100 disease-causing mutations have been identified in the AT gene, *SERPINC1*, found on 1q23-q25 not far from the factor V gene. Due to the wide variety of mutations and murky genotype-phenotype correlations, AT assays are preferable and molecular testing is not widely available. Nonetheless, there are 2 general classes of mutation: those resulting in the absence (quantitative) of AT (type I), and those resulting in a dysfunctional (qualitative) form of AT (type II). Heterozygotes for the type I mutation have decreased AT, and homozygotes have no AT. The type I mutations are either frameshift or complete gene deletions. Type II mutations are generally single-nucleotide point mutations and may be further subdivided into those affecting the heparin binding domain and those affecting the thrombin binding domain.

Protein C & protein S deficiency

Protein C is activated in vivo by thrombin-thrombomodulin complexes. APC proteolytically cleaves factors Va and VIIIa into the inactive forms Vi and VIIIi. Protein S is the cofactor for protein C.

The incidence of protein C or protein S deficiency in the general population is estimated between 1 in 200 and 1 in 500, and each is responsible for 1-5% of thrombophilia. Both are autosomal dominant conditions. Heterozygotes have a 5-7× increased risk of thrombosis and are at risk for coumadin induced skin necrosis. Homozygotes present as newborns with purpura fulminans, a rapidly fatal form of DIC that requires immediate treatment with anticoagulation and FFP. Acquired protein C deficiency may result from coumadin therapy, liver disease, and pregnancy.

Warfarin (Coumadin), a mainstay of treatment for thrombophilia, must be used with caution; it must be started at very low doses in conjunction with unfractionated or LMW heparin to prevent skin and fat necrosis. Alternatively, long term low dose subcutaneous mucosal or cutaneous LMW heparin may be used. Protein C concentrates have been developed for treatment in deficiency states.

A wide variety of disease-causing mutations have been identified, and for this reason molecular testing is not widely available. Where available, direct DNA sequencing is required. The protein S gene is found on 3p11.1-q11.2. The protein C gene is on 2q13-q14.

Both functional (coagulation based) and antigenic (immunologic) assays are available for proteins C and S. Functional assays are preferred for screening. Protein C activity levels in healthy adults range from 70-140% and increase slightly with age. Protein C levels in heterozygous protein C deficiency usually fall below 55% but sometimes fall into an indeterminate zone between 55-70%. In these patients, it may be helpful to document 2 low levels on separate occasions. Protein C activity levels in newborns are normally around 20-40%.

The deficiencies of protein C may be classified as type I (quantitative) or type II (qualitative). Type I deficiency, in which both qualitative and quantitative results are low, is by far the most common. In type II deficiency, there is a normal antigenic level of the protein but reduced activity, and detecting the relatively uncommon type II deficiency is the reason for the widespread recommendation that a functional assay be used for screening.

Deficiencies of protein S come in 3 varieties. About 60% of protein S in plasma is bound to C4b binding protein. In addition to functional and antigenic assays, free and total antigenic assays are available. Thus 3 types of protein S deficiency states can be identified: type I is a global quantitative defect, type II is a qualitative defect (the functional activity of protein S is decreased, but the antigen levels are normal), and type III is characterized by decreased free protein S. Type I is by far the most common. There is more overlap between normal and abnormal ranges for protein S than protein C, so that repeat sampling on separate occasions is advised. Protein S in healthy newborns is ~15-30% of normal. Levels of protein S are normally slightly lower in females than males, and an acquired

form of protein S deficiency can occur during both pregnancy and oral contraceptives use. Normal ranges for protein S activity in pregnancy are as follows: 1st trimester—50-100%; 2nd trimester—25-75%; 3rd trimester—20-50%. Protein S is reduced in HIV infection. In contrast to antithrombin, levels of both protein S and protein C increase in nephrotic syndrome.

MTHFR gene mutation & hyperhomocysteinemia

Homocysteine is an amino acid that is formed in the breakdown of proteins. It is normally not an end-product in itself, but rather is a temporary intermediary in the interconversion of methionine and cysteine, both of which can then go on to be used for other purposes. Whenever the utilization of methionine or cysteine is blocked, excess homocysteine may lead to hyperhomocysteinemia.

A point of possible confusion is the relationship between homocystinuria and hyperhomocysteinemia. Homocystinuria is a manifestation of extreme hyperhomocysteinemia (>100 µmol/L) that leads to a syndrome characterized by overflow of homocysteine into the urine (homocystinuria), mental retardation, ectopia lentis, premature atherosclerosis, and thrombosis. This syndrome is most commonly caused by homozygous cystathionine-β-synthase deficiency or homozygous methylenetetrahydrofolate reductase (MTHFR) deficiency and is extremely rare. Mild to moderate hyperhomocysteinemia (16-100 µmol/L) is not associated with a recognizable clinical syndrome, is quite common, and is the subject of this section.

Mild to moderate hyperhomocysteinemia affects 5-7% of the population and is considered an independent risk factor for both atherosclerosis and recurrent arteriovenous thromboembolism. Hyperhomocysteinemia is present in up to 40% of patients with premature atherosclerosis and ~15-20% of those with thrombophilia. Hyperhomocysteinemia is classified as mild (16-24 µmol/L), moderate (25-100 µmol/L), or severe (>100). It is usually diagnosed by measuring plasma levels of homocysteine using high pressure liquid chromatography. Very mild defects can be detected by demonstrating an abnormal increase in plasma homocysteine after an oral methionine load. Elderly patients, smokers, and patients with renal failure frequently have elevated plasma homocysteine concentrations in the absence of vitamin deficiencies. Deficiency of folate, B_6, and B_{12} are common acquired causes of hyperhomocysteinemia.

The most common inherited cause of mild to moderate hyperhomocysteinemia is heterozygosity for the *MTHFR* gene mutation, followed by heterozygous cystathionine-β-synthase deficiency. The *MTHFR* gene is located at 1p36.3. The mutated form of the *MTHFR* gene is called the T allele and results in an alanine to valine substitution at amino acid 677 (C677T). The alanine to valine substitution at amino acid 677 results in thermolability of the MTHFR protein and loss of activity. Testing for the mutation is clinically available. People who have elevated homocysteine on the basis of the *MTHFR* mutation can often achieve normal homocysteine with folate and/or B_6 supplementation.

Paroxysmal nocturnal hemoglobinuria (PNH)

PNH (discussed on p 227) is associated with thromboembolic events and, to a much lesser extent, bleeding. Despite this, when subjected to such measures of global platelet function as thromboelastography and aggregometry, a marked reduction of platelet reactivity is observed. This is compounded by the frequent development of thrombocytopenia. For these reasons, it is thought that the thrombotic tendency in PNH is based upon some alteration in the coagulation system.

Heparin cofactor II (HC-II) deficiency

HC-II is an inhibitor of coagulation that, like AT, is activated by heparin. Thrombotic tendencies are associated with levels <60% HC-II activity, but HC-II deficiency appears to be a rare cause of unexplained thrombosis (around 1%). HC-II activity has been studied in patients with nephrotic syndrome and found to remain normal, in contrast to AT activity, which is commonly decreased in nephrotic syndrome.

Factor XII deficiency

Despite the fact that factor XII is active in the intrinsic clotting pathway, and deficiency in factor XII leads to tremendous prolongation in the aPTT, this condition virtually never causes a bleeding diathesis. Instead, patients with factor XII deficiency present with thrombosis, both arterial and venous. Among factor XII deficient patients, there is a 2-10% incidence of thrombosis, often with a presentation of myocardial infarctions in a young adult. There appear to be several disease-causing mutations in the factor XII gene. Most of them affect the serine protease domain.

The aPTT is often >100 seconds, while the PT and TT are normal. When the 1:1 mix is performed, there is initial correction, followed by prolongation after a 10 minute incubation. The aPTT can be corrected by exposure to glass. While F XII initiates the intrinsic coagulation system in vitro, it is believed to be uninvolved in coagulation in vivo. Deficiencies in prekallikrein and high-molecular-weight-kininogen are also not associated with clinical bleeding.

Elevated plasminogen activator inhibitor type 1 (*PAI-1* gene polymorphisms)

PAI-1 is the major physiologic inhibitor of fibrinolysis (inhibitor of clot lysis). In the process of fibrinolysis, tissue plasminogen activator (tPA) converts plasminogen to plasmin, and plasmin degrades fibrin. PAI-1 inhibits tPA, and in the proper quantity it is a crucial part of the delicate balance between fibrin formation and fibrin degradation. Too much PAI-1 prevents fibrinolysis, promoting thrombophilia, and too little PAI-1 promotes bleeding.

The *SERPINE1* gene on chromosome 7q21.3-q22 encodes plasminogen activator inhibitor-1 (PAI-1). PAI-1 levels are under numerous influences, some of them genetic, and certain polymorphisms in the *PAI-1* gene have been associated with increased blood concentrations. Other influences on PAI-1 are clearly at work, however. Raised blood levels of insulin are associated with elevated PAI-1 levels, and patients with insulin resistance (eg, type 2 diabetes) tend to have increased PAI-1. Elevated PAI-1 causes a thrombophilic state, especially

associated with arterial thrombotic events such as myocardial infarction.

In the clinical laboratory, PAI-1 is usually measured by immunoassay, but a functional assay is also available. Importantly, PAI-1 displays diurnal variation, with highest plasma concentration in the morning (important for result interpretation but also possibly related to the higher early morning incidence of myocardial infarctions). Standardization is best achieved by drawing samples between 0800-0900 (and certainly not outside 0700-1000). This will be compared with normal ranges based on 0800-0900 samples. Further, PAI-1 is an acute phase reactant and may be elevated following a thrombotic event. It is best to wait ≥2 weeks after an event before testing, and testing for PAI-1 is best performed parallel with a C-reactive protein as a "control" for the acute phase. Plasminogen activator inhibitor type 1 (PAI-1) antigen essentially parallels activity, and all the caveats regarding PAI-1 activity apply. Low levels of PAI-1 suggest the very rare familial PAI-1 deficiency, a cause of hemophilia.

Antiphospholipid (APL) syndrome: anticardiolipin antibody (ACA) & lupus anticoagulant (LAC) t5.15

The antiphospholipid (APL) syndrome encompasses 2 similar but distinct clinical syndromes

1. lupus anticoagulant (LAC) syndrome
2. anticardiolipin antibody (ACA) syndrome

t5.15 Anticardiolipin antibody vs lupus anticoagulant

Feature	ACA syndrome	LAC syndrome
Prevalence	+++	+
Thrombosis	+	+
Fetal wastage	+	+
Thrombocytopenia	+/−	+/−
Arterial thrombosis	+	−
Venous thrombosis	+	+
Prolongation of the aPTT	−	+
Associated with livedo reticularis	+	−
Associated with lupus (secondary APL)	10-20%	10-20%
Otherwise healthy (primary APL)	80%	80%
Warfarin for long term prophylaxis	Often ineffective	Effective

The 2 share some features. Both may be found in association with systemic lupus erythematosus (secondary APL syndrome), but both are most commonly seen in otherwise healthy individuals (primary APL syndrome). Both may also be associated with HIV, malignancy, and nonlupus collagen vascular diseases. Both may be caused by medication. Drugs associated with APL syndromes are phenytoin, quinidine, hydralazine, procainamide, phenothiazines, interferon (IFN) α, and cocaine. Both ACA and LAC syndromes are causes of thrombosis, and both have been implicated as causes of pulmonary hypertension. Both ACA and LAC syndromes are associated with a fetal wastage syndrome of frequent abortion (particularly in the first trimester) recurrent fetal wastage (second and third trimesters), placental vasculopathy (infarction, decidual vasculopathy, thrombosis, perivillous fibrinoid change), and variable maternal thrombocytopenia. In patients affected by fetal wastage syndrome, anticoagulant therapy can increase the chances of a term delivery from<50% to >75%. Low dose aspirin and subcutaneous heparin have been used in this regard. Thrombocytopenia is associated with both APL syndromes, occurring in around 50% of patients with the secondary APL syndrome and <10% of those with primary APL syndrome. Most individuals with ACA antibodies do not have a LAC, and most with the LAC do not have ACA. Overall, ~80% of patients with APS have ACA, ~20% have LAC.

Some features are more or less unique to the ACA syndrome. The ACA syndrome is a cause of both venous and arterial thrombosis. ACA antibodies have been associated with premature coronary atherosclerosis, early angioplasty failure (re-stenosis), and early coronary artery bypass graft occlusion. Some ACAs are associated with the dermatological manifestation of livedo reticularis. ACAs have also been associated with a unique, transient, postpartum syndrome of fever, pleuritic chest pain, pleural effusion, patchy pulmonary infiltrates, cardiomyopathy, and ventricular arrhythmias, presenting 2-10 days postpartum. Many patients with ACA syndrome fail warfarin therapy (>60%), and one should exclude anticardiolipin antibodies in a patient with warfarin failure.

The LAC syndrome causes mainly venous thrombosis. Secondary LAC syndrome may be associated with arterial thrombosis on occasion. LAC often first comes to clinical attention as a result of a prolonged PTT. This is an in vitro artifact, and LAC is not associated with bleeding.

Testing for APL is indicated in patients with unexplained thrombosis, lupus, recurrent pregnancy loss (more than one loss of anatomically normal fetus after 10 weeks gestation or 2 or more spontaneous abortions prior to 10th week), and primary pulmonary hypertension. Some would add livedo reticularis as an indication. In systemic lupus erythematosus (SLE), the incidence of thrombosis is very high, possibly as high as 2% per year. APL antibodies in SLE are a risk factor for premature coronary atherosclerosis, increased incidence of renal disease, and cerebrovascular events. With regard to cerebrovascular lupus, SLE should always be considered in the differential diagnosis of a young patient with neurologic disorders, and the histopathology of brains affected in lupus shows bland thrombosis, without vasculitis or immune complexes. Like all autoantibodies, APL antibodies increase with age, and APL antibodies are a treatable and common contributing factor in thrombophilia of the elderly. APL antibodies have been shown to play a major (possibly causative) role in ~10% of cases of so-called primary pulmonary hypertension. Women who have experienced 1st trimester abortion, particularly if recurrent, and women who have experienced 2nd or 3rd trimester fetal loss should be screened. Evaluation of such patients includes, in addition to the serum assays described below, careful examination of the placentas associated with their prior adverse events, with particular attention being paid to the existence of placental vasculopathy. The finding of a placental infarct in a 1st trimester placenta is distinctly unusual and should make the suspicion of APA syndrome very high.

In order to diagnose the antiphospholipid syndrome, one must demonstrate either anticardiolipin (ACA) antibody or lupus anticoagulant (LAC) on 2 separate occasions (8-12 weeks apart). Lupus anticoagulant tests are clot-based assays, based upon the observation that LACs can prolong phospholipid-dependent clotting times. Characteristically, as is typical of inhibitors, there is failure of the clotting time to correct in a 1:1

mix. Some weak inhibitors will correct in the 1:1 and may be only detected with a 4:1 mix. In order to confirm the diagnosis of LAC, one must demonstrate both prolongation of a phospholipid-dependent clotting time and correction of the clotting time with excess phospholipid. Either the activated partial thromboplastin time (aPTT) or the dilute Russell viper venom time (DRVVT) may be used for this purpose. Some LACs do not prolong the PTT at all but will prolong the DRVVT, which is more sensitive to LAC. In patients receiving oral anticoagulation, the plasma should be mixed with normal plasma (to correct factor deficiencies) before testing. Also notable, assays for factors XII, XI, IX, and VII may yield artifactually low values in the presence of LAC—dilution of the test plasma (ie, dilution of the inhibitor) causes the measured level of these factors to approach the normal range.

Anticardiolipin antibody tests are ELISA-based. Patients with low-titer IgG (<1:40) or who have solely IgM are not at significant risk for thrombosis, but both types of patients have a high risk of developing high titer IgG later, at which time they are at risk. Thus, the presence of low titer IgG or of IgM alone is an indication for serial testing. Some have recommended that ACA should be tested in a $\beta 2$ glycoprotein I (β2-GPI)-dependent manner. Many anticardiolipin antibodies are directed against cardiolipin bound to β2-GPI, and while other ACAs and ACA assays exist, it appears that those specific for the β2-GPI-linked antigen correlate most strongly with thrombotic risk. The significance of non-β2-GPI-linked ACAs remains unclear. Syphilis, Q fever, and HIV infection can produce a false positive ACA test (usually an IgM ACA). Furthermore, the anticardiolipin antibody may produce a false positive syphilis test (RPR).

Patients with thrombosis and antiphospholipid antibodies need long term anticoagulant therapy, and treatment should be stopped only if the antibody becomes persistently undetectable for a continuous period of 4-6 months.

Platelet glycoprotein polymorphisms

Glycoprotein IIIa is part of the glycoprotein IIb/IIIa complex, a platelet-surface receptor that binds fibrinogen and vWF. GPIIb/IIa forms the basis for the CD41/CD61 antigen. The components of the IIb/IIIa complex are both encoded on chromosome 17q. The 2 alleles at the IIIa locus are PLA1 (HPA-1a) and PLA2 (HPA-1b). The difference between PLA1 and PLA2 is a single nucleotide and single amino acid. The PLA2 allele has been associated with premature myocardial infarction as well as stent re-occlusion.

Glycoprotein IIb of the GPIIb/IIIa complex has 2 common alleles: Bak^a (HPA-3a) and Bak^b (HPA-3b). Again, a single nucleotide substitution separates these molecules. At amino acid position 843, an isoleucine is present in Bak^a, and a serine is present in Bak^b. Thus far, there does not seem to be a prothrombotic risk in either allele.

Glycoproteins Ib, V, and IX form a complex that acts as the platelet vWF receptor (and the CD42 antigen). The polymorphisms in this complex are mainly found within GPIb. Amino acid 145 determines whether the HPA^{2A} (threonine) or HPA^{2B} (methionine) antigen is expressed. HPA^{2A} is present in ~90% of the population, and HPA^{2B} in 10%. Furthermore, the PGIb protein normally has a certain number of leucine rich repeats within its extracellular domain. The number of these can vary, resulting in additional polymorphism (variable number of tandem repeats or VNTR). The impact of these polymorphisms on thrombotic risk is unknown.

The Ia/IIa complex forms a receptor for collagen. The Ia molecule, the product of a very large gene on 5q, has numerous polymorphisms. One of these, a threonine substitution at amino acid 807, is present in ~35% of the population and seems to be associated with thrombosis.

Wien-Penzing defect

The Wien-Penzing defect is extremely rare. It is caused by an inherited deficiency in the lipoxygenase metabolic pathway. Compensatory increases in cyclooxygenase pathway products, including thromboxane, prostaglandin E2, and prostaglandin D2, are thought to underlie the thrombotic tendency. Wien-Penzing-like defect arising in association with myeloproliferative neoplasms is much more common than the inherited defect. Patients suffer from early myocardial infarction.

Sticky platelet syndrome

Sticky platelet syndrome (SPS) is a recently described cause of arterial and venous thrombosis. Its exact incidence is unknown. The greatest chance of finding it is in young patients with cerebrovascular events. About half present with venous thrombi, and half with arterial thrombi, most commonly cerebrovascular events (>50%). The laboratory diagnosis relies upon the demonstration of hyperaggregation patterns in platelet aggregation studies using epinephrine and ADP. Low dose acetylsalicylic acid (ASA) is the recommended treatment. This has been demonstrated to normalize SPS aggregation patterns.

Heparin induced thrombocytopenia (HIT)

HIT is a potentially life threatening condition that must be considered in patients with new onset thrombocytopenia. Treatment is relatively simple: discontinuation of heparin. It is the management of suspected HIT that is somewhat complicated, because it depends upon the level of suspicion combined with a small number of suboptimal tests, in the face of the extreme expense of heparin alternatives.

If HIT is suspected, pending the results of laboratory assays, a decision must be made regarding the patient's anticoagulation. If suspicion of HIT is high (see below), or if an arterial thrombosis occurs, heparin in all its forms should be discontinued. Management of anticoagulation depends upon the use of argatroban, danaparoid, lepirudin, or other agents with no crossreactivity with the HIT antibodies. Warfarin should be avoided because of the risk of microvascular thrombosis. Platelet transfusions are contraindicated. Many clinicians will cautiously continue the use of heparin if suspicion is low, pending the results of laboratory tests. Even in the face of a positive PF4 antibody test, given its low precision, some will discontinue heparin only grudgingly if conditions do not seem appropriate for HIT.

2 types of HIT were delineated, and the distinction still has merit. Type 1 HIT occurs early during heparinization, and the platelet count diminishes very mildly. In typical type 1 HIT, the platelet count decreases by day 1 or 2 of heparinization,

and the platelet count does not decrease beyond 50% of baseline. Type 1 HIT arises in ~5% of heparinized patients, poses no danger to the patient, is not immune mediated, and is not a contraindication to future heparin use. In Type 2 HIT, a drop in platelets is usually noted after day 7 of heparinization, and the platelet count is usually <50% of baseline. Type 2 HIT is immune mediated, and thrombosis is an enormous risk. The incidence in heparinized patients is around 1%.

HIT causes both arterial and venous thromboses, and bleeding is not usually a problem. Arterial thrombosis often involves the extremities (5-10%), the central nervous system (3-5%), or the heart, causing myocardial infarction (3-5%). Venous thrombosis manifests as lower-limb deep-vein thrombosis (50%), pulmonary embolism (25%), upper limb deep-vein thrombosis (10%), or adrenal hemorrhagic necrosis. Microvascular thrombosis may occur, particularly in patients treated with coumadin, and it is for this reason that coumadin is relatively contraindicated in HIT. Erythematous plaques or skin necrosis may form at the site of subcutaneous heparin injection.

Knowledge of the prototypical course of HIT type 2 is necessary in order to arrive at the proper level of suspicion, or pretest probability. While certain risk factors for HIT have been recognized, none has translated meaningfully into predictive models. Risk factors for HIT include surgery (3-5× risk as compared to medical patients), and female gender (2× risk). The most important variables to note are the time of onset, magnitude of platelet diminution, and presence of thrombosis. Onset of type 2 HIT is typically between 5-10 days following the start of heparinization. Rapid-onset HIT may be seen in those exposed to heparin within the recent past (30 days). The HIT syndrome can occur after cessation of heparin therapy, for up to 3 weeks; thus, patients may suffer a thrombotic event after discharge from a hospitalization during which they were exposed to heparin. This delayed-onset HIT is often quite severe. Furthermore, re-exposure to heparin while anti-PF4 antibodies are still present (within up to 124 days) may produce a rapid onset of HIT syndrome. However, once anti-PF4 antibodies disappear, there does not appear to be an anamnestic response. The biggest risk factor, of course, is exposure to unfractionated heparin. But this may be more difficult to discover than it seems, as heparin permeates a vast number of medical interventions. Furthermore, though lower, there is a risk in patients treated only with LMWH. So any exposure to the heparin antigen, including the use of heparin-coated (hep-locked) intravenous catheters, must be queried. Lastly, HIT is associated with a typical platelet count nadir that is 50% or less of baseline, but usually not extremely low and rarely below $20 \times 10^9/L$. Some patients with baseline normal to high platelet counts may not exceed the lower limit of normal. A 4-point scoring system, sometimes called the "4 Ts," has been developed that can be applied to the diagnosis of HIT.

Type 2 HIT is mediated by antibodies against the complex of platelet factor 4 (PF4) and heparin. PF4 is a product of platelet α granules that is released by activated platelets; once released, PF4 normally binds noncovalently to the platelet surface. In the presence of heparin, heparin-PF4 complexes form, which then bind to the platelet surface. If there are circulating anti-PF4/heparin antibodies, these bind to the heparin-PF4 complex whose location on the surface of the platelet permit association of the Fc portion of the antibody with the platelet's Fc receptor. Binding of the immunoglobulin Fc to the platelet Fc receptor results in platelet activation.

Most rapid laboratory tests for HIT are based upon identification of PF4 antibodies in blood. The anti-PF4 antibody test by ELISA is reported to be around 90% sensitive and 95% specific, and that by the more rapid immunoflocculation technique are around 85% specific. Once antibodies are formed, they are detectable (by ELISA) for a median duration of 85 days (up to 124 days) and functionally active (by SRA) for a median of 50 days (up to 64 days). The serotonin release assay (SRA) is the gold standard test but not widely available. The heparin induced platelet aggregation assay (HIPA) essentially involves a platelet aggregation study in which heparin is added as the "agonist." Enhanced aggregation with heparin is abnormal. This test is considered to be around 95% specific but its sensitivity ranges from 30-80%.

Thrombotic thrombocytopenia purpura (TTP)

TTP is a syndrome resulting from the widespread formation of microvascular platelet thrombi, particularly affecting the central nervous system, kidneys, gastrointestinal tract, and other organs. It presents with a classic pentad that includes thrombocytopenia, microangiopathic hemolytic anemia, neurologic abnormalities, renal abnormalities, and fever. Platelets usually number <20,000 /µL, and schistocytes are numerous in the peripheral smear. The serum LD is very high, often >1,000 IU/dL, a feature that is used diagnostically and to follow course and therapy.

TTP is usually an idiopathic and isolated event. In some cases of idiopathic TTP, there is recurrence. Familial TTP (Upshaw-Schulman syndrome) is typically chronic and relapsing. Some cases of TTP have been associated with medications, pregnancy, and hematopoietic stem cell transplantation; this group is referred to as "secondary TTP." Medications associated with secondary TTP include ticlopidine, clopidogrel (Plavix), cyclosporine, tacrolimus, interferon, mitomycin, gemcitabine, cisplatin, and bleomycin.

When the sera of patients with TTP were initially studied in the 1980s, it was noted that there were abnormally large circulating multimers of vWF. The usually predominant small multimers were absent. Recall that vWF is released into the circulation as large multimers which are subsequently broken down, with the result being that serum vWF is found in a range of sizes, predominantly dimers. Recently, the role of a circulating vWF cleaving protease—known as ADAMTS-13—has been elucidated. It is the function of ADAMTS-13 to cleave larger multimers into smaller ones. It is known that a large number of those with sporadic TTP, and nearly all those with familial TTP, are deficient in ADAMTS-13. Secondary TTP is not strongly associated with deficiency of ADAMTS-13. Familial TTP is caused by mutations in the gene encoding ADAMTS-13. In sporadic TTP, this deficiency may be the result of autoimmunity mediated by anti-ADAMTS-13 antibodies.

Platelet transfusions are contraindicated in TTP. Daily plasmapheresis with replacement of FFP is the mainstay of therapy. Before pathogenesis of TTP was understood, plasma transfusion was known to be beneficial; we now believe that this is because of the presence of normal vWF multimers in the transfused plasma. Before the advent of transfusion therapy

for TTP, death was the likely outcome. We know from early case series that the mortality rate exceeded 90%. It must therefore have been stunning news in the 1970s when 8 of a series of 14 patients survived when treated with exchange transfusion. In some of these cases, neurologic deficits remitted during the transfusion. It later became clear that the key element was the replacement of patient plasma with normal plasma—albumin replacement was ineffective, and simple transfusion of normal plasma was less effective. Plasmapheresis is not effective in secondary TTP.

When should plasmapheresis be initiated, and when can it be stopped? TTP must often be managed before the diagnosis is certain and often as soon as the diagnosis is considered. Generally, TTP is considered likely enough to treat when a patient presents with microangiopathic hemolytic anemia and thrombocytopenia which cannot be otherwise explained; ie, after exclusion of other causes of microangiopathic hemolytic anemia (eg, DIC, HELLP). The other 3 features of the classic pentad—neurologic changes, renal insufficiency, and fever—are helpful if present, but they are signs of the end-organ damage one wishes to avoid. So treatment is ideally instituted prior to these findings.

LD is markedly elevated in TTP, often in excess of 1,000 IU/dL. The LD level in DIC is not usually this high. Schistocyte number is often higher in TTP as well. Schistocytes exceeding 1% of red cells suggests TTP, but these may not emerge until 24 hours after clinical presentation, so serial smears should be observed if schistocytes are initially absent or low in number. In one study, schistocytes were found in 58% of normal adults, with a mean of 0.05% of all red cells, range of 0-0.27%. In patients with chronic renal failure, 93% had schistocytes, with a mean of 0.21% and a range of 0-0.6% of all red cells. In this same study, 100% of TTP patients had schistocytes, with mean of 5% and range of 1.1-9.4%. Coagulation parameters in TTP, including PT and PTT, are normal in contrast to DIC.

A test for ADAMTS-13 is often not readily available, nor can it exclude sporadic TTP. While severe ADAMTS-13 deficiency (<5% activity) is present in nearly all cases of familial TTP, it is present in only ~75% of patients with sporadic TTP. Patients with secondary TTP only rarely have ADAMTS-13 deficiency. Nonetheless, there is value in performing the test. It has been shown that the likelihood of relapse correlates with the magnitude of the ADAMTS-13 nadir. The presence of anti-ADAMTS-13 antibodies also is predictive of relapse. Furthermore, it appears that the level of ADAMTS-13 following recovery can predict relapse; lower levels being predictive of relapse. Patients with TTP and normal ADAMTS-13 still benefit from plasmapheresis, nearly as much as patients with ADAMTS-13-deficient TTP.

Hemolytic uremic syndrome (HUS)

HUS is another syndrome of microvascular platelet thrombi, with effects that are limited to the renal circulation. While there may be little etiologic commonality between HUS and TTP, they share the features of renal impairment and thrombotic microangiopathy, making distinction difficult. HUS usually occurs as a single episode that follows exposure to the Shiga toxin as a result of enteric infection with *S dysenteriae* or *E coli* O157:H7. A rare recurring form of HUS has been associated with deficiency in factor H (in the complement pathway). A deficiency in ADAMTS-13 has not been found in HUS. Neither plasma exchange nor any other specific therapy has been effective for HUS, other than supportive care and antimicrobials.

It can be difficult to distinguish HUS from TTP. Predominant renal impairment favors HUS, while the presence of neurologic impairment suggests TTP. The presence of antecedent diarrheal illness favors HUS. In unclear cases, it is best to treat as if the patient has TTP.

Thrombocytosis

While it is known that the risk of thrombotic events is increased by thrombocytosis, there is not a linear relationship. Moreover, patients with reactive thrombocytosis generally do not display a significantly increased risk of thrombosis (the exception being patients with significant underlying atherosclerotic vascular disease). In contrast, thrombocytosis that is caused by a myeloproliferative disorder is strongly associated with both thrombosis and hemorrhage. This association is not limited to essential thrombocythemia; in fact, polycythemia vera has possibly the highest rate of thrombosis.

Therapeutic agents & monitoring
Anticoagulants

Warfarin (Coumadin)

Warfarin inhibits posttranslational modification of the vitamin K-dependent coagulation factors: II, VII, IX, and X. Importantly, the anticoagulant factors C & S are also vitamin K-dependent and have shorter half lives than most of the vitamin K-dependent procoagulants. Therefore, initiation of warfarin therapy is associated with a brief but dangerous thrombophilic state that may manifest as the syndrome of warfarin skin necrosis. This temporary thrombophilia is more pronounced in patients who are congenitally deficient in factor C or S. Furthermore, warfarin anticoagulation is not immediate and may require a week or more for therapeutic effect. To prevent warfarin skin necrosis, and to provide immediate anticoagulation, treatment is usually initiated with concomitant heparin anticoagulation.

Initiation of warfarin therapy usually begins with 5 mg or 10 mg doses, concurrently given with heparin. Unfractionated heparin, administered intravenously in the inpatient setting, is the traditional form of heparinization, but in some instances outpatient initiation with low molecular weight heparin (LMWH) can be used. Heparin is continued for ~5 days or until the target international normalized ration (INR) is reached.

The response to warfarin differs from patient to patient and from time to time within individual patients, necessitating close serial INR monitoring. The anticoagulant effect of warfarin depends upon age, race, comorbidity, diet, concomitant medication use, and genetics. Cholestyramine and some antibiotics inhibit absorption, blunting warfarin effect. Many agents, including metronidazole, TMP-SMT, cimetidine, and omeprazole inhibit warfarin metabolism, thus enhancing its effect. Amiodarone directly potentiates (augments) the effect of warfarin. Other agents, by way of upregulation of the cytochrome p450 system, stimulate metabolism and thereby reduce the warfarin effect; these include barbiturates, carbamazepine (tegretol), rifampin, and alcohol. Dietary intake of vitamin K, found in green leafy vegetables, can alter the warfarin effect. Liver disease may affect the anticoagulant effect of warfarin in unpredictable ways. Comorbidities that affect warfarin anticoagulation include heart failure, abnormal thyroid function, and malignancy.

The 2 genes with greatest impact upon warfarin are *VKORC1* and *CYP2C9*. *VKORC1* encodes vitamin K epoxide reductase (VKOR) that is the principal target of warfarin. *CYP2C9* encodes 2C9, a p450 enzyme that is principally responsible for warfarin metabolism. There has been much debate regarding the necessity of testing for polymorphisms at these loci, with one large prospective European study recently demonstrating that *CYP2C9* and *VKORC1* can reliably predict optimal dosing. There are 2 common alleles for *CYP2C9*— CYP2C9*2 and CYP2C9*3—both of which encode a hypofunctional 2C9 enzyme and enhanced warfarin sensitivity. At the *VKORC1* locus, a common variant in the promoter sequence, c.-1639G>A, results in diminished gene expression and enhanced warfarin sensitivity. Other *VKORC1* variants result in warfarin resistance.

The prothrombin time (PT) test with INR modification is the most common method for monitoring warfarin therapy (see p 302). The PT responds to reduction of 3 of the 4 vitamin K-dependent factors (II, VII, X). Note that during the first few days of warfarin therapy, the prolongation of the PT reflects mainly a reduction of factor VII and only later also reflects a reduction of factors X and II. A particular target INR, often of 2.0-3.0, has been determined for most indications.

Warfarin reversal may be needed for patients with supratherapeutic INR and bleeding t5.16. The most conservative approach, often applied to patients with INR <9.0 who do not have significant bleeding, is to omit 1 or several doses and resume therapy at a lower dose when the INR is in the therapeutic range. In some patients this is supplemented with oral vitamin K, particularly if the patient is at increased risk for bleeding. For patients with very high INR (>20) or with serious bleeding, discontinue warfarin therapy and administer vitamin K by slow IV infusion, supplemented with fresh plasma or prothrombin complex concentrate, depending on the urgency of the situation.

For planned invasive procedures, warfarin may be discontinued 4 days before surgery and replaced with heparin. Heparin can be discontinued hours before surgery. This is commonly referred to as "bridge" therapy. As with initiation of warfarin therapy, bridge therapy may involve either unfractionated heparin or LMWH.

t5.16 Warfarin reversal (American College of Chest Physician guidelines)

Clinical situation	Guidelines
INR elevated but <5 No significant bleeding	Lower the dose or omit the next dose Resume warfarin at a lower dose when INR therapeutic
INR 5-9 No significant bleeding	Hold warfarin Monitor INR Resume warfarin at a lower dose when INR is therapeutic
Increased risk for bleeding or Minor bleeding evident	Hold warfarin Give vitamin K 1-2.5 mg orally Monitor INR & resume at lower dose
Rapid reversal for surgery	Hold warfarin Give vitamin K 2.5-5 mg orally (expect reduced INR in 24 hours) If INR still high at 24 hours, additional vitamin K 1-2.5 mg orally can be given
INR >9 No significant bleeding	Hold warfarin Give vitamin K 2.5-5 mg orally (expect reduced INR in 24-48 hours) Monitor INR more often & give additional vitamin K if necessary Resume therapy at a lower dose when the INR is within therapeutic range
Serious bleeding at any INR elevation or INR >20	Hold warfarin Give vitamin K 10 mg slow IV infusion (can be repeated every 12 hours) Supplement with fresh frozen plasma (1-2 units) if needed, up to 20 mL/kg (FFP can be repeated every 6-12 hours) Consider factor supplementation (prothrombin complex concentrate, factor VIIa) for life threatening bleed
Elective surgery	Management depends upon the risk of bleeding & risk of thromboembolism (see t5.18, t519) Low risk of bleeding/any risk of thromboembolism: Warfarin should be continued as usual, assuming that the patient is within the desired therapeutic range High & intermediate risk of bleeding/low risk of thromboembolism: bridge therapy is not routinely recommended. Warfarin should be held beginning 4-5 days preoperatively. INR is tested 1 day before surgery. If still >1.5, then a low dose of vitamin K should be given (1-2 mg, orally). Alternatively, warfarin can be discontinued 2 days preoperatively, with administration of vitamin K (2.5 mg, orally) 2 days preoperatively, with the expectation that the patient will be sub-therapeutic for only 1-2 days. The maintenance dose of warfarin is resumed postoperatively and supplemented with low dose heparin (5000 U) or LMWH administered subcutaneously every 12 hours, if necessary. Warfarin should be restarted 12-24 hours after surgery (evening after surgery or next morning), assuming there is no evidence of ongoing bleeding. High & intermediate risk of bleeding/moderate risk of thromboembolism: bridge therapy is recommended (see t5.17; options include therapeutic-dose subcutaneous LMWH, therapeutic-dose intravenous UFH, or low dose subcutaneous LMWH; therapeutic-dose subcutaneous LMWH is recommended High & intermediate risk of bleeding/high risk of thromboembolism: bridge therapy is recommended. Options include therapeutic-dose subcutaneous LMWH or therapeutic-dose intravenous UFH; LMWH is recommended over UFH In patients given therapeutic-dose subcutaneous LMWH as bridging therapy, it is recommended that the last dose be given 24 hours prior to surgery In patients given intravenous UFH as bridging therapy, it is recommended that the infusion be stopped ~4 hours prior to surgery
Urgent surgery	For surgery that can be delayed by 24 hours, vitamin K 2.5-5.0 mg (orally) is recommended For immediate surgery, either plasma or prothrombin concentrate in addition to low dose oral vitamin K

t5.17 Suggested bridge therapy protocol

7 days preoperative	Stop any aspirin therapy Check INR
4-5 days preoperative	Stop warfarin
2-3 days preoperative	Start heparin/LMWH
1 day preoperative	Give last dose of heparin/LMWH 12-24 hours before procedure Check INR; if 1.5 or higher, give vitamin K (1 mg, orally)
Day of surgery or 1 day postoperative & when hemostasis achieved	Resume warfarin in evening Restart heparin/LMWH therapeutic dosage or prophylactic dosage (procedures with high risk of bleeding)
1 day postoperative	Continue regular warfarin dosage Continue heparin/LMWH
2-10 days postoperative	Check INR Stop heparin/LMWH when INR is 2.0 or higher

t5.18 Risk stratification for thromboembolism

Low risk	Atrial fibrillation without major risk factors (age >65 years, diabetes mellitus, coronary artery disease, or hypertension) for stroke (CHADS score 0-2) Single VTE >12 months earlier & no high risk features (active malignancy, multiple episodes of VTE, known thrombophilic state) Bileaflet aortic valve without atrial fibrillation & no other risk factors for stroke (prior stroke, prior TIA, hypertension, diabetes, CHF, age >75 years)
Moderate risk	Atrial fibrillation with CHADS score 3-4 VTE within past 3-12 months & a "nonsevere" thrombophilia (factor V Leiden heterozygote, prothrombin mutation heterozygote) Bileaflet aortic valve with atrial fibrillation, prior stroke, prior TIA, hypertension, diabetes, CHF, or age >75 years
High risk	Atrial fibrillation with history of stroke, history of TIA, rheumatic heart disease, or CHADS score 5-6 VTE within 3 months or with "severe" thrombophilia (protein C deficiency, protein S deficiency, AT deficiency, APL syndrome, or combined abnormalities) VTE >3 months earlier with high risk features (active malignancy, multiple episodes of VTE, known thrombophilic state) Any mitral valve prosthesis, older (first-generation) ball/cage or tilting disc aortic valves, or valve with recent (within 6 mo) stroke or TIA

t5.19 Risk stratification for bleeding

Low risk	Arthrocentesis, most dental procedures, ophthalmic procedures (cataract, trabeculectomy, vitreoretinal), dermatologic procedures, most upper & lower gastrointestinal endoscopy with or without biopsy
Moderate risk	Most orthopedic surgery, most laparotomies, axillary node dissection, dilatation & curettage, hydrocele repair, pacemaker insertion, internal cardiac defibrillator insertion, endarterectomy, noncataract eye surgery (complex lid, lacrimal, orbital), extensive dental surgery (multiple tooth extractions), hemorrhoidectomy, angiography, PTCA, some GI endoscopy (upper endoscopy with sphincterotomy, lower endoscopy with polypectomy especially if >2 cm or sessile), bronchoscopy, small biopsies (prostate, bladder, thyroid, breast, lymph node, pancreas)
High risk	Cardiac surgery (bypass, valve), AAA repair, peripheral arterial bypass, neurosurgery, most oncologic surgery, major orthopedic surgery (hip or knee replacement), prostate surgery (including TURP), renal biopsy, reconstructive plastic surgery

Unfractionated heparin (UH)

UH is a heterogeneous mixture of mucopolysaccharides, ranging widely in size, that is derived from mast cell rich mammalian sources such as pig intestine. Heparin binds to AT, enhancing several-fold the capacity of AT to inactivate thrombin and factor Xa, in addition to factors IXa, XIa, and XIIa. To a similar extent, heparin activates heparin cofactor II (HCII), also an inhibitor of thrombin.

Heparin is not absorbed orally and must be administered parenterally. Usually an intravenous bolus is followed by a continuous intravenous infusion. Within the blood stream, heparin binds to a number of plasma proteins and cell surfaces, reducing in a somewhat unpredictable manner its bioavailability and its anticoagulant activity. Heparin is cleared by the kidneys.

Heparin therapy has an anticoagulant effect that is difficult to predict, and monitoring is required. The aPTT is the preferred test to monitor heparin therapy, but the anti-Xa assay may also be used. Because of varying sensitivities to heparin, in-house aPTT assays should be calibrated according to a standard anti-Xa curve. Generally, a therapeutic range of 1.5-2.5× control for aPTT compares with a range of 0.3-0.7 IU/mL for anti-Xa.

Heparin resistance refers to the requirement of unusually high doses of heparin (>35,000 U/day) to achieve therapeutic aPTT prolongation. The most common cause for this is AT deficiency, but additional considerations are high factor VIII or fibrinogen levels. One should measure anti-Xa activity in these patients. In the case of AT deficiency, resistance reflected in the aPTT truly reflects an in vivo failure of anticoagulation, and the anti-Xa will be correspondingly sub-therapeutic. In the other instances, high factor VIII and fibrinogen may shorten the in vitro aPTT and mask appropriate in vivo anticoagulation. In these instances, therefore, one should consider using the anti-Xa assay for monitoring.

Heparin reversal is generally straightforward. If time permits, simply discontinuing heparin generally results in normalization of the aPTT within 30 minutes to 1 hour. In more urgent situations, intravenous protamine sulfate is administered. Adverse reactions include hypotension, bradycardia, and anaphylaxis.

Adverse reactions with heparin, in addition to the enhanced risk of bleeding, include HIT (see p 319), elevated liver function tests, and osteoporosis with long term use.

Low molecular weight heparin (LMWH)

LMWH is prepared from UH through chemical processing. The advantage of LMWH is reduced need for close monitoring. Its smaller size reduces the nonspecific binding to serum proteins and cells, resulting in a predictable high recovery and bioavailability. Like UH, LMWH interacts with AT to inactivate both Xa and thrombin. Like UH, parenteral administration is required, and LMWH is usually given subcutaneously. By this route, it has a longer half life than intravenous UH, ~4-8 hours.

The LMWH agents include enoxaparin, dalteparin, nadroparin, tinzaparin, and danaparoid. Danaparoid is considered a "heparinoid," because it is a mixture of glycosaminoglycans, including heparan sulfate, dermatan sulfate, and chondroitin sulfate; ie, it contains no actual heparin. Nonetheless, it is similar to the other LMWH in its mechanism of action and clinical utility.

There is debate regarding the need for LMWH monitoring. It is certainly not required in all patients. Some advise monitoring in severely obese patients, pregnant patients, and patients with renal failure. In such instances, the anti-factor Xa assay is used. Blood should be drawn 4 hours after injection.

Protamine sulfate does not neutralize LMWH as effectively as UH. Furthermore, because of the prolonged absorption of LMWH into the blood from subcutaneous sites, a second or third dose of protamine is often required.

The frequency of HIT is lower with LMWHs than with UH. The risk of osteoporosis is likewise reduced.

Fondaparinux (Arixtra)

Fondaparinux, sometimes called a direct Xa inhibitor, is a synthetic analogue of heparin designed to be richly endowed with the AT binding pentasaccharide moiety that was discovered to be the operant component of UH. It binds AT and promotes inactivation of Xa, but its small size is incapable of enhancing AT in its inactivation of thrombin. Fondaparinux is monitored using an anti-Xa assay. Unlike UH and LMWH, fondaparinux cannot be reversed with protamine. The half life is between 17 and 21 hours. It can be administered subcutaneously or intravenously. Fondaparinux does not crossreact with HIT antibodies and does not cause HIT.

Direct thrombin inhibitors (DTI)

Direct thrombin inhibitors (DTI) inhibit thrombin without an intermediary, such as AT. The first-discovered DTI, hirudin, was isolated from the salivary glands of the leech H medicinalis. Recombinant forms of hirudin were developed and marketed as lepirudin (United States) and desirudin (Europe). Currently, the DTIs include lepirudin, desirudin, bivalirudin, argatroban, ximelagatran, and melagatran. Antibodies develop in a significant minority of patients exposed to hirudin and its recombinant analogs; while these do not cause clinical problems per se, they may prolong the half life of the drug. In addition, anaphylaxis can occur if patients with antibodies are re-exposed.

Renally cleared DTIs include hirudin, lepirudin, and desirudin. In patients with renal insufficiency, reduced dose and/or monitoring is advised. Argatroban is a hepatically metabolized DTI and the agent of choice in patients with severe renal insufficiency. The aPTT is used for monitoring, when required, for all DTIs. The dose-response curve is nonlinear. A more linear response can be demonstrated with the ecarin clotting time, but this test is neither widely available nor standardized. Bivalirudin is metabolized largely by peptidases and is only partially reliant on renal clearance. Bivalirudin has a half life of 25 minutes, the shortest of all the DTIs. When given in high doses, such as in the cardiac catheterization laboratory, bivalirudin is monitored with the activated clotting time (ACT). In lower doses, it can be monitored with the aPTT. All of the DTIs prolong the PT/INR, but the effect is variable.

Argatroban is widely used for prevention of thrombosis in patients with HIT. Often, because the thrombotic risk in HIT may persist for months, patients must be transitioned to warfarin. This is complicated by the tendency of DTIs to prolong the PT/INR. 2 options have been proposed in this setting. First, a chromogenic Xa assay is recommended to monitor warfarinization. Second, it has been found that a conversion factor can be used—with an INR of 4.0 in patients on combined argatroban/warfarin corresponding to an INR of 2.0 for patients solely on warfarin.

New oral anticoagulants

For many years, warfarin was the only available oral anticoagulant. When an alternative was required, as in pregnant women, only subcutaneous LMWH was available. Recently, several new oral anticoagulants have been introduced which work predominantly as inhibitors of Xa or thrombin.

Apixaban and rivaroxaban are direct Xa inhibitors which can be taken orally. They achieve peak plasma concentration within 3-4 hours and have a half life of ~12 hours. Dabigatran is a direct thrombin inhibitor. Peak concentrations are achieved in 1-2 hours, with a half life of 18 hours. All of these agents prolong the PTT, but the optimal monitoring modality has not been established.

Antiplatelet agents

Aspirin

Aspirin (acetylsalicylic acid), once a quaint analgesic, has emerged as a major pharmacologic agent in the secondary prevention of cardiovascular events. The effectiveness of aspirin in prevention of cardiovascular events has been well documented in numerous trials, and in a recent meta-analysis, a 22% reduction in death and serious vascular events was attributed to aspirin.

At usual doses (75-325 mg/day) aspirin exerts antiplatelet effects through the selective irreversible inhibition of platelet cyclooxygenase (COX-1), which is operant in the cascade that produces thromboxane A2 (TXA2). TXA2 causes platelet activation and local vasoconstriction. Decreased TXA2 leads to reduced platelet aggregation in vivo and in vitro. Note that at high doses (>1,000 mg/day), aspirin begins to inhibit endothelial cyclooxygenase (COX-2), reducing the production of prostacyclin. Prostacyclin is itself an inhibitor of platelet aggregation and a potent vasodilator. Thus, such high doses of aspirin would be expected to have reduced efficacy in clot prevention.

In some patients, aspirin does not exert antiplatelet effects, a condition called aspirin resistance. Aspirin resistance should be distinguished from aspirin intolerance. Aspirin intolerance (aspirin allergy) is a condition that is usually found in patients with a history of atopic disorders and nasal polyps, in whom aspirin may induce bronchospasm. Aspirin resistance is estimated to affect 25% of adults. It may be tested by platelet aggregation in response to the agonist arachidonic acid or with the VerifyNow aspirin assay, but a standard definition for aspirin resistance does not exist. In clinical practice, such assays are most often used to verify that the effect of aspirin has abated prior to an elective procedure.

Thienopyridines

Ticlopidine (Ticlid) and clopidogrel (Plavix) exert their effect through blockade of the P2Y12 receptor that mediates ADP induced platelet activation. Both ticlopidine and clopidogrel are prodrugs that must be metabolically activated by hepatic cytochrome P450 enzymes; thus, their onset is delayed. For this reason, aspirin is preferred in the setting of acute myocardial infarction.

While bleeding is the major side effect, Ticlid has been associated with cytopenias and thrombotic thrombocytopenic purpura. The hematologic complications usually occur within the first few months of treatment.

As with aspirin, some patients are resistant to thienopyridines. Resistance appears to be largely related to polymorphisms in cytochrome P450 enzymes. Both platelet aggregometry and the VerifyNow P2Y12 assay can assess the extent of platelet inhibition. As with aspirin, these assays can also be used to detect reversal of inhibition prior to elective surgery. The PFA-100 assay is insensitive to the P2Y12 antagonists.

Dipyridamole

Dipyridamole is a platelet inhibitor that, through the downstream effects of phosphodiesterase inhibition, reduces intracellular calcium concentrations. In combination, dipyridamole and low dose aspirin are marketed as Aggrenox. It is used occasionally in secondary stroke prevention.

GPIIb/IIIa receptor antagonists

Inhibitors of the platelet glycoprotein GPIIb/IIIa include abciximab (ReoPro), eptifibatide (Integrilin), and tirofiban (Aggrastat). The GPIIb/IIIa receptor binds fibrinogen and vWF on the surfaces of activated platelets. Thus, these agents induce an acquired Glanzmann thrombasthenia-like state, in which platelet aggregation studies demonstrate impaired aggregation to all agonists except ristocetin. GPIIb/IIIa antagonists are used most often in acute coronary syndrome (ACS). While these agents have a shared mechanism of action, they are structurally distinct. As the name abciximab would imply, it is a humanized murine monoclonal antibody directed against the GPIIb/IIIa receptor. Eptifibatide and tirofiban a small synthetic polypeptides. All of the GPIIb/IIIa antagonists are administered parenterally, with an intravenous bolus followed by continuous infusion. In addition to bleeding, thrombocytopenia may result from the GPIIb/IIIa inhibitors.

References

Adcock DM, Fink L, Marlar RA [1997] A laboratory approach to the evaluation of hereditary hypercoagulability. *Am J Clin Pathol* 108:434-449. PMID:9322598.

Adcock DM [2002] Factor VIII inhibitors in patients with hemophilia A. *Clin Hemostasis Rev* 16:1.

Ananyeva NM, Lacroix-Desmazes S, Hauser CAE, Shima M, Ovanesov MV, Khrenov AV, Saenko EL [2004] Inhibitors in hemophilia A: mechanisms of inhibition, management and perspectives. *Blood Coagul Fibrinolysis* 15(2):109-124. PMID:15090997.

Andrew M, Paes B, Milner R, Johnston M, Mitchell L, Tollefsen DM, Powers P [1987] development of the human coagulation system in the full-term infant. *Blood* 70:165-172. PMID:3593964.

Ansell J, Hirsh J, Hylek E, et al [2008] Pharmacology and management of the vitamin K antagonists: American College of Chest Physicians evidence-based clinical practice guidelines (8th edition). *Chest* 133:160S-198S PMID:18574265.

Antithrombotic Trialists' Collaboration [2002] Collaborative meta-analysis of randomised trials of antiplatelet therapy for prevention of death, myocardial infarction, and stroke in high risk patients. *BMJ* 324:71-86. PMID:18574265.

Ariëns RAS, Lai TS, Weisel JW, Greenberg CS, Grant PJ [2002] Role of factor XIII in fibrin clot formation and effects of genetic polymorphisms. *Blood* 100:743-754. PMID:12130481.

Baron JM,Baron BW [2005] Thrombotic thrombocytopenic purpura and its look-alikes. Clinical advances in hematology & oncology. 3(11):868-874. PMID:16491632.

Bayston TA and Lane DA [1997] Antithrombin: molecular basis of deficiency. *Thromb Haemost* 78(1):339-343. PMID:9198176.

Behrens WE [1975] Mediterranean macrothrombocytopenia. *Blood* 46:199-208. PMID:1095094.

Bernard GR, Margolis BD, Shanies HM, et al [2004] Extended evaluation of recombinant human activated protein C United States Trial (ENHANCE US): a single-arm, phase 3B, multicenter study of drotrecogin alfa (activated) in severe sepsis. *Chest* 125:2206-2216. PMID:15189943.

Bernard GR, Vincent JL, Laterre PF [2001] Efficacy and safety of recombinant human activated protein C for severe sepsis. *N Engl J Med* 344:699-709. PMID:11236773.

Blackall DP, Uhl L, Spitalnik SL [2001] Cryoprecipitate-reduced plasma: rationale for use and efficacy in the treatment of thrombotic thrombocytopenic purpura. *Transfusion* 41:840-844. PMID:11399830.

Bukowski RM, Hewlett JS, Harris JW, et al [1976] Exchange transfusions in the treatment of thrombotic thrombocytopenic purpura. *Semin Hematol* 13:219-232. PMID:779037.

Burns ER, Lou Y, Pathak A [2004] Morphologic diagnosis of thrombotic thrombocytopenic purpura. *Am J Hematol* 75:18-21. PMID:14695628.

Casonato A, Pontara E, Sartorello F, Cattini MG, Gallinaro L, Bertomoro A, Rosato A, Padrini R, Pagnan A [2006] Identifying type Vicenza vWD. *J Lab Clin Med* 147:96-102. PMID:16459168.

Catto AJ, Kohler HP, Coore J, et al [1999] Association of a common polymorphism in the factor XIII gene with venous thrombosis. *Blood* 93(3):906-908. PMID:9920839.

Cervera R, Piette JC, Font J, et al [2002] Antiphospholipid syndrome: clinical and immunologic manifestations and patterns of disease expression in a cohort of 1,000 patients. *Arthritis Rheum* 46(4):1019-1027. PMID:11953980.

Chang S, Tillema V, Scherr D [2002] A percentage correction formula for evaluation of mixing studies. *Am J Clin Pathol* 117:62-73. PMID:11789732.

Cines DB, Blanchette VS [2002] Immune thrombocytopenic purpura. *New Engl J Med* 346:995-1008. PMID:11919310.

Cuker A, Connors JM, Levy BD, Loscalzo J [2009] Clinical problem solving: a bloody mystery. *New Engl J Med* 361:1887-1894. PMID:19890132.

Cunningham MT, Brandt JT, Laposata M, Olson JD [2002] Laboratory diagnosis of dysfibrinogenemia. *Arch Pathol Lab Med* 126(4):499-505. PMID:11900586.

Danilenko-Dixon DR, Van Winter JT, Homburger HA [1996] Clinical implications of antiphospholipid antibodies in obstetrics. *Mayo Clin Proc* 71:1118-1120. PMID:8917300.

De Moerloose P, Reber G, Perrier A, Perneger T, Bounameaux H [2000] Prevalence of factor V Leiden and prothrombin G20210A mutations in unselected patients with venous thromboembolism. *Br J Haematol* 110(1):125-129. PMID:10930988.

De Stefano V, Martinelli I, Mannucci PM, Paciaroni K, Chiusolo P, Casorelli I, Rossi E, Leone G [2000] The risk of recurrent deep venous thrombosis among heterozygous carriers of both factor V Leiden and the G20210A prothrombin mutation. *N Engl J Med* 342(3):214-215. PMID:10477778.

Delanghe JR, Langlois MR, De Buyzere ML, Torck MA [2007] Vitamin C deficiency and scurvy are not only a dietary problem but are codetermined by the haptoglobin polymorphism. *Clin Chem* 53(8):1397-1400. PMID:17644791.

DeRossi SS and Glick MG [1996] Bleeding time: an unreliable predictor of clinical hemostasis. *J Oral Maxillofac Surg* 54(9):1119-20. PMID:8811825.

Dhainaut JF, Shorr AF, Macias WL, et al [2005] Dynamic evolution of coagulopathy in the first day of severe sepsis: relationship with mortality and organ failure. *Crit Care Med* 33:341-348. PMID:15699837.

Douketis JD, Berger PB, Dunn, AS, et al [2008] The perioperative management of antithrombotic therapy: American College of Chest Physicians evidence-based clinical practice guidelines (8th edition). *Chest* 133:299-339S PMID:18574269.

Douketis JD, Johnson JA, Turpie AG [2004] Low-molecular-weight heparin as bridging anticoagulation during interruption of warfarin: assessment of a standardized periprocedural anticoagulation regimen. *Arch Intern Med* 164:1319-26. PMID:15226166.

Drachman JG [2004] Inherited thrombocytopenia: when a low platelet count does not mean ITP. *Blood* 103:390-398. PMID:14504084.

Dumenco LL, Blair AJ, Sweeney JD [1998] The results of diagnostic studies for thrombophilia in a large group of patients with a personal or family history of thrombosis. *Am J Clin Pathol* 110:673-682. PMID:9802354.

Elliot MA, Tefferi A [2004] Thrombosis and haemorrhage in polycythemia vera and essential thrombocythaemia. *Brit J Haematol* 128:275-290. PMID:15667529.

Emilia G, Longo G, Luppi M, Gandini G, Morselli M, Ferrara L, Amarri S, Cagossi K, Torelli G [2001] *Helicobacter pylori* eradication can induce platelet recovery in idiopathic thrombocytopenic purpura. *Blood* 97:812-814. PMID:11157503.

Eriksson BI, Quinlan DJ, Weitz JI [2009] Comparative pharmacodynamics and pharmacokinetics of oral direct thrombin and factor xa inhibitors in development. *Clin Pharmacokinet* 48(1):1-22. PMID:19071881.

Fabris F, Ahmad S, Cella G, Jeske WP, Walenga JM, Fareed J [2000] Pathophysiology of HIT. *Arch Pathol Lab Med* 124:1657-1666. PMID:11079020.

Franchini M, Lippi G [2008] Acquired factor VIII inhibitors. *Blood* 112:250-255. PMID:18463353.

Franchini M, Manzato F [2004] Update on the treatment of disseminated intravascular coagulation. *Hematology* 9(2): 81-85. PMID:15203862.

Francis CW [2002] Plasminogen activator inhibitor-1 levels and polymorphisms. *Arch Pathol Lab Med* 126: 1401-1404. PMID:12421149.

Frost SD, Brotman DJ, Michota FA [2003] Rational use of D-dimer measurement to exclude acute venous thromboembolic disease. *Mayo Clin Proc* 78:1385-1391. PMID:14601697.

Furlan M, Robles R, Galbusera M, Remuzzi G, Kyrle PA, Brenner B, Krause M, Scharrer I, Aumann V, Mittler U, Solenthaler M, Lämmle B [1998] vWF-cleaving protease in thrombotic thrombocytopenic purpura and the hemolytic-uremic syndrome. *New Engl J Med* 339:1578-1584. PMID:9828245.

Garay SM, Gardella JE, Fazzini EP, Goldring RM [1979] Hermansky-Pudlak syndrome: pulmonary manifestations of a ceroid storage disorder. *Am J Med* 66:737-747. PMID:443250.

Garcia D, Libby E, Crowther MA [2010] The new oral anticoagulants. *Blood* 115(1):15-20. PMID:19880491.

Geiger J, Teichmann L, Grossmann R, et al [2005] Monitoring of clopidogrel action: comparison of methods. *Clin Chem* 51(6):957-965. PMID:15817818.

Gewirtz AS, Miller ML, Keys TF [1996] The clinical usefulness of the preoperative bleeding time. *Arch Pathol Lab Med* 120(4):353-356. PMID:8619746.

Gill JC, Endres-Brooks J, Bauer PJ, Marks WJ Jr, Montgomery RR [1987] The effect of ABO blood group on the diagnosis of vWD. *Blood* 69(6):1691-1695. PMID:3495304.

Gladding P, Webster M, Ormiston J, et al [2008] Antiplatelet drug nonresponsiveness. *Am Heart J* 155:591-599. PMID:18371464.

Griffin JH, Evatt B, Wideman C, Fernandez JA [1993] Anticoagulant protein C pathway defective in the majority of thrombophilic patients. *Blood* 82:1989-1994. PMID:8400251.

Grunewald M, Grunewald A, Schmid A, Schopflin C, Schauer S, Griesshammer M, Koksch M [2004] The platelet function defect of paroxysmal nocturnal haemoglobinuria. *Platelets* 15(3):145-154. PMID:15203716.

Hanley JP [2004] Warfarin reversal. *J Clin Pathol* 57:1132-1139. PMID:15509671.

Hassell K [2005] The management of patients with HIT who require anticoagulant therapy. *Chest* 127(2):1S-8S PMID:15706025.

Heath KE, Campos-Barros A, Toren A, Rozenfeld-Granot G, Carlsson LE, Savige J, Denison JC, Gregory MC, White JG, Barker DF, Greinacher A, Epstein CJ, Glucksman MJ, Martignetti JA [2001] Nonmuscle myosin heavy chain IIA mutations define a spectrum of autosomal dominant macrothrombocytopenias: May-Hegglin anomaly and Fechtner, Sebastian, Epstein, and Alport-like syndromes. *Am J Hum Genet* 69:1033-1045. PMID : 11590545.

Heim SW, Schectman JM, Siadaty MS, Philbrick JT [2004] D-dimer testing for deep venous thrombosis: a metaanalysis. *Clin Chem* 50(7):1136-1147. PMID:15142977.

Hirsh J, Bauer KA, Donati MB, et al [2008] Parenteral anticoagulants: American College of Chest Physicians evidence-based clinical practice guidelines (8th edition). *Chest* 133:141S-l59S PMID:18574264.

Hirsh J, Dalen JE, Aiuleison DR, Foller U, Btissei H, Anftell J, Deykin D [2001] Oral anticoagulants: mechanism of action, clinical effectiveness, and optimal therapeutic range. *Chest* 119:8S-21S PMID:11157640.

Hirsh J, Fuster V, Ansell J, Halperin JL [2003] American Heart Association/American College of Cardiology Foundation guide to warfarin therapy. *Circulation* 107:1692-1711. PMID:12668507.

Hohlfeld P, Forestier F, Kaplan C, Tissot JD, Daffos F [1994] Fetal thrombocytopenia: a retrospective survey of 5,194 fetal blood samplings. *Blood* 84(6): 1851-1856. PMID:8080991.

Hosler GA, Cusumano AM, Hutchins GM [2003] Thrombotic thrombocytopenic purpura and HUS are distinct pathologic entities. *Arch Pathol Lab Med* 127:834-839. PMID:12823037.

Hovens M, Snoep J, Eikenboom J, et al [2007] Prevalence of persistent platelet reactivity despite use of aspirin: a systematic review. *Am Heart J* 153:175-181. PMID:17239674.

Hoyer LW [1994] Hemophilia A. *N Engl J Med* 330(1):38-47. PMID:8259143.

Iacoviello L, Di Castelnuovo A, de Knijff P, et al [1998] Polymorphisms in the coagulation factor VII gene and the risk of myocardial infarction. *N Engl J Med* 338(2):79-85. PMID:9420338.

Ivandic BT, Giannitsis E, Schlick P, et al [2007] Determination of aspirin responsiveness by use of whole blood platelet aggregometry. *Clin Chem* 53(4):614-619. PMID:17332149.

Jafri SM [2004] Periprocedural thromboprophylaxis in patients receiving chronic anticoagulation therapy. *Am Heart J* 147:3-15. PMID:14691412.

Jensen R [2001] The antiphospholipid antibody syndrome. *Clin Hemostasis Rev* 15.

Jorquera JI, Montoro JM, Fernandez MA [1994] Modified test for activated protein C resistance. *Lancet* 344:1162-1163. PMID:7864945.

Kane WH, Davie EW [1988] Blood coagulation factors V and VIII: structural and functional similarities and their relationship to hemorrhagic and thrombotic disorders. *Blood* 71(3):539-555. PMID:3125864.

Kankirawatana S, Berkow RL, Marques MB [2006] A neonate with bleeding and multiple factor deficiencies. *Lab Med* 37(2):95-97.

Kapiotis S, Quehenberger P, Jilma B, Handler S, Pabinger-Fasching I, Mannhalter C, Speiser W [1996] Improved characteristics of APC-resistance assay: coatest APC resistance by predilution of samples with factor V deficient plasma. *Am J Clin Pathol* 106(5):588-593. PMID:8929467.

Karpatkin S [2004] Autoimmune thrombocytopenias. *Autoimmunity* 34(4):363-368. PMID:15518060.

Kelley MJ, Jawien W, Ortel TL, Korczak JF [2000] Mutation of MYH9, encoding non-muscle myosin heavy chain A, in May-Hegglin anomaly. *Nature Genet* 26:106-108. PMID:10973260.

Kelton JG, Warkentin TE [2008] HIT: a historical perspective. *Blood* 112(7):2607-2615. PMID:18809774.

Kelton JG, Warkentin TE [1995] Diagnosis of HIT. *Am J Clin Pathol* 104:611-613. PMID:8526201.

Kempton CL, White GC [2009] How we treat a hemophilia A patient with a factor VIII inhibitor. *Blood* 113:11-17. PMID:18820129.

Key NS, McGlennen RC [2002] Hyperhomocysteinemia and thrombophilia. *Arch Pathol Lab Med* 126:1367-1374. PMID:12421143.

Kitchens CS, Alving BM, Kessler CM, Eds. [2002a] *Consultative Hemostasis and Thrombosis,* Philadelphia: WB Saunders Company.

Kitchens CS [2002b] The contact system. *Arch Pathol Lab Med* 126:1382-1386. PMID:12421145.

Kjeldsberg CR, Perkins SL [2010] *Practical Diagnosis of Hematologic Disorders*, 5th ed. Chicago, ASCP Press, Vol 1. ISBN:978-089189-5718.

Kohda K, Kuga T, Kogawa K, Kanisawa Y, Koike K, Kuroiwa G, Hirayama Y, Sato Y, Matsunaga T, Niitsu Y [2002] Effect of *Helicobacter pylori* eradication on platelet recovery in Japanese patients with chronic idiopathic thrombocytopenic purpura and secondary autoimmune thrombocytopenic purpura. *Br J Haematol* 118:584 PMID:12139750.

Kojouri K, Vesely SK, Terrell DR, George JN [2004] Splenectomy for adult patients with idiopathic thrombocytopenic purpura: a systematic review to assess long term platelet count responses, prediction of response, and surgical complications. *Blood* 104:2623-2634. PMID:15217831.

Kottke-Marchant KK, Duncan A [2002a] Antithrombin deficiency: issues in laboratory diagnosis. *Arch Pathol Lab Med* 126:1326-1336. PMID:12421140.

Kottke-Marchant KK, Corcoran G [2002b] The laboratory diagnosis of platelet disorders: an algorithmic approach. *Arch Pathol Lab Med* 126:133-146. PMID:11825107.

Laposata M, Green D, Van Cott EM, et al [1998] College of American Pathologists conference XXXI on laboratory monitoring of anticoagulant therapy: the clinical use and laboratory monitoring of low-molecular weight heparin, danaparoid, hirudin and related compounds, and argatroban. *Arch Pathol Lab Med* 122(9):799-807. PMID:9740137.

Laposata M, Van Cott EM, Lev M [2007] Case records of the Massachussetts General Hospital: a 40 year old woman with epistaxis, hematemesis, and altered mental status. *New Engl J Med* 356(2):174-182. PMID:17215536.

Lederer DJ, Kawut SM, Sonett JR, Vakiani E, Seward SL Jr, White JG, Wilt JS, Marboe CC, Gahl WA, Arcasoy SM [2005] Successful bilateral lung transplantation for pulmonary fibrosis associated with the Hermansky-Pudlak syndrome. *J Heart Lung Transplant* 24:1697-1699. PMID:16210104.

LeGal G, Righini M, Roy P, Sanchez O, Aujesky D, Bounameaux H Perrier A [2006] Prediction of pulmonary embolism in the emergency department: the revised Geneva score. *Ann Int Med* 144:165-171. PMID:16461960.

Lehman CM, Blaylock RC, Alexander DP, Rodgers GM [2001] Discontinuation of the bleeding time test without detectable adverse clinical impact. *Clin Chem* 47:1204-1211. PMID:11427450.

Leung A, Huang CK, Muto R, et al [2007] CYP2C9 and VKORC1 genetic polymorphism analysis might be necessary in patients with factor V Leiden and prothrombin gene G2021A mutation(s). *Diagn Mol Pathol* 16:184-186. PMID:17721328.

Levi M, TenCate H [2002] Disseminated intravascular coagulation. *New Engl J Med* 341:586-592. PMID:10451465.

Levi M [2007] Disseminated intravascular coagulation. *Crit Care Med* 35(9):2191-2195. PMID:17855836

Levine JS, Branch DW, Rauch J [2002] The antiphospholipid syndrome. *New Engl J Med* 346:752-763. PMID:11882732.

Lind SE [1991] The bleeding time does not predict surgical bleeding. *Blood* 77:2547-2552. PMID:2043759.

Ma J, Hennekens CH, Ridker PM, et al [1999] A prospective study of fibrinogen and risk of myocardial infarction in the physician's health survey. *J Am Coll Cardiol* 33(5):1347-1352. PMID:10193737.

Macy PA [2003] Identification and clinical significance of platelet antibodies. *Clin Hemostasis Rev* 17:5.

Mannucci PM, Duga S, Peyvandi F [2004a] Recessively inherited coagulation disorders. *Blood* 104:1243-1252. PMID:15138162.

Mannucci PM [2004b] Treatment of vWD. *N Engl J Med* 351:683-694. PMID:15306670.

Matsubara K, Fukaya T, Nigami H, Harigaya H, Hirata T, Nozaki H, Baba K [2004] Age-dependent changes in the incidence and etiology of childhood thrombocytosis. *Acta Haematol* 111:132-137. PMID:15034233.

McGlennen RC, Key NS [2002] Clinical and laboratory management of the prothrombin G20210A mutation. *Arch Pathol Lab Med* 126:1319-1324. PMID:12421139.

Meijers JC, Tekelenburg WLH, Bouma BN, et al [2000] High levels of coagulation factor XI as a risk factor for venous thrombosis. *N Engl J Med* 342(10):696-701. PMID:10706899.

Mhawech P, Saleem A [2000] Inherited giant platelet disorders: classification and literature review. *Am J Clin Pathol* 113:176-190. PMID:10664620.

Michelson AD [1998] Platelet function in the newborn. *Semin Thromb Hemost* 24(6):507-512. PMID:10066145.

Miller JL [1996a] Blood coagulation and fibrinolysis. In: *Clinical Diagnosis and Management by Laboratory Methods, 19th ed*. Philadelphia: WB Saunders Company.

Miller JL [1996b] Blood platelets In: *Clinical Diagnosis and Management by Laboratory Methods, 19th ed*. Philadelphia: WB Saunders Company.

Miller JL [1996c] Platelet-type vWD. *Thromb Haemost* 75(6):865-869. PMID:8822577.

Moake JL, Rudy CK, Troll JH, et al [1982] Unusually large plasma factor VIII:vWF multimers in chronic relapsing thrombotic thrombocytopenic purpura. *N Engl J Med* 307:1432-1435. PMID:6813740.

Moake JL [2002a] Thrombotic microangiopathies. *New Engl J Med* 347:589-600. PMID:12192020.

Moake JL [2002b] TTP and the HUS. *Arch Pathol Lab Med* 126:1430-1433. PMID:12421153.

Moeller A, Weippert-Kretschmer M, Prinz H, Kretschmer V [2001] Influence of ABO blood groups on primary hemostasis. *Transfusion* 41:56-60.

Moll S, Ortel TL [1997] Monitoring warfarin therapy in patients with lupus anticoagulants. *Ann Intern Med* 127(3):177-185. PMID:9245222.

Nair S, Ghosh K, Kulkarni B, Shetty S, Mohanty D [2002] Glanzmann thrombasthenia: updated. *Platelets* 13:387-393. PMID:12487785.

Neerman-Arbez M, de Moerloose P, Bridel C, Honsberger A, Schonborner A, Rossier C, Peerlinck K, Claeyssens S, Di Michele D, d'Oiron R, Dreyfus M, Laubriat-Bianchin M, Dieval J, Antonarakis SE, Morris MA [2000] Mutations in the fibrinogen Aα gene account for the majority of cases of congenital afibrinogenemia. *Blood* 96:149-152. PMID:10891444.

Norman KE, Cotter MJ, Stewart BJ [2003] Combined anticoagulant and antiselectin treatments prevent lethal intravascular coagulation. *Blood* 101:921-928. PMID:12393622.

Nutescu EA, Shapiro NL, Chevalier A [2008] New anticoagulant agents: direct thrombin inhibitors. *Cardiol Clin* 26:169-187. PMID:18406993.

O'Shea J, Sherlock M, Philip R [2005] Thrombocytosis in childhood [letter]. *Acta Haematol* 113:212 PMID:15870494.

Olson JD, Arkin CF, Brandt JT [1998] College of American Pathologists conference XXXI on laboratory monitoring of anticoagulant therapy: laboratory monitoring of UH therapy. *Arch Pathol Lab Med* 122(9):782-798. PMID:9740136.

Passam FH, Krilis SA [2004] Laboratory tests for the antiphospholipid syndrome: current concepts. *Pathology* 36(2):129-138. PMID:15203748.

Peershke EIB, Castellone DD, Ledford-Kraemer M, et al [2009] Laboratory assessment of factor VIII inhibitor titer. *Am J Clin Pathol* 131:552-558. PMID:19289591.

Pollak ES, Russell TT, Ptashkin B, et al [2006] Asymptomatic factor VII deficiency in African Americans. *Am J Clin Pathol* 126:128-132. PMID:16753603.

Portielje J, Westendorp R, Kluin-Nelemans H, Brand A [2001] Morbidity and mortality in adults with idiopathic thrombocytopenic purpura. *Blood* 97:2549-2554. PMID:11313240.

Press RD, Bauer KA, Kujovich JL, Heit JA [2002] Clinical utility of factor V Leiden (R506Q) testing for the diagnosis and management of thromboembolic disorders. *Arch Pathol Lab Med* 126:1304-1318. PMID:12421138.

Rao AK, Niewiarowski S, Guzzo J, et al [1981] Antithrombin III levels during heparin therapy. *Thromb Res* 24:181-186. PMID:6800057.

Rees DC, Cox M, and Clegg JB [1995] World distribution of factor V Leiden. *Lancet* 346:1133-1134. PMID:7475606.

Ridker PM, Miletich JP, Hennekens CH, et al [1997] Ethnic distribution of factor V Leiden in 4047 men and women. *JAMA* 277(16):1305-1307. PMID:9109469.

Rodgers RP, Levin J [1990] A critical reappraisal of the bleeding time. *Semin Thromb Hemost* 16(1):1-20. PMID:2406907.

Roelse J, Koopman R, Büller H, Berends F, ten Cate JW, Mertens K, van Mourik JA [1994] Association of idiopathic venous thromboembolism with single point-mutation at Arg506 of factor V. *Lancet* 343:1535-1539. PMID:7911872.

Rozman P [2002] Platelet antigens: the role of human platelet alloantigens (HPA) in blood transfusion and transplantation. *Transpl Immunol* 10:165-181. PMID:12216947.

Rubbia-Brandt L, Neerman-Arbez M, Rougemont AL, et al [2006] Fibrinogen gamma375 Arg-Trp mutation (fibrinogen aguadilla) causes hereditatry hypofibrinongenemia, hepatic endoplasmic reticulum storage disease, and cirrhosis. *Am J Surg Pathol* 30(7):906-911. PMID:16819336.

Ruggeri ZM, Pareti factor I, Mannucci PM, Ciavarella N, Zimmerman TS [1980] Heightened interaction between platelets and factor VIII/vWF in a new subtype of vWD. *N Engl J Med* 302:1047-1051. PMID:6767976.

Sadler JE [2003] Aortic stenosis, von Willebrand factor, and bleeding. *N Engl J Med* 349;4:323-325. PMID:12878737.

Sadler JE [2008] Von Willebrand factor, ADAMTS13, and thrombotic thrombocytopenic purpura. *Blood* 112(1):11-18. PMID:18574040.

Schinella RA, Greco MA, Cobert BL, Denmark LW, Cox RP [1980] Hermansky-Pudlak syndrome with granulomatous colitis. *Ann Intern Med* 92:20-23. PMID:7350869.

Schrecengost JE, LeGallo RD, Boyd JC, et al [2003] Comparison of diagnostic accuracies in outpatients and hospitalized patients of D-dimer testing for the evaluation of suspected pulmonary embolism. *Clin Chem* 49(9):1483-1490. PMID:12928229.

Segal JB, Eng J, Tamariz LJ, Bass EB [2007] Review of the evidence on diagnosis of deep venous thrombosis and pulmonary embolism. *Ann Fam Med* 5:63-73. PMID:17261866.

Seligsohn U, Lubetsky A [2001] Genetic susceptibility to venous thrombosis. *New Engl J Med* 344:1222-1231. PMID:11309638.

Seri M, Cusano R, Gangarossa S, et al [2000] Mutations in MYH9 result in the May-Hegglin anomaly, and Fechtner and Sebastian syndromes. *Nat Genet* 26(1):103-105. PMID:10973259.

Shetti S, Ghosh K [2008] Reduced clinical severity in a mutationally well-characterized cohort of severe hemophilia with associated thrombophilia. *Am J Clin Pathol* 130:84-87. PMID:18550475.

Strobl FJ, Hoffman S, Huber S, et al [1998] Activated protein C resistance assay performance: improvement by sample dilution with factor V-deficient plasma. *Arch Pathol Lab Med* 122(5):430-433. PMID:9593344.

Svensson PJ, Dahlbäck B [1994] Resistance to activated protein C as a basis for venous thrombosis. *N Engl J Med* 330(8):517-522. PMID:8302317.

Taylor FBJ, Toh CH, Hoots WK, et al [2001] Towards definition, clinical and laboratory criteria, and a scoring system for disseminated intravascular coagulation. *Thromb Haemost* 86:1327-1330. PMID:11816725.

Tollefson DM [2002] Heparin cofactor II deficiency. *Arch Pathol Lab Med* 126:1394-1400. PMID:12421148.

Triplett DA [2002] Antiphospholipid antibodies. *Arch Pathol Lab Med* 126:1424-1433. PMID:12421152.

Tsai HM, Lian EC [2002] Antibodies to vWF-cleaving protease in acute thrombotic thrombocytopenic purpura. *New Engl J Med* 339:1585-1594. PMID:9828246.

Upshaw JD Jr [1978] Congenital deficiency of a factor in normal plasma that reverses microangiopathic hemolysis and thrombocytopenia. *N Engl J Med* 298:1350-1352. PMID:651994.

Van Cott EM, Laposata M, Prins MH [2002] Laboratory evaluation of hypercoagulability with venous or arterial thrombosis. *Arch Pathol Lab Med* 126:1281-1294. PMID:12421136.

Van Oerle R, van Pampus L, Tans G, et al [1997] The clinical application of a new specific functional assay to detect the factor V (Leiden) mutation associated with activated protein C resistance. *Am J Clin Pathol* 107(5):521-526. PMID:9128263.

Vincentelli A, Susen S, LeTourneau T, Six I, Fabre O, Juthier F, Bauters A, Decoene C, Goudemand J, Prat A, Jude B [2003] Acquired von Willebrand syndrome in aortic stenosis. *N Engl J Med* 349:343-349. PMID:12878741.

Wadelius M, Chen LY, Lindh JD et al [2009] The largest prospective warfarin-treated cohort supports genetic forecasting. *Blood* 113:784-792. PMID:18574025.

Warkentin TE, Kelton JG [2001a] Delayed onset HIT and thrombosis. *Ann Intern Med* 135:502-506. PMID:11578153.

Warkentin TE, Kelton JG [2001b] Temporal aspects of HIT. *New Engl J Med* 344:1286-1292. PMID:11320387.

Warkentin TE [2002] Platelet count monitoring and laboratory testing for HIT. *Arch Pathol Lab Med* 126:1415-1422. PMID:12421151.

Warkentin TE [2005a] HIT. *Dis Mon* 51:141-149. PMID:15900266.

Warkentin TE [2005b] New approaches to the diagnosis of HIT. *Chest* 127(2):35S-45S PMID:15706029.

Warren BL, Eid A, Singer P [2001] High-dose antithrombin III in severe sepsis: a randomized controlled trial. *JAMA* 1869-1878. PMID:11597289.

Weiss EJ, Bray PF, Tayback M, Schulman SP, Kickler TS, Becker LC, Weiss JL, Gerstenblith G, Goldschmidt-Clermont PJ [1996] The platelet glycoprotein IIIa polymorphism PLA2: an inherited platelet risk factor for coronary thrombotic events. *N Engl J Med* 334:1090-1094. PMID:8598867.

Wildenberg SC, Fryer JP, Gardner JM, Oetting WS, Brilliant MH, King RA [1998] Identification of a novel transcript produced by the gene responsible for the Hermansky-Pudlak syndrome in Puerto Rico. *J Invest Dermatol* 110:777-781. PMID:9579545.

Wilson DB, Gard KM [2003] Evaluation of an automated, latex-enhanced turbidimetric D-dimer test (advanced D-dimer) and usefulness in the exclusion of acute thromboembolic disease. *Am J Clin Pathol* 120:930-937. PMID:14671982.

Zehnder JL, Benson RC [1996] Sensitivity and specificity of the APC resistance assay in detection of individuals with factor V leiden. *Am J Clin Pathol* 106(1):107-111. PMID:8701918.

Zhou L, Schmaier AH [2005] Platelet aggregation testing in platelet-rich plasma: description of procedures with the aim to develop standards in the field. *Am J Clin Pathol* 123:172-183. PMID:15842039.

Zotz RB, Winkelmann BR, Nauck M, Giers G, Maruhn-Debowski B, März W, Scharf RE [1998] Polymorphism of platelet membrane glycoprotein IIIa: human platelet antigen 1b (HPA-1b/PLA2) is an inherited risk factor for premature myocardial infarction in coronary artery disease. *Throm Haemost* 79:731-735. PMID:9569182.

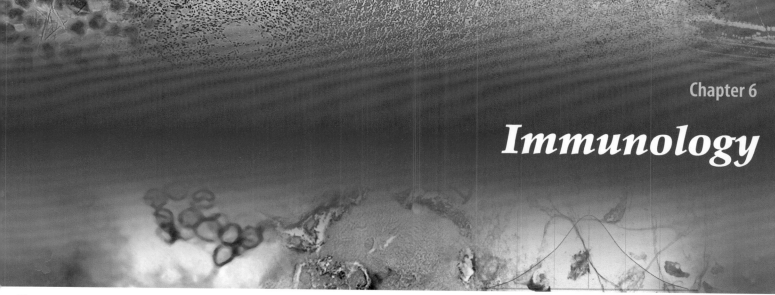

Chapter 6

Immunology

Immune system

Proper function of the immune system requires the complex interplay of the cellular and humoral components. Dysregulation of any of these components can create pathology in the form of hypersensitivity, autoimmunity, or immunodeficiency.

Cellular constituents

Stem cells

Lymphoid stem cells differentiate into lymphoid progenitor cells of 3 cell types: T lymphocytes, B lymphocytes, and natural killer (NK) lymphocytes. The myeloid stem cells differentiate into histiocytes, monocytes, dendritic cells, mast cells, neutrophils, eosinophils, basophils, megakaryocytes and erythrocytes.

B cells

B cells originate and mature in the marrow in a stepwise process t6.1. During this process they undergo rearrangement of their immunoglobulin genes.

t6.1 B & T cell maturation sequences

B cell stage	Definition	T cell stage	Definition
Lymphoid stem cell	CD34+, TdT+, HLA-DR+	Lymphoid stem cell	CD34+, TdT+, HLA-DR+
Pro-B cell (pre-pre-B cell)	CD34+, TdT+, HLA-DR+, CD19+, CD10+, Ig H chain rearranging	Prothymocytes	CD34+, TdT+, CD7+
Pre-B cell	CD34−, TdT−, HLA-DR+, CD19+, CD10+, CD20+, cytoplasmic μ heavy chains+Ig L chain rearranging	Immature/common thymocytes	CD34−, TdT+, CD1+, CD2+, cytoplasmic CD3+ (surface CD3−), CD5+, CD7+, CD4 & CD8+, TCR rearranged
B cell	All of the above plus surface Ig, CD21+, CD22+	Mature thymocyte	All of the above, except: TdT− & CD1− Surface CD3 becoming +, CD4 or CD8+
Plasma cell	Loss of B cell markers (CD19−, CD20−) & cytoplasmic (not surface) Ig+	Mature T cell	All of the above, except surface CD3+

Immunoglobulin (Ig) molecules consist of 4 polypeptide chains, including 2 heavy chains and 2 light chains, bound together by disulfide bonds. Light chains have 2 domains: 1 variable and 1 constant. Heavy chains have 4-5 domains: 1 variable and 3-4 constants f6.1. The terminal constant region may insert into the membrane of B cells or, if free in serum, is called the Fc portion. This Fc may bind to Fc receptors (FcR) on the surfaces of phagocytic cells. Mast cells bear an Fcε receptor that renders them capable of binding IgE. The variable regions of a light and heavy chain combine to form the antigen binding site, the paratope. This recognizes a specific molecular structure, the epitope, which is often an amino acid sequence of a larger molecule or cell. An antigen therefore may contain several epitopes.

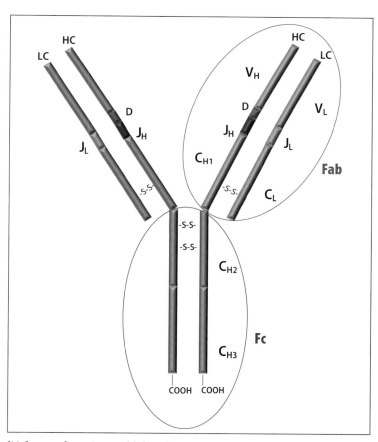

f6.1 Structure of serum immunoglobulin molecules, which are composed of 2 light chains (LC) & 2 heavy chains (HC), linked by disulfide bonds (-S-S-). Light chains are composed of a N-terminal variable region (V_L), a J chain (J_L), and a C-terminal constant region (C_L). Heavy chains are made up of an N-terminal variable region (V_H), D chain, J chain, and several constant regions (C_{H1}-C_{H3}).

Immunoglobulin genes that encode light chains are found on chromosomes 2 (κ) and 22 (γ). Genes for the heavy chains (γ, α, μ, δ, ε) are found on chromosome 14. During B cell development, these genes are physically rearranged. This process begins when the variable regions for both the light and heavy chain genes rearrange. The final variable region gene is created when separate V and J (light chain) or V, D, and J (heavy chain) segments are brought together (rearranged) in a fashion that has tremendous built-in randomness. The rearranged variable region gene sequence is then joined to a light chain or heavy chain constant region gene sequence. The latter is always initially a μ heavy chain gene, resulting in a completed gene that encodes an IgM protein with some particular epitope specificity.

Mature B cells coexpress surface IgM and IgD. The randomness that is built into rearrangement leads to a population of B cells with a nearly infinite variety of variable regions; ie, specificities for a nearly infinite variety of antigens. Up to this point, the process proceeds without antigen stimulation. Subsequent differentiation of the IgM+/IgD+ mature B cells awaits stimulation by an antigen which is complementary to the antigen binding site (paratope) of the surface Ig. Once stimulated by antigen in the presence of T_h cells the mature B cells proliferate and each progeny B cell rearranges its DNA yet again, rejoining their prefabricated variable genes with a different heavy chain gene (isotype switch). During this isotype switch, additional variability is created, leading to a group of B cells having an array of epitope specificities very nearly approximating that of the parent B cell, some having greater and some lesser affinity for the initiating antigen.

Since any protein can be an epitope, the variable end of the antibody itself may act as one. An epitope formed by the variable end of an Ig molecule is referred to as an idiotope (idiotype), and antiidiotope (idiotype) antibodies may be formed against it. Furthermore, there are 5 Ig classes, based on the heavy chain isotype: IgG, IgA, IgM, IgD, and IgE (listed in order of serum concentration). There are also 2 light chain isotypes (κ and λ). There are 4 subclasses of IgG: IgG1, IgG2, IgG3, IgG4. There are 2 subclasses of IgA: IgA1, IgA2 t6.2.

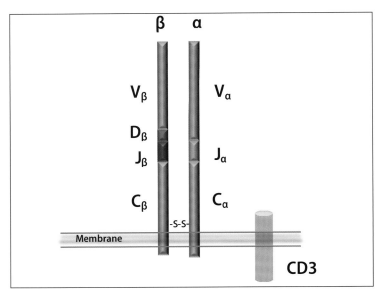

f6.2 T cell receptor molecules are transmembrane protein dimers that are noncovalently associated with CD3 molecules. In this case, an αβ TCR is illustrated, which is composed of 2 chains of similar length attached by disulfide bonds. There is significant homology with the immunoglobulin molecule.

T cell receptor (TCR) genes (α, β, γ, δ) are present on chromosome 7. The diversity of these TCR proteins is created by rearrangement of the genes in a fashion similar to the immunoglobulins.

T cells differentiate into several types that are separable on the basis of cell surface antigens. T-helper (T_h) cells are the pivotal cells in most immune responses and bear the antigen CD4. T-suppressor (T_s), and T-cytotoxic (T_c) cells bear the antigen CD8. The usual CD4:CD8 ratio is ~2:1.

T cell receptors (TCR) are found on the surfaces of T cells. TCRs are highly analogous to immunoglobulin f6.2, but unlike Ig can only respond to epitopes presented in conjunction with MHC/HLA molecules. CD4+ (T_h) cells must have the antigen presented in conjunction with class II MHC molecules (they are said to be class II MHC restricted), while CD8+ (T_c) cells must have the antigen presented in conjunction with class I MHC molecules (class I restricted). Each TCR is composed of a pair of equally-sized chains. Each chain has variable and constant domains. There are 2 classes of TCR: TCR αβ (composed of one α and one β chain) and TCR γδ. Like immunoglobulin, TCRs get the variability in the variable domains from the randomness built into the rearrangement of the V, D, and J segments of the variable region gene. But there is an additional degree of variability created by the terminal deoxynucleotidyl transferase (TdT) enzyme which randomly adds nucleotides into the gene.

We are thus endowed with lymphocytes that can recognize any antigen we may one day encounter. Exposure to that antigen in postnatal life causes proliferation of clones whose TCR/Ig receptor most closely recognizes the antigen. During this proliferation, more variety arises during the process of isotype switching, leading to more clones with greater or lesser antigen specificity.

Most (>95%) T lymphocytes have TCR αβ. A small percentage of T lymphocytes have a TCR γδ. TCR γδ cells are found in greatest number in mucosal surfaces and skin. TCR is expressed in noncovalent association with the CD3 molecule.

t6.2 Immunoglobulin classes

Ig class	Form found in blood	Average concentration in serum	Activates complement	Notes
IgG	Monomers (2 binding sites)	120 mg/dL	+ (classic pathway)	4 subclasses, IgG1–IgG4; IgG4 lowest in concentration
IgA	Dimers (4 binding sites)	30 mg/dL	+ (alternate pathway)	2 subclasses, IgA1–IgA2; IgA2 lowest in concentration
IgM	Pentamers (10 binding sites)	15 mg/dL	+ (classic pathway)	
IgD	Bound to B cells	0.3 mg/dL	–	
IgE	Bound to mast cells	0.0005 mg/dL	–	

T cells

T cells undergo stepwise maturation in the thymus. Under normal conditions, T lymphocytes outnumber B lymphocytes in blood by a ratio of ~2:1 and represent ~65% of circulating lymphocytes. T cells are primarily found in paracortical areas of lymph nodes and within periarteriolar lymphatic sheaths in the spleen.

The CD3 protein assists with transmembrane signaling when an antigen binds to the TCR.

NK cells

NK cells represent ~10% of peripheral blood lymphocytes. They are a subset of lymphocytic cells that bear neither the TCR nor Ig. The TCR and Ig genes are in the germline (nonrearranged) state. NK cells lack surface CD3, and express CD16, CD56, and CD57. CD16 is the receptor for the Fc portion of γ heavy chains (FcγR). Through binding of opsonized cells with this receptor, they mediate antigen dependent cellular cytotoxicity (ADCC); through this mechanism they are instrumental in combating viral infection and tumor cells. NK cells secrete IFN-γ and are morphologically recognizable in peripheral blood as large granular lymphocytes (LGLs).

Antigen presenting cells

Antigen presenting cells (monocytes, macrophages, histiocytes) are thought to originate in the marrow and include a wide variety of organ-specific cell types. Within this rubric are monocyte-macrophage cells, the Küpffer cell of hepatic sinusoids, the Hofbauer cell within placental villi, the interdigitating reticulum cell (IRC) of the interfollicular portions of lymph nodes, the dendritic reticulum cell (DRC) of germinal centers, and the Langerhans cells found in such places as the epidermis and lung. All of these cell types share phagocytic properties and certain cell antigens: MHC class II antigens, CD68 (KP-1), and lysozyme. All except the monocyte-macrophage cells have S100 and CD1a. T cells are not stimulated by soluble antigens, therefore, antigens are internalized by phagocytosis then processed and presented on the cell surface in association with MHC molecules. Stimulation of the remaining immune system begins with this process. Antigen-presenting cells also secrete IL-1 as a mechanism for modulating the inflammatory response.

Granulocytes

Neutrophils are attracted by cytokines, particularly IL-8, and upon arrival are stimulated to release their granules into the surroundings. The granules contain toxic substances and enzymes that degrade tissue indiscriminately. Neutrophils are also capable of limited phagocytic activity.

Basophils and mast cells have Fcε receptors upon their surfaces and are thus able to bind IgE. If antigen (allergen) is present, the surface IgE may become crosslinked. This activates the cell to release histamine and other substances which mediate hypersensitivity.

IL-5, secreted by T lymphocytes, specifically stimulates the terminal differentiation release of eosinophils. A sub-subset of CD4+ T cells called T$_h$2 cells stimulate both the production of IgE (secrete IL-4) and eosinophilic infiltration (secrete IL-5), particularly in the setting of parasitic infections.

Complement

Effect of formed complement

The attachment of the complement protein C3b to a foreign substance (opsonization) leads to phagocytosis. The attachment of the complex of complement proteins C5-9 (membrane

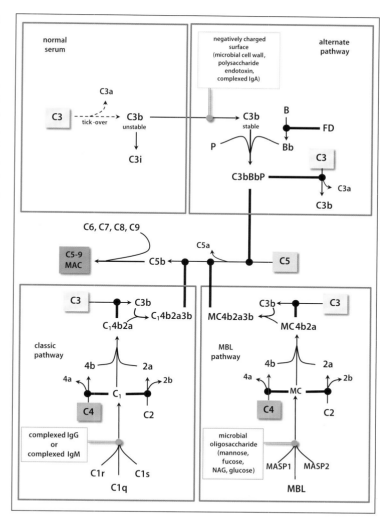

f6.3 Complement cascades: Classical, alternate & MBL (mannan binding lectin). All of the pathways converge, by way of their individual C5 convertases, upon C5 which initiates the formation of the membrane-attack complex (MAC). The original complement components are denoted C1-C9. C1 is a complex composed of C1q, C1r & C1s. Additional proteins, particularly those active in the alternate pathway, are called "factors," including factor B & factor D. Proteolysis results in fragments of the original proteins that are typically called "a" & "b" as in C3a & C3b. An inactive fragment is denoted 'I' as in C3i (or sometimes iC3b). MASP = MBL-associated serine protease

attack complex) leads directly to the lysis of membrane-bound structures (cells, bacteria). Lastly, the complement proteins C3a and C5a (anaphylatoxins) promote the release of histamine from basophils.

Complement pathways

There are 3 distinct pathways to complement activation, including the classic pathway, the alternate pathway, and the mannan binding lectin (MBL) pathway. These 3 pathways converge to activate C5 thereby assembling the membrane attack complex (MAC) **f6.3**.

The *classic pathway* can be activated by IgM and certain subclasses of IgG (IgG1, IgG2, IgG3). It is the Fc portion of the Ig molecule that interacts with C1q to initiate this process. Activated C1 catalyzes the association of C4 and C2 to make C4b2a (the C3 convertase of the classic pathway). This molecule (C4b2a) is capable of converting C3 into C3b and C3a. The now abundantly available C3b associates with C4b2a to make C4b2a3b (the C5 convertase of the classic pathway) causing deposition of the terminal complement components on the target surface.

The *alternate pathway* can be activated by bacterial cell walls, venoms, endotoxin, or complexed IgA. Initiation of this pathway is through deposition of C3b onto any of these substances; C3b is being produced at low levels at all times in peripheral blood as a result of a "tick-over" phenomenon in which minute amounts of C3 are constantly converted to C3a and C3b. C3b binds to an amide or hydroxyl group, present on the surface of bacteria, in venom, endotoxin, or complexed IgA, to prevent its degradation. Normally C3b is rapidly inactivated by factor I, unless a suitable surface is present to prevent it and promote the association of C3b with factor B to make C3bBb. Factor D cleaves the factor B to form the surface bound convertase (the C3 convertase of the alternate pathway) which is further stabilized by properdin to prolong the half life of the C3 convertase. This molecule (C3bBb) is capable of converting more C3 to C3b and C3a, thereby amplifying the reaction. The now abundantly available C3b associates with C3bBb and properdin (P) to make C3bBb3b, stabilized by P, sometimes written C3b(2)BbP (the C5 convertase of the alternate pathway).

The *mannan binding lectin pathway* is a recently described pathway that uses mannose binding lectin or mannose binding protein, formed in the liver, to bind onto the surfaces of microbes. MBL is capable of recognizing pathogenic carbohydrates but not carbohydrates found on mammalian glycoproteins, allowing for discrimination between self and nonself. Once the proteins bind, they undergo a conformational change allowing them to associate with 3 MBL associated serine proteases, MASP-1, MASP-2, and MASP-3 to activate the complement cascade. After activation, MASP-2 cleaves C4 and C2 to generate C4b2a, the C3 convertase, thereby activating C3.

The end result of the alternative, classic and MBL pathways is to converge on activating C3 to allow for assembly of the membrane attack complex by producing C5 convertase (a molecule capable of converting C5 into C5b and C5a). Once C5b is formed, it quickly complexes (on the surface of adjacent cells, eg, bacteria, transfused red cells) with C6, C7, C8 and C9 to form C5b6789 (the membrane attack complex or MAC). Note that C3a and C5a are formed as by-products of the above reactions. These 2 molecules are known as *anaphylatoxins*, because they are capable of increasing vascular permeability and causing vasodilation. C3b alone, like IgG, coats the surfaces of cells and acts as an opsonin. That is, it interacts with receptors on phagocytic cells, leading to ingestion of the bound cell.

MHC complex & HLA antigens

HLA proteins are encoded by genes located within the major histocompatibility complex (MHC). The MHC complex is a cluster of genes located sequentially on chromosome 6p. Genes encoding the HLA molecules are the most polymorphic loci in the human genome, with some loci having >300 alleles. These genes have been categorized into 3 groups—class I, class II, and class III. Also embedded in the MHC region are the genes for hereditary hemochromatosis and 21-hydroxylase. These and the MHC genes are such closely linked loci that are inherited en bloc from each parent, with little to no crossing over.

Class I genes are distributed among 3 loci, termed HLA-A, HLA-B, and HLA-C. Each locus has multiple possible alleles, termed, eg, HLA-A1, HLA-A2. These genes encode the HLA class I antigens which are heterodimer molecules composed of one heavy chain and one light chain. The heavy chain is a transmembrane glycosylated polypeptide composed of 3 α domains. It is noncovalently associated with a light chain that is a single molecule of α_2-microglobulin. Somatic cells that express foreign antigen on their surface in conjunction with class I MHC molecules invite destruction from T_c (CD8+) cells. This is important in mounting an immune response against viral infection. Class I antigens are found on the surfaces of most nucleated cells in the body.

Class II genes are distributed among 3 loci, termed HLA-DR, HLA-DP, and HLA-DQ. For each locus, there are several possible alleles, termed, eg, HLA-DR3, HLA-Dw2. These genes encode HLA class II antigens which consist of 2 polypeptide chains, α and β, each with 2 domains similar to the immunoglobulin light chains, in addition to a transmembrane domain. Antigen-presenting cells (APCs) present antigen to T_h (CD4+) cells in association with class II MHC antigens. HLA class II antigens are constitutively expressed on B lymphocytes, monocytes, macrophages, and dendritic cells. T lymphocytes normally do not express class II antigens unless they become activated.

Class III genes largely encode non-HLA antigens, most of which still have something to do with immunity. Class III genes include genes for complement proteins, the *NOTCH-4* gene, the tumor necrosis factor (TNF) genes, and others.

Since each MHC complex is closely linked and inherited en bloc, each parental chromosome can be thought of as a haplotype. Thus, the chance that 2 siblings are HLA identical is essentially 25%. The formula to calculate the probability of having at least 1 HLA matched sibling with n siblings is: $1-(0.75)^n$. Therefore, the chance of having an HLA identical sibling increases with the number of siblings: with 1 sibling, the chance is 25%; with 2, it is ~45%; and with 3 it is nearly 60%; however, the probability of having an HLA identical sibling never reaches 100%.

Evaluation of immune function
Screening tests
History & physical examination

The history provides clues to the presence and nature of a primary immunodeficiency. Primary immunodeficiencies disproportionately affect males, since the majority of disorders are X-linked. Patients with immunoglobulin or B cell defects report recurring bacterial infections of the upper and lower respiratory tract, ultimately resulting in bronchiectasis, or recalcitrant intestinal infection; eg, with *Giardia lamblia*. T cell deficiencies usually result in susceptibility to viral and fungal opportunistic infections. Mucocutaneous candidiasis is an indication of defective T cell function. Phagocyte defects are associated with *Staphylococcus* species and other catalase positive organisms. Terminal complement deficiencies present with severe infections due to encapsulated organisms such as *Streptococcus pneumoniae* or *Neisseria meningitides*. Since many of the primary immunodeficiencies present in the infection-prone period of childhood, it is difficult to determine who needs special evaluation. In general, children with frequent or prolonged infections, infections involving unusual agents or unusual sites should be investigated. Furthermore, children with chronic diarrhea and/or failure to thrive should be evaluated.

The physical examination may reveal the constitutional effects of immunodeficiency, such as growth retardation, so monitoring height and weight are important in these patients. Palpation of the peripheral lymph nodes may reveal small or undetectable nodes in some of the B cell defects; alternatively, nodes may be significantly enlarged in common variable immunodeficiency or chronic granulomatous disease. Petechiae, and easy bruisability are seen in Wiskott-Aldrich syndrome. Also note in the medical record the results of any pulmonary function tests or radiographic examinations that are available.

Global tests of immune system

The white cell count, differential and peripheral smear examination for morphology should be undertaken first. Absolute lymphopenia is more common in T cell defects, since they compromise the majority of circulating peripheral lymphocytes, and is uncommon in B cell defects. Lymphocyte subsets are easily enumerated by flow cytometry, providing absolute number of B cells, T cells, CD8+ T cells, and CD4+ T cells. Absolute neutropenia may suggest inherited (constitutional) or acquired (autoimmune, drug) neutropenia. Thrombocytopenia may suggest such things as Wiskott-Aldrich syndrome.

Immunoglobulins should be assessed, since antibody deficiencies are one of the most common immune defects. Quantitative immunoglobulins (IgG, IgA, IgM) and subclasses should be measured and compared to age-matched controls, since levels progressively increase with age in children. Evaluation of isohemagglutinin titers against blood groups is an alternative; however, testing is not valid until 4-6 months of age due to the persistence of maternal antibody. Some normal children have low concentration of isohemagglutinin titers until 5-10 years of age.

Radiologic imaging may disclose characteristic bony abnormalities. Infantile onset adenosine deaminase deficiency presents with hip or rib defects identified on x-ray. Patients with either T or B cell defects have metaphyseal defects and dwarfism. Hyper IgM syndrome can present with diffuse osteoporosis; patients suffer from fractures with minor trauma and have midline bony defects. Computed tomography (CT) and magnetic resonance imaging (MRI) can assess soft tissue abnormalities in patients with immunodeficiencies. Bronchiectasis or chronic pulmonary fibrosis can develop over time in patients with B cell deficiency. Chronic interstitial pneumonia and absence of a thymus can be identified in patients with T cell defects.

Since many patients with B or T cell deficiencies have longstanding pulmonary infections, they may exhibit obstructive or restrictive patterns on pulmonary function tests. Therefore, even with a normal imaging study of the lungs, pulmonary function testing should be performed.

Specific tests

Testing B cell function

The total immunoglobulin (Ig) level and levels of various Ig classes serve as global reflections of B cell function. The patient's specific antibody may be measured when such levels are borderline. For example, anti-pneumococcal antibody may be measured pre- and post-immunization. Enzyme linked immunosorbent assays (ELISAs) available in most commercial labs can test for vaccine responses to tetanus, diphtheria, *Haemophilus*, and pneumococcus in children who have been routinely immunized. In this regard, it is useful to recall that antibodies raised to protein antigens require orchestration of T and B cell function, whereas B cells are capable of autonomous production of antibody to carbohydrate antigen. A poor response to a protein antigen such as tetanus or diphtheroid toxoid could indicate either a B cell or a T cell defect. On the other hand, a poor reaction to carbohydrate antigens (such as pneumococcal or meningococcal vaccine or ABO antigens) is purely indicative of a B cell defect.

The most common isolated isotype deficiency is IgA deficiency, with an incidence of 1 in 700 people of European ancestry. IgG subclass deficiency (eg, IgG2 deficiency) may also occur and can result in serious bacterial infections, even when the overall IgG level is normal. Total IgE testing has been advocated to exclude a list of uncommon conditions, all of which are associated with high IgE: parasitic infection, Churg-Strauss syndrome, hyper-IgE (Job) syndrome, IgE myeloma, and Hodgkin lymphoma. IgE is not uniformly elevated in allergic states, and therefore is not a useful screening test in that setting.

RAST (radio-allergosorbent test) is an allergen-specific IgE measurement that can be useful to evaluate allergy, principally for inhaled allergens. RAST is used to determine levels of specific serum IgE antibodies by adding serum to a particular antigen, such as ragweed, complexed to a solid phase, followed by the addition of radiolabeled anti-IgE antibody. Remember that hereditary angioedemia (angioedema without urticaria) is not a true IgE mediated allergic reaction, nor is chronic urticaria, so RAST testing is not useful in these scenarios. Also, specified suspected antigens must be identified, and RAST is therefore not a screening test.

Testing T cell function

A gross estimation of circulating T cells is obtained from the blood total lymphocyte count, since most circulating lymphocytes are T cells. By flow cytometry, the proportion of all lymphocyte subsets, including T cell subsets can be determined. The total CD3+ count is the most accurate way to enumerate T cells. The ratio of CD4:CD8 cells is normally around 2:1. Deviation from this ratio, particularly a decrease, is found in T cell immunodeficiency states.

A test of delayed-type hypersensitivity (DTH) is the usual screening test for T cell function. A tuberculin skin test is the classic example of this phenomenon. Antigen is inoculated subcutaneously and the skin is observed for the development of a lesion, usually by 24-48 hours, indicative of T cell activation. More than one antigen should be incorporated in this testing. Caution should be exercised when interpreting the results in infants or young children, since they may not have had sufficient exposure to an antigen to mount an immune response.

Proliferation assays can be performed by exposing T cells to mitogens, which are plant substances that stimulate both helper and suppressor T cells, such as phytohemagglutinin or concanavalin A. Proliferation is measured by the uptake of radioactive DNA precursors (tritiated thymidine) and indicates there may be adequate numbers of T cells but does not assess their ability to clear these infectious organisms.

Testing NK cell function

By flow cytometry, NK cells (CD3−, CD16+, CD56+, CD57+) can easily be enumerated. Isolated NK cell deficiency is rare. Severe herpesvirus infections have been reported in this context.

NK cell function can be assessed by chromium release assays; however, this is labor intensive and utilizes undesirable radioactive materials. A colorimetric substrate to detect granzyme B, a serine protease present in the granules of NK cells and cytotoxic T cells can be used to assess NK cell function. Flow cytometry has been used with a variety of cell surface markers, fluorescent tags, degranulation and other cellular parameters to differentiate living and dead cells.

Testing neutrophil function

An excellent screening test for neutrophils is simply the absolute neutrophil count and peripheral smear, since most inherited defects in this arm of the immune system have readily identifiable numerical and/or morphologic findings. In addition, one can specifically look at chemotaxis, phagocytosis, or oxidative burst functions with various assays. One such assay is the nitroblue tetrazolium (NBT) assay in which yellow NBT dye is added to neutrophils which are then stimulated. Cells capable of a normal oxidative burst will reduce the yellow NBT to a purple-blue formazan (f) precipitate, and are said to be f+. Normal individuals will have nearly 100% f+ cells. An abnormal result, with perhaps <10% f+ cells, is expected in chronic granulomatous disease (CGD), in which deficiency of NADPH oxidase prevents the oxidative burst. These patients are predisposed to infections with catalase positive organisms, which can survive intracellular ingestion and proliferate.

The NBT test has been replaced in some laboratories with a flow cytometry test that detects intracellular oxidation of products such as dihydrorhodamine 123. When these products are oxidized they will fluoresce and are objectively evaluated by the instrumentation, an improvement over the subjective interpretation of the NBT dye test.

Myeloperoxidase staining can disclose myeloperoxidase deficiency, an autosomal recessive trait which produces at most mild immunodeficiency.

Testing complement

The CH50 test is a functional assay of the classic complement pathway, in which total hemolytic activity is measured. This test is performed by preparing doubling dilutions of the patient's serum and then adding immunoglobulin-coated sheep RBCs. The complement in the patient's serum will bind to the immune complexes on the sheep RBCs and cause lysis. The endpoint of the assay is the dilution of the patient's serum

causing 50% lysis of the immunoglobulin-coated sheep red cells and the result is expressed as the reciprocal of this dilution. Absence of 1 of the 9 complement components will lead to a CH50 of 0; however, a normal value will not rule out the possibility of reduced quantities of individual complement components. If this is suspected, antigenic assays of individual components should be performed.

Antigenic assays are undertaken for quantitation of specific complement components. Individual radial diffusion methods or nephelometric methods are predominantly used to assess C3 and C4 levels. C3 levels are used to look at the alternate pathway. Decreased levels of C3 reflect either primary C3 deficiency or activation of the alternate complement pathway. Levels of C4 or C1q are typically used to look at the classic pathway.

HLA testing

HLA testing does not normally have a role in the evaluation of immunodeficiency; instead, it is used primarily in pretransplantation compatibility testing, platelet refractoriness, paternity/ forensic identity testing, and the evaluation of HLA-linked autoimmune disorders.

The *complement dependent cytotoxicity (CDC)* assay is the gold standard for detecting HLA antigens, detecting HLA antibodies, or performing HLA crossmatching for determining solid organ transplant compatibility. For the detection of antigens, the CDC assay is performed upon lymphocytes separated as a buffy coat from peripheral blood. HLA antisera are incubated with patient lymphocytes, in the presence of excess complement, followed by the addition of dye. If the antiserum binds to the corresponding antigen present on the cells it will form an immune complex, causing complement to bind and lyse the lymphocytes. Microscopic examination shows either

1. intact lymphocytes that repel the dye (a negative reaction), indicating they had no attached antibody or activated complement and therefore no damage to their membrane

2. damaged lymphocytes which have internalized the dye (a positive reaction) indicating antibody was bound, complement was activated and the membrane was lysed

Fluorescent dyes can also be used if a fluorescence microscope is available. HLA class II antigen typing can only be performed on B cells, since they are the only leukocyte in the peripheral circulation to express these antigens. Magnetic beads coated with monoclonal antibodies are used to isolate a B cell population for testing. *For the detection of HLA antibodies*, patient serum is incubated with lymphocytes of known HLA type, and a similar procedure is carried out. The patient's serum can be run against a panel of known lymphocytes to determine the panel reactive antibody (PRA) level (see below).

Mixed lymphocyte culture (MLC) is an assay capable of detecting HLA class II (HLA-D) differences among potential donor and recipient. Recall that class II molecules are numerous on the surface of B cells but not on resting T cells, so a B cell enrichment step is needed. Prospective donor and recipient B lymphocytes are cultured together. They proliferate if stimulated by one another's HLA dissimilarities. At the end of the incubation period, the assay is pulsed with radioactive thymidine to determine the extent of DNA synthesis, a reflection of the amount of proliferation and thus the amount of incompatibility. By first subjecting the donor T lymphocytes to irradiation (rendering them incapable of proliferation), the reaction can be made more specific for recipient intolerance of the potential donor. This test detects mainly HLA class II differences which are of paramount importance, second only to ABO compatibility, in organ transplantation. This test is influenced by transfusion, health status and disease state of the patient, therefore, it has been largely replaced by DNA methods.

Crossreactive antigen groups (CREGs)

In the early stages of HLA typing, testing was performed by serologic techniques. Human antisera are capable of binding to more than one HLA allelic product (serologic crossreactivity). Serologic crossreactivity between alleles of HLA-A and HLA-B loci are used to cluster molecules within the same crossreactive antigen groups (CREGs). This phenomenon can be explained by the sharing of amino acid sequences among the HLA molecules within a CREG, but there is considerable overlap in the CREG groupings. More precise DNA-based methods allowed for appropriate identification of HLA alleles and demonstrated the necessity for a systemic and logical format for naming HLA alleles.

Public antigens

HLA antigens contain common amino acid sequences that are present in many different HLA antigens but demonstrate common reactivities. These "public" antigens are present in the less variable regions of the HLA molecule. For example, HLA-Bw4 and HLA-Bw6 are 2 public antigens that are present in almost all HLA-B molecules with only a few exceptions. If a patient lacks one of these public antigens and becomes immunized during pregnancy or transfusion, it appears as multiple discrete HLA antibodies. These antibodies can impact patient responses to platelet transfusion or their ability to receive a compatible solid organ transplant.

DNA assays have become widespread in HLA typing. PCR testing has the advantage of eliminating many of the biologic uncertainties of the "serologic" techniques described above. Furthermore, it can resolve HLA types with much greater specificity than the serologic techniques. The DNA is ordinarily obtained from nucleated cells circulating in the peripheral blood and only requires a small quantity of whole blood, 0.2-1.0 mL. *Sequence specific primers (SSP)* are used to amplify HLA alleles of interest for additional study. If the allele(s) are present, the amplified product can be identified as a band on gel electrophoresis and the genotype is confirmed. *Sequence specific oligonucleotides (SSOP)* is a molecular technique that detects different alleles at a locus by probes that recognize HLA allele specificities. The oligonucleotides hybridize to denatured PCR-amplified DNA attached to a solid support. The oligonucleotides are tagged with an enzyme that will then cleave a substrate to produce a colored product or light (chemiluminescence). Lastly, *sequence based testing (SBT)*, essentially nucleic acid sequencing, is used to characterize new alleles. These techniques can be applied to amplified DNA to determine the identity of the alleles. For example, if looking for HLA-B27, the patient's HLA-B locus can first be nonspecifically amplified then treated with HLA-B27-specific oligonucleotide probe to see if hybridization occurs. Alternatively, HLA-B27-specific primer sequences can be used in the amplification step; the presence of an identifiable band on gel electrophoresis after PCR confirms HLA-B27. Lastly, an unknown allele can be directly sequenced and compared to known sequences.

Transplantation specific considerations
Transplantation testing

Panel reactive antibody (PRA) tests are used to monitor patients who are waiting for a transplant. These patients may be sensitized to HLA antigens either through transfusion of donor blood products, pregnancy, or previous organ transplantation. PRA assesses the proportion of the donor population that the patient's HLA antibodies will react against, giving some guidance to the rate of compatibility of an unrelated donor organ. For example if the patient has a PRA of 80%, this indicates the patient is highly sensitized and has about a 20% chance of compatibility with an unrelated donor organ that becomes available. This highly sensitized patient will have difficulty finding a compatible organ. Most organ transplant services require monthly PRAs for patients waiting on the transplant list, and the PRA value is used as part of the decision making process for organ assignment to recipients. PRAs can be assessed by several different testing methods such as ELISA, CDC, flow cytometry and Luminex.

HLA matching for transplantation usually involves matching ≥3 loci: HLA-A, HLA-B, and HLA-DR. Since each person has 2 alleles (one on each 6p) for each locus, there are 6 possible alleles. The potential recipient may have been sensitized to these and other not normally tested alleles through pregnancy or transfusion; thus, even when there appears to be a perfect 6 of 6 match, an in vitro assessment of compatibility (a crossmatch) is still necessary.

The CDC crossmatch can detect preexisting HLA alloantibodies in the serum of the potential recipient that have specificity for HLA antigens in the potential donor. These preformed HLA antibodies are the mediators of so-called hyperacute rejection, in which the transplanted organ is rapidly destroyed by circulating antibodies, often before the surgery is complete. The CDC crossmatch is performed by incubating donor lymphocytes (separated into B and T lymphocytes or unseparated) with recipient serum in the presence of excess complement. An auto-crossmatch is performed to control for autoantibodies (which do not appear to impact transplant survival). Positive results of a CDC crossmatch between donor and recipient indicate an incompatibility, and the organ should not be transplanted into the patient. A positive CDC crossmatch is an excellent predictor of hyperacute rejection if solid organ transplantation occurs.

The flow cytometric crossmatch is a more sensitive test than the CDC assay and allows for detection of lower titers for both complement dependent and complement independent recipient antibodies to the donor graft than the CDC assay. This assay can be performed before or after solid organ transplantation. Flow cytometry detects recipient antibodies to donor B and T cells based on the differential expression of HLA class molecules on these cells. Donor lymphocytes are incubated with anti-CD3 or anti-CD20, each with a different fluorescent tag, and recipient serum. The cells are washed and fluorescein isothiocyanate conjugated (FITC) anti-human-IgG or IgM is added to the lymphocytes. The cells are then analyzed by flow cytometry which measures the fluorescent intensity of the tags present and the cells are gated on histograms based on their forward scatter. A 40 channel mean fluorescence shift is considered a positive result.

Luminex technology uses polystyrene microspheres or beads which are embedded with a unique fluorochrome and are coated with specific HLA molecules. The beads are incubated with recipient serum and then a fluorescent labeled anti-human globulin is added to bind with any patient HLA antibody coating the microspheres. The instrument uses cell sorting to detect immune complexes on the bead and also identifies the unique fluorochrome of the specific bead to determine the HLA antigen specificity of the antibody. The reactions are quantified as mean fluorescence intensity (MFI) and each medical center determines thresholds for assessing donor organ compatibility. Luminex has been correlated with flow crossmatches and CDC testing. Luminex values above 5,000 MFI correlates with a positive T cell and B cell flow crossmatch and values >10,000 MFI correlates with a positive CDC, indicating hyperacute rejection is likely if the organ is transplanted to the patient.

For renal transplantation, organs should be ABO-compatible, HLA-A, HLA-B, and HLA-DR matched (6 of 6 ideally), and crossmatch compatible. The CDC crossmatch is most commonly performed but flow cytometric crossmatches are more sensitive and are better at predicting acute rejection and delayed graft function after transplant. A positive T cell flow crossmatch with IgG antibodies indicates there are antibodies to HLA class I antigens and is associated with higher rejection rates and lower graft survival after kidney transplant. Therefore, more aggressive immunosuppression therapies are used, including plasmapheresis and IVIg. Detection of IgG antibodies to B cells and IgM antibodies to B or T cells is more significant when specifically directed against donor HLA class I or II antigens.

For transplantation of heart, lung, and liver, such stringency is not required, and ABO compatibility is the main determinant for donor selection. HLA typing may be performed but is not a requirement.

HLA typing resolution requirements for allogenic progenitor cell transplants are more stringent than for renal transplants. Higher resolution DNA allele typing for HLA class I and class II loci is required to match the donor and recipient for progenitor cell transplants. Potential donors are typed for HLA-A, B, C, DR and DQ alleles and sometimes for HLA-DP alleles. It is optimal to match the donor and recipient alleles at the HLA-A, B, C and DRB1 loci. Although HLA matched related siblings are the best choice for allogenic transplants, there is increasing use of HLA matched unrelated donors registered in the National Marrow Donor Program. Now with T cell depletion of HPC products, there is more use of umbilical cord HPCs and HPC grafts from HLA mismatched donors.

Transplant rejection

Hyperacute rejection occurs within hours of transplantation and is mediated by preformed high titer antibodies to ABO or HLA antigens expressed by donor graft endothelium. Immunoglobulin is deposited along vessel walls, inducing

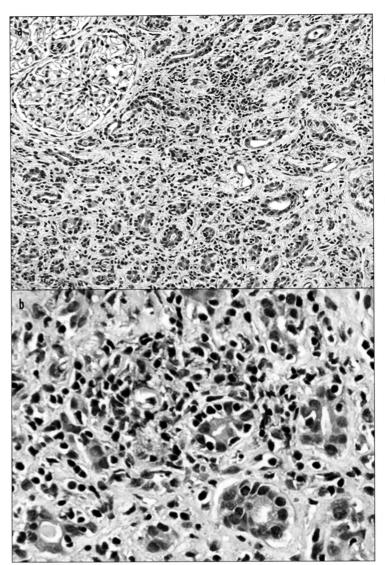

f6.4 Acute cellular rejection of kidney a, characterized by lymphocytic infiltrate with interstitial edema; at high magnification b, there is evidence of tubulitis, a lesion consisting of T lymphocytes infiltrating into renal tubular epithelium

complement-mediated vascular injury. The result is the formation of fibrin and platelet thrombi, causing ischemic necrosis. This can occur as soon as the vascular connections are made and the organ may become mottled and dusky during the surgical procedure. This type of rejection is resistant to therapy and can only be prevented with pretransplant screening and crossmatching techniques. A positive CDC crossmatch correlates well with increased risk of hyperacute rejection.

Acute cellular rejection evolves over days to weeks after transplant and is mediated by T cells. Recipient T cells recognize foreign HLA antigens and stimulate a powerful cellular cytotoxic response. Histologically, a lymphocytic infiltrate is seen within graft epithelium (tubulitis) and endothelium (endothelitis), along with interstitial edema f6.4. By immunohistochemistry, a mixture of CD4+ and CD8+ T cells is identified. Acute cellular rejection responds to therapy if recognized early and treated with combination immunosuppressive pharmacologic agents such as steroids, cyclosporine, and antithymocyte globulin (ATG) therapy.

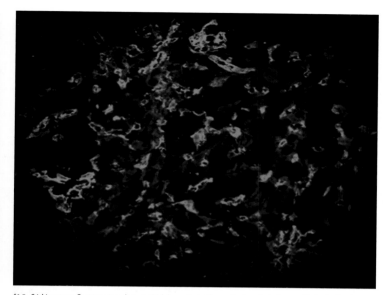

f6.5 C4d immunofluorescence detects C4d deposits in the cortical peritubular capillaries indicating the presence of alloantibodies against HLA antigens on the peritubular capillary endothelium; normal kidneys demonstrate C4d deposition in glomeruli only

Acute humoral rejection presents within days to weeks after transplantation and is mediated by antibody. Like hyperacute rejection, the endothelium is the primary target, with resulting injury taking 1 of 2 forms. First, there may be a pattern similar to hyperacute rejection, with fibrinoid necrosis and neutrophilic infiltration of vessel walls and resulting graft infarct. Second, there may be a more insidious vascular subendothelial intimal thickening with more protracted graft ischemia. Patients who are HLA alloimmunized as a result of pregnancy or transfusion are at significantly higher risk. In either case, immunohistochemistry demonstrates deposition of C4d in vessel walls f6.5. Acute humoral rejection is associated with a higher risk of death and graft failure than acute cellular rejection and requires the addition of specific antihumoral interventions such as plasmapheresis and IVIg.

Chronic rejection is mediated by a combination of lymphocytes and antibodies over months to years, leading to eventual graft failure. Histological findings include interstitial fibrosis, arteriolosclerosis of vessels and complement deposits in peritubular vessels.

Graft vs host disease (GVHD)

There are 3 requisites for the development of GVHD: immunocompetent donor T cells, immunosuppressed recipient, and antigenic differences between donor and recipient. Immunocompetent donor T cells, present in the graft, target "foreign" antigens in the recipient. While HLA matching is important for prevention of GVHD, even HLA-identical transplants have an incidence of GVHD >20%, presumably due to non-HLA antigens.

Acute GVHD is traditionally defined as that occurring within the first 100 days after transplant, with most cases presenting within the first 30 days. The 3 main targets of acute GVHD are the epithelium of the skin, intestinal tract, and hepatobiliary tract. Skin involvement is initially characterized by an erythematous, pruritic rash, histologically demonstrating characteristic erythema multiforme-like apoptosis

that is most pronounced at the bases of rete ridges. Intestinal tract involvement presents with diarrhea. Histologically, colon biopsies show ectatic crypts with attenuated enterocytes, crypt abscesses, and striking apoptosis within the crypt epithelium. The small bowel may show similar features, with villous blunting. Liver involvement presents with jaundice, histologically characterized by mononuclear portal inflammatory infiltrates with endothelialitis, ductitis, and ductopenia.

Chronic GVHD occurs after the first 100 days and may follow the acute form or may start insidiously de novo. Chronic GVHD affects the skin, hepatobiliary tract, intestinal tract, and the mucosa of the mouth, vagina, eye, and respiratory tract. These patients experience extensive cutaneous sclerosis that resembles progressive systemic sclerosis. They may experience esophageal strictures, bronchiolitis obliterans, scarring ocular lesions, and chronic liver damage.

The greater the HLA disparity between the donor and recipient, the greater the risk of GVHD. The risk is reduced when receiving stem cell/bone marrow graft from a related donor, particularly a sibling, since many of the HLA antigens are shared.

This is different from transfusion associated GVHD (TA-GVHD) in which the main target of the attack is the bone marrow. The rate of death in TA-GVHD is >90% due to aplastic anemia and can be prevented by irradiating lymphocyte containing blood products in immunocompromised patients.

Primary immunodeficiency disorders
B cell defects
General features

Defective B cell function is characterized by recurrent bacterial sinopulmonary infections and recalcitrant intestinal infections; opportunistic fungal and viral infections are not typical. B cell defects often present at or after 6 months of age, due to persistence of maternal antibodies in the infant serum.

Bruton (X-linked) agammaglobulinemia

Patients with X-linked agammaglobulinemia (XLA) present with recurrent bacterial infections, particularly related to encapsulated bacteria such as pneumococcus and haemophilus, beginning around 6 months of age. This may lead to eventual bronchiectasis. Affected individuals have largely normal immunity against most viral and fungal pathogens; however, they show susceptibility to polio, hepatitis, and enteroviruses, possibly due to defective IgA at the mucosal surface. They also suffer from a high incidence of lymphoid neoplasms and autoimmune diseases.

Serum immunoglobulin levels (IgG, IgA, and IgM) are markedly reduced, as is the number of circulating mature CD19+ B cells. Differential diagnostic considerations in the infant include protein losing states, severe malnutrition, and transient hypogammaglobulinemia. In contrast to these conditions, patients with XLA demonstrate diminished responses to vaccine and failure to develop blood group antibodies. Interestingly, severe neutropenia occurs in some patients, often in the presence of severe sepsis.

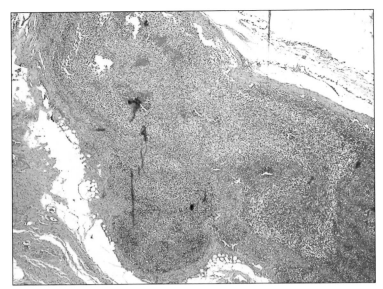

f6.6 Lymph node in Bruton agammaglobulinemia; note the absence of lymphoid follicles

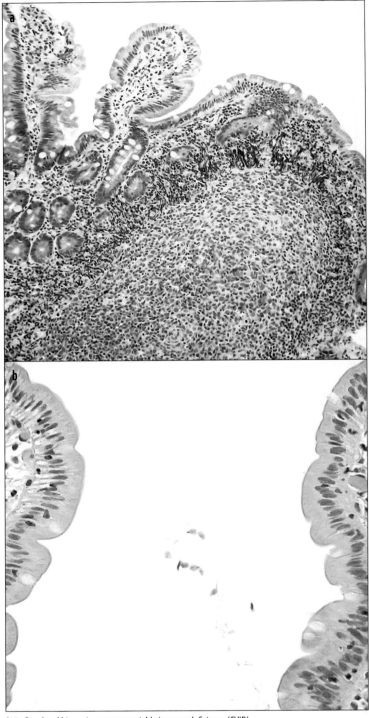

f6.7 Duodenal biopsy in common variable immunodeficiency (CVID)
a Note pronounced lymphoid follicular hyperplasia with germinal center formation
b At higher power, plasma cells are absent; *Giardia* was present on the luminal surface

Pre-B cells are found in lymph nodes and bone marrow where they do not mature normally. Lymph nodes f6.6 and tonsils are rudimentary, lacking germinal centers and plasma cells. An upper endoscopy and duodenal biopsy may be performed for evaluation of chronic diarrhea. When reviewing such a biopsy, particularly in a child or young adult, it is important to look for organisms such as *Giardia*; however, it is also important to ensure that there are plasma cells in the lamina propria. The absence of plasma cells in the intestinal mucosa is distinctly abnormal and should prompt evaluation for a B cell defect.

The responsible gene, *BTK*, is found on the X chromosome. It encodes a tyrosine kinase called Btk (Bruton tyrosine kinase). Genetic testing is clinically available.

Common variable immunodeficiency (CVID)

The clinical severity and age of onset for CVID are somewhat variable; the typical onset is around the second or third decade. Most patients suffer from recurrent upper and lower respiratory tract infections (*Streptococcus pneumoniae, Haemophilus influenzae*, and *Mycoplasma*), intestinal bacterial overgrowth, and intestinal *Giardia lamblia* infection. The development of bronchiectasis is extremely common.

CVID is characterized by low serum immunoglobulin (IgG, IgM, and IgA) and variable T cell deficiency. A normal number of B cells are found in blood and tissue, but these cells lack the capacity to differentiate into plasma cells. Germinal centers are hyperplastic; the typical small bowel morphology f6.7 includes pronounced reactive follicular lymphoid hyperplasia in the face of a distinctly low number of plasma cells.

Multiple genetic defects are associated with CVID, and molecular analysis is not required for diagnosis. Molecular testing in this condition is utilized to exclude other immune deficiencies arising from known genetic defects.

Selective IgA deficiency

Patients with selective IgA deficiency suffer from recurrent respiratory and gastrointestinal bacterial infections, a high incidence of autoimmunity, and are at risk for anaphylaxis due to transfusion of IgA-containing blood products. Decreased levels of IgA is the sole laboratory finding.

Selective IgA deficiency is the most common inherited immunodeficiency disease, affecting around 1 in 700 people. The first identified mutation in this disorder was discovered in the tumor necrosis factor receptor family member "transmembrane activator and calcium-modulator and cyclophilin ligand interactor" (TACI), which mediates isotype switching in B cells. It is unclear if this genetic mutation is the causative defect in this disorder since it has also been identified in patients with CVID.

Hyper-IgE syndrome (Job syndrome)

Hyper-IgE syndrome presents with recurrent staphylococcal infection, coarse facial features, and elevated IgE t6.3. Infections begin in infancy and take the form of staphylococcal skin, lung, and joint infection. Affected persons have abnormally high serum IgE, high levels of specific IgE antistaphylococcal antibody, eosinophilia and eczema. The level of other immunoglobulin classes is normal, but in some cases IgD is elevated along with IgE.

Hyper-IgE syndrome has both autosomal dominant and autosomal recessive forms. Autosomal dominant hyper-IgE syndrome has been related to dominant-negative mutations of the signal transducer and transcription activator 3 (STAT3). 2 patients with autosomal recessive hyper-IgE syndrome have been identified with a homozygous null mutation in tyrosine kinase 2 (TYK2).

t6.3 Immunodeficiency syndromes with abnormal IgE levels

Increased IgE	Wiskott-Aldrich syndrome
	Job syndrome (hyper-IgE syndrome)
	Nezelof syndrome
Decreased IgE	Bruton agammaglobulinemia
	Ataxia-telangiectasia

T cell defects

General features

Defective T cell function is characterized by susceptibility to chronic viral, fungal, and protozoal infections. T cell disorders often engender a certain degree of B cell dysfunction because of their role in orchestrating B cell activities. T cell defects tend to present at an earlier age, often in the neonatal period.

DiGeorge syndrome

In DiGeorge syndrome there is failure of the 3rd and 4th pharyngeal pouches to adequately develop, resulting in a hypoplastic or aplastic thymus and parathyroids. Other structures forming at this stage in embryogenesis are often affected, resulting in anomalies of the great vessels, typical facies (hypertelorism, low set ears, mandibular hypoplasia), bifid uvula, and a higher than usual incidence of esophageal atresia. DiGeorge syndrome frequently presents in the neonatal period as hypocalcemic tetany.

Partial DiGeorge syndrome, resulting from variable hypoplasia of the thymus and parathyroid glands, is more common than complete DiGeorge syndrome in which these structures are entirely aplastic. Complete DiGeorge syndrome accounts

for only 1% of all cases. 1/3 of infants with complete DiGeorge syndrome have the CHARGE sequence (coloboma, heart defect, choanal atresia, retardation of development, genital hypoplasia, and ear anomalies).

Thymic hypoplasia results in a T cell defect. These patients have an increased susceptibility to opportunistic pathogens such as fungi, viruses, and *Pneumocystis jirovecii*, and increased risk of transfusion associated graft vs host disease.

Laboratory findings include deficient numbers of CD3+ cells, thereby creating similar effects on the T cell subsets, CD4+ and CD8+ cells. Secondary to hypoplastic parathyroids, affected individuals also suffer from hypocalcemia and may present with neonatal tetany. Histologically, lymph node paracortical areas are depleted, and poorly developed periarteriolar lymphatic sheaths (PALS) are found in the spleen.

Variable microdeletions involving chromosome 22q11.2 are associated with DiGeorge syndrome, velocardiofacial syndrome (VCFS), Shprintzen syndrome, and occasionally isolated conotruncal cardiac defects, while deletions on 10p13p14 (DiGeorge syndrome II locus) have also been associated with the phenotypic features of DiGeorge syndrome (DiGeorge syndrome II). A dual-probe FISH assay is available for these loci, with a sensitivity of ~95%. Most will demonstrate a deletion of 22q11, with the deletion of 10p13p14 being rare. DiGeorge syndrome does not display Mendelian inheritance and occurs sporadically. Some cases have been associated with in utero exposure to Accutane.

Severe combined immunodeficiency (SCID)

SCID is a syndrome characterized by decreased or absent T cell function, low or undetectable immunoglobulin levels, and thymic dysplasia. This results in severe, life threatening, immunodeficiency that presents early in life with severe infections, diarrhea, and wasting. If transfused with nonirradiated blood, infants are at risk for graft vs host disease. SCID is only treatable by bone marrow transplantation.

A large number of genetic defects can produce the SCID phenotype. Just over half of cases are X-linked recessive (SCID-X1) and caused by a defect in a polypeptide chain shared by the receptors for IL-2, IL-4, and others. Many of the remaining cases are autosomal recessive and caused by a variety of defects, including deficiency in the enzyme adenosine deaminase (ADA), JAK3 deficiency, purine nucleoside phosphorylase (PNP) deficiency, CD3 deficiency, and RAG1/RAG2 deficiency.

Hyper-IgM syndrome (X-linked immunodeficiency with hyper-IgM)

In the hyper-IgM syndrome, there appears to be impaired isotype class switching in B cells, such that non-IgM antibody classes (IgG, IgA, IgE) are lacking, with compensatory increase in IgM. The lack of IgA and IgG imparts a clinical picture similar to Bruton agammaglobulinemia. Unlike Bruton there is a normal number of circulating B lymphocytes.

An X-linked inherited T cell disorder forms the basis for hyper-IgM syndrome. The defect is in the gene that encodes CD154, the T cell ligand for the B cell receptor CD40.

Wiskott-Aldrich syndrome (WAS)

WAS is an X-linked inherited disorder that presents with the triad of eczema, thrombocytopenia, and immunodeficiency. The immunodeficiency is predominantly humoral in nature, with failure to mount antibody responses to a variety of polysaccharide antigens (T cell independent) and inability to produce an anamnestic response to polypeptide antigens (T cell dependent). Affected individuals have increased susceptibility to infection by pneumococci and other encapsulated bacteria, *Pneumocystis jirovecii*, and herpesvirus. In addition, there is a 12% incidence of fatal malignancies.

The platelets are morphologically small and functionally deficient. It has also been noted that there is loss of the CD43 antigen on circulating leukocytes and platelets, and there is a reduced number of circulating CD3+ T cells.

The *WAS* gene is located on the X chromosome. A variety of mutations may occur in *WAS*, some producing Wiskott-Aldrich syndrome, and others producing X-linked thrombocytopenia and X-linked congenital neutropenia. Wiskott-Aldrich syndrome protein (WASP) refers to the product of the *WAS* gene. WASP is found mainly within hematopoietic cells and appears to be responsible for the cytoskeletal malleability that is necessary for physiologic activities.

Ataxia-telangiectasia

Ataxia-telangiectasia (Louis-Bar syndrome) is characterized by cerebellar ataxia, oculocutaneous telangiectasia, recurrent sinopulmonary infections, and a high incidence of malignancies. The immunodeficiency is a combined T cell and B cell defect. IgA is usually deficient, and there is impaired antibody response to pneumococcal vaccine. The lifetime risk for malignancy is 38%, and hematolymphoid malignancies account for most of these.

Laboratory abnormalities include deficient IgA, along with very high serum AFP and CEA for unknown reasons. On MRI, the cerebellum is frequently small. There is a radiosensitive assay that determines the survival of lymphoid cells following irradiation, and this is abnormal in >95% of affected individuals.

Ataxia-telangiectasia is an autosomal recessive disease caused by mutations in the *ATM* gene, on 11q22.3. *ATM* encodes the Atm protein kinase, an enzyme involved in DNA repair. An immunoblotting assay is available for the Atm protein in nuclear lysate, as well as assays for Atm kinase activity. Routine cytogenetics can detect the t(7;14) in ~10% of cases, an anomaly that affects the TCR gene and IgH gene.

Chronic mucocutaneous candidiasis

Chronic mucocutaneous candidiasis is a highly selective defect in T cell immunity to candidal infection that leads to chronic, recalcitrant, mucocutaneous candidal infections. Affected individuals often have associated endocrinopathies and a variety of autoimmune disorders such as autoimmune hemolytic anemia, idiopathic thrombocytopenic purpura, rheumatoid arthritis and autoimmune neutropenia. Mutations are found in autoimmune regulator gene (AIRE), which is localized to chromosome 21q22.3

Duncan disease (X-linked lymphoproliferative disease)

Duncan disease typically presents as a fulminant and often fatal immune response to Epstein-Barr virus (EBV) infection. The result of EBV infection in these patients varies, from fulminant hemophagocytic syndrome to fulminant hepatic failure to the development of a neoplastic B cell proliferation. Even before EBV infection occurs, affected individuals often have a common variable immunodeficiency-like immune system defect. The median survival is ~10 years of age.

Notable laboratory abnormalities include an inverted CD4:CD8 ratio in the peripheral blood and hypogammaglobulinemia, with or without decreased B-, T-, or NK-subsets. Flow cytometry to measure the surface expression of SAP can be used for screening, but it is not a confirmatory assay.

The underlying genetic abnormality is found in the *SH2D1A* gene, found at Xq25, which codes for an SH2 domain on a signal transducing protein called SLAM-associated protein (SAP). The SAP protein plays an important role in signaling events to activate T- and NK cells. Direct sequence analysis is clinically available.

Neutrophil/phagocytic defects

General features

Defects in phagocytosis lead to particular susceptibility to infections with staphylococci, *E coli*, *S pneumoniae*, *P aeruginosa*, *S marcescens*, and *C albicans*.

Chronic granulomatous disease (CGD)

CGD results from defective intracellular oxidative killing of ingested organisms, most commonly resulting from deficiency of NADPH oxidase. The disease is characterized by chronic suppurative infections with catalase positive bacteria, especially staphylococci, enterobacter, and aspergillus. Such individuals almost never have streptococcal infections. Common sites of infection include the lung, skin and bone, associated with unusual organisms such as *Serratia*. At the sites of infection, there is extensive granuloma formation.

The screening test is the nitroblue tetrazolium (NBT) test, in which phagocytic cells with normal oxidative function can convert the yellow dye to a blue product. Oxidative burst can also be measured by chemiluminescence or flow cytometry. Affected leukocytes are also deficient in C3b receptors. Red cells often bear the McLeod phenotype (absence of Kell antigen, Kx).

CGD has been associated with several genetic defects. About 65% of cases have X-linked inheritance and are caused by genetic defects that encode gp91, a component of the cytochrome p245 molecule. The remaining cases have autosomal recessive inheritance and a variety of genetic defects.

Chédiak-Higashi syndrome

Chédiak-Higashi is an autosomal recessive condition that presents as neutropenia, recurrent infection, thrombocytopenia, and oculocutaneous albinism. Some patients demonstrate peripheral nerve defects and periodontal disease. The basic abnormality is defective degranulation, resulting in severe pyogenic infections. In late stages, an accelerated phase may develop, characterized by lymphoma-like proliferations within viscera.

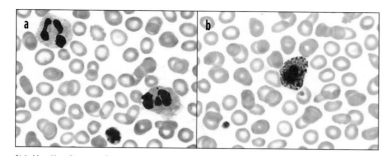

f6.8 May-Hegglin anomaly
a Prominent Döhle bodies within granulocytes, in addition to an enlarged platelet
b Döhle body within a basophil

Affected patients demonstrate normal immunoglobulin levels but mild neutropenia and platelet dysfunction. Granulocytes, lymphocytes, and monocytes show giant cytoplasmic granules, representing abnormally fused primary and secondary granules. The underlying defect is an autosomal recessive mutation in the lysosomal trafficking regulator (*CHS1/LYST*) gene at 1q42.1-2

Other neutrophil/phagocyte defects

May-Hegglin anomaly is an autosomal dominant condition manifesting as Döhle-like bodies in granulocytes and monocytes, variably sized platelets, and thrombocytopenia f6.8. The Döhle-like bodies can be abolished by addition of ribonuclease. About half of patients have an abnormal bleeding history, but bleeding complications have only been documented when the platelet count falls below 80,000. Platelet aggregation studies are usually normal, and there does not appear to be much of an immune defect.

Alder-Reilly anomaly is mainly a morphologic finding. It is an autosomal dominant condition manifesting as large azurophilic granules resembling toxic granulation in all white blood cells. There is an association with mucopolysaccharidoses.

Pelger-Huët anomaly is an autosomal dominant disorder with dysfunctional segmentation of neutrophils. Bilobed neutrophils are seen rather than normally segmented forms. In homozygotes, monolobated neutrophils (Stodtmeister cells) are seen. Functionally, the cells are normal.

Jordan anomaly is characterized by vacuolization of leukocyte cytoplasm by fat vacuoles.

Complement deficiencies

Deficiency of classic pathway components (C1q, C2, C4) is primarily manifested by autoimmune phenomena such as lupus.

Deficiency of C2 and C3 leads to recurrent infections with Gram+ encapsulated organisms. C3 deficiencies are also associated with Gram– septicemia.

Deficiency of membrane attack complex components (C5-C9), also referred to as terminal complement components, leads to recurrent serious systemic infections, especially due to *N meningitidis* and *N gonorrhea*.

C1 esterase inhibitor (C1 Inh) deficiency & hereditary angioedema (HAE)

Angioedema refers to abrupt-onset of swelling within skin and mucous membranes, including that of the upper aerodigestive tract and gastrointestinal tract. The swelling is nonpruritic, nonpitting and usually nonerythematous. Many of these features contrast with urticaria, swelling that is restricted to skin, erythematous, and pruritic. The distinction is confusing, because most cases of urticaria are accompanied by angioedema (called urticaria/angioedema), whereas true angioedema occurs without urticaria.

A variety of conditions cause angioedema. Angioedema that is accompanied by urticaria is usually caused by allergy. Isolated angioedema, however, is found only in a small number of circumstances. These include ACE inhibitor therapy, NSAID or aspirin therapy, acquired C1 Inh deficiency (autoimmune-mediated), and inherited C1 Inh deficiency. Inherited C1 esterase inhibitor (C1 Inh) deficiency is an autosomal dominant disorder also called *hereditary angioedema (HAE).*

Classic HAE displays a fairly characteristic temporal and spatial pattern of edema episodes. On average, women have more severe disease than men, and patients with an early onset of symptoms have more severe disease than those with late onset. For most with HAE the pattern is as follows: a symptom-free infancy and early childhood is followed by the onset of clinical symptoms in late childhood or adolescence. After onset, the disease persists for the life of the patient, with critical and inter-critical periods. With regard to the spatial pattern, swelling is seen most consistently in the skin (upper extremity more than lower) and intestinal tract (causing abdominal pain episodes). Laryngeal edema, though classic and potentially lethal, is present in only ~1% of episodes but has a lifetime incidence of ~50%. Facial swelling is rare, and while there is swelling of the soft palate and uvula, it spares the tongue.

In the past, acute episodes were treated with infusions of donor plasma; however, recombinant C1 inhibitor concentrate became available in 2008 and is now the first line therapy for these patients. 2 other first line therapies include a kallikrein inhibitor (ecallantide) and a bradykinin B2 receptor (icatibant) antagonist. Ecallantide is a first line therapy for acute laryngeal edema or acute gastrointestinal attacks and blocks the production of bradykinin by inhibiting plasma kallikrein. Icatibant is structurally similar to bradykinin and competitively antagonizes the bradykinin B2 receptor. Androgenic agents (danazol, oxandrolone and methyltestosterone) are used as prophylaxis to prevent relapse. These agents may be effective because they increase levels of aminopeptidase P, which inactivates kinins, or by increasing hepatic production of C1 INH or some other undetermined mechanism.

There are 2 major forms of HAE, one in which C1 Inh is absent (type I) and another in which C1 Inh is present but functionally defective (type II). A third type of HAE has been described that is not associated with C1-INH deficiency, and its underlying mechanism is unknown. Urinary histamine levels and serum C1 levels are elevated during attacks, while serum CH50, C4, and C2 are decreased. Between attacks, C4 is always low, while C2 levels are normal.

Autoimmunity & rheumatologic disease
Pathophysiology
Tolerance

The acquisition of self-tolerance occurs during fetal development in the thymus, a process whereby self-reactive T and B cells are selectively destroyed. Developing T and B cells undergo rearrangement of their TCR and Ig genes with nearly an infinite degree of randomness leading to a large variety of antigenic specificities. In the fetal thymus, however, the entire array of self antigens are presented to developing lymphocytes, and those whose surface TCR or Ig has avidity for the expressed antigens are either removed from the population or rendered ineffective.

Autoimmunity

Autoimmunity occurs when there is a breakdown in self-tolerance, such that an immune reaction is raised against self antigens. The response may be humoral, mediated by circulating autoantibodies, or cellular, mediated by T cells. The major histocompatibility complex (MHC) and encoded human leukocyte antigens (HLA) play a role in autoimmunity, thought to be on the basis of the hapten mechanism. Foreign antigens are presented to lymphocytes on the surfaces of antigen-presenting cells in conjunction with HLA proteins. The hapten theory holds that a foreign antigen closely presented in conjunction with a self HLA antigen may promote the proliferation of lymphocyte clones with sufficient avidity for the self antigen alone that autoimmunity ensues. This may explain the association of certain autoimmune disorders with antecedent infection or drug exposure (drug induced lupus; rheumatic fever).

MHC disease associations

There are a remarkable number of diseases associated with the MHC genes. Most of these are autoimmune in nature. Incomplete penetrance complicates assigning modes of inheritance and predicting who may be affected by disease. Some MHC-associated diseases are monogenic, such as hereditary hemochromatosis and 21-hydroxylase deficiency. Most are polygenic, being influenced by a variety of haplotypes t6.4. The best- and longest-known of these is the association of ankylosing spondylitis with HLA-B27; so strong is the association that a negative test for HLA-B27 essentially excludes the diagnosis from consideration.

t6.4 HLA disease associations

Polygenic disease	MHC gene association
Hereditary hemochromatosis	HLA-A3
21-hydroxylase deficiency	HLA-C4
Ankylosing spondylitis	HLA-B27
Behçet disease	HLA-B51
Celiac sprue	HLA-DQ2, DQ8 (specific alleles: DRB1*0301, DQB1*0201, DQA1*0501, DRB1*0701, DQB1*0201, DQA1*0501)
Diabetes mellitus (DM), type 1	Increased incidence of DM: HLA-DR3 or DR4, (specific alleles: DQB1*0302, DQA1*0301); (specific alleles with decreased incidence: DRB1*1501, DQB1*0602)
Multiple sclerosis	HLA-DRB1; HLA-DQB1 (specific alleles: DRB1*1501, DQB1*0602, DQA1*0102)
Narcolepsy	HLA-DQ6 (specific allele: DQB1*0602)
Rheumatoid arthritis (RA)	HLA-DR4 (specific alleles: DRB1*0401; DRB1*0404; DRB1*0405; DRB1*0408)

Predisposing factors

Autoimmune diseases are most prevalent in women of reproductive age. Exceptions worth noting are ankylosing spondylitis, which affects males more often than females, and Sjögren syndrome, which affects postmenopausal females. In addition, several diseases, most notably rheumatoid arthritis (RA), are typically more severe when they affect males.

Triggering agents include both microorganisms and medications. Infection with Coxsackie B virus is thought to provoke some cases of insulin dependent diabetes mellitus (IDDM), while hepatitis B viral (HBV) infection can trigger polyarteritis nodosum (PAN), and *K pneumonia* infection may provoke ankylosing spondylitis. The drug methyldopa can lead to autoimmune hemolytic anemia, and penicillamine is linked to systemic vasculitis. Procainamide, hydralazine, & isoniazid are associated with drug induced lupus.

Notes on laboratory testing
General laboratory abnormalities in autoimmune disease

Common findings in these patients include anemia of chronic disease and elevation of acute phase reactants. It is usual to find normochromic, normocytic anemia. Platelets may be elevated, as an acute phase reactant, or reduced because of immune thrombocytopenic purpura. There may be leukocytosis or leukopenia, and lupus in particular is associated with lymphopenia. The aPTT may be prolonged if there is a lupus anticoagulant.

Markers of injury specific to the targeted organ are abnormal. For example, liver function tests are abnormal in autoimmune hepatitis, thyroid function tests are abnormal in Hashimoto thyroiditis, and creatinine levels are raised in glomerulonephritis caused by a myriad of immune mediated diseases.

Nonspecific inflammatory markers include CRP, ESR, ferritin, and fibrinogen. These are sensitive markers that can be used to exclude an inflammatory condition such as systemic autoimmune disease. Furthermore, the ESR has been used to monitor disease activity in autoimmune conditions such as rheumatoid arthritis. Complement levels can serve as markers of disease activity in immune complex deposition disorders such as lupus.

Synovial fluid & synovial tissue analysis

Synovial fluid analysis is discussed on p 61.

The major cytologic patterns observed are mononuclear cell-predominant, neutrophil-predominant, histiocyte-predominant, and pauci-inflammatory. Pauci-inflammatory synovia is typical of degenerative joint disease, in which the predominant features are collagen degeneration and subchondral cysts. The mononuclear pattern is typical of RA and RA-like conditions. Histiocyte-predominant infiltrates are typical of pigmented villonodular synovitis (PVNS) and response to foreign material (eg, prosthesis). Lastly, neutrophil-predominant synovia typifies septic arthritis and gout.

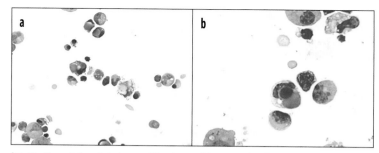

f6.9 LE cells consisting of a leukocyte with an ingested degenerated nucleus

Lupus erythematosus (LE) cells f6.9 are neutrophils with ingested lymphocyte nuclei; the lymphocyte nucleus should be devoid of chromatin detail and stain pink in Wright stained preparations. These may be seen in pleural effusions, joint effusions, or bone marrow aspirates. LE cells provide strong evidence for SLE. The "tart" cell mimics the LE cell but retains chromatin detail, and chromatin stains blue-purple.

Histologically, RA and RA-like conditions (psoriatic arthritis, ankylosing spondylitis, reactive arthritis) demonstrate marked papillary synovial hyperplasia and usually dense infiltrate of lymphocytes and plasma cells. Often there are nodular lymphoid aggregates within which there may be germinal centers. On the synovial surface, there is often fibrin deposition. Note that the histiocyte rich pattern is characterized by mono- and multi-nucleated, typically foamy or pigmented, histiocytes. The presence of well-formed epithelioid granulomas suggests tuberculous arthritis, fungal arthritis, or sarcoidosis.

Autoantibody detection by immunofluorescence

Direct immunofluorescence (DIF) involves incubating cryostat sections of patient tissue with fluorescein-labeled anti-human globulin (AHG). Positive DIF tests confirm the in vivo presence of bound autoantibodies in the patient's tissues. Examples include skin IF (eg, for SLE, dermatitis herpetiformis), and renal IF (for glomerulonephritides).

Indirect immunofluorescence (IIF) involves incubating patient serum with cells/tissue known to contain specific antigens, then adding fluorescein-labeled anti-human globulin (AHG). Positive IIF tests confirm the presence of *circulating autoantibodies*. ANA screening is customarily performed by IIF.

Antinuclear antibodies (ANA)

ANA may be detected by IIF, incubating patient serum with HEp-2 cells. Patient serum is screened at a starting dilution of 1:40. After incubation, the slides are rinsed and then fluorescein-labeled AHG and counterstain are added. The slides are examined using a fluorescence microscope for presence and pattern of fluorescence both in the mitotically active and resting cells f6.10 t6.5. All positives are repeated using serial dilutions to determine the titer of the autoantibody.

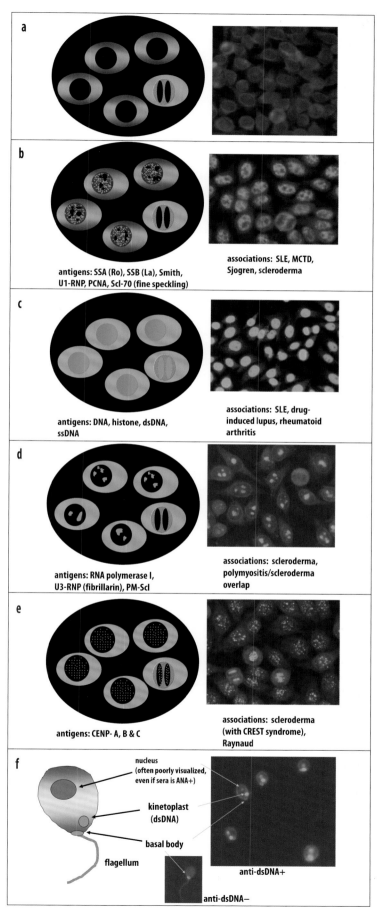

f6.10 ANA patterns: a negative, b speckled, c homogeneous, d nucleolar, e centromere f anti-dsDNA quantitation with *Crithidia luciliae*

t6.5 ANA patterns

Fluorescent staining pattern	Antigen specificity & disease associations
Homogeneous or peripheral (rim pattern), mitoses +	Fluorescent mitotic figures distinguish this from a finely speckled pattern
	Homogeneous pattern: indicate antibodies to ssDNA & histone
	Rim pattern: indicate anti-dsDNA, which are antibodies to nuclear envelope antigens or lamins
	Disease associations: suggestive of SLE, especially if titer is high. Low titer homogeneous pattern: Sjögren syndrome, mixed connective tissues disease (MCTD) & rheumatoid arthritis
	Rim pattern: Primary biliary cirrhosis, chronic liver disease, drug induced SLD
Speckled (mitoses−)	Anti-Sm, RNP, Scl-70, Ro/SS-A, La/SS-B, PCNA (extractable nuclear antigens)
	Disease associations: this pattern occurs in CREST, SLE, mixed connective tissue disease (MCTD), Sjögren syndrome, rheumatoid arthritis & scleroderma
Nucleolar (mitoses−)	Antibodies to RNA polymerase I & proteins of small nucleolar RNP complex (fibrillin, hU3-55K, Mpp10) Th/To, B23, PM-Scl & NOR-90
	Disease associations: Scleroderma
Centromere (mitoses+ in centromeric pattern)	Antibodies to centromeres of chromosomes, specifically on active centromere proteins: CENP-A, CENP-B, CENP-C
	Disease associations: CREST (50-80% patients are positive), idiopathic Raynaud phenomenon (25% patients are positive)

CREST= syndrome of calcinosis, Raynaud, esophageal sclerosis, sclerodactyly & telangiectasia

The ANA test has sensitivity for lupus of around 99%; thus, a negative ANA virtually excludes systemic lupus erythematosus (SLE). ANA is not specific for SLE, however, and specificity depends upon both pretest probability and titer. ~20% of normal adults have an ANA titer of 1:40, and up to 5% have a positive ANA with a titer of 1:160. When a cutoff titer of 1:40 is used, the specificity is around 80%. When 1:160 is used, the specificity is around 95%. The number of false positives increases with age. Non-SLE conditions associated with a positive ANA t6.6 include other autoimmune diseases (Sjögren syndrome, scleroderma, rheumatoid arthritis), multiple sclerosis, infection, malignancy, and fibromyalgia.

t6.6 Frequency of ANA in various conditions

Condition	Approximate frequency (%)
Systemic lupus erythematosus	≈100%
Progressive systemic sclerosis	95
Polymyositis/dermatomyositis	60
Sjögren syndrome	60
Drug induced lupus	100 (by definition)
Mixed connective tissue disease	100 (by definition)
Antiphospholipid antibody syndrome	40
Rheumatoid arthritis	40
Normal adults	10 (at cutoff of 1:80)

When a positive ANA is detected, additional testing can help confirm the diagnosis of SLE, particularly testing for anti-double stranded (ds) DNA, anti-Smith (Sm), and antiphospholipid antibodies; however, these tests have lower sensitivity for SLE. Both anti-dsDNA and anti-Sm antibodies are highly specific markers for SLE and an increase in the titer of anti-dsDNA is predictive of disease flare. Anti-dsDNA is found in 70-95% of SLE cases while anti-Sm, antiribonucleoprotein (RNP), Anti-SS-A/Ro and Anti-SS-B/La are each found in only 30-40% of active cases of SLE.

Other ANAs may point to non-SLE collagen vascular diseases. High titer anti-RNP (>1:10,000) antibodies are characteristic of mixed connective tissue disease (MCTD), particularly if unaccompanied by other ANAs. Anti-RNP is commonly seen in SLE, but titers are usually modest. Anti-SS-A/Ro & Anti-SS-B/La antibodies present with negative dsDNA & Sm are compatible with Sjögren syndrome. Anti-Scl-70 (anti-topoisomerase 1) is seen exclusively in progressive systemic sclerosis (PSS). Anti-centromere antibodies are strongly suggestive of CREST syndrome (calcinosis, Raynaud, esophageal sclerosis, sclerodactyly & telangiectasia) and are occasionally seen in PSS and Raynaud syndrome. Drug induced lupus is usually negative for dsDNA, Sm, and RNP but is characterized by positive ANA and antihistone antibodies directed at the H2A-H2B dimer complex.

The terms "extractable nuclear antigens" and "signal recognition particles" refer to subgroups of ANAs. Extractable nuclear antigens include Smith (Sm), ribonucleoprotein (RNP), SSA (Ro), and SSB (La). They are called extractable because they are extractable in neutral buffers. Signal recognition particles (SRP) include Jo-1 and PM/Scl. SRPs are strongly associated with inflammatory myositis.

Anti-dsDNA detection by immunofluorescence relies upon the presence of dsDNA in the kinetoplast of the organism *Crithidia luciliae*. Anti-dsDNA can be detected by IIF assay using patient serum and the substrate *Crithidia luciliae*.

Antibodies to cytoplasmic constituents

Screening for antibodies to cytoplasmic constituents is performed by IIF using rat tissue as substrate. Patient serum diluted to 1:40 is incubated with prepared tissues consisting of rat liver, kidney, and stomach which are "sandwiched" together. After washing, fluorescein-labeled AHG and counterstain are added to the slide. The slide is examined for fluorescence t6.7 and all positives are titered. In certain instances, this approach has been replaced with ELISA.

t6.7 Cytoplasmic antibodies

Cytoplasmic antibody	Fluorescent staining pattern	Disease associations
Anti-mitochondrial antibody (AMA)	Cytoplasm of gastric parietal cells, renal tubular cells & hepatocytes	Primary biliary cirrhosis
Anti-smooth muscle antibody (ASMA)	Gastric smooth muscle & renal parenchymal arteries	Autoimmune hepatitis
Antiparietal antibody (APA)	Gastric parietal cells	Pernicious anemia, atrophic gastritis
Anti-liver kidney microsomal (LKM)	Cytoplasm of hepatocytes & renal tubular cells	Autoimmune hepatitis
p-ANCA	Perinuclear staining of neutrophils	Primary sclerosing cholangitis, Ulcerative colitis, microscopic polyangiitis, polyarteritis nodosum (PAN)
c-ANCA	Cytoplasmic staining of neutrophils	Wegener granulomatosis, microscopic polyangiitis

Anti-mitochondrial antibody (AMA) demonstrates reactivity with the cytoplasm of gastric parietal cells, renal tubular cells, and hepatocytes. AMA is directed against a mitochondrial antigen from the inner mitochondrial membrane, called M2, which is thought to be dihydrolipoamide acetyltransferase, a component of the pyruvate dehydrogenase enzyme complex. AMA is associated with primary biliary cirrhosis (PBC). Anti-M2 mitochondrial antibodies are found in ~90% of patients with PBC and is highly (~95-99%) specific. M1 has been found in syphilis, M5 in collagen vascular diseases, M6 in isoniazid induced hepatitis, and M7 in cardiomyopathy.

Anti-smooth muscle antibody (ASMA) produces a reaction with the smooth muscle of the gastric tissue and renal arterioles in the rat tissue "sandwich." Anti-liver kidney microsomal (anti-LKM) antibody reacts with the cytoplasm of hepatocytes and renal tubular epithelial cells. Both ASMA and anti-LKM are associated with autoimmune hepatitis.

Antineutrophil cytoplasmic antibody (ANCA) refers to a pattern of reactivity obtained when patient sera are incubated with alcohol-fixed neutrophils. The IIF technique involves incubating patient serum with alcohol-fixed neutrophils, adding fluorescein-labeled AHG and counterstain. The slide is examined for presence and type (cytoplasmic or perinuclear) of fluorescence. All positive ANCA results are titered, and testing for ANAs is performed on all positives to exclude a false positive ANCA due to the presence of ANAs. Cytoplasmic ANCA (cANCA) appears as a cytoplasmic granular pattern with perinuclear accentuation. The cANCA antibody has been demonstrated to have antiproteinase 3 (PR3) specificity. cANCA is positive in ~90% of Wegener granulomatosis. It is highly specific (95-99%) for Wegener, and c-ANCA titers can be used to monitor disease activity. Perinuclear ANCA (pANCA) is characterized by predominantly perinuclear immunofluorescence, and has predominantly antimyeloperoxidase (MPO) activity. pANCA is less specific than cANCA but still has clinical utility, since it is seen in a small number of disorders: microscopic polyangiitis (MPA), polyarteritis nodosum (PAN), primary sclerosing cholangitis (PSC) and ulcerative colitis (UC).

Detection of antithyroid antibodies by immunofluorescence is similar. Incubate serum with cryostat sections of thyroid and fluorescein-labeled AHG. Fluorescence that highlights follicular epithelial cell cytoplasm but does not stain the nuclei is consistent with antithyroid peroxidase (anti-microsomal) antibody. Fluorescence that highlights follicular content on methanol fixed tissue is consistent with antithyroglobulin. Hashimoto thyroiditis is characterized by anti-microsomal and antithyroglobulin antibodies. Long-acting thyroid stimulating (LATS) antibody is not identified in Hashimoto but is instead a feature of Graves disease. A subset of Graves disease is found in association with anti-microsomal or antithyroglobulin antibodies.

Automated methods for autoantibody detection

Automated techniques such as EIA are supplanting fluorescence-based testing in many laboratories. The main advantage is ease of use and interpretation, and many of the antibodies detectable by IIF have now been developed on this platform t6.8. In the typical scenario, patient serum is incubated in a well that is coated with reagent antigen. Dilutions are carried out by the instrument. Bound antibodies are detected via enzyme linked anti-human immunoglobulin. The main disadvantage of the EIA techniques is suboptimal specificity.

t6.8 Review of clinically useful autoantibodies & specificities

Antibody	Clinical utility
Anti-dsDNA	Also called anti-native DNA, has high specificity for SLE. The substrate, *Crithidia luciliae*, is a flagellate with a giant mitochondrion that contains double stranded DNA concentrated in an area called the kinetoplast. Antibodies to ssDNA do not react with *C luciliae*.
Anti-Jo1	Also called anti-tRNA synthetase Polymyositis (PM), especially PM with pulmonary fibrosis
Antihistone	High specificity for drug induced systemic lupus; associated drugs include hydralazine, procainamide, isoniazid, dilantin, methyldopa & penicillin
Extractable nuclear antigens	A number of antigens, the so-called extractable nuclear antigens (ENAs), are present in the extract of calf thymus. ENAs typically give a speckled pattern on fluorescent ANA testing. ENAs include Smith, ribonucleoprotein (RNP), SS-A (Ro) & SS-B(La).
Anti-Smith (Sm)	Virtually diagnostic of SLE
Anti-RNP	Mixed connective tissue disease (MCTD), especially if ANA is negative
Anti-nucleolar	Scleroderma (PSS)
Anti-SS-B /anti SS-A	SS-A (Ro) is present in 70% of patients with Sjögren syndrome & 30% of patients with SLE. SS-B(La) is present in 50% of patients with Sjögren & 15% of patients with SLE. Anti-SS-A/SS-B are highly prevalent in neonatal lupus. Patients who are ANA+, SS-A+ but SS-B− are very likely to have lupus nephritis.
Anti-mitochondrial (AMA)	AMA is detected in 85% of patients with primary biliary cirrhosis (PBC). AMA is reactive with the cytoplasm of parietal cells of the stomach & renal tubular cells in the mouse stomach/kidney substrate.
Anti-smooth muscle (ASMA)	Lupoid (autoimmune) hepatitis is characterized by titers of >1:80. ASMA are specifically directed at F-actin. ASMA are detected on the mouse stomach/kidney substrate where they are reactive with the muscle underlying the gastric mucosa.
Anti-LKM	Autoimmune hepatitis
Anti-microsomal	High specificity (90%) & sensitivity (95%) for Hashimoto disease, although up to 50% of patients with Graves disease will have antibodies.
Antiendomysial antibody	Endomysin is present in the reticular investment of muscle fibers. Antiendomysial antibodies are IgA antibodies. They are highly sensitive & specific for celiac sprue & dermatitis herpetiformis. Antibody titers respond to a gluten-free diet.
Antigliadin	Celiac sprue
Anti-tissue transglutaminase (tTG)	Celiac sprue
Anti-GBM	Goodpasture syndrome; the epitope is the M2 subunit of type IV collagen (GBM = glomerular basement membrane)
Anti-IF	Polymyositis/dermatomyositis (IF = intermediate filament)
Anti-Scl-70	Anti-Scl-70 antibody is an antitopoisomerase Ig seen in 20% of patients with scleroderma
Anti-PM1	Overlap syndrome with overlapping features of scleroderma & dermatomyositis
cANCA	High specificity for Wegener syndrome; cANCA is antiproteinase 3 (PR3)
pANCA	Microscopic polyangiitis, Churg-Strauss
Anti-thyroglobulin	Hashimoto disease
Thyroid-stimulating antibody	Also called LATS, it is present in 90% of individuals with Graves disease
Anti-RNA polymerase 3	Scleroderma (PSS)
Anti-topoisomerase (Scl-70)	Scleroderma (PSS)
Anti-ribosomal P	PM, DM
Rheumatoid factor (RF)	Rheumatoid arthritis
Anti-CCP	Rheumatoid arthritis

Other tests for autoimmune diseases

Rheumatoid factor (RF) is an autoantibody that binds to the Fc portion of the IgG molecule. While an excellent marker for rheumatoid arthritis (RA), RF can be found in healthy adults and a wide range of non-RA disease conditions. The most common non-RA conditions in which RF is found include other rheumatologic diseases, chronic infection, acute viral infection, and hematolymphoid neoplasms. In such conditions, RF is often of low affinity and of the IgM isotype. When more than 1 isotype of RF is present, specificity is higher. RF is detected by a variety of methods sensitive to the formation of antigen-antibody complexes between RF and IgG. Agglutination assays using sheep red blood cells or latex particles coated with IgG particles are commonly used. Agglutination assays are generally reported as a titer (the lowest titer that produces agglutination). Nephelometry and ELISA are usually reported in international units (IU). With the ELISA assays, the isotype (IgM, IgG, IgA) can be determined.

Anticitrullinated protein (anti-CCP) antibodies have greater specificity and sensitivity for RA than RF. Anti-CCP antibodies are usually detected by ELISA. One second generation ELISA test claims 98% specificity with 70% sensitivity for the diagnosis of RA. These antibodies recognize the proteins with the amino acid citrulline, the result of posttranslational modification of arginine; citrulline is found in a variety of connective tissue proteins, including filaggrin (anti-CCP sometimes called antifilaggrin), vimentin, and collagen.

Angiotensin converting enzyme (ACE) is an enzyme that is predominantly tissue bound (>90%) in the endothelial membranes of the body and much lower levels are present in plasma. Both the testes and lungs are tissues with high concentrations of ACE. In pulmonary endothelium it functions to convert angiotensin I to angiotensin II, the active form of the hormone. ACE is an extremely useful test in the evaluation of patients with suspected sarcoidosis, in which it is nearly always elevated when the disease is active. The more organs involved and more active granulomas are present, the higher the elevations of ACE levels. More mature and inactive granulomas produce lower amounts of ACE. Inactive sarcoidosis is associated with normal levels of ACE. Other causes of elevated ACE are primary biliary cirrhosis (PBC), Gaucher disease, and leprosy. All of these have in common the formation of granulomas; however, most other granulomatous diseases are not associated with an elevated ACE.

Autoimmune diseases

Systemic lupus erythematosus (SLE)

SLE is a fairly common disorder with protean manifestations, entering into the differential diagnosis of a multitude of clinical presentations. Disease activity waxes and wanes, and disease activity can generally be tracked by complement levels, reflecting the immune complex nature of the disease. Therapy primarily involves immunosuppression.

Like most autoimmune conditions, females are disproportionately affected, with the female to male ratio ~8-9:1. Most patients are initially diagnosed between the ages of 15 and 45 years. The overall prevalence in the population is nearly 1%, with ~3-fold greater prevalence in African Americans.

Presentation is variable from patient to patient t6.9, and many patients initially or perpetually have limited manifestations. The 1982 American College of Rheumatology criteria, revised in 1997 t6.10, were intended for research purposes; 4 of 11 must be fulfilled for the diagnosis of SLE. In practice nearly half of patients diagnosed with SLE fail to fulfill these criteria. A negative ANA test essentially excludes lupus, but ANA is not specific for lupus, and other autoantibodies may be present t6.11.

t6.9 Frequency of findings in SLE

Finding	Frequency (%)
Rash	90
Arthralgia	75
Neurologic	65
Serositis	60
Hematologic (anemia, thrombocytopenia)	60
Raynaud phenomenon	45
Vasculitis	40
Glomerulonephritis	30
Endocarditis	15

t6.10 1997 update of the 1982 criteria for systemic lupus erythematosus

1. Malar rash
2. Discoid rash
3. Photosensitivity
4. Oral ulcers
5. Arthritis (involving 2 or more peripheral joints)
6. Serositis (pleuritis, pericarditis)
7. Renal dysfunction (proteinuria >0.5 g/day or >3+ or cellular casts)
8. Neurologic dysfunction (seizures or psychosis)
9. Hematologic disorder (hemolytic anemia with reticulocytosis or leukopenia <4,000/mm^3 or lymphopenia <1,500/mm^3 or thrombocytopenia <100,000/mm^3)
10. Autoantibodies (anti-dsDNA or anti-Sm or antiphospholipid antibodies [IgG or IgM anticardiolipin antibodies or lupus anticoagulant] or false positive serologic test for syphilis known to be positive for ≥6 months & confirmed by *Treponema pallidum* immobilization or the fluorescent treponemal antibody absorption test)
11. Antinuclear antibody (ANA): positive with an elevated titer in the absence of drugs associated with drug induced lupus

t6.11 Autoantibodies in SLE

Antibody	Frequency in SLE (%)
ANA	>99
Anti-dsDNA	40-90
Anti-single strand DNA	70
Anti-Ro (SSA)	24-60
Anti-La (SSB)	9-35
Anti-Sm	15-35
Anti-RNP	35
Anticardiolipin and/or LAC	25
Anti-ribosomal P	10

Prominent among the manifestations are *constitutional symptoms*, including fatigue, fevers, and weight loss. *Cutaneous manifestations* are present in most patients, classically consisting of the butterfly pattern facial rash distributed over the malar and nasal prominences and sparing of the nasolabial folds. A wide variety of other cutaneous and mucosal manifestations may be observed, including discoid skin lesions, which generally occur in a separate subset of patients who may have limited disease (discoid lupus). Scarring alopecia is a typical feature of discoid lupus. Lupus panniculitis presents as tender firm subcutaneous nodules. Mucosal ulcerations may occur within the buccal mucosa. Cutaneous eruptions are photo-sensitive. *Arthralgia* is often accompanied by nonerosive arthritis, distributed over the proximal interphalangeal and metacarpophalangeal joints of the hands. In the *heart*, the most common finding is pericarditis, a manifestation of the widespread serositis that typifies SLE. Endocarditis is a well known complication, but it has only recently become apparent that endarteritis, with premature atherosclerosis, is a common complication as well. Endocarditis in SLE (Libman-Sacks endocarditis) consists of subendocardial fibrous lesions usually found on the atrial aspect of the mitral valve leaflets. Lupus may cause conduction disturbances, most commonly an atrioventricular block, particularly in neonatal cases. *Serositis (pleuritis)* is the most frequent pulmonary manifestation. *Anemia* is found in ~50% of patients and may be related to anemia of chronic disease and/or direct antiglobulin test (DAT) (Coombs) positive hemolytic anemia. *Thrombocytopenia* is found in ~30% of cases and reflects immune thrombocytopenic purpura. Lastly, leukopenia, reflecting primarily *lymphopenia*, is sometimes found and should be present on ≥2 or more occasions to meet the outlined criteria. SLE must be considered in a wide range of *neuropsychiatric* presentations. The most common manifestation is cognitive dysfunction, followed by psychosis, seizures, stroke, and transverse myelitis. Antiphospholipid antibodies, including anticardiolipin antibody and lupus anticoagulant, are nearly always present in patients with CNS findings. Neuropathologic studies in patients with CNS lupus have found a bland, noninflammatory vasculopathy involving the small vessels of the cerebral cortex. Actual vasculitis is rare.

A common and dreadful complication is lupus nephritis. Clinical glomerulonephritis is found in up to 75% of patients during the course of the illness, and histopathologic findings are present in up to 100%. Mesangial deposition of immune complexes is believed to be the earliest change and, when isolated, represents the most benign form of lupus nephritis. Deposition provokes mesangial cell proliferation and a histopathologic picture resembling mesangial glomerulonephritis. Subendothelial immune complex deposition results in a global proliferative and exudative lesion. Subepithelial immune complex deposition results in a membranous-type glomerulonephritis with nephrotic-range proteinuria.

The question of whether pregnancy exacerbates lupus is unsettled, but there is no doubt that lupus increases the likelihood of unfavorable fetal outcome. There is a higher likelihood of fetal loss, premature labor, preeclampsia, intrauterine growth restriction, and fetal distress in pregnant women with lupus.

Drug induced lupus differs from primary lupus, in that it generally follows a benign course. Agents associated with drug induced lupus include procainamide, hydralazine, quinidine, isoniazid, and interferon-α. Drug induced lupus is notable for a very low incidence of serious visceral manifestations (especially low incidence of renal and neurologic manifestations). It manifests primarily with rash, serositis, and arthritis. It has been noted that the medications associated with drug induced lupus are ones that are metabolized by acetylation, and lupus is induced primarily in patients with a genetic paucity of hepatic N-acyltransferase ("slow acetylators") but patients with high levels of the enzyme ("rapid acetylators") are not protected against developing a positive ANA. Antihistone

antibodies are the hallmark of drug induced lupus and are present in >95% of patients. These are usually directed against the H2A-H2B dimer complex protein of the histone which is more specific than other histone antibodies found in other conditions such as SLE or autoimmune hepatitis.

The differential diagnosis of lupus is broad and includes infections, especially gonococcal and parvoviral. Parvovirus B19 can produce a transient illness that fulfills the diagnostic criteria for SLE, including the presence of diagnostic autoantibodies. Antibodies that have been documented in parvovirus B19 include anti-dsDNA, anti-RNP, and antiphospholipid antibodies.

Rheumatoid arthritis

RA is the most common cause of chronic inflammatory arthritis, but its clinical manifestations extend far beyond the joint space. Extra-articular manifestations include interstitial lung disease, pleuritis, endocarditis, and systemic vasculitis. The overall incidence of RA is 0.5-0.8%, with women affected about twice as often as men, and initial onset of symptoms between the ages of 30 and 50 years. There is an increased incidence of RA in patients with HLA DR4.

RA presents with polyarticular discomfort and constitutional symptoms. Unknown triggers lead to an inflammatory reaction within the subsynovial connective tissue, leading to the accumulation of T cells, B cells, plasma cells, and histiocytes. These eventually organize into a pannus at the periphery of the joint space, where they cause destruction to the articular cartilage, joint capsule, and adjoining tendons. Joint involvement is bilateral and symmetric, and the particular joints affected are highly characteristic. RA typically affects the joints of the wrist, the metacarpophalangeal, metatarsophalangeal, and proximal interphalangeal joints, sparing the distal interphalangeal joints. The spine is usually spared, with the exception of the C1-C2 joint, which may cause major instability requiring external fixation. The large joints are often spared early but may be involved late. Weakening of the joint capsule may lead to cyst formation, such as Bakers cyst near the knee joint. A typical symptom is morning stiffness or "gelling" after extended periods of inactivity. The appearance of the hands is characteristic, with tendon swelling and muscle atrophy combining to produce ulnar deviation of the metacarpophalangeal joints, and angulation of the fingers classically described as swan-neck and boutonnieres deformities.

Extra-articular manifestations are somewhat more common in males and in patients with high-titer RF. These include subcutaneous nodules composed of necrotizing granulomatous lesions, pleuritis, pericarditis, vasculitis, endocarditis, interstitial lung disease, and amyloidosis. Rheumatoid pleuritis and pericarditis have a typical appearance. Fluid samples demonstrate a paucity of mesothelial cells and abundance of fibrinoid material. There may be slender histiocytes, some of which are multinucleated, and neutrophils. The fluid is yellow–green and usually fulfills the Light criteria for an exudate. Glucose levels are low, protein levels high, and pH low, thus entering into the differential diagnosis with empyema. Pleural biopsies show that the mesothelium is effaced and replaced with layers of fibrin surrounded by perpendicularly oriented palisading histiocytes. Essentially, the pleural space has been turned into a large rheumatoid nodule. There may be a variety of hematologic findings, most commonly anemia of chronic disease. The triad of RA, splenomegaly, and neutropenia, classically called Felty syndrome, may be a form of large granular lymphocyte leukemia.

Both the C-reactive protein and ESR are elevated at presentation and may be used to monitor disease activity. RA is a common cause of anemia of chronic disease, and platelets are often mildly elevated as an acute phase reactant. The rheumatoid factor (RF) test is the classic diagnostic test, but up to 30% of patients initially have a negative RF. Furthermore, RF is nonspecific and found in up to 1% of the healthy adult population and a higher number of patients with non-RA conditions such as SLE, Sjögren syndrome, sarcoidosis, lymphoma, and infection. The anti-cyclic citrullinated peptide (anti-CCP) antibody is significantly more specific than RF and with new generation ELISA testing the sensitivity has improved. Synovial fluid analysis is notable for elevated white count with preponderance of neutrophils and low glucose (with negative cultures and no crystals).

Seronegative spondyloarthropathies

The seronegative spondyloarthropathies are a group of distinct entities that have symptoms in common with RA but are RF-negative. These include ankylosing spondylitis, reactive arthritis (previously Reiter syndrome), and psoriatic arthritis. All seronegative spondyloarthropathies are more common in males and in persons with the class I human leukocyte antigen allele HLA B27.

Clinically, ankylosing spondylitis commonly affects the sacroiliac joints and uveal tract. There is a tendency for new bone formation at the site of pannus formation (ankylosis), and the points of tendon insertion are frequently involved (enthesitis). The overall incidence of ankylosing spondylitis is 0.2%, and among those with HLA-B27 the incidence is 2%. Ankylosing spondylitis presents with lower back pain that typically is worse after prolonged inactivity and improved by exercise. Range of motion may be limited by ankylosis.

Psoriatic arthritis occurs in ~5% of patients with psoriasis. Reactive arthritis is a seronegative spondyloarthropathy that is provoked by antecedent mucosal infection, typically urethritis (*Chlamydia*) or gastroenteritis (*Shigella*, *Salmonella*, *Yersinia*, and *Campylobacter*). It was initially described in 1916 by Hans Reiter in a soldier who developed the triad of urethritis, uveitis, and symmetrical arthritis after an episode of dysentery. Later unethical experimentation during the second world war led to his eponymous recognition falling into disfavor.

Celiac disease

Celiac disease has world-wide distribution and may arise at any time after eating begins. Many cases present in the pediatric age group, but new diagnoses are frequently made in the elderly. The disorder is precipitated by gluten ingestion, the major protein in wheat and other grains, causing a sensitivity which induces mucosal damage in the gut and eventual malabsorption.

In the United States, the estimated incidence is 1 in 100. Celiac disease tends to cluster within families, and there is a strong association with HLA-DQ2 and HLA-DQ8. This genetic predisposition is most common in Caucasians of northern European descent, particularly the Welsh. While the link is

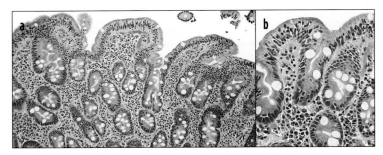

f6.11 Celiac sprue showing a blunted villi, b increased intraepithelial lymphocytes

strong among relatives of affected individuals, it is far from autosomal. Furthermore, while >90% of cases arise in HLA-DQ2/8+ patients, only ~10% of those with this HLA type have disease.

Often, celiac disease arises in patients with other autoimmune conditions. The best known of these associations is with type 1 diabetes mellitus, but there is also a strong association with autoimmune liver disease. There is an increased incidence of celiac disease in patients with IgA deficiency, cystic fibrosis, Turner syndrome, and Down syndrome.

The typical patient presents with malabsorptive diarrhea, but there are a variety of other presentations, including unexplained weight loss, bloating, steaorrhea, idiopathic short stature in children, iron deficiency, folate deficiency, and osteoporosis. Increasingly, patients are identified by screening of high risk populations (first-degree relatives of index cases or patients with other autoimmune conditions).

Celiac disease affects both intestinal and extra-intestinal sites. Histologically, the duodenum is the site of greatest activity f6.11. In fully developed lesions, there is villous atrophy, intraepithelial lymphocytosis, and crypt hyperplasia. Many of those affected have only an increase in intraepithelial lymphocytes without architectural change; however, this finding alone is nonspecific. Furthermore, many with histologic findings have no symptoms. After prolonged inflammation, there is a risk of malnutrition (a common cause of idiopathic short stature and unexplained iron deficiency anemia) and the development of lymphoma (enteropathy-associated T cell lymphoma). Extra-intestinal manifestations include arthritis and dermatitis herpetiformis.

Serologic markers of celiac sprue include antigliadin, antiendomysium, antireticulin and anti-tissue transglutaminase (tTG) antibodies. IgA anti-tTG is considered the best first-line test, the reported sensitivity and specificity being 95% and 90%, respectively. Antiendomysial antibody has sensitivity of ~80-85% but specificity of >99%; it is a more subjective immunofluorescence test than anti-tTG and for that reason is considered a second-line test. By comparison, antigliadin has lower sensitivity and specificity than both assays. Because of the high incidence of IgA antitransglutaminase antibodies in patients with chronic liver diseases (particularly among those with autoimmune liver diseases) the specificity of this antibody in the setting of chronic liver disease is low. There appears to be an increased incidence of IgA deficiency in celiac disease; thus, some authors recommend excluding IgA deficiency first. In cases of known or suspected IgA deficiency, one can test for IgG anti-tTG, but the sensitivity and specificity are not as good as for the IgA test. In serologically murky cases, upper endoscopy with small bowel biopsy is recommended. Antitransglutaminase antibodies, antiendomysial antibodies and antigliadin antibodies vary with exposure to gluten, but none correlates with mucosal recovery in celiac disease. Tests of mucosal absorption, such as the D-xylose absorption test, may be useful in this regard. Transthyretin (a rapidly responsive indicator of nutritional status) correlates very well with mucosal recovery. Lastly, HLA testing may be undertaken with the understanding that nearly all affected individuals have HLA DQ2 or DQ8 but most patients with these alleles are unaffected; thus, only a negative test is informative.

Inflammatory bowel disease

The most useful serologic marker for ulcerative colitis (UC) has been pANCA by IIF. Its sensitivity for UC is ~70% and its specificity 90%. Positive IIF for pANCA is also found in primary sclerosing cholangitis, some cases of autoimmune hepatitis, and microscopic polyangiitis. The particular antigen targeted by pANCA in UC is unknown, so there is not an ELISA-based substitute for IIF testing.

The autoantibodies with promise in diagnosing Crohn disease (CD) include pancreatic antibodies (PAB) and anti-*Saccharomyces cerevisiae* antibody (ASCA). PAB are highly specific (95%) but have low sensitivity, being present in 30% of cases. ASCA is an antibody against the yeast used to make beer and bread, and it can help distinguish irritable bowel syndrome from inflammatory bowel disease. It is found in ~65% of patients with CD and up to 5% of normal adults. It is also found in ~15% of patients with UC and celiac sprue.

The overall performance of autoantibodies fails to provide a viable alternative to endoscopy and biopsy. Even panels of antibodies achieve a sensitivity of only around 80% and do not permit confident distinction of CD from UC. These tests may have utility in sorting out patients with indeterminate colitis and in preventing unnecessary colonoscopy in small children, but this has yet to be proven.

Progressive systemic sclerosis (scleroderma)

Progressive systemic sclerosis (PSS) typically presents with Raynaud phenomenon and scleroderma. Some patients experience widespread disease involving the GI tract, heart, lungs, and kidneys. Leading causes of death include pulmonary hypertension and renal crisis, the latter a form of hypertensive emergency.

The major forms of PSS are diffuse cutaneous PSS (widespread scleroderma and visceral involvement), limited cutaneous PSS (limited scleroderma, limited to no visceral involvement), and localized scleroderma (including, eg, linear scleroderma, morphea).

Diffuse cutaneous PSS is characterized by sclerosis of skin that extends beyond the distal extremities, usually involving both acral and trunk areas, in conjunction with Raynaud phenomenon. There is nail fold capillary dilatation and destruction and tendon friction rubs. Visceral involvement takes the form of interstitial lung disease, oliguric renal failure, diffuse disease of the gastrointestinal tract, and cardiac involvement. Patients with diffuse cutaneous PSS are usually positive anti-Scl-70 and negative anti-centromere antibodies.

Limited cutaneous PSS (CREST syndrome) usually manifests as scleroderma limited to the distal extremities, without cardiac, renal or pulmonary involvement. The manifestations are usually limited to those described by the CREST acronym: calcinosis, Raynaud, esophageal sclerosis, sclerodactyly, and telangiectasia. Dermal sclerosis typically remains confined to the hands and feet but may involve the face and forearms. Raynaud phenomenon often precedes skin changes by several years.

The major autoantibodies associated with PSS, aside from the nonspecific ones such as ANA, include anti-centromere, anti-Scl-70 (antitopoisomerase), anti-U1-RNP (antifibrillarin), anti-RNA polymerase 3, anti-Th/To, and anti-Pm/Scl. Anti-Th/To and anti-Pm-Scl are responsible for anti-nucleolar reactivity identified as specific for PSS. Anti-RNA polymerase 3, anti-U3-RNP, and anti-Scl-70 (antitopoisomerase) are associated with diffuse cutaneous SS. Anti-centromere, anti-Th/To, anti-U1-RNP, and anti-Pm/Scl are associated with limited cutaneous (CREST) SS.

The clinical differential diagnosis includes several unusual disorders of skin, all of which are negative for the PSS-associated autoantibodies. These include scleredema, scleromyxedema, nephrogenic systemic sclerosis, and eosinophilic fasciitis. Each has a sufficiently characteristic clinical setting to render clinical distinction easier than histopathologic distinction. Scleredema is associated with diabetes or *S pyogenes* infection. Scleromyxedema is found in patients with monoclonal gammopathy. Nephrogenic systemic sclerosis arises in patients with renal impairment who are exposed to gadolinium. Lastly, eosinophilic fasciitis is found in association with peripheral blood eosinophilia.

IgG4-related sclerosing disease

For decades, pathologists have been aware of the morphologic similarities amongst an anatomically diverse group of fibroinflammatory lesions, including sclerosing mediastinitis, idiopathic retroperitoneal fibrosis, Riedel thyroiditis, sclerosing cholangitis, orbital pseudotumor, and sclerosing pancreatitis. This entity came into focus in 2001 when Hamano et al reported finding elevated serum IgG4 levels in sclerosing pancreatitis that was successfully treated with corticosteroids; simultaneous with clinical improvement they noted decreasing serum IgG4 levels. Subsequently, an increase in both tissue and serum IgG4 has been documented in many of these morphologically similar conditions, including IgG4 associated cholangitis, autoimmune hepatitis, Sjögren syndrome, nephritis, and retroperitoneal fibrosis. This disease entity is collectively known as IgG4-related systemic disease.

Sclerosing (autoimmune) pancreatitis was first reported in 1961 by Sarles and colleagues, who suggested an autoimmune underpinning. But interest waned, partially because of the apparent rarity of this lesion. The impression of rarity resulted from difficulty in imaging the pancreas, coupled with the disparate nomenclature of subsequent case reports ("lymphoplasmacytic sclerosing pancreatitis," "nonalcoholic duct-destructive pancreatitis," "sclerosing pancreaticocholangitis," "autoimmune chronic pancreatitis"). Later, high resolution imaging techniques made sclerosing pancreatitis re-appear in seemingly epidemic fashion, and in 1995 Yoshida and colleagues described the clinical characteristics of the disease, renaming it "autoimmune pancreatitis." Autoimmune pancreatitis presents as a sonolucent mass, often with segmental

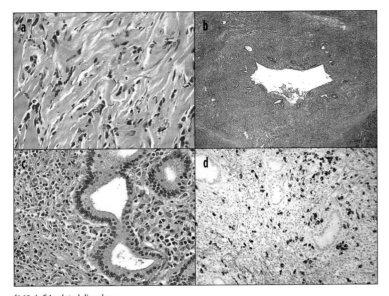

f6.12 IgG4-related disorders
a Idiopathic retroperitoneal fibrosis, consisting of dense collagenous sclerosis in association with an infiltrate of lymphocytes & plasma cells
b Autoimmune pancreatitis, showing ductocentric inflammation
c Autoimmune pancreatitis, showing a dense lymphoplasmacytic inflammatory infiltrate
d Autoimmune pancreatitis, immunohistochemical staining for IgG4

narrowing of the pancreatic duct, and obstructive jaundice; ie, the presentation is similar to that of pancreatic adenocarcinoma. Preoperative distinction of these 2 lesions is possible through fine needle aspiration or core biopsy. Such specimens may display a lymphoplasmacytic infiltrate, rich in IgG4+ plasma cells (>10×-20/40× objective HPF, looking in the densest areas which tend to be periductal). Elevated numbers of IgG4+ plasma cells have also be documented in periampullary biopsies and regional lymph nodes.

While the pancreas is most commonly affected, the liver, biliary tree, salivary glands, lymph nodes, prostate, retroperitoneal soft tissue, and kidneys can also be affected. Biopsies display a lymphoplasmacytic infiltrate, rich in IgG4-producing plasma cells as identified by immunohistochemistry stains. All tend to be tumefactive lesions with infiltrative margins that entrap, surround, and distort anatomic structures and appear histologically as parallel arrays of dense keloidal collagen, nodular lymphoid aggregates, and interstitial plasma cells f6.12.

Elevation of serum IgG4 is found in most (>90%) cases. In normal individuals, IgG4 is present in concentrations lower than any other IgG subclass, representing ~5% of total IgG, with upper limit of normal often reported as 135 mg/dL. However, one study found mild IgG4 elevation in some patients with pancreatic cancer. The level of IgG4 in all of these patients with pancreatic cancer was <200 mg/dL; thus, 135-200 mg/dL may be a range in which to exercise caution.

The importance of recognizing this entity is that patients with IgG4 related systemic disease benefit from corticosteroid therapy and surgery may be avoided.

Autoimmune hepatitis

Autoimmune hepatitis (AIH) has a peak incidence at 35 years old and is more common in females. It is a heterogenous group of disorders with an unknown etiology. The disease has been categorized into Type I and Type II with described subtypes that are still under discussion.

Clinical symptoms may range from asymptomatic to fulminant hepatic failure. Those who present with acute hepatitis complain of nonspecific constitutional symptoms such as fatigue, lethargy, malaise, arthralgias, amenorrhea, nausea, pruritus and anorexia. As the disease progresses they may develop jaundice due to worsening liver function.

Laboratory findings include hypergammaglobulinemia attributed to polyclonally increased IgG and abnormal liver function tests, including prolonged PT/INR and raised AST and ALT, out of proportion to alkaline phosphatase and bilirubin. Viral hepatitis serologies are negative. Circulating autoantibodies differ among the subtypes. In AIH Type I, ANA and anti-smooth muscle antibody (SMA) are typical. 30% of adults and 60% of children with Type I AIH have antibodies to a soluble liver protein (anti-SLP). AIH Type II is characterized by anti-liver kidney microsomal antibody (LKM1), an antibody against CYP 2D6. ANA/ASMA and LKM1 tend to be mutually exclusive, and are rarely both positive in an individual patient. In many cases there is associated extrahepatic autoimmunity, especially ulcerative colitis, arthritis, immune thrombocytopenic purpura (ITP), autoimmune hemolytic anemia (AIHA), thyroiditis, and diabetes.

Histologically, AIH is characterized by chronic portal hepatitis rich in plasma cells, with characteristically brisk limiting plate necrosis. Hepatocyte rosettes are typical, and bile ducts are usually spared.

Primary biliary cirrhosis

Primary biliary cirrhosis (PBC) is commonly diagnosed in asymptomatic patients who are found to have abnormal liver function tests or abnormal cholesterol panel. When symptomatic, the most common complaint is pruritus or fatigue. Jaundice is a late finding and rarely present at the time of diagnosis.

Liver function test abnormalities have a cholestatic pattern, with prominence of alkaline phosphatase and GGT. Median serum bilirubin at diagnosis is 1.0 mg/dL. Anti-mitochondrial antibodies (AMA), subtype M2, are present in >95% of cases and are virtually diagnostic for PBC. The original technique for AMA detection consisted of indirect immunofluorescence using rat kidney, stomach, and liver as substrate. AMA+ sera coarsely stain renal tubules (sparing glomeruli), gastric parietal cells, and hepatocytes. It is important to note that LKM1 reactivity is easy to confuse with AMA reactivity. It was later determined that the AMA target antigens are part of an enzyme housed within the inner mitochondrial membrane. HEp-2 cells may also be used to detect AMA, giving a coarse cytoplasmic reaction (concomitant ANA, which are frequently present, can be determined by this technique). Unlike other autoantibodies, AMA titer provides no additional information and remains stable in individual patients over time. 2 additional antibodies, IgG anti-sp100 and IgG anti-gp210, are highly specific for PBC, though only ~20-30% sensitive. Lastly, polyclonal hyper-immunoglobulin M has been observed in PBC.

Histopathologically, PBC presents as a portal lymphoplasmacytic infiltrate with direct bile duct infiltration and progressive bile duct destruction (chronic nonsuppurative destructive cholangitis).

Autoimmune cholangitis

Autoimmune cholangitis is a chronic cholestatic process with a clinical presentation and histologic features similar to PBC but the AMA is negative. Instead, these patients have serologic findings that are similar to AIH type I and test positive for antinuclear antibodies (ANA) and/or anti-smooth muscle autoantibodies (ASMA). Some have termed this condition AMA-negative PBC. IgG and IgM levels are just slightly elevated.

Primary sclerosing cholangitis (PSC)

PSC typically presents in males with a history of an inflammatory bowel disease. Approximately 50% of patients with PSC have ulcerative colitis (UC), while PSC is seen in only ~5% of patients with UC.

Clinically, PSC presents with fatigue, fever, chills, night sweats, pruritus, and possibly right upper quadrant pain. Patients are found to have elevated alkaline phosphatase, and increased aminotransferases with or without hyperbilirubinemia. ANA or p-ANCA may be positive, but AMA is negative.

Imaging studies are pivotal in diagnosing PSC. Cholangiography demonstrates beading pattern of bile ducts due to focal strictures.

Sjögren syndrome

Sjögren syndrome (SS) is a chronic inflammatory condition that is marked by dryness of the eyes, mouth and other mucous membranes. It may be primary, or it can be associated with other systemic autoimmune diseases (secondary SS), particularly RA, primary biliary cirrhosis, systemic lupus erythematosus (SLE) or systemic sclerosis.

Anti-SS-A/Ro and anti-SS-B/La antibodies are characteristic of SS. The presence of either anti-SS-A/Ro or anti-SS-B/La has a sensitivity and specificity of around 95%. While anti-SS-A/Ro antibodies are seen in ~60% of Sjögren syndrome and 35% of SLE patients, anti-SS-B/La is seen in 40% and 15%, respectively. When anti-SS-A/La is identified with anti-SS-B/LA, this is indicative of primary SS. Neither antibody is useful to follow disease activity.

In certain circumstances, biopsy confirmation of Sjögren syndrome is needed. Minor salivary glands from the lip are usually submitted. Affected glands are infiltrated with aggregates of lymphocytes. Sjögren syndrome is supported by the presence of >1 inflammatory focus/4 mm^2 of salivary tissue, with a focus defined as an aggregate of least 50 mononuclear inflammatory cells.

Vasculitis

Like many autoimmune disorders, the vasculitides can present in nonspecific fashion, and the diagnosis can be missed or delayed. Often systemic vasculitis presents with nonspecific constitutional symptoms or organ dysfunction. One should always consider vasculitis with certain characteristic presentations, including new onset chronic sinusitis in the older adult, unexplained hematuria, pulmonary hemorrhage, palpable purpura, or mononeuritis multiplex. The vasculitis syndromes can be roughly divided into those with fairly precise serologic markers and those without; fortunately, those without serologic markers have highly characteristic clinical features t6.12. As general pathologists, we must be vigilant to identify vasculitis. Skin biopsies, upper airway biopsies, medical lung biopsies, renal biopsies, nerve biopsies, and resections of ischemic tissue, especially bowel, all offer an opportunity to make this diagnosis.

t6.12 Vasculitides

Syndrome	Serologic marker	Clinical features
Giant cell arteritis	None	Older adults
		Temporal headache, tender temporal artery
		May have visual symptoms, jaw claudication, polymyalgia rheumatica
Takayasu arteritis	None	Children & adolescents
		Pulseless disease (decreased arterial pulses)
		Blood pressure difference between extremities
		Angiography diagnostic
Kawasaki syndrome	None	Children
		Fever of ≥4 days duration
		Erythema of palms & soles
		Desquamation within 5 days of fever onset
		Bilateral conjunctivitis
		Cracking of lips & strawberry tongue
		Cervical lymphadenopathy
Cogan syndrome	None	Keratitis
		Vestibulo-auditory symptoms
Behçet disease	None	Oral ulcers, genital ulcers, uveitis; pathergy test positive
Henoch-Schönlein purpura	None	Children
		Lower extremity palpable purpura, abdominal pain, nephritis
Buerger disease	None	Young adult smokers
		Upper extremity ischemia
Polyarteritis nodosum	None/HBV±	Widespread effects, sparing lungs
Microscopic polyangiitis	pANCA	Widespread effects
Churg-Strauss syndrome	pANCA	Widespread effects; eosinophilia
Wegener granulomatosis	cANCA	Widespread effects
Goodpasture	Anti-GBM	Mainly lung & kidneys affected
Cryoglobulinemia	Cryoglobulins	Widespread effects
Syphilis	RPR	Widespread effects, can mimic Takayasu
Rheumatoid or other collagen vascular disease associated	eg, RF, ANA, RPR	Widespread effects

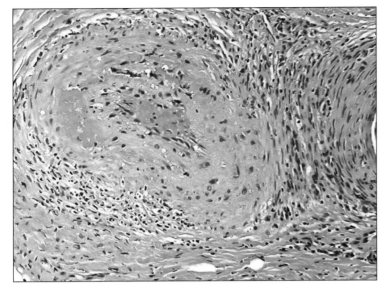

f6.13 Polyarteritis nodosa (PAN) demonstrating the typical lesion, consisting of segmental fibrinoid necrosis of the vessel wall; a similar appearance may be seen in Wegener granulomatosis & microscopic polyangiitis

Polyarteritis nodosa (PAN)

PAN is a multisystem vasculitis or medium-sized arteries that usually spares the lungs. Renal involvement may take the form of cortical infarcts. Mononeuritis multiplex is the usual peripheral nerve presentation. Mesenteric vasculitis may result in "intestinal angina" (abdominal pain provoked by consumption of food) or ischemic bowel. There are multiple cutaneous manifestations, including subcutaneous nodules, cutaneous ulcers, digital necrosis, and livedo reticularis.

Biopsy of nerve or other affected tissue shows segmental fibrinoid necrosis f6.13 of inflamed arterial walls, with a predilection for branch points. The segmental nature of involvement, with active and healing lesions next to normal segments of blood vessel, is highly characteristic of PAN. This is reflected in the typical findings on angiogram, consisting of segmental narrowing and aneurysms.

Laboratory findings include those that indicate chronic inflammation, including normochromic anemia, neutrophilia, hypoalbuminemia, hypergammaglobulinemia, and raised erythrocyte sedimentation rate (ESR). Autoantibodies, including ANA or RF, may be found in 10-40% of patients. There are no diagnostic serologic findings, but a significant minority of patients are seropositive for HBV.

Microscopic polyangiitis (MPA)

MPA was initially thought a variant of PAN, but several important differences were observed that led researchers in the 1950s to recognize MPA as a distinct entity. Chief among these are pulmonary involvement and renal glomerular involvement, with sparing of medium-sized arteries in favor of small arterioles and venules. Later, the presence of pANCA came to define MPA as one of the ANCA-associated vasculitides, along with Wegener granulomatosis (WG) and Churg-Strauss. In its classic form, MPA causes a systemic vasculitic syndrome dominated by the effects of pulmonary capillaritis and renal glomerulonephritis; thus, it is also within the group of pulmonary–renal syndrome-producing vasculitides, along with Wegener and Goodpasture.

Renal involvement is characterized by rapidly progressive glomerulonephritis (RPGN), that histologically is notable for focal segmental necrotizing glomerulonephritis. When this pattern is observed, the differential diagnosis rests upon the immunofluorescence. Linear IgG reactivity defines Goodpasture syndrome, and the lack of immunofluorescence reactivity defines "pauci-immune" focal necrotizing glomerulonephritis, implying MPA and WG. A combination of clinical and serologic features can distinguish MPA (pANCA+, anti-MPO) from WG (cANCA+, anti-PR3).

Pulmonary involvement typically manifests as pulmonary hemorrhage with hemoptysis, histologically associated with intraalveolar hemorrhage with capillaritis. Patients may undergo bronchoalveolar lavage (BAL), where numerous siderophages are found. Unlike WG, granulomas and geographic necrosis are not typical features; the histologic features of Goodpasture, though, may be indistinguishable from MPA.

Wegener granulomatosis (WG)

In its classic form, WG presents with involvement of the upper respiratory tract, lower respiratory tract, and kidneys. Patients present with otitis media, sinusitis, nasal obstruction or ulceration with bleeding. Some patients develop destructive nasal lesions that obliterate the supporting cartilage, leading to the saddle nose deformity typical of lethal midline granuloma. Common pulmonary symptoms include pulmonary infiltrates, nodules, hemoptysis, or pleuritis. Although only a small portion of patients with WG present with renal disease, most will develop glomerulonephritis at some time during the course of this disease.

Like MPA, the typical renal lesion is focal segmental necrotizing glomerulonephritis f6.14, pauci-immune type. In the lung, patients may develop masses that are often interpreted as malignant radiographically. They often also develop pulmonary hemorrhage with capillaritis. In addition to these characteristic findings, there is usually widespread systemic vasculitis in a PAN-like pattern, and all of the features of PAN may be observed in WG.

Laboratory findings include normochromic anemia, moderate leukocytosis, and thrombocytosis. Elevated BUN and creatinine signify renal involvement. Renal sediment is notable for hematuria with red cell casts. Complement levels are normal, and there may be hypergammaglobulinemia with increased IgA levels. ANCA is positive in a cytoplasmic pattern (cANCA) with anti-PR3 activity by ELISA. About half of patients are RF positive. Anti-GBM antibodies are negative

Churg-Strauss syndrome (allergic angiitis & granulomatosis)

Churg-Strauss syndrome (CSS) develops slowly >3-5 years, initially presenting as adult-onset asthma and, when fully developed, a fulminant vasculitis syndrome. Early symptoms emanate from the upper and lower respiratory tract, consisting of sinusitis, wheezing, and expiratory rales. In essence, this first (prodromal) stage has features typical of asthma. Over time, patients develop peripheral eosinophilia, which may be associated with eosinophilic tissue infiltration of lung and GI tract. Pulmonary eosinophil infiltration takes the form of transient pulmonary infiltrates (Loeffler syndrome) that tend to be peripheral (reverse CHF pattern), while GI infiltrates present with nonspecific symptoms exacerbated by consumption. Finally, systemic vasculitis sets in, presenting with a myriad of typical vasculitic findings such as mononeuropathy multiplex, fixed pulmonary infiltrates, ischemic bowel, and palpable purpura. Cardiac involvement is the major cause of death, taking the form of congestive cardiomyopathy due to myocarditis. In a patient presenting with vasculitis, peripheral eosinophilia and a history of asthma have 99% specificity for Churg-Strauss syndrome.

Laboratory findings include leukocytosis with eosinophilia in excess of $1.5 \times 10^3/\mu L$. Serum complement levels are normal. Serum pANCA (anti-MPO) is positive in most cases.

Histopathologically, biopsies of involved tissue demonstrate necrotizing (fibrinoid) vasculitis and necrotizing granulomas, within which there are variably degenerating eosinophils (allergic granulomas). In the kidney, the typical finding is focal segmental necrotizing glomerulonephritis, similar to that seen in Wegener. In nerve biopsies, vasculitis is seen within epineural vessels.

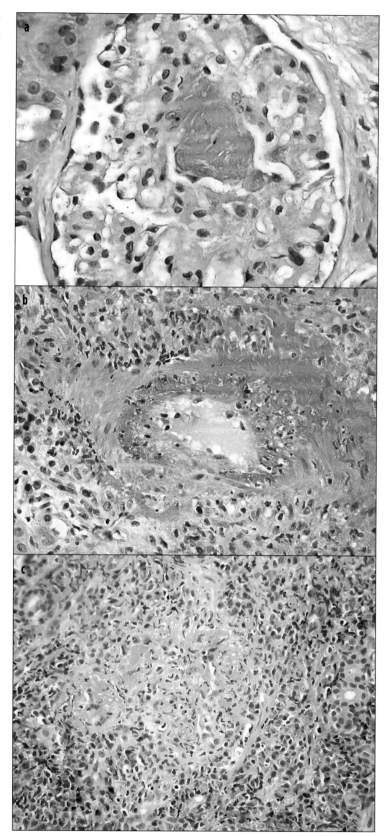

f6.14 Wegener granulomatosis
a glomerulus involved by focal segmental necrotizing glomerulonephritis seen in Wegener, Goodpasture & microscopic polyangiitis
b arterial involvement in Wegener, which has an appearance similar to PAN
c nasal biopsy in Wegener

Behçet disease (BD)

As it was originally described, Behçet disease (BD) is the triad of recurrent oral aphthous ulcers, genital aphthous ulcers, and uveitis. It is in fact a multisystem disease largely mediated by vasculitis. The incidence of BD is highest in the Middle East, Far East, and Mediterranean, and the incidence is fairly low in Europe and North America. To date, there is no specific autoantibody test for Behçet. HLA-B51 has been reported to be present in the majority of Turkish and Japanese patients, in whom there is a 6-fold increased risk of BD. The pathergy test (development of erythema, induration, and pustule ~2 mm or more in size at the site of a needle stick ~48 hours later) is among the diagnostic criteria. In some Middle Eastern populations the pathergy test is actually quite specific for the diagnosis of BD.

Giant cell arteritis (temporal arteritis)

Giant cell arteritis (GCA) is characterized by inflammation of large and medium-sized branches of the aorta with predilection for the extracranial branches of the carotid artery. GCA is the most common vasculitis in adult patients, and elderly adults are mainly affected. Prompt diagnosis and treatment is necessary to prevent ischemic complications, particularly blindness. Headache is the main presenting symptom, and is characteristically of sudden onset and temporal. While the temporal artery is often involved, any branch of the aorta, and indeed the aorta itself, may be targeted. Ischemic sequelae include jaw claudication, loss of vision or diplopia, and stroke, in particular in the vertebrobasilar territory. About 5-10% of patients with biopsy-proven GCA present without obvious vascular manifestations. These patients with subclinical (silent) GCA, may present with only polymyalgia rheumatica (PMR) or fever of unknown origin.

The temporal artery biopsy remains the gold standard diagnostic modality for GCA f6.15. Despite variable reported sensitivity ranging from 30-90%, the specificity is nearly 100%. The procedure has low associated morbidity, and a positive biopsy removes all doubt regarding the need for treatment. A negative biopsy allows cessation of corticosteroids in low-risk patient. The difficulty arises when a patient strongly suspected of having GCA has a negative biopsy. The false negativity rate is affected by the size of the specimen and the initiation of corticosteroid therapy prior to biopsy. In one study, of patients treated with high dose corticosteroids prior to biopsy, the sensitivity of biopsy was 78% in patients treated for <2 weeks, 65% in patients treated for 2-4 weeks, and 40% in patients treated for >4 weeks prior to biopsy. Therefore, while it should be noted that corticosteroids can alter the histologic picture, the evidence supports prompt treatment of patients with suspected GCA with no loss of enthusiasm for biopsy.

The histopathologic diagnosis of GCA begins with proper specimen handling. The entire specimen should be submitted, cutting the vessel into 2 mm segments along its length. 5-10 levels of each tissue block should be reviewed. The diagnostic findings include chronic inflammation within the wall of the vessel, generally centered upon the elastic laminae, with or without giant cells. Chronic inflammation in branch vessels only is considered suggestive of GCA. There may be

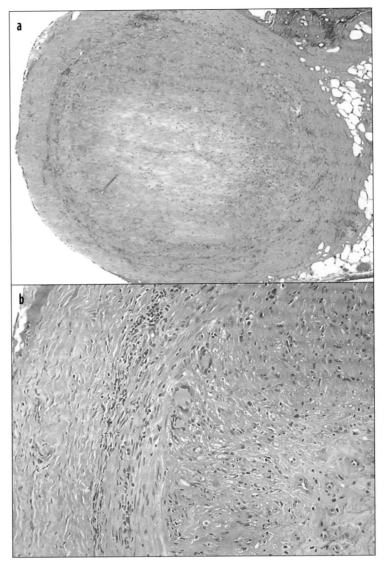

f6.15 Temporal arteritis
a Low power image demonstrating mural inflammation & luminal occlusion by intimal hyperplasia
b High power image of the inflammatory population, composed of lymphocytes & multinucleated giant cells that are centered upon the elastic lamina

secondary changes, including mural fibrosis and reduplication of the elastic laminae, but without inflammation, the diagnosis should be withheld. Chronic perivascular inflammation, without mural inflammation, is not evidence of GCA.

GCA is tightly associated with polymyalgia rheumatica, which is characterized by pain in the proximal muscles of the shoulder, hip, and torso. Like GCA, patients are older adults with marked elevation in ESR. A brisk response to corticosteroids is typical and in some cases aids in the diagnosis. Skeletal muscle biopsies are essentially normal.

Several nonspecific laboratory abnormalities are found at the time of presentation. The CBC often demonstrates anemia of chronic disease with reactive thrombocytosis. The ESR is elevated in 95-100% of cases. An ESR >50 mm/h is one of the American College of Rheumatology criteria for GCA.

Takayasu arteritis

Takayasu is histopathologically identical to GCA and shares a similar arterial distribution. While Takayasu is less likely to involve the temporal artery, both diseases may involve the major branches of the aortic arch, so that the distinction between these entities rests largely upon patient age. GCA is generally confined to patients over the age of 40 years, and Takayasu is found in patients younger than 40. Note that vasculitic involvement of the arch and its branches also raises the possibility of syphilis.

Also called "pulseless disease" because of its tendency to occlude branches of the aortic arch, Takayasu may be found anywhere in the world. It is most common in Japan, China, and India, with areas of high prevalence in Mexico. Takayasu is relatively uncommon in North America and Europe. The median age of onset is 25 years, with women affected much more often than men (M:F ratio 8:1).

Symptoms usually begin abruptly, consisting initially of fever, malaise, weight loss and night sweats. There may be symptoms related to ischemia of affected organs. During the chronic obliterative stage of their disease, patients may have decreased or absent pulses of affected arteries. Characteristic angiography findings confirm the clinical diagnosis. Laboratory findings are nonspecific, consisting of normochromic anemia with mild leukocytosis, raised ESR, and hypergammaglobulinemia with hypoalbuminemia. Biopsy is seldom undertaken.

Buerger disease (thromboangiitis obliterans)

Buerger disease presents with symptoms of arterial insufficiency affecting the distal upper and lower extremities. Symptoms include claudication progressing to digital ischemia. The disease was first described in 1879, with the advent of the widespread smoking of cigarettes in the western world, because Buerger disease typically occurs in young male smokers.

3 pathologic phases are identified. In the acute phase, inflammatory thrombi develop in the arteries and veins of the distal extremities. The intermediate (subacute) phase is characterized by progressive organization of the thrombus. Lastly, in the chronic phase organized thrombus and vascular fibrosis remains.

The inflammation in thromboangiitis obliterans is really centered upon the intima, with formation of inflammatory cell rich intravascular thrombi. The thrombi may contain neutrophils and multinucleate giant cells but the vessel wall is free of inflammation. The mural layers (internal elastic lamina, muscle coats) remain intact, in contrast to atherosclerosis and other vasculitides. There are no specific serologic markers.

Kawasaki disease (mucocutaneous lymph node syndrome)

Kawasaki disease is found only in children, with mean age at onset of 2-3 years. It begins with high fevers, and within days to weeks the characteristic features emerge, including palmar erythema with desquamation of the fingertips, cervical adenopathy, conjunctivitis, strawberry tongue, and cracked lips. The child appears quite ill but will recover, except for the small number of patients who develop coronary involvement, which can lead to aneurysmal dilation, thrombosis, myocardial infarction, and death (1-2% of untreated patients). It is for this reason that echocardiography is mandatory in all cases. There are no specific serologic markers.

Henoch-Schönlein purpura (HSP)

HSP is a subgroup of hypersensitivity vasculitis and a disease of children that presents with the triad of palpable purpura on the lower extremities, abdominal pain, and glomerulonephritis. Most patients initially present with gastrointestinal signs and symptoms such as nausea, vomiting, blood or mucus in the stool.

Laboratory findings include leukocytosis but normal platelet count despite purpura. The ESR is elevated. Skin biopsy shows leukocytoclastic vasculitis with IgA deposition by IF. The renal biopsy findings are similar to those for IgA nephropathy.

Inflammatory myopathies

Inflammatory myopathies typically present with proximal symmetrical muscle weakness, elevated serum creatine kinase, and characteristic EMG findings. Several distinct categories are recognized, including connective tissue disease-associated myositis, malignancy-associated myositis, polymyositis (PM), dermatomyositis (DM) and inclusion body myositis (IBM).

Dermatomyositis and polymyositis are often considered together, but there are important differences. What they share is a tendency towards symmetric proximal muscle weakness and a characteristic set of serologic markers, including anti-Jo1, anti-SRP, and anti-PM/Scl antibodies. Dermatomyositis is associated with a highly characteristic heliotrope rash and Gottron papules, and typical perifascicular atrophy on muscle biopsy, often with a paucity of mononuclear inflammation. Polymyositis lacks the rash and demonstrates a pronounced mononuclear cell infiltrate on muscle biopsy. Lung involvement is frequent in both polymyositis and dermatomyositis and is a major cause of morbidity and mortality. While a certain amount of pulmonary insufficiency is attributable to respiratory muscle dysfunction, there is histologic evidence of insterstitial lung disease in many patients. The histologic features are nonspecific, mimicking other primary interstitial lung diseases, primarily nonspecific interstitial pneumonitis (NSIP).

In some newer classifications of myositis, an emphasis on the serologic picture has identified an "antisynthetase syndrome," defined by the presence of antibodies against aminoacyl-tRNA synthetases, most commonly anti-Jo1. This syndrome is characterized by a distinct set of clinical features, including myositis (either dermatomyositis or polymyositis), interstitial lung disease, Raynaud phenomenon, fever during flares, polyarthralgia, and so-called mechanic's hands (scaling and fissuring of the skin of the fingers, most pronounced on the radial aspect).

IBM is the most common inflammatory myopathy in older adults. It is important to distinguish from the others because of resistance to corticosteroid treatment. A characteristic feature of its presentation is difficulty with fine motor skills of the hands. This is because IBM typically involves 2 main muscle groups—the quadriceps and forearm flexors. Dysphagia may arise in up to half of patients. Unlike other forms of myopathy, IBM is characteristically asymmetric. There is no specific serologic test, making muscle biopsy mandatory in many cases. Characteristic histologic features include myositis (mononuclear cell infiltration of myopathic muscle), eosinophilic intracellular inclusions, rimmed vacuoles, and intracellular amyloid material in Congo Red stained sections. Electron microscopy demonstrates 15-21 nm tubulofilamentous inclusions.

Secondary myositis that is seen in association with other connective tissue diseases typically arises in SLE, RA, Sjögren syndrome, and progressive systemic sclerosis (scleroderma).

While the ideal muscle biopsy is taken from a muscle that is moderately weak (neither entirely unaffected nor entirely atrophic), many general surgeons simply select the quadriceps. In all forms of myositis, the muscle biopsy demonstrates myopathic changes, including combined fibrillar degeneration and regeneration, often within a background of necrotic fibrils. To a variable degree, there are endomysial mononuclear cell infiltrates that encircle individual nonnecrotic myofibrils. Dermatomyositis is notable for a paucity of intramuscular mononuclear inflammation; instead, perivascular inflammatory infiltrates (without vasculitis) are found in association with perifascicular atrophy. In contrast, polymyositis, secondary myositis, and IBM demonstrate pronounced mononuclear infiltration, predominantly by CD8+ T cells and macrophages. It is important not to over-interpret mononuclear inflammation that surrounds necrotic fibers, a feature that may be seen in noninflammatory disorders such as facioscapulohumeral or Duchenne muscular dystrophy. IBM has the further specific features noted above.

Autoantibodies are infrequent in cancer-associated myositis and IBM. Anti-synthetases (eg, anti-Jo-1, anti-PL-7) are the most common autoantibody found and imply a high likelihood of pulmonary interstitial fibrosis. Anti-SRP is found mainly in PM (rather than DM) patients and is associated with a high frequency of cardiac involvement, HLA-DR5, and a very poor prognosis. Anti-Mi-2 is associated almost exclusively with DM and tends to have a good prognosis.

Myasthenia gravis (MG)

MG presents as muscle weakness and fatigue. Typical signs include ptosis, diplopia, and fatiguable muscle weakness. The diagnosis is supported by the characteristic EMG finding of progressive decrement in muscle action potential on repetitive stimulation, a Tensilon test showing a dramatic response to cholinesterase inhibitor, and characteristic autoantibodies.

There are 5 clinical types of MG, including early onset, late onset, thymoma associated, ocular, and seronegative. Early onset MG affects primarily females <40 who tend to have thymic follicular hyperplasia; whereas late onset MG affects predominantly males >40 with no thymic pathology. Thymoma associated MG has no age or sex predilection.

Antibodies to the muscle acetylcholine receptor (AChR) are present in 75-95% of patients with MG, and false positives are extremely rare t6.13. Particularly in thymoma-associated disease, antibodies to skeletal muscle components (ryanodine receptor and titin) can be found. Recently, antibodies to MuSK have been found in a proportion of patients with AChR antibody negative ("seronegative") MG. MuSK is a tyrosine kinase that is restricted to the neuromuscular junction, and antibodies to MuSK appear to define a steroid-refractory form of MG seen in younger females with frequent bulbar manifestations.

t6.13 Myasthenia gravis testing

Type	Anti-AChR	Anti-titin	Anti-MuSK
Early-onset	+	–	–
Late-onset	+	+	–
Thymoma-associated	+	+	–
Ocular	+/–	–	–
Seronegative	–	–	+/–

Treatment involves thymectomy, particularly in patients <60 years old. Immunosuppression starts with prednisone and intravenous immunoglobulins and in selected cases plasma exchange.

Familial Mediterranean fever (FMF)

Familial Mediterranean fever (FMF) is the prototype for a recently elucidated group of "auto-inflammatory fever syndromes." This group of disorders is characterized by anomalies in the innate immune system and in most cases is caused by mutations in the genes encoding the pyrin family of proteins. Other members of this group include the hyper immunoglobulin D fever syndrome, familial cold urticaria syndrome, and Muckle-Wells syndrome.

In FMF, symptoms usually arise by the age of 10 years, consisting of paroxysmal attacks of fever and pain. The pain is derived from inflammation of one of the serosal membranes (peritoneum, pleura, synovium, or tunica vaginalis); thus, typical presentations include peritonitis, pleuritis, arthritis, or acute orchitis. Between attacks, patients are asymptomatic, but systemic amyloidosis with renal failure is a noted complication of untreated FMF. Amyloidosis is of the amyloid A (AA) type.

FMF is an autosomal recessive disorder mainly found among people whose ethnicity can be traced to the Mediterranean basin, including Sephardic Jews, Armenians, Greeks, Italians, Turks, and Arabs. The first report of the disease was in a Sephardic Jewish family in North Africa. The gene responsible for FMF, *MEFV* (chromosome 16), encodes a protein known as pyrin/marenostrin. The protein can normally be found only in neutrophils where it is thought to play an antiinflammatory role. More than 100 *MEFV* mutations have been described in association with FMF, most occurring within exon 10.

Laboratory findings include neutrophilia and elevation of acute phase reactants such as CRP. Serum amyloid A (SAA) may be elevated and, if so, discriminates FMF from much of what is in the differential diagnosis (eg, functional abdominal pain, surgical acute abdomen). Diagnosis is largely based upon clinical findings.

Treatment reduces the incidence of febrile/painful episodes and largely prevents amyloidosis in FMF. Colchicine is currently the mainstay of treatment.

Hypersensitivity reactions

Classically defined hypersensitivity reactions are the basis of all autoimmune diseases.

Type I hypersensitivity (immediate-type hypersensitivity)

Type I hypersensitivity is the result of antigen binding to IgE on the surfaces of mast cells (bound by the $F_c\epsilon R$). IgE induced crosslinking of $F_c\epsilon R$ results in degranulation, with release of histamine, heparin, serotonin, arachidonate.

Examples of type I hypersensitivity include anaphylaxis, urticaria, asthma, and eczema. Anaphylactoid reactions result from mast cell degranulation without IgE intermediation (heat, cold, trauma). Hereditary angioedema (HAE) also has nothing to do with IgE and is caused by deficiency of C1 esterase inhibitor (C1Inh).

Anaphylaxis

Anaphylaxis is mediated primarily by IgE. After exposure to certain allergens, some patients for unclear reasons mount an anamnestic IgE response. Formed IgE becomes bound to $F_c\epsilon R$ (the Fc epsilon receptor) on the surfaces of mast cells and basophils. Re-exposure to antigen may result in crosslinking of bound IgE on the cell surface, causing degranulation.

Serum (or plasma) levels of tryptase are recommended in laboratory diagnosis of anaphylaxis. Note that tryptase levels are chronically elevated in patients with systemic mastocytosis. Tryptase may be measured as total tryptase or mature tryptase. Total tryptase levels generally reflect the mast cell burden within the body (as in mastocytosis), while mature tryptase more closely reflects mast cell degranulation. Serum tryptase levels peak ~60-90 minutes after the onset of anaphylaxis and persist for several hours. Plasma *histamine* levels peak more quickly than tryptase, at ~10 minutes after the onset of anaphylaxis. Levels return to normal within an hour. The urinary histamine, however, may be elevated for 24 hours.

While the tryptase and histamine are helpful tests, the laboratory can be of most help in excluding conditions that mimic anaphylaxis. For example, carcinoid syndrome can be excluded by measuring urinary HIAA, serum serotonin, and other analytes. A peculiar form of histamine poisoning (scombroidosis) may result from ingestion of spoiled fish and can clinically resemble anaphylaxis. It is due to the production of histamine by bacteria within the fish. Elevated histamine, without elevated tryptase, and perhaps a history of several people affected together, point to this diagnosis. Similar conditions that can mimic anaphylaxis and be distinguished through laboratory testing include hereditary angioedema (C1q deficiency), urticarial vasculitis, pheochromocytoma, and hyper-IgE (Job) syndrome.

Type II hypersensitivity (antibody-mediated cellular cytotoxicity)

Type II hypersensitivity is produced by antibody-antigen binding that leads to tissue damage mediated by opsonization. Examples include Goodpasture syndrome, myasthenia gravis, immune hemolysis, and erythroblastosis fetalis.

Type III hypersensitivity

Type III hypersensitivity is mediated by the formation of immune complexes as a result of antibody-antigen interaction with activation of complement. Examples include SLE, Henoch-Schönlein purpura (HSP), serum sickness, post-streptococcal glomerulonephritis (PSGN), membranous glomerulonephritis (MGN), and the Arthus reaction.

Type IV hypersensitivity (delayed-type hypersensitivity)

Type IV is mediated by T cells reacting to antigen, usually with granuloma formation. The classic example is the tuberculin skin test.

References

Abril A, Calamia KT, Cohen MD [2003] The Churg Strauss syndrome (allergic granulomatous angiitis): review and update. *Semin Arthritis Rheum* 33:106-114. PMID:14625818.

AGA Institute [2006] AGA Institute medical position statement on the diagnosis and management of celiac disease. *Gastroenterology* 131:1977-1980. PMID:17087935.

Aghamohammadi A, Farhoudi A, Moin M, Rezaei N, Kouhi A, Pourpak Z, Yaseri N, Movahedi M, Gharagozlou M, Zandieh F, Yazadni F, Arshi S, Zadeh I, Ghazi B, Mahmoudi M, Tahaei S, Isaeian A [2005] Clinical and immunological features of 65 Iranian patients with common variable immunodeficiency. *Clin Diagn Lab Immunol* 12:825-832. PMID:16002630.

Al-Araji A, Kidd, DP [2009] Neuro-Behçet disease: epidemiology, clinical characteristics, and management. *Lancet Neurol* 8:192-204. PMID:19161910.

Anderlini P, Korbling M, Dale D, Gratwohl A, Schmitz N, Stroncek D, Howe C, Leitman S, Horowitz M, Gluckman E, Rowley S, Przepiorka D, Champlin R [1997] Allogeneic blood stem cell transplantation: considerations for donors. *Blood* 90:903 PMID:9242518.

Balbir-Gurman A, Yigla M, Nahir AM, Braun-Moscovici Y [2006] Rheumatoid pleural effusion. *Semin Arthritis Rheum* 35:368-378. PMID:16765714.

Balmer P, North J, Baxter D, et al [2003] Measurement and interpretation of pneumococcal IgG levels for clinical management. *Clin Exp Immunol* 133:364-369. PMID:12930362.

Barrett DJ, Lee CG, Ammann AJ, Ayoub EM [1984] IgG and IgM pneumococcal polysaccharide antibody responses in infants. *Pediatr Res* 18:1067-1071. PMID:6514433.

Baumgart KW, Britton WJ, Kemp A, et al [1997] The spectrum of primary immunodeficiency disorders in Australia. *J Allergy Clin Immunol* 100:415-423. PMID:9314356.

Bogdanos D, Baum H, Vergani D [2003] Anti mitochondrial and other autoantibodies. *Clin Liver Dis* 7:759-777. PMID:14594130.

Bork K, Barnstedt SE, Koch P, Traupe H [2000] Hereditary angioedema with normal C1-inhibitor activity in women. *Lancet* 356:213-217. PMID:10963200.

Bork K, Meng G, Staubach P, Hardt J [2006] Hereditary angioedema: new findings concerning symptoms, affected organs, and course. *Am J Med* 119:267-274. PMID:16490473.

Bourne HC, Weston S, Prasad M, Edkins E, Benson EM [2004] Identification of WASP mutations in 10 Australian families with Wiskott-Aldrich syndrome and X-linked thrombocytopenia. *Pathology* 36(3):262-264. PMID:15203732.

Bowen, T, Cicardi, M, Farkas, H, et al [2010] 2010 international consensus algorithm for the diagnosis, therapy, and management of hereditary angioedema. *Allergy, Asthma Clin Immunol* 6:24 PMID:20667127.

Bruton OC [1952] Agammaglobulinemia. *Pediatrics* 9:722-728. PMID:14929630.

Buckley RH [2000] Primary immunodeficiency diseases due to defects in lymphocytes. *N Engl J Med* 343:1313-1324. PMID:11058677.

Buerger L [1908] Thrombo-angiitis obliterans: a study of the vascular lesions leading to presenile spontaneous gangrene. *Am J Med Sci* 136:567-580.

Carlucci F, Tabucchi A, Aiuti A, Rosi F, Floccari F, Pagani R, Marinello E [2003] Capillary electrophoresis in diagnosis and monitoring of adenosine deaminase deficiency. *Clin Chem* 49:1830-1838. PMID:14578314.

Chaabouni HB, Ksantini M, M'rad R, et al [2005] MEFV mutations in Tunisian patients suffering from familial Mediterranean fever. *Semin Arthritis Rheum* 36:397-401. PMID:17276496.

Cheuk W, Yuen HKL, Chu SYY, et al [2008] Lymphadenopathy of IgG4-related sclerosing disease. *Am J Surg Pathol* 32(5):671-681. PMID:18344866.

Choi S, Lee S, Khang S, Jeon S [2010] IgG4-related sclerosing pachymeningitis causing spinal cord compression. *Neurology* 75:1388-1390. PMID:20938032.

Corcoran GM, Prayson RA, Herzog KM [2001] The significance of perivascular inflammation in the absence of arteritis in temporal artery biopsy specimens. *Am J Clin Pathol* 115:342-347. PMID:11242789.

Cunningham-Rundles C, Bodian C [1999] Common variable immunodeficiency: clinical and immunological features of 248 patients. *Clin Immunol* 92:34-48. PMID:10413651.

Cunningham-Rundles C [2002] Hematologic complications of primary immune deficiencies. *Blood Rev* 16:61-64. PMID:11913998.

Davidson A, Diamond B [2001] Autoimmune diseases. *N Engl J Med* 345:340-350. PMID:11484692.

Delves PJ, Roitt IM [2000] The immune system. First of two parts. *N Engl J Med* 343:37-49. PMID:10882768.

Delves PJ, Roitt IM [2000] The immune system. Second of two parts. *N Engl J Med* 343:108-117. PMID:10891520.

Derry J, Kerns J, Weinberg K [1995] *WASP* gene mutations in Wiskott-Aldrich syndrome and X-linked thrombocytopenia. *Hum Mol Genet* 4:1127-1135. PMID:8528199.

Deshpande V, Mino-Kenudson M, Brugge WR, et al [2005] Endoscopic ultrasound guided fine needle aspiration biopsy of autoimmune pancreatitis. *Am J Surg Pathol* 29(11):1464-1471. PMID:16224213.

Deshpande V, Gupta R, Sainani N, et al [2011] Subclassification of autoimmune pancreatitis: a histologic classification with clinical significance. *Am J Surg Pathol* 35(1):26-35. PMID:21164284.

Devriendt K, Kim AS, Mathijs G, Frints SGM, Schwartz M, Van den Oord JJ, Verhoef GEG, Boogaerts MA, Fryns J-P, You D, Rosen MK, Vandenberghe P [2001] Constitutively activating mutation in WASP causes X-linked severe congenital neutropenia. *Nat Genet* 27:313-317. PMID:11242115.

Dickey W, Hughes DF, McMillan SA [2000] Disappearance of endomysial antibodies in treated celiac disease does not indicate histological recovery. *Am J Gastroenterol* 95:712-714. PMID:10710062.

Dubinsky MC, Ofman JJ, Urman M, et al [2001] Clinical utility of serodiagnostic testing in suspected pediatric inflammatory bowel disease. *Am J Gastroenterol* 96:758-65. PMID:11280547.

Eiermann TH, van Bekkum DW, Vriesendorp HM, Machida U, Kami M, Hirai H, Bolan CD, Leitman SF, Sasazuki T, Juji T, Kodera Y, Aversa F, Martelli MF, Reisner Y [1999] Hematopoietic stem-cell transplantation for acute leukemia. *N Engl J Med* 340(10):809-812. PMID:10075527.

Erlich H, Opelz G and Hansen J [2001] HLA DNA typing and transplantation. *Immunity* April;14(4):34-56. PMID:11336680.

Ewen C, Kane KP, Shostak I, et al [2003] A novel cytotoxicity assay to evaluate antigen-specific CTL responses using a colorimetric substrate for granzyme B *J Immunol Methods* 279:89-101. PMID:12738362.

Farrell RF, Kelly CP [2002] Celiac sprue. *New Engl J Med* 346:180-188. PMID:11796853.

Fleisher TA [2003] Evaluation of suspected immunodeficiency. *MLO Med Lab Obs* February;35(2):10-21. PMID:12624871.

Frank MM [2008] Hereditary angioedema. *J Allergy Clin Immunol* 121:S398-401. PMID:18241690.

Gennery AR, Cant AJ [2001] Diagnosis of severe combined immunodeficiency. *J Clin Pathol* 54:191-195. PMID:11253129.

Genta MS, Genta RM, Gabay C [2006] Systemic rheumatoid vasculitis: a review. *Semin Arthritis Rheum* 36:88-98. PMID:17023257.

Gerlach JA [2002] Human leukocyte antigen molecular typing: how to identify the 1250+ alleles out there. *Arch Pathol Lab Med* 126:281-4. PMID:11860300.

Germenis AE, Yiannaki EE, Zachou K, Roka V, Barbanis S, Liaskos C, Adam K, Kapsoritakis AN, Potamianos S, Dalekos GN [2005] Prevalence and clinical significance of immunoglobulin A antibodies against tissue transglutaminase in patients with diverse chronic liver diseases. *Clin Diagn Lab Immunol* 12:941-948. PMID:16085912.

Gonzalez-Gay MA, Lopez-Diaz MJ, Barros S, Garcia-Porrua C, Sanchez-Andrade A, Paz-Carreira J, Martin J, Llorca J [2005] Giant cell arteritis laboratory tests at the time of diagnosis in a series of 240 patients. *Medicine* 84(5):277-290. PMID:16148728.

Hamano H, Kawa S, Horiuchi A, Unno H, Furuya N, Akamatsu T, Fukushima M, Nikaido T, Nakayama K, Usuda N, Kiyosawa K [2001] High serum IgG4 concentrations in patients with sclerosing pancreatitis. *N Engl J Med* 344:732-738. PMID:11236777.

Hong R [1998] The DiGeorge anomaly (CATCH 22, DiGeorge/velocardiofacial syndrome). *Semin Hematol* 35:282-290. PMID:9801257.

Hoppner M, Luhm J, Schlenke P, et al [2002] A flow-cytometry based cytotoxicity assay using stained effector cells in combination with native target cells. *J Immunol Methods* 267:157-163. PMID:12165437.

Illoh OC [2004] Current applications of flow cytometry in the diagnosis of primary immunodeficiency diseases. *Arch Pathol Lab Med* 128:23-31. PMID:14692816.

Imai K, Nonayama S, Ochs HD [2003] *WASP* (Wiskott-Aldrich Syndrome Protein) gene mutations and phenotype. *Curr Opin All Clin Immunol* 3:427-436. PMID:14612666.

Imai K, Morio T, Zhu Y, Jin Y, Itoh S, Kajiwara M, Yata J, Mizutani S, Ochs HD, Nonoyama S [2004] Clinical course of patients with *WASP* gene mutations. *Blood* 103(2):456-464. PMID:12969986.

Itoh S, et al [1998] Autoantibodies against a 210kDa glycoprotein of the nuclear pore complex as a prognostic marker in patients with primary biliary cirrhosis. *J Gastroenterol Hepatol* 13:257-65. PMID:9570238.

Jin Y, Mazza C, Christie JR, Giliani S, Fiorini M, Mella M, Gandellini F, Stewart DM, Zhu Q, Nelson DL, Notarangelo LD, Ochs HD [2004] Mutations of the Wiskott-Aldrich Syndrome Protein (WASP): hotspots, effect on transcription, and translation and phenotype/genotype correlation. *Blood* 104(13):4010-4019. PMID:15284122.

Kamisawa T, Okamoto A, Funata N [2005] Clinicopathologic features of autoimmune pancreatitis in relation to elevation of serum IgG4. *Pancreas* 31(1):28-31. PMID:15968244.

Kamradt T, Mitchison NA [2001] Tolerance and autoimmunity. *N Engl J Med* 344:655-664. PMID:11228281.

Kaplan AP, Greaves MW. Angioedema. *J Am Acad Dermatol* 2005;53(3):373-388. PMID:16112343.

Karcher DS, McPherson RA [2011] Cerebrospinal, synovial, serous body fluids and alternative specimens. In: McPherson RA, Pincus MR, eds. *Henry's Clinical Diagnosis and Management by Laboratory Methods*, 22nd ed. Philadelphia: Saunders; 480-506.

Kavanaugh A, Tomar R, Reveille J, Solomon DH, Homburger HA [2000] Guidelines for clinical use of the antinuclear antibody test and tests for specific autoantibodies to nuclear antigens. *Arch Pathol Lab Med* 124:71-82. PMID:10629135.

Keren DF [2002] Antinuclear antibody testing. *Clin Lab Med* 22:447-474. PMID:12134471.

Kitagawa S, Zen Y, Harada K, et al [2005] Abundant IgG4-positive plasma cell infiltration characterizes chronic sclerosing sialadenitis (Kuttner's tumor). *Am J Surg Pathol* 29:783-791. PMID:15897744.

Kniker WT, Lesourd BM, McBryde JL, Corriel RN [1985] Cell-mediated immunity assessed by multitest CMT skin testing in infants and preschool children. *Am J Dis Child* 139:840-845. PMID:4025264.

Kobashigawa J, Mehra M, West L, et al [2009] Report from a consensus conference on the sensitized patient awaiting heart transplantation. *J Heart Lung Transplant* 28:213-225. PMID:19285611.

Kojima M, Sipos B, Klapper W, et al [2007] Autoimmune pancreatitis: frequency, IgG4 expression, and clonality of T and B cells. *Am J Surg Pathol* 31(4):521-528. PMID:17414098.

Kuijpers TW, Weening RS, Roos D [1999] Clinical and laboratory work-up of patients with neutrophil shortage or dysfunction. *J Immunol Methods* 232:211-229. PMID:10618522.

Lane HC, Depper JM, Greene WC, et al [1985] Qualitative analysis of immune function in patients with the acquired immunodeficiency syndrome: evidence for a selective defect in soluble antigen recognition. *N Engl J Med* 313:79-84. PMID:2582258.

Lekstrom-Himes JA, Gallin JI [2000] Primary immunodeficiency diseases due to defects in phagocytes. *N Engl J Med* 343:1703-1714. PMID:11106721.

Levine JS, Branch DW, Rauch J [2002] The anti phospholipid syndrome. *N Engl J Med* 346:752-763. PMID:11882732.

Lieberman P [2006] Anaphylaxis. *Med Clin N Am* 90:77-95. PMID:16310525.

Lindegren ML, Kobrynski L, Rasmussen SA [2004] Applying public health strategies to primary immunodeficiency diseases: a potential approach to genetic disorders. *MMWR Recomm Rep* 53(RR-1):1-29. PMID:14724556.

Llorente MJ, Sebastian M, Fernandez-Acenero MJ, et al [2004] IgA antibodies against tissue transglutaminase in the diagnosis of celiac disease: concordance with intestinal biopsy in children and adults. *Clin Chem* 50(2):451-453. PMID:14752021.

Lobo PI, Spencer C, Gorman J, Pirsch G [1981] Critical appraisal of complement dependent microlymphocytotoxicity assay for detecting donor-specific alloantibody pretransplant—importance of indirect immunofluorescence as a superior alternative. *Human Immunol* 2(1):55-64. PMID:7024219.

Loyd JE, Tillman BF, Atkinson JB, et al [2005] Mediastinal fibrosis complicating histoplasmosis. *Medicine* 1988; 67:295-310. PMID:3045478.

Lutskiy MI, Rosen FS, Remold-O'Donnell E. Genotype-proteotype linkage in the Wiskott-Aldrich syndrome. *J Immunol* 175(2):1329-1336. PMID:16002738.

Majeed HA, El-Khateeb M, El-Shanti H, et al [2005] The spectrum of familial Mediterranean fever gene mutations in Arabs: report of a large series. *Semin Arthritis Rheum* 34:813-818. PMID:15942916.

Marsh SGE [2000] Nomenclature for factors of the HLA system: update March 2000. *Tissue Antigens* 56:103-4. PMID:10958365.

Masi AT, Hunder GG, Lie JT, et al [1990] The American College of Rheumatology 1990 criteria for the classification of Churg-Strauss syndrome (allergic granulomatosis and angiitis). *Arthritis Rheum* 33:1094-1100. PMID:2202307.

McMillan SA, Dickey W, Douglas JP, Hughes DF [2001] Transthyretin values correlate with mucosal recovery in patients with coeliac disease taking a gluten free diet. *J Clin Pathol* 54:783-786. PMID:11577127.

Mitchinson MJ [1970] The pathology of idiopathic retroperitoneal fibrosis. *J Clin Pathol* 23(8):681-689. PMID:5488039.

Moder KG [1996] Use and interpretation of rheumatologic tests: a guide for clinicians. *Mayo Clin Proc* 71:391-396. PMID:8637264.

Montano-Loza AJ, Lalor E, Mason AL [2008] Recognizing immuno-globulin G4-related overlap syndromes in patients with pancreatic and hepatobiliary disease. *Can J Gastroenterol* 22:840-846. PMID:18925309.

Nakamura M, et al [2007] Anti-gp210 and anti centromere antibodies are different risk factors for the progression of primary biliary cirrhosis. *Hepatology* 45:118-27. PMID:17187436.

Narváez J, Bernad B, Roig-Vilaseca D, et al [2007] Influence of previous corticosteroid therapy on temporal artery biopsy yield in giant cell arteritis. *Semin Arthritis Rheum* 37:13-19. PMID:17360027.

Notohara K, Burgart L, Lawrence J, Yadav D, Chari S, Smyrk TC [2003] Idiopathic chronic pancreatitis with periductal lymphoplasmacytic infiltration: clinicopathologic features of 35 cases. *Am J Surg Pathol* 27(8):1119-1127. PMID:12883244.

O'Gorman MR, Corrochano V [1995] Rapid whole-blood flow cytometry assay for diagnosis of chronic granulomatous disease. *Clin Diagn Lab Immunol* 2:227-232. PMID:7697534.

Olin J [2000] Thromboangiitis obliterans (Buerger's disease). *New Engl J Med* 343(12):864-869. PMID:10995867.

Padeh S, Berkun Y [2007] Auto-inflammatory fever syndromes. *Rheum Dis Clin N Am* 33:585-623. PMID:17936178.

Panush RS, Paraschiv D, Dorff RE [2003] The tainted legacy of Hans Reiter. *Semin Arthritis Rheum* 32:231-236. PMID:12621586.

Passam FH, Diamantis ID, Perisinaki G, Saridaki Z [2004] Intestinal ischemia as the first manifestation of vasculitis. *Semin Arthritis Rheum* 34:431-441. PMID:15305242.

Picard C, Puel A, Bustamante J, Ku C, Casanova J [2003] Primary immuno-nodeficienies associated with pneumococcal disease. *Curr Opin All Clin Immunol* 3:451-459. PMID:14612669.

Poggio ED, Augustine JJ, Clemente M, et al [2007] Pretransplant cellular alloimmunity as assessed by a panel of reactive T cells assay correlates with acute renal graft rejection. *Transplantation* 83(7):847-52. PMID:17460554.

Pope JE, Krizova A, Garg AX, et al [2007] *Campylobacter* reactive arthritis: a systematic review. *Semin Arthritis Rheum* 37:48-55. PMID:17360026.

Raina A, Krasinskas AM, Greer JB, et al [2008] Serum immunoglobulin G fraction 4 levels in pancreatic cancer: elevations not associated with autoimmune pancreatitis. *Arch Pathol Lab Med* 132:48-53. PMID:18181673.

Sanders DB, El-Salem K, Massey JM, McConville J, Vincent A [2003] Clinical aspects of MuSK antibody positive seronegative MG. *Neurology* 60:1978-1980. PMID:12821744.

Sarkar K, Miller FW [2004] Autoantibodies as predictive and diagnostic markers of idiopathic inflammatory myopathies. *Autoimmunity* 37(4):291-294. PMID:15518044.

Sarles H, Sarles JC, Muratore R, et al [1961] Chronic inflammatory sclerosis of the pancreas—an autonomous pancreatic disease? *Am J Dig Dis* 6:688-698. PMID:13746542.

Sategna-Guidetti C, Grossa S, Bruno M, et al [1996] Reliability of immunologic markers of celiac sprue in assessment of mucosal recovery after gluten withdrawal. *J Clin Gastroenterol* 23:101-104. PMID:8877634.

Schwartz RS [2003] Diversity of the immune repertoire and immuno-regulation. *N Engl J Med* 348:1017-1026. PMID:12637612.

Schwartz LB [2006] Diagnostic value of tryptase in anaphylaxis and mastocytosis. *Immunol Allergy Clin N Am* 2006; 26:451-463. PMID:16931288.

Scornik JC, Clapp W, Patton R, et al [2001] Outcome of kidney transplants in patients known to be flow cytometry crossmatch positive. *Transplantation* 71:1098-1102. PMID:11374409.

Sepehr A, Mino-Kenudson M, Ogawa F, et al [2008] IgG4+ to IgG+ plasma cells ratio of ampulla can help differentiate autoimmune pancreatitis from other "mass forming" pancreatic lesions. *Am J Surg Pathol* 32(12):1770-1778. PMID:18779730.

Sève P, Ferry T, Koenig M, et al [2004] Lupus-like presentation of parvovirus B19 infection. *Semin Arthritis Rheum* 34:642-648. PMID:15692957.

Simons ER [2008] Anaphylaxis. *J Allergy Clin Immunol* 121:S402-407. PMID:18241691.

Soliotis FC, Moutsopoulos HM [2004] Sjögren's syndrome. *Autoimmunity* 37(4):305-307. PMID:15518047.

Specks U, Homburger HA [1994] Anti-neutrophil cytoplasmic antibodies. *Mayo Clin Proc* 69:1197-1198. PMID:7967783.

Stiehm ER, Conley ME [1996] Immunodeficiency disorders: general considerations. In: Stiehm ER ed. *Immunologic Disorders of Infants and Children,* 4th ed. Philadelphia: WB Saunders; 201-252. ISBN:978-0721649481.

Steen VD [2005] Autoantibodies in systemic sclerosis. *Semin Arthritis Rheum* 35:35-42. PMID:16084222.

Sweinberg SK, Wodell RA, Grodofsky MP, et al [1991] Retrospective analysis of the incidence of pulmonary disease in hypogammaglobulinemia. *J Allergy Clin Immunol* 88:96-104. PMID:2071789.

Thiele DL [2005] Autoimmune hepatitis. *Clin Liver Dis* 9:635-646. PMID:16207568.

Thomas R [2004] Celiac disease. *Adolesc Med Clin* 15(1):91-103. PMID:15272258.

Tursi A, Brandimarte G, Giorgetti GM [2003] Lack of usefulness of anti-transglutaminase antibodies in assessing histologic recovery after gluten-free diet in celiac disease. *J Clin Gastroenterol* 37:387-391. PMID:14564185.

Vergani D, Mieli-Vergani G [2004] Autoimmune hepatitis and sclerosing cholangitis. *Autoimmunity* 37(4):329-332. PMID:15518053.

Vermeire S, Vermeulen N, Van Assche G [2008] (Auto)antibodies in inflammatory bowel diseases. *Gastroenterol Clin N Am* 37:429-438. PMID:18499029.

Vincent A, Rothwell P [2004] Myasthenia gravis. *Autoimmunity* 37(4):317-319. PMID:15518050.

Walport MJ [2001a] Complement. First of 2 parts. *N Engl J Med* 344:1058-1066. PMID:11287977.

Walport MJ [2001b] Complement. Second of 2 parts. *N Engl J Med* 344:1140-1144. PMID:11297706.

Weening JJ, D'Agati VD, Schwartz MM, et al [2004] The classification of glomerulonephritis in systemic lupus erythematosus revisted. *Kidney Int* 65:521-30. PMID:14717922.

Weiler CR, Bankers-Fulbright JL [2005] Common variable immunodeficiency: test indications and interpretations. *Mayo Clin Proc* 80(9):1187-1200. PMID:16178499.

Weinberger HW, Ropes MW, Kulka JP, et al [1962] Reiter's syndrome, clinical and pathologic observations: a long term study of 16 cases. *Medicine* 41:35-91. PMID:14038032.

Welsh JP, Skvarka CB, Ko C, Cusack CA [2007] Mystery of the silk road. *Am J Med* 120:322-324. PMID:17398224.

Wen L, Atkinson JP, Giclas PC [2004] Clinical and laboratory evaluation of complement deficiency. *J Allergy Clin Immunol* 113:585-593. PMID:15100659.

Winkelstein JA, Marino MC, Ochs H, Fuleihan R, Scholl PR, Geha R, Stiehm ER, Conley ME [2003] The X-linked hyper-IgM syndrome: clinical and immunologic features of 79 patients. *Medicine.* Nov;82(6):373-84. PMID:14663287.

Yoshida K, Toki F, Takeuchi T, et al [1995] Chronic pancreatitis caused by an autoimmune abnormality. Proposal of the concept of autoimmune pancreatitis. *Dig Dis Sci* 40(7):1561-1568. PMID:7628283.

Zandman-Goddard G, Chapman J, Shoenfeld Y [2007] Autoantibodies involved in neuropsychiatric SLE and anti phospholipid syndrome. *Semin Arthritis Rheum* 36:297-315. PMID:17258299.

Zen Y, Kasahara Y, Horita K, Miyayama S, Miura S, Kitagawa S, Nakanuma Y [2005] Inflammatory pseudotumor of the breast in a patient with a high serum IgG4 level: histologic similarity to sclerosing pancreatitis. *Am J Surg Pathol* 29:275-278. PMID:15644785.

Zhang L, Notohara K, Levy MJ, et al [2007] IgG4-positive plasma cell infiltration in the diagnosis of autoimmune pancreatitis. *Mod Pathol* 20:23-28. PMID:16980948.

Zhu Q, Watanabe C, Liu T, Hollenbaugh, Blaese RM, Kanner SB, Aruffo A, Ochs HD [1997] Wiskott-Alrich syndrome/X-linked thrombocytopenia: WASP gene mutations, protein expression, and phenotype. *Blood* 90:2680-2689. PMID:9326235.

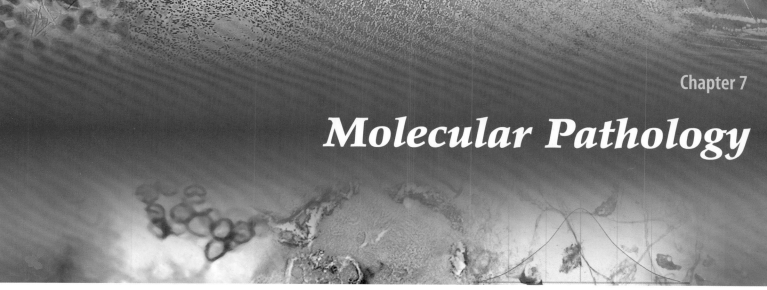

Chapter 7

Molecular Pathology

Molecular biology
The structure of nucleic acids (DNA & RNA)

Nucleotides

Deoxyribonucleic acid (DNA) and ribonucleic acid (RNA) are chains of nucleotides. Each nucleotide has 3 major parts, including a pentose sugar, either ribose (RNA) or deoxyribose (DNA), a phosphate group, and a nitrogenous base. Each carbon of the pentose ring can be numbered starting with the one bound to the nitrogenous base (the one-prime or 1' carbon), with subsequent carbons numbered according to its clockwise position relative to the 1' carbon. Both ribose and deoxyribose have a 3' hydroxyl group which is critical for the formation of the phosphodiester bond. The difference between ribose and deoxyribose is the presence of a 2' hydroxyl group in ribose f7.1. This is important because it allows RNA to form a unique 2'-5' phosphodiester bond, critical for posttranscriptional mRNA splicing.

The nitrogenous base is bound to the initial (1') carbon of the pentose ring. Bases are categorized according to whether there is a heterocyclic 6-member ring (pyrimidines) or a pyrimidine ring fused to an imidazole ring (purines). The pyrimidine bases of significance to the nucleic acid are cytosine, thymine, and uracil, while the purine bases are adenine and guanine f7.2. Nonnucleotide purines include caffeine and theobromine. Uracil is unique to RNA, where it substitutes for thymine.

The final component needed to make a nucleotide is the phosphate group that binds to the 5' carbon of the pentose ring. The nomenclature for each of the nucleotides includes the name of the nitrogenous base followed by triphosphate. For example dATP is adenosine triphosphate f7.3, the "d" prefix signifying deoxyribose. Nucleotides are central to cellular

f7.2 Nitrogenous bases

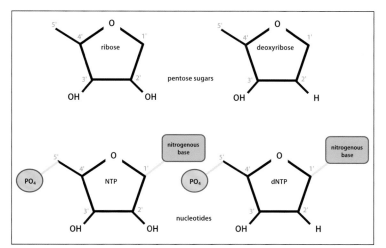

f7.1 Nucleotides; the core of a nucleotide is the pentose sugar, either ribose (upper left) or deoxyribose (upper right); the difference between ribose & deoxyribose is the presence of a 2' hydroxyl group in ribose To complete the nucleotide, a phosphate group & a nitrogenous base are added; ribonucleotide is shown in the lower left & deoxyribonucleotide in the lower right

f7.3 Adenosine triphosphate

ISBN 978-089189-5985

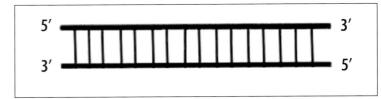

f7.4 Phosphodiester bond

A:T base pair (2 H⁺ bonds)   G:C base pair (3 H⁺ bonds)

f7.5 Hydrogen bonds formed between purines & pyrimidines

5'   3'
3'   5'

f7.6 Antiparallel strands

metabolism, with purines ATP and GTP additionally serving as critical sources of energy utilized in catalytic reactions.

The phosphodiester bond

Formed from the hydrolysis of the 5′ triphosphate of one nucleotide and the 3′ hydroxyl group of another, the phosphodiester bond is the backbone of the nucleic acid strand f7.4. The process of sequential addition of bases is called polymerization, a process that results in the production of a phosphodiester-bonded oligonucleotide while also producing pyrophosphate, which is composed of the 2 remaining phosphate groups of the triphosphate. Since the bond occurs between the 5′ phosphate and the 3′ OH of the subsequent base the process of polymerization is said to be directional from 5′ to 3′. This is important when replication and transcription are later discussed.

Double stranded DNA (hydrogen bonding)

The Watson and Crick model was built piecemeal upon previous data. Erwin Chargaff calculated that the proportion of guanine and cytosine in a DNA molecule were equivalent, similarly for adenine and thymine. From this they were able to infer that one strand of the molecule interacted with the other through the nitrogenous bases. The structure was solved with the critical piece of information from the X-ray crystallography studies of Rosalind Franklin—that the bases were oriented inward. This allowed for base pairing through hydrogen bonding of adjacent complementary bases f7.5. Cytosine/guanine base pairs share 3 hydrogen bonds, while adenine/thymine pairs share 2.

The melting temperature of a double stranded segment of nucleic acid is defined as the point at which 50% of the sequence is single stranded. Therefore, all things being equal

the temperature must be higher for equivalent length cytosine/guanine rich sequences relative to adenine/thymine rich sequences due to the presence of an additional hydrogen bond. In addition to hydrogen bonding the purine and pyrimidine rings are planar or flatly arranged within the double stranded nucleic acid, allowing for "stacking" or stable interactions between bases located above and below the paired bases. Another characteristic of the double stranded DNA is the so-called "antiparallel" arrangement where one strand in the 5′ to 3′ direction base pairs with the other strand arranged in a 3′ to 5′ direction f7.6.

The double stranded DNA twists across itself in a double helical structure. In B-form (the most common physiological form) the double-prime helix measures 2 nm across with 10 nucleotides/complete helical turn. Each turn measures 3.4 nm in length. Due to the helical nature of the double stranded DNA, 2 grooves are formed f7.7. Based on size the grooves can be categorized as either major or minor. Each major groove on one side of the double helix is faced by a minor groove on the other while on the same side of the helix each groove alternates.

Types of nucleic acids

Deoxyribonucleic acid (DNA) is the molecule responsible for the majority of inherited information. It is predominantly double stranded and further compacted into higher order structures to form the total genetic information of an organism, the genome. With each cell division the entirety of the genome must be replicated.

RNA is virtually identical to DNA with the exceptions noted previously. RNA is inherently less stable than DNA and has a relatively shorter half life. This lack of stability is

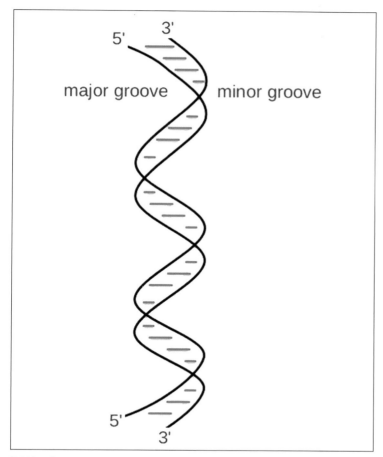

5'
3'

major groove   minor groove

5'
3'

f7.7 Major & minor grooves in double stranded DNA

Nucleic acid-modifying enzymes

Polymerase

A polymerase is an enzyme that catalyzes the formation of a phosphodiester bond between adjacent single nucleotides or between a nucleotide chain and a single nucleotide. DNA polymerase catalyzes the formation of DNA molecules, while RNA polymerase catalyzes RNA molecule production. There are different subtypes of each enzyme. RNA polymerase I produces rRNA, RNA polymerase II produces mRNA and miRNA, and RNA polymerase III produces the tRNA.

Ligase

Ligase catalyzes the formation of the phosphodiester bonds between ends of adjacent nucleotide chains.

Nuclease

Nucleases catalyze the enzymatic cleavage of the phosphodiester bond. There are 2 main types of nucleases—endonucleases, which can cleave within nucleic acid chains and exonucleases, which require a free end of a nucleic acid chain to catalyze cleavage. Restriction endonucleases are a notable type of endonuclease which cut in a palindromic sequence specific fashion. Furthermore, nucleases can be classified according to what type of nucleic acid they cleave, ie, deoxyribonuclease (DNase) and ribonuclease (RNase).

Mitochondrial DNA

The mitochondrion is a highly specialized organelle responsible for the production of ATP via oxidative phosphorylation. In addition, mitochondria play a role in programmed cell death (apoptosis). Lastly mitochondria have a role in degradation of reactive oxygen species, the urea and Krebs cycles, and fatty acid oxidation. Nearly every cell has numerous (dozens to hundreds of) mitochondria.

Mitochondrial genome

The mitochondrial genome is composed of 1 to several 16 kilobase circular double stranded DNA molecules. There are 37 genes present that encode components of the oxidative phosphorylation complex subunits, as well as tRNAs and rRNAs utilized in the translation of mitochondrial genes. Replication of the mitochondrial genome occurs independently of the nuclear genome. Importantly, not all proteins in the mitochondrion are encoded by the mitochondrial genome, with many encoded in the cell nucleus.

Heteroplasmy/homoplasmy

Since almost all cells have numerous mitochondria it is possible that when a progenitor cell divides, the daughter cells may end up with an uneven distribution of the mitochondria. A mutation that arises in a single mitochondrion could lead to the condition of heteroplasmy, or a nonhomogeneous distribution of mitochondrial alleles (remember that mitochondrial genomic replication occurs separately from the nuclear genome). The "normal" situation of all mitochondria in a cell being genetically identical is referred to as homoplasmy. This is important in disorders of mitochondria and may explain the relative penetrance of some disorders (and consequent

mostly due to the relative abundance of RNAse enzymes that degrade RNA. There are many different types of RNA, each with a unique role. Ribosomal RNA (rRNA) plays a structural and catalytic role within ribosomes in the translation of mRNA into amino acid chains. Messenger RNA (mRNA) is involved in transferring the information present in DNA into amino acid sequences (proteins). MicroRNAs (miRNA) are short fragments of RNA transcribed by RNA polymerase II that have a role in the regulation of mRNA levels and consequently protein expression. The term "heterogeneous nuclear RNAs (hnRNA)" refers to the sum of miRNA and mRNA. Transfer RNA (tRNA) performs the function of delivering specific amino acids to the ribosome for addition to a growing peptide chain. tRNAs are named according to the amino acid they bind. There is a dedicated group of tRNAs for each of the 20 amino acids used in protein synthesis. Each of these can exist in 2 main forms: aminoacylated (amino acid attached) or nonacylated. Aminoacylation refers to the addition of an aminoacyl group to the tRNA molecule, resulting in a tRNA with covalently bound amino acid at the 3' end. Transfer RNAs are designated as follows, using alanine as an example: alanine tRNA or tRNA^{Ala} (for the nonacylated form), alanyl-tRNA or Ala-tRNA or Ala-tRNA^{Ala} (aminoacylated form).

variable severity) in the context of dosage of mutant mitochondria. It is also notable that since there are multiple copies of the mitochondrial genome within each mitochondrion, there can be heteroplasmy at the level of the individual organelle.

Maternal inheritance

In gametogenesis the complement of mitochondria in an embryo comes almost exclusively from the egg. As a result mitochondrial genetic information in a developing embryo is predominantly of maternal origin. This explains the unusual pattern in the pedigree of most mitochondrial disorders as being inherited from the mother's side only and affecting male and female offspring equally. Additionally, one can utilize mitochondrial genetic information as a marker of maternal inheritance.

Fundamentals of expression

Cell signaling basics

The interaction between a cell and its surroundings is mediated through a complex web of interacting signalling pathways. These pathways translate changes in the extracellular environment into a functional response, usually in the form of altered gene expression. In broad terms signalling begins at the cell surface with soluble ligands binding the extracellular portion of a cell surface receptor. Cell surface receptors often have extracellular and intracellular portions with a transmembrane region in between. As a consequence of binding ligand the extracellular signal is transmitted through modification of the intracellular portion of the receptor. Modification of the intracellular portion leads to recruitment of proteins to further transmit the signal. In some signalling pathways, such as the Jak-Stat pathway, proteins recruited to the cell surface receptor actually are modified to enter the nucleus and bind DNA regulatory regions affecting gene expression. In other pathways, such as the EGFR pathway a cascade of kinases (enzymes that phosphorylate proteins) eventually phosphorylate a protein (or regulatory protein) that can then enter the nucleus, bind regulatory regions in genes and affect gene expression in either a positive or negative manner.

Genes

Genes are encoded as DNA nucleotide sequences that are utilized mainly to produce proteins that have either a structural or enzymatic function. One interesting feature of inheritance is that defects in structural genes tend to show dominant inheritance, while defects in enzymatic genes usually show recessive inheritance.

It was once thought that for each gene there was exactly 1 possible gene product. This concept of "1 gene = 1 protein" is now debunked as we know that through alternate splicing or the use of different transcription start sites, multiple different proteins can be products of the same gene.

A gene is any segment of DNA that can be *transcribed* into RNA. Most RNA transcripts are subsequently *translated* into protein, but some remain as RNA (noncoding RNA, eg, as miRNA, tRNA). The first portion of a gene, that is typically located the farthest "upstream" in the extreme 5' end, is the promoter sequence. Following the promoter is the coding region (the portion of the gene that is actually transcribed

into RNA). Most genes contain both exons (portions of the coding sequence that are ultimately translated into protein) and introns (untranslated sequences). The exon is composed of a specific sequence of nucleotides, functionally divided into trinucleotides (codons) that encode a specific amino acid. The smallest known human gene, encoding one of the histones, consists of 1 exon (no introns) and around 500 nucleotides. In contrast, the largest known gene, which encodes the protein dystrophin, has 70 exons, 70 introns, and around 2.5 million nucleotides (2,500 kilobases).

Transcription & its regulation

Differentiation, the process by which an undifferentiated cell becomes a specialized cell, has its basis largely in the regulation of gene expression. The set of genes undergoing active expression in a hepatocyte is very different from the set being expressed in a myocyte, for example. Likewise, cell activation is largely based upon the regulation of expression. Thus, a hepatocyte that has undergone induction as a result of exposure to phenytoin is expressing a different set of genes than the unstimulated hepatocyte. The control of gene expression takes place in 4 main points:

1. gene transcription, which can be upregulated or downregulated by a variety of mechanisms

2. mRNA splicing, which can proceed in a variety of alternate ways resulting in a variety of mature mRNA sequences

3. mRNA translation into protein, wherein the interfering action of miRNA is felt

4. protein degradation, which can be modified to proceed at variable rates

Transcription is the process whereby RNA is made from a DNA template. Transcription, like DNA replication, occurs in the 5' to 3' direction. The vast majority (up to 75%) of transcription involves the production of the ribosomal RNAs. The remaining types of RNA (tRNA, miRNA, and mRNA) account for the remaining transcription activity. The strand of DNA from which the transcript derives is referred to as the "sense" strand, while noncoding DNA strand is the "antisense" strand. The process of transcription begins at the TATA box, a 6 nucleotide (TATAAA) sequence located 25 bases upstream from the transcription start site. The TATA binding protein binds to the TATA box and initiates the formation of the transcriptional machinery which contains multiple factors including RNA polymerase. Polymerization occurs until the transcript reaches an AAUAAA sequence and the process terminates. The primary transcript contains both coding sequence (exons), as well as noncoding sequence (introns). A significant portion of the control of gene expression occurs at the level of transcription. The DNA to be transcribed must be "unpacked" from the highly complex 3-dimensional structure of the chromosome and "melted" into 2 single strands for this process to work. Initiation of transcription is a complex multistep process involving recruitment of factors to access the DNA template and to assemble the transcriptional machinery. Gaining access to the tightly packed chromatin involves a concerted effort between numerous factors with both positive and negative regulatory roles.

Splicing happens in the nucleus following transcription. Small nuclear ribonucleoproteins or snRNPs (proteins with a ribonucleic acid component) form the subunits of the spliceosome complex. A 5′ splice donor site, usually a GU set of bases, and a 3′ splice acceptor site, usually an AG sequence, are almost always present at the start and end of introns. The spliceosome complex binds the pre-mRNA and catalyzes the formation of a 2′ to 5′ lariat structure on an invariate branch site adenine residue. The lariat structure is subsequently spliced out and the ends of exons joined. The use of different splice acceptor sites is the basis of alternative splicing, producing different mature mRNAs from the same gene leading to greatly increased genetic diversity from a limited number of genes. In fact the vast majority of genes with multiple exons undergo alternative splicing events. Mutations in the splice acceptor, splice donor, or branch site can lead to aberrant splicing. In addition mutations that lead to the formation of novel splice donor or acceptor sites can cause the formation of alternative splicing and the inclusion of intronic sequence in mature mRNAs. Often intronic sequences are rich in stop codons, so this scenario frequently results in premature translation termination.

After splicing the maturing mRNA undergoes modification of the 5′ nucleotide by guanylyltransferase. A methylated guanine residue is added to the 5′ end through a 5′ to 5′ bond. This methylguanine "cap" has several functions for the nascent mRNA: facilitating nuclear export, ensuring stability when exported to the cytoplasm for translation, and promoting translation. The third major posttranscriptional modification of the mRNA is the addition of the poly-A tail to the 3′ end of the transcript. Similar to the 5′ cap the 3′ poly A (adenine) tail functions to maintain the integrity of the transcript, facilitate nuclear export, and promote translation of the mRNA. A series of proteins recognize an AAUAAA sequence in the 3′ untranslated region of the transcript and perform the cleavage and polyadenylation of the nascent mRNA.

Epigenetic regulation is a recently discovered mechanism by which gene expression is controlled. In a loose sense, epigenetic regulation refers to any factor not encoded in the DNA that affects gene expression. It generally follows 2 attributes: it can be reversed and it can be inherited. One notable example is DNA methylation. The methylation of nucleotides, most often affecting cytosine moieties located within cytosine-phosphate-guanine (CpG) islands, results in gene silencing. This it does through recruitment of proteins that are capable of prohibiting transcription. Methylation is not an all-or-none phenomenon, with the degree of silencing correlating with the number of methylated nucleotides. Methylation forms the basis for imprinting. In many different kinds of cancer it has been shown that the aberrant methylation of tumor suppressor gene promoters contributes to oncogenesis. Another common example of epigenetic regulation is histone acetylation. The nucleosome structure provides a physical barrier to transcription. The interaction between the positively charged histones and the negatively charged nucleic acid is the basis of this barrier. Transcription factors work to upregulate gene expression through several different mechanisms, including recruitment of proteins capable of acetylating histones. The effect of histone acetylation is "loosening" of the stable nucleic acid-histone interaction by decreasing the positive charge on

first position	second position				third position
	U	**C**	**A**	**G**	
U	phenylalanine	serine	tyrosine	cysteine	U
	phenylalanine	serine	tyrosine	cysteine	C
	leucine	serine	STOP	STOP	A
	leucine	serine	STOP	tryptophan	G
C	leucine	proline	histidine	arginine	U
	leucine	proline	histidine	arginine	C
	leucine	proline	glutamine	arginine	A
	leucine	proline	glutamine	arginine	G
A	isoleucine	threonine	asparagine	serine	U
	isoleucine	threonine	asparagine	serine	C
	isoleucine	threonine	lysine	arginine	A
	methionine	threonine	lysine	arginine	G
G	valine	alanine	aspartic acid	glycine	U
	valine	alanine	aspartic acid	glycine	C
	valine	alanine	glutamic acid	glycine	A
	valine	alanine	glutamic acid	glycine	G

f7.8 Triplet codons

the histones. As a result the DNA is more accessible to the machinery of transcription. Conversely, the recruitment of histone deacetylating proteins leads to the repression of gene expression.

Translation & its regulation

Translation refers to the process of building a polypeptide based upon the sequence of the mRNA. Mature mRNAs are exported from the nucleus into the cytoplasm for translation. The 5′ methylguanine cap acts as a recognition sequence for ribosomal proteins. Ribosomes are riboproteins composed of ribosomal RNA and proteins. There are 2 major subunits in eukaryotes, a 60s subunit that binds tRNAs and amino acids, and a smaller 40s subunit that binds mRNA. The initiation of translation is mediated by a number of eukaryotic initiation factors (eIFs) which regulate the formation of the ribosome and the binding of mRNA to the assembled ribosomal complex.

The addition of peptides begins with the 5′ initiator codon, the initial AUG of the mRNA encoding methionine. Charged tRNAs covalently bonded to specific amino acids contain recognition "anticodon" sequences complementary to the codon sequences of the mRNA. These triplet codons are specific for different tRNAs and consequently different amino acids. Since there are 64 possible codons, but only 20 amino acids there is redundancy built into the codons f7.8. The third base of the codon is less specific than the first 2 and is referred to as the "wobble" position. Formation of the peptide bond (the bond between amino acids in the growing peptide chain) is performed by catalytic ribonucleotides, so-called "ribozymes." Sequential addition of amino acids continues until the translational machinery encounters one of the stop codons (UAG, UAA, UGA). When this happens a release factor initiates the dissolution of the ribosome complex and subsequent freeing of the newly-formed peptide. It is important to note that some ribosomes are free and some are bound to the rough endoplasmic reticulum (RER). Those bound to the RER secrete their peptides into the endoplasmic reticulum where they are often posttranslationally modified (glycosylation for example) and destined either for export from the cell or packaging within lysosomes.

MicroRNAs (miRNAs) are a member of a family of short interfering RNAs. These RNAs, through complementary antisense base pairing to nascent RNA transcripts, control translation. It is estimated that there are >1,000 miRNAs involved with regulating >1/2 of the human genes. MicroRNAs are transcribed in a manner very similar to mRNAs by RNA polymerase II, including the addition of the 5' cap and 3' poly A tail. The precursor miRNA forms a self-paired double stranded RNA molecule with a hairpin loop at the end. This precursor is processed in the nucleus by a complex of proteins including Drosha and DGCR8 which remove the unpaired ends containing the 5' cap and 3' tail. The mature miRNA is exported from the nucleus where it is further processed by Dicer which removes the hairpin loop. The double stranded miRNA loses one of the strands to RNase while the other strand is incorporated into the riboprotein RNA induced silencing complex (RISC). The single miRNA strand can bind to the complementary 3' untranslated region of mRNA and modify expression through several different mechanisms. Most commonly the RISC complex inhibits protein translation, but it can also affect DNA methylation, histone modification, or degradation of mRNA transcripts.

Basics of protein structure
Primary structure (peptide bonds & amino acids)
The peptide bond is the basis of primary protein structure. As mRNA is translated from individual amino acids based on the triplet codon and specific complementary tRNA into a nascent polypeptide chain, it is the peptide bond that holds those amino acids together. The primary structure of a protein is simply the amino acid sequence as it is translated. The carboxyl group of the preceding amino acid forms a covalent bond with the amino group of the subsequent amino acid. This is the peptide bond and the structure formed from these linked amino acids is a polypeptide. The directionality of translation is amino group to carboxyl group. The folding structure of the globular protein is determined by the composition of the side chains of each amino acid and the energy minimization of packing each of those residues into a 3-dimensional molecule. Forces such as ionic interactions, van der Waals forces, and hydrogen bonds primarily between individual amino acid side chains affect the folding of the protein and the subsequent formation of higher-order structure.

Secondary structure
Secondary structure refers to the conserved basic structures that peptides form. The 2 most common of these structures are the α helix and the β strand. The α helix forms when hydrophobic side chains can be buried within the globular protein away from interactions with water. α helix requires relatively "flexible" side chains and certain amino acids, such as proline cannot be included based on the structure of their

side chains. β strands are less strict in the amino acids that can be involved. They are basically "stretched out" peptide sequences that fit like puzzle pieces (in a hydrogen bonding sense of the term) with each other to make β-sheets, or β-pleated sheets. Depending on the orientation of the adjacent strands the sheets can be referred to as being either parallel (amino terminus lines up with adjacent amino terminus of the peptide chain) or antiparallel (amino terminus lines up with the carboxy terminus of the adjacent chain). These secondary structures can then form more complex arrangements, such as the β stranded Greek key or the α helical helix-loop-helix.

Higher-order structure
The elements of tertiary and quaternary structure involve interactions between amino acids (tertiary) or protein subunits (quaternary). Tertiary structure refers to the packed conformation of secondary structures that the globular protein assumes based on minimization of potential interactions between the solute and the hydrophobic sides and/or the interactions between amino acid side chains themselves. Importantly, disulfide bonds between sulfur-containing amino acids (methionine and cysteine) are considered to be tertiary structure. Quaternary structure is the interaction of protein subunits to create a novel complex. A number of different kinds of bonds can hold the subunits together. A classic example is the 4 globin subunits that form the protein core of hemoglobin.

DNA replication & cell division
DNA replication
Cell division requires the synthesis of a complete copy of the genome. The process involves opening up the coiled double helical DNA to expose single stranded DNA templates for making new copies and occurs during the S phase of the cell cycle. Replication in this manner is referred to as "semiconservative" because each copy of the newly replicated DNA contains one new and one "conserved" strand.

DNA helicase and DNA topoisomerase are the major proteins involved in unwinding and opening the double helix to allow replication to occur. Single stranded binding protein prevents the replication bubble from reforming double stranded DNA. Multiple sites (AT rich "origins") along the DNA molecule undergo replication simultaneously, resulting in several replication bubbles. The replication fork f7.9 is the point at which the single stranded ends of the replication bubble meet to become double stranded. Since DNA polymerase requires

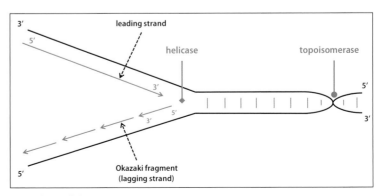

f7.9 Replication fork

a primer to extend, the enzyme primase synthesizes short complementary RNA primers on the single stranded DNA. DNA polymerase then catalyzes strand synthesis in the 5' to 3' direction. Because of this unidirectional activity one strand is produced in an uninterrupted fashion (the "leading" strand), while another requires multiple primers and a discontinuous production of copied DNA (the "lagging" strand). The short new copies of DNA on the lagging strand are referred to as Okazaki fragments. Once synthesis is completed the RNA primers are removed by RNase and DNA is synthesized in the gaps followed by ligation of the gaps between the primer replacement sites and the Okazaki fragments. DNA polymerase is capable of incredible fidelity, producing <1 misincorporated base per 1×10^7 properly incorporated bases.

Cell cycle

The cell cycle refers to the processes in the cell that dictate cell division. The entire process is mediated by cyclins and cyclin-dependent kinases, which are furthermore tightly regulated by a number of different proteins in response to environmental stimuli. There are several phases to the cell cycle, the interphase composed of 2 gap periods, G1 and G2, and the synthesis (S) phase. Additionally, between the 2 gap phases is the mitotic phase, further subdivided into prophase, metaphase, anaphase, and telophase.

Terminally-differentiated (and therefore incapable of dividing) cells are in a phase referred to the G0 phase. "Entry" into the cell cycle takes place with the cell entering the G1 phase with a diploid (2N) number of chromosomes. Following G1 the cell enters the synthesis phase where the chromosomes multiply to produce a tetraploid (4N) complement. Once the cell has replicated, the progression through the subsequent G2 phase and entry into mitosis is less tightly regulated.

Mitosis begins with prophase where the centrioles move to opposite poles in the nucleus and the microtubule apparatus begins to form. In metaphase the nuclear envelope disappears and chromosomes begin to condense and align with the central metaphase plate. This is the period of maximal chromosome condensation, explaining why karyotype analysis relies on the "metaphase spread" of chromosomes. Anaphase follows with separation of sister chromatids (duplicated chromosomes). Finally the chromosomes are located at the opposite poles during telophase. Shortly thereafter the nuclear envelope reforms and cytokinesis physically divides the cell in 2.

Meiosis

Meiosis is a related process that occurs only in the germ cells of the testis and ovaries. It provides the haploid gametes required for fertilization. Meiosis starts with a single diploid precursor cell and ends with 4 haploid daughter cells. The first part of meiosis is preceded by DNA replication raising the DNA content from 2N to 4N. The 4 chromatids of each chromosome are composed of 2 copies each of maternal and paternal chromosomes, joined at the centromere.

The first phase of meiosis I is prophase I, where the chromosomes form synaptic connections to each other, facilitating homologous recombination and exchange of genetic information between the maternal and paternal chromosomes. In the ovary primary oocytes arise from oogonium and arrest at prophase I, entering the dictyotene stage unique to oocytes. This

phase completes shortly before birth. It isn't until puberty that oocytes "reawaken" and a few each month complete meiosis I to form the secondary oocyte and first polar body. The secondary oocyte enters meiosis II and arrests at metaphase II, where it will remain until fertilized. Spermatogenic meiosis is more straightforward, beginning at puberty and ceaselessly creating more spermatozoa throughout the male lifetime.

Nondisjunction refers to aberrant separation of chromosomes during meiosis. It most commonly occurs during meiosis I, but can also occur during meiosis II and results in aneuploidy (a multiple of chromosomes other than an even multiple of 23). Nondisjunction during meiosis I leads to all 4 daughter germ cells being aneuploid, while nondisjunction during meiosis II generally leads to half normal gametes and half aneuploid.

Classification of genetic anomalies
Classification schemes

Mutations can be classified according to a number of schemes. First, it is important to recognize that strictly speaking a mutation refers to a genetic change with a deleterious outcome. If there is a genetic change that is not deleterious (and it is present in ≥1% of the population) the term "polymorphism" is used. Mutations can be categorized according to the effect of the mutation on the function of the protein, structure of the gene, or the overall effect on the organism.

Function

Mutations can be categorized as to the effect on the function of the protein: loss of function, gain of function. One type of gain of function mutation, the dominant-negative mutation, results in a novel protein that inhibits the action of the native protein or operates in a manner that overcomes the native protein's function.

Structure

Mutations may be categorized according to the change they produce on the gene, eg, point mutations, insertion mutations, deletion mutations, inversions, translocations. Point mutations can be further subcategorized according to their effect. Nonsense mutations result in premature truncation of translation, missense mutations lead to changes in amino acid sequence, and silent mutations change the nucleic acid sequence but do not result in the productions of either a stop codon or different amino acid. Point mutations of splicing donor or acceptor sequences can cause splice site mutations. Any mutation that leads to a change in the reading frame of the ribosome in translation is called a frameshift mutation. The most common mutations to cause frameshift are insertions and deletions.

Effect on organism

Finally, one can categorize mutations according to the change in the fitness of an organism that they produce. Deleterious mutations negatively affect the organism's fitness, while beneficial mutations result in increased fitness. As the more fit organism has a better chance to reproduce, the mutation has a greater chance of being passed on.

Concepts in human genetics
Chromosome structure & nomenclature

If a single copy of the human genome were stretched out it would be nearly 1 meter long (0.3 nm/nucleotide multiplied by 3.2 billion). The packaging of 3.2 billion nucleotides into the nucleus of a single cell requires an incredible measure of organized compaction. In addition, the packaged DNA has to be nearly instantly accessible for the cell to respond to environmental stimuli and change gene expression patterns.

The first level of compaction is the nucleosome. A nucleosome is composed of an octameric complex of positively-charged core histone proteins, 2 each of histones 2A, 2B, 3, and 4. Wrapped around this core complex is 146 bases of DNA. In between adjacent nucleosomes is a short linker of ~20-50 bases. Each sequential nucleosome is linked one to another by the linker histone, H1. The negative charge on the DNA is the basis of the attraction to the positively charged histones. Modifications to the charge on histones (primarily through acetylation) affect the binding properties of the DNA "loosening" the attraction and making DNA available for transcription (nucleosomes are a physical barrier to transcription). The nucleosomes have been shown to "slide" or move translationally to accommodate transcription. In addition transcription factors often recruit and form complexes with proteins with histone acetylation activity, facilitating histone modification and transcription. This "beads on a string" assembly is further compacted by stacking of the nucleosomes into the 30 nm chromatin fiber with 6 nucleosomes/turn. 50-fold higher compaction is accomplished with looping, followed by twenty-fold more with loops into minibands. Finally, the end result is the chromosome.

In the metaphase of the cell cycle the chromosome achieves maximal compaction. During the interphase there is a degree of relaxation of condensation. However, certain regions of the chromosome called heterochromatin retain constitutively higher levels of compaction. Conversely, euchromatin is associated with increased expression of genes and lighter compaction.

Molecular techniques
Karyotyping/G-banding

The early attempts to identify chromosomes were based on the length of each chromosome, from the longest (chromosome 1) to the shortest (chromosome 22, which actually is not the shortest, that is 21; but at the time it was thought to be the shortest). Subsequent efforts focused on staining of metaphase chromosomes with Giemsa stain (G-banding), quinacrine (Q-banding), or a number of techniques to produce a reverse staining pattern to G-banding (R-banding). G-banding regions that stain more intensely (AT rich) or less intensely (GC rich) are used to distinguish chromosomal identity, regions, bands, and sub-bands.

In relation to the centromere most chromosomes are divided into a short p arm and a longer q arm. Different types of chromosomes are classified by the location of the centromere.

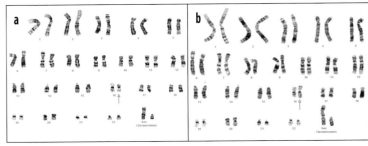

f7.10 Conventional cytogenetics; G-banded karyograms demonstrating a inv16 & b t(16;16) in 2 cases of acute myeloid leukemia

Chromosomes with roughly equivalent-length arms are called metacentric, ones with longer q than p arms are submetacentric, and those without significant p arms are called acrocentric. The acrocentric chromosomes contain short areas in place of p arms that encode the majority of rRNAs and are often the site of translocations.

The regions of the individual arms are numbered in relationship to the centromere. The first region away from the centromere is labeled "1" and depends on whether it resides on the p arm (p1) or the q arm (q1). Each region is further divided into bands and possibly, sub-bands. The nomenclature used is [chromosome][arm][region][band][sub-band]. For example "sub-band 3 of band 1 in region 2 on the long arm of chromosome 18" where the *BCL2* locus resides is written as 18q21.3. Higher resolution imaging of Giemsa stained chromosomes leads to more precise banding.

The metaphase spread stained chromosome image is referred to as a karyogram f7.10, while its interpretation is the karyotype. The normal human male karyotype is 46,XY; normal female is 46,XX with 46 referring to the total number of chromosomes and XX or XY the set of sex chromosomes.

Basic techniques in molecular pathology

Molecular pathology is most broadly defined as the investigation of disease through nucleic acid-based testing. The collection of sufficient and intact nucleic acid from a number of different specimens is a critical element in molecular pathology. Once nucleic acid is isolated it can be studied. There are a number of techniques that effectively amplify either the amount of nucleic acid or the signal from the nucleic acid present. Sometimes there is also a need to modify or manipulate the nucleic acid that has been isolated.

Specimen requirements & isolation of nucleic acid

Nucleic acid can be extracted from a number of different specimens including whole blood and blood products, tissue (either fresh, fresh-frozen, or formalin-fixed), body fluids (eg, pleural fluid, cerebrospinal fluid, urine), swabs of body sites (buccal epithelium), wounds, or hair root. Formalin fixation results in the crosslinking of nucleic acid to protein and subsequently leads to nucleic acid fragmentation. For this reason amplification and analysis of DNA from formalin-fixed tissue is best limited to short (<300 base pairs) sequences. Certain specimens should be avoided, such as heparin-containing blood; heparin has been shown to inhibit the polymerase chain reaction. In addition fixatives such as Bouin or Zenker should be avoided as they introduce chemicals, such as mercury in the case of Bouin, that interfere with common nucleic acid extraction protocols.

While both liquid phase and solid phase extraction techniques have proven successful in the isolation of nucleic acid, solid phase extraction is preferred due to its ease of use and scalability. The majority of liquid phase nucleic acid isolation techniques take advantage of the chemistry of the phosphate backbone. As a strong acid, nucleic acid is soluble in water up to a relatively high concentration and can be selectively precipitated with alcohol. The protocols for most of these nucleic acid isolation techniques first involve disrupting cell and nuclear membranes, preferentially degrading or precipitating proteins, centrifugation or extraction to separate the nucleic acid in aqueous phase from the cell membranes and precipitated protein, then isolating the nucleic acid from water via the alcohol precipitation and dehydration. For solid phase extraction, nucleic acid selectively adsorbs to a selective matrix (eg, silica) which is bound to an immobile solid, such as plastic or magnetic beads or a filter membrane. The initial procedures are similar to liquid phase extraction, except the precipitated nucleic acid binds to the silica under high ionic strength (low stringency) conditions and can be washed and subsequently eluted with a low ionic strength eluant.

Due to its structure and the near omnipresence of RNases, RNA is less stable than DNA. For these reasons the conditions under which one prepares RNA must be more strict than for DNA. Tissue must be better preserved, inhibitors of RNase and RNase-free products and supplies should be used. As DNA preparation often involves the use of RNase to degrade unwanted RNA, it is important to separate supplies and equipment used for DNA preparation from that which is used to prepare RNA.

Once isolated, nucleic acid can be verified through spectrophotometric absorption at 260 nm. Nucleic acid absorbs light at 260 nm wavelength (ultraviolet) stoichiometrically so that 1 unit of absorbance equals 50 μg/mL of double stranded DNA or 40 μg/mL of RNA. Protein absorbs light maximally at 280 nm, so that purity of DNA can be assessed with a ratio of absorbance at 260 nm to 280 nm. A ratio of <1.8 is considered to be relatively pure and free from contaminating protein.

DNA amplification

With only 5-10 pg (trillionths of a gram) of DNA per cell there is a need to increase the limited amount of assayable material to facilitate detection. There are several techniques to do so, employing amplification of either the target (usually via synthesis, such as polymerase chain reaction) or the signal (such as with branched DNA detection). Each technique has its limitations and benefits. Target amplification is plagued by contamination, which is subsequently amplified. Signal amplification suffers from greater failure rates than target amplification.

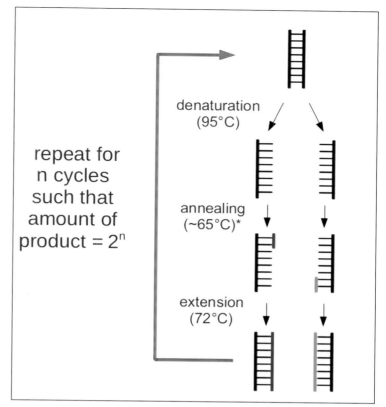

repeat for n cycles such that amount of product = 2^n

denaturation (95°C)

annealing (~65°C)*

extension (72°C)

f7.11 Polymerase chain reaction

Target amplification is the most commonly utilized technique for nucleic acid detection. Of the techniques, polymerase chain reaction (PCR) is the most prevalent. Other systems have evolved, some with benefits over PCR, including isothermal techniques of strand-displacement amplification, nucleic acid sequence-based amplification, transcription-mediated amplification, and loop-mediated isothermal amplification. Because the techniques are based on isothermal amplification they do not require a specialized thermal cycler like PCR does.

While the concept of amplifying DNA with DNA polymerase and a set of primers was first proposed >10 years before PCR was invented, the DNA polymerase would be denatured after each cycle and had to be reintroduced after cooling. Thus, there was no "chain" reaction, only a series of tedious single reactions prone to contamination. The giant leap into PCR was enabled by the discovery of a DNA polymerase that is stable under high temperatures. The polymerase of *Thermus aquaticus* (Taq), a microbe that lives and thrives near deep sea geothermal vents, is such a polymerase. Taq polymerase allowed the reaction to be started and finished in a closed, temperature cycling system.

The basic principle of PCR is the cyclic polymerization of DNA copies f7.11. The starting ingredients must contain at least a DNA template of interest, a set of complementary primers, a variety of dNTPs, and a heat stable polymerase. Most polymerases are dependent on exogenous divalent magnesium cation. Additional buffering or denaturing agents can be added as needed. The initial step, denaturation at 95°C, splits the double stranded DNA into single strands to facilitate the

ISBN 978-089189-5985

second step, annealing. In the annealing phase the temperature is lowered to one that favors annealing of the sequence specific primers. Primers must be carefully chosen so that melting temperatures of each are similar and so that there are no sequence similarities between the pairs, which can lead to inhibitory primer-dimer formation. The exact temperature for annealing is dependent on the characteristics of the primers. Following annealing the temperature is again raised to 72°C in order to facilitate polymerization along the single stranded DNA template. Once extension is complete the process begins anew with 95°C denaturation. Each cycle of PCR amplifies the DNA 2-fold. To represent the amount of DNA produced under optimal conditions the equation $[DNA] = 2^n$, where n=number of cycles. Therefore, a 10-fold amplification takes place every 3.3 cycles ($2^{3.3}=10$). Following that arithmetic, if there are 100 copies in cycle 7 then there will be 1,000 copies in cycle 10.

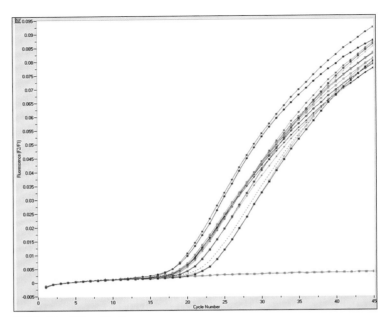

f7.12 Real time PCR amplification

Methylation-specific PCR

Methylation of genes is associated with repression of gene expression. There are a number of ways to detect whether or not a gene is methylated. One such technique is methylation-specific PCR. Methylated cytosine residues in the presence of sodium metabisulfite are reduced to uracil. After pretreatment with metabisulfite, PCR primers that are specific to a sequence containing uracils in the place of cytosines are utilized to selectively amplify the methylated sequence.

Reverse transcriptase PCR

As a single stranded unstable molecule, RNA cannot be directly amplified in a PCR reaction. However, through the use of reverse transcriptase a DNA copy can be produced from an RNA template. Subsequently a second DNA strand is synthesized from the first cDNA strand and a double stranded DNA representation of the RNA is produced. This double stranded DNA can then be used as a template for PCR. Some systems use a single step process where a heat stable DNA polymerase with reverse transcriptase activity (rTth polymerase, for example) is used. The RNA can be added to a closed system, reverse-transcribed, and then followed by PCR. Some systems use a 2-step process where the cDNA is first produced and then manually added to a PCR reaction.

Real time PCR

One of the most significant contributions of PCR to clinical assays is in the form of real time PCR. Real time, or quantitative PCR enables detection of synthesized DNA as it is being produced. It is this detection during the process that enables quantitation. "Usual" end stage PCR exhausts starting materials (primers, dNTPs) after a set number of cycles and fails to further amplify (the plateau phase). By monitoring amplification during the logarithmic stage, one can directly compare different samples. The cycle at which amplification enters the logarithmic phase is directly dependent on the amount of starting template. This point is referred to as the crossing threshold (Ct) f7.12. Following the equation mentioned previously (2^n), every 3.3 cycles is equivalent to a 10-fold difference in starting template. As expected the more starting material the sooner the reaction will enter the logarithmic phase of amplification. Several different detection systems have been employed including non sequence specific binding of nascent double stranded DNA by fluorescent intercalating dyes and sequence specific probes.

Melting point analysis

Increased specificity of PCR product identification can be achieved with melting point analysis. Following PCR with either nonhydrolyzable probes or intercalating dye analysis of the PCR product can be performed. It is important to note that when hydrolyzable probes are used melting curve analysis cannot be performed. The procedure involves measuring fluorescence while incrementally increasing the reaction temperature. The melting point of a PCR product is defined as the point at which 50% of the product is single stranded. On a plot of fluorescence vs temperature the melting point is the point of the maximal change in rate of melting f7.13. This melting point is dependent on a number of characteristics of the product, eg, length, G:C content, amount of mismatch. When plotted as the first derivative of fluorescence change a single specific peak can be identified for any given amplicon. Mismatches in the amplicon or the probe will result in shifted melting points.

Transcription-mediated amplification (TMA) & nucleic acid sequence-based amplification (NASBA)

TMA and NASBA are related techniques for isothermal amplification of RNA targets. They are primarily used for infectious disease applications, such as the detection of *Mycobacterium tuberculosis*. The principle in each technique is similar, utilizing specific sequences that are recognized by bacteriophage RNA polymerase in order to make more RNA copies. They differ in that NASBA uses a separate RNase H enzyme to degrade the RNA in an RNA:DNA hybrid, whereas that activity is present in the reverse transcriptase in TMA. The RNA copies produced can then be probed with specific probes, usually fluorescently labeled. The techniques are diagrammed in f7.14.

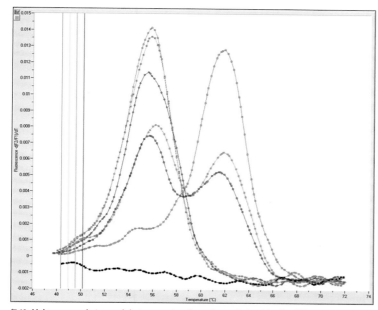

f7.13 Melt-curve analysis reveals heterozygosity of samples as distinguished by differing melting temperatures

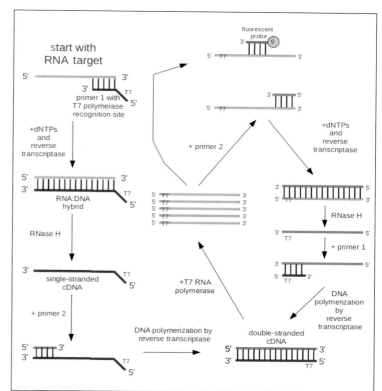

f7.14 Transcription mediated amplification (TMA) & nucleic acid sequence-based amplification (NASBA)

Multiplex ligation-dependent probe amplification (MLPA)

MLPA is an ingenious method to interrogate multiple (sometimes several hundred) mutations at the same time. The technique utilizes numerous specific probes varying in the length of an extragenetic stuffer sequence, but each containing gene-specific sequence and sequence shared with all the other probes for PCR. For each possible mutation there is a specific probe and an adjacent anchor probe separated by a single base. Only when the 2 probes anneal adjacent to each other are they able to be subsequently ligated and then amplified with probe-specific primers. Variations in the technique are useful for determination of single nucleotide polymorphisms/mutations, dosage and copy number, and methylation status.

Digital PCR

Digital PCR is a technique based on ± amplification (hence the digital). It is a nanoscale approach to quantitation of nucleic acids through partitioning of a sample into very small individual reactions. By diluting the nucleic acid sufficiently the amplification of a single copy of a target DNA allows very precise quantitation.

Bead based technology

Bead based technology allows for simultaneous amplification and subsequent separation of amplification products. Using principles pioneered with flow cytometry, beads that differentially fluoresce can be coated with any number of reagents, allowing for high throughput and multiplexed reactions.

Mass spectrometry

Some of the techniques with the highest multiplexing capacity rely on chemical analysis. With mass spectrometry one can separate particles based on their individual mass to charge ratios. A sample is ionized by any one of a number of techniques into component charged particles which travel through a magnetic field toward a detector in a reproducible manner and rate according to their mass to charge ratio. Therefore, any quantitative or qualitative change to a particle's identity is detectable. Large scale multiplexed analysis of sequence mutations has been performed using mass spectrometry.

Signal amplification

Techniques that aim to detect nucleic acid by amplification of a signal rather than amplification of the starting material have been historically less susceptible to spurious results due to contamination. However, they are usually not as sensitive. One can amplify either the probe (the cleavase reaction or ligation amplification reaction) or the signal itself (the branched DNA or hybrid capture techniques).

The cleavase technique is capable of multiplexing and is exquisitely sensitive. The principal is hybridization of a specific probe with a sequence of interest that is already bound to a second sequence specific probe thus creating a unique triplex structure. The triplex is recognized by cleavase, an endonuclease specific for the triplex structure. Upon cleavage, a specific probe sequence is released. The probe can be directly detected (via release of a quencher from a fluorophore-labeled fragment by cleavase) or detected with an additional probe-specific secondary probe.

Ligation amplification employs a thermostable ligase and allows the discrimination of DNA sequences differing in only a single base pair. The principle of LCR is based on the ligation of 2 adjacent oligonucleotide primers, which have been designed to hybridize with the target DNA such that the 3′ end of one sits immediately adjacent to the 5′ end of the next, and the point where they meet is the location of a known potential single base pair difference in the targeted sequence. This single base pair difference may define 2 different alleles or 2 different bacterial species. If the nucleotide in the target DNA is complementary to that of the 3′ end of the upstream primer, then the 2 primers will be joined by DNA ligase. If not, ligase cannot complete the joining of the 2 primer strands. 4 separate probes are utilized for each double stranded DNA. The double stranded target DNA is denatured with heating then cooled to 65°C so that the primers can be annealed. Each strand binds to a set of probes. If there is any mismatch at the 3′ end of one of the probes adjacent to the 5′ end of the second probe, then ligation cannot occur. After multiple cycles of denaturation, annealing, and ligation only the sequence without the aforementioned mismatch, if present, will be amplified.

Branched DNA amplifies the signal from a nucleic acid molecule through an elaborate multilayered branching mechanism. A capture probe is bound to a solid support, usually either beads or the wells of a plate. A hybrid probe called an extender is designed to hybridize to a nucleic acid of interest as well as the capture probe. As a result target nucleic acid is immobilized on the solid support. To this immobilized complex a second hybrid probe called a label extender is bound. The label extender recognizes both the target nucleic acid and a molecule called a preamplifier. Once the preamplifier is bound to the label extender the preamplifier molecule acts as the trunk of a tree on which an amplifier molecule forms the branches. The amplifier molecule in addition to recognizing the preamplifier also is studded with numerous biotin molecules. The biotin molecules are each recognized by a streptavidin-fluorophore conjugate which when excited fluoresces like the lights on a tree.

Hybrid capture uses a similar approach as branched DNA, but with fewer steps. A series of RNA probes directed against specific DNA sequences is incubated with specific antibodies that recognize RNA:DNA hybrid molecules. A sandwich approach is employed—immobilize these antibodies to the wells of a plate, bind hybrid DNA:RNA molecules, then recognize with a conjugated antihybrid antibody.

Restriction enzymes

Restriction enzymes are bacterial endonucleases (enzymes that cut within a DNA strand) that recognize and cleave specific DNA sequences. The endonucleases are named according to the genus, species, and strain from which they were isolated,

HindIII is from *H influenza* and EcoRI is from *E coli*. Each endonuclease in addition to recognizing a specific sequence will cleave in a particular fashion to leave either a 5′ overhang, blunt ends, or a 3′ overhang. Overhangs can be useful for many purposes, such as cloning or labeling a fragment by filling in the overhang with a labeled nucleotide. Because of their sequence specific cleavage activity, restriction endonucleases are used to cleave DNA in a predictable manner. Mutations in sequence sites can result in either loss or gain of a recognition sequence. This property is exploited in other assays, such as the Southern blot or the restriction fragment length polymorphism (RFLP) assay. Furthermore, methylation status of a gene can be deduced from whether the sequence is protected from endonuclease digestion.

Blotting (Southern, northern, western)

The process of transferring nucleic acid or protein to a solid support is referred to as blotting. The naming is dependent on the type of molecule being transferred. DNA is Southern blotted, RNA is northern blotted, and protein is western blotted. Hybrids of these exist, such that southwestern blotting is blotting of proteins that bind DNA and northwestern blots are for proteins that bind RNA. Direct application of the nucleic acid or protein is referred to as dot blotting. For the most part the molecules of interest are first separated from other molecules through gel electrophoresis. The gel is then blotted to a solid support membrane through either capillary or electrophoretic action. Once transferred, the molecules on the membrane can be probed. The presence of a signal and its location on the membrane when hybridized to the probe characterize the molecule of interest.

DNA sequencing

Most commercial applications of sequencing are based on monitoring and controlling the synthesis of a copy of a DNA strand. Previous techniques that depended on biochemical degradation of DNA in a specific fashion are no longer widely used.

Sanger dideoxy sequencing

One of the longest lasting sequencing technologies, dideoxy sequencing is elegant and simple. The principle is to perform in vitro DNA replication with a radiolabeled primer, but to terminate replication selectively at each different base. Initially, 4 different reactions were performed, one for each of the bases. In each reaction deoxynucleotides were added, but for each different tube one of the bases was added in a mix of deoxynucleotide and dideoxynucleotide. Since a dideoxynucleotide lacks the 3′ hydroxyl needed to form the phosphodiester bond replication ceases. As a result in each tube there would be a mix of synthesized nascent DNA strands, each terminated wherever the dideoxynucleotide was incorporated. Subjecting this mix to electrophoresis through a polyacrylamide gel would separate the DNA strands by length and provide a ladder, each rung representing an aborted replication due to incorporation of a chain terminating dideoxynucleotide. When each of the 4 reactions was run next to one another the sequence of the target could be read from the bottom of the autoradiograph

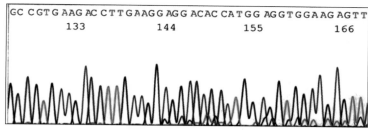

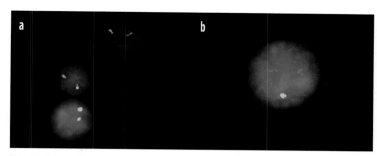

f7.15 Dideoxysequencing: capillary electrophoresis with fluorescence detection of differentially-labeled dideoxy NTPs in cycle sequencing assay; the presence of an additional sequence signal indicates a mixed sample

f7.16 Break apart probes consist of 2 differently colored probes that hybridize with DNA sequences on either side of a breakpoint in a gene; rearrangement splits the normal (fusion) signal into separate orange & green signals
Dual-color break apart probes are useful for detecting translocations that may have multiple translocation partners or inversions in single chromosomes, FISH break apart probes for IgH rearrangement
a In normal nuclei the IGH break apart probe generates 2 fusion signals (red-green or yellow), indicating 2 normal (un-rearranged) IgH genes on chromosomes 14
b In cells with IgH rearrangement, the most commonly pattern is 1 red-green or yellow fusion (retained normal IgH), 1 red & 1 green signal (the latter 2 representing the broken apart or rearranged IgH)

(shortest fragments) to the top (longest fragments). This technique was greatly simplified (and improved) through the use of dideoxynucleotides conjugated to different fluorophores. The reactions could be run through a single polymer matrix capillary and the identity of each fluorophore determined as it migrated past a fixed detector f7.15. This allowed for a single reaction, no radioactivity, and greater length of sequence read.

Pyrosequencing (single base extension)

Pyrosequencing relies on quantitative measurement of the pyrophosphate that is released whenever a trinucleotide phosphate is incorporated into a phosphodiester bond. Since the pyrophosphate is released in a stoichiometric amount in relation to the number of bases incorporated, the sequence of a target DNA can be inferred. By sequentially adding each base, a single-base extension reaction will occur whenever the appropriate complementary base is added. When this single base is incorporated a stoichiometric amount of pyrophosphate is released. The released pyrophosphate can be measured, usually through a secondary light-producing reaction. If a string of identical bases is encountered in a sequence then there will be stoichiometrically more pyrophosphate released than if there was a single base. Pyrosequencing is a rapid, inexpensive, and sensitive method of sequencing best utilized to analyze sequences close to the primer. For this reason it is most often used for point mutation or single nucleotide polymorphism characterization.

Hybridization techniques (FISH, CGH, array CGH)

Fluorescent in situ hybridization (FISH) f7.16-f7.18 is a versatile test. Many variations of FISH exist, especially in the area of probe design. Alternatives to fluorescent detection, such as chromogenic (CISH) or silver particles (SISH) exist. Advantages of in situ hybridization include the ability to use numerous different samples such as interphase cells, the ability to interrogate individual cells in a background of other cells, the ability to separate signals in space, the ability to quantitate signals, and the ability to detect multiple signals in a single specimen. There are 3 major types of probes used in conventional FISH analysis—chromosome enumeration probes, locus-specific probes, and sets of probes that cover entire chromosomes used for chromosome "painting." Chromosome enumeration probes are targeted to repeat regions present in the centromeric

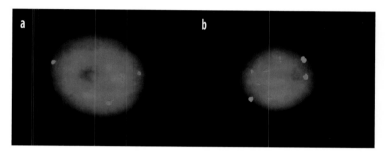

f7.17 Enumeration (CEP) probes are chromosome specific probes that hybridize to highly repetitive human satellite DNA sequences, usually located near the centromere; in this example, probes for chromosome 9 & 11 show a normal chromosome number in a & polysomy in b

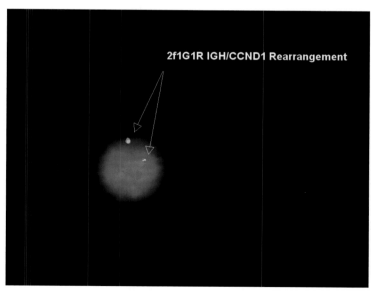

f7.18 Dual color dual fusion FISH is similar to dual color single fusion FISH, except the probe spans across the gene target. Thus, when rearrangement occurs, the probe splits, and translocation results in a dual orange/green (fusion) signal, 1 on each derivative chromosome. This probe greatly reduces the number of normal nuclei exhibiting abnormal signal patterns, and is advantageous in detecting low levels of nuclei possessing a simple balanced translocation. In this figure, an example of *IgHC-CCND1* fusion is demonstrated.

region of the chromosome. They are often used in combination with locus-specific probes to determine identity and copy number of individual chromosomes. In the case of translocations the locus-specific probes can be further subdivided into whether the goal is to detect fusion genes or breaks in genes. Fusion probes are useful for well defined translocations with conserved break/fusion points. Either dual color, single fusion (2 different colors for the normal genes become a single third color when fused) or dual color, dual fusion (2 different colors for the normal genes become 2 different colors representing the fusion gene and the derivative gene left behind). Single fusion probes are useful when the translocation is represented in a large number of cells, but is subject to false positives when there are a lower percentage of cells with the defined translocation. In that case dual color, dual fusion probes are most helpful. On the other hand if there is a gene that is more promiscuous and involved in several different translocations a break apart probe is a better choice. With break apart probes a single normal signal is "broken" into 2 separate (separated by space) different colored signals.

Comparative genomic hybridization (CGH) is a hybridization technique that provides pan-genomic chromosomal copy number information, providing information about copy losses and gains in chromosomes and subchromosomal regions. The most common uses for CGH are with genetic characterization of chromosomal anomalies in developmentally delayed, dysmorphic, or autistic children with no recognized karyotypic abnormalities or for the characterization of chromosomal gains and losses in cancer cells relative to noncancer cells. In the instance of cancer, CGH probes are made from the entire genome of the cancer cells as well as the normal genome. Each set of probes (cancer vs noncancer) is differentially labeled (usually by fluorescent colors). The sets of probes are hybridized to a metaphase spread of normal human chromosomes on a slide. Competition for binding sites on the metaphase chromosomes between the cancer probes and the noncancer probes creates a pattern where cancer probes are over-represented in regions that are amplified and underrepresented in deletions. CGH can determine whether entire chromosomes or regions of chromosomes are either amplified or deleted. It is important to realize that CGH can only detect quantitative differences between normal and "nonnormal." It cannot detect balanced translocations or any other nonquantitative abnormalities.

The term "array" CGH refers to a similar technique wherein, instead of hybridization to metaphase human chromosomes, the differentially-labeled probes are hybridized to an array representing the entire human genome or a focal region of interest. From this a plot of amplifications and deletions can be precisely mapped to regions of chromosomes.

Applications

Parentage, forensic identity & chimerism using short tandem repeats

Short tandem repeats (STRs) are sequences of DNA that consist of a run of repeated dinucleotides or trinucleotides. The length (copy number) of these STRs is stably inherited and is normally stable from cell to cell, while it is different from person to person. The STR haplotype of an individual is based on the set of chromosomes that they inherit, a copy of one STR

allele from each parent. For this reason a panel of STRs can be used to determine parentage. Similarly, a panel can be used for identification of remains for forensic purposes, and for the assessment of chimerism in transplant recipients.

Note that expansion of STRs within coding sequences is a mechanism of disease in several different conditions, known as trinucleotide repeat disorders, such Huntington disease. In addition, differing length of STRs in different cells from the same patient indicates anomalies in mismatch repair genes, such as in Lynch syndrome.

Haplotyping using single-nucleotide polymorphisms

Single nucleotide polymorphisms (SNPs) are single base pair differences that cause variability in the sequences between individuals. SNPs usually meet 2 criteria—they are present in ≥1% of the population and do not cause disease. SNPs are present on average in 1 of every 1,000 bases. The grand total of an individual's SNPs is referred to as the haplotype. Certain portions of a haplotype are traceable and useful as a sort of genetic family tree. Haplotypes are similar within a population and may partially account for the geographic predisposition to certain diseases, traits, or responses to medications. Genome-wide array studies have shown that certain SNPs are associated with increased or decreased predisposition to certain specified diseases. The International HapMap Project published in 2009 is an attempt to begin to characterize some of this variation by comparing the haplotypes of certain chromosomes and SNPs between and within widely dispersed populations.

Whole-genome applications

While the characterization of SNPs in an individual holds promise for unlocking some of the secrets within the genome, SNP haplotyping only scratches the surface. The "holy grail" is the personalized genome, a sequencing of the entire genetic composition of an individual. In 2000 the first draft sequences of the haploid genome were published, and by 2007 the first full sequence of a diploid genome was published. The technology necessary for the accomplishment of such feats relies on a few basic principles—fragmenting the genome into smaller pieces, sequencing these pieces by parallel in vitro synthesis, and compilation of the sequenced fragments into a single contiguous uninterrupted sequence using powerful computing techniques.

Next generation sequencing or high-throughput sequencing refers to the powerful techniques used to elucidate large genomic sequences. Most of these techniques are founded on the principles defined above—massive parallel in vitro sequencing, sensitive detection and separation of individual signals, and subsequent computerized assembly of all the contiguous sequences (contigs). There are now several different platforms that are capable of sequencing entire genomes, but almost all of them are based on the principles previously mentioned.

It is clear that whole genome sequencing would enable greater resolution of the genetic variation than SNP haplotyping. However, there exists significant variation that genome sequencing is unable to resolve. Current techniques of genomic sequencing rely on "averaging," that is populations of sequence are analyzed in parallel and the resultant average signal is reported. The next major step in the evolution of genomic sequencing will involve so-called "deep sequencing." Deep sequencing refers to a greater depth of coverage of sequence thereby allowing resolution of subpopulations within the sequence. On average deep sequencing provides 7-10 fold coverage of a specific sequence to allow for the characterization of sequence in greater detail.

Pharmacogenomics

Pharmacogenomics is the study of multiple genetic factors that influence an individual's response to a drug (pharmacokinetics) or a drug's effect on an individual (pharmacodynamics). Strictly speaking, pharmacogenetics is a subset of pharmacogenomics and usually refers to a single gene or group of related genes and their influence(s) on the above-mentioned factors.

One of the most important concepts in pharmacogenomics is genetic polymorphism. There can be polymorphism in regulatory or coding regions of genes whose products are involved with drug metabolism that affect the response that a particular drug elicits. It is often said that the purpose of pharmacogenomics is to ensure that any given individual gets the right drug in the right amount to elicit the desired response and minimize undesired ones.

Of the genes involved with drug metabolism members of the cytochrome P450 (CYP) family hold an exalted position, estimated to be involved in the metabolism of ~3/4 of medications. The nomenclature for *CYP* genes is standardized so that the name reflects the supergene family (CYP), the family, the subfamily, the isoenzyme, and the allelic variant. For example the wild type (*1) allele of the 2 family, D subfamily, 6 isoenzyme is transcribed as CYP2D6*1. The purpose of the gene products of the CYP family is the oxidative metabolism of toxins, which includes drugs. It is important to realize that polymorphisms in CYP not only affect the inactivation and clearance of drugs, but can also affect the activation of a prodrug, as is the case with the CYP2D6 metabolism of codeine to the active metabolite morphine. The different alleles are categorized as to whether they result in poor metabolizers, intermediate metabolizers, extensive metabolizers, or ultrarapid metabolizers. It follows that a poor metabolizer will experience increased toxic effects from drugs whose clearance is regulated by CYP and decreased response to prodrugs activated by CYP. CYP2D6 polymorphisms also have a role in the metabolism of tricyclic antidepressants, such as nortriptyline. CYP2C9 plays an important role in the metabolism of warfarin and phenytoin. There are several alleles of CYP2C9 associated with reduced activity including the more common *2 and *3 alleles. The CYP2C19 gene product is responsible for the metabolism of omeprazole, phenytoin, and diazepam. Certain polymorphisms of CYP2C19 lead to decreased activity and subsequent increased toxicity. These polymorphisms are most common in Asians.

The target of warfarin is inhibition of the vitamin-K epoxide reductase (*VKORC1*). The *VKORC1* gene product is involved in the metabolism of vitamin K, a key cofactor in γ-carboxylation of the vitamin K-dependent coagulation factors (factors II, VII, IX, X, protein C, and protein S). Polymorphisms in the gene named H1 and H2 are associated with enhanced sensitivity to warfarin. The H7, H8, and H9 haplotypes are associated with decreased sensitivity to warfarin (warfarin resistance).

N-acetyltransferase is central for the metabolism of isoniazid, some polymorphisms result in increased or decreased activity. Some strains of *M tuberculosis* express NAT leading to isoniazid resistance.

Administered as prodrugs for chemotherapy, thiopurines are activated by hypoxanthine guanine phosphoribosyl transferase (*HGPRT*). Thiopurine methyltransferase (*TPMT*) inactivates thiopurines. Polymorphisms in the *TPMT* gene have been identified associated with increased activity (reduced therapeutic effect) or decreased activity (increased toxicity).

Methylene tetrahydrofolate reductase (*MTHFR*) is inhibited by the antimetabolite methotrexate. The most common polymorphisms of *MTHFR*, C677T and A1298C are both associated with an increased incidence of methotrexate toxicity (and increased homocysteine levels).

Practical aspects of molecular pathology
Legislation & oversight

In 2003, CLIA regulations were revised to include specific requirements for the clinical cytogenetics laboratory. Laboratories conducting molecular genetic testing were not specifically addressed, but such testing is generally considered "high complexity" under CLIA regulations. Proficiency testing surveys are available for some of the more common molecular tests, but in many instances molecular laboratories must implement an alternative plan to verify accuracy at least twice annually, in order to be in compliance with CLIA regulations. One limitation of proficiency testing surveys in molecular pathology is that the survey material often consists of purified DNA, such that the process of extracting and isolating DNA is not assessed.

Legislation regarding consent for molecular genetic testing is the responsibility of the individual states. At this time, informed consent for genetic testing is required by law in Alaska, Alabama, Florida, Georgia, Massachusetts, Michigan, Nebraska, New Mexico, New York, South Carolina, South Dakota, and Vermont. Some of the states explicitly define what information must be given in the informed consent, while others do not. CLIA regulations do not specifically require that the laboratory document informed consent for requested tests. The responsibility of informed consent rests with the ordering physician.

Furthermore, some states have passed legislation to protect genetic information beyond the protections offered by federal law (HIPAA) of health information in general. This treatment of genetic information has been termed "genetic exceptionalism," defended upon the basis of the uniquely predictive and personal nature of genetic information. Some states have defined genetic information as "personal property." Passed into federal law in 2008, the Genetic Information Nondiscrimation Act (GINA) protects individuals from discrimination for employment or group health insurance (but not life or disability insurance) based on the results of genetic testing.

Genetic counseling

Genetic counseling is an important facet of molecular testing. The implications of inherited disease are far-reaching to both family members and the tested (proband) individual. In addition to consent for genetic testing, it is appropriate to send patients for genetic counseling to explain the ramifications of a potential test result and the significance of a negative result. Genetic counselors are usually masters-level subject matter experts in risk assessment and counseling. Risk assessment calculations are made based on pedigreed family history, personal medical history, and the results of genetic or genomic tests. Based on this information genetic counselors utilize Bayesian calculations to assess for residual risk.

Bayesian calculations take into account prior probability and conditional probability of a particular finding to generate a joint probability and posterior probability. Intuitively, it makes sense that a negative test result from a particular test with a defined sensitivity does not imply a zero risk. A residual risk exists because the test does not detect all potentially affected individuals. It also stands to reason that the sensitivity of a test varies with the population being tested and as a result so does the residual risk. Bayesian calculations are a way of assigning a quantitative value to that residual risk. The residual risk is what is left over after one calculates the probability of a test result being "meaningful" (ie, does it separate "disease" from "nondisease").

Patterns of inheritance

Inherited vs acquired genetic disorders

Disorders that result from a gene defect are generally considered genetic disorders. These are not all inherited disorders. Many genetic defects are sporadic; that is, the defect is absent in both the paternal and maternal genome and is somehow acquired during oogenesis, spermatogenesis, or early embryogenesis. For most genetic disorders, there are both inherited and sporadic forms, the latter termed "simplex" cases. Such sporadic defects are usually "germline" nevertheless; that is, the defect is present in all cells of the organism. Other genetic defects arise within a differentiated cell; such "somatic" defects are not found in germline DNA and are unlikely to be passed on to offspring.

Inheritance patterns

Autosomal dominant disorders have the following features: at least 1 parent is usually affected; males and females are affected with equal frequency, and both males and females have a 50% chance of transmitting the condition to offspring. Of course, sporadic examples of autosomal dominant conditions need not follow these rules. Autosomal dominant conditions are modified by penetrance and expressivity. Penetrance refers to the proportion of patients with the mutation who manifest a phenotypic abnormality. Genetic defects that always result in abnormal phenotype are said to have 100% penetrance. Expressivity refers to the severity and range of manifestations. Autosomal dominant genetic defects often involve genes that encode structural proteins, receptor proteins, or transmembrane channels.

Autosomal recessive disorders have the following features: generations are skipped (parents are usually unaffected, but both parents are implied carriers), males and females are equally affected, and if a couple has an affected child, the likelihood of a second affected child is 25%. Rare autosomal recessive genetic defects rely heavily upon consanguinity for survival in the population. In general, autosomal recessive conditions do not vary in terms of penetrance or expressivity. Autosomal recessive genetic defects usually involve genes that encode enzymes.

X-linked recessive disorders are expressed almost exclusively in males. Females may be affected in regions of very high mutant gene frequency, such that a homozygous female becomes a statistical likelihood. Females may also be affected on the basis of asymmetric lyonization or Turner syndrome (monosomy X). Males cannot pass the trait to their male offspring, but their daughters are obligate carriers. Females have a 50% chance of passing the trait to their male offspring (who will be affected) and to their female offspring (who will be carriers).

Genetics of nonneoplastic disease
Renal
Inherited nephritic syndrome

Inherited nephritic syndrome is caused primarily by mutations in the genes encoding type IV collagen. At the severe end of the spectrum is Alport syndrome, which presents with the triad of glomerulonephritis, sensorineural hearing loss, and ocular (corneal, lenticular, and macular) lesions. Initially presenting with hematuria, a manifestation of glomerulonephritis, Alport syndrome will progress eventually to end stage renal disease. ~80% of cases have a pattern of X-linked recessive inheritance, with most remaining cases autosomal recessive. Carrier females for the X-linked trait often manifest asymptomatic hematuria.

The simplest way of making the diagnosis of Alport syndrome is through examination of skin or renal biopsies. The absence of immunohistochemical staining for the α_5 chain of type IV collagen—$\alpha_5(IV)$—supports the diagnosis. In fact, immunohistochemical staining of kidney often shows complete absence of α_3, α_4, and α_5 chains of type IV collagen. The immunohistochemical tests are imperfect, with normal staining seen in up to 20% of cases. Glomerular examination by electron microscopy (EM) shows a thin, disrupted, and inhomogeneous lamina densa, sometimes appearing multilaminar f7.19, that entraps rounded electron-dense bodies. EM may show scalloping of the epithelial aspect of the glomerular basement membrane.

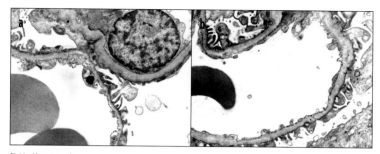

f7.19 Alport syndrome
a Glomerular basement membrane thinning
b Typical splitting & splintering of the glomerular basement membrane

X-linked recessive Alport syndrome is caused by mutations in the *COL4A5* gene on Xp22.3, which encodes the α_5 chain of type IV collagen. There are >400 documented pathogenic mutations in *COL4A5*, including missense, splice site, and deletion mutations. The 3 most common mutations in adult-onset Alport syndrome are point mutations, c.4692G>A, c.4946T>G, and c.5232G>A.

A milder disorder known as benign familial hematuria or thin basement membrane disease may represent a heterozygous variant of Alport syndrome. This manifests as persistent hematuria, without proteinuria or progression to renal failure. There is normal staining for α_3, α_4, and α_5 chains. Electron microscopy displays the diffuse uniform thinning of glomerular basement membranes that defines this entity.

Inherited nephrotic syndrome

Nephrotic syndrome is a common pediatric illness, characterized by massive proteinuria, edema, hypoalbuminemia, and hyperlipidemia. The most common cause of childhood nephrotic syndrome is minimal change disease, an acquired condition that usually arises between the ages of 1-10 years. Minimal change disease is exquisitely sensitive to steroids. As a result, children with nephrotic syndrome are often treated empirically with steroids, and improvement is taken as presumptive evidence of minimal change disease. In those who do not improve, other possibilities are considered, and a biopsy may be undertaken.

Congenital nephrotic syndrome is defined as nephrotic syndrome detected before 3 months of age. This is only rarely caused by minimal change disease. Congenital nephrotic syndrome may present just after birth but often begins in utero. Typical findings include dependent edema (dorsum for a neonate), abdominal distension, and a large placenta. There is marked (nephrotic range) proteinuria, hypoalbuminemia, and hyperlipidemia. The differential diagnosis must include certain perinatal infections (rubella, toxoplasmosis, syphilis, cytomegalovirus) and a group of inherited disorders (inherited nephrotic syndromes) t7.1.

t7.1 Inherited nephrotic syndrome

Congenital nephrotic syndrome of the Finnish type	*NPHS1* (19q13.1) gene, which encodes nephrin Nephrin is a key component of the glomerular slit diaphragm Affected children born with markedly enlarged placenta Massive proteinuria begins in utero, nephrotic syndrome by 1 month of age Electron microscopy is notable for an abnormal variation in the size of the slit pores (the space between podocyte foot processes) & rarefaction of the slit diaphragms
Pierson syndrome	*LAMB2* (3p21) gene, which encodes β_2 laminin β_2 laminin is a component of the glomerular basement membrane Associated with microcoria (fixed, narrow, pupils) Death within several months Renal biopsy shows mesangial sclerosis & crescents
Nail-patella syndrome	*LMX1B* (9q34.1) gene, which encodes a transcription factor that regulates transcription of COL4A3 Autosomal dominant disorder manifesting with skeletal & ocular anomalies, abnormalities of the nails & renal disease (variable) Renal biopsy shows basement membrane expansion by fibrillary collagen deposits
Denys-Drash syndrome/Frasier syndrome	*WT1* gene (11p13) Wilms tumors, male pseudohermaphroditism & rapidly progressive renal failure Renal biopsy shows mesangial sclerosis Frasier syndrome similar but less severe, associated with gonadoblastoma
Familial autosomal dominant focal segmental glomerulosclerosis	*ACTN4* gene, which encodes α-actinin *TRPC6* gene, which encodes transient receptor potential cation channel 6 Onset of nephrotic syndrome in adolescence or young adulthood
Familial autosomal recessive corticosteroid-resistant nephrotic syndrome	*NPHS2* gene, which encodes podocin Onset of proteinuria in early childhood Renal biopsy initially resembles mimimal change disease but transforms into focal segmental glomerulosclerosis

One of the more common causes of inherited nephrotic syndrome is *congenital nephrotic syndrome of the Finnish type*, which is due to mutations in the gene *NPHS1* located on chromosome 19q13.1 and encoding the protein nephrin. Nephrin plays a key role in the establishment of the glomerular slit diaphragm. Pierson syndrome (not to be confused with the mitochondrial disorder "Pearson syndrome"), is another cause of congenital nephrotic syndrome that is associated with microcoria. Mutations in the gene *LAMB2* on chromosome 3p21 lead to deficiencies in the β_2-laminin protein, a key component of the glomerular basement membrane. Nail-patella syndrome is an autosomal dominant disorder involving the *LMX1B* gene on chromosome 9q34.1. The *LMX1B* gene product is a transcription factor that regulates expression of the *COL4A3* gene. Patients present with skeletal, ocular, and nail abnormalities along with nephrotic syndrome. Those who do have renal involvement (variable) have ultrastructural evidence of fibrillary collagen deposits in the basement membrane. Denys-Drash syndrome is one of many disorders associated with mutations in the *WT1* gene on 11p13. Those affected have a high incidence of Wilms tumor, male pseudohermaphroditism, and rapidly progressive renal failure (usually leading to end stage renal disease by age 3). Also associated with mutations of *WT1* is Frasier syndrome, which has a slower progression to renal failure and an increased incidence of gonadoblastoma.

Inherited tubular disorders

Renal Fanconi syndrome refers to a type of proximal tubular dysfunction for which there are numerous causes, both inherited and acquired t7.2. Generalized proximal tubular dysfunction manifests as glycosuria, amino aciduria, phosphaturia, hypokalemia, and metabolic acidosis (bicarbonate wasting). Phosphaturia can cause rickets in children and osteomalacia in adults. Most of the acquired causes are toxic in nature (myeloma kidney, heavy metals, and urate nephropathy). Inherited causes include cystinosis, tyrosinemia, and galactosemia, which cause secondary tubular damage, and direct inheritance of tubular defects, such as Dent disease (X-linked recessive defect in the *CLCN5* gene encoding a chloride channel).

t7.2 Causes of tubular dysfunction

Inherited	Acquired
Cystinosis	Myeloma kidney
Tyrosinemia type I	Urate nephropathy
Galactosemia	Heavy metal toxicity
Glycogen storage disease	Amyloidosis
Hereditary fructose intolerance	Collagen vascular diseases
Wilson disease	Renal transplant rejection
Idiopathic renal Fanconi syndrome	Medication (antineoplastic agents, antiretroviral
Dent disease	agents, aminoglycosides)

Polycystic kidney disease

Autosomal recessive polycystic kidney disease (ARPKD)

The manifestations of ARPKD typically begin in utero. The first manifestation may be oligohydramnios, the result of diminished urine output. Hypertension and respiratory distress are often present at birth, the latter a result of pulmonary hypoplasia as part of the oligohydramnios sequence. The kidneys have radially oriented cysts, consisting of ectatic elongated collecting ducts, maintaining their overall reniform shape f7.20. More than half of cases progress to end stage renal disease within the first decade. ARPKD must be distinguished from congenital cystic renal dysplasia and the rare infantile/ in utero presentation of ADPKD.

Patients with ARPKD almost always have hepatic involvement that becomes problematic only in those who survive into adulthood. The morphologic features are those of typical biliary plate malformations, consisting of ectatic portal bile ducts, circumferential proliferation of ductules, and periportal fibrosis.

More than 95% of cases have mutations of the *PKHD1* gene on chromosome 6p. The gene is large, without significant common, mutations, so direct sequencing is impractical. Mutation scanning is the preferred technique for identifying mutants.

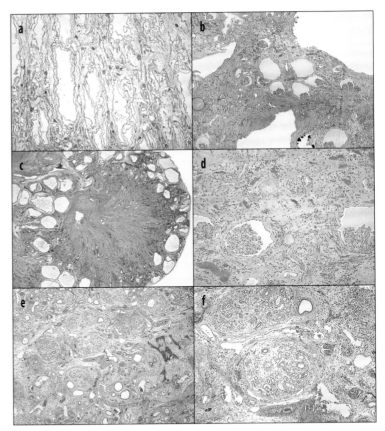

f7.20 Cystic renal diseases
a Autosomal recessive polycystic kidney disease demonstrates radiating elongated cystic tubules
b Autosomal dominant polycystic kidney disease demonstrates variably sized cysts with prominent glomerulocystic changes
c Rarely, autosomal dominant polycystic kidney disease may present in a neonate or fetus; in contrast to cystic renal dysplasia, the overall corticomedullary interface is vaguely preserved & glomerulocystic lesions are evident
d Glomerulocystic renal disease, which may be a variant of autosomal dominant polycystic kidney disease
e & f Cystic renal dysplasia is markedly disorganized renal parenchyma with fibroblastic mesenchymal cuffs of stroma; cartilage may be present

Autosomal dominant polycystic kidney disease (ADPKD)

ADPKD typically becomes evident in adulthood. It is more common than ARPKD, with an estimated prevalence of 1 in 500 births. There is essentially 100% penetrance by the 5th decade, and ~1/2 of patients have progressed to end stage renal disease by age 60. Symptoms such as impaired urine concentrating ability (isosthenuria) and hypertension often precede renal failure by decades. Flank pain is common and may be caused by cyst hemorrhage, cyst infection, intracystic tumor, and renal stones (the prevalence of renal stones is 20%, usually in the form of calcium oxalate or urate stones).

The cysts in ADPKD are both cortical and medullary, markedly enlarging and distorting the kidney f7.20. There has been debate regarding susceptibility to renal cell carcinoma (the only cystic disease unequivocally associated with an increased risk is that associated with long term dialysis), but when tumors occur they occur at a younger than usual age, are often multicentric or bilateral, and are very difficult to detect.

In 75% of cases, there is hepatic involvement in the form of polycystic liver disease. Mitral valve prolapse is identified in up to 25% of cases, pancreatic cysts in ~10%, and intracranial berry aneurysms in 10-20%.

Approximately 85% or cases result from mutations in *PKD1* on chromosome 16p13. The *PKD1* gene is located adjacent to *TSC2*, one of the genes involved with tuberous sclerosis, and there have been reports of a contiguous gene syndrome when both genes are affected. The remaining 15% of cases are due to mutations in the *PKD2* gene. The diagnosis can be confirmed with imaging studies alone, for which specific criteria exist; however, these findings are often not fully penetrant until about the age of 30-50, so molecular testing may be needed if earlier diagnosis is desired. When sufficient relatives are available and willing to be tested, the diagnosis can be made with linkage analysis. Informative microsatellites are adjacent to the *PKD1* and *PKD2* genes, which can be exploited for this purpose. Direct sequencing of the large *PKD1* and *PKD2* genes is difficult but can detect up to 85% of disease causing mutations.

Cystic renal dysplasia (multicystic dysplastic kidney)

Cystic renal dysplasia (multicystic dysplastic kidney) is a fairly common cause of flank masses in infants. It is a non-inherited (sporadic) disorder that may result from in utero ureteral obstruction. Kidneys are distinctly nonreniform in shape and contain a mixture of cysts and loose mesenchyme, with the latter sometimes containing cartilage. Sometimes the disease affects only a segment of the kidney, but usually the entire kidney is involved, and occasionally it is bilateral. Sometimes, cystic renal dysplasia is found as a component of a larger syndrome, the Meckel-Gruber syndrome. Meckel-Gruber syndrome is a rare autosomal recessive disorder that is associated with a wide and variable range of anomalies. The most consistent of these are polycystic kidney disease, polydactyly, and occipital encephalocele. Variable features of Meckel-Gruber syndrome include cleft palate, ductal plate malformations of the liver, and cardiac abnormalities. The syndrome is uniformly fatal as a result of pulmonary hypoplasia or renal failure. The incidence is ~1 in 100,000.

Glomerulocystic kidney disease (GCKD)

Glomerulocystic kidney disease (GCKD) is a rare disorder that presents in the neonatal period with large palpable flank masses. It may be very difficult to distinguish, clinically and radiographically, from ARPKD; however, it appears to be more related genotypically to ADPKD. Microscopic examination shows dilation of Bowman capsule and renal dysplasia f7.20.

Nephronophthisis (juvenile nephronophthisis, medullary sponge kidney)

Nephronophthisis is an autosomal recessive inherited cause of medullary sponge kidney, a disorder with cysts at the corticomedullary junction. It is a member of the family of ciliopathies, defects in cilia function. Multiple genes have been implicated, including *NPHP* genes 1-8, having phenotypes that differ primarily by the age of onset.

Sporadic & multifactorial congenital renal disorders

Potter sequence

Potter sequence refers to the numerous, often lethal, effects of low urine output in utero. Urine is important for maintaining an adequate volume of amniotic fluid, and it is the inhalation and exhalation of amniotic fluid that promotes growth and differentiation of the lungs. Furthermore, amniotic fluid protects the developing fetus from compression by the surrounding uterus. Thus, any condition that markedly reduces urine volume can lead to a syndrome characterized by pulmonary hypoplasia and a typical physical appearance, known as Potter sequence (or Potter syndrome). The most common causes of Potter sequence include bilateral renal agenesis, urine outflow obstruction (posterior urethral valves), prune belly syndrome, bilateral cystic renal dysplasia, and autosomal recessive polycystic kidney disease. Aside from ARPKD, these disorders are largely sporadic or multifactorial.

Bilateral renal agenesis

Bilateral renal agenesis occurs with a frequency of ~1 in 3,000 births, and it is the cause of ~1 in 5 cases of the Potter sequence. It is quickly fatal, owing to pulmonary hypoplasia. Bilateral renal agenesis is often suspected when fetal ultrasound (performed for evaluation of oligohydramnios) fails to visualize a bladder (contracted due to lack of urine) or kidneys. It is thought to result from an event that interrupts development of the renal bud during the first trimester. Some cases have been associated with mutations in transcription factors or homozygosity for severely deleterious mutations in *WT-1*. Some cases occur in families with a high rate of other urologic anomalies, including unilateral renal agenesis.

Prune belly syndrome (Eagle-Barrett syndrome)

The prune belly syndrome consists of the triad of abdominal wall muscle flaccidity, urinary tract dilation, and bilaterally undescended testes. Though the genetic basis is unknown, it is thought that prune belly syndrome is an inherited disorder. Prune belly syndrome is rare and affects mostly males. It is believed that a severe urethral obstruction occurs early in fetal life, possibly due to the transient existence of an obstructing urethral membrane that subsequently recanalizes. Early obstruction is thought to impair the development of the abdominal wall musculature. Reestablishment of urinary outflow permits the development of adequate (though hypoplastic) lungs and kidneys. Nonetheless, the kidneys have some degrees of dysplasia, the prostatic urethra, bladder and ureters are massively dilated, and the testes are usually intraabdominal. The bladder empties incompletely because its muscle, like that of the abdominal wall, is relatively flaccid.

Posterior urethral valves

Posterior urethral valves are the most common cause of severe urinary obstruction in the neonate, affecting predominantly males. Posterior urethral valves are membranous cusps of tissue that form in the prostatic urethra and, while having a slit-like aperture, cause obstruction. Ultimately, this leads to hydronephrosis and/or renal dysplasia, in addition to the other features of Potter sequence.

Cardiovascular

Channel conduction disorders

Brugada syndrome

In Southeast Asia, where it is most prevalent, Brugada syndrome has been called by a variety of names, including the "sleep death" (Laos), "sudden and unexpected death in sleep" (Japan), and "to rise and moan in sleep" (Philippines). As implied by the foregoing, the disease is most prevalent in Southeast Asia and presents in otherwise healthy young men as sudden death during sleep. A characteristic ECG pattern includes right bundle branch block with ST segment elevation in the right chest leads V1-V3. Brugada syndrome, in ~1 in 4 cases, is caused by a mutation in the sodium channel gene *SCN5A* on chromosome 3p21; in all, mutations in 8 genes (*SCN5A, GPD1L, CACNA1C, CACNB2, SCN1B, KCNE3, SCN3B, HCN4*) are known to cause Brugada syndrome. Interestingly, mutations in *SCN5A* are also responsible for one type of the long QT syndrome (LQT type 3).

Arrhythmogenic right ventricular dysplasia (ARVD; Uhl anomaly)

ARVD accounts for ~20% of sudden cardiac death in young adults. Unlike Brugada syndrome, sudden cardiac death in ARVD is most likely to occur during physical activity. The characteristic histologic features include fibrous and fatty replacement of the right ventricular myocardium f7.21. Most cases are diagnosed between the ages of 15 and 40 years, most commonly as a result of sudden cardiac death, syncope, right heart failure, or an episode of ventricular tachycardia. A right bundle branch block and/or T-wave inversion in leads V1–V3 are common during episodes of ventricular tachycardia. Some advocate formal invasive electrophysiologic (EP) testing, MRI, and/or right ventricular endomyocardial biopsy for definitive diagnosis. A number of genes have been associated with ARVD including the cardiac ryanodine receptor gene *RYR2* (*ARVD2*) on 1q, the *DSP* (*ARVD9*) gene on 6p for desmoplakin, and *PKP2* (*ARVD8*), also on 6p, that encodes plakophilin-2. Naxos disease (named for the Greek island on which it was discovered) is a form of ARVD associated with cutaneous manifestations and wooly hair.

Long QT (LQT) syndromes

The majority of inherited cardiac conduction disorders are categorized as LQT syndromes. The QT interval is the section on the ECG tracing between the QRS complex (left ventricular contraction) and the T wave (cardiac repolarization). The length of the QT interval is somewhat variable from person to person and within an individual over time. The QT interval increases with decreasing heart rate as well, and the QT interval must be corrected for heart rate (QTc). Physiologically, the QT interval reflects the time it takes for ion channels to open, and not surprisingly many of the molecular causes of a prolonged QT interval are due to defects in genes encoding ion channels.

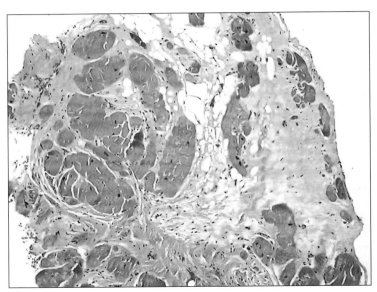

f7.21 Arrhythmogenic right ventricular dysplasia, endomyocardial biopsy; in addition to fatty change, there is prominent of stromal fibrosis

Patients with a persistently prolonged QT interval are prone to develop ventricular arrhythmias, including the type of ventricular tachycardia known as torsade de pointes. Ventricular arrhythmias may manifest as syncope or sudden cardiac death. The QT interval is determined by a variety of acquired and genetic influences t7.3.

t7.3 Causes of long QT interval

Inherited	Acquired
Romano-Ward syndrome	Hypokalemia
Jervell Lange-Nielsen syndrome	Hypomagnesemia
Andersen-Tawil syndrome	Hypercalcemia
	Medications (tricyclic antidepressants, phenothiazines, macrolide antibiotics, class IA antiarrhythmics, class III antiarrhythmics)

The inherited long QT syndromes have traditionally been divided, according to clinical presentation, into the Romano-Ward syndrome (autosomal dominant, no hearing loss) and the Jervell Lange-Nielsen syndrome (autosomal recessive, with hearing loss). More recently, there has been a tendency to classify them according to their genotype: *LQTS1* through *LQTS7* t7.4.

t7.4 Genes underlying inherited long QT syndromes

LQT1 (KCNQ1)	11p15.5 Encodes a portion of a voltage-gated potassium channel Most commonly mutated gene in the long QT syndrome Exercise (especially swimming)-triggered arrhythmias
LQT2 (KCNH2, HERG)	7q35-36 Encodes a second voltage-activated potassium channel Second most commonly affected gene in LQTS Auditory stimulus- or emotional stimulus-triggered arrhythmias
LQT3 (SCN5A)	3p21-25 Sleep-triggered arrhythmias
LQT4 (ANKB)	4q25-27
LQT5 (KCNE1)	21q22.1
LQT6 (MiRP1, KCNE2)	21q22.1
LQT7 (KCNJ2)	Encodes portions of a channel shared with skeletal muscle Mutations cause Andersen-Tawil syndrome (triad of episodic paralysis, long QT interval & dysmorphic features)

Despite autosomal inheritance there is a 2:1 female predominance in clinically significant long QT syndrome. Even in normal adults, the QT interval is somewhat longer in women than in men. Furthermore, estrogen appears to downregulate the implicated channels on cardiac myocytes. Thus, the disease has greater *penetrance* in females. In general, heterozygous mutations in these genes cause Romano-Ward syndrome, and homozygous (or compound heterozygous) mutations cause JLNS. 2 of the known genes (*KCNQ1* and *KCNH2*) encode voltage-gated potassium channels, and *SCN5A* encodes a sodium channel. *ANKB* encodes an ion channel anchor, a protein that associates noncovalently with ion channels. Interestingly, each of the mutations are associated with different stimuli that lead to sudden cardiac arrhythmias—mutations in *KCNQ1* are associated with swimming, mutations in *KCNQ2* with auditory stimuli, and *SCN5A* mutations with arrhythmias while sleeping.

Myocardial disorders

Dilated (congestive) cardiomyopathy

The causes of dilated cardiomyopathy have been traditionally listed as infection (coxsackie B, Chagas disease, diphtheria, HIV), sarcoidosis, toxin (alcohol, adriamycin), pregnancy, and idiopathic. The idiopathic group has always been large, comprising 1/3 of cases. It is now known that nearly all idiopathic cases result from genetic defects.

X-linked dilated cardiomyopathy is associated with mutations of the dystrophin gene, the same gene implicated in Duchenne and Becker muscular dystrophy (in which heart failure is common in those who survive to adulthood). Autosomal dominant dilated cardiomyopathy has been associated with a large number of mutations, most commonly in the *MYH7* gene encoding β-myosin heavy chain (also involved in some cases of hypertrophic cardiomyopathy).

Hypertrophic cardiomyopathy (idiopathic hypertrophic subaortic stenosis)

Hypertrophic cardiomyopathy is one of the most common causes of sudden cardiac death in young adults, with an incidence approaching 1 in 500. Gross examination of the heart reveals myocardial hypertrophy with disproportionate thickening of the ventricular septum as compared with the left ventricular free wall (asymmetric septal hypertrophy). The sonographic and gross anatomic findings can be closely mimicked by amyloidosis and hypertensive heart disease. Histologically, hypertrophic cardiomyopathy displays myocyte hypertrophy, myofiber disarray with prominent myocyte branching, and interstitial fibrosis. Most of the mutations that cause hypertrophic cardiomyopathy are in genes encoding sarcomeric structural proteins, the most commonly affected gene being *MYH7* on 14q, and the most commonly implicated mutation is the R403Q mutation. The pattern of inheritance is autosomal dominant.

Restrictive cardiomyopathy

Restrictive cardiomyopathy is overwhelmingly an acquired condition, caused by such things as radiation therapy, amyloidosis, and sarcoidosis. There are rare inherited causes of restrictive cardiomyopathy, including inherited metabolic diseases and endocardial fibroelastosis, a rare X-linked recessive condition.

Familial isolated cardiac amyloidosis

Mutations in the transthyretin (*TTR*) gene cause most cases of familial cardiac amyloidosis. One mutation, V30M, is present in 30-45% of affected individuals. The clinical spectrum of transthyretin-associated amyloidosis may include peripheral neuropathy, leptomeningeal amyloidosis, and cardiomyopathy. Isolated cardiac amyloidosis is what has in the past been referred to as *senile cardiac amyloidosis*; likewise, isolated leptomeningeal amyloidosis has been called *cerebral amyloid angiopathy*.

Transthyretin amyloidosis displays autosomal dominant inheritance. The disease shows pockets of high prevalence in Portugal, Sweden, Japan, and parts of Africa. The frequency of *TTR* amyloidosis ranges from ~1 in 500 in northern Portugal to ~1 in 100,000 among Caucasian Americans; it is estimated to be much higher in African Americans.

Structural cardiac disorders as a part of a larger genetic syndrome

Structural cardiac anomalies are a common feature of genetic multisystem disease t7.5. There are cardiac anomalies associated with single gene mutations, including mutations in *TBX-5* (Holt-Oram syndrome), *TBX-1* (DiGeorge syndrome), *PTPN11* (Noonan syndrome), and *JAG1* (Alagille syndrome). Chromosomal anomalies such as Down syndrome and Turner syndrome have notable cardiac features. Microdeletion syndromes, such as DiGeorge and Williams syndromes also have a high incidence of structural cardiac defects. The majority of structural cardiac abnormalities, however, are multifactorial.

t7.5 Structural cardiac defects in multisystem genetic disorders

Category	Genetic defect	Notes
Single gene mutation	NKX2-5	The NKX2-5 gene on chromosome 5q34 encodes a transcription factor that is expressed very early in cardiogenesis & appears to be responsible for activating transcription of most genes involved in the process. Mutations in NKX2-5 have been identified in patients with a large variety of structural malformations.
Single gene mutation	GATA-4	GATA-4, a gene located on 8p, encodes a transcription factor that is important in cardiac embryogenesis. Rare kindreds have been identified that carry germline GATA-4 mutations & have autosomally inherited septal defects, especially ostium secundum atrial septal defects.
Single gene mutation	TBX-5	TBX-5 (12q) mutations are responsible for most cases of Holt-Oram syndrome (heart-hand syndrome), an autosomal dominant disorder combining characteristic heart & upper limb anomalies. Upper limb malformations may involve the radius, thumb phalanges, or carpal bones & they range from severe (phocomelia) to minimal (subtle carpal bone deformities). These are usually bilateral & symmetrical & if asymmetrical, the left is more severely affected. Cardiac malformations most commonly take the form of septal defects, especially secundum atrial septal or muscular ventricular septal defects.
Single gene mutation	TBX-1	TBX-1 is found on 22q & is contained within the region commonly deleted in DiGeorge syndrome (see below).
Single gene mutation	PTPN11	Noonan syndrome consists of right-sided heart defects, most commonly pulmonic stenosis. Hypertrophic cardiomyopathy is the second most common finding. Lymphatic malformations are also common. While the incidence of Noonan syndrome in the population is only ~1 in 1,500, the incidence amongst children with congenital heart disease may be as high as 1 in 100. Prolonged coagulation times are frequently observed, due to a wide range of defects (eg, vWD phenotypes, factor V deficieny, factor VIII deficiency). PTPN11 has also been implicated in some examples of LEOPARD syndrome & juvenile myelomonocytic leukemia (JMML).
Single gene mutation	JAG1	Alagille syndrome is an autosomal dominant condition caused by mutations in JAG1. Best known for its association with bile duct paucity, Alagille syndrome (arteriohepatic dysplasia) is also a disease of blood vessels & the heart. Most commonly affected is the pulmonary circulation, in the form of pulmonary artery stenosis. Other defects include tetralogy, atrial septal defects, ventricular septal defects, aortic stenosis & coarctation.
Structural chromosomal disorder	Trisomy 21 (Down syndrome)	Structural cardiac anomalies in >1/2 of cases. The classic association is malformation of the endocardial cushion, resulting most commonly in a membranous ventricular septal defect. This is followed in frequency by patent ductus arteriosus, atrial septal defect & atrioventricular septal defect.
Structural chromosomal disorder	45,X (Turner syndrome)	Cardiac anomalies are present in up to 1/2 of cases. Bicuspid aortic valve is the most common defect, followed by coarctation of the aorta. Aortic root dilation is common & may lead to aortic dissection.
Microdeletions & sequences	22q11 microdeletion	Di George syndrome (velocardiofacial syndrome, Shprintzen syndrome) is associated with cardiac anomalies in most cases (75% of affected individuals), especially the conotruncal malformations. These include tetralogy of Fallot, interrupted aortic arch, ventricular septal defects & truncus arteriosus. Among the several genes wiped out by this microdeletion, TBX1 is believed to be responsible for the cardiac anomalies.
Microdeletions & sequences	7q11.23 microdeletion	Williams syndrome is characterized by dysmorphic facial features, mental retardation, short stature, hypercalcemia, abnormalities of connective tissue (hernias, diverticula, joint laxity, skin laxity) & structural cardiac & vascular defects. The most distinctive cardiac anomaly is supravalvar aortic stenosis (hourglass stenosis). Many of the findings in Williams syndrome can be attributed to deletion of the elastin gene.
Multifactorial	Many	The vast majority of structural cardiac anomalies are "multifactorial" in origin. That is, while a Mendelian pattern of inheritance is inapparent & a specific genetic defect has not been found, there is clustering within families & around particular exposures. Furthermore, it is known that offspring of consanguineous parents are strongly predisposed to "multifactorial" structural cardiac anomalies. Structural cardiac anomalies are prominent among the multifactorial disorders, others being pyloric stenosis, cleft lip & cleft palate.

Endocrine

Adrenal cortex

Congenital adrenal hyperplasia

Congenital deficiency of one of the enzymes in the steroid hormone biosynthetic pathway leads to (1) diminished cortisol and/or mineralocorticoid and (2) excess of precursors, many of which have androgenic properties. The disorder gets its name from the massive adrenal hyperplasia that results from hypersecretion of adrenocorticotrophic hormone (ACTH) in response to low levels of serum cortisol.

There is a broad range of clinical severity that can best be understood based upon 3 principles. First, mild enzyme deficiency affects mainly the production of cortisol, while severe deficiency impairs both cortisol and mineralocorticoid (aldosterone) production. Thus, mild deficiencies result in the so-called simple virilizing form of the disease, while severe enzyme deficiencies result in the salt-wasting form of disease. Second, the most profound consequences of hypocortisolism for the developing fetus is not the paucity of cortisol itself but rather the very high ACTH that drives the build-up of androgens. Third, males and females have differing reactions to androgen. Accordingly, there are several potential phenotypes:

1. a female who is virilized at birth or becomes virilized shortly thereafter

2. a female with precocious puberty

3. a male with pseudoprecocious puberty (the external appearance of puberty)

4. an infant with salt-losing crisis (similar to an Addisonian crisis)

Serum 17-hydroxyprogesterone (17-OHP), a precursor in the cortisol biosynthetic pathway, is elevated in all forms of CAH. 17-OHP can be measured by immunoassay, which can be performed on dried blood spots for neonatal screening. Since some neonates may present in the first days of life with adrenal insufficiency crisis, early knowledge of the diagnosis can be extremely beneficial.

21-hydroxylase deficiency is the most common cause of CAH. It is responsible for ~90% of cases and has an estimated incidence of 1 in 10,000-1 in 25,000. 21-hydroxylase (also called CYP21A2 and P450C21) is a cytochrome P-450 enzyme found within the smooth endoplasmic reticulum. The gene encoding 21-hydroxylase is CYP21. CYP21 is located at 6p21 and is thus within the HLA locus, adjacent to genes that encode complement protein C4. Nearby is a gene known as *CYP21P*, a pseudogene (nontranscribed gene) with >95% homology with *CYP21* but rendered nonfunctional by virtue of several nucleotide differences. The most common disease-causing mutations are (1) large *CYP21* gene deletions and (2) gene conversions—recombinations between *CYP21* and *CYP21P*, converting CYP21 into a nonfunctional allele. Several additional point mutations have been described. Different mutations have different phenotypic effect, with some causing complete enzyme deficiency and others causing only impaired enzyme activity. Molecular testing of the *CYP21* gene is clinically available. Directed mutation analysis for a set of common mutations can detect >95% of abnormal alleles. One common approach is the use of Southern blot analysis with restriction enzymes. Restriction enzymes produce predictable digestion fragments which can be compared to known standards and to an internal standard (*CYP21P*). PCR is problematic because of simultaneous amplification of *CYP21P*. Prenatal diagnosis may permit prenatal treatment through the administration of corticosteroids, leading to suppression of ACTH secretion.

11-hydroxylase deficiency is the second most common cause of CAH (5-7% of cases). It is caused by mutations in the *CYP11B1* gene located on chromosome 8q24 and is especially prominent in North African Jews. Unlike 21-hydroxylase deficiency, a salt-wasting form of 11-hydroxylase deficiency is very uncommon; however, hypertension is much more commonly seen in 11-hydroxylase deficiency. Findings indicative of androgen excess are equally common in both conditions.

Androgen insensitivity syndrome

Androgen insensitivity syndrome is an X-linked recessive disorder that affects genotypic males (46,XY). There are different degrees of severity, ranging from testicular feminization at birth to adult infertility, with phenotypes described as complete, partial, or mild androgen insensitivity syndrome. In complete androgen insensitivity, the external genitalia resemble that of a female, while at the opposite end of the spectrum the external genitalia may be ambiguous or male-appearing. Often a mass is detected in the inguinal canal, representing undescended testes. There may be rudimentary müllerian structures (ovary, fallopian tubes, uterus). Serum testosterone is normal to elevated, and there is normal conversion of testosterone to dihydrotestosterone, with normal or elevated serum luteinizing hormone (LH). The workup begins with a karyogram indicating a 46,XY karyotype t7.6. Following this direct sequencing of the androgen receptor (*AR*) gene on the X chromosome will demonstrate mutations in >95% of cases with complete insensitivity. Mutation detection rate drops to 40% in cases of partial or mild insensitivity.

t7.6 Definitions relating to hermaphroditism & pseudohermaphroditism

Genotypic sex	Determined by the status of the Y chromosome—the presence of a single Y chromosome (regardless of the number of X chromosomes) is definitive of a genotypic male
Gonadal sex	Depends upon the histologic nature of the gonads. The Y chromosome, in particular the SRY gene, influences the genital primordium to develop into testes; in the absence of a Y chromosome, the gonadal primordium will develop into ovaries.
Phenotypic sex	Refers to the appearance of the external genitalia, which may be ambiguous
True hermaphrodite	The term implies the presence of both ovarian & testicular tissue, either separately or within the same gonadal structure (ovotestis). This is an extremely rare condition in which the genotype is usually 46,XX, but by FISH, transposed *SRY* gene material can nearly always be found. In some cases, in fact, true hermaphroditism is associated with 46,XX/46,XY mosaicism. A 46,XY genotype is not associated with true hermaphroditism.
Pseudohermaphroditism	Refers to discordance between phenotypic sex & gonadal/genotypic sex. The presumed sex is that indicated by the gonadal histology; thus, male pseudohermaphrodites have a Y chromosome & testes, but the external genitalia (and often the genital ducts) are either ambiguous or feminized. There are a wide variety of causes, the most common of which are the androgen insensitivity syndromes (testicular feminization). Female pseudohermaphrodites have no Y chromosome (usually 46,XX), ovaries & external genitalia that are either ambiguous or male-appearing (virilized). Female pseudohermaphroditism is caused by excessive exposure to androgens during fetal development, most commonly due to congenital adrenal hyperplasia (CAH).

Steroid sulfatase deficiency

Prolonged or nonprogressive labor, unresponsive to oxytocin, may be the first sign of steroid sulfatase deficiency. After birth, cholesterol sulfate begins to accumulate in the blood and in tissues such as the cornea and skin. In skin, it appears to prevent the dissolution of desmosomal attachments (desquamation), leading to the X-linked ichthyosis (scaly skin) phenotype. Ichthyosis becomes apparent shortly after birth. Corneal opacities develop somewhat later. Males have a high incidence of cryptorchidism, which leads to a higher incidence of germ cell tumors. It is the function of steroid sulfatase to remove sulfate moieties from steroid sulfates (including cholesterol sulfate), thus converting them to biologically active forms. The gene for steroid sulfatase (*STS*) is located on the short arm of the X chromosome (Xp22.3). In nearly 90% of cases, steroid sulfatase deficiency is due to a complete *STS* gene deletion, sometimes including the entire distal short arm of the X chromosome. Most of the remaining patients have single point mutations within the *STS* gene. The diagnosis may be made in several ways. The enzyme may be specifically assayed in samples of peripheral blood leukocytes or skin. Elevated cholesterol sulfate levels may be demonstrated in serum or skin. Lastly, the gene deletion may be demonstrated by FISH.

Pituitary gland

Kallmann syndrome

Kallmann syndrome most often affects men and can present with hypogonadotropic hypogonadism and anosmia. The hormone most commonly deficient is luteinizing hormone releasing hormone. Kallmann syndrome can be inherited as X-linked, autosomal dominant, or autosomal recessive. Most X-linked cases (and 15% of cases overall) are due to mutations in the *KAL1* gene on Xp22.3, close to steroid sulfatase.

Isolated growth hormone deficiency

Multiple inherited isolated pituitary hormone deficiencies have been described, the most common of which is isolated growth hormone (GH) deficiency. It may be inherited as an X-linked, autosomal recessive, or autosomal dominant condition. Autosomal recessive GH deficiency is usually the result of mutations in growth hormone releasing hormone, autosomal dominant GH deficiency is associated with mutations in the growth hormone gene, and the X-linked form with mutations in the *BTK* gene. *BTK* is the gene associated with Bruton agammaglobulinemia, and indeed many affected individuals are also immunocompromised.

Parathyroid gland

Inheritance of isolated parathyroid anomalies is extremely rare. More often, parathyroid abnormalities are inherited as part of a larger syndrome, such as the DiGeorge syndrome.

Pseudohypoparathyroidism

Pseudohypoparathyroidism encompasses multiple diseases all sharing peripheral resistance to parathyroid hormone (PTH). Patients present with hypocalcemia despite elevated parathyroid hormone. Infantile tetany is often the presenting feature. Older children display short stature, a round face, dimpling of the dorsum of the hand, brachydactyly (characteristically, the second digit is spared, such that it is longer than the third), dystrophic soft tissue calcification and heterotopic ossification. Albright hereditary osteodystrophy (pseudohypoparathyroidism type IA) is an autosomal dominant disorder caused by inactivating mutations of the *GNAS1* gene encoding the α subunit of the stimulatory G protein. The PTH receptor is coupled to a G-protein to facilitate transmembrane signaling, usually through activation of adenylate cyclase and the production of the second messenger, cyclic adenosine monophosphate (cAMP). Mutations in the G-protein lead to defective signal transduction.

McCune-Albright syndrome

Gain of function mutations of the *GNAS1* gene can lead to McCune-Albright syndrome. These types of mutations, when inherited as a germline disorder, are incompatible with life; consequently all McCune-Albright cases are inherited as somatic mosaics. The severity of the disorder can be highly variable depending on the extent of tissues affected by the mutation, ranging from fully developed McCune-Albright syndrome to isolated fibrous dysplasia. McCune-Albright syndrome consists of café au lait spots, polyostotic fibrous dysplasia, precocious puberty, and other endocrine anomalies. Precocious puberty is a feature mainly of females with the syndrome, with many achieving puberty by the age of 3 years. Levels of LH and FSH are low.

Familial hypocalcuric hypercalcemia (benign familial hypercalcemia)

Familial hypocalcuric hypercalcemia is an autosomal dominant disorder presenting with isolated hypercalcemia, with normal parathyroid glands and normal serum parathyroid hormone levels. Importantly, subtotal parathyroidectomy has no effect on calcium levels. The condition is caused by mutations in a G-protein gene that leads to lack of parathyroid response to elevated serum calcium.

Thyroid gland

Congenital hypothyroidism

Congenital hypothyroidism is a common disorder affecting 1 in 3,000-4,000 live births. Fetal development is usually unaffected, because of a maternal supply of thyroid hormone. Post-natal thyroid deficiency can lead to abnormal brain development and can be easily treated. Because of this, all newborns in the United States are tested for congenital hypothyroidism.

The vast majority (90%) of cases is associated with thyroid hypoplasia or aplasia, often the result of maternal autoantibodies. A number of genes have been associated with inherited cases of congenital hypothyroidism including *PAX-8* and *TSHR*, defects of which lead to defective gland formation. Mutations in these genes usually are inherited in an autosomal recessive manner and lead to defective thryoid hormone production despite seemingly normal thyroid development. Pendred syndrome, an autosomal recessive condition due to mutations in the gene *SLC26A4*, presents with sensorineural hearing loss and goiter, often with hypothyroidism.

Diabetes mellitus

Type I (insulin-dependent) diabetes mellitus (DM1)

DM1 is an autoimmune disease, and there are certain HLA genotypes that are associated with a higher than average incidence of disease. HLA-DR3 and HLA-DR4 heterozygotes have a 2-3-fold increased risk over average risk of developing IDDM. Homozygotes have a 10-fold increased risk. First-degree relatives of affected persons have a higher-than-average risk of developing type 1 DM, siblings have a 5-10% chance of developing it, and identical twins have ~60% concordance.

There is a variety of rare monogenetic causes of diabetes mellitus. Pancreatic agenesis is extremely rare, thought to be the result of sporadic mutations within transcription factor genes. Agenesis causes absolute insulin deficiency, a form of type 1 diabetes mellitus. Mutations in the insulin receptor gene (particularly in association with inherited leprechaunism or Rabson-Mendenhall syndrome) can cause insulin resistance. Inherited leprechaunism is characterized by intrauterine growth retardation, post-prandial hyperglycemia, and fasting hypoglycemia. There is marked peripheral insulin resistance, with profoundly elevated serum insulin. Rabson-Mendenhall syndrome is similar to inherited leprechaunism but with acanthosis nigricans and other anomalies. Cystic fibrosis leads to progressive pancreatic insufficiency, both exocrine and endocrine, with many who survive into the teenage years and nearly all who survive into adulthood developing type 1 diabetes mellitus.

Maturity onset diabetes of the young (MODY)

Maturity onset diabetes of the young (MODY) derives its name from traditional systems of diabetes classification in which type 1 was generally classified as juvenile onset diabetes and type 2 was usually classified as maturity onset diabetes. It was recognized that a subset of children with diabetes had a clinical picture resembling maturity onset diabetes—in that they were noninsulin dependent—and these cases were named MODY. MODY is a form of noninsulin dependent (type 2) diabetes with autosomal dominant inheritance that usually arises in childhood. It is responsible for ~5% of type 2 cases. Affected individuals are rarely obese. There are in fact multiple genotypic forms of MODY. Accounting for the vast majority of cases are: *GCK/MODY2* (glucokinase), *HNF4a/MODY1* (hepatocyte nuclear factor 4 α), *HNF1a/MODY3* (hepatocyte nuclear factor 1 α), *IPF1/MODY4* (insulin promoter factor 1), and *HNF1b/MODY5* (hepatocyte nuclear factor 1 β).

Gastrointestinal, hepatobiliary & pancreatic

Hirschsprung disease

Throughout the length of the colon, with the exception of the last 1-2 cm of rectum, clusters of ganglion cells can normally be found within the muscularis mucosa (Meissner submucosal plexus) and muscularis propria (Auerbach myenteric plexus). Embryologically, primitive cells destined to develop into ganglion cells emerge from the neural crest and migrate to the developing bowel, populating it proximally to distally. An interruption in this process, therefore, always affects the distal-most portions of bowel. Hirschsprung disease results from such an interruption, and indeed the distal-most colon (rectum) is always involved with or without a variable length of more proximal colon. Hirschsprung disease is an example of a neurocristopathy, a disease caused by abnormal migration of neural crest cells during fetal development. As was the outcome of the cases described by Harald Hirschsprung in the 19th century, untreated disease results in death in infancy from toxic megacolon.

Hirschsprung disease is classified according to the length of colon involved. Most cases are restricted to the rectum or rectosigmoid and considered short-segment Hirschsprung disease. Some cases involve only the very distal rectum and are considered ultrashort segment Hirschsprung disease. In ~15%, the aganglionosis extends proximal to the splenic flexure (long-segment Hirschsprung disease). Rare cases (<5%) involve the entire colon (total colonic aganglionosis). Short-segment disease is 4 times more common in males than in females, whereas the numbers are essentially equal for long-segment Hirschsprung disease.

Hirschsprung disease usually presents as failure to pass meconium (meconium ileus) within the first 48 hours of life. Those with very short affected segments may be capable of passing meconium, and will present somewhat later with constipation or other evidence of altered bowel motility. Other congenital causes of meconium ileus must be considered, including cystic fibrosis, intestinal atresia, and imperforate anus. Definitive diagnosis requires a biopsy, taken >2 cm from the dentate line (the normally aganglionic segment should not be biopsied). In affected individuals, one finds an absence of ganglion cells in association with axonal hypertrophy.

A structural chromosomal abnormality is present in ~10% of cases, most commonly trisomy 21. Single gene defects known to cause Hirschsprung disease are not found on 21, however, and include deleterious mutations in the *RET* gene (10q11.2), *GDNF* gene (5p), and *EDNRB* gene (13q). Note that some *RET* protooncogene gain of function mutations result in the MEN2A syndrome, while other *RET* mutations lead to MEN2B, neither of which is associated with Hirschsprung disease, in which there are loss of function *RET* mutations. In addition, Hirschsprung disease is often a component of a larger syndrome, such as neurofibromatosis type 1 (NF1), multiple endocrine neoplasia type 2A (MEN2A), Waardenburg syndrome, congenital central hypoventilation (Haddad) syndrome, familial dysautonomia (Riley-Day) syndrome, and Smith-Lemli-Opitz syndrome.

Osler-Weber-Rendu syndrome (hereditary hemorrhagic telangiectasia)

This is a condition in which vascular walls are structurally abnormal, leading to recurrent episodes of bleeding, and it may initially be taken to represent a coagulation disorder. The initial manifestation in most patients, beginning in childhood, is epistaxis. In adolescence or young adulthood, skin lesions appear, taking the form of telangiectasias on the face, lips, ears, and chest. Similar lesions can be found on the oral mucosa. In the 4th or 5th decade, GI bleeding arises, resulting from bleeding telangiectasias or arteriovenous malformations. Arteriovenous malformations may also form within the brain, lung, or liver.

Osler-Weber-Rendu syndrome is an autosomal dominant disorder with a frequency of ~1 in 5,000. It can be caused by mutations in either the *ENG* gene or the *ACVRL1* gene. *ENG* is found at 9q34 and encodes endoglin. *ACVRL1* is found at 12q and encodes a serine/threonine protein kinase receptor. About 80% of all disease-causing mutations can be detected by direct sequence analysis.

Microvillus inclusion disease (MID)

MID is a cause of chronic malabsorptive malnutrition in infants. It is considered the most common cause of malabsorption to present in the neonatal period. It is inherited as an autosomal recessive trait. Characteristically, the wall of the small intestine is paper thin. Small bowel biopsy shows villus blunting, with overall mucosal atrophy, and characteristic apical intracellular inclusions. Ultrastructurally, these consist of vesicles of invaginated brush border constituents, and traditionally ultrastructural examination has been required for the diagnosis. There are several histochemical and immunohistochemical alternatives to electron microscopy. PAS staining, polyclonal CEA, and CD10 normally highlight the brush border of intestinal epithelia in a linear apical pattern. All have also been shown to highlight the microvillus inclusions in MID by displaying cytoplasmic staining in a globular or grainy pattern.

Multifactorial disorders & syndromic disorders affecting the GI tract

Esophageal atresia

The overall incidence of congenital structural anomalies of the esophagus is ~1 in 3,000 live births, most of these taking the form of esophageal atresia, with or without a tracheoesophageal fistula (TEF). Over 90% of cases are part of a larger syndrome, especially the VACTERL sequence (vertebral, anal, cardiac, tracheal, esophageal, renal, and limb). There are several forms of TEF, the most common being the distal-type (90% of cases) which communicates between the trachea and the distal end of the esophagus (distal to the stenosis). Esophageal atresia most often comes to clinical attention by producing polyhydramnios (amniotic fluid is normally swallowed by the fetus). Alternatively, it may present as difficulty with feeding. The atresia is confirmed by failure to pass a nasogastric tube, and the presence of a distal TEF is confirmed by the radiographic presence of a gastric gas bubble (which would be absent without a distal TEF).

Pyloric stenosis

Anatomically, pyloric stenosis results from hypertrophy of the smooth muscle surrounding the pyloric channel. It presents in infants, usually between 1 and 6 weeks of age, with projectile vomiting following meals. The pyloric valve may be palpable as mass (olive) in the epigastrium. The diagnosis can usually be confirmed by imaging. Dye studies reveal a classic string sign, and ultrasound gives a typical double-track sign; however these findings are not 100% specific (being potentially produced by pylorospasm); thus, strict quantitative ultrasound criteria have been adopted. Surgical intervention (eg, pyloromyotomy) is highly successful.

While a strict Mendelian pattern of inheritance is not observed, familial clustering is, and concordance among identical twins is ~50%. Furthermore, pyloric stenosis is often present in association with Turner syndrome, trisomy 18, Cornelia de Lange syndrome, and Hirschsprung disease. The overall incidence is ~1 in 300 live births. The incidence is highest among Caucasians, especially those of northern European descent, and males are disproportionately affected (4:1). Interestingly, first-born children are more likely to be affected than their siblings. The pathogenesis is presently considered multifactorial.

Intestinal atresia

Intestinal atresia is among the most common congenital defects of the GI tract, with an incidence of around 1 in 500-1 in 1,000 live births. The term refers to a segment of stenotic intestine, thought to be the result of a failure of recanalization of the bowel at around 10 weeks. The affected segment is present in the form of a solid cord. A vascular insult may underlie this failure. The most common location is the ileum, followed by jejunum and duodenum. Most cases of intestinal atresia are isolated defects, but ~30% of cases are associated with Down syndrome. With regard to Mendelian disorders, atresia is seen frequently in Feingold syndrome, a rare autosomal dominant disorder characterized by duodenal atresia, microcephaly, and limb malformations.

Abdominal wall defects: omphalocele & gastroschisis

Omphalocele and gastroschisis are congenital abdominal wall defects which must be distinguished from one another, as their clinical implications are markedly different. The location of a gastroschisis is typically just to the right of the umbilicus. It is composed of loops of intestine without covering. In contrast an omphalocele is located in the midline, essentially within the umbilical cord. Omphalocele is composed of multiple viscera, including intestine, liver, and spleen, and it is covered by a membrane composed of peritoneum and amnion. Abdominal wall defects occur sporadically, but gastroschisis is strongly associated with *decreased* maternal age. Importantly, the incidence of additional congenital anomalies is very high in association with omphalocele (60%) but relatively low in association with gastroschisis (10%). Furthermore, anomalies associated with gastroschisis are largely intestinal, whereas omphalocele is often associated with major cardiac defects, chromosomal anomalies (trisomy 21, trisomy 18, trisomy 13), or the Beckwith-Wiedemann syndrome. Abdominal wall defects can be diagnosed prenatally. Often there is an elevated maternal serum α fetoprotein (MSAFP) on routine prenatal screening, being much higher in gastroschisis than in omphalocele.

Autoimmune enteric diseases: celiac sprue, Crohn disease & ulcerative colitis

Celiac sprue is an autoimmune condition provoked by gluten. HLA-DQ2 allele is present in ~95% of patients with celiac sprue (as compared to around 30% of the general population). HLA-DQ8 is present in most of the remaining cases. Only ~1% of those with HLA DQ2 or DQ8 type have disease, however. HLA typing may have some utility in patients with equivocal biopsy and serology. Those negative for DQ2 and DQ8 are extremely unlikely to have celiac sprue. The incidence depends upon how the disease is defined. Those with symptomatic celiac sprue represent only a small fraction of those with serologic or histologic findings consistent with it. In the United States, the incidence of clinically significant celiac sprue is ~1 in 7,000, but the incidence based upon serologic studies is as high as 1 in 1,000. While the disease is present worldwide, it is relatively infrequent in sub-Saharan African, Chinese, and Japanese populations. Concordance for celiac sprue among identical twins is ~70%.

Chronic idiopathic inflammatory bowel disease (IIBD) encompasses 2 distinct clinicopathologic syndromes: Crohn disease (CD) and ulcerative colitis (UC). CD can affect any part of the intestine, and is characterized by discontinuous, transmural inflammatory lesions sometimes having a granulomatous component. UC affects the rectum and sometimes proximal portions of the colon, always in a continuous fashion (at least initially), with inflammation that is superficial and not associated with granulomas. Familial clustering has long been noted in cases of Crohn disease. The rate of concordant disease among siblings is ~15-30%. The relative risk among first-degree relatives is 15× that of the general population, and the concordance among identical twins approaches 70%. Furthermore, Ashkenazi Jews have a relative risk of ~4-fold that of the general population. Several susceptibility genes have been identified, including the *NOD2/CARD15* gene (IBD1 locus) on chromosome 16 and the *OCTN* gene (IBD5 locus) on 5q31. Interestingly, consistent associations with HLA polymorphisms have not been demonstrated in Crohn disease. Familial clustering is evident in ulcerative colitis as well; however, the concordance rate for identical twins is only ~15-20% (much lower than Crohn). A sibling of an affected individual has a ~10% chance of being affected. Several susceptibility genes have been explored, including the IBD2 locus on chromosome 12. Both UC and Crohn disease appear to be influenced by polymorphisms in the *MDR1* (multidrug resistance 1) gene. In particular, a C3435T polymorphism appears to be associated with both diseases.

Biliary fibrocystic diseases (Caroli disease & congenital hepatic fibrosis)

The conditions in this category are considered disorders of the ductal plate (ductal plate malformations). In fact, the classic histologic finding in congenital hepatic fibrosis—a sleeve-like annular bile duct encircling a central core of connective tissue—is the normal appearance of the fetal liver at around 10 weeks. In the normal course of events, this ductal plate becomes reorganized into the portal triad as we

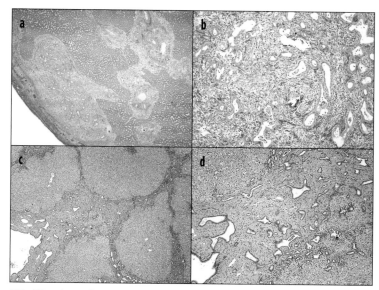

f7.22 Biliary plate malformations
a Trichrome stained section demonstrating mildly ectatic interlobular bile ducts with associated dense fibrosis in Caroli disease
b Biliary microhamartoma may be seen alone or in association with malformation syndromes
c & d Congenital hepatic fibrosis

normally envision it. This process is thought to be interrupted in ductal plate malformations. Biliary fibrocystic diseases are associated with autosomal recessive polycystic disease, nephronophthisis, and mutations in the *PKHD1* gene on 6p. This gene encodes a protein called fibrocystin (polyductin) which is thought to be involved in the normal embryogenesis of the bile ducts and renal tubules.

Caroli disease is characterized by segmental dilation of the intrahepatic bile ducts (and to a lesser extent extrahepatic ducts), not related to obstruction. Dilation may be fusiform early, but in its mature form is saccular. Stone formation and recurrent bouts of bacterial cholangitis typically complicate this syndrome. Caroli disease can be diagnosed with ultrasound or endoscopic retrograde cholangiopancreatography (ERCP), showing the typical saccular or fusiform dilations in the intrahepatic bile ducts (without evidence of an obstruction). The liver biopsy may show features of ascending cholangitis. Strictly defined, Caroli disease is a term that refers to bile ductular ectasia without the other findings of congenital hepatic fibrosis **f7.22**. Congenital hepatic fibrosis (CHF) is characterized by enlargement of portal tracts by interstitial fibrosis within which there are segmentally dilated and abnormally shaped (sleeve-like) bile ducts. The result is biliary obstruction and portal hypertension.

Autosomal dominant polycystic kidney disease has associated hepatic cysts (and von Meyenburg complexes) in ~1/2 of patients. These differ from Caroli and CHF in that they are usually simple cysts, not in continuity with the ductal system. These are much more prominent in affected females.

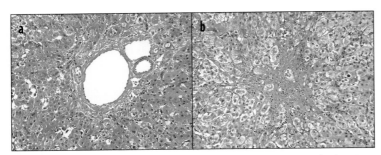

f7.23 Alagille syndrome; portal triads with pauci-inflammatory bile duct loss; surrounding hepatic parenchyma is notable for cholestasis & feathery degeneration

Syndromic paucity of bile ducts (Alagille syndrome, arteriohepatic dysplasia)

Alagille syndrome is an autosomal dominant disorder characterized by a set of dysmorphic features in association with a noninflammatory loss of interlobular bile ducts f7.23. Mutations in the *JAG1* gene, responsible for encoding the protein Jagged1, have been identified in around 70% of cases. Jagged1 is a signaling protein involved in fetal development, serving as a ligand for Notch receptors. Genetic anomalies range from point mutations to entire gene deletion. A small percentage of patients with this syndrome have instead a mutation in the *NOTCH2* gene.

Alagille syndrome usually presents with cholestasis, often in the neonatal period. Total bilirubin is elevated (~50:50 conjugated:unconjugated), and there is elevated alkaline phosphatase. Additional features include facial dysmorphism (broad forehead, widely spaced eyes, small mandible, prominent ears, imparting an overall triangular profile), butterfly vertebrae, posterior embryotoxon of the eye, and congenital heart disease (especially peripheral pulmonic stenosis).

At very early stages, the liver biopsy shows hepatitis resembling neonatal (giant cell) hepatitis. The number of bile ducts is normal at birth and progressively diminishes thereafter (hence the alternate designation—the disappearing bile duct syndrome). The characteristic paucity of bile ducts (duct to portal tract ratio <1:2) may not be apparent until after 6 months of age. Histologic examination shows no evidence of ductal inflammation and no injury to existing ducts. It is thought that the mechanism underlying bile duct paucity is the failure of ducts to continue to elongate following birth. The differential diagnosis for paucity of interlobular bile ducts in infancy includes congenital rubella syndrome and α_1 antitrypsin deficiency.

Hereditary hemochromatosis (HH)

The basic defect in HH is enhanced intestinal iron absorption. The normal adult absorbs only a small percentage of ingested iron, amounting to ~1-2 mg/day. Absorption is regulated by the demand for iron, through a feedback loop which is interrupted in HH. The mechanisms for this have not been fully elucidated, but a protein hormone called hepcidin appears to be involved. Hepcidin is synthesized in the liver at a rate influenced by iron stores, and it exerts an inhibitory effect upon iron absorption. In HH, hepcidin levels are low. Iron absorption is in excess of what can be utilized by

the reticuloendothelial system. The result is iron deposition within hepatocytes, pancreas, pituitary, synovium, heart, and skin. This causes damage to the liver (usually pauci-inflammatory fibrosis progressing to cirrhosis), pancreas (fibrosis with impairment of islet cell function leading to diabetes), pituitary gland (hypogonadotrophic hypogonadism leading to infertility—not much direct impact on the gonads), joints (osteoarthritis), heart (dilated or restrictive cardiomyopathy), and skin (bronzing secondary to increased melanin). Regardless of genotype, women are half as likely as men to develop complications of hemochromatosis.

HH is an autosomal recessive-inherited disorder that in most cases is caused by defects in the *HFE* gene, which is located within the major histocompatibility complex coding region on 6p21.3. The product of the *HFE* gene is involved with regulating iron uptake in the intestine. There is a wide variety of known *HFE* gene mutations, most clinically insignificant. The most common clinically significant mutation, C282Y disrupts a conserved disulfide bond leading to misfolding and accumulation of protein in the Golgi. The second most common mutation, H63D, is less likely to cause clinically significant disease. Neither of the mutations have a high penetrance. Genes other than *HFE*, such as those encoding the transferrin receptor (*TFR2*) and ferritin heavy chain (*FTH1*) have been implicated in hemochromatosis as well t7.7. Genes encoding hepcidin (*HAMP*) and hemojuvulin (*HFE2*) are associated with juvenile-onset hemochromatosis. Clinically affected individuals are most often (60-90%) homozygous for the C282Y mutation, and most of the remaining cases are due to compound heterozygosity for C282Y and the H63D mutation.

t7.7 Hemochromatosis associated genes

Gene	Location	Disease
HFE (most common variants: C282Y, H63D)	6p21.3	Hereditary hemochromatosis
HFE2 (hemojuvlin)	1q21	Juvenile hemochromatosis A
HAMP (hepcidin)	19q13	Juvenile hemochromatosis B
TFR2 (transferrin receptor)	7q22	Hemochromatosis type 3
FTH1 (ferritin heavy chain)	11q13	Familial iron overload

Hereditary hemochromatosis is the most common inherited disorder in northern Europeans with a prevalence similar to cystic fibrosis of 1-300 in American Caucasians. The H63D mutation (or polymorphism) is quite common in Caucasians, being present in 25% of the population. It only causes disease when co-inherited with a C282Y mutation (compound heterozygote); however, the compound heterozygotes represent ~2% of the population, and only a small minority of them will develop clinical disease. Even in those homozygous for C282Y, clinically significant hemochromatosis arises at a low rate. Homozygotes for H63D are clinically well. Simple heterozygotes for either C282Y or H63D are generally healthy, with the following caveats: many have abnormal serum iron studies reflecting some degree of iron overload, and there is a greater likelihood of progression in other forms of hepatic injury, such as steatohepatitis.

Screening involves serum iron studies, especially percent transferrin saturation and ferritin (both elevated in HH). A transferrin saturation ≥45% has a sensitivity of >95%, and this

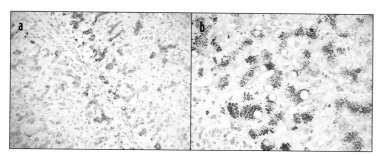

f7.24 Hereditary hemochromatosis
a Prussian blue stained section in which a longitudinally oriented portal tract runs diagonally, demonstrating zone 1-predominant siderosis
b At high magnification, there is an abundance of iron that is predominantly within hepatocytes, rather than primarily within Kupffer cells (as may be seen in secondary forms of siderosis)

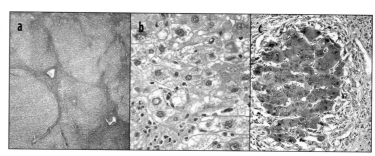

f7.25 Wilson disease
a Cirrhotic liver of a patient with Wilson disease
b At high magnification, the findings include inflammation, pseudoglycogenated nuclei & focal pigment deposition
c Copper staining highlights abundant copper within hepatocytes

is the most widely recommended single screening assay (suggested cutoffs vary from 45-60%, and an elevated value should be repeated). However, specificity is hampered by a number of causes of secondary siderosis, including steatohepatitis, chronic hemolytic anemia, dietary iron overload (eg, excessive iron supplementation, Bantu siderosis), chronic transfusions, sideroblastic anemia, and porphyria cutanea tarda. The traditional confirmatory test has been liver biopsy with either qualitative or quantitative iron assessment. The liver biopsy displays increased hepatocellular iron f7.24, particularly when stained with Prussian blue, with the greatest deposition in periportal (zone 1) hepatocytes. Semiquantitative iron grading (0-4+ scale) correlates extremely well with hepatic iron quantitation, especially at the extremes (0-1+ and 4+). Hepatic iron can be measured quantitatively by atomic absorption spectrophotometry, and expressed either as the hepatic iron concentration (μmol/g of dry liver weight) or as the hepatic iron index (hepatic iron concentration divided by age in years). A normal hepatic iron index is <1.1, and >1.9 is considered diagnostic of HH. The value of the hepatic iron index once cirrhosis is established is lower. Confirmation by molecular methods may substitute for liver biopsy in appropriate settings. The molecular diagnosis of HH is an excellent example of the application of targeted mutation analysis. Since nearly all affected persons have either C282Y or H63D, it is cost effective to look for only these 2 alleles.

Wilson disease (hepatolenticular degeneration)

Wilson disease may present in one of 3 ways—liver disease, neuropsychiatric disease, or hemolysis. These manifestations usually begin by young adulthood. Hepatitis in Wilson disease often presents acutely with jaundice and abdominal pain, but it may present with chronic hepatitis. Kayser-Fleischer rings often develop in association with neurologic disease. The neurologic manifestations, which formed the basis for the first description by Samuel Alexander Kinnier Wilson in 1912, are protean and may include movement disorders (dysarthria, tremors, rigidity, bradykinesia, and abnormal gait) and psychosis. It is important to think of Wilson disease when examining a liver biopsy from a young adult with hepatitis. The liver biopsy shows glycogenated nuclei, steatosis, and inflammation that may mimic the pattern of chronic viral

hepatitis f7.25. Fibrosis ultimately leads to cirrhosis. Unlike liver iron stains, hepatic copper stains are somewhat unreliable in comparison with formal hepatic copper quantitation (which is considered the gold standard). Furthermore, the finding of stainable copper is highly nonspecific and may be seen in steatohepatitis and cholestasis.

The plasma ceruloplasmin may serve as a screening test. Low levels are found in Wilson disease, but there are several causes of falsely elevated and falsely depressed levels. In fully established Wilson disease, the serum copper is elevated; however, at various stages, the copper may be low, normal, or high. The urinary copper excretion is usually elevated.

Wilson disease is caused by mutations in the *ATP7B* gene, which encodes an ATPase utilized in copper binding to ceruloplasmin. The *ATP7A* gene is mutated in Menkes kinky hair syndrome as well. Inheritance is autosomal recessive, and the disease is rare, with a frequency of ~1 in 30,000.

α_1 antitrypsin deficiency

The *SERPINA1* (*PI*) gene on chromosome 14q31-32.3 is the site of moderate polymorphism. Most healthy adults are homozygous for the M allele (denoted Pi-MM). ~10% of the population is heterozygous for M and some other allele, of which there are ~75 t7.8. The alleles are named according to the electrophoretic mobility of the encoded protein, from fastest (A) to slowest (Z). The wild-type allele is denoted M. α_1 antitrypsin deficiency is usually caused by homozygosity for the Z allele (Pi-ZZ).

t7.8 *SERPINA1* (PI) gene alleles

Genotype	Prevalence	Approximate AAT (mg/dL)
MM	90%	150-350
MS	6%	125-300
MZ	5%	100-200
SS	<1%	100-200
SZ	<1%	75-120
ZZ	<1%	20-50

The Z allele is transcribed normally but polymerizes post-translationally within the endoplasmic reticulum. The paucity of functional α_1 antitrypsin leads to an imbalance in the normal remodeling enzymes and as a result, damage to the lung. Its accumulation within hepatocytes leads to inflammation and

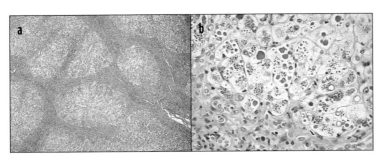

f7.26 α₁ antitrypsin (AAT) deficiency
a Cirrhotic liver in a patient with AAT deficiency
b Abundant red globules are seen in PAS-diastase stained sections, most numerous in periportal hepatocytes

fibrosing liver disease, eventuating in cirrhosis f7.26. AAT deficiency presents as neonatal hepatitis in a significant portion of patients. Others are spared as neonates and may present instead with early onset emphysema, cirrhosis, hepatocellular carcinoma, or panniculitis. There appears to be an increased incidence of Wegener granulomatosis and other vasculitides. In contrast to usual-type emphysema which is centro-acinar and upper lobe-predominant, AAT-associated emphysema has panacinar histopathology and basilar predominance.

The Z allele (Glu342Lys) has a frequency in the US population of ~1-2%. In Europe, the allele frequency is highest in the North (5% in Scandinavians) and lowest in the South (1% of Italians). The S allele (Glu264Val) has the opposite distribution: 10% in southern Europe, 5% in the north. Nearly all clinically relevant AAT deficiency is associated with at least one copy of the Z allele. The vast majority of affected patients have either PI-ZZ or PI-SZ. The S allele is by itself incapable of causing clinical disease, though homozygosity for S leads to modest reductions in plasma AAT. AAT deficiency is thus inherited as an autosomal recessive trait. AAT is a member of the serpin family of protease inhibitors, related to C1 esterase inhibitor and antithrombin, that are highly conformation-dependent and exquisitely sensitive to specific amino acid substitutions within the "hinge" regions. The conformational effects of disease-causing mutations lead to polymerization of AAT within hepatocytes. This mechanism of organ damage caused by conformation-driven intracellular accumulation has been termed "conformational disease" and is a mechanism shared with Alzheimer and Pick diseases.

Bilirubin excretion disorders

Bilirubin conjugation disorders (Gilbert & Crigler-Najjar syndromes)

Conjugation disorders result from deficient bilirubin glucoronosyl transferase, the product of the *UGT1A1* gene. The result is impaired hepatic conjugation of bilirubin, leading to increased levels of unconjugated bilirubin and jaundice.

Gilbert syndrome is caused by mutations in the 5′ TATA box of the promoter for the *UGT1A1* gene, resulting in mildly deficient bilirubin conjugation. This anomaly is fairly common, estimated to affect ~5% of the population. Clinically, Gilbert syndrome is benign, manifesting as mild hyperbilirubinemia provoked by physiologic stress (eg, fasting, infection).

Crigler-Najjar is more severe and caused by mutations in the coding sequence of the *UGT1A1* gene. In Type I Crigler-Najjar, there is no detectable glucuronosyl transferase activity,

leading to severe jaundice beginning in the neonatal period, often complicated by kernicterus. In Type II Crigler-Najjar (also called Arias syndrome), there is some glucuronosyl transferase activity, usually <10% of normal, and jaundice presents somewhat later.

Bilirubin secretion disorders (Dubin-Johnson & Rotor syndromes)

The secretion disorders result from defective secretion of conjugated bilirubin into the canaliculus. The effect of this is mild conjugated hyperbilirubinemia. Dubin-Johnson syndrome is caused by mutations in the *MRP2* (multidrug resistance protein 2) gene that encodes the canalicular multispecific organic anion transporter (cMOAT). This is associated with heavily pigmented but otherwise undamaged hepatic parenchyma. Rotor syndrome is similar to Dubin-Johnson, but does not produce hepatic parenchymal pigmentation.

Inherited pancreatitis

Inherited pancreatitis can be classified into 4 distinct categories

1. cystic fibrosis

2. those associated with metabolic disorders such as hypercalcemia or hyperlipidemia

3. single gene defects such as mutations in the *PRSS1* gene (cationic trypsinogen) or *SPINK1* gene (pancreatic secretory trypsin inhibitor)

4. part of another multisystem inherited disorder (eg, Pearson syndrome)

Cystic fibrosis

Cystic fibrosis (CF) is a multisystem disorder resulting from mutations in the cystic fibrosis transmembrane receptor (*CFTR*) gene on chromosome 7q31.2. This gene is very large, composed of 27 exons, and a wide range of mutations are possible. Over 1,000 distinct mutations have been described. The *CFTR* gene encodes a chloride channel and is expressed in multiple tissues, including upper and lower respiratory tract, gastrointestinal tract, skin adnexa, hepatobiliary system, pancreas, and male reproductive tract. A pattern of protein expression reflects the systems affected by the disease.

Cystic fibrosis is the most common autosomal recessive condition among Caucasians, with a carrier frequency approaching 1 in 25. CF affects ~1 in 2,000 live births. Among other ethnicities the incidence is lower.

The earliest sign of CF is often a meconium ileus. Later manifestations may include chronic pancreatitis, unexplained malnutrition/failure to thrive, rectal prolapse, nasal polyps, and male infertility caused by congenital bilateral absence of the vas deferens (CBAVD). Liver disease results from biliary obstruction, leading to focal or generalized cirrhosis f7.27. Recurrent bacterial bronchitis and pneumonia may lead to bronchiectasis f7.28; pulmonary infection in childhood that is caused by *S aureus*, *B cepacia* or *P aeruginosa* is strong presumptive evidence of CF. In particular, mucoid forms of *Pseudomonas* are considered strongly suggestive of CF. CF is responsible for many cases of sinusitis and nasal polyps, particularly when these are seen in children. Lastly, as a direct consequence of

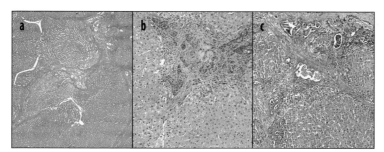

f7.27 Cystic fibrosis with severe hepatic involvement
a Low magnification view showing biliary pattern cirrhosis
b & c Intermediate magnification view showing obstructive biliary changes in the portal triads

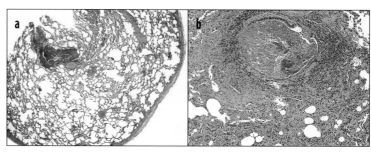

f7.28 Cystic fibrosis with mild pulmonary involvement
a Low magnification view showing bronchiolocentric inflammatory changes
b Bronchiolitis with inspissated luminal mucus

the ion channel disorder, CF can lead to severe salt loss and hyponatremia t7.9.

t7.9 Most common presentations of cystic fibrosis (in order of decreasing frequency)

Recurrent pneumonia and/or bronchiectasis

Unexplained malnutrition or failure to thrive

Meconium ileus

Hyponatremia, especially with hypochloremia & metabolic alkalosis

Rectal prolapse

Unexplained chronic diarrhea

Refractory sinusitis or asthma

Nasal polyps in childhood

Chronic, recurrent, pancreatitis

Hepatic disease (focal biliary obstruction, unexplained jaundice)

Male infertility

The above generalities notwithstanding, in any given case certain organs may be relatively spared; conversely, there are cases in which manifestations are restricted to a single organ. For example, some cases of CF present only as idiopathic pancreatitis. In some males, only the function of the vas deferens is affected; congenital bilateral absence of vas deferens (CBAVD) occurs frequently in isolation, without multisystem disease. These variations are thought to be the result of differing *CFTR* mutations as well as the effects of other inherited (modifier genes) or environmental influences. The severity of lung disease, for example, varies tremendously, even among those with identical *CFTR* genotype. The MPO activity within circulating neutrophils is known to vary among individuals, and the MPO activity has been shown to correlate with the FEV1/FVC in CF patients. Another example is a locus on chromosome 19 that appears to be strongly associated with meconium ileus. The degree of both pulmonary and hepatic involvement seems to vary with the α_1 antitrypsin genotype. Interestingly, it has been found that among alcoholics who develop chronic calcifying pancreatitis, CFTR mutations are quite common.

The diagnosis of CF can be established, in a patient with suggestive clinical features, with one of the following: molecular testing, 2 consecutive abnormal pilocarpine iontophoresis sweat chloride tests, or an abnormal transepithelial nasal potential difference (NPD) measurement. Many states have implemented newborn screening for CF. The method commonly employed for this is an immunoreactive trypsinogen (IRT) assay, performed on blood spots. IRT levels are elevated in cystic fibrosis until the age of ~2 months. This finding must

be confirmed by another modality and should not be used after ~2 months of age. The sweat test is difficult to perform reproducibly. Positive results should be confirmed with a repeat test, and negative tests should be repeated if suspicion is high. False positive and false negative results are common. Increased potential (voltage) differences across nasal epithelium has been used to confirm the diagnosis in patients with borderline sweat tests. Heterozygotes are asymptomatic and, to date, there is no test capable of detecting them aside from DNA studies.

Several multiple-mutation targeted mutation analysis panels are clinically available, generally probing for between 20 and 25 common mutations. Such panels are capable of detecting ~90% of cases overall. The most common disease-causing mutation is ΔF508 (present in ~70% of affected individuals) t7.10.

t7.10 Most common *CFTR* gene mutations

Mutation	Frequency in affected persons
ΔF508	66.0%
G542X	2.4%
G551D	1.6%
N1303K	1.3%
W1282X	1.2%
R553X	0.7%

The ΔF508 mutation is a 3-nucleotide deletion of codon 508, leading to in-frame loss of a single phenylalanine (F) at position 508. The mutation results in a protein that, though functional, is rapidly degraded. About 5-10% of *CFTR* mutations are due to premature truncation, and these are particularly common in Ashkenazi Jews. The W1282X mutation, a truncating mutation, occurs in 60% of the Ashkenazi Jews with CF. The American College of Medical Genetics recommends testing with a 23-mutation panel with reflex testing for an additional allele in the presence of certain mutant alleles. These alleles were chosen because they are present in ≥0.1% of the populations being tested. The post-test probability of CF with negative test result varies depending upon the ethnicity of the patient tested. *CFTR* mutation testing is most common in the Ashkenazi Jewish population and is one of the 4 recommended genetic disorders in the recommended testing panel for this population (including Canavan disease, Tay-Sachs disease, and familial dysautonomia).

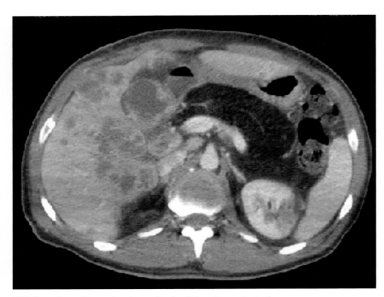

f7.29 Shwachman-Diamond syndrome showing fatty metamorphosis of pancreas

Pearson syndrome

Pearson syndrome is an extremely rare cause of chronic pancreatitis showing autosomal dominant inheritance and an association with marrow failure. Despite its rarity, the disease is fascinating as it is a chromosomal breakage syndrome affecting the mitochondrial DNA. The marrow shows sideroblastic anemia with vacuolization of precursors, and the pancreas shows fibrosis typical of chronic pancreatitis. The molecular defect is a microdeletion within the mitochondrial DNA.

Pancreatic lipomatosis syndromes (Shwachman-Diamond & Johanson-Blizzard syndromes)

While generally thought of as a bone marrow failure syndrome, nearly all patients with Shwachman-Diamond syndrome also suffer from exocrine pancreatic insufficiency, on the basis of fatty metamorphosis f7.29. Note that this syndrome is distinct from Blackfan-Diamond syndrome (pure red cell aplasia, no pancreatic disease). The hematologic findings include cyclic neutropenia, eventually leading to aplastic anemia, myelodysplasia, and possibly acute leukemia. Neutropenia leads to recurrent infections, particularly skin infections, osteomyelitis, otitis media, and sinusitis. Pancreatic insufficiency may manifest itself in infancy as steatorrhea, malabsorption, and malnutrition. The histologic features are similar to those seen in Johanson-Blizzard syndrome (described next): the acini are devoid of exocrine cells and replaced with adipose tissue. The islets are preserved and disposed in a background of adipose tissue (pancreatic lipomatosis). Unlike chronic pancreatitis, there is no fibrosis. Interestingly, over time some patients begin to develop some exocrine pancreatic function, and their symptoms improve. The syndrome is caused by mutations in a gene known as *SBDS* (Shwachman-Bodian-Diamond syndrome). While the function of the gene is unknown, mutations in it appear to arise as a result of exchange of genetic material with a nearby pseudogene (*SBDSP*) in a manner similar to the mechanism of mutation in congenital adrenal hyperplasia (gene conversion).

Johanson-Blizzard syndrome is characterized by hypoplasia of the nasal alae, pancreatic exocrine insufficiency, hypothyroidism, and deafness. Like Shwachman-Diamond syndrome, there is lipomatous change in the pancreas (replacement of acini with adipocytes), with preservation of the pancreatic ducts and islets.

Neuromuscular

Central neurodegenerative disease

Alzheimer disease

Alzheimer disease is classified as early onset (presentation prior to 60 years of age) and usual (or late) onset. About 5% of cases have early onset, and ~1/2 of these are familial or so-called early onset familial Alzheimer disease (EOFAD). One of the consistent findings in Alzheimer disease is accumulation of a type of amyloid (Aβ amyloid), which is derived from amyloid precursor protein (APP), the gene for which (*APP*) is found on chromosome 21. Histopathologic features of Alzheimer disease are universal in those with trisomy 21 by the age of 40 years, thought to be because of amplification of the *APP* gene. In addition to *APP* gene mutations, EOFAD may be caused by mutations in *PSEN1* or *PSEN2*. *PSEN1* is found at 14q24 and encodes presenilin 1. *PSEN2* is on 1q and encodes presenilin 2. Lastly, there is an association of usual (late) onset Alzheimer disease with the E4 allele at the *APOE* gene locus at 19q13.2.

Familial Pick disease (Frontotemporal dementia with Parkinsonism)

Pick disease disproportionately involves the frontal cortex; thus, disinhibition is a prominent feature. Subcortical involvement is also present, leading to Parkinson-like rigidity and bradykinesia. The onset of symptoms is often in the mid 40s, and the disease progresses to dementia and death, frequently within 10 years. The characteristic anatomic finding is cortical atrophy that is distinctly limited to the fronto-temporal region. Histologically, argyrophilic intraneuronal inclusions (Pick bodies) and achromatic neurons (Pick cells) are found in these regions. The gene implicated is *MAPT*, on 17q, which encodes the microtubule-associated protein tau. The tau protein is a member of the microtubule associated protein (MAP) family that is found mainly within neurons. Disease-associated mutations appear to exert their effects through causing altered binding of the tau protein to the microtubule. Pick disease is an example of so-called tauopathy; other conditions associated with tau abnormalities include Alzheimer disease, progressive supranuclear palsy, and dementia pugilistica.

Parkinson disease & Lewy body disease

Parkinson disease is the most common cause of Parkinsonism, a movement disorder characterized by bradykinesia, rigidity, and resting tremor. Dementia is a feature in a significant proportion of cases. Lewy body disease is a term that denotes clinical dementia in conjunction with the histopathologic finding of Lewy bodies; thus, Lewy body disease encompasses both dementia associated with Parkinson disease and isolated dementia with Lewy bodies f7.30. There

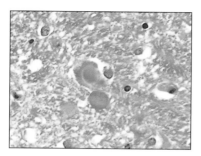

f7.30 Lewy body

is a clinical continuum between these entities, with most cases exhibiting variable degrees of the characteristic clinical features: progressive and fluctuating cognitive impairment, Parkinsonism, delusions, and visual hallucinations. The Lewy body is the unifying histopathologic feature of this group of diseases. The distribution of Lewy bodies correlates reasonably well with the clinical manifestations; thus, Lewy bodies within the neocortex correlate with dementia and neuropsychiatric manifestations, and Lewy bodies within the subcortical white matter correlate with the movement disorder. Some cases of Parkinson disease are familial, and genetic anomalies have been identified in these families in genes denoted as *PARK1* through *PARK8*.

Huntington disease (HD)

HD is a prototypical triplet repeat disorder (trinucleotide repeat disorder). Inherited as an autosomal dominant condition, HD is associated with an expanded CAG repeat in the coding sequence for the *HTT* gene on the end of the short arm of chromosome 4. *HTT* encodes a protein called huntingtin. The disease affects the caudate nucleus and putamen, presenting with choreiform movements, hemiballismus, dementia, and psychosis. As is typical of trinucleotide repeat disorders, anticipation is noted (earlier presentation and/or more severe disease in successive generations). The age of onset and severity of symptoms is dependent on the number of triplet repeats, which tends to increase with successive generations. When there are <28 repeats, a normal phenotype results. Between 28 and 35 repeats is considered an intermediate allele (premutation) with those harboring the repeats usually unaffected. 36-40 repeats causes an allele with reduced penetrance; some are mildly affected, and some are unaffected. Individuals with >40 repeats are almost uniformly affected. Imaging (CT & MRI) shows a highly characteristic atrophy of the caudate and putamen. Median survival is ~15 years after onset. There appears to be a strong correlation between paternal inheritance and early disease onset. Nearly all cases of juvenile-onset HD have both numerous CAG repeats and paternal inheritance.

Cerebral autosomal dominant arteriopathy with subcortical infarctions & leukoencephalopathy (CADASIL)

CADASIL is an inherited autosomal dominant condition caused by mutations in the *NOTCH3* gene on chromosome 19p13.2-p13.1. Patients present at a mean age of 45 years with with migraine headaches accompanied by auras, transient ischemic attacks, and stroke-like events, progressing eventually to dementia. The dementia is subcortical in nature, characterized by disturbances of memory, motivation, and mentation. MRI reveals multiple hyperintense lesions within the periventricular white matter (particularly in the frontal lobes), basal ganglia, and brain stem. Highly characteristic are subcortical lacunar lesions, appearing as grouped lacunar lesions arranged linearly at the gray-white interface. The underlying pathophysiology is related to abnormal vasculature within the white matter and basal ganglia. The vessels therein demonstrate granular eosinophilic medial deposits. Vascular occlusion leads to multiple lacunar infarctions. Similarly affected vessels can be found in the skin, such that skin biopsies may be used for diagnosis.

Pantothenate kinase-associated neurodegeneration (formerly Hallervorden-Spatz syndrome)

Pantothenate kinase-associated neurodegeneration (PKAN) is a disease in which there is abundant deposition of iron in the basal ganglia, resulting in choreoathetosis, dystonia, rigidity, and pigmentary retinopathy. Systemic iron metabolism is normal. Onset is usually in childhood, and MRI shows a classic "eye of the tiger" sign, in which the globus pallidus has a central region of hyperintensity and a rim of hypointensity. The sign is apparently quite sensitive and specific. Histopathologically, there is rust-brown discoloration in the globus pallidus and substantia nigra, due to accumulated iron. Within areas of iron accumulation one can find axonal spheroid bodies. The responsible gene is *PANK2*, found at 20p13, which encodes pantothenate kinase 2.

Copper storage defects (Menkes disease, Occipital horn syndrome, Wilson disease)

Underlying these diseases are defects in the copper-transporting ATPase genes, *ATP7A* and *ATP7B*. The defects result in imbalances in copper metabolism—both accumulation of copper in tissues and reduced availability of copper for copper-dependent enzymes such as dopamine β hydroxylase (DBH) and lysyl oxidase. Menkes disease is caused by mutations in *ATP7A* and presents as cognitive neurologic impairment and characteristic hair changes (lightly colored, short, coarse, twisted and sparse) in an infant. When examined microscopically, the hair shaft displays pili torti (180° twists), trichoclasis (transverse breaks), and trichoptilosis (longitudinal splits). Occipital horn syndrome presents with calcifications at the sites of attachment of the trapezius and sternocleidomastoid muscles to the occipital bone (occipital horns), along with laxity of skin and joints, bladder diverticula, inguinal hernias, vascular tortuosity, and dysautonomia. Wilson disease, due to mutations in *ATP7B* presents with endocrine, hepatic, and dermatologic findings. Neurologic (cognitive decline and inco-ordination) and psychiatric findings are common.

Familial prion disease (familial Creutzfeldt-Jakob disease, Gerstmann-Sträussler-Scheinker disease, fatal familial insomnia)

Mutations in the *PRNP* gene (chromosome 20p) are associated with a variety of disease phenotypes, including familial Creutzfeldt-Jakob disease, Gerstmann-Sträussler-Scheinker disease, and fatal familial insomnia. Features common to all include dementia, myoclonus, ataxia, dysarthria, autosomal dominant inheritance, and onset in adulthood. The familial Creutzfeldt-Jakob disease phenotype usually presents between the age of 30 and 50 with dementia, ataxia and myoclonus. Death occurs within a few months to a few years. The brain biopsy shows typical spongiform change. The familial Gerstmann-Sträussler-Scheinker syndrome phenotype also presents between 30-50, initially with cerebellar dysfunction. Dementia occurs at a later stage, and the course is slower, with death in 7-10 years. Amyloid plaques are more common than spongiform change. Fatal familial insomnia presents in adulthood with the insidious onset of insomnia. Over time, autonomic disturbances and ataxia develop, and dementia arises late in the course of disease.

Kuru, the original prion disease, was found in those who acquired prions through the practice of cannibalism in New Guinea. Sporadic (acquired) prion diseases are far more common than the familial types, with features that are fairly similar. Initially these acquired disorders were thought to be the result of infection with virus, but it slowly became apparent that an infectious protein particle was responsible. The infectious protein, or prion, was found to be a misfolded variant of a protein normally expressed by the human *PRNP* gene (whose function is uncertain). The misfolded protein is hypothesized to act as a catalyst to change the conformation of the normally produced protein such that it, too, becomes misfolded. The misfolded proteins accumulate extracellularly and eventually lead to the spongiform degeneration. In the case of inherited disorders, mutations in the gene encoding the prion protein (known as PrP) are thought to lead to increased susceptibility to form the misfolded conformation.

Peripheral neuropathy

The hereditary peripheral neuropathies are generally classified as to whether they primarily affect sensory and motor neurons (HSMN) or whether they affect primarily sensory and autonomic neurons (HSAN). The spinal muscular atrophies (SMA) form a third category, affecting lower motor neurons. A prototypic HSMN disorder is Charcot-Marie-Tooth disease, and a prototypic HSAN is familial dysautonomia.

Charcot-Marie-Tooth (CMT)

Charcot-Marie-Tooth (CMT) is an autosomal dominant inherited disorder affecting both sensory and motor neurons. The most common form is CMT type 1, which is associated with peripheral nerve demyelination. The neuropathy most often affects legs, hands, and feet, presenting with weakness, atrophy, and anesthesia. Biopsy of the nerve shows prominent onion bulb formation, and muscle biopsy findings are typical of denervation atrophy. The most common genetic basis for type 1 CMT is duplication of a 1.5 Mb region of DNA on 17p12 containing the *PMP22* gene and subsequent dosage effects. Incidentally, a 1.5 Mb deletion at this site causes hereditary neuropathy with pressure palsies (HNPP). Type 2 CMT is less common and is associated with axonal degeneration instead of demyelination.

Familial dysautonomia (Riley-Day syndrome)

Familial dysautonomia is an autosomal recessive condition primarily affecting individuals of Ashkenazi Jewish descent. The American Congress of Obstetricians and Gynecologist's (ACOG) recommended panel for carrier screening in Ashkenazi Jews includes familial dysautonomia, cystic fibrosis, Bloom syndrome, and Canavan syndrome. Familial dysautonomia presents with autonomic, sensory, and motor deficits including decreased pain sensation, altered temperature sensation, and decreased deep tendon reflexes. Autonomic dysfunction presents as episodic hemodynamic instability, abnormal gastric motility, profuse sweating, and insensitivity to hypercapnia. Mutations in the gene *IKBKAP* on chromosome 9q31 are responsible for the disorder with 2 founder mutations accounting for >99% of cases.

Spinal muscular atrophy (SMA)

The SMAs are a family of disorders presenting with lower motor neuron deficits, all inherited in autosomal recessive fashion. SMA type 1 (Werdnig-Hoffmann disease) is the most severe. Infants with SMA type 1 present with hypotonia, and death usually follows within 2 years. Type 2 SMA has later onset and presents with gross motor skill delay and death shortly thereafter. SMA type 3 presents in childhood, but affected individuals are usually able to ambulate. Type 4 SMA or "adult-type" can be exceptionally subtle and difficult to diagnose. Mutations in the gene, survival motor neuron 1 (*SMN1*) are responsible for all of the SMAs. A nearly-identical gene, *SMN2*, which likely arose via a duplication mechanism, is located adjacent to the *SMN1* locus on chromosome 5. Since the SMAs are all caused by loss of *SMN1*, it is the role of *SMN2* to determine the severity of the disease. Mutations in the intron 6 or exon 7 of *SMN2* lead to altered splicing, decreased SMN2 and more severe disease.

Skeletal muscle diseases
Duchenne & Becker muscular dystrophy (dystrophinopathies)

With 79 exons, the *DMD* gene on chromosome Xp21.2 encodes the largest known human protein with a mass of >2,000 kDa. Mutations in the *DMD* gene cause a family of X-linked recessive diseases known as the dystrophinopathies. The most common of these are Duchenne muscular dystrophy, Becker muscular dystrophy, and X-linked cardiomyopathy. Patients with dystrophinopathies uniformly have elevated creatine kinase levels at the time of presentation.

Duchenne muscular dystrophy presents in early childhood (before age 5) as progressive skeletal muscle weakness, delays in gross motor skill development, and calf hypertrophy. Weakness is symmetrical and begins with the proximal muscles, as is typical for primary myopathic processes. Patients are wheelchair-bound by age 12. The majority (>90%) of patients also have a cardiomyopathy, and the most common causes of

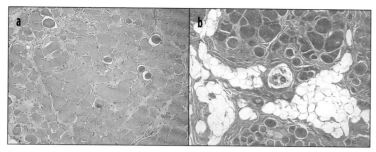

f7.31   Duchenne muscular dystrophy with a rounded atrophic fibers & b fatty infiltration

death are dilated cardiomyopathy and pneumonia. The incidence is ~1 in 3,500 live births, making it the most common inherited muscular dystrophy. Up to 1/3 of cases are the result of sporadic mutations. Skeletal muscle biopsy shows variation in fiber size and scattered hypereosinophilic small rounded fibers f7.31. When normal skeletal muscle is stained by immunohistochemistry, dystrophin is found coating the inner aspect of the cell membrane; in DMD, dystrophin staining is absent. A mosaic pattern of staining is described in female carriers.

Becker muscular dystrophy is much less than Duchenne. The presentation is usually later than Duchenne, less severe, and more slowly progressive. By definition patients with Becker muscular dystrophy are ambulatory at or after 16 years of age.

A small group of patients with *DMD* gene mutations manifest only dilated cardiomyopathy (X-linked dilated cardiomyopathy). It appears that this syndrome is caused by mutations within the dystrophin gene promoter region and that the isolated heart involvement results from so-called phenotypic rescue mediated by alternate promoters in skeletal muscle.

A 200-kB region spanning exon 45 (and the flanking introns 44 and 45) is the major site of *DMD* gene deletions. Another major group of deletions is found at the 5′ end. The reading frame hypothesis has been proposed to explain the differences between Duchenne and Becker muscular dystrophy. It is thought that mutations which alter the reading frame, leading to protein truncation, result in the more severe DMD phenotype, whereas those that do not alter the reading frame result in the BMD phenotype. About 10% of cases are due to partial gene duplications. These are distributed within the same regions in which deletions are found. Because of the large size of the gene, scanning technologies, such as multiplex ligation-dependent probe amplification (MLPA) or multiplex PCR are most commonly utilized, but these techniques are insensitive to duplications. Deletions are common, especially deletion of exon 45.

Myotonic muscular dystrophy (MMD)

Myotonic dystrophy is an autosomal dominant inherited trinucleotide repeat disorder. As is common in trinucleotide repeat disorders, MMD displays anticipation (progressive severity with successive generations). MMD is the most common muscular dystrophy presenting in adults (and second behind the dystrophinopathies in children). Unlike Duchenne and Becker muscular dystrophy, myotonic dystrophy can also exhibit smooth muscle effects, such as bowel dysmotility, and

nonmuscular features such as cataracts, cardiac conduction abnormalities, and endocrine disorders. In fact, cataracts may be the only manifestation in minimally affected patients, and those with the full syndrome often have ancestors with early onset cataracts. The other unusual feature is that skeletal muscle, while weak, is persistently contracted (myotonic).

The majority of cases of myotonic dystrophy are caused by expansion of a CTG repeat in the *DMPK* gene (type 1) or the *CNBP* gene (type 2). Less than 35 repeats is considered normal, >50 repeats is highly associated with disease, while the intermediate number of repeats is associated with a premutation allele.

Other dystrophies

Fascioscapulohumeral muscular dystrophy presents with facial and scapular muscle weakness. This gives rise to a distinctive appearance, with gaping mouth, eyelid droop, decreased facial expression, sloping shoulders, and scapular winging. In addition to these features, patients often have cardiac conduction defects, retinal changes, and sensorineural hearing loss. Fascioscapulohumeral muscular dystrophy shows an autosomal dominant pattern of inheritance. The genetic defect is located at 4q35, in a region that normally contains a large number of repeats of a single DNA sequence (called D4Z4). Disease is associated with <11 D4Z4 repeats.

Inclusion body myositis (IBM) can be sporadic or inherited in an autosomal recessive fashion. IBM presents as distal muscle weakness (different from most myopathic processes that cause proximal weakness). IBM classically presents in young adulthood with weakness of the anterior tibialis muscle, resulting in foot drop and gait disturbances, progressing later to involve the hands. Diagnosis is most often made on frozen muscle biopsy where the characteristic features of vacuoles rimmed with basophilic granular material. A single founder effect mutation in the *GNE* gene on chromosome 9p is responsible for the majority of cases.

The finding of nemaline rods in muscle biopsy specimens define the class of diseases known as the nemaline rod myopathies. The nemaline rods are sarcoplasmic rod-like inclusions seen in trichrome stained sections but not seen in H&E stained sections. The rods contain the same lattice-like structure as the Z-discs, appear to be in continuity with them, and are composed of Z-disc proteins such as α-actinin. Mutations in the genes for many structural sarcomeric proteins have been found to cause nemaline rod myopathy, including actin and troponin.

Limb-girdle muscular dystrophies are a collection of diseases caused by mutations in a number of genes but all having features consistent with a myopathy: symmetric and proximal muscle weakness, elevated creatine kinase, and muscle biopsy results consistent with myopathic changes. These patients present in a fashion similar to the dystrophinopathies but fail to demonstrate defective or deficient dystrophin.

Malignant hyperthermia (MH)

Prior to its recognition there was a very high mortality rate in patients with malignant hyperthermia when exposed to inhalational anesthetics. Hypercarbia while under anesthesia is often the first sign and results from a physiologic response to systemic lactic acidosis. If untreated, MH progresses to rhabdomyolysis, hyperkalemia, disseminated intravascular coagulation, and congestive heart failure. The early recognition and use of dantrolene has reduced mortality significantly. Defective RYR1 calcium channels resulting in uncontrolled release of calcium from the sarcoplasmic reticulum are the cause of malignant hyperthermia. The excess calcium causes muscle contraction which leads to consumption of ATP and ultimately, anaerobic metabolism. Dantrolene inhibits the prolonged RYR1 calcium channel opening in response to inhaled anesthesia. Functional testing (caffeine/halothane contracture test) on muscle biopsy specimens can confirm the diagnosis but lacks specificity. Genetic testing of the *RYR1* gene is complicated by the large number of causal mutations that could be present, many of which are unique within families.

Congenital hearing loss

It is estimated that fully 1% of human genes are associated with hearing. With that many genes (several hundred) it stands to reason that there would be many different causes of inherited hearing loss. Congenital hearing loss can be classified as either syndromic or nonsyndromic or alternatively, as sensorineural, conductive, or central. The categorizations are not exclusive and there can be overlap. Congenital hearing loss is quite common, affecting almost 1 in 1,000 births. Up to 1/2 of these cases are estimated to have a genetic cause. Most of the congenital cases of hearing loss are nonsyndromic. Congenital hearing loss is most often detected in the newborn period because of universal hearing screening. This is significant because early intervention, such as with cochlear implants is the key to proper speech development.

Mutations of the *GJB2* gene are the most common cause of nonsyndromic congenital hearing loss. Depending on the nature of the change, mutations in *GJB2* can be inherited as autosomal dominant or autosomal recessive conditions. The most common mutation of *GJB2* is the 35delG mutation, accounting for 2/3 of the cases in Caucasians. In other ethnic groups other mutations predominate (eg, 235delC in Chinese). The *GJB2* gene encodes connexin26, a protein involved in the formation of cochlear gap junctions. Mutations affect the ability of the gap junctions to exchange ions and therefore transmit the electrical impulses that the cochlea is supposed to transduce from sound waves. Neither balance through the vestibular system nor conduction from the auditory nerve is affected by mutant connexin26.

Syndromic hearing loss is sometimes difficult to distinguish from nonsyndromic in the newborn period due to the later development of some of the symptoms, such as the renal problems with Alport syndrome, retinitis in Usher syndrome, long QT interval in Jervell and Lange-Nielsen syndrome, or goiter in Pendred syndrome. Waardenburg syndrome is the most common type of autosomal dominant syndromic hearing loss. The syndrome consists of sensorineural hearing loss and pigmentary abnormalities of the skin, eyes (heterochromia iridis), and hair (white forelock). Usher syndrome is the most common type of autosomal recessive syndromic hearing loss. It consists of sensorineural hearing loss and retinitis pigmentosa (RP), ultimately leading to blindness. It is the most common cause of combined deafness and blindness.

Disorders of mitochondria
Background

Because of the central role of mitochondria in the aerobic (oxidative) production of energy (ATP), tissues with high energy requirements are most severely affected by mitochondrial dysfunction. These tissues include the brain, myocardium, and skeletal muscle. Thus, mitochondrial disorders result in a heterogeneous constellation of finding within the neuromuscular and cardiovascular systems. Typical findings include ophthalmoplegia, ptosis, retinopathy, optic atrophy, skeletal myopathy, cardiomyopathy, sensorineural deafness, and encephalopathy.

Some proteins expressed in mitochondria are encoded by the mitochondrial genome, and some are encoded by the nuclear genome. Thus, mitochondrial disorders may follow either mitochondrial (maternal) inheritance or Mendelian inheritance patterns. Those that arise from mitochondrial gene mutations tend to arise in adulthood while those related to mutations in nuclear genes tend to manifest earlier in life.

Mitochondrial inheritance, also called maternal inheritance, is simple in some respects but complicated in others. The sperm provides the fertilized ovum with no mitochondria. All mitochondria, and therefore all mitochondrial DNA (mtDNA), are passed on to the offspring from the mother. Furthermore, only affected daughters can pass an mtDNA trait on to the next generation. What complicates this simple scheme is that, unlike the nucleus which contains 2 copies of each chromosome for a total of 46 discrete DNA molecules, each mitochondrion contains thousands of DNA molecules. Thus, whereas a mutation in nuclear DNA can be present in 1 or 2 of 2 gene copies, a mutation may be present in the mitochondrial genome in a very wide range of dilutions. These mutations become clinically significant when they reach a certain concentration (the threshold effect). Also, when mitochondria divide (in order to provide sufficient mitochondria for both products of a cell division) these mtDNA molecules are randomly divided among the newly formed mitochondria, such that different cells (and different tissues) can end up with genetically very different mitochondria, a situation called heteroplasmy. The cells of normal individuals usually contain a single clone of mitochondria (with identical genomes, inherited from the mother, aka homoplasmy). Heteroplasmy is the basis for the broad phenotypic variability observed in mitochondrial disease.

Mitochondrial diseases should be considered in the differential diagnosis of any unexplained multilevel neuromuscular disorder. Screening tests include plasma or CSF lactic acid, ketones, acylcarnitines, and urinary organic acids. If these are abnormal, one should next consider muscle biopsy. The muscle biopsy classically contains ragged red fibers (trichrome stain). The succinate dehydrogenase stain, in addition to highlighting the muscle fibers, shows stronger than usual staining in blood vessels, due to an abundance of mitochondria. Ultrastructural examination shows characteristic (parking lot) inclusions.

Structural mitochondrial DNA defects
Kearns-Sayre syndrome & Pearson syndrome

These syndromes have in common a basis in major structural defects—gross deletions or large rearrangements—in mtDNA. Such defects are usually sporadic (de novo), but they are sometimes maternally derived. Heteroplasmy leads to the variety of clinical presentations. Kearns-Sayre syndrome most often presents before the age of 20 and patients usually display pigmentary (salt and pepper) retinopathy, external ophthalmoplegia, elevated CSF protein, cerebellar ataxia, cardiac conduction block, sensorineural hearing loss, skeletal myopathy, diabetes mellitus, and hypoparathyroidism. Progressive external ophthalmoplegia (PEA) and maternally inherited diabetes mellitus (MIDM) are syndromes that present after the age of 20 with the limited manifestations that their names describe. Pearson syndrome presents in childhood and is uniformly fatal. Its manifestations include sideroblastic anemia, progressing to pancytopenia, and pancreatic exocrine insufficiency.

MELAS

Mitochondrial encephalopathy with lactic acidosis and stroke-like episodes (MELAS) presents in childhood, often between 2-10 years of age. Initial development is normal, but this is followed by progressive neurologic deterioration. This deterioration begins with stroke-like neurologic deficits (transient hemiparesis or cortical blindness), often accompanied by seizures. Additional features are diabetes mellitus, cardiomyopathy, sensorineural hearing loss, pigmentary retinopathy, cerebellar ataxia, and lactic acidosis (causing easy fatigability). Notably, stroke-like episodes are associated with lesions on MRI that are inconsistent with a vascular distribution. The basal ganglia often show calcifications. MELAS is caused by mutations in the *MT-TL1* gene, which is located within the mitochondrial genome and encodes tRNALeu. Since a single mutation—an A to G substitution at nucleotide 3243 (A3243G)—is responsible for >80% of cases, this disease lends itself to targeted mutation analysis.

MERRF

Myoclonic epilepsy with ragged red fibers (MERRF) manifests as myoclonic seizures, cerebellar ataxia, dementia, optic atrophy, sensorineural hearing loss, skeletal myopathy, and cardiomyopathy. In some cases, there are symmetrical lipomas affecting the neck and shoulders. Like MELAS, a single mutation is responsible for >80% of cases—an A to G substitution at nucleotide 8344 (A8344G)—in the mitochondrial *MT-TK* gene which encodes tRNALys. Targeted mutation analysis for this and 2-3 other mutations can detect >90% of cases.

MNGIE

Mitochondrial neurogastrointestinal encephalomyopathy (MNGIE) is inherited as an autosomal recessive trait and is caused by nuclear DNA mutations. It presents in late childhood, adolescence, or early adulthood (average 19 years of age) and is characterized by episodes of abdominal pain accompanied by nausea, vomiting and/or diarrhea. These symptoms are the result of a functional bowel obstruction (pseudo-obstruction). In addition, there are neurologic manifestations that include progressive external ophthalmoplegia, leukodystrophy, skeletal myopathy, and peripheral neuropathy.

Leigh syndrome

Leigh syndrome presents in childhood, usually before the second birthday, initially with failure to thrive, developmental delay, hypotonia, and eventual developmental regression, external ophthalmoplegia, optic atrophy, and seizures. Death results from pneumonia or apnea. Also called subacute necrotizing encephalomyelitis, Leigh syndrome is characterized by scattered but symmetric foci of spongy degeneration and vascular proliferation, located predominantly within the cerebellum, basal ganglia, and thalamus. Leigh syndrome is genetically heterogeneous, being caused by mutations in several mitochondrial and nuclear genes.

Microdeletion disorders t7.11

t7.11 Microdeletion syndromes

Syndrome	Aberration	Manifestations
DiGeorge syndrome, Catch 22 syndrome, CHARGE sequence, velo-cardiofacial syndrome	22q11.2	Thymic aplasia/hypoplasia (immunodeficiency), parathyroid aplasia/hypoplasia (hypocalcemia, tetany), abnormal facial features, mental retardation, conotruncal cardiac anomalies
Cri du chat	5p15.2	Abnormal (cat) cry, microcephaly, mental retardation
Kallman	Xp22.3	Anosmia, hypogonadism
Prader-Willi	15q11.2 (paternal)	Hyperphagia, obesity, hypogonadism, mild mental retardation
Angelman	15q11.2 (maternal)	Hyperactivity, inappropriate laughter, aphasia, ataxia, mental retardation, seizures
Smith-Magenis syndrome	17p11.2	Moderate mental retardation, prominent forehead, flat, broad midface, self-mutilating behavior, disturbed REM sleep
Williams syndrome	7q11.23	Elfin-like facies, abnormal dentation, growth deficiency, heart malformations, infantile hypercalcemia, mental retardation
Wolf syndrome	4p deletion	Intrauterine growth retardation, heart malformations, microcephaly, cleft lip & palate, broad nasal root, severe mental retardation
Miller-Dieker syndrome	17p13	Microcephaly, type I lissencephaly, heart malformations, renal malformations, seizures, prominent forehead, vertical furrowing of brow
CHARGE sequence	22q11.2	Coloboma, heart malformations, choanal atresia, genital hypoplasia, deafness, mental retardation

Solid tumors & inherited tumor syndromes
Gastrointestinal tract tumors
Colorectal adenocarcinoma

Up to 10% of colorectal carcinomas are associated with inherited germline mutations. The genes involved in such cases are often the same genes that are mutated, on an acquired (somatic) basis, in sporadic colorectal carcinoma. In both inherited and sporadic cases, there are 2 major molecular pathways to colorectal carcinoma. The first begins with defects in the adenomatous polyposis coli (*APC*) gene, and the second begins with defects in one of the mismatch repair (*MMR*) genes.

ISBN 978-089189-5985

APC-associated sporadic & inherited tumors

Mutations involving the *APC* gene (5q) are responsible for the majority of sporadic colorectal carcinomas. The molecular sequence begins with mutations in the *APC* gene, but additional mutations are required for the development of malignancy, including mutation of (or loss of heterozygosity of) the second *APC* gene. With regard to the initial *APC* mutation, most of these occur in a region of the gene known as MCR (major cluster region), found between codons 1061 and 1309. Such mutations usually result in protein truncation. Next, a series of additional mutations occurs, nearly always including mutation of the *KRAS* gene. Additional anomalies common to tumors deriving from this pathway include mutations of *TP53* and *DCC* (deleted in colon cancer, 18q). A small minority of adenomas and colon cancers has a normal *APC* genotype and in fact has mutations in β-*catenin* which render the β-*catenin* product resistant to the action of normal APC protein.

APC functions as a tumor suppressor gene, negatively regulating the expression of genes involved in proliferation. Under normal conditions, an enterocyte may be found in the stimulated or unstimulated state; stimulation arises when a transmembrane receptor (called Frizzled protein) binds its ligand (Wnt protein). In the cytoplasm of unstimulated cells, the APC gene product binds to β-catenin, promoting the eventual degradation of β-catenin through ubiquitin-dependent proteolysis. Signaling through the frizzled receptor by the ligand Wnt leads to initiation of the Wnt (wingless-type) signaling pathway. APC undergoes a conformational change, rendering it incapable of regulating β-catenin. Increased β-catenin is translocated to the nucleus, and through interaction with the TCF protein causes increased expression of genes involved in proliferation, including *CMYC* and *BCL1*. Permanent loss of *APC* through mutation leads to unregulated proliferation by ligand-independent de-repression of β-catenin signaling.

The histologic sequence of progression starts with tubular, tubulovillous, or villous adenoma f7.32. With acquisition of additional genetic anomalies, there is progression to adenoma with high grade dysplasia and eventual carcinoma. Invasive carcinoma developing from the APC pathway, whether sporadic or inherited, has characteristic clinicopathologic features. Tumors tend to arise in the left colon, with nearly 60% of lesions presenting in the rectosigmoid colon. Due in part to the narrowness of the lumen in this segment of colon, tumors tend to grow circumferentially and present as annular "napkin-ring" lesions that may cause obstruction. Endophytic (invasive) growth is usually out of proportion to exophytic growth. The neoplastic cells are columnar and pseudostratified and form lumens with central necrosis admixed with the karyorrhectic debris of degenerating neutrophils (so-called dirty necrosis) f7.33. The advancing edge of the tumor is usually infiltrative, and peritumoral lymphocytes are not a prominent feature.

Germline mutations of the *APC* gene are associated with several tumor syndromes, the most common of which is *familial adenomatous polyposis (FAP)*. By the age of 20 most patients with FAP have formed at least 1 adenomatous polyp

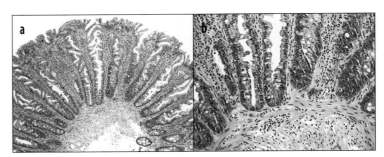

f7.32 Hyperplastic polyp; serration is luminal predominant, sparing the base of the crypts that narrow to pinpoint lumens

and, by definition, >100 adenomatous polyps by age 35. Most patients with FAP have developed invasive adenocarcinoma by the age of 50. Overall, FAP is estimated to cause ~1% of all cases of colorectal carcinoma. In addition, there is an increased incidence of gastric fundic gland polyps and small intestinal polyps (especially duodenal ampullary adenomas) with a slightly increased risk of small bowel adenocarcinoma, ampullary adenocarcinoma, thyroid cancer, and fibromatosis (desmoids). The recommended treatment for FAP is prophylactic colectomy in young adulthood.

Attenuated FAP is associated with mutations at the 5' or 3' end of the gene and is characterized by fewer polyps and a slower progression to invasive colorectal carcinoma. *Gardner syndrome* consists of the features of FAP in addition to epidermal cysts, mandibular or maxillary osteomas, deep (desmoid) fibromatoses, and congenital hypertrophy of the retinal pigmented epithelium (CHRPE). *Turcot syndrome*, the association of adenomatous polyposis and tumors of the central nervous system, may be caused either by *APC* gene mutations or *MMR* gene mutations. The CNS tumor most commonly seen in *APC*-associated Turcot syndrome is medulloblastoma. In *MMR*-associated Turcot syndrome, glioblastoma multiforme arises.

FAP and related disorders are caused by inherited germline mutations, but up to 1/3 of cases are due to sporadic germline mutations. Since the mutation is germline, it is present in all the cells of the body, so diagnosis of the syndrome can be confirmed with *APC* analysis on peripheral blood. Mutations in *APC* are not well-conserved and the gene is rather large, making confirmation by sequencing difficult. Mutation scanning approaches or in vitro protein truncation testing can be utilized to detect these mutations.

Mismatch repair-associated sporadic & inherited tumors

Mutations in mismatch repair (MMR) genes underlie ~15% of colorectal carcinomas. Acquired (somatic) aberrations account for ~95% of cases, and inherited (germline) mutations ~5%.

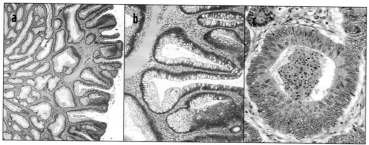

f7.33 APC pathway tumors
a & b Tubular adenoma, in which adenomatous change takes the form of luminal-predominant hyperchromatic proliferative pseudostratified enterocytes with nuclear enlargement
c Invasive adenocarcinoma consists of an infiltrative proliferation of glandular structures similarly having pseudostratified cells, with central "dirty" necrosis

The *MMR* genes encode a variety of enzymes involved in correcting errors in DNA replication, by removing single base pair mismatches and replacing the proper nucleotide. The nomenclature of MMR proteins derives from early studies involving the analogous repair process in bacteria, known as the mutator pathway. In the mutator mechanism, 2 proteins called MutS and MutL mediate the necessary repair functions. Human proteins with homology to the bacterial proteins, when discovered, were called either MutS homologs (MSH) or MutL homologs (MLH). Presently, 9 human homologs are recognized, including the MutS homologs *MSH2, MSH3, MSH4, MSH5,* and *MSH6,* and the MutL homologues *MLH1, MLH3, PMS1,* and *PMS2.* The MMR proteins work as dimers, the predominant dimers being MSH2/MSH6 and MLH1/PMS2. Unlike mutations in *APC* which play a direct role in carcinogenesis, defects in mismatch repair proteins play an indirect role by creating an environment in which the mutation rate is high; subsequent oncogenic mutations typically involve *BRAF, KRAS,* and *p16INK4a.*

Microsatellite instability (MSI) is a surrogate marker for MMR protein dysfunction and can be found in both inherited and sporadic cases. MSI is not by itself pathologic, nor is it a step in the carcinoma sequence. MSI is defined as the expansion or contraction of the normally stable microsatellite repeat sequences. By stable, what is meant is that from one cell to another within an individual, the length of the sequences is the same. The repeat nature of the microsatellites makes them prone to errors in replication. Under normal conditions these errors are repaired by the mismatch repair system. However, when there are defects in mismatch repair these repeat sequences are susceptible to instability.

As in *APC*-associated tumors, stepwise histologic progression exists in tumors associated with defects in MMR. The noninvasive precursor lesion is most often the sessile serrated adenoma **f7.33**, which is most commonly located in the right colon. Invasive tumors with MMR defects tend to present as large exophytic masses in the right colon. Histologically, they often present as mucinous (colloid) carcinomas **f7.33**. The degree of differentiation varies, from well differentiated gland-forming tumors to poorly differentiated

trabecular tumors, and some have a significant signet ring cell component. Importantly, the gland-forming MMR tumors lack central "dirty" necrosis. MMR tumors have prominent tumor-infiltrating lymphocytes (TIL) and/or a peritumoral "Crohn-like" nodular lymphoid reaction. A "pushing" rather than infiltrating tumor margin is characteristic. Because of this circumscribed appearance, a usually high nuclear grade, and infiltrating lymphocytes, the tumors have been described as medullary-like (referring to medullary breast carcinoma). Individual histologic features, as described above, predict MSI with moderate specificity and sensitivity. The most accurate morphologic predictor of MSI in several studies has been tumor-infiltrating lymphocytes (TILs).

Inherited defects in *MMR* genes cause several autosomal dominant syndromes with overlapping clinical features. Lynch syndrome is caused by germline mutations in MMR genes, with *MLH1* and *MSH2* mutations accounting for 90% of clinically recognized cases. The term hereditary nonpolyposis colorectal cancer (HNPCC) is often used interchangeably with the term Lynch syndrome but is misleading in several respects. First, it discounts the strong predisposition to noncolonic tumors, and second, ignores the existence of a precursor polyp (serrated adenoma). Lynch syndrome is an autosomal dominant condition that demonstrates incomplete penetrance. Penetrance is highest with mutations in *MLH1* or *MSH2.* Individuals with *MSH6* or *PMS2* mutations often do not fulfill the Amsterdam criteria and tend to present at an older age with mainly extracolonic tumors.

As noted previously, some cases of Turcot syndrome are associated with *MMR* gene mutations. The MMR-associated Turcot syndrome most commonly presents with glioblastoma multiforme, unlike the FAP-associated Turcot syndrome that presents with medulloblastoma. Muir-Torre syndrome is another subtype of Lynch syndrome, in which skin tumors (sebaceous tumors and keratoacanthomas) are a prominent feature.

The mechanism of *MMR* gene inactivation differs in familial and sporadic MMR tumors. Lynch syndrome is caused by germline mutations in the *MMR* coding sequence. Such mutations are seldom found in sporadic MMR tumors, in which the coding sequences in the *MMR* genes are normal in the vast majority of cases. Instead, the molecular defect in sporadic MMR tumors is hypermethylation of the promoter region of one of the *MMR* genes, leading to reduced transcription. The *MLH1* gene promoter contains CpG islands found to be heavily methylated in most sporadic MMR colon cancers. Of course, in order to cause tumorigenesis, promoter hypermethylation must affect both copies of the gene. The cause of this hypermethylation is presently unknown.

Algorithm-based testing is becoming more prominent in the workup of cases of mismatch repair. Many large institutions have turned to testing all cases of colorectal carcinoma for defects in mismatch repair in light of findings from the EGAPP group which estimated 30% of cases are missed with Amsterdam/Bethesda criteria-directed testing. In addition

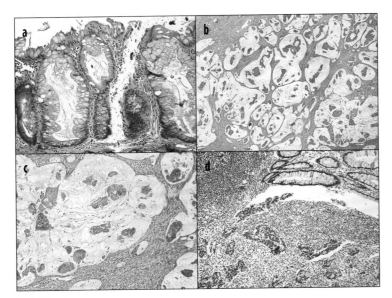

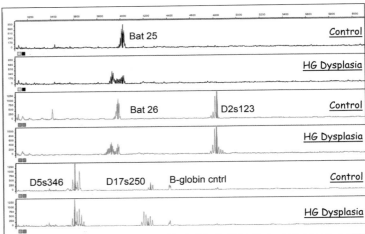

f7.35 Microsatellite instability assay in a case of high grade dysplasia
Compared with normal tissue, new stutter peaks are present in the high grade dysplasia in all 5 markers, indicating it was microsatellite unstable high; the peaks patterns in the high grade dysplasia differ from the pattern in the invasive adenocarcinoma

f7.34 MSI pathway tumors
a Serrated adenoma, in which adenomatous change takes the form of serrated proliferative enterocytes in a pattern superficially resembling hyperplastic polyp; in contrast to hyperplastic polyp, serration asymmetrically involves individual crypts & affects the bases of crypts, which are therefore ectatic at their bases
b & c Invasive adenocarcinoma often has mucinous differentiation (colloid carcinoma)
d Immunohistochemical staining for MMR proteins (in this case MSH1) shows strong nuclear expression (no loss of MMR protein), with positive internal control in both background enterocytes & lymphocytes

t7.12 MMR gene assessment by immunohistochemistry

Mutation	MLH1 (IHC)	MSH2 (IHC)	MSH6 (IHC)	PMS2 (IHC)
MLH1	−	+	+	−
MSH2	+	−	−	+
MSH6	+	+	−	+
PMS2	+	+	+	−

recent studies have shown that screening all colon cancers for Lynch syndrome is cost-effective. There are several approaches to testing. One is to perform immunohistochemical staining for the 4 most common mismatch repair proteins (MLH1, MSH2, MSH6, PMS2) on tumor tissue f7.34. Absence of staining indicates defective protein expression. Care must be utilized in the interpretation of staining. It is hypothesized that since the proteins function as heterodimers, a mutation of the dominant protein in the dimer should also be reflected as loss of staining in the partner. Presumably, there is stabilization of the protein due to its interaction with the partner protein. For example germline mutation of *MLH1* will show lack of staining for MLH1, but will also show lack of staining for PMS2 t7.12. The converse is not true—mutation of *PMS2* causes lack of staining for PMS2 but intact MLH1. In addition lack of staining for MLH1 does not necessarily imply mutation of the protein. The most common reason for MLH1 underexpression is methylation of the promoter (commonly seen in sporadic tumors with the MMR phenotype). The next step in the algorithm for cases lacking MLH1 and PMS2 staining is often testing for BRAF mutations. MLH1 mutation and BRAF mutation are almost always mutually exclusive, so that the presence of the BRAF mutation effectively eliminates inherited defects in MMR. Some also propose to test *MLH1* promoter for hypermethylation at this point as well. For cases with a high clinical suspicion of inherited MMR (such as those fulfilling clinical criteria) that fail to show defects in the MMR proteins tested by immunohistochemistry, it is recommended that MSI testing be performed.

A minimum panel of 5 markers, including 2 mononucleotide (BAT25 and BAT26) and 3 dinucleotide microsatellites has been proposed by the National Cancer Institute to be sensitive and specific for the diagnosis of microsatellite instability. DNA from tumor tissue is compared to normal tissue or peripheral blood f7.35. Instability in the tumor of ≥2 markers (or 30% of markers in an alternate panel) is classified as MSI-H (MSI-high) f7.36. If only 1 marker (or <30%) is unstable the tumor is classified as MSI-L (MSI-low). If none of the markers are unstable the tumor is classified as microsatellite stable (MSS). Since 15% of sporadic cancers are associated with MSI, the presence of MSI is not definitive for a diagnosis of Lynch syndrome. Full-gene sequencing for mutations in *MMR* genes is the definitive assay.

Full-gene sequencing is the test of choice in patients with clinical evidence of Lynch syndrome and demonstrated MSI and/or immunohistochemical evidence of defective mismatch repair proteins. Immunohistochemistry is an effective screening assay as it directs which genes should be sequenced for mutations. In addition the screening for relatives of patients with Lynch syndrome cannot be accomplished with MSI or IHC because presumably there is no tumor to test and therefore either sequencing or mutation scanning technologies should be employed.

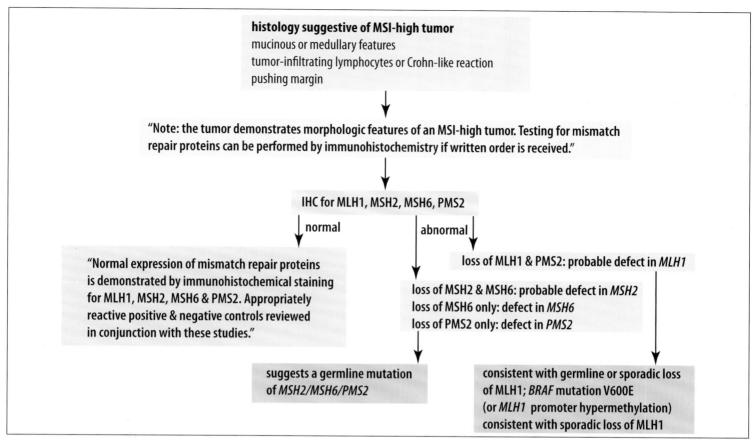

histology suggestive of MSI-high tumor
mucinous or medullary features
tumor-infiltrating lymphocytes or Crohn-like reaction
pushing margin

"Note: the tumor demonstrates morphologic features of an MSI-high tumor. Testing for mismatch repair proteins can be performed by immunohistochemistry if written order is received."

IHC for MLH1, MSH2, MSH6, PMS2

normal

abnormal

"Normal expression of mismatch repair proteins is demonstrated by immunohistochemical staining for MLH1, MSH2, MSH6 & PMS2. Appropriately reactive positive & negative controls reviewed in conjunction with these studies."

loss of MLH1 & PMS2: probable defect in *MLH1*

loss of MSH2 & MSH6: probable defect in *MSH2*
loss of MSH6 only: defect in *MSH6*
loss of PMS2 only: defect in *PMS2*

suggests a germline mutation of *MSH2/MSH6/PMS2*

consistent with germline or sporadic loss of MLH1; *BRAF* mutation V600E (or *MLH1* promoter hypermethylation) consistent with sporadic loss of MLH1

f7.36   One algorithmic option for evaluation of suspected MSI

Targeted therapy in colorectal carcinoma

Amplification of *EGFR* is known to play a role in colorectal carcinoma development. When the EGF ligand binds the EGFR at the cell surface, there is intracellular auto-phosphorylation of specific serine and threonine residues, with phosphate groups taken from ATP. This autophosphorylation leads to the productive interaction with RAS (*KRAS* gene product). The cascade of activation continues with downstream activation of RAF (*BRAF* gene product) which eventually transduces signals to the nucleus and results in the induction of specific genes.

Specific anti-EGFR agents have been used with success in the treatment of metastatic or unresectable colorectal carcinomas. There are 2 categories of agents with anti-EGFR activity. One consists of small-molecule tyrosine kinase inhibitors (gefitinib and erlotinib) whose mechanism of action involves competitive blocking of adenosine triphosphate (ATP) in the ATP binding site of the EGFR molecule. These have shown benefit in non-small cell lung cancer but have not been useful in colorectal carcinoma. The second category consists of anti-EGFR monoclonal antibodies (cetuximab; Erbitux) that inhibit EGFR by binding to its extracellular domain. Monoclonal antibody anti-EGFR agents have shown benefit in colorectal carcinoma; however, from the initial trials with these agents it became clear that there exists a subset of tumors that do not respond to anti-EGFR therapy. Subsequent investigation into the mechanism of resistance demonstrated that many of these tumors harbor specific mutations in the signaling molecules *BRAF* and *KRAS*. Specific testing is now required to determine eligibility for these agents. *KRAS* mutations of codons 12 and/or 13 are associated with poor response to anti-EGFR therapy. Similarly, the most common *BRAF* mutation, V600E, is associated with nonresponse to monoclonal antibody inhibitors.

KRAS mutations cause constitutive KRAS protein activation. Such mutations lead to EGFR-independent signaling; as a result, EGFR inhibition is not effective in tumors harboring these mutations, which are found in ~30-40% of colorectal carcinomas. To date, only wild-type *KRAS* is definitely associated with response to EGFR inhibition. The most common *KRAS* mutations occur in codons 12 or 13 of exon 2. The American Society of Clinical Oncology (ASCO) recommends that *KRAS* mutation testing be performed before initiating therapy with anti-EGFR monoclonal antibody.

Testing for *BRAF* mutations should only be pursued in tumors determined to be wild-type for *KRAS*. Mutations in *BRAF* are mutually exclusive with mutations in *KRAS*, and *BRAF* mutations are independently associated with poor prognosis and resistance to anti-EGFR antibody treatment.

Cetuximab was initially approved for patients whose tumors express EGFR by IHC (~75% of colorectal carcinoma). It was later demonstrated, however, that many EGFR-negative tumors also respond to cetuximab; therefore, EGFR testing is no longer required.

Targeted therapy in gastric & gastroesophageal junction cancer

Recently, there has been renewed hope in the treatment of advanced gastric cancer, on the basis of Her2/Neu inhibition with trastuzumab (Herceptin). Like its cousin EGFR, the HER2 protein is a cell surface receptor that, when it binds ligand, initiates an intracellular cascade that proceeds through RAS, RAF, and MAPK. Like breast cancer, ~20% of gastric cancers and 30% of gastroesophageal junction tumors overexpresses HER2. In patients studied in the ToGA trial the addition of trastuzumab, compared to chemotherapy alone, resulted in significantly improved survival. Unlike breast cancer, however, HER2 overexpression by either FISH or IHC is evidence of likely response. Thus, many laboratories test with one modality or the other initially, followed by the second modality if results are negative.

IHC for *HER2* in gastric cancer is interpreted somewhat differently as well. First, criteria differ between small biopsy specimens and resection specimens. Second, instead of the circumferential membranous staining observed in breast cancer, basolateral membranous staining is typical of gastric cancer, with no staining along the apical (luminal) border. In gastric cancer, a grade of 1+ is achieved if 10% of tumor cells stain. The distinction between 1+, 2+, and 3+ depends upon the intensity of staining t7.13. Lastly, Her2 expression in gastric cancer is patchy; and in small biopsy specimens grading is assessed according to tumor cell clusters, defined as a group of ≥5 tumor cells.

t7.13 Grading of Her2 in gastric cancer

Grade	Small biopsy specimen	Resection specimen
0+ (Negative)	No expression	Expression in <10% of tumor cells
1+ (Negative)	Any tumor cell cluster (≥5 cells) with faint or barely perceptible staining	Faint or barely perceptible staining in ≥10% of tumor cells in any part of the membrane
2+ (Equivocal)	Any tumor cell cluster with weak to moderate basolateral or lateral membranous staining	Weak to moderate staining in ≥10% of tumor cells in basolateral or lateral membranes
3+ (Positive)	Any tumor cell cluster with strong basolateral or lateral membranous staining	Strong complete staining in ≥10% of tumor cells in basolateral or lateral membranes

Other gastrointestinal tract tumor syndromes

Juvenile polyposis is an autosomal dominant condition associated with a moderately increased risk of colorectal cancer, but its foremost expression is the juvenile polyp. These are found in the stomach, small intestine, and large intestine. The juvenile polyp is a particular histologic type of polyp with a smooth outer contour, cystically dilated mucus-filled glands lined by nonadenomatous enterocytes, and a dense collagenous stroma permeated by inflammatory cells. Most affected individuals have some polyps by the age of 20, but the number of polyps developed over a lifetime is highly variable, ranging from 1 to >100. The lifetime risk of malignancy ranges from 9-50%, and most of these are colorectal adenocarcinomas. Several potential genes have mutations that are implicated in juvenile polyposis, including *BMPR1A* and *SMAD4*.

Peutz-Jeghers syndrome (PJS) is an autosomal dominant condition that presents with mucocutaneous pigmentation and hamartomatous intestinal polyps. There is a significantly

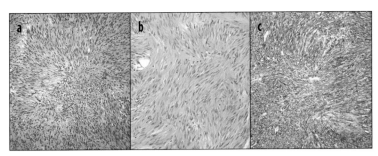

f7.37 Gastrointestinal stromal tumor (GIST)
a & b The tumors have a variety of appearances, ranging from myoid to neuroid to epithelioid
c Strong & diffuse expression of CKIT (CD117)

increased risk for malignancy, including a 120 fold increased risk of pancreatic cancer. Rare tumors that are unique to Peutz-Jeghers syndrome include the sex cord tumor with annular tubules (SCTAT) of the ovary, adenoma malignum (minimal deviation adenocarcinoma) of the cervix, and the calcifying Sertoli cell tumor of the testis. There is a high incidence of nasal polyposis in some patients with PJS; PJS and cystic fibrosis should be considered in pediatric patients presenting with nasal polyps. Intestinal hamartomatous polyps arise most commonly in the small intestine, but can also be found in the stomach and large intestine. They begin to appear around the age of 10 years. Lined by mucinous epithelium, the distinguishing feature of the Peutz-Jeghers polyp is stroma built of thin complexly branching muscle bundles with an arborizing appearance. Up to 75% of cases are due to mutations in the gene *STK11/LKB1* on chromosome 19p.

Hereditary diffuse gastric cancer is associated with the development of diffuse (signet ring) gastric adenocarcinoma at a young age. E-cadherin, a protein involved in cell to cell adhesion, is encoded by the *CDH1* gene found on 16q. Germline mutations in the *CDH1* gene are the cause of hereditary diffuse gastric cancer. Interestingly, decreased expression of E-cadherin by immunohistochemistry is noted in diffuse gastric cancer, whether inherited or sporadic.

Gastrointestinal stromal tumor (GIST)

GIST is the most common mesenchymal neoplasm of the GI tract. The cell of origin is the interstitial cell of Cajal, a specialized mesenchymal cell with dual myoid and neural differentiation. GIST may occur anywhere in the GI tract but is most commonly found in the stomach, where it presents as a mural-based submucosal nodule. The morphology ranges from spindled, in which either myoid or neural differentiation may predominate, to epithelioid f7.37. Every GIST has metastatic potential, and the behavior of any individual GIST is best predicted according to size and mitotic rate.

The concept of GIST has evolved over the past several decades. Until recently, such tumors were classified as leiomyomas or, occasionally, as nerve sheath tumors, depending upon the predominant differentiation noted immunohistochemically and ultrastructurally. The unifying term "stromal tumor" was introduced in 1983 by Mazur and Clark and was buttressed by the finding that all such tumors, whether predominantly myoid or predominantly neural, express CD34. CD34 became the defining marker of GIST for a time until activating mutations and overexpression of *KIT* were noted. Since that time, KIT (c-kit) immunohistochemistry has become the key diagnostic test for such tumors, and pharmacologic therapy targeted to KIT has become the mainstay of therapy. Most GISTs show strong and diffuse cytoplasmic staining. Many also demonstrate paranuclear dot-like (Golgi-pattern) staining, and a small number have only dot-like staining. GISTs that are KIT-weak or KIT-negative (up to 5% of GISTs) are likely to harbor *PDGFRA* mutations, but PDGFRA immunohistochemistry is unreliable. Rare adult GISTs and most pediatric GISTs are negative for both KIT and PDGFRA.

While mutation analysis for *CKIT* or *PDGFRA* mutations is generally not needed to confirm the diagnosis or predict the biologic behavior, mutation analysis can be helpful in the prediction of response to tyrosine kinase inhibitors. GISTs are most often associated with a gain of function mutation in *KIT* exon 11, a mutation type that is highly associated (up to 85%) with imatinib response. Mutations in exons 9, 13, and 17 are somewhat less likely (40-50%) to be imatinib sensitive. Tumors with no *KIT* mutation (wild-type) may be imatinib sensitive in up to 30% of cases. Mutations in *PGFRA* are most commonly found in exons 18, 12 and 14. The most common *PDGFRA* mutation (D842V) is completely insensitive to imatinib, while others may be responsive.

GIST may be a feature of Carney triad (GIST, pulmonary chondromas, extra-adrenal paragangliomas) and neurofibromatosis, type 1 (NF1). In addition, inherited germline mutations in *KIT* have been identified in familial GIST syndrome. Patients with NF1 may have multiple GISTs in the small intestine that are notable for KIT overexpression despite unmutated *KIT* and *PDGFRA* genes.

Pancreatic tumors
Ductal adenocarcinoma
Risk to individuals whose first-degree relative has pancreatic ductal adenocarcinoma is double that of the general population. The risk increases exponentially when there is >1 affected first-degree relative. Several syndromic predispositions to pancreatic cancer are known. Of them the one with the greatest risk to develop pancreatic cancer is Peutz-Jeghers syndrome (PJS) where the risk is >100-fold greater than that of the general population. PJS is an autosomal dominant condition caused by mutations in the gene *STK11/LKB1* on chromosome 19. Pancreatic involvement may present with precursor lesions, such as intraductal papillary mucinous neoplasm (IPMN), or with fully developed invasive adenocarcinoma. The familial atypical mole melanoma syndrome (FAMM syndrome) is an autosomal dominant condition associated with a 50-fold increased risk for pancreatic adenocarcinoma. Germline mutations in the *P16/CDKN2A* gene are responsible for FAMM. Hereditary pancreatitis, due to mutations in either *PRSS1* or *SPINK1* is an autosomal dominant condition with a 50-fold increased risk of developing pancreatic adenocarcinoma. Patients typically present with a history of multiple bouts of pancreatitis beginning at an early age. Familial adenomatous polyposis (FAP), hereditary breast and ovarian cancer syndrome (*BRCA2* mutations), ataxia telangiectasia, and Lynch syndrome are all associated with increased risk of pancreatic cancer, ranging from 2 to 10-fold.

Whether sporadic or inherited, pancreatic ductal adenocarcinoma arises through progression of nonneoplastic epithelium through dysplasia, in situ carcinoma, and eventual invasive carcinoma, in parallel with conserved genetic changes. The vast majority of pancreatic ductal adenocarcinomas (95%) contain a *KRAS* mutation, usually point mutations in codons 12 and 13, which is considered to be an early promoter of carcinogenesis. Such mutations are present in a large proportion of pancreatic intraepithelial neoplastic (PanIN) lesions. Subsequent to activating *KRAS* mutations, many tumors develop inactivating mutations in tumor suppressors, such as *P16/CDKN2A* (also present in 95% of tumors) and *TP53* (present in up to 75% of tumors). Roughly parallel to the development of inactivating mutations in tumor suppressor genes, pancreatic tumors tend to also have abnormal telomerase activity and telomere shortening. As intraepithelial neoplasia progresses to higher-grade lesions, >1/2 contain mutations of *SMAD4*. Aberrant methylation is observed in the majority of pancreatic tumors, associated with increased expression of genes encoding DNA methyltransferase enzymes. In pancreatic cancer (and many other cancers) increased methylation of the regulatory regions (CpG islands) near tumor suppressors leads to decreased expression. Many of the tumor suppressors mutated in pancreatic cancer (p16, p53, SMAD4) also have demonstrated increased methylation of the regulatory CpG islands. Contemporaneous hypomethylation and upregulation of protooncogenes, such as *SOCS1*, an inhibitor of JAK/STAT signaling, is observed in high grade lesions. Lastly, there is altered miRNA expression pattern, as is seen in a variety of cancers. Gene regulation through miRNAs can take many forms including direct control of mRNA translation into protein. In pancreatic cancer specifically, miR-21 and miR-155 have been shown to be abnormally expressed in precursor PanIN lesions.

Neuroendocrine tumors (islet cell tumors)
Multiple endocrine neoplasia 1 (MEN1) is caused by mutations in the *MEN1* gene on chromosome 11q13, which encodes the tumor suppressor menin. Patients with MEN1 are at risk for the development of multiple endocrine tumors, usually of the pituitary, parathyroid, and pancreas. Other syndromes associated with an increased risk for the development of pancreatic endocrine tumors include neurofibromatosis 1 (NF1), von Hippel-Lindau syndrome, and tuberous sclerosis.

Hepatobiliary tumors
Hepatocellular carcinoma (HCC)
HCC is predominantly associated with environmental exposures, most commonly chronic viral infection (HBV, HCV). Risk factors for sporadic HCC, in addition to chronic viral hepatitis, include aflatoxin consumption in food and exposure to thorotrast, cycasin, pyrrolizidine alkaloids, and vinyl chloride. A variety of inherited conditions cause increased susceptibility to HCC. These include hereditary hemochromatosis, tyrosinemia, glycogen storage disease (types 1 and 2), α_1-antitrypsin deficiency, Wilson disease, porphyria cutanea tarda, and galactosemia.

Whether provoked by inherited or environmental influences, most HCC arises within a background of cirrhosis. Cirrhotic nodules are formed from the propagation of individual hepatocytes, and the cirrhotic liver is the site of intense hepatocytic proliferative activity. Intense proliferation provides an opportunity for errors in DNA replication, particularly within the background of oxidative stress that is common to many of the underlying disorders. The acquisition of mutations within regenerative nodules gives rise to dysplastic nodules, the precursor of hepatocellular carcinoma.

The molecular events underlying HCC are incredibly complex and differ significantly from one case to the next. For example, HBV induced HCC is strongly associated with *TP53* alterations, but these are present in only a minority of non-HBV tumors. Furthermore, HBV-driven tumors quite often have portions of the HBV genome incorporated into the host cell genome, but this is not seen in HCV-driven tumors. Expression of the HBV gene *HBX* leads to suppression of the p53 protein. In all, dozens of genetic alterations have been described in HCC, and subsets of these are found together in individual cases. Nascent efforts to sub-classify HCC on the basis of the molecular substrate are under way.

The approach to treatment of HCC has traditionally relied upon surgical resection, when feasible, and locoregional ablation. Sorafenib, a tyrosine kinase inhibitor (TKI), was the first molecular targeted therapy to be approved for the systemic treatment of HCC. Unlike most TKI therapy, sorafenib is not targeted at the neoplastic hepatocytes; instead, its target is the endothelial cells involved in angiogenesis.

Cholangiocarcinoma

Risk factors for both intrahepatic and extrahepatic cholangiocarcinoma include infection with liver fluke (*Clonorchis sinensis*, *Opisthorchis viverrinii*), primary sclerosing cholangitis, Caroli disease, choledochal cysts, thorotrast exposure, and a variety of genetic polymorphisms. Risk factors mainly for intrahepatic cholangiocarcinoma include hepatolithiasis, HCV and HBV infection, and hepatic schistosomiasis. Risk factors for extrahepatic cholangiocarcinoma include duct obstruction (choledocholithiasis), and obesity.

Virtually 100% of cholangiocarcinomas harbor telomerase abnormalities. Mutations in many of the same genes involved with the development of HCC can also be seen in cholangiocarcinoma including WNT pathway factors, p53, and p16, with similar patterns of epigenetic inhibition. Mutations in *EGFR* have been found in a minority (~10%) of cases of cholangiocarcinoma and <5% of hepatocellular carcinoma cases. Targeted small molecule inhibitor therapy, similar to lung adenocarcinoma harboring amenable *EGFR* mutations of EGFR-mutant cholangiocarcinoma has shown some early success.

Breast cancer

HER2 (Neu, ERB-B2)

The HER2 receptor is a member of the epidermal growth factor receptor (EGFR) family. About 20% of breast cancers exhibit overexpression of the HER2 receptor, usually through a mechanism of gene amplification. Amplification of *HER2* is associated with high nuclear grade, increased mortality rate, and increased rate of recurrence; however, the addition of anti-Her2 (trastuzumab) to adriamycin based chemotherapy mitigates these aggressive features.

With regard to the correlation of histology with Her2 status, a few generalizations can be made. As noted, Her2+ tumors tend to have a higher nuclear grade; grade 1 tumors are rarely Her2+, and the vast majority of Her2+ tumors have a grade of 3.

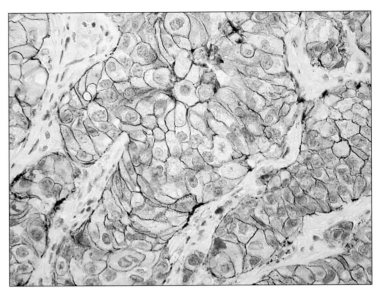

f7.38 Her2 by immunohistochemistry, showing circumferential membranous staining

Furthermore, Her2 overexpression is seen almost exclusively in invasive ductal carcinoma of the usual type. Her2 is rarely overexpressed in ductal carcinoma variants such as mucinous (colloid) and tubular carcinoma, and within the spectrum of lobular carcinoma is seen mainly in pleomorphic variants, if at all.

Much hinges upon the result of Her2 testing. Therapeutic benefits can be great; however, a course of therapy is extremely expensive, and there is a risk of serious cardiotoxicity. As with all tests, the pathologist must ensure the validity of the result through meticulous control of the conditions under which the test is performed and interpreted. At the very least, one should participate in interlaboratory proficiency testing and conform to guidelines published jointly by the American Society of Clinical Oncologists (ASCO) and the College of American Pathologists (CAP).

In assessing Her2 expression by IHC, only circumferential membranous staining f7.38 is considered. Expression is usually reported as 0-3+, depending upon the proportion of cells displaying strong circumferential membranous staining. Scores of 0 and 1+ are considered negative, 3+ is positive, and 2+ is equivocal. A 3+ result is defined as strong circumferential staining in >30% of tumor cells. An equivocal result (2+) is defined as complete circumferential membrane staining, that is either nonuniform or weak, in >10% of tumor cells. Occasionally, a 2+ result can be due to strong membranous staining in >10% but <30% of tumor cells. 1+ is defined as weak incomplete (noncircumferential) staining in any proportion of tumor cells. Strong (3+) IHC staining is closely associated with amplification of HER2. Equivocal staining (2+) is associated with HER2 amplification ~25% of the time, and such results are an indication for FISH testing. Negative (0+) or very weak (1+) staining is very infrequently associated with HER2 amplification.

HER2 amplification by FISH is determined by calculating the ratio of signals from HER2 (located on chromosome 17) to a chromosome enumeration probe (CEP) for chromosome 17 f7.39. Amplification is defined as a ratio >2.2; a negative result

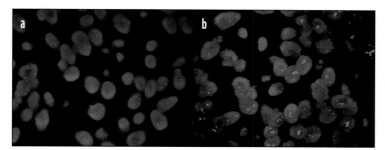

f7.39 Her2 by fluorescence in situ hybridization (FISH)
a The ratio of Her2 signals (red) & chromosome 17 signals (green) is 1.0; no amplification is present
b Large clusters of Her2 signals (red) are present in this case with Her2 amplification

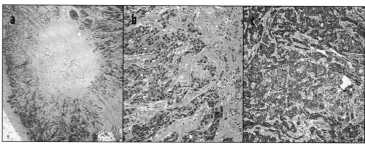

f7.40 Basal-like invasive breast carcinoma
a Low magnification view shows a somewhat circumscribed tumor with central collagenous scarlike zone
b Intermediate magnification shows that the tumor is composed of high grade epithelial cells arranged in somewhat syncytial trabecular groups
c Strong & diffuse expression of CK5/6

is a ratio <1.8. Equivocal FISH results (ratio between 1.8 and 2.2) should be repeated or more cells counted. If repeatedly equivocal FISH results are obtained, IHC should be considered (if not already done).

TP53 tumor suppressor gene

The *TP53* gene (17p) encodes the transcription factor p53. It is the normal function of p53 to bind to several specific DNA sequences and enhance their transcription. The genes it normally enhances—such as those which promote apoptosis and others which inhibit entry into the cell cycle—work in concert to control cell division. Clinically significant *TP53* mutations usually affect the DNA binding domain and result in loss of specificity of p53 protein; thus, this effective promoter of transcription becomes less inclined to promote its usual targets and becomes free to activate other genes.

Mutated *TP53* encodes a p53 protein that is resistant to degradation (so-called TP53 stabilized mutant protein); thus *TP53* mutations, though associated with decreased p53 functional activity, are associated with increased p53 immunohistochemical (IHC) staining.

In breast cancer, *TP53* mutations correlate with tumor aggressiveness, higher tumor grade, and lower rates of ER/PR expression. There is some evidence that *TP53* mutation may reduce the efficacy of chemotherapeutic agents whose mechanism of action involves the induction of apoptosis; eg, adriamycin, 5-fluorouracil (5-FU).

Steroid receptors

The steroid receptors ER and PR, like all steroid receptors, reside within the nucleus and, when bound to steroid hormone, activate transcription of specific genes. There is an α form and a β form for both ER and PR. In the case of ER, these are encoded by separate largely homologous genes. In contrast, PRα and PRβ are encoded by the same gene, one with more 3′ (amino-terminal) material than the other. In routine immunohistochemical assays for ER, only ERα is measured; whereas the PR assay measures both PRα and PRβ.

A clinical response to hormonal therapy (tamoxifen, aromatase inhibitors, or LHRH agonists) is largely, but not entirely, dependent upon the expression of steroid hormone receptors. In fact, ~70% of tumors expressing both ER and PR will respond to hormonal therapy, and only ~5% of tumors negative for ER and PR will respond. ER+, PR– tumors respond at roughly the same rate as those positive for both; however, ER–, PR+ tumors respond in only ~15% of cases.

BRCA-associated tumors

~1/2 of familial breast cancer is caused by inherited defects in one of the *BRCA* genes. In most of the remaining familial cases, no defined genetic defect has been identified.

There are 2 *BRCA* genes, *BRCA1* located on chromosome 17q21, and *BRCA2* on chromosome 13q12-13. Each encodes a tumor suppressor protein. Each of the genes is large, with thousands of described mutations, making mutation detection difficult. *BRCA* mutations are especially prevalent in the Ashkenazi Jewish population. A quarter of Ashkenazi women with breast cancer harbor *BRCA* mutations. Within this population, mutation detection is facilitated by a small number of founder mutations that account for 90% of all cases: 185delAG mutation in *BRCA1*, 5385insC mutation in *BRCA1*, and 6174delT mutation of *BRCA2*.

A mutated *BRCA* gene (*BRCA1* or *BRCA2*) is expressed in an autosomal dominant fashion, with high penetrance. In families harboring germline *BRCA* gene mutations, there are often 2 or more generations of women with premenopausal breast cancer, sometimes arising bilaterally. In addition, there is an increased risk of neoplasms of the ovary, fallopian tube, colon, uterus, and pancreas. In particular, the *BRCA2* 6174delT mutation is strongly associated with familial pancreatic cancer. In families with *BRCA2* mutations, there is a high rate of prostate cancer. *BRCA* mutations increase the lifetime risk of breast cancer to 80%, compared to the 10% risk seen in the general population. Such mutations increase the risk of ovarian cancer to 50%, especially *BRCA1* mutations. The lifetime risk of breast cancer in a male who carries a *BRCA* mutation is ~6%; *BRCA2* carries a higher male breast cancer risk than does *BRCA1*.

About 5% of all women with breast cancer and 25% of Ashkenazi Jewish women with breast cancer have a germline *BRCA* mutation. Additionally, in a woman with breast cancer who is found to harbor a *BRCA* mutation, the risk of cancer developing in the contralateral breast is 25%. *BRCA*-associated breast cancers often have distinctive though not entirely specific histologic features. The tumors tend to have a high nuclear grade, a central acellular scar-like zone, pushing rather than infiltrating margins, and tumor-infiltrating lymphocytes (medullary carcinoma-like histology) **f7.40**. They are most negative for ER, PR, and HER2 (triple-negative), negative for luminal cytokeratins (CK8/18), and positive for basal cell markers (CK5/6). This constellation of findings has been described as the basal-like phenotype. While typical of *BRCA*-associated tumors, basal-like carcinoma is frequently seen sporadically.

Other inherited influences upon breast cancer

Germline mutations in *P53* (Li-Fraumeni syndrome), *PTEN* (Cowden syndrome), *CDH1* (hereditary diffuse gastric cancer syndrome), and *STK11* (Peutz-Jeghers syndrome) are associated with an increased risk of breast cancer.

Molecular classification of breast carcinoma (gene expression profiling)

It has long been acknowledged that certain histologic subtypes of breast cancer demonstrate particular clinical courses, while some seemingly histologically disparate tumors behave similarly. In addition it is known that the benefit of adjuvant chemotherapy is variable between patients. Classification of breast carcinomas by gene expression patterns and the utilization of gene expression panels to make clinical decisions have gained support as a means to better characterize tumors and better predict their behavior. Some of the first work was done with predictive quantitative multigene panels. In an effort to stratify patients who would derive the most benefit from adjuvant hormone therapy, panels of genes including proliferation markers, hormone receptors and some downstream targets of hormone receptors, and genes associated with metastatic disease among others were constructed. Given the quantitative basis the results are given as a quantitative "score." Patients with certain test values are predicted to derive the most benefit from hormone therapy while others less so. Since the initial description of this test many others with similar testing strategies have evolved with likely more in the future. The design of markers to determine whether any individual tumor will respond to a particular chemotherapeutic regimen, such as the quantitative multigene assays previously described, is a form of supervised (directed) classification. If a large panel of expressed genes is grouped according to their expression patterns (eg, upregulated, downregulated), this is referred to as unsupervised classification.

Unsupervised classification of gene expression by mathematical tools such as hierarchical clustering allows patterns to evolve and groups to form based on shared molecular expression features. Surprisingly, once tumors are grouped into clusters the gene expression patterns within these groups is fairly consistent. In addition the expression pattern of most genes is consistent between groups. There are, however, genes that can be used to distinguish certain groups with high reproducibility. The most basic groups based on hierarchical clustering are

1. luminal—expressing low molecular-weight cytokeratins (CK8/18), harboring a favorable outcome, and most often associated with ER positivity

2. basal-like—expressing high molecular-weight cytokeratins (CK5/17 or 5/6), having a poor prognosis, often ER– and high nuclear grade, but sensitive to chemotherapy

3. HER2+—also associated with a poor prognosis and sensitivity to chemotherapy, almost always associated with amplified HER2

It is clear depending on the nature of the clustering that some of these groups may have subgroups (luminal-A, luminal-B, luminal-C) but the significance of these subgroups is unclear in relationship to the parent group. Note also that "basal-like" and "triple-negative" are not synonymous terms. While most basal-like tumors are in fact triple-negative, a wide variety of triple-negative tumors do not have basal-like features.

Predictive panels to determine response to chemotherapy also promise to improve response to particular agents. By testing tumors for genes that are associated with response to individual agents, such as tamoxifen or one of the taxols it can be predicted whether a patient may respond and a tailored chemotherapeutic regimen can be designed. A further challenge is to combine the results of prognostic and predictive panels to determine whether a patient with a certain molecular expression group responds to a particular chemotherapeutic reagent.

Much is still unknown, particularly about how robust molecular classification will be, but the promise exists for tailoring therapeutic options and prognosis based on gene expression patterns. Of note, it has recently been demonstrated that a combination of morphology and immunohistochemical analysis can be used to derive results comparable to those obtained by gene expression profiling t7.14.

t7.14 Breast cancer subtyping by morphology & IHC

Subtype	Morphology	ER, PR, Her2	Other IHC	Notes
Luminal A	Low grade ductal, NOS	ER+, PR±, Her2–	Low Ki67 CK8/18+	Sensitive to endocrine therapy, variable response to chemotherapy, overall good prognosis
Luminal B	High grade ductal, NOS	ER+, PR±, Her2+	Mod to high Ki67 CK8/18+	Tend to be sensitive to endocrine therapy, variable response to chemotherapy, more aggressive than luminal A
Her2+		ER–, PR–, Her2+	High Ki67	Sensitive to trastuzumab
Basal-like		Triple negative	High Ki67 CK5/6+, P63+	Resistant to everything, require aggressive chemotherapy BRCA1-related
Triple-negative		Triple negative		

Genitourinary tumors

Renal cell carcinoma syndromes

Von Hippel-Lindau syndrome (VHL syndrome) is an autosomal dominant condition causing predisposition to a variety of tumors, including clear cell renal cell carcinoma, hemangioblastoma of the central nervous system (cerebellum, retina, or spinal cord), pheochromocytoma, pancreatic islet cell tumors and cysts, cystadenomas of the epididymis or broad ligament, and the papillary tumor of endolymphatic sac origin. Germline mutations in the gene *VHL* located on chromosome 3p25-26 account for the majority of cases. Alteration of 3p is extremely common in sporadic clear cell renal cell carcinoma. A form of the syndrome having all the usual features except pheochromocytoma is known as type 1 VHL. It is associated with nonproduction of the VHL gene product, resulting from gene deletion or missense mutation. Forms of the syndrome with a high risk of pheochromocytoma are known as type 2 VHL, and these are associated with missense mutations. The *VHL* gene product is a part of a ubiquitin-dependent complex that is responsible for the degradation of the hypoxia inducible factor (HIF-1). Increased HIF-1 leads to increased angiogenesis and promotion of tumor growth.

Birt-Hogg-Dubé syndrome is an autosomal dominant condition predisposing to renal cell carcinoma. Skin lesions and spontaneous pneumothorax complete the diagnostic triad. Skin manifestations include multiple fibrofolliculomas, trichodiscomas, and acrochordons, especially affecting the head, neck, and upper trunk. The lung contains numerous cystic parenchymal spaces in addition to blebs and bullae, causing recurrent spontaneous pneumothorax. The spontaneous pneumothoraces tend to involve the lower lobes of the lung, unlike most other conditions that predispose to pneumothorax (α_1 antitrypsin deficiency, lymphangiomyomatosis, Langerhans cell histiocytosis, Ehlers-Danlos syndrome, Marfan syndrome). The renal tumors tend to be bilateral and multifocal and have features of a combined chromophobe renal cell carcinoma and oncocytoma f7.41. Mutations of the *BHD* (*FLCN*) gene on chromosome 17p11.2 encoding the protein folliculin are responsible for the syndrome.

Familial clear cell renal cell carcinoma is associated with mutations of 3p and lacks the other features of the VHL syndrome. A hereditary form of papillary renal cell carcinoma is associated with bilateral papillary renal cell carcinomas and gain of function mutations of the protooncogene *C-MET* on chromosome 7q31. *C-MET* functions in a manner similar to C-KIT, with mutation resulting in a constitutively activated tyrosine kinase. Tuberous sclerosis is associated with increased incidence of renal cell carcinoma, but is much more commonly associated with the renal angiomyolipoma.

Sporadic renal cell carcinoma

The most common type of renal cell carcinoma t7.15 is conventional clear cell carcinoma. Portions of the short arm of chromosome 3 are deleted in most cases. 3 particular loci are disproportionately affected: 3p14, 3p25.3 (the location of the *VHL* gene), and 3p21.3. Only a small percentage of cases have 3p anomalies as the sole abnormality; most tumors start with 3p mutations and collect additional ones, commonly in 14q, 9p, 8p, and 6q. Furthermore, del(3p) by itself has no impact

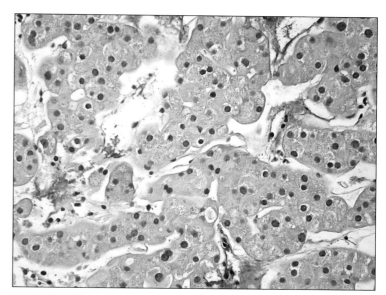

f7.41 Birt-Hogg-Dubé syndrome-associated renal tumor

upon prognosis, while loss of 14q, 9p, and 8p each correlates with higher stage and a worse prognosis.

Papillary renal cell carcinoma accounts for ~15% of renal cell carcinomas. Like many of the nonclear variants, the gross appearance is that of a uniform brown tumor. Papillary renal cell carcinoma is often multifocal. There are 2 histologic subtypes—type 1, characterized by bland cuboidal cells on tubular or papillary formations, and type 2, which has larger pseudostratified cells lining papillary cores. The vascular cores in each tend to have foamy interstitial macrophages. Type 2 papillary RCC is more often associated with multiple chromosomal anomalies, but both can be associated with loss of the Y chromosome and gains of chromosomes 7 and 17 (similar to urothelial carcinoma). These chromosomal abnormalities help differentiate papillary RCC from the histologically similar mucinous tubular and spindle cell carcinoma of the kidney.

t7.15 2004 WHO classification of renal tumors (modified)

Tumor	Immunophenotype	Genetic anomalies	Behavior
Clear cell renal cell carcinoma	CD10+, vimentin+, RCC Ag+	del(3p)	Aggressive
Papillary renal cell carcinoma	CD10+, vimentin+, AMACR+, CK7+	Loss of Y, gains of 7 & 17	Indolent
Chromophobe renal cell carcinoma	CD10−/+, vimentin−, CD117+, CK7+	Loss of Y, 1, 2, 6, 10, 13, 17 & 21	Indolent
Collecting (Bellini) duct carcinoma	CD10−, vimentin−, high MW keratin+	del(1q)	Aggressive
Renal medullary carcinoma	CD10−, vimentin−, CEA+	Unknown	Aggressive
Xp11.2 translocation carcinoma	TFE3+ (nuclear) CD10+	Xp11.2 translocation	Indolent
Oncocytoma	CD10−/+, vimentin±, CK7 rare focal +, CD117+	Highly variable: loss of 1, 14. t(5;11)	Benign
Mucinous, tubular & spindle cell carcinoma	CD10−, vimentin+	Loss of 1, 4, 6, 8, 13, 14	Indolent
Angiomyolipoma	HMB45+	LOH at *TSC2* on 16p	Benign

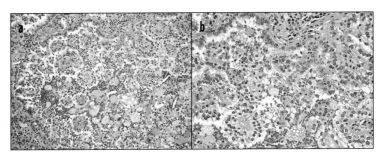

f7.42 Renal carcinoma with Xp11.2 translocation

Chromophobe RCC has clear to microvacuolated cytoplasm and distinct "plant cell" borders. Hale colloidal iron and CD7 preferentially stain chromophobe RCC and help to distinguish it from oncocytoma. CD117 helps to distinguish it from clear cell RCC. Most chromophobe RCCs are hypodiploid with common losses of multiple chromosomes including Y, 1, 2, 6, 10, 13, 17, and 21.

Renal carcinoma with Xp11.2 translocation most commonly affects children and young adults. The tumor has a distinctive appearance with alveolar (nested) and papillary architecture, clear cells, and psammoma bodies f7.42. Based upon the foregoing, therefore, TFE3-associated carcinoma should be thought of whenever

1. a diagnosis of a RCC with a mixed histologic pattern is entertained

2. any RCC is seen in a child

The tumor is characteristically negative for EMA (a marker uniformly positive in conventional clear cell carcinoma) but positive for CD10. Translocations of the transferrin receptor *TFE3* gene is responsible for the disease. Several Xp11.2 abnormalities have been described in connection with these tumors, including t(X;1)(p11.2;q21), producing the *TFE3-PRCC* fusion gene, t(X;17)(p11.2;q25), producing *TFE3-ASPL*, and t(X;1)(p11.2;p34), producing *TFE3-PSF*. The *TFE3-ASPL* gene fusion of t(X;17) is also seen in alveolar soft part sarcoma (ASPS); however, a key difference is that the translocation in ASPS is an unbalanced one, while that in renal carcinoma is balanced. The *TFE-ASPL* renal tumors characteristically present at advanced stage but, like ASPS, follow an indolent course marked by very late relapses/metastases. Renal cell carcinomas with t(6;11)(p11.2;q12) involves the *TFEB* gene which is closely related in function to the *TFE3* gene. The resulting tumor is essentially identical to Xp11.2 tumors.

Wilms tumor

Nephroblastoma or Wilms tumor is most often caused by a mutation in the *WT1* gene on chromosome 11p13. Wilms tumor is a feature of WAGR syndrome, which is caused by a microdeletion that involves the *WT1* gene and adjacent *PAX6* gene. Loss of *PAX6* is associated with the aniridia of WAGR syndrome.

Prostate cancer

When studied by conventional cytogenetics, most prostatic adenocarcinomas have a normal karyotype. However, numerous small abnormalities are demonstrable by FISH or comparative genomic hybridization (CGH), the most common of which is loss of 8p. More recently, a recurrent translocation t(4;6)(q22;q15) has been demonstrated. Found in ~10% of cases, this translocation creates the fusion transcript *TMPRSS2:ERG*, and is associated with high stage at presentation, high tumor volume, and high baseline PSA levels. Several oncogenes are overexpressed in prostatic adenocarcinoma, *MYC* and *BCL2* especially, and many cases demonstrate mutations in *PTEN*, *GSTP1*, and *P53*.

Some genes overexpressed in carcinoma have been exploited for diagnostic purposes. The prostate cancer 3 (*PCA3*) gene encodes a nontranslated transcript called DDT3 that is excreted in urine. The DDT3 transcript is elevated in >95% of prostate cancers (by 66-fold on average). The gene encoding PSA, *KLK3*, is not overexpressed (increased PSA in cancer is probably caused by increased release of the protein into the extracellular matrix). Using quantitative reverse transcriptase PCR, the quantity of the PCA3 transcript can be measured and compared to the urine PSA (to correct for the number of prostatic cells obtained).

About 5% of cases are associated with a strong family history. The proportion may be as high as 40% in cases diagnosed before age 55. Presently, most cases are thought to be linked to the *RNASEL* gene (encoding ribonuclease L). Additionally, families with germline mutations of the *BRCA1* or *BRCA2* genes have a higher rate of prostatic adenocarcinoma.

From a practical standpoint, specimen identity testing is occasionally required in the practice of prostate pathology and other types of biopsy pathology. Specimen identity testing refers to the use of molecular techniques to ensure that a specimen belongs to a particular patient. Most pathologists are familiar with the uniquely alarming circumstance in which cancer cannot be found in a prostatectomy after a positive biopsy. Often the issue can be resolved with thorough sectioning, but there are rare cases in which even after exhaustive efforts one is left with the predicament of an unequivocally positive biopsy and a negative prostate gland. In 1995, Goldstein referred to this situation as the "vanishing cancer" phenomenon. While there are a number of possible explanations, one that must occasionally be entertained is a specimen mix-up. One approach to this problem is the comparison of DNA microsatellites, either between biopsy and patient or between biopsy and prostatectomy. Microsatellites are regions of the genome composed of a short repetitive sequence; eg, a run of adenine bases, a run of alternating cytosine-adenine (CA) couplets. They are usually found in noncoding segments of DNA, and each person inherits, for every microsatellite locus, one maternal and one paternal allele. The parental alleles are usually of differing length (heterozygous), but they are occasionally the same (homozygous); within a particular person, every cell in the body has microsatellites of equal length. From person to person, microsatellites are usually of different lengths, and, particularly if several microsatellite loci are looked at simultaneously, they can be used to very reliably distinguish one person from another. This analysis can be performed on formalin-fixed, paraffin-embedded tissue from which DNA is extracted. The recovered DNA is subjected to multiplex (multiple primers) PCR designed to amplify several microsatellite markers. The amplified products can be subjected to electrophoresis on a gel and analyzed visually. The pattern derived from a prostate biopsy should match exactly that obtained from the prostatectomy.

Urothelial (transitional cell) carcinoma

Biologically speaking there appear to be ≥2 distinct pathways to arrival at urothelial carcinoma. The first pathway leads to the development of low grade papillary transitional cell carcinoma, with almost no metastatic potential. Low grade lesions may occasionally be a precursor to high grade tumors, but mainly serve as a marker of risk. The other pathway involves high grade papillary carcinoma and flat urothelial carcinoma in situ, each of which may give rise to a high grade invasive tumor. The low grade tumors often have loss of *P16* on chromosome 9p21 and mutations in the *FGFR3* gene. While high grade tumors frequently have loss of *P16*, they usually lack *FGFR3* mutations. Instead they demonstrate inactivation of *P53*, chromosomal instability, and an often complex karyotype with gains or losses of 6p, 7, 9, and 17. Diagnosis has been facilitated with a recent application of FISH technology to urine specimens in patients with microhematuria or recurrent tumors. Enumeration probes for chromosomes 3, 7, and 17 along with a locus-specific indicator for the *P16* gene on 9p21 form the basis of the UroVysion assay. Examination of cytologically abnormal cells for quantitation of FISH signals provides high specificity and sensitivity. In initial reports, specificity approached 100%, with positive FISH results in some patients preceding the development of clinically apparent tumor ("anticipatory positives"). Subsequent studies have not confirmed this degree of specificity.

Testicular tumors

Several chromosomal regions, including the Y chromosome gr/gr deletion have been shown to be associated with an inherited risk of developing testicular germ cell tumors. No clear candidate genes involved with an inherited predisposition for testicular have been yet identified.

The majority of germ cell tumors are associated with gains of chromosome 12p, most often as an isochromosome, i(12p). Gain of 12p can be seen in all types of germ cell tumors and may represent an early step in tumor development. *CKIT* mutations are frequent in seminoma, as a result of which many seminomas exhibit strong immunohistochemical staining for c-kit (CD117). The membranous staining pattern is strongly associated with seminoma, other staining patterns can be found in nonseminomatous germ cell tumors.

Soft tissue & bone

Tumors of ectodermal or epithelial origin often demonstrate one or several gene mutations, but with rare exception they lack specific chromosome structural rearrangements. In contrast, tumors of mesodermal origin, including the hematolymphoid system, soft tissue, and bone, often demonstrate specific and reproducible structural rearrangements, such as translocations t7.16.

t7.16 Molecular features of soft tissue tumors

Tumor	Most common rearrangement(s)	Genes
Chondroid lipoma	t(11;16)(q13;p12-13)	C11orf95/MKL2
Schwannoma	del(22q12)	NF2
Ewings/PNET	t(11;22)(q24;q12)	EWS/FLI1
	t(21;22)(q22;q12)	EWS/ERG
	t(7;22)(p22;q12)	EWS/ETV1
	t(17;22)(q21;q12)	EWS/ETV4
	t(2;22)(q33;q12)	EWS/FEV
Neuroblastoma	del(1p), +17	n-MYC
Alveolar rhabdomyosarcoma	t(2;13)(q35;q14)	PAX3/FOXO1
	t(1;13)(p36;q14)	PAX7/FOXO1
Alveolar soft part sarcoma	der(17)t(X;17)(p11;q25)	ASPSCR1/TFE3
Desmoplastic small round cell tumor	t(11;22)(p13;q12)	EWS/WT1
Myxoid & round cell liposarcoma	t(12;16)(q13;p11)	FUS/DDIT3
Low grade fibromyxoid sarcoma, hyalinizing spindle cell tumor with giant rosettes	t(7;16)(q33;p11)	FUS/CREB3L2
Dermatofibrosarcoma protuberans, giant cell fibroblastoma	t(17;22)(q22;q13)	COL1A1/PDGFB
Infantile fibrosarcoma, congenital mesoblastic nephroma	t(12;15)(p12;q25)	ETV6/NTRK3
Myxoid chondrosarcoma, extraskeletal	t(9;22)(q22;q12)	EWS/NR4A3
Liposarcoma	t(12;16)(q13;p11)	FUS/CHOP
Angiomatoid fibrous histiocytoma	t(12;22)(q13;q12)	EWS/ATF1
	t(2;22)(q33;q12)	EWS/CREB1
Clear cell sarcoma	t(12;22)(q13;q12)	EWS/ATF1
	t(2;22)(q33;q12)	EWS/CREB1
Synovial sarcoma	t(X;18)(p11.2;q11.2)	SSX1/SYT
	t(X;18)(p11.2;q11.2)	SSX2/SYT
Inflammatory myofibroblastic tumor	t(1;2)(q25;p23)	TPM3/ALK
	t(2;19)(p23;p13)	TPM4/ALK

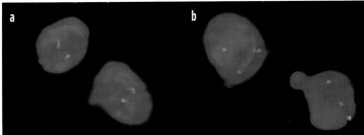

f7.44 Ewing sarcoma FISH utilizing dual color break apart probes; the red & green probes flank the region of known breakpoints
a A normal nucleus contains 2 red-green fusion signals (2F)
b An abnormal nucleus demonstrates 1 red-green fusion signal & separate red & green signals (1R,1G,1F)

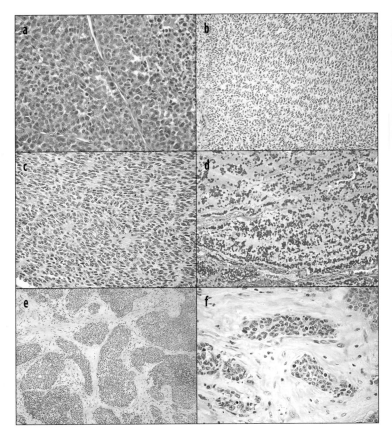

f7.43 Ewing family tumors
a-c Ewing sarcoma/PNET
d Extraskeletal myxoid chondrosarcoma
e & f Intraabdominal desmoplastic small round cell tumor

Ewing sarcoma family of tumors

Ewing sarcoma f7.43 is a member of a large family of tumors, all of which have fusion genes involving the *EWS* gene. Ewing sarcoma is one of the most common soft tissue tumors of children, accounting for 20% of soft tissue tumors in this population. Primitive neuroectodermal tumor (PNET) is essentially identical to Ewing sarcoma with the addition of neuroectodermal features as demonstrated by histologic, immunohistochemical, or ultrastructural means.

The *EWS* gene often undergoes translocation to a member of the ETS transcription family f7.44. The ETS sites function as DNA binding domains; thus, such translocations localize the strong transcriptional activation domain of the EWS to ETS inducible genes. Almost 95% of cases of Ewing sarcoma express a particular translocation of the *EWS* gene on chromosome 22q12 to the *FLI1* gene on 11q24. There is some variation in the exact breakpoints but most commonly the breaks occur between exon 7 of *EWS* and exon 6 of *FLI1*. Less common (5% of cases) is the t(21;22)(q22;q12) translocation of *EWS* with *ERG*. Rare cases have been associated with the translocations t(7;22), t(17;22), t(2;22), inversion of 22q, and even a non-*EWS* translocation of t(16;21)(p11;q22) resulting in a *TLS-ERG* fusion. The *TLS* gene shares extensive homology with *EWS*. Additional cytogenetic abnormalities (most often gains of 1q, 8, 12) can be found in 1/2 of the cases of Ewing sarcoma and portend a poor prognosis. Genetic diagnosis can be made with RT-PCR, which provides high sensitivity and specificity when primers and probes to cover all the different breakpoints are used. Other common modalities used for diagnosis include karyotyping, FISH with EWS break apart probes, or Southern blotting.

Intraabdominal desmoplastic small round cell tumor is a recently described tumor, most commonly presenting as an abdominal mass in a young male. It is consistently associated with the translocation t(11;22)(p13;q12) fusing the genes *EWS* with *WT1*. The tumor appears histologically as a small round blue cell tumor; its only distinctive feature is growth within strikingly desmoplastic stroma. A unique immunohistochemical profile usually aids in identifying this tumor, which is found to be NSE+, EMA+, keratin+ and desmin+ in the vast majority of cases.

Clear cell sarcoma of tendons and aponeuroses (malignant melanoma of soft parts) is another member of the *EWS* tumor family. Aside from presenting in the deep soft tissue of young adults, it shares many histomorphologic, immunohistochemical, and ultrastructural features with melanoma. Unlike malignant melanoma, nearly 90% of cases of clear cell sarcoma are associated with a specific translocation, t(12;22)(q13;q12) fusing *EWS* to the transcription factor *ATF1*. There are 3 major fusion protein subtypes involved, the major one involving exon 8 of *EWS* to exon 4 of *ATF1*.

Extraskeletal myxoid chondrosarcoma is another member of the EWS family of tumors. It is a rare tumor whose chondroid differentiation is subtle, consisting largely of a cording pattern of growth. Extraskeletal myxoid chondroscarcoma is commonly associated with the translocation t(9;22)(q22;q12) that fuses the *EWS* gene with the *CHN* (TEC) gene. The remaining cases are found to harbor 1 of 2 additional translocations, t(9;12)(q22;q11) that fuses *CHN* to *TAF2N*, or t(9;15)(q22;q21) that fuses *CHN* to the gene *TCF12* These translocations are specific for extraskeletal myxoid chondrosarcoma and have not been seen with any other chondroid related tumors.

Neuroblastoma

Neuroblastoma f7.45 is the most common malignancy in patients under the age of 5 years. It presents as an abdominal mass or a posterior mediastinal mass, as it usually arises from the adrenal medulla or sympathetic chain. Amplification of the *MYCN* (n-Myc) protooncogene is found in 30% of neuroblastomas and is a marker of aggressive behavior. The mechanism of amplification is primarily as extrachromosomal

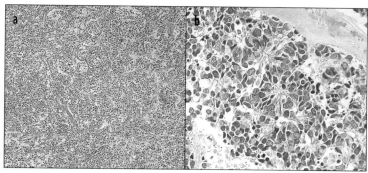

f7.45 Adrenal neuroblastoma

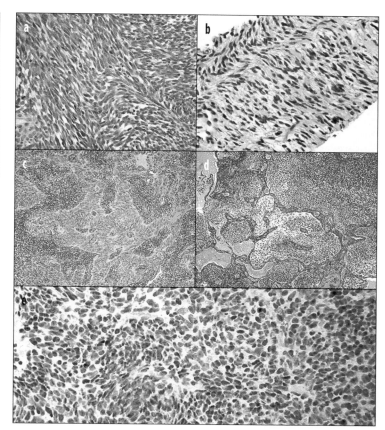

f7.46 Synovial sarcoma
a & b Monophasic synovial sarcomas
c & d Biphasic synovial sarcomas
e Immunohistochemical expression of TLE1

double minutes, though in some cases there is in situ gene duplication and in others gene duplication and insertion into random chromosomes, leading to segmental chromosome gain that may be visible as homogeneously staining regions (HSRs). Greater than 10-fold amplification is correlated with poor prognosis. The overall proportion of tumors with this degree of *MYCN* amplification is 30%, but 40% in high stage tumors and only 10% in low stage tumors. Several modalities are available for detecting *MYCN* duplication, including FISH, CISH, Southern blotting, and quantitative RT-PCR. In addition to *MYCN* amplification, neuroblastomas may display aneuploidy and/or a complex set of structural chromosomal anomalies. Abnormalities of 17q23 are present in >50% of cases, deletion of 1p36 in 30-40%, and deletion of 11q23 in 40-50%. The 1p deletion is associated with poor prognosis. The DNA content (ploidy) of the tumor has been shown to correlate with outcome, particularly in infants. Those with hyperdiploid tumors (DNA index >1.0) have a more favorable outcome (similar to what is seen in acute lymphoblastic lymphoma).

Rhabdomyosarcoma

While there are several subtypes of rhabdomyosarcoma, the only one that is consistently associated with a chromosomal rearrangement is alveolar rhabdomyosarcoma (ARMS), in which is found the *PAX-FOXO1* (formerly *FKHR*) fusion. Approximately 60% of cases are associated with t(2;13)(q35;q14) which fuses *PAX3* with *FOXO1*, while ~20% of cases are associated with t(1;13)(p36;q14), fusing *PAX7* with *FOXO1*. Similar to *EWS-FLI*, the fusion protein in ARMS joins the DNA binding region of the *PAX* genes with the transcriptional activation region of *FOXO1*. The breakpoints in the translocations associated with alveolar rhabdomyosarcoma are consistent, involving intron 7 of *PAX3* or *PAX7* with intron 1 of *FOXO1*. Amplification of the *PAX7-FOXO1* fusion gene is seen in a majority of cases with the t(1;13) translocation and to a much lesser extent with the *PAX3-FOXO1* fusion from t(2;13).

Detection of the fusion gene for diagnosis is limited by the sensitivity of RT-PCR for nucleic acid isolated from fixed tissue (~50%) and the relative high incidence (up to 20%) of tumors that fail to demonstrate the presence of a translocation. Detection of the translocation, however, is very specific as it has not been demonstrated in any other tumor type. Despite the ability to detect both fusion genes with a primer set that contains a single primer to both *PAX3* and *PAX7* conserved sequence, it is important to identify the *PAX* fusion gene. Tumors associated with the *PAX3* translocation are associated with a very poor prognosis (<10% survival at 4 years), while tumors harboring *PAX7* have a relatively favorable prognosis.

Synovial sarcoma

Synovial sarcoma f7.46 is a tumor with a predilection for young adults and adolescents. Typically arising within the para-articular deep soft tissue in an extremity, these tumors can be either monophasic or biphasic. Monophasic tumors are highly cellular spindle cell lesions without the characteristic herringbone features of fibrosarcoma. Biphasic tumors are less common and in addition to a spindle cell component also have an epithelial component composed of glands or papillary structures. In 90% of synovial sarcomas is associated the characteristic t(X;18)(p11;q11) translocation. Most commonly the translocation is not the sole abnormality and aneuploidies of 3–, 7+, 8+, and 12+ have been described. The genes involved are the *SSX* genes (predominantly *SSX1*, *SSX2*, and *SSX4*) on the X chromosome and *SS18* (also known as *SYT* or *SSXT*) on chromosome 18. The most common fusion, *SS18-SSX1* accounts for 2/3 of cases, while *SS18-SSX2* accounts for most of the remaining cases. Rare case reports exist describing the *SS18-SSX4* fusion. TLE1 immunohistochemistry, which shows strong nuclear reactivity in synovial sarcoma, can act as a surrogate marker, though TLE1 expression is not entirely specific.

Low grade fibromyxoid sarcoma (LGFMS)/hyalinizing spindle tumor with giant rosettes

These tumors f7.47 are now considered extremes of the morphologic spectrum of tumors with the translocation t(7;16) (q34;p11). The translocation produces a fusion gene of the 5' transcriptional activation domain of *TLS* with the 3' DNA binding and leucine zipper region of the *CREB3L2* gene. Another related translocation t(11;16)(p11;p11) of *TLS* with *CREB3L1* has to be found in a small minority of cases.

Tumors of adipocytes

Most lipomas are associated with complex cytogenetic anomalies, often involving high mobility group protein genes, such as *HMGA2* on chromosome 12q13-q15. The most common translocation is t(3;12)(q29;q15) fusing the genes *HMGA2* and *LPP*. Rearrangements of the chromosome 8q12 region with the *PLAG2* gene underlie a significant portion of lipoblastomas. An additional mechanism for *PLAG2* overexpression occurs in ~20% of lipoblastomas with chromosome 8 polysomy.

Well differentiated liposarcoma and atypical lipomatous tumor involve alterations of the region 12q14-q15 and take the form of supernumerary ring chromosomes, translocations, or giant marker chromosomes with amplifications.

The most common rearrangement observed in myxoid and round cell liposarcoma is t(12;16)(q13;p11) which makes a fusion gene of *TLS* (previously called *FUS*) on 16p11 with *DDIT3* (previously known as *CHOP* or *GADD153*) on 12q13. Less common is the translocation t(12;22)(q13;q12) which fuses *DDIT3* with the promiscuous *EWS*.

Osteochondromatosis

Osteochondromatosis is an autosomal dominant condition with a hereditary predisposition to the formation of multiple bony exostoses (osteochondromas), differing from solitary sporadic osteochondromas in their location and malignant potential. In patients with osteochondromatosis, osteochondromas develop on the femur in 70% of cases. While this site is typical for sporadic osteochondromas, syndromic lesions tend to be bilateral and symmetrical. Furthermore, osteochondromas are found in uncommon sites such as the forearm, scapula, pelvis, vertebrae, phalanges, wrist, and ankle. Sarcomatous change occurs in ~1% of cases. Other frequent bony lesions include short stature, bone deformities, and premature osteoarthritis. The most common mutation associated with osteochondromatosis affects the gene *EXT1* on chromosome 8q (70%), with the remaining cases attributed to the *EXT2* gene on 11p.

Head & neck tumors

Squamous cell carcinoma

More than 95% of head and neck malignancies are squamous cell carcinomas. The risk factors for head and neck squamous cell carcinoma have traditionally been tobacco and alcohol. Increasingly, human papillomavirus (HPV) is being recognized as causing a subset of head and neck squamous cell carcinomas. HPV-driven tumors often arise in younger patients who are nonsmokers, and their behavior is more indolent. HPV status and smoking history may in fact be stronger predictors of long term outcome than traditional TNM staging. As rates of smoking have been decreasing, HPV-associated

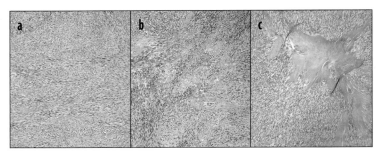

f7.47 Low grade fibromyxoid sarcoma (LGFMS)—hyalinizing spindle tumor with giant rosettes (HSTGR) spectrum tumors
a Tumor with predominantly LGFMS features
b Tumor showing intermediate features
c Tumor with predominantly HSTGR features

carcinoma has become relatively more prevalent. High risk serotypes, especially HPV 16, are typically involved.

In smoking-associated squamous cell carcinoma, the most common molecular anomalies are found in the tumor suppressor genes, including loss of genetic material in 3p, 9p, and 17p (*TP53* locus). Overexpression of p53 by immunohistochemistry is associated with poor prognosis. EGFR is overexpressed in the majority of tobacco related head and neck squamous cell carcinoma; however, EGFR genetic anomalies are uncommon. Neither molecular nor immunohistochemical assessment of EGFR status correlates with response to anti-EGFR therapy.

HPV-associated squamous cell carcinoma (HPV-SCC) is usually found in the oropharynx, including base of tongue and tonsils. Up to 70% of squamous cell carcinomas in these sites are positive for HPV. Tumors of the oral tongue have a low incidence of HPV. HPV-SCC is significantly more likely to have nonkeratinizing and basaloid histology. As in cervical HPV-driven SCC, integration of portions of the HPV genome, including *HPVE6* and *HPVE7*, leads to suppression of p53 and Rb and overexpression of p16. TP53 is un-mutated and not overexpressed by immunohistochemistry. Immunohistochemistry for p16 is commonly used as a surrogate for HPV infection. Up to 15% of p16+ tumors show no evidence of HPV infection by in situ hybridization. Some studies have shown that these apparently HPV–/p16+ tumors behave similarly to HPV+/ p16+ tumors. P16 overexpression appears to be a more useful marker than HPV in situ hybridization.

Salivary gland tumors

The most common malignant tumor of the salivary glands is mucoepidermoid carcinoma (MEC). The translocation t(11;19)(q21;p13) fusing the transcriptional activators *MECT2* on chromosome 19 to *MAML2* on chromosome 11. This translocation can be found by cytogenetic analysis in ~1/2 of cases, especially the low and intermediate-grade tumors. RT-PCR detection is more sensitive and can detect the translocation in almost 90% of cases. The presence of the translocation in Warthin tumors is controversial.

The most common benign salivary gland tumor is pleomorphic adenoma (PA). The majority of cases have demonstrable karyotypic abnormalities, most commonly rearrangements of 8q12 involving the gene *PLAG1*. Translocation t(3;8) of *PLAG1* to the β-catenin gene, *CTNNB1*, is the most common, followed by the translocation t(5;8) of *PLAG1* to *LIFR*, the leukemia inhibitory factor receptor. The end result of these translocations is the overexpression of *PLAG1*. Some tumors demonstrate *PLAG1* overexpression in the absence of demonstrable chromosomal abnormalities. The second most common gene involved with PA is *HMGA2* on chromosome 12q15. It is most commonly rearranged as t(3;12), resulting in fusion of *HMGA2* with *FHIT* (fragile histidine triad).

NUT midline carcinoma is a tumor uniquely defined by its molecular features. Rearrangements in the *NUT* (nuclear protein in testis) gene on chromosome 15q14 are definitive for the tumor, as demonstrated by either RT-PCR or FISH. Most cases exhibit the translocation t(15;19)(q14;p13.1), fusing the *NUT* gene to *BRD4*. Because of the reliance on the molecular features for accurate diagnosis the tumor is often misdiagnosed. Most often they are poorly differentiated tumors with abrupt keratinization that are easily confused with other small blue cell tumors. Currently, promising results are being seen with immunohistochemistry using a NUT-specific antibody, which may facilitate accurate diagnosis.

Thyroid

Familial thyroid carcinoma

The cardinal manifestations of multiple endocrine neoplasia type 1 (MEN 1; Wermer syndrome) are parathyroid adenomas, pituitary adenomas, and pancreatic islet cell tumors. The most common and earliest manifestation is usually primary hyperparathyroidism, caused by a PTH-secreting pituitary adenoma. Most of the pituitary tumors are prolactinomas. Pancreatic tumors often produce gastrin (gastrinomas) or insulin (insulinomas). Nonendocrine lesions in MEN1 include facial angiofibromas, collagenomas, lipomas, and meningiomas. A predisposition exists to endocrine tumors in the lung, adrenal cortex, thymus, and gastrointestinal tract. The *MEN1* gene on chromosome 11q13 encodes the protein menin and 90% of the time a germline *MEN1* mutation can be found in patients with MEN 1 syndrome. Somatic *MEN1* mutations are found in 15-20% of sporadic parathyroid adenomas, islet cell tumors, and gastrinomas.

Mutations in the *RET* protooncogene on chromosome 10q are a feature common to multiple endocrine neoplasia type 2A (MEN2A; Sipple syndrome), MEN2B, and familial medullary thyroid carcinoma (FMTC). The 3 syndromes—MEN2A, MEN2B, and FMTC—have some things in common, all imparting a high risk for medullary thyroid carcinoma, all autosomal dominant, and all due to a *RET* gene mutation. These features alone comprise FMTC. These features plus pheochromocytoma and parathyroid adenoma comprise the MEN2A syndrome; and these plus pheochromocytoma, mucosal neuromas, ganglioneuromatous intestinal polyps, and Marfanoid body habitus comprise MEN2B. While the histology of medullary thyroid carcinomas f7.48 is not particularly distinctive in these syndromes, the appearance of the background thyroid is: C-cell hyperplasia and numerous microscopic foci of medullary carcinoma. MEN2A is caused by mutations affecting exons 10-11 of the *RET* gene, most often affecting a particular cysteine residue (634 Cys). MEN2B is most often due to a *RET* mutation affecting exon 16, encoding the tyrosine kinase domain. FMTC is caused by *RET* mutations affecting other cysteine residues, particularly 609, 611, 618, and 620 Cys. Mutations of the *RET* gene are associated with Hirschsprung disease (often gain of function), and almost 1/2 of sporadic papillary thyroid carcinoma. About

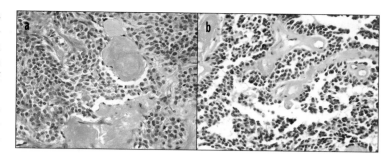

f7.48 Medullary carcinoma of thyroid

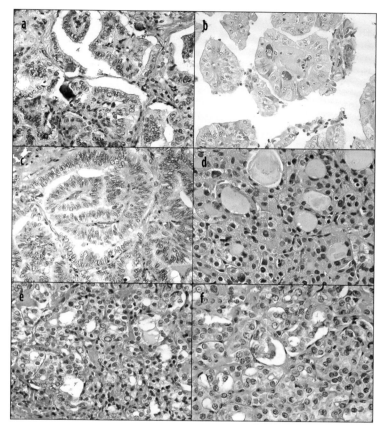

f7.49 Papillary carcinoma
a Classic papillary carcinoma, papillary variant
b Tall cell variant
c Columnar variant
d-f Follicular variant

40% of sporadic papillary thyroid carcinomas have somatic mutations in *RET*.

Papillary thyroid carcinoma

Papillary thyroid carcinoma (PTC) is the most common sporadic cancer of the thyroid, accounting for >75% of all thyroid malignancies. Mutations in *BRAF*, *RET*, and *RAS*, all of which are capable of causing unregulated MAPK stimulation, have been found in PTC in mutually exclusive distribution.

The most common mutation found in PTC is the *BRAF* V600E mutation, which is seen in almost 1/2 of cases. *BRAF* mutation is found with highest frequency in conventional (60%) and tall cell (80%) variants of PTC f7.49, and it is found in only 10% of follicular variant. Several studies have demonstrated that the accuracy of thyroid FNA diagnosis can be significantly improved by adding *BRAF* testing. In this setting, the *BRAF* mutation appears to have a specificity of >99% for PTC. Lastly, *BRAF* mutation serves as a prognostic marker, with BRAF positive PTCs demonstrating more aggressive behavior.

There are several structural chromosomal rearrangement involving the *RET* gene that result in marked *RET* overexpression. Collectively, these rearrangements are denoted *RET/PTC*, but individual rearrangement partners are termed *PTC1* through *PTC11*. The vast majority of PTCs harboring such a rearrangement have either *RET/PTC1* or *RET/PTC3*, with *PTC1* being the *CCDC6* gene and *PTC3* the *NCOA4* gene. Nonclonal *RET/PTC* rearrangements can be found in benign thyroid tissue, and clonal rearrangements are found in 20-30% of PTCs, being more common in radiation-associated PTC and in PTC arising in children. Tumors with RET/PTC have classic architecture and a high rate of lymph node metastases.

Nearly all PTCs with *RAS* mutations have follicular architecture (follicular variant of PTC). Interestingly, nearly 1/2 of follicular carcinomas also have *RAS* mutations, as do 1/3 of follicular adenomas. *RAS* mutations appear to correlate with metastatic potential, especially to bone.

Skin tumors

Basal cell carcinoma (BCC)

BCC, the most common cutaneous malignancy, often appears on sun-damaged skin in adults. Several inherited disorders are associated with an increased risk of basal cell carcinoma. Gorlin syndrome (nevoid basal cell carcinoma syndrome) is due to germline mutations in the *PTCH* gene. The protein product of the *PTCH* gene is involved in sonic-hedgehog (SHH) signaling, functioning as an inhibitor of signal transduction. Mutations in *PTCH* lead to SHH-independent signaling. PTCH mutations are found in a high proportion of sporadic BCC.

Xeroderma pigmentosa-affected individuals are prone to several different types of cutaneous malignancies, including BCC and squamous cell carcinoma.

Melanoma

Less common than either squamous cell carcinoma or basal cell carcinoma but accounting for far more morbidity and mortality than the 2 combined, melanoma is one of the worst human cancers. Emerging molecular data suggests that the entity we had been referring to as melanoma may actually represent a class of tumors sharing similar morphologic features. It is difficult to predict behavior of the tumors as metastatic disease can occur with even thin melanomas. Even molecular characterization of melanoma is fraught with difficulty as many of the changes seen in melanoma, such as *BRAF* mutations, are present in benign melanocytic nevi.

Increased risk for the development of cutaneous melanoma can be due to several factors—fair skin and a tendency to freckle, having multiple nevi, environmental exposure (deep sunburns), and familial predisposition. The latter is a feature of several familial melanoma syndromes, including familial atypical mole and melanoma (FAMM) syndrome. It is estimated that ~10% of melanoma is due to a familial predisposition. Dysregulation of p16, the product of the gene *CDKN2A* (cyclin-dependent kinase inhibitor 2A) underlies FAMM. Another form of familial melanoma is based upon defects in the *CDK4* gene on chromosome 12q14, which functions as an oncogene in the retinoblastoma pathway.

In sporadic melanoma, comparative genomic hybridization (CGH) studies have elucidated certain reproducible chromosomal gains and losses that may help to differentiate Spitz nevi and other ambiguous melanocytic tumors from melanomas, while also demonstrating that different types of melanomas have different genetic anomalies with which they are often associated. Based on the array CGH findings a refined set of 4 FISH probes has shown initially promising results in differentiation of melanocytic.

Approximately 1/3 of mucosal and acral melanomas are associated with mutations in *C-KIT*. This presents an attractive therapeutic target since *C-KIT*-mutation tumors may respond to the tyrosine kinase inhibitor imatinib. Additionally, strong immunohistochemical staining for c-kit has been shown to have a close association with mutation status, opening a potential screening test for *C-KIT* mutation analysis.

Mutations in *BRAF* are more closely associated with cutaneous melanoma. Specifically, *BRAF* mutations (pV600E predominantly) are common in cutaneous melanomas that are not associated with sun damage. The *BRAF* pV600E mutation results in a constitutively active protein that sends proliferative signals to the nucleus in the absence of mitogen activation. Successes in the treatment of metastatic melanoma with a specific small molecule inhibitor of BRAF kinase herald a new era in therapy.

An additional issue with molecular testing in melanoma is lymph node evaluation. As lymph node status is a major determinant in prognosis, accurate assessment for the presence of melanoma is critical. With current histomorphologic and immunohistochemistry techniques it is clear that some potentially microscopically-positive lymph nodes are going undetected because a significant number of node-negative cases develop recurrent disease. Specific mRNA markers for the detection of melanoma have been developed for paraffin-embedded tissue and show some promise in detecting occult metastatic melanoma in these lymph nodes.

Dermatofibrosarcoma protuberans (DFSP)

Like many other soft tissue tumors, DFSP is associated with a characteristic chromosomal translocation. Fusion of the type I collagen α-1 chain gene, *COL1A1*, to the platelet derived growth factor β-chain gene, *PDGFB*, either via linear translocation (most common) or supernumerary ring chromosome formation is the hallmark of DFSP. While there are several specific breakpoints leading to translocation heterogeneity, the fusion gene is present in almost all cases of DFSP. In addition, the same translocation is seen in the pediatric giant cell fibroblastoma tumor, providing evidence that in fact that DFSP and giant cell fibroblastoma are the same tumor with different ages of presentation.

Central nervous system tumors

Gliomas

Diffuse gliomas (astrocytoma & oligodendroglioma)

The most common primary neoplasms of the central nervous system (CNS) are the diffuse gliomas (astrocytoma and oligodendroglioma). Diffuse gliomas are categorized by the WHO into grades II through IV, with grade I lesions being benign well-circumscribed tumors. Grade IV glioma, also called glioblastoma multiforme (GBM), may arise de novo (primary GBM) or from preexisting grade II/III glioma (secondary GBM). Primary GBM is a rapidly progressive tumor that generally arises in older patients, while secondary GBM arises in younger patients and has a somewhat more protracted clinical course. The accumulated evidence suggests that a small number of genetic events gives rise to grade II glioma, and a series of additional genetic events accrues in the progression from grade II to grade IV glioma.

Early events in tumorigenesis include mutations in the *IDH1* and/or *IDH2* genes. *IDH* mutations are rare in tumors outside the CNS and, importantly, not found in benign CNS conditions such as reactive gliosis. Direct (Sanger) sequence analysis is generally required to detect *IDH* mutations, but recently a promising new immunohistochemical marker has become available. A divergence in paths occurs somewhat later, with tumors acquiring 17p13 (*TP53*) anomalies differentiating into grade II astrocytomas, and those developing 1p and/or 19q deletions differentiating into grade II oligodendroglioma. Note that both types of glioma retain their original *IDH* mutations. Additional anomalies are found in grade III lesions, including deletion of 9p and *CDKN2*. Lastly, progression to grade IV glioma (secondary GBM) is usually marked by the loss of material from 10q. As might be expected, primary GBM often lacks many of these early abnormalities, demonstrating instead amplification of *EGFR*, mutation of *PTEN*, and loss of 10q.

About 1/3 of astrocytomas harbor mutations in *TP53*. *TP53* mutations are rare in oligodendrogliomas. As expected, Li-Fraumeni syndrome (germline *TP53* mutation) is associated with the development of astrocytoma. Immunohistochemical evidence of p53 nuclear accumulation correlates well with *TP53* mutation status. Furthermore, *TP53* mutations are operant in the development of secondary GBM but are not found commonly in secondary GBM in which *EGFR* amplification is found. *EGFR* amplification and *TP53* mutations rarely co-exist in these tumors. EGFR immunohistochemistry is an effective means of assessing for *EGFR* mutation status. *EGFR* mutated tumors display aggressive behavior, are associated with a small cell phenotype, but respond to small molecule EGFR kinase inhibitors.

Because of their infiltrative nature, surgical cure is often difficult to achieve. Adjuvant chemotherapy and radiation therapy have an important role, and in general oligodendrogliomas respond better to adjuvant therapy. Therefore it is important to distinguish between astrocytoma and oligodendroglioma t7.17. While many oligodendrogliomas are quite straightforward, presenting as a proliferation of cells with rounded nuclear contours and perinuclear halos within a background of arborizing "chicken-wire" capillaries, a significant number of cases have borderline or mixed features. Fortunately, the loss of the

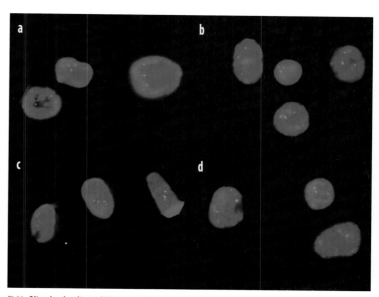

f7.50 Oligodendroglioma FISH; in a & b there is a red marker for 1p & a green marker for 1q
a There is a normal 2 red, 2 green (2R2G) signal, indicative of retention of 1p
b There is only 1 red signal (1R2G) indicating 1p deletion
Likewise, in c & d red (19q) & green (19p) markers are used to assess the status of 19q, with
c a normal result & d 19q deletion

1p and 19q are very specific for oligodendroglioma f7.50. The frequency 1p/19q co-deletion is up to 90% in grade II oligodendrogliomas, 60% in grade III (anaplastic) oligodendrogliomas, and up to 50% in mixed oligoastrocytomas. The presence of the combined loss of 1p/19q is important, as these tumors tend to respond better to chemotherapy (including temazolamide) and have an overall better prognosis than oligodendrogliomas (and astrocytomas) lacking these genetic anomalies. PCR-based assays for microsatellite regions within 1p and 19q or locus-specific FISH probes can be used to assess for loss of heterozygosity.

t7.17 Oligodendroglioma vs astrocytoma

	Oligodendroglioma	Astrocytoma
Imaging	Peripheral (cortical), well demarcated, calcified	Central (subcortical), infiltrative
Histology	Round, regular nuclei Paucity of glial processes Perineural satellitosis Microcysts filled with mucin	Elongated, irregular nuclei Abundant glial processes
WHO types	Grade II (oligodendroglioma) Grade III (anaplastic oligodendroglioma)	Grade II (low grade astrocytoma) Grade III (anaplastic astrocytoma) Grade IV (GBM)
IHC	Not generally useful, although astrocytomas are more likely to express strong GFAP & p53, with considerable overlap	
Genetics (by LOH or FISH)	Loss of 1p in 80% Loss of 19q in 80% Loss of 1p & 19q in 60-80% Losses in 9p & 10q increase with grade No EGFR amplification	Loss of 1p in 30-40% Loss of 19q in 10-15% Loss of 1p & 19q in 5% Losses in 9p & 10q increase with grade EGFR amplification in high grade astrocytomas (esp GBM)
Prognosis	Better, with combined loss of 1p & 19q associated with chemosensitivity	Worse, with unclear significance of combined loss of 1p & 19q cases

The *MGMT* (O⁶-methylguanine-DNA methyltransferase) gene, which is involved in DNA repair, plays an interesting role in glioma management. In some but not all gliomas, the *MGMT* gene undergoes epigenetic silencing through promoter hypermethylation. The status of the *MGMT* gene profoundly impacts clinical response to treatment with temozolomide and radiotherapy; that is, an unsuppressed *MGMT* gene can mitigate the DNA-damaging effect of combined therapy, thus rescuing the tumor cells from harm. The mechanism of action of temozolomide, an alkylating agent, is the addition of a methyl group to the O^6-position of nucleotide guanine residues, which results in DNA damage; the MGMT protein is capable of repairing this damage. In 2006, Hegi et al reported that, in GBM patients treated with temozolomide and XRT, 49% of those with methylated *MGMT* were alive at 2 years, compared to 15% of those with unmethylated *MGMT*. The status of the *MGMT* gene can be assessed by a variety of methods, including methylation-specific PCR.

Pilocytic astrocytoma

The *BRAF* gene, encoding the MAPK pathway protein RAF, is involved in tumorigenesis throughout the body. In many tumors, *BRAF* activation arises as a result of a point mutation, most commonly the *BRAF* V600E mutation. In pilocytic astrocytoma, *BRAF* mutation appears to be the sole inciting genetic event. Both *BRAF* point mutations and *BRAF* gene duplication have been found. *BRAF* anomalies are found in up to 80% of pilocytic astrocytomas, but they are rare in diffuse astrocytomas.

Retinoblastoma

Retinoblastoma is a rare tumor closely associated with mutations of the *RB1* gene on chromosome 13q14. Over 90% of cases of retinoblastoma are sporadic, the remainder are associated with an inherited defect in one copy of the *RB1* gene. The presence of bilateral retinoblastomas in a young patient should raise suspicion of an inherited cause. Patients with inherited mutations in *RB1* are at high risk for later development of osteosarcoma, pineal gland tumors, and primitive neuroectodermal tumors (PNETs).

Meningioma

Monosomy of chromosome 22 is the most common abnormality found in meningiomas, and this was one of the first chromosomal rearrangements described in solid tumors. The key region appears to be 22q12.2 where the *NF2* gene is located. Recall that meningioma is one of the features of the NF2 syndrome (caused by germline *NF2* mutations). Merlin is the protein encoded by the *NF2* gene. Merlin is found in the cell membrane where its function is to mediate cell-cell contact and cell contact inhibition.

The frequency of *NF2* anomalies varies from one histologic variant to the next. *NF2* abnormalities are found in 80% of transitional and fibroblastic meningiomas but in only 25% of meningothelial meningiomas and in virtually no secretory meningiomas. The overall rate is ~50%.

NF2 anomalies are an early event in tumorigenesis and that additional molecular defects underlie tumor progression. Higher grade (atypical and anaplastic) meningiomas are found to have *NF2* abnormalities at roughly the same rate as low grade meningiomas, but have additional complex anomalies, including numerous genetic gains and losses. The losses involve 1p, 9p, 14, and others, and the gains include 1q, 9q, and others. In fact, del 1p is the second most common chromosomal abnormality found in meningiomas. Deletion of 14 (monosomy 14) and/or deletion of 9p21 have been associated with shortened survival.

Particular histologic subtypes are thought to have a higher rate of progression, including clear cell, chordoid, rhabdoid, and papillary. With regard to the more aggressive subtypes, only chordoid meningioma so far appears to have a molecular signature. An unbalanced translocation—der(1)t(1;3)(p12-13;q11)—has been found in this variant and preliminarily promises to be a specific marker.

Embryonal tumors

Embryonal tumors belong to a group defined by the presence of undifferentiated-appearing small blue cells, which account for the majority of primary pediatric brain tumors. 3 of the embryonal tumors—medulloblastoma, primitive neuroectodermal tumor, and atypical teratoid/rhabdoid tumor—have characteristic molecular alterations.

Medulloblastoma is a tumor of the posterior fossa affecting the cerebellum with a tendency to metastasize within the CNS. There are several subtypes with varying histologic appearances and prognoses. Certain inherited tumor predisposition conditions are associated with a higher risk of developing medulloblastoma, including Turcot syndrome secondary to mutations in *APC*, Gorlin syndrome, and Li-Fraumeni syndrome. In sporadic medulloblastoma, the most common aberration, seen in 1/2 of tumors, is isochromosome 17q. The alteration most strongly associated with prognosis is loss of chromosome 17p, present in 1/3 of tumors. Loss of 17p is associated with more aggressive tumor behavior, shortened survival, and a relatively poor response to chemotherapy.

Atypical teratoid/rhabdoid tumor (AT/RT) is a particularly aggressive pediatric CNS tumor that usually affects the very young (<2 years old). AT/RT is prone to extensive metastatic disease and lack of response to chemotherapy. Loss of the *SMARCB1* gene on chromosome 22q11.2, which encodes INI1, is found in majority of AT/RTs. The INI1 protein is a component of a SWI/SNF chromatin remodeling complex involved in DNA replication and transcription. Loss of INI1 enables confident distinction from other related and similar-appearing tumors, such as medulloblastoma or PNET, as this mutation is not frequently seen in either. Immunohistochemistry for INI1 is available, as are FISH probes for the affected region on chromosome 22.

Pulmonary tumors

Lung carcinoma can be divided histologically into 2 major categories: small cell lung cancer (SCLC) and for lack of a better name, non-small cell lung cancer (NSCLC). The latter group encompasses the majority of lung tumors and includes adenocarcinoma and squamous cell carcinoma. For many years there was little or no clinical benefit obtained from efforts to distinguish among non-small cell carcinoma types. Studies published in 2004 and 2006 changed this, as it became clear that patients with squamous cell carcinoma might suffer fatal hemorrhagic complications if treated with antiangiogenesis agents such as bevacizumab (Avastin). As a result of this finding, it became critical to distinguish squamous cell carcinoma from other varieties of non-small cell lung cancer. For poorly differentiated tumors, an immunohistochemical panel can be helpful in this regard; eg, a panel consisting of CK5/6 and P63 (both positive in squamous cell carcinoma) vs TTF1 and BerEP4 (both positive in adenocarcinoma).

A demand for even sharper distinction among non-small cell carcinomas emerged as a result of success with EGFR-targeted therapy in some patients. In particular, it seems that adenocarcinomas show the best response to these agents, and further histologic subtyping of adenocarcinoma can roughly predict response. Tumors with a lepidic component are likely to have EGFR-susceptible mutations, as are tumors with predominantly micropapillary or solid growth patterns. There appears to be no correlation, positive or negative, with acinar growth, and tumors with mucinous differentiation and enteric differentiation are very unlikely to respond.

Mutation analysis is the best predictor of response. 3 genes in particular have been shown to be frequently mutated in lung adenocarcinoma—*EGFR*, *KRAS*, and *ALK*—all mutually exclusive of one another.

EGFR mutations in this setting most commonly affect exons 18 through 21, which encodes a portion of the tyrosine kinase domain. In particular, one common mutation in exon 21 consists of a leucine to arginine substitution at amino acid 858 (L858R). Also frequent is a deletion in exon 19. These anomalies have the result of constitutive activation and signaling. Adenocarcinomas with these mutations are most commonly seen in patients with specific demographic features—young Asian females and/or never-smokers. Anti-EGFR agents come in 2 varieties, including small molecular tyrosine kinase inhibitors (EGFR-TKIs) such as gefitinib (Iressa) and erlotinib (Tarceva), and anti-EGFR monoclonal antibodies such as cetuximab (Erbitux). Tumors with mutations in exons 18 through 21 have a high likelihood of response to EGFR-TKIs but are unlikely to respond to anti-EGFR monoclonal antibodies. *EGFR* status by immunohistochemistry and FISH has not reliably predicted response, and at this time mutation analysis by PCR is recommended, targeting exons 18-21. As discussed below, mutations in the genes encoding downstream proteins in the EGFR signaling cascade (*KRAS*, *BRAF*) are found exclusively in tumors that lack *EGFR* mutations. Lastly, some patients develop secondary resistance to anti-EGFR therapy. Secondary resistance is associated with certain additional mutations in *EGFR* (T790M) as well as mutations in other genes such as *MET*.

KRAS mutations can lead to signaling downstream and independent of EGFR. There is a very high *KRAS* mutation rate in mucinous adenocarcinoma (75%) as compared to non-mucinous adenocarcinoma (45%). Since they are mutually exclusive, the presence of *KRAS* mutations would theoretically be associated with nonresponsiveness to anti-EGFR therapy (as is the case in colon cancer); on the contrary, this has not consistently proven to be the case. While *KRAS* mutations do appear to predict lack of response to EGFR-TKIs (gefitinib, erlotinib), there is no correlation with response to anti-EGFR monoclonal antibodies (cetuximab).

The small percentage of lung adenocarcinomas not associated with *EGFR* or *KRAS* mutations may have mutations in the anaplastic lymphoma kinase gene, *ALK*. While uncommon in lung cancer overall (1-5%), *ALK* rearrangements have been described in up to 20% of high-stage tumors. ALK, another receptor tyrosine kinase, was originally identified as part of the t(2;5)(p23;35) translocation in anaplastic large cell lymphomas and subsequently shown to be rearranged in inflammatory myofibroblastic tumor. Oncogenic *ALK* fusion genes are ones that result in overexpression and constitutive activation *ALK*. In non-small cell lung cancer, the *EML4-ALK* translocation (and less commonly, *TFG-ALK* and *KIF5-ALK*) causes the formation of a fusion gene of the transcription activation domain of *ALK* with the dimerization domain of *EML4*, leading to constitutive activation. The translocation is the result of an interstitial inversion in the short arm of chromosome 2. So far, it appears that IHC correlates poorly with response to small-molecule ALK-TKIs, and FISH is recommended.

Reduced expression of the miRNA, let-7 is a stage-independent poor prognostic finding. It is hypothesized that one of the targets of let-7-mediated control of gene expression, RAS may be the effector molecule for this poor prognosis. Other miRNAs, including the miR-17-92 cluster and miR-31 act as oncogenes and have been demonstrated to be aberrantly expressed in a number of non-small cell lung cancer cases.

Gynecologic tumors
Inherited gynecologic tumor syndromes

Most of the cases of inherited predisposition to gynecologic tumors are due to germline mutations in mismatch repair proteins (Lynch syndrome) or mutations in BRCA1/BRCA2 (hereditary breast and ovarian cancer). Peutz-Jeghers can present with particular gynecologic manifestations, such as adenoma malignum of the cervix and ovarian sex cord tumor with annular tubules (SCTAT).

Lynch syndrome is caused by an inherited germline mutation in the gene for one of the proteins involved in mismatch repair, most commonly *MLH1*, *MSH2*, or *MSH6*. Women with Lynch syndrome have a nearly 50% lifetime risk of endometrial cancer (often of the lower uterine segment) and a 10% risk of an epithelial ovarian cancer. The risk for endometrial cancer in Lynch syndrome is equivalent to the risk for colorectal carcinoma. Ovarian cancer in Lynch syndrome tends to present at an early age, usually before 50, and is often of the clear cell type. While most screening guidelines (Bethesda, Amsterdam) are focused more on colorectal carcinoma, there are also guidelines proposed by Society of Gynecologic Oncologists that address screening for an increased risk of endometrial and ovarian carcinoma. Similar to colorectal carcinoma it has been proposed that universal screening of all endometrial carcinomas for defects in mismatch repair be performed.

Hereditary Breast/Ovarian Cancer (HBOC) is caused by mutations in the tumor suppressor genes *BRCA1* or *BRCA2*. It is estimated that a patient with *BRCA* mutations has a 10-fold increased risk of developing an epithelial ovarian carcinoma, and ~10% of ovarian cancers are caused by underlying *BRCA* mutations. The majority of high grade serous ovarian carcinomas due to mutations in *BRCA* also harbor mutations in *P53*. These high grade or type II serous carcinomas are different from low grade or type I serous carcinoma in behavior, appearance, and underlying mutations. Type I tumors are less likely to be associated with mutations in *BRCA*, instead harboring mutations in *KRAS* or *BRAF*. Recently it has become clear that these high grade tumors in *BRCA* patients arise from a precursor lesion in the fallopian tube, serous tubal intraepithelial carcinoma (STIC). STIC lesions often predate high grade serous tumors and have similar mutations in *P53*. Prophylactic bilateral salpingo-oophorectomy is reported to reduce the risk of developing pelvic cancer by as much as 90%.

Cervix

In the United States, the incidence of invasive cervical cancer is relatively low due to the success of Pap screening. Still, in some countries of southern Asia, central America, and sub-Saharan Africa cervical cancer is still for women the most common cause of death from cancer. The most common cause of cervical carcinoma is human papillomavirus (HPV) infection.

HPV is a double stranded DNA virus with many different serologic subtypes. These subtypes are grouped according to their risk for developing squamous carcinoma. The HPV types that are considered carcinogenic are referred to as high risk HPV (HRHPV) and include HPV 16, 18, 31, 33, 35, 39, 45, 51, 52, 56, 58, 59, 68, 73, and 82. Others, such as 6 and 11 are extremely common causes of human infection but do not pose a great cancer risk. The likelihood of malignant transformation appears to relate to 2 variables:

1. the ease with which the viral genome becomes integrated into the host genome

2. the particular gene sequence (alleles) of the viral E6 and E7 genes

That is, HPV infections that result in benign processes are usually associated with an episomal viral DNA, whereas HPV infections that result in malignancy are usually associated with integration of the viral DNA into the host genome. Such integration results in unchecked transcription of 2 viral genes in particular—E6 and E7—that trigger malignant transformation. The E6 and E7 gene products act through several mechanisms, important among them being the inhibition of the retinoblastoma (Rb) and p53 tumor suppressor proteins. The E6 protein is known to bind to the p53 protein, leading to its subsequent degradation through the ubiquitin pathway. The E7 protein interacts with the Rb-E2F complex, blocking Rb inhibition. Uninhibited, E2F can function as a transcriptional activator of the genes involved in cell cycle progression. This biphasic attack on the regulatory apparatus of the cell leads to unregulated cell division. Various serotypes differ in the effectiveness of their respective E6 and E7 proteins to abrogate cellular regulatory machinery. A surrogate marker of unregulated cell cycle progression, p16, can be used to detect cells that may be infected with high risk HPV subtypes.

The approach most widely advocated for HPV screening is cervical cytology. When a cytologic diagnosis of either low- or high grade squamous intraepithelial lesion (LSIL or HSIL) is rendered, colposcopy is indicated. When a cytologic diagnosis of atypical squamous cells (ASC) is rendered, molecular testing for the presence of high risk HPV (HRHPV) is indicated, followed by colposcopy and biopsy if this is positive. In all 3 instances, the purpose of colposcopy is to exclude a high grade lesion. Several assays are currently available for the molecular detection of HPV in cervical samples, most of which are performed on the same liquid-based collection system used to prepare the slide for cytologic screening. The most common assay is a solution-phase hybridization using labeled RNA probes. Successful hybridization of the probes (with any viral DNA present in the sample) is detected by enzymatic reaction. This assay may be used to detect HRHPV specifically, or it may be used to detect low-risk HPV. Such assays have much higher sensitivity than cytology, but they are positive in a large number of women with no lesion (low specificity); hence the recommendation for testing only in the presence of an atypical cytology.

Endometrium

Type I endometrial adenocarcinomas, including those with endometrioid, mucinous, and secretory morphology, are often estrogen-dependent and low grade. Type I tumors typically demonstrate mutations in mismatch repair genes, with associated microsatellite instability, and mutations in *PTEN*, *KRAS*, and *CTNNB1* (β-catenin). Type II tumors, serous papillary and clear cell carcinoma, are high grade estrogen unresponsive tumors. These tumors are more likely to have mutations of *HER2* and *P53*.

Endometrial stromal tumors arise from the mesenchymal stroma of the uterus. The translocation t(7;17)(p15;q21) has been found in a significant number of cases of endometrial stromal sarcoma (ESS). The translocation creates a chimeric protein between the *JAZF1* gene on chromosome 7 and the *JJAZ1* on chromosome 17. The translocation is found in the majority of cases of ESS, but has also been found in a number of endometrial stromal nodules and neoplastic undifferentiated endometrial sarcomas, thereby limiting its diagnostic specificity for ESS.

Gestational trophoblastic disease

Partial moles are most commonly derived from the fertilization of an egg by 2 sperm. Partial mole is triploid (usually 69, XXY) and may be found in association with a triploid fetus. Complete moles are derived from the fertilization of a blighted ovum (one without genetic material), either by a single sperm followed by duplication of genetic material or by 2 sperm. Complete moles are diploid, but composed entirely of paternal genetic information. Historically, morphology and ploidy analysis has been used to distinguish between the complete and partial mole. Chromosomal enumeration can distinguish partial moles from hydropic abortuses. However, hydropic products of conception can resemble complete molar pregnancies, and both are diploid.

Immunohistochemical stains for a paternally-imprinted gene, *P57* have shown promise as a way of distinguishing complete molar pregnancies. Complete moles show no staining for *P57*, while the nuclei of intermediate trophoblastic cells will stain in a partial mole or hydropic pregnancy. In addition, STR analysis of potential molar pregnancies has been used for classification purposes. By comparing the STR haplotype of the presumed molar pregnancy to maternal tissue or blood one can determine the origin of the genetic material in the products of conception. If a diploid conceptus has evidence of maternal STRs, then one can exclude a complete mole.

Other tumor syndromes

Tuberous sclerosis complex (Bourneville syndrome)

Named for 2 cardinal features of the disorder, the tuber-like lesions of the cerebral cortex and the periventricular calcification, tuberous sclerosis presents with a myriad of findings. The Tuberous Sclerosis Alliance has proposed criteria for the clinical diagnosis of tuberous sclerosis. The major criteria include facial angiofibroma ("adenoma sebaceum"), subungual or periungual fibroma ("Koenen tumor"), 3 or more hypomelanotic macules ("ash leaf spots"), connective tissue nevus ("Shagreen patch"), retinal hamartomas, cerebral cortical tuber, subependymal nodule, subependymal giant cell astrocytoma, cardiac rhabdomyomas, lymphangioleiomyomatosis (LAM) f7.51, and renal angiomyolipoma. Minor criteria include dental enamel pits, hamartomatous rectal polyps, bone cysts, cerebral white matter radial migration lines, gingival fibromas, nonrenal hamartomas, retinal achromic patch, cutaneous symmetric hypopigmented macules, and multiple renal cysts.

As is evident from the listed criteria, tuberous sclerosis is a multisystem disorder with a predilection to development of mainly benign lesions characterized by a variety of mostly benign tumors. There is, however, an increased risk of malignant renal neoplasms, including clear cell renal cell carcinoma.

TSC is caused by autosomal dominant inheritance or sporadic mutation in 1 of 2 genes. Most (80%) cases are due to mutations in the *TSC1* gene, located on chromosome 9q34, which encodes the protein hamartin. The remaining cases are due to mutations in the *TSC2* gene, located on chromosome 16p13, which encodes the protein tuberin. ~60% of TSC cases arise sporadically, reflecting the high rate of de novo mutations.

Nevoid basal cell carcinoma syndrome (Gorlin Goltz syndrome)

Nevoid basal cell carcinoma syndrome, as first described by Gorlin and Goltz, is characterized primarily by odontogenic keratocysts, multiple basal cell carcinomas, and bifid ribs. Additional anatomic findings may include calcification of the falx cerebri, palmoplantar pits, and frontal bossing with coarse facies. The tumor predisposition also includes a high rate of medulloblastoma, rhabdomyosarcoma, and meningioma. In a large study of affected individuals, features present in >1/2 of patients included palmar pits, odontogenic keratocysts, basal cell carcinomas, and calcification of the falx cerebri. Anomalies in the *PTCH1* gene on chromosome 9q22.3 underlie nearly all cases of Gorlin-Goltz syndrome. Mutations in the *PTCH1* gene are inherited in an autosomal dominant manner; penetrance approaches 100%, but expression is variable.

Neurofibromatosis type 1 (NF1; von Recklinghausen disease)

NF1 is caused by mutations in the *NF1* gene encoding neurofibromin on chromosome 17q11.2. Neurofibromatosis is inherited in an autosomal dominant fashion, although 1/2 of cases are sporadic. It is most often diagnosed by a constellation of clinical features. These features, codified in an NIH consensus statement in 1988, include the presence of 6 or more café au lait spots, 2 or more neurofibromas or any single plexiform neurofibroma, groin/axilla freckling (Crowe sign), 2 or

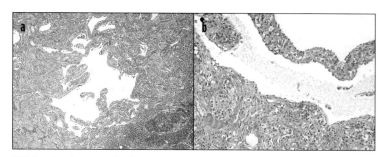

f7.51 Lymphangiomyomatosis of lung

more ocular Lisch nodules, one of the distinctive bony lesions (eg, dysplasia of the sphenoid wing), and a first degree affected relative.

In childhood, NF1 initially presents with multiple café au lait spots and intertriginous (groin, axilla) freckling. Neurofibromas typically begin to emerge in adolescence or early adulthood (diagnosis is often delayed into the second decade as a result). Many women with NF1 experience a rapid increase in the number and size of neurofibromas during pregnancy. Ocular Lisch nodules are fairly common but innocuous. Inconsistent features include vertebral dysplasia, sphenoid wing dysplasia, scoliosis, bone cortical thinning, pseudarthrosis, mental retardation, pulmonic stenosis, and NF1 vasculopathy. The latter most often manifests as renal artery stenosis (arterial dysplasia), with associated hypertension. An appearance resembling Noonan syndrome is seen in ~12% of individuals with NF1.

NF1 results in a predisposition toward certain tumors, including malignant peripheral nerve sheath tumor (MPNST), optic glioma, leukemia, medulloblastoma, pheochromocytoma, ampullary adenocarcinoma of the small intestine, and breast cancer. The lifetime risk for MPNST is 10%. Optic gliomas nearly always take the form of pilocytic astrocytomas and may cause visual loss.

Most mutations of the *NF1* gene result in protein truncation and loss of function of the *NF1* tumor suppressor gene. Most clinically significant *NF1* mutations are nonsense mutations, missense mutations, or microdeletions that, while distributed throughout the gene, cause protein truncation. Discrete point mutations are responsible for only ~10% of cases. Thus, while there are an enormous variety of mutations, the laboratory can screen for ~80% of them with protein truncation tests. FISH can detect the 5-10% of cases that are caused by microdeletions (conventional cytogenetic testing is not sensitive enough). Genetic testing is primarily indicated for prenatal testing and rarely for confirmation in individuals who do not fulfill the diagnostic criteria.

Neurofibromatosis type 2 (NF2; bilateral acoustic neuroma syndrome)

Mutations in the *NF2* gene on chromosome 22q, which encodes the protein merlin, is the cause of NF2. Up to 1/3 of NF2 cases are sporadic (simplex) cases. Much about the nomenclature of this syndrome is confusing. NF2 is characterized by bilateral vestibular nerve (not acoustic nerve) schwannomas (neither neurofibromas nor neuromas occur), and it has almost no relationship to NF1. The disease first manifests around the age of 20, and nearly all affected individuals have bilateral vestibular schwannomas by the age of 30. Early detection is important, to prevent deafness. Schwannomas may arise in association with other nerves as well, and there is an increased tendency to develop meningiomas, ependymomas, and pilocytic astrocytomas.

Li-Fraumeni syndrome

Mutations in the tumor suppressor gene *TP53* (p53) are found in ~50% of malignancies, regardless of type, and are the most common genetic anomaly found in malignant tumors. An inherited (germline) mutation in *TP53* causes Li-Fraumeni syndrome; as might be predicted, Li-Fraumeni is associated with a tendency to develop numerous widespread malignancies,

Early reports focused on the association of Li-Fraumeni syndrome with a number of tumors, including osteosarcoma, soft tissue sarcoma, breast cancer, adrenal cortical carcinoma, and acute leukemia. It seems now that there is no limit to the variety of tumors, however, with well-documented documented increased risk for gastric adenocarcinoma, colorectal carcinoma, pancreatic carcinoma, esophageal carcinoma, germ cell tumors, melanoma, Wilms tumor, and malignancy of the central nervous system. Perhaps the only characteristic features of Li-Fraumeni are (1) that any given tumor type arises at a younger age than would be expected for a sporadic tumor of the same type, and (2) that multiple disparate tumors may arise in the same person. About 40% of those with Li-Fraumeni have developed a malignancy by the age of 20 years, 60% by age 40, and 90% by age 60.

Especially concerning for Li-Fraumeni is the appearance of adrenocortical carcinoma in a young adult; >1/2 such cases are associated with Li-Fraumeni syndrome. Adrenocortical carcinoma is rare overall, and they often occur in children with Li-Fraumeni syndrome. Thus, the occurrence of an adrenocortical carcinoma in a child or young adult is sufficient indication for Li-Fraumeni testing.

About 85% of cases are due to *TP53* mutations (chromosome 17p); mutations in the *CHEK2* gene (whose product is one of the intracellular targets of p53) has been identified in a minority of cases. While there are a variety of *TP53* mutations, most arise between exons 4 through 9 (or amino acids 91 through 309). This permits good (95%) sensitivity for sequencing analyses confined to this portion of the gene.

Immunohistochemistry can be performed for p53 expression. Most mutated forms of p53, though nonfunctional as tumor suppressor proteins, have a prolonged half life within the cell (the mutated forms are able to avoid protein degradation). Thus, tumors with *TP53* mutations (and *decreased* p53 activity) have overexpression of p53.

Aniridia/WAGR syndrome

Aniridia may be a sporadic or inherited trait, usually occurring as an isolated finding; however, in some it occurs as part of a Mendelian syndrome that includes Wilms tumor, aniridia, genitourinary anomalies, and mental retardation (WAGR syndrome). The WAGR syndrome is a contiguous gene syndrome in which a microdeletion spanning 11p13 affects several genes. In ~20-30% of cases, the deletion is detectable by high-resolution chromosome studies. FISH studies, utilizing several probes that span the affected band, can also be diagnostically useful.

Beckwith-Wiedemann syndrome

Beckwith-Wiedemann syndrome can be caused by any one of several defects, the common thread being abnormal transcription of genes within the 11p15.5 band. 11p normally is an imprinted domain (expression depends upon whether inherited from the mother or from the father), one in which maternally derived alleles are preferentially expressed. Several genes are located within 11p, including:

1. *KCNQ1*, encoding a potassium channel, and the same gene implicated in Romano-Ward and Jervell Lange-Nielsen syndromes
2. *IGF2*, encoding an insulin-like growth factor (IGF)
3. *H19*, encoding a nontranslated mRNA
4. *CDKN1C*, encoding a cyclin-dependent kinase inhibitor

Embryonal tumors (Wilms tumor and hepatoblastoma, in particular) occur with a high rate in Beckwith-Wiedemann syndrome. The syndrome may become apparent in utero, with a fetus that is large for gestational age (LGA) and has polyhydramnios. At birth, the placenta is large, and the umbilical cord is abnormally long. Additional features that may be identified at birth include macrosomia, macroglossia, hemihypertrophy (asymmetric growth), omphalocele (exomphalos), and anterior ear creases or pits. A peculiar adrenocortical cytomegaly has been described in patients with Beckwith-Wiedemann, and renal anomalies (renal medullary dysplasia, nephrocalcinosis, medullary sponge kidney, and nephromegaly) are very common.

About 80% of cases are inherited, and the remaining are sporadic (simplex) cases. Beckwith-Wiedemann is primarily a clinical diagnosis. The molecular diagnosis is problematic, as no single finding defines it. Conventional cytogenetics can identify an anomaly at 11p15 in only ~1% of cases. FISH can identify another 1-2%. Methylation assays are capable of finding abnormalities in >1/2 of patients (either gain or loss of methylation). Uniparental disomy studies can identify abnormalities in ~15% of cases. Lastly, a single gene defect in *CDKN1C* appears to underlie around 10% of simplex cases and up to 40% of familial cases.

Chromosomal breakage syndromes

Among this group of disorders, which are usually transmitted in an autosomal recessive fashion, the unifying feature is a tendency in cell culture to exhibit elevated rates of chromosomal breakage or instability. Underlying this tendency are defects in DNA repair mechanisms, and the clinical effect is a predisposition to cancer. Chromosomal breakage disorders are numerous and include Bloom syndrome, ataxia telangiectasia, Nijmegen syndrome, Fanconi syndrome, and xeroderma pigmentosa. This group of disorders should be conceptually distinguished from the trinucleotide repeat disorders associated with the presence of "fragile sites" which do not cause a cancer predisposition.

Xeroderma pigmentosa (XP) is characterized by a 1,000-fold increased risk of cutaneous malignancy, including basal cell carcinoma, squamous cell carcinoma, and melanoma, resulting from extreme sensitivity to ultraviolet (UV) light. Freckling begins by the age of 2 years, and a cutaneous tumor typically arises by the age of 20 years. XP is caused by autosomal recessive inheritance of a mutation in one of the genes of the nucleotide excision repair complementation groups, including *XPA* through *XPG*, whose function is to repair UV induced DNA damage. Some forms of XP are associated with neurologic deficits and others with ocular manifestations. Affected patients must assiduously avoid UV light exposure.

PTEN-related disorders: Cowden syndrome, Bannayan-Riley-Ruvalcaba syndrome & Proteus syndrome

This family of disorders is associated with mutations in the gene *PTEN* on 10q23. PTEN, which stands for phosphatase and tensin homolog, encodes a phosphatidylinositol 3,4,5-trisphosphate 3-phosphatase negatively regulating a key compound in the AKT signaling pathway. All the PTEN-related disorders demonstrate a tendency to form hamartomatous tumors.

In Cowden syndrome these are most commonly hamartomatous intestinal polyps. In addition there can be multiple lipomas and fibromas, malformations of the genitourinary tract, and mucocutaneous lesions such as facial trichilemmomas, papillomas, palmoplantar keratoses, and palmoplantar hyperkeratotic pits. Microcephaly and mental retardation are common, and these are strongly associated with cerebellar dysplastic gangliocytoma (Lhermitte-Duclos lesion) f7.52, which is considered pathognomonic. Patients with Cowden syndrome are at an increased risk of carcinoma, including follicular carcinoma of the thyroid gland and carcinomas of the breast, colon, and endometrium.

Bannayan-Riley-Ruvalcaba syndrome has a different presentation with macrocephaly and mental retardation, high birth weight, myopathy, joint hypermobility, pectus excavatum, and scoliosis. Associated tumors include hamartomatous intestinal polyps and pigmented macules of the glans penis.

As the name suggests, Proteus syndrome has a highly variable presentation and demonstrates a pattern of affected individuals consistent with mosaicism; ie, some organs are heavily affected whereas others are entirely spared. Some examples of the syndrome manifest connective tissue nevi (considered pathognomonic), asymmetric limb growth, skull hyperostosis, megaspondylodysplasia of the vertebrae, or visceral overgrowth (especially of spleen and thymus).

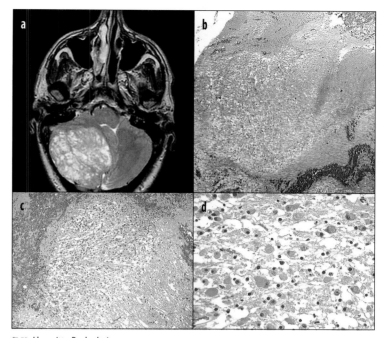

f7.52 Lhermitte-Duclos lesion
a MRI shows cerebellar thickening with enlarged folia & cystic-appearing areas
b-d Histology demonstrates a thickened molecular & internal granular area in which there are nodular collections of dysplastic ganglion cells

Carney complex

Carney complex is an autosomal dominant condition also known as LAMB syndrome (an acronym denoting lentigines, atrial myxoma, and blue nevi) or NAME syndrome (nevi, atrial myxoma, myxoid neurofibroma, and ephelides). Cutaneous lentigines (simple lentigos) are the most common presenting finding, located on the face (particularly the oral and conjunctival mucosa), vagina, and penis. Blue nevi, are common, particularly the cellular blue nevus. Cardiac myxomas occur frequently, at a young age, and may affect any chamber. In addition to the previously mentioned features, there may also be myxomas of the breast, female genital tract, and skin, as well as endocrine tumors such as follicular adenomas of the thyroid gland, pituitary adenomas, and primary pigmented nodular adrenocortical disease (PPNAD), which presents as Cushing disease. Large cell calcifying Sertoli cell tumors arise in most affected males. Note that this unusual tumor is also seen in Peutz-Jeghers syndrome; however, the SCTAT of Peutz-Jeghers is not seen in females with Carney complex. Psammomatous melanotic schwannoma, rare as a sporadic tumor, is common in the Carney complex. Nearly 1/2 the cases of Carney complex are due to mutations in the *PRKAR1A* gene on 17q24. No other genes have yet to be implicated in the remaining cases. Note that the similarly named Carney triad is an entirely different syndrome (triad of gastric GIST, pulmonary chondroma, and extraadrenal paraganglioma).

References

Online references

Association of Molecular Pathology (www.amp.org)

The Association for Molecular Pathology is a professional society dedicated to promulgation of molecular and genetic testing. Their website provides information about the profession of molecular pathology and information for other physicians as well as the public on public policy, testing, education, and other relevant interests to molecular pathology.

Gene Tests (www.genetests.org)

GeneTests.org provides information to physicians and other interested individuals about genetic disease and testing. The website provides informational review materials about selected genetic diseases and has a large database of testing laboratories and the tests that they offer.

Online Mendelian Inheritance in Man (www.ncbi.nlm.nih.gov/omim)

The National Center for Biotechnology Information (NCBI) at the National Library of Medicine has many resources for genetic information. The Online Mendelian Inheritance in Man (OMIM) database is an attempt to correlate genotypic information (eg, sequence, inheritance patterns) with phenotypic information (physical manifestations). The NCBI also has a large database of SNPs and their associated phenotypes.

Literature references

Aaltonen LA, Salovaara R, Kristo P, et al [1998] Incidence of hereditary nonpolyposis colorectal cancer and the feasibility of molecular screening for the disease. *N Engl J Med* 338:1481-7. PMID:9593786.

Aarnio M, Mecklin JP, Aaltonen LA, et al [1995] Lifetime risk of different cancers in hereditary non-polyposis colorectal cancer (HNPCC) syndrome. *Int J Cancer* 64:430-3. PMID:8550246.

Ackerman MJ, Clapham DE [1997] Ion channels---basic science and clinical disease. *N Engl J Med* 336:1575-86. PMID:9164815.

Ackerman MJ, Siu BL, Sturner WQ, Tester DJ, Valdivia CR, Makielski JC, Towbin JA [2001] Postmortem molecular analysis of SCN5A defects in sudden infant death syndrome. *JAMA* 286:2264-9. PMID:11710892.

Adams PC, Deugnier Y, Moirand R, Brissot P [1997] The relationship between iron overload, clinical symptoms, and age in 410 patients with genetic hemochromatosis. *Hepatology* 25(1):162-166. PMID:8985284.

Adams D, Samuel D, Goulon-Goeau C, et al [2000] The course and prognostic factors of familial amyloid polyneuropathy after liver transplantation. *Brain* 123:1495-504. PMID:10869060.

Adeva M, El-Youssef M, Rossetti S, et al [2006] Clinical and molecular characterization defines a broadened spectrum of autosomal recessive polycystic kidney disease (ARPKD). *Medicine* 85:1-21. PMID:16523049.

Ahmad F, Li D, Karibe A, et al [1998] Localization of a gene responsible for arrhythmogenic right ventricular dysplasia to chromosome 3p23. *Circulation* 98:2791-5. PMID:9860777.

Albers S, Levy HL, Irons M, et al [2001] Compound heterozygosity in 4 asymptomatic siblings with medium-chain acyl-CoA dehydrogenase deficiency. *J Inherit Metab Dis* 24:417-8. PMID:11486912.

Albright F, Butler AM, Hampton AO, Smith PH [1937] Syndrome characterized by osteitis fibrosa disseminata, areas of pigmentation and endocrine dysfunction, with precocious puberty in females: Report of 5 cases. *N Engl J Med* 216: 727-746.

Alcalai R, Metzger S, Rosenheck S, Meiner V, Chajek-Shaul T [2003] A recessive mutation in desmoplakin causes arrhythmogenic right ventricular dysplasia, skin disorder, and woolly hair. *J Am Coll Cardiol* 42:319-27. PMID:12875771.

Algar E, Brickell S, Deeble G, Amor D, Smith P [2000] Analysis of CDKN1C in Beckwith Wiedemann syndrome. *Hum Mutat* 15:497-508. PMID:10862080.

Allinen M, Huusko P, Mantyniemi S, Launonen V, Winqvist R [2001] Mutation analysis of the CHK2 gene in families with hereditary breast cancer. *Br J Cancer* 85:209-12. PMID:11461078.

Altiok S. Molecular markers in cervical cytology [2003] *Clin Lab Med* 23:709-728. PMID:14560536.

Amberla K, Waljas M, Tuominen S, et al [2004] Insidious cognitive decline in CADASIL. *Stroke* 35:1598-602. PMID:15143298.

Ando Y, Nakamura M, Araki S [2005] Transthyretin related familial amyloidotic polyneuropathy. *Arch Neurol* 62:1057-62. PMID:16009758.

Andre F, Pusztai L [2006] Molecular classification of breast cancer: implications for selection of adjuvant chemotherapy. *Nat Clin Prac Onc* 3(11):621-632. PMID:17080180.

Ang KK, Harris J, Wheeler R, Weber R, et al [2010] Human papillomavirus and survival of patients with oropharyngeal cancer. *N Engl J Med.* 363(1):24-35. PMID:20530316.

Angrist M, Bolk S, Thiel B, et al [1995] Mutation analysis of the RET receptor tyrosine kinase in Hirschsprung disease. *Hum Mol Genet* 4:821-30. PMID:7633441.

Angrist M, Bolk S, Halushka M, et al [1996] Germline mutations in glial cell line derived neurotrophic factor (GDNF) and RET in a Hirschsprung disease patient. *Nat Genet* 14:341-4. PMID:8896568.

Antonescu CR, Tschernyavsky SJ, Woodruff JM, et al [2002] Molecular diagnosis of clear cell sarcoma: detection of EWS-ATF1 and MITF-M transcripts and histopathological and ultrastructural analysis of 12 cases. *J Mol Diag* 4:44-52. PMID:11826187.

Antzelevitch C, Brugada P, Brugada J, Brugada R, Towbin JA, Nademanee K [2003] Brugada syndrome 1992 2002: a historical perspective. *J Am Coll Cardiol* 41:1665-71. PMID:12767644.

Aono S, Adachi Y, Uyama E, et al [1995] Analysis of genes for bilirubin UDP-glucuronosyltransferase in Gilbert's syndrome. *Lancet* 345(8955):958-9. PMID:7715297.

Argani P, Antonescu CR, Couturier J, et al [2002] PRCC-TFE3 renal carcinomas morphologic, immunohistochemical, ultrastructural, and molecular analysis of an entity associated with the t(X;1)(p11.2;q21). *Am J Surg Pathol* 26(12): 1553-1566. PMID:12459622.

Argani P, Lae M, Hutchinson B, et al [2005] Renal carcinomas with the t(6;11)(p21;q12): clinicopathologic features and demonstration of the specific alpha-tfeb gene fusion by immunohistochemistry, RT-PCR, and DNA PCR. *Am J Surg Pathol* 29:230-240. PMID:15644781.

Argov Z, Eisenberg I, Grabov-Nardini G, Sadeh M, Wirguin I, Soffer D, Mitrani-Rosenbaum S [2003] Hereditary inclusion body myopathy: the Middle Eastern genetic cluster. *Neurology* 60:1519-1523. PMID:12743242.

Ariyurek Y, Lantinga-van Leeuwen I, Spruit L, Ravine D, Breuning MH, Peters DJ [2004] Large deletions in the polycystic kidney disease 1 (PKD1) gene. *Hum Mutat* 23:99 PMID:14695542.

Ars E, Kruyer H, Morell M, Pros E, Serra E, Ravella A, Estivill X, Lazaro C [2003] Recurrent mutations in the NF1 gene are common among neurofibromatosis type 1 patients. *J Med Genet* 40:e82 PMID:12807981.

Aylward EH, Li Q, Stine OC, et al [1997] Longitudinal change in basal ganglia volume in patients with Huntington's disease. *Neurology* 48:394 9 PMID:9040728.

Aylward EH, Sparks BF, Field KM, et al [2004] Onset and rate of striatal atrophy in preclinical Huntington disease. *Neurology* 63:66-72. PMID:15249612.

Bacon BR, Powell LW, Adams PC, et al [1999] Molecular medicine and hemochromatosis: at the crossroads. *Gastroenterology* 116:193-207. PMID:9869618.

Balakumaran BS, Febbo PG [2006] New insights into prostate cancer biology. *Hematol Oncol Clin N Am* 20:773-796. PMID:16861114.

Bane AL, Beck JC, Bleiweiss I, et al [2007] BRCA2 mutation-associated breast cancers exhibit a distinguishing phenotype based on morphology and molecular profiles from tissue microarrays. *Am J Surg Pathol* 31:121-128. PMID:17197928.

Bang YJ, Van Cutsem E, Feyereislova A, et al [2010] Trastuzumab in combination with chemotherapy vs chemotherapy alone for HER2-positive advanced gastric or gastro-oesophageal junction cancer (ToGA): a phase 3, open-label, randomised controlled trial. *Lancet* 376: 687-697. PMID:20728210.

Barhanin J, Lesage F, Guillemare E, Finc M, Lazdunski M, Romey G [1996] KVLQT1 and IsK (minK) proteins associate to form the IKs cardiac potassium current. *Nature* 384:78-80. PMID:8900282.

Baser ME, Kuramoto L, Joe H, et al [2004] Genotype-phenotype correlations for nervous system tumors in neurofibromatosis 2: a population-based study. *Am J Hum Genet* 75:231-9. PMID:15190457.

Baser ME, Friedman JM, Evans DG [2006] Increasing the specificity of diagnostic criteria for schwannomatosis. *Neurology* 66:730-2. PMID:16534111.

Basson CT, Cowley GS, Solomon SD, et al [1995] The clinical and genetic spectrum of the Holt-Oram syndrome (heart-hand syndrome). *N Engl J Med* 330:885-91. PMID:8114858.

Bates MD, Balistreri WF [2004] The liver and biliary system. In: *Nelson Textbook of Pediatrics*, 17th ed. Philadelphia: Saunders, Elsevier Science.

Belz MM, Fick-Brosnahan GM, Hughes RL, et al [2003] Recurrence of intracranial aneurysms in autosomal-dominant polycystic kidney disease. *Kidney Int* 63:1824-30. PMID:12675859.

Ben-Yosef T, Ness SL, Madeo AC, Bar-Lev A, Wolfman JH, Ahmed ZM, Desnick RJ, Willner JP, Avraham KB, Ostrer H, Oddoux C, Griffith AJ, Friedman TB [2003] A mutation of PCDH15 among Ashkenazi Jews with the Type 1 Usher syndrome. *N Engl J Med* 348:1664-70. PMID:12711741.

Bennett MJ, Rinaldo P, Millington DS, Tanaka K, Yokota I, Coates PM [1991] Medium-chain acyl-CoA dehydrogenase deficiency: post-mortem diagnosis in a case of sudden infant death and neonatal diagnosis of an affect sibling. *Pediatr Pathol* 11:889-95. PMID:1775402.

Benson MD [1996] Leptomeningeal amyloid and variant transthyretins. *Am J Pathol* 148:351-4. PMID:8579096.

Berg AO, Armstrong K, Botkin J, et al [2009] Recommendations from the EGAPP Working Group: genetic testing strategies in newly diagnosed individuals with colorectal cancer aimed at reducing morbidity and mortality from Lynch syndrome in relatives. *Genet Med* 11(1):35-41. PMID:19125126.

Bergmann C, Senderek J, Kupper F, et al [2004a] PKHD1 mutations in autosomal recessive polycystic kidney disease (ARPKD). *Hum Mutat* 23:453-63. PMID:15108277.

Bergmann C, Senderek J, Schneider F, et al [2004b] PKHD1 mutations in families requesting prenatal diagnosis for autosomal recessive polycystic kidney disease (ARPKD). *Hum Mutat* 23:487-95. PMID:15108281.

Bergmann C, Senderek J, Windelen E, et al [2005] Clinical consequences of PKHD1 mutations in 164 patients with autosomal-recessive polycystic kidney disease (ARPKD). *Kidney Int* 67:829-48. PMID:15698423.

Berko BA, Swift M [1987] X-linked dilated cardiomyopathy. *N Engl J Med* 316:1186-91. PMID:3574369.

Bernier FP, Spaetgens R [2006] The geneticist's role in adult congenital heart disease. *Cardiol Clin* 24: 557-569. PMID:17098511.

Bernstein D [2004] Congenital heart disease. In: *Nelson Textbook of Pediatrics*, 17th ed. Philadelphia: Saunders, Elsevier Science.

Bertram L, Tanzi RE [2004] Alzheimer's disease: one disorder, too many genes? *Human Molecular Genetics* 13(Review Issue 1):R135-R141 PMID:14764623.

Beutler E, Felitti VJ, Koziol JA, Ho NJ, Gelbart T [2002] Penetrance of 845G→A (C282Y) HFE hereditary haemochromatosis mutation in the USA. *Lancet* 359:211-8. PMID:11812557.

Bhaijee F, Pepper DJ, Pitman KT, Bell D [2011] New developments in the molecular pathogenesis of head and neck tumors: a review of tumor-specific fusion oncogenes in mucoepidermoid carcinoma, adenoid cystic carcinoma, and NUT midline carcinoma. *Ann Diagn Pathol* 15(1):69-77. PMID:21238915.

Bhatia E, Durie P, Zielenski J, et al [2000] Mutations in the cystic fibrosis transmembrane regulator gene in patients with tropical calcific pancreatitis. *Am J Gastroenterol* 95(12):3658-9. PMID:11151920.

Biaggioni I, Goldstein DS, Atkinson T, Robertson D [1990] Dopamine-beta-hydroxylase deficiency in humans. *Neurology* 40:370-3. PMID:2300263.

Biegel JA, Conard K, Brooks JJ [1993] Translocation (11;22)(p13;q12): primary change in intraabdominal desmoplastic small round cell tumor. *Genes Chromosomes Cancer* 7:119-21. PMID:7687454.

Biesecker LG, Happle R, Mulliken JB, et al [1999] Proteus syndrome: diagnostic criteria, differential diagnosis, and patient evaluation. *Am J Med Genet* 84:389-95. PMID:10360391.

Bijwaard KE, Fetsch JF, Przygodzki R, et al [2002] Detection of SYT-SSX fusion transcripts in archival synovial sarcomas by real time reverse transcriptase-polymerase chain reaction. *J Mol Diag* 4:59-64. PMID:11826189.

Birch JM, Alston RD, McNally RJ, Evans DG, Kelsey AM, Harris M, Eden OB, Varley JM [2001] Relative frequency and morphology of cancers in carriers of germline TP53 mutations. *Oncogene* 20:4621-8. PMID:11498785.

Bird TD [2005a] Genetic factors in Alzheimer's disease. *N Engl J Med* 352(9):862-864. PMID:15745976.

Bird TD [2005b] Myotonic dystrophy type 1 (Steinert's disease). *GeneTests.Org*. 22 November.

Birt AR, Hogg GR, Dube WJ [1977] Hereditary multiple fibrofolliculomas with trichodiscomas and acrochordons. *Arch Dermatol* 113:1674-1677. PMID:596896.

Boardman LA, Thibodeau SN, Schaid DJ, et al [1998] Increased risk for cancer in patients with the Peutz-Jeghers syndrome. *Ann Intern Med* 128:896-9. PMID:9634427.

Boardman LA, Couch FJ, Burgart LJ, et al [2000] Genetic heterogeneity in Peutz-Jeghers syndrome. *Hum Mutat* 16:23-30. PMID:10874301.

Boehmer AL, Brinkmann O, Bruggenwirth H, et al [2001] Genotype vs phenotype in families with androgen insensitivity syndrome. *J Clin Endocrinol Metab* 86:4151-60. PMID:11549642.

Boerkoel CF, Takashima H, Garcia CA, et al [2002] Charcot-Marie-Tooth disease and related neuropathies: Mutation distribution and genotype-phenotype correlation. *Ann Neurol* 51:190-201. PMID:11835375.

Boito CA, Melacini P, Vianello A, et al [2005] Clinical and molecular characterization of patients with limb-girdle muscular dystrophy type 2I. *Arch Neurol* 62:1894-9. PMID:16344347.

Boles RG, Buck EA, Blitzer MG, et al [1998] Retrospective biochemical screening of fatty acid oxidation disorders in postmortem livers of 418 cases of sudden death in the first year of life. *J Pediatr* 132:924-33. PMID:9627580.

Bonnardeaux A, Bichet DG [2004] Inherited disorders of the renal tubule. In: *Brenner & Rector's The Kidney*. Philadelphia: Elsevier.

Bonneau D, Longy M [2000] Mutations of the human PTEN gene. *Hum Mutat* 16:109-22. PMID:10923032.

Boocock GR, Morrison JA, Popovic M, Richards N, Ellis L, Durie PR, Rommens JM [2003] Mutations in SBDS are associated with Shwachman-Diamond syndrome. *Nat Genet* 33:97-101. PMID:12496757.

Bosma PJ, Chowdhury JR, Bakker C, et al [1995] The genetic basis of the reduced expression of bilirubin UDP-glucuronosyltransferase 1 in Gilbert's syndrome. *N Engl J Med* 333(18):1171-5. PMID:7565971.

Brandi ML, Gagel RF, Angeli A, et al [2001] Guidelines for diagnosis and therapy of MEN type 1 and type 2. *J Clin Endocrinol Metab* 86:5658-71. PMID:11739416.

Brandt J, Bylsma FW, Gross R, Stine OC, Ranen N, Ross CA [1996] Trinucleotide repeat length and clinical progression in Huntington's disease. *Neurology* 46:527-31. PMID:8614526.

Branski D, Fasano A, Troncone R [2006] Latest developments in the pathogenesis and treatment of celiac disease. *J Pediatr* 149:295-300. PMID:16939736.

Brauckhoff M, Gimm O, Hinze R, Ukkat J, Brauckhoff K, Dralle H [2002] Papillary thyroid carcinoma in patients with RET protooncogene germline mutation. *Thyroid* 12:557-61. PMID:12193298.

Breitner JC [1996] APOE genotyping and Alzheimer's disease. *Lancet* 347:1184-5. PMID:8609780.

Brett M, Persey MR, Reilly MM, et al [1999] Transthyretin Leu12Pro is associated with systemic, neuropathic and leptomeningeal amyloidosis. *Brain* 122(2):183-90. PMID:10071047.

Brown GJ, St John DJ, Macrae FA, Aittomaki K [2001] Cancer risk in young women at risk of hereditary nonpolyposis colorectal cancer: implications for gynecologic surveillance. *Gynecol Oncol* 80:346-9. PMID:11263929.

Bruder E, Passera O, Harms D, et al [2004] Morphologic and molecular characterization of renal cell carcinoma in children and young adults. *Am J Surg Pathol* 28:1117-1132. PMID:15316311.

Brugada P, Brugada J [1992] Right bundle-branch block, persistent ST segment elevation and sudden cardiac death: a distinct clinical and electrocardiographic syndrome. A multicenter report. *J Am Coll Cardiol* 20:1391-6. PMID:1309182.

Brugada J, Brugada R, Brugada P [2003] Determinants of sudden cardiac death in individuals with the electrocardiographic pattern of Brugada syndrome and no previous cardiac arrest. *Circulation* 108:3092-6. PMID:14623800.

Brugge KL, Nichols SL, Salmon DP, et al [1994] Cognitive impairment in adults with Down's syndrome: similarities to early cognitive changes in Alzheimer's disease. *Neurology* 44:232-8. PMID:8309564.

Brunelli M, Eble JN, Zhang S, et al [2005] Eosinophilic and classic chromophobe renal cell carcinomas have similar frequent losses of multiple chromosomes from among chromosomes 1, 2, 6, 10, and 17, and this pattern of genetic abnormality is not present in renal oncocytoma. *Mod Pathol* 18:161-169. PMID:15467713.

Bulaj ZJ, Griffen LM, Jorde LB, et al [1996] Clinical and biochemical abnormalities in people heterozygous for hemochromatosis. *N Engl J Med* 335:1799-805. PMID:8943161.

Burdick JS, Tompson ML [2006] Anatomy, histology, embryology, and developmental anomalies of the pancreas. In: *Sleisenger & Fordtran's Gastrointestinal and Liver Disease*, 8th ed. Philadelphia: Saunders Elsevier.

Burgart LJ [2005] Testing for defective DNA mismatch repair in colorectal carcinoma: a practical guide. *Arch Pathol Lab Med* 129:1385-1389. PMID:16253016.

Burger B, Uhlhaas S, Mangold E, et al [2002] Novel de novo mutation of MADH4/SMAD4 in a patient with juvenile polyposis. *Am J Med Genet* 110:289-91. PMID:12116240.

Burstein HJ [2005] The distinctive nature of HER2-positive breast cancers. *N Engl J Med* 353(16):1652-1654. PMID:16236735.

Burt MJ, George PM, Upton JD, et al [1998] The significance of haemochromatosis gene mutations in the general population: implications for screening. *Gut* 43:830-6. PMID:9824612.

Bushby KM, Thambyayah M, Gardner-Medwin D [1991] Prevalence and incidence of Becker muscular dystrophy. *Lancet* 337:1022-4. PMID:1673177.

Bushby KM [1999] Making sense of the limb-girdle muscular dystrophies. *Brain* 122(8):1403-20. PMID:10430828.

Butnor KJ, Guinee DG [2006] Pleuropulmonary pathology of Birt-Hogg-Dubé syndrome. *Am J Surg Pathol* 30:395-399. PMID:16538061.

Buxbaum JN, Tagoe CE [2000] The genetics of the amyloidoses. *Annu Rev Med* 51:543-69. PMID:10774481.

Buzza M, Dagher H, Wang YY, Wilson D, Babon JJ, Cotton RG, Savige J [2003] Mutations in the COL4A4 gene in thin basement membrane disease. *Kidney Int* 63:447-53. PMID:12631110.

Campbell R, Gosden CM, Bonthron DT [1994] Parental origin of transcription from the human GNAS1 gene. *J Med Genet* 31:607-614. PMID:7815417.

Carney JA, Hruska LS, Beauchamp GD, Gordon H [1986] Dominant inheritance of the complex of myxomas, spotty pigmentation, and endocrine overactivity. *Mayo Clin Proc* 61:165-72. PMID:3945116.

Carney JA [2005] Familial multiple endocrine neoplasia: the first 100 years. *Am J Surg Pathol* 29:254-274. PMID:15644784.

Carrell RW, Lomas DA [1997] Conformational disease. *Lancet* 350:134-8. PMID:9228977.

Carrell RW, Lomas DA [2002] Alpha 1-antitrypsin deficiency: a model for conformational diseases. *N Engl J Med* 346(1):45-53. PMID:11778003.

Carter BS, Beaty TH, Steinberg GD, Childs B, Walsh PC [1992] Mendelian inheritance of familial prostate cancer. *Proc Natl Acad Sci USA* 89:3367-3371. PMID:1565627.

Casey M, Mah C, Merliss AD, et al [1998] Identification of a novel genetic locus for familial cardiac myxomas and Carney complex. *Circulation* 98:2560-6. PMID:9843463.

Celli J, van Bokhoven H, Brunner HG [2003] Feingold syndrome: clinical review and genetic mapping. *Am J Med Genet* 122:294-300. PMID:14518066.

Chabriat H, Levy C, Taillia H, et al [1998] Patterns of MRI lesions in CADASIL. *Neurology* 51:452-7. PMID:9710018.

Chapusot C, Martin L, Puig PL, et al [2004] What is the best way to assess microsatellite instability status in colorectal cancer? Study on a population base of 462 colorectal cancers. *Am J Surg Pathol* 28:1553-1559. PMID:15577673.

Cheadle JP, Reeve MP, Sampson JR, Kwiatkowski DJ [2000] Molecular genetic advances in tuberous sclerosis. *Hum Genet* 107:97-114. PMID:11030407.

Chen Q, Zhang D, Gingell RL, et al [1999] Homozygous deletion in KVLQT1 associated with Jervell and Lange-Nielsen syndrome. *Circulation* 1999;99:1344-7. PMID:10077519.

Chen L, Lee L, Kudlow BA, et al [2003] LMNA mutations in atypical Werner's syndrome. *Lancet* 362:440-5. PMID:12927431.

Cheng H, Xu C, Costa DB, Powell CA, Halmos B [2010] Molecular testing in lung cancer: the time is now. *Curr Oncol Rep* 12:335-348. PMID:20623207.

Cheung PK, McCormick C, Crawford BE, Esko JD, Tufaro F, Duncan G [2001] Etiological point mutations in the hereditary multiple exostoses gene EXT1: a functional analysis of heparan sulfate polymerase activity. *Am J Hum Genet* 69:55-66. PMID:11391482.

Chung EB, Enzinger FM [1983] Malignant melanoma of soft parts: a reassessment of clear cell sarcoma. *Am J Surg Pathol* 7:405-413. PMID:6614306.

Church J, Simmang C [2003] Practice parameters for the treatment of patients with dominantly inherited colorectal cancer (familial adenomatous polyposis and hereditary nonpolyposis colorectal cancer). *Dis Colon Rectum* 46:1001-12. PMID:12907889.

Cohen MS, Moley JF [2003] Surgical treatment of medullary thyroid carcinoma. *J Intern Med* 253:616-26. PMID:12755957.

Collins MT, Sarlis NJ, Merino MJ, et al [2003] Thyroid carcinoma in the McCune-Albright syndrome: contributory role of activating G(s)-alpha mutations. *J Clin Endocr Metab* 88:4413-4417. PMID:12970318.

Connors LH, Lim A, Prokaeva T, Roskens VA, Costello CE [2003] Tabulation of human transthyretin (TTR) variants, 2003. *Amyloid* 10:160-84. PMID:14640030.

Corrado D, Basso C, Schiavon M, Thiene G [1998] Screening for hypertrophic cardiomyopathy in young athletes. *N Engl J Med* 339:364-9. PMID:9691102.

Cossu-Rocca P, Eble JN, Delahunt B, Zhang S, Martignoni G, Brunelli M, Cheng L [2006] Renal mucinous tubular and spindle carcinoma lacks the gains of chromosomes 7 and 17 and losses of chromosome Y that are prevalent in papillary renal cell carcinoma. *Mod Pathol* 19:488-493. PMID:16554730.

Cox GF, Kunkel LM [1997] Dystrophies and heart disease. *Curr Opin Cardiol* 12:329-43. PMID:9243091.

Cunningham JM, Kim CY, Christensen ER, et al [2001] The frequency of hereditary defective mismatch repair in a prospective series of unselected colorectal carcinomas. *Am J Hum Genet* 69:780-90. PMID:11524701.

Curless RG [2001] Use of "unidentified bright objects" on MRI for diagnosis of neurofibromatosis 1 in children. *Neurology* 55:1067-8. PMID:11061281.

Curran ME, Splawski I, Timothy KW, Vincent GM, Green ED, Keating MT [1995] A molecular basis for cardiac arrhythmia: HERG mutations cause long QT syndrome. *Cell* 80:795-803. PMID:7889573.

Cuthbert AP, Fisher SA, Mirza MM, et al [2002] The contribution of NOD2 gene mutations to the risk and site of disease in inflammatory bowel disease. *Gastroenterology* 122:867-74. PMID:11910337.

Czene K, Hemminki K [2003] Familial papillary renal cell tumors and subsequent cancers: A nationwide epidemiological study from Sweden. *J Urol* 169:1271-5. PMID:12629341.

Dacic S [2011] Molecular diagnostics of lung carcinomas. *Arch Pathol Lab Med* 135:622-629. PMID:21526960.

Dadras SS [2011] Molecular diagnostics in melanoma—current status and perspectives. *Arch Pathol Lab Med* 135:860-869. PMID:21732775.

Davenport M, Tizzard SA, Underhill J, et al [2006] The biliary atresia splenic malformation syndrome: a 28-year single-center retrospective study. *J Pediatr* 149:393-400. PMID:16939755.

Davies S, Ramsden DB [2001] Huntington's disease. *Mol Pathol* 54:409-413. PMID:11724916.

de Die-Smulders CE, Howeler CJ, Thijs C, et al [1998] Age and causes of death in adult-onset myotonic dystrophy. *Brain* 121(8):1557-63. PMID:9712016.

De Gobbi M, Roetto A, Piperno A, et al [2002] Natural history of juvenile haemochromatosis. *Br J Haematol* 117:973-9. PMID:12060140.

De Jonghe P, Timmerman V, Ceuterick C, et al [1999] The Thr124Met mutation in the peripheral myelin protein zero (MPZ) gene is associated with a clinically distinct Charcot-Marie-Tooth phenotype. *Brain* 122(2):281-90. PMID:10071056.

de Sanctis C, Lala R, Matarazzo P, et al [1999] McCune-Albright syndrome: a longitudinal clinical study of 32 patients. *J Pediat Endocr Metab* 12:817-826. PMID:10614538.

DeAngelis LM [2001] Medical progress: brain tumors. *N Engl J Med* 344(2):114-123. PMID:11150363.

DeBella K, Szudek J, Friedman JM [2000a] Use of the national institutes of health criteria for diagnosis of neurofibromatosis 1 in children. *Pediatrics* 105:608-14. PMID:10699117.

DeBella K, Poskitt K, Szudek J, Friedman JM [2000b] Use of "unidentified bright objects" on MRI for diagnosis of neurofibromatosis 1 in children. *Neurology* 54:1646-51. PMID:10762507.

del Castillo I, Villamar M, Moreno-Pelayo MA, et al [2002] A deletion involving the connexin 30 gene in nonsyndromic hearing impairment. *N Engl J Med* 346:243-9. PMID:11807148.

Delahunt B, Eble JN [1997] Papillary renal cell carcinoma: a clinicopathologic and immunohistochemical study of 105 tumors. *Mod Pathol* 10:537-44. PMID:9195569.

DeLeeuw WJ, Dierssen J, Vasen HF, et al [2001] Prediction of a mismatch repair gene defect by microsatellite instability and immunohistochemical analysis in endometrial tumours from HNPCC patients. *J Pathol* 192:328-35. PMID:11054716.

DeLeng WWJ, Westerman AM, Weterman MA, et al [2007] Nasal polyposis in Peutz-Jeghers syndrome: a distinct histopathological and molecular genetic entity. *J Clin Pathol* 60:392-396. PMID:16775120.

Dell KM, Avner ED [2006] Autosomal recessive polycystic kidney disease. *GeneTests.Org.* 21 March.

Deutsch E, Maggiorella L, Eschwege P, Bourhis J, Soria JC, Abdulkarim B [2004] Environmental, genetic, and molecular features of prostate cancer. *Lancet Oncol* 5:303-13. PMID:15120667.

Dichgans M, Mayer M, Uttner I, et al [1998] The phenotypic spectrum of CADASIL: clinical findings in 102 cases. *Ann Neurol* 44:731-9. PMID:9818928.

DiFonzo A, Rohe CF, Ferreira J, et al [2005] A frequent LRRK2 gene mutation associated with autosomal dominant Parkinson's disease. *Lancet* 365:412-5. PMID:15680456.

Dim DC, Cooley LD, Miranda RN [2007] Clear cell sarcoma of tendons and aponeuroses. *Arch Pathol Lab Med* 131:152-156. PMID:17227118.

Dische FE, Weston MJ, Parsons V [1985] Abnormally thin glomerular basement membranes associated with hematuria, proteinuria or renal failure in adults. *Am J Nephrol* 5:103-9. PMID:3887920.

Dong SM, Lee EJ, Jeon ES, Park CK, Kim KM [2005] Progressive methylation during the serrated neoplasia pathway of the colorectum. *Mod Pathol* 18:170-178. PMID:15389252.

Downs-Kelly E, Yoder BJ, Stoler M, Tubbs RR, Skacel M, Grogan T, Roche P, Hicks DG [2005] The influence of polysomy 17 on HER2 gene and protein expression in adenocarcinoma of the breast: a fluorescent in situ hybridization, immunohistochemical, and isotopic mRNA in situ hybridization study. *Am J Surg Pathol* 29:1221-1227. PMID:16096413.

Drumm ML, Konstan MW, Schluchter MD, et al [2005] Genetic modifiers of lung disease in cystic fibrosis. *N Engl J Med* 353:1443-53. PMID:16207846.

Du M, Zhou W, Beatty LG, Weksberg R, Sadowski PD [2004] The KCNQ1OT1 promoter, a key regulator of genomic imprinting in human chromosome 11p15.5. *Genomics* 84:288-300. PMID:15233993.

Duffy MJ [2005] Predictive markers in breast and other cancers: a review. *Clin Chem* 51(3):494-503. PMID:15637130.

Dürr A, Cossee M, Agid Y, Campuzano V, Mignard C, Penet C, Mandel JL, Brice A, Koenig M [1996] Clinical and genetic abnormalities in patients with Friedreich's ataxia. *N Engl J Med* 335:1169-75. PMID:8815938.

Eble JN, Sauter G, Epstein JI, Sesterhenn IA, eds. [2004] *Tumours of the Urinary System and Male Genital Organs.* Lyon: IARC Press.

Ebly EM, Parhad IM, Hogan DB, Fung TS [1994] Prevalence and types of dementia in the very old. *Neurology* 44:1593-600. PMID:7936280.

Ellis I [2004] Genetic counseling for hereditary pancreatitis—the role of molecular genetics testing for the cationic trypsinogen gene, cystic fibrosis and serine protease inhibitor Kazal type 1. *Gastroenterol Clin N Am* 33:839-854. PMID:15528021.

Eng C, Mulligan LM [1997] Mutations of the RET protooncogene in the multiple endocrine neoplasia type 2 syndromes, related sporadic tumours, and Hirschsprung disease. *Hum Mutat* 9:97-109. PMID:9067749.

Enzinger F [1968] Clear cell sarcoma of tendons and aponeuroses: an analysis of 21 cases. *Cancer* 18:1163-1172. PMID:14332545.

Esteller M, Garcia-Foncillas J, Andion E, et al [2000] Inactivation of the DNA repair gene MGMT and the clinical response of gliomas to alkylating agents. *N Engl J Med* 343(19):1350-1354. PMID:11070098.

Estivill X, Fortina P, Surrey S, et al [1998] Connexin-26 mutations in sporadic and inherited sensorineural deafness. *Lancet* 351:394-8. PMID:9482292.

Evans HL [1987] Low grade fibromyxoid sarcoma: a report of 2 metastasizing neoplasms having a deceptively benign appearance. *Am J Clin Pathol* 88:615-9. PMID:3673943.

Evans HL [1993] Low grade fibromyxoid sarcoma: a report of 12 cases. *Am J Surg Pathol* 17:595-600. PMID:8333558.

Evans DG, Sainio M, Baser ME [2000] Neurofibromatosis type 2. *J Med Genet* 37:897-904. PMID:11106352.

Fabrizi GM, Cavallaro T, Angiari C, et al [2004] Giant axon and neurofilament accumulation in Charcot-Marie-Tooth disease type 2E. *Neurology* 62:1429-31. PMID:15111691.

Falk RJ, Jennette JC, Nachman PH [2004] Primary glomerular disease. In: *Brenner & Rector's The Kidney.* Philadelphia: Elsevier.

Farazi TA, Spitzer JI, Morozov P, Tuschl T [2011] miRNAs in human cancer. *J Pathol* 223:102-115. PMID:21125669.

Farfel Z, Bourne HR, Iiri T [1999] The expanding spectrum of G protein diseases. *N Eng J Med* 340:1012-1020. PMID:10099144.

Farrer M, Chan P, Chen R, et al [2001] Lewy bodies and parkinsonism in families with parkin mutations. *Ann Neurol* 50:293-300. PMID:11558785.

Farshid G, Balleine RL, Cummings M, Waring P [2006] Morphology of breast cancer as a means of triage of patients for BRCA1 genetic testing. *Am J Surg Pathol* 30:1357-1366. PMID:17063074.

Ferner RE [2007] Neurofibromatosis 1 and neurofibromatosis 2: a twenty-first century perspective. *Lancet Neurol* 6:340-51. PMID:17362838.

Filla A, De Michele G, Cavalcanti F, et al [1996] The relationship between trinucleotide (GAA) repeat length and clinical features in Friedreich ataxia. *Am J Hum Genet* 59:554-60. PMID:8751856.

Finckh U, Alberici A, Antoniazzi M, et al [2000] Variable expression of familial Alzheimer disease associated with presenilin 2 mutation M239I. *Neurology* 54:2006-8. PMID:10822446.

Finsterer J, Stollberger C [2003] The heart in human dystrophinopathies. *Cardiology* 99:1-19. PMID:12589117.

Fitze G, Appelt H, Konig IR, et al [2003] Functional haplotypes of the RET protooncogene promoter are associated with Hirschsprung disease (HSCR). *Hum Mol Genet* 12:3207-14. PMID:14600022.

Fontaine G, Fontaliran F, Frank R [1998] Arrhythmogenic right ventricular cardiomyopathies: clinical forms and main differential diagnoses. *Circulation* 97:1532-5. PMID:9593556.

Forest MG [1998] Prenatal diagnosis, treatment, and outcome in infants with congenital adrenal hyperplasia. *Curr Opin Endocrinol Diab* 4:209-217.

Forsmark CE [2006] Chronic pancreatitis. In: *Sleisenger & Fordtran's Gastrointestinal and Liver Disease,* 8th ed. Philadelphia: Saunders Elsevier.

Forster LF, Defres S, Goudie DR, Baty DU, Carey FA [2000] An investigation of the Peutz-Jeghers gene (LKB1) in sporadic breast and colon cancers. *J Clin Pathol* 53:791-793. PMID:11064676.

Fox NC, Kennedy AM, Harvey RJ, et al [1997] Clinicopathological features of familial Alzheimer's disease associated with the M139V mutation in the presenilin 1 gene. *Brain* 120 (3):491-501. PMID:9126060.

Fradet Y, Saad F, Aprikian A, et al [2004] UPM3, a new molecular urine test for the detection of prostate cancer. *Urology* 64:311-316. PMID:15302485.

Francannet C, Cohen-Tanugi A, Le Merrer M, Munnich A, Bonaventure J, Legeai-Mallet L [2001] Genotype-phenotype correlation in hereditary multiple exostoses. *J Med Genet* 38:430-4. PMID:11432960.

Franchini M, Veneri D [2005] Recent advances in hereditary hemochromatosis. *Ann Hematol* 84(6):347-352. PMID:15747119.

Frank TS [1999] Laboratory determination of hereditary susceptibility to breast and ovarian cancer. *Arch Pathol Lab Med* 123:1023-1026. PMID:10539900.

Frank-Raue K, Hoppner W, Frilling A, et al [1996] Mutations of the ret protooncogene in German multiple endocrine neoplasia families: relation between genotype and phenotype. *J Clin Endocrinol Metab* 81:1780-3. PMID:8626834.

Frederick J [2006] Pick disease: a brief overview. *Arch Pathol Lab Med* 130:1063-1066. PMID:16831037.

Friedman JM, Birch PH [1997] Type 1 neurofibromatosis: a descriptive analysis of the disorder in 1,728 patients. *Am J Med Genet* 70:138-43. PMID:9128932.

Friedman JM [2007] Neurofibromatosis 1. *Gene Tests Gene Reviews;* Online.

Gabriel JM, Erne B, Pareyson D, Sghirlanzoni A, Taroni F, Steck AJ [1997] Gene dosage effects in hereditary peripheral neuropathy: expression of peripheral myelin protein 22 in Charcot-Marie-Tooth disease type 1A and hereditary neuropathy with liability to pressure palsies nerve biopsies. *Neurology* 49:1635-40. PMID:9409359.

Gaffney D, Fell GS, O'Reilly D [2000] Wilson's disease: acute and presymptomatic laboratory diagnosis and monitoring. *J Clin Pathol* 53:807-812. PMID:11127261.

Ganz T [2003] Hepcidin, a key regulator of iron metabolism and mediator of anemia of inflammation. *Blood* 102(3):783-788. PMID:12663437.

Garcia-Barcelo M, Sham M, Lee W, et al [2004] Highly recurrent RET mutations and novel mutations in genes of the receptor tyrosine kinase and endothelin receptor B pathways in Chinese patients with sporadic Hirschsprung disease. *Clin Chem* 50(1):93-100. PMID:14633923.

Garcia-Castro M, Reguero JR, Batalla A, et al [2003] Hypertrophic cardiomyopathy: low frequency of mutations in the myosin heavy chain (MYH7) and cardiac troponin T (TNNT2) genes among Spanish patients. *Clin Chem* 49(8):1279-1285. PMID:12881443.

Garg V, Kathiriya IS, et al [2003] GATA4 mutations cause human congenital heart defects and reveal an interaction with TBX5. *Nature* 424:443-7. PMID:12845333.

Gariepy E [2004] Developmental disorders of the enteric nervous system: Genetic and molecular bases. *J Pediatr Gastroenterol Nutr* 39:5-11. PMID:15187773.

Garner HP, Phillips JR, Herron JG, et al [2004] Peroxidase activity within circulating neutrophils correlates with pulmonary phenotype in cystic fibrosis. *J Lab Clin Med* 144:127-33. PMID:15454881.

Gath R, Goessling A, Keller KM, et al [2001] Analysis of the RET, GDNF, EDN3, and EDNRB genes in patients with intestinal neuronal dysplasia and Hirschsprung disease. *Gut* 48:671-5. PMID:11302967.

Gerami P, Zembowicz A [2011] Update on fluorescence in situ hybridization in melanoma—state of the art. *Arch Pathol Lab Med* 135:830-837. PMID:21732770.

Gershoni-Baruch R, Lerner A, Braun J, et al [1990] Johanson-Blizzard syndrome: Clinical spectrum and further delineation of the syndrome. *Am J Med Genet* 35:546-51. PMID:2185632.

Gerstenblith MR, Goldstein AM, Tucker MA [2010] Hereditary genodermatoses with cancer predisposition. *Hematol Oncol Clin N Am* 24:885-906. PMID:20816579.

Gerull B, Heuser A, Wichter T, et al [2004] Mutations in the desmosomal plakophilin-2 are common in arrhythmogenic right ventricular cardiomyopathy. *Nat Genet* 36:1162-4. PMID:15489853.

Ghiggeri GM, Caridi G, Magrini U, et al [2003] Genetics, clinical and pathological features of glomerulonephrites associated with mutations of nonmuscle myosin IIA (Fechtner syndrome). *Am J Kidney Dis* 41:95-104. PMID:12500226.

Giardiello FM, Brensinger JD, Tersmette AC, et al [2000] Very high risk of cancer in familial Peutz-Jeghers syndrome. *Gastroenterology* 119:1447-53. PMID:11113065.

Gologan A, Sepulveda AR [2005a] Microsatellite instability and DNA mismatch repair deficiency testing in hereditary and sporadic gastrointestinal cancers. *Clin Lab Med* 25:179-196. PMID:15749237.

Gologan A, Krasinskas A, Hunt J, Thull DL, Farkas L, Sepulveda AR [2005b] Performance of the revised Bethesda guidelines for identification of colorectal carcinomas with a high level of microsatellite instability. *Arch Pathol Lab Med* 129:1390-1397. PMID:16253017.

Gorlin RJ, Goltz RW [1960] Multiple nevoid basal-cell epithelioma, jaw cysts and bifid rib. A syndrome. *N Engl J Med* 262:908-912. PMID:13851319.

Gras E, Matias-Guiu X, Catasus L, Arguelles R, Cardona D, Prat J [2000] Application of microsatellite PCR techniques in the identification of mixed up tissue specimens in surgical pathology. *J Clin Pathol* 53:238-240. PMID:10823148.

Greenberg DA [1997] Calcium channels in neurological disease. *Ann Neurol* 42:275-82. PMID:9307247.

Greenson JK, Bonner JD, Ben-Yzhak O, et al [2003] Phenotype of microsatellite unstable colorectal carcinomas well differentiated and focally mucinous tumors and the absence of dirty necrosis correlate with microsatellite instability. *Am J Surg Pathol* 27(5):563-570. PMID:12717242.

Griggs RC, Askanas V, DiMauro S, et al [1995] Inclusion body myositis and myopathies. *Ann Neurol* 38:705-13. PMID:7486861.

Grody WW [1999] Cystic fibrosis: molecular diagnosis, population screening, and public policy. *Arch Pathol Lab Med* 123:1041-1046. PMID:10539904.

Groisman GM, Amar M, Livne E [2002] CD10: A valuable tool for the light microscopic diagnosis of microvillous inclusion disease (familial microvillous atrophy). *Am J Surg Pathol* 26(7):902-907. PMID:12131157.

Gryfe R, Kim H, Hsieh ETK, et al [2000] Tumor microsatellite instability and clinical outcome in young patients with colorectal cancer. *N Engl J Med* 342:69-77. PMID:10631274.

Guay-Woodford LM, Desmond RA [2003] Autosomal recessive polycystic kidney disease: the clinical experience in North America. *Pediatrics* 111:1072-80. PMID:12728091.

Gubler MC, Knebelmann B, Beziau A, et al [1995] Autosomal dominant Alport syndrome: immunohistochemical study of type IV collagen chain distribution. *Kidney Int* 47:1142-7. PMID:7783412.

Guilford PJ, Hopkins JB, Grady WM, et al [1999] E-cadherin germline mutations define an inherited cancer syndrome dominated by diffuse gastric cancer. *Hum Mutat* 14:249-55. PMID:10477433.

Gulley ML, et al [2007] Clinical laboratory reports in molecular pathology. *Arch Path Lab Med* 131:852-863. PMID:17550311.

Gupta M, Djalilvand A, Brat DJ [2005] Clarifying the diffuse gliomas: an update on the morphologic features and markers that discriminate oligodendroglioma from astrocytoma. *Am J Clin Pathol* 124:755-768. PMID:16203285.

Gutmann DH, Aylsworth A, Carey JC, et al [1997] The diagnostic evaluation and multidisciplinary management of neurofibromatosis 1 and neurofibromatosis 2. *JAMA* 278:51-7. PMID:9207339.

Gutmann DH [1998] Recent insights into neurofibromatosis type 1: clear genetic progress. *Arch Neurol* 55:778-80. PMID:9626767.

Guttmacher A, Collins FS [2002] Genomic medicine—a primer. *N Engl J Med* 347(19):1512-1520. PMID:12421895.

Haas M [2006] Thin glomerular basement membrane nephropathy: incidence in 3471 consecutive renal biopsies examined by electron microscopy. *Arch Pathol Lab Med* 130:699-706. PMID:16683888.

Hahn SA, Bartsch DK [2005] Genetics of hereditary pancreatic carcinoma. *Clin Lab Med* 25:117-133. PMID:15749235.

Hall JG [1990] Genomic imprinting: review and relevance to human diseases. *Am J Hum Genet* 46:857-873. PMID:2187341.

Halvarsson B, Lindblom A, Johansson L, Lagerstedt K, Nilbert M [2005] Loss of mismatch repair protein immunostaining in colorectal adenomas from patients with hereditary nonpolyposis colorectal cancer. *Mod Pathol* 18:1095-1101. PMID:15731775.

Hamilton SR, Liu B, Parsons RE, et al [1995] The molecular basis of Turcot's syndrome. *N Engl J Med* 332:839-47. PMID:7661930.

Hampe J, Grebe J, Nikolaus S, et al [2002a] Association of NOD2 (CARD 15) genotype with clinical course of Crohn's disease: a cohort study. *Lancet* 359:1661-5. PMID:12020527.

Hampe J, Frenzel H, Mirza MM, et al [2002b] Evidence for a NOD2-independent susceptibility locus for inflammatory bowel disease on chromosome 16p. *Proc Natl Acad Sci* 99(1):321-6. PMID:11752413.

Hampel H, Frankel WL, Martin E, et al [2005] Screening for the Lynch syndrome (hereditary nonpolyposis colorectal cancer). *N Engl J Med* 352:1851-60. PMID:15872200.

Happle R [1986] The McCune-Albright syndrome: a lethal gene surviving by mosaicism. *Clin Genet* 29:321-324. PMID:3720010.

Harris PC, Torres VE [2006] Autosomal dominant polycystic kidney disease. *GeneTests.Org*. 6 June.

Hartmann LC, Schaid DJ, Woods JE, et al [1999] Efficacy of bilateral prophylactic mastectomy in women with a family history of breast cancer. *N Engl J Med* 340:77-84. PMID:9887158.

Hateboer N, Dijk MA, Bogdanova N, et al [1999] Comparison of phenotypes of polycystic kidney disease types 1 and 2. *Lancet* 353:103-7. PMID:10023895.

Hattori T, Takei Y, Koyama J, Nakazato M, Ikeda S [2003a] Clinical and pathological studies of cardiac amyloidosis in transthyretin type familial amyloid polyneuropathy. *Amyloid* 10:229-39. PMID:14986482.

Hattori N, Yamamoto M, Yoshihara T, et al [2003b] Demyelinating and axonal features of Charcot-Marie-Tooth disease with mutations of myelin related proteins (PMP22, MPZ and Cx32): a clinicopathological study of 205 Japanese patients. *Brain* 126:134-51. PMID:12477701.

Hawley RJ, Milner MR, Gottdiener JS, Cohen A [1991] Myotonic heart disease: a clinical follow-up. *Neurology* 41:259-62. PMID:1992371.

Hayflick SJ, Westaway SK, Levinson B, et al [2003] Genetic, clinical, and radiographic delineation of Hallervorden-Spatz syndrome. *N Engl J Med* 348:33-40. PMID:12510040.

Heckmann JM, Low WC, de Villiers C, et al [2004] Novel presenilin 1 mutation with profound neurofibrillary pathology in an indigenous Southern African family with early onset Alzheimer's disease. *Brain* 127:133-42. PMID:14570818.

Hedenfalk I, Duggan D, Chen Y, et al [2001] Gene-expression profiles in hereditary breast cancer. *N Engl J Med* 344:539-48. PMID:11207349.

Hedera P, Turner RS [2002] Inherited dementias. *Neurol Clin N Am* 20:779-808. PMID:12432830.

Hegi ME, Diserens AC, Gorlia T, et al [2005] MGMT gene silencing and benefit from temozolomide in glioblastoma. *N Engl J Med* 352(10):997-1003. PMID:15758010.

Hill DA, O'Sullivan MJ, Zhu X, et al [2002] Practical application of molecular genetic testing as an aid to the surgical pathologic diagnosis of sarcomas: a prospective study. *Am J Surg Pathol* 26(8):965-977. PMID:12170083.

Hisada M, Garber JE, Fung CY, Fraumeni JF Jr, Li FP [1998] Multiple primary cancers in families with Li-Fraumeni syndrome. *J Natl Cancer Inst* 90:606-11. PMID:9554443.

Hitchins MP, Wong JJL, Suthers G, Suter CM, Martin DIK, Hawkins NJ, Ward RL [2007] Inheritance of a cancer-associated MLH1 germline epimutation. *N Engl J Med* 356:697-705. PMID:17301300.

Holt M, Oram S [1960] Familial heart disease with skeletal malformations. *Br Heart J* 22:236-42. PMID:14402857.

Hong S-M, Park JY, Hruban R, Goggins M [2011] Molecular signatures of pancreatic cancer. *Arch Pathol Lab Med* 135:716-727. PMID:21631264.

Hoogerwaard EM, Bakker E, Ippel PF, et al [1999] Signs and symptoms of Duchenne muscular dystrophy and Becker muscular dystrophy among carriers in The Netherlands: a cohort study. *Lancet* 353:2116-9. PMID:10382696.

Howe JR, Mitros FA, Summers RW [1998] The risk of gastrointestinal carcinoma in familial juvenile polyposis. *Ann Surg Oncol* 5:751-6. PMID:9869523.

Hoyme HE, Seaver LH, Jones KL, Procopio F, Crooks W, Feingold M [1998] Isolated hemihyperplasia (hemihypertrophy): report of a prospective multicenter study of the incidence of neoplasia and review. *Am J Med Genet* 79:274-8. PMID:9781907.

Hsieh K, Albertsen PC [2003] Populations at high risk for prostate cancer. *Urol Clin N Am* 30:669-676. PMID:14680306.

Huang FD, Chen J, Lin M, Keating MT, Sanguinetti MC [2001] Long-QT syndrome-associated missense mutations in the pore helix of the HERG potassium channel. *Circulation* 104:1071-5. PMID:11524404.

Hudson BG, Tryggvason K, Sundaramoorthy M, Neilson EG [2003] Alport's syndrome, Goodpasture's syndrome, and type IV collagen. *N Engl J Med* 348:2543-56. PMID:12815141.

Hulot JS, Jouven X, Empana JP, Frank R, Fontaine G [2004] Natural history and risk stratification of arrhythmogenic right ventricular dysplasia/cardiomyopathy. *Circulation* 110:1879-84. PMID:15451782.

Hunt JL [2011] An update on molecular diagnostics of squamous and salivary gland tumors of the head and neck. *Arch Pathol Lab Med* 135:602-609. PMID:21526958.

Hwang PJ, Kousseff BG [2004] Omphalocele and gastroschisis: an 18-year review study. *Genet Med* 6(4):232-6. PMID:15266212.

Igbokwe A, Lopez-Terrada DH [2011] Molecular testing of solid tumors. *Arch Pathol Lab Med* 135:67-82. PMID:21204713.

Iino H, Simms L, Young J, et al [2000] DNA microsatellite instability and mismatch repair protein loss in adenomas presenting in hereditary non-polyposis colorectal cancer. *Gut* 47:37-42. PMID:10861262.

Ikeda S [2004] Cardiac amyloidosis: heterogenous pathogenic backgrounds. *Intern Med* 43:1107-14. PMID:15645642.

Imboden M, Swan H, Denjoy I, et al [2006] Female predominance and transmission distortion in the long-QT syndrome. *N Engl J Med* 355:2744-51. PMID:17192539.

Inabnet WB, Caragliano P, Pertsemlidis D [2000] Pheochromocytoma: inherited associations, bilaterality, and cortex presentation. *Surgery* 128:1007-11. PMID:11114636.

Inoue K, Shimotake T, Inoue K, Tokiwa K, Iwai N [1999] Mutational analysis of the RET protooncogene in a kindred with multiple endocrine neoplasia type 2A and Hirschsprung's disease. *J Pediatr Surg* 34:1552-4. PMID:10549772.

Inoue K, Shimotake T, Iwai N [2000] Mutational analysis of RET/GDNF/NTN genes in children with total colonic aganglionosis with small bowel involvement. *Am J Med Genet* 93:278-84. PMID:10946353.

Ionasescu VV, Ionasescu R, Searby C, Neahring R [1995] Dejerine-Sottas disease with de novo dominant point mutation of the PMP22 gene. *Neurology* 45:1766-7. PMID:7675244.

Irobi J, De Jonghe P, Timmerman V [2004] Molecular genetics of distal hereditary motor neuropathies. *Hum Mol Genet* 13(Review Issue 2):R195-R202 PMID:15358725.

Ishibashi-Ueda H, Imakita M, Yutani C, Takahashi S, Yazawa K, Kamiya T, Nonaka I [1990] Congenital nemaline myopathy with dilated cardiomyopathy: an autopsy study. *Hum Pathol* 21:77-82. PMID:2295510.

Jääskeläinen J, Mongan NP, Harland S, Hughes IA [2006] 5 novel androgen receptor gene mutations associated with complete androgen insensitivity syndrome. *Hum Mutat* 876:Online PMID:16470553.

Jacobson DR, Pastore RD, Yaghoubian R, et al [1997] Variant-sequence transthyretin (isoleucine 122) in late-onset cardiac amyloidosis in black Americans. *N Engl J Med* 336:466-73. PMID:9017939.

Janssen JC, Beck JA, Campbell TA, Dickinson A, Fox NC, Harvey RJ, Houlden H, Rossor MN, Collinge J [2003] Early onset familial Alzheimer's disease: mutation frequency in 31 families. *Neurology* 60:235-9. PMID:12552037.

Jarvinen HJ, Aarnio M, Mustonen H, et al [2000] Controlled 15-year trial on screening for colorectal cancer in families with hereditary nonpolyposis colorectal cancer. *Gastroenterology* 118:829-34. PMID:10784581.

Jennings L, Van Deerlin VM, Gulley ML [2009] Recommended principles and practices for validating clinical molecular pathology tests. *Arch Path Lab Med* 133:743-755. PMID:19415949.

Jervell A, Lange-Nielsen F [1957] Congenital deaf-mutism, functional heart disease with prolongation of the Q-T interval and sudden death. *Am Heart J* 54:59-68. PMID:13435203.

Jimenez RE, Wallis T, Tabasczka P, Visscher DW [2000] Determination of Her-2/Neu status in breast carcinoma: comparative analysis of immunohistochemistry and fluorescent in situ hybridization. *Mod Pathol* 13(1):37-45. PMID:10658908.

Joensuu H, Roberts PJ, Sarlomo-Rikala M, Andersson LC, Tervahartiala P, Tuveson D, Silberman SL, Capdeville R, Dimitrijevic S, Druker B, Demetri G [2001] Effect of the tyrosine kinase inhibitor STI571 in a patient with a metastatic gastrointestinal stromal tumor. *N Engl J Med* 344(14):1052-1056. PMID:11287975.

Johnson CA, Gissen P, Sergi C [2003] Molecular pathology and genetics of congenital hepatorenal fibrocystic syndromes. *J Med Genet* 40:311-9. PMID:12746391.

Johnson DH, Fehrenbacher L, Novotny WF, et al [2004] Randomized phase II trial comparing bevacizumab plus carboplatin and paclitaxel with carboplatin and paclitaxel alone in previously untreated locally advanced or metastatic nonsmall-cell lung cancer. *J Clin Oncol* 22(11):2184-2191. PMID:15169807.

Jones NL, Hofley PM, Durie PR [1994] Pathophysiology of the pancreatic defect in Johanson-Blizzard syndrome: a disorder of acinar development. *J Pediatr* 125:406-8. PMID:8071749.

Jones TD, Eble JN, Cheng L [2005] Application of molecular diagnostic techniques to renal epithelial neoplasms. *Clin Lab Med* 25:279-303. PMID:15848737.

Jones JS [2006] DNA-based molecular cytology for bladder cancer surveillance. *Urology* 67(Suppl 3A):35-47. PMID:16530074.

Joutel A, Dodick DD, Parisi JE, Cecillon M, Tournier-Lasserve E, Bousser MG [2000] De novo mutation in the Notch3 gene causing CADASIL. *Ann Neurol* 47:388-91. PMID:10716263.

Kamath BM, Piccoli DA [2003] Heritable disorders of the bile ducts. *Gastroenterol Clin North Am* 32:857-75. PMID:14562578.

Kamboh MI [2004] Molecular genetics of late-onset Alzheimer's disease. *Ann Hum Genet* 68:381-404. PMID:15225164.

Kamisago M, Sharma SD, DePalma SR, et al [2000] Mutations in sarcomere protein genes as a cause of dilated cardiomyopathy. *New Engl J Med* 343:1688-96. PMID:11106718.

Kashtan CE [1999] Alport syndrome: an inherited disorder of renal, ocular, and cochlear basement membranes. *Medicine* 78:338-60. PMID:10499074.

Kashtan CE [2004] Diagnosis of Alport syndrome. *Kidney Int* 66:1290-1. PMID:15327435.

Kauff ND, Satagopan JM, Robson ME, et al [2002 Risk-reducing salpingo-oophorectomy in women with a BRCA1 or BRCA2 mutation. *N Engl J Med* 346:1609-15. PMID:12023992.

Kazama Y, Watanabe T, Kanazawa T, et al [2006] Mucinous colorectal cancers with chromosomal instability. A biologically distinct and aggressive subtype. *Diagn Mol Pathol* 15:30-34. PMID:16531766.

Keating MT, Atkinson D, Dunn C, Timothy K, Vincent GM, Leppert M [1991] Linkage of a cardiac arrhythmia, the long QT syndrome, and the Harvey ras-1 gene. *Science* 252:704-6. PMID:1673802.

Keegan E, Killeen AA [2001] An overview of molecular diagnosis of steroid 21-hydroxylase deficiency. *J Mol Diagn* 3(2):49-54. PMID:11393164.

Kelley TW, Tubbs RR, Prayson RA [2005] Molecular diagnostic techniques for the clinical evaluation of gliomas. *Diagn Mol Pathol* 14:1-8. PMID:15714057.

Kimonis VE, Goldstein AM, Pastakia B, et al [1997] Clinical manifestations in 105 persons with nevoid basal cell carcinoma syndrome. *Am J Med Genet* 69(3):299-308. PMID:9096761.

Kirk JMW, Brain CE, Carson DJ, et al [1999] Cushing's syndrome caused by nodular adrenal hyperplasia in children with McCune-Albright syndrome. *J Pediat* 134:789-792. PMID:10356155.

Knebelmann B, Breillat C, Forestier L, et al [1996] Spectrum of mutations in the COL4A5 collagen gene in X-linked Alport syndrome. *Am J Hum Genet* 59:1221-32. PMID:8940267.

Ko JM, Fisher DE [2010] A new era: melanoma genetics and therapeutics. *J Pathol* 223:241-250. PMID:21125678.

Kobayashi S, Boggon TJ, Dayaram T, et al [2005] EGFR mutation and resistance of non-small-cell lung cancer to gefitinib. *N Engl J Med* 352:786-92. PMID:15728811.

Kovacs K, Giannini C, Scheithauer BW, et al [1997] Pituitary changes in ataxia-telangiectasia syndrome: an immunocytochemical, in situ hybridization, and DNA cytometric study of 3 cases. *Endocr Pathol* 8:195-203. PMID:12114723.

Krajewski KM, Lewis RA, Fuerst DR, et al [2000] Neurological dysfunction and axonal degeneration in Charcot-Marie-Tooth disease type 1A. *Brain* 123(7):1516-27. PMID:10869062.

Krause DS, Van Etten RA [2005] Tyrosine kinases as targets for cancer therapy. *N Engl J Med* 353:172-87. PMID:16014887.

Kriaucionis S, Bird A [2003] DNA methylation and Rett syndrome. *Hum Mol Gen* 12(Review Issue 2):R221-R227 PMID:12928486.

Kruse R, Rutten A, Lamberti C, et al [1998] Muir-Torre phenotype has a frequency of DNA mismatch-repair-gene mutations similar to that in hereditary nonpolyposis colorectal cancer families defined by the Amsterdam criteria. *Am J Hum Genet* 63:63-70. PMID:9634524.

La P, Tan LK, Chen B [2005] Correlation of HER-2 status with estrogen and progesterone receptors and histologic features in 3,655 invasive breast carcinomas. *Am J Clin Pathol* 123:541-546. PMID:15743737.

Laakso M, Loman N, Borg A, Isola J [2005] Cytokeratin 5/14-positive breast cancer: true basal phenotype confined to BRCA1 tumors. *Mod Pathol* 18:1321-1328. PMID:15990899.

Ladabaum U, Wang G, Terdiman J, et al [2011] Strategies to identify the Lynch syndrome among patients with colorectal cancer: a cost-effectiveness analysis. *Ann Intern Med* 155:69-79. PMID:21768580.

Lae ME, Roche PC, Jin L, Lloyd RV, Nascimento AG [2002] Desmoplastic small round cell tumor. A clinicopathologic, immunohistochemical, and molecular study of 32 tumors. *Am J Surg Pathol* 26(7):823-835. PMID:12131150.

LaFranchi S [2004] Disorders of the thyroid gland. In: *Nelson Textbook of Pediatrics*, 17th ed. Philadelphia: Saunders, Elsevier Science.

Laitinen PJ, Brown KM, Piippo K, et al [2001] Mutations of the cardiac ryanodine receptor (RyR2) gene in familial polymorphic ventricular tachycardia. *Circulation* 103:485-90. PMID:11157710.

Lancaster JM, Powell CB, Kauff ND, et al [2007] Society of Gynecologic Oncologists Education Committee statement on riskassessment for inherited gynecologic cancer predispositions. *Gynecol Oncol* 107:159-62. PMID:17950381.

Lane KL, Shannon RJ, Weiss SW [1997] Hyalinizing spindle cell tumour with giant rosettes: A distinctive tumor closely resembling low grade fibromyxoid sarcoma. *Am J Surg Pathol* 21:1481-8. PMID:9414192.

Lang AE, Lozano AM [1998] Parkinson's disease: second of 2 parts. *N Engl J Med* 339:1130-43. PMID:9770561.

Lantermann A, Hampe J, Kim WH, et al [2002] Investigation of HLA-DPA1 genotypes as predictors of inflammatory bowel disease in the German, South African, and South Korean populations. *Int J Colorectal Dis* 17(4):238-44. PMID:12073072.

Ledbetter DJ [2006] Gastroschisis and omphalocele. *Surg Clin N Am* 86:249-260. PMID:16580922.

Lee HH, Chang JG, Tsai CH, Tsai FJ, Chao HT, Chung BC [2000] Analysis of the chimeric CYP21P/CYP21 gene in steroid 21-hydroxylase deficiency. *Clin Chem* 46(5):606-611. PMID:10794740.

Leemans CR, Braakhuis BJM, Brakenhoff RH [2011] The molecular biology of head and neck cancer. *Nat Rev Cancer* 11:9-21. PMID:21160525.

Lefevre M, Couturier J, Sibony M, Bazille C, Boyer K, Callard P, Vieillefond A, Allory Y [2005] Adult papillary renal tumor with oncocytic cells: clinicopathologic, immunohistochemical, and cytogenetic features in 10 cases. *Am J Surg Pathol* 29:1576-1581. PMID:16327429.

Legoix P, Sarkissian HD, Cazes L, Giraud S, Sor F, Rouleau GA, Lenoir G, Thomas G, Zucman-Rossi J [2000] Molecular characterization of germline NF2 gene rearrangements. *Genomics* 65:62-6. PMID:10777666.

Lewis JS Jr, Thorstad WL, Chernock RD, Haughey BH, Yip JH, Zhang Q, El-Mofty SK [2010] P16+ oropharyngeal squamous cell carcinoma: an entity with a favorable prognosis regardless of tumor HPV status. *Am J Surg Pathol* 34(8):1088-96. PMID:20588174.

Li FP, Fraumeni JF Jr [1969] Soft-tissue sarcomas, breast cancer, and other neoplasms. A familial syndrome? *Ann Intern Med* 71:747-52. PMID:5360287.

Li M, Squire JA, Weksberg R [1998a] Molecular genetics of Wiedemann-Beckwith syndrome. *Am J Med Genet* 79:253-9. PMID:9781904.

Li H, Chen Q, Moss AJ, Robinson J, Goytia V, Perry JC, et al [1998b] New mutations in the KVLQT1 potassium channel that cause long QT syndrome. *Circulation* 97:1264-9. PMID:9570196.

Li M, Squire J, Shuman C, Fei YL, Atkin J, Pauli R, Smith A, Nishikawa J, Chitayat D, Weksberg R [2001] Imprinting status of 11p15 genes in Beckwith-Wiedemann syndrome patients with CDKN1C mutations. *Genomics* 74:370-6. PMID:11414765.

Li SC, Burgart L [2007] Histopathology of serrated adenoma, its variants, and differentiation from conventional adenomatous and hyperplastic polyps. *Arch Pathol Lab Med* 131:440-445. PMID:17516746.

Lin AE, Herring AH, Scharenberg K [1999] Cardiovascular malformations: changes in prevalence and birth status, 1972-1990. *Am J Med Genet* 84:102 PMID:10323733.

Lippa CF, Swearer JM, Kane KJ, Nochlin D, Bird TD, Ghetti B, Nee LE, St George-Hyslop P, Pollen DA, Drachman DA [2000] Familial Alzheimer's disease: site of mutation influences clinical phenotype. *Ann Neurol* 48:376-9. PMID:10976645.

Litman RS, Rosenberg H [2005] Malignant hyperthermia: update on susceptibility testing. *JAMA* 293:2918-2924. PMID:15956637.

Loke J, MacLennan DH [1998] Malignant hyperthermia and central core disease: disorders of calcium release channels. *Am J Med* 104:470-486. PMID:9626031.

Longacre TA, Fenoglio-Preiser CM [1990] Mixed hyperplastic adenomatous polyps/serrated adenomas: a distinct form of colorectal neoplasia. *Am J Surg Pathol* 14:524-537. PMID:2186644.

Lonser RR, Kim J, Butman JA, Vortmeyer AO, Choo DI, Oldfield EH [2004] Tumors of the endolymphatic sac in von Hippel-Lindau disease. *N Engl J Med* 350:2481-6. PMID:15190140.

Loukola A, Salovaara R, Kristo P, et al [1999] Microsatellite instability in adenomas as a marker for hereditary nonpolyposis colorectal cancer. *Am J Pathol* 155:1849-53. PMID:10595914.

Lovicu M, Dessi V, Zappu A, De Virgiliis S, Cao A, Loudianos G [2003] Efficient strategy for molecular diagnosis of Wilson disease in the Sardinian population. *Clin Chem* 49(3):496-498. PMID:12600964.

Lu J, Getz G, Miska EA, et al [2005] MicroRNA expression profiles classify human cancers. *Nature*. 2005; 435(7043):834-8. PMID:15944708.

Lucking CB, Durr A, Bonifati V, et al [2000] Association between early onset Parkinson's disease and mutations in the parkin gene. *N Engl J Med* 342:1560-7. PMID:10824074.

Lumbroso S, Paris F, Sultan C [2004] Activating Gs-alpha mutations: Analysis of 113 patients with signs of McCune-Albright syndrome. *J Clin Endocr Metab* 89:2107-2113. PMID:15126527.

Lupski JR, Chance PF, Garcia CA [1993] Inherited primary peripheral neuropathies: molecular genetics and clinical implications of CMT1A and HNPP. *JAMA* 270:2326-30. PMID:8230595.

Lynch HT, de la Chapelle A [2003] Hereditary colorectal cancer. *N Engl J Med* 348:919-932. PMID:12621137.

Machin P, Catasus L, Pons C, et al [2002] Microsatellite instability and immunostaining for MSH-2 and MLH-1 in cutaneous and internal tumors from patients with the Muir-Torre syndrome. *J Cutan Pathol* 29:415-20. PMID:12139636.

Mack DR, Forstner GG, Wilschanski M, Freedman MH, Durie PR [1996] Shwachman syndrome: exocrine pancreatic dysfunction and variable phenotypic expression. *Gastroenterology* 111:1593-602. PMID:8942739.

Mais, DD, Nordberg, M [2008] *Quick Compendium of Molecular Pathology*. Chicago: ASCP Press.

Mak V, Zielenski J, Tsui LC, Durie P, Zini A, Martin S, Longley TB, Jarvi KA [2000] Cystic fibrosis gene mutations and infertile men with primary testicular failure. *Hum Reprod* 15(2):436-9. PMID:10655318.

Mantovani G, Romoli R, Weber G, et al [2000] Mutational analysis of GNAS1 in patients with pseudo-hypoparathyroidism: Identification of 2 novel mutations. *J Clin Endocr Metab* 85:4243-4248. PMID:11095461.

Mantovani G, Maghnie M, Weber G, et al [2003] Growth hormone-releasing hormone resistance in pseudohypoparathyroidism type 1a: New evidence for imprinting of the Gs-alpha gene. *J Clin Endocr Metab* 88:4070-4074. PMID:12970263.

Mao R, Nelson L, Kates R, et al [2002] Prenatal diagnosis of 21-hydroxylase deficiency caused by gene conversion and rearrangements: pitfalls and molecular diagnostic solutions. *Prenat Diagn* 22:1171-6. PMID:12478627.

Margallo-Lana M, Morris CM, Gibson AM, et al [2004] Influence of the amyloid precursor protein locus on dementia in Down syndrome. *Neurology* 62:1996-8. PMID:15184603.

Markus HS, Martin RJ, Simpson MA, Dong YB, Ali N, Crosby AH, Powell JF [2002] Diagnostic strategies in CADASIL. *Neurology* 59:1134-8. PMID:12395806.

Marrosu MG, Vaccargiu S, Marrosu G, Vannelli A, Cianchetti C, Muntoni F [1998] Charcot-Marie-Tooth disease type 2 associated with mutation of the myelin protein zero gene. *Neurology* 50:1397-401. PMID:9595994.

Mastrianni JA, Nixon R, Layzer R, Telling GC, Han D, DeArmond SJ, Prusiner SB [1999] Prion protein conformation in a patient with sporadic fatal insomnia. *N Engl J Med* 340:1630-8. PMID:10341275.

Mastrianni JA, Roos RP [2000] The prion diseases. *Semin Neurol* 20:337-52. PMID:11051298.

Mathew CG, Lewis CM [2004] Genetics of inflammatory bowel disease: progress and prospects. *Hum Mol Genet* 13:R161-R168 PMID:14764625.

Mattman A, Huntsman D, Lockitch G, et al [2002] Transferrin receptor 2 (TfR2) and HFE mutational analysis in non-C282Y iron overload: identification of a novel TfR2 mutation. *Blood* 100:1075-1077. PMID:12130528.

Mayeux R, Saunders AM, Shea S, et al [1998] Utility of the apolipoprotein E genotype in the diagnosis of Alzheimer's disease. *N Engl J Med* 338:506-11. PMID:9468467.

Mazur MT, Clark HB [1983] Gastric stromal tumors. Reappraisal of histogenesis. *Am J Surg Pathol* 7(6):507-19. PMID:6625048.

McCandless SE, Millington DS, Andresen BS, et al [2002] Clinical findings in MCAD patients heterozygous for the common mutation identified by MS/MS newborn screening. *Am J Hum Genet* 71(Suppl):419.

McCarthy TV, Quane KA, Lynch PJ [2000] Ryanodine receptor mutations in malignant hyperthermia and central core disease. *Hum Mutat* 15:410-417. PMID:10790202.

McCarthy MI [2004] Progress in defining the molecular basis of type 2 diabetes mellitus through susceptibility-gene identification. *Hum Mol Genet* 13, Review Issue:R33-R41 PMID:14722160.

McGarrity TJ, Kulin HE, Zaino RJ [2000] Peutz-Jeghers syndrome. *Am J Gastroenterol* 95:596-604. PMID:10710046.

Medeiros F, Corless CL, Duensing A, et al [2004] KIT-negative gastrointestinal stromal tumors. Proof of concept and therapeutic implications. *Am J Surg Pathol* 28:889-894. PMID:15223958.

Mercado AB, Wilson RC, Cheng KC, et al [1995] Prenatal treatment and diagnosis of congenital adrenal hyperplasia owing to steroid 21-hydroxylase deficiency. *J Clin Endocrinol Metab* 80:2014-20. PMID:7608248.

Miettinen M, Sobin LH, Lasota J [2005] Gastrointestinal stromal tumors of the stomach: a clinicopathologic, immunohistochemical, and molecular genetic study of 1765 cases with long term follow-up. *Am J Surg Pathol* 29:52-68. PMID:15613856.

Miettinen M, Lasota J [2006] Gastrointestinal stromal tumors: review on morphology, molecular pathology, prognosis, and differential diagnosis. *Arch Pathol Lab Med* 130:1466-1478. PMID:17090188.

Misago N, Narisawa Y [2000] Sebaceous neoplasms in Muir-Torre syndrome. *Am J Dermatopathol* 22:155-61. PMID:10770437.

Moers AM, Landsvater RM, Schaap C, et al [1996] Familial medullary thyroid carcinoma: not a distinct entity? *Am J Med* 101:635-41. PMID:9003111.

Moirand R, Adams PC, Bicheler V, Brissot P, Deugnier Y [1997] Clinical features of genetic hemochromatosis in women compared with men. *Ann Intern Med* 127:105-10. PMID:9229998.

Monnier N, Romero NB, Lerale J, et al [2000] An autosomal dominant congenital myopathy with cores and rods is associated with a neomutation in the RYR1 gene encoding the skeletal muscle ryanodine receptor. *Hum Mol Genet* 9:2599-608. PMID:11063719.

Moskaluk CA [2005] Vanishing prostate cancer syndrome: symptom of a larger clinical issue. *Am J Surg Pathol* 29:561-563. PMID:15767813.

Mullis PE [2007] Genetics of growth hormone deficiency. *Endocrinol Metab Clin N Am* 36:17-36. PMID:17336732.

Mura C, Raguenes O, Ferec C [1999] HFE mutation analysis in 711 hemochromatosis probands: evidence for S65C implication in mild form of hemochromatosis. *Blood* 93:2502-5. PMID:10194428.

Nagel M, Nagorka S, Gross O [2005] Novel COL4A5, COL4A4, and COL4A3 mutations in Alport syndrome. *Hum Mutat* 26 PMID:15954103.

National Institutes of Health Consensus Development Conference [1988] Neurofibromatosis. Conference statement. *Arch Neurol* 45:575-578. PMID:3128965.

Nault JC, Zucman-Rossi J [2011] Genetics of hepatobiliary carcinogenesis. *Semin Liver Dis* 31:173-187. PMID:21538283.

Nelson WG, DeMarzo AM, DeWeese TL [2001] The molecular pathogenesis of prostate cancer: focus on the earliest steps. *Eur Urol* 39:8-11. PMID:11340278.

Netto GJ, Saad RD [2006] Diagnostic molecular pathology: an increasingly indispensable tool for the practicing pathologist. *Arch Pathol Lab Med* 130:1339-1348. PMID:16948522.

Neumann HP, Eng C, Mulligan LM, et al [1995] Consequences of direct genetic testing for germline mutations in the clinical management of families with multiple endocrine neoplasia, type II. *JAMA* 274:1149-51. PMID:7563486.

Neumann HP, Bausch B, McWhinney SR, et al [2002] Germ-line mutations in nonsyndromic pheochromocytoma. *N Engl J Med* 346:1459-66. PMID:12000816.

Newman EA, Mulholland MW [2006] Prophylactic gastrectomy for hereditary diffuse gastric cancer syndrome. *J Am Coll Surg* 202:612-617. PMID:16571431.

Ng B, Connors LH, Davidoff R, Skinner M, Falk RH [2005] Senile systemic amyloidosis presenting with heart failure: a comparison with light chain-associated amyloidosis. *Arch Intern Med* 165:1425-9. PMID:15983293.

Nichols L, Dickson G, Phan PG, Kant JA [2006] Iron binding saturation and genotypic testing for hereditary hemochromatosis in patients with liver disease. *Am J Clin Pathol* 125:236-240. PMID:16393683.

Nielsen P, Carpinteiro S, Fischer R, et al [1998] Prevalence of the C282Y and H63D mutations in the HFE gene in patients with hereditary haemochromatosis and in control subjects from Northern Germany. *Br J Haematol* 103(3):842-845. PMID:9858243.

Nigro JM, Takahashi MA, Ginzinger DG, et al [2001] Detection of 1p and 19q loss in oligodendroglioma by quantitative microsatellite analysis, a real time quantitative polymerase chain reaction assay. *Am J Pathol* 158:1253-1262. PMID:11290543.

Nikiforov YE [2011] Molecular diagnostics of thyroid tumors. *Arch Pathol Lab Med* 135:569-577. PMID:21526955.

Nilsson O, Tisell LE, Jansson S, Ahlman H, Gimm O, Eng C [1999] Adrenal and extra-adrenal pheochromocytomas in a family with germline RET V804L mutation. *JAMA* 281:1587-8. PMID:10235148.

Nishino I, Noguchi S, Murayama K, et al [2002] Distal myopathy with rimmed vacuoles is allelic to hereditary inclusion body myopathy. *Neurology* 59:1689-93. PMID:12473753.

Numakura C, Lin C, Oka N, Akiguchi I, Hayasaka K [2000] Hemizygous mutation of the peripheral myelin protein 22 gene associated with Charcot-Marie-Tooth disease type 1. *Ann Neurol* 47:101-3. PMID:10632107.

O'Brien MJ, Yang S, Clebanoff JL, et al [2004] Hyperplastic (serrated) polyps of the colorectum: relationship of CpG island methylator phenotype and K-ras mutation to location and histologic subtype. *Am J Surg Pathol* 28:423-434. PMID:15087661.

O'Brien MJ, Yang S, Mack C, et al [2006] Comparison of microsatellite instability, CpG island methylation phenotype, BRAF and KRAS status in serrated polyps and traditional adenomas indicates separate pathways to distinct colorectal carcinoma end points. *Am J Surg Pathol* 30:1491-1501. PMID:17122504.

Oakley GJ, Tubbs RR, Crowe J, et al [2006] HER-2 amplification in tubular carcinoma of the breast. *Am J Clin Pathol* 126:1-4. PMID:16753605.

Oda T, Elkahloun AG, Pike BL, et al [1997] Mutations in the human Jagged1 gene are responsible for Alagille syndrome. *Nat Genet* 16:235-42. PMID:9207787.

Ogino S, Leonard DGB, Rennert H, Wilson RB [2002] Spinal muscular atrophy genetic testing experience at an academic medical center. *J Mol Diagn* 4(1):53-58. PMID:11826188.

Ogino S, Brahmandam M, Cantor M, et al [2006] Distinct molecular features of colorectal carcinoma with signet ring cell component and colorectal carcinoma with mucinous component. *Mod Pathol* 19:59-68. PMID:16318624.

Oncel M, Church JM, Remzi FH, Fazio VW [2005] Colonic surgery in patients with juvenile polyposis syndrome: a case series. *Dis Colon and Rectum* 48:49-56. PMID:15690657.

Ong AC, Harris PC [2005] Molecular pathogenesis of ADPKD: the polycystin complex gets complex. *Kidney Int* 67:1234-47. PMID:15780076.

Paner GP, Lindgren V, Jacobson K, et al [2007] High incidence of chromosome 1 abnormalities in a series of 27 renal oncocytomas: cytogenetic and fluorescence in situ hybridization studies. *Arch Pathol Lab Med* 131:81-85. PMID:17227127.

Pang S [1997a] Congenital adrenal hyperplasia. *Endocrinol Metab Clin North Am* 26:853-91. PMID:9429863.

Pang S, Shook MK [1997b] Current status of neonatal screening for congenital adrenal hyperplasia. *Curr Opin Pediatr* 9:419-23. PMID:9300201.

Parham DM, Ellison DA [2006] Rhabdomyosarcomas in adults and children: an update. *Arch Pathol Lab Med* 130:1454-1465. PMID:17090187.

Parisi MA, Kapur RP [2000] Genetics of Hirschsprung disease. *Curr Opin Pediatr* 12:610-7. PMID:11106284.

Parkes M, Barmada MM, Satsangi J, et al [2000] The IBD2 locus shows linkage heterogeneity between ulcerative colitis and Crohn disease. *Am J Hum Genet* 67:1605-10. PMID:11078482.

Parman Y, Plante-Bordeneuve V, Guiochon-Mantel A, Eraksoy M, Said G [1999] Recessive inheritance of a new point mutation of the PMP22 gene in Dejerine-Sottas disease. *Ann Neurol* 45:518-22. PMID:10211478.

Patel RM, Downs-Kelly E, Weiss SW, et al [2005] Dual-color, break-apart fluorescence in situ hybridization for EWS gene rearrangement distinguishes clear cell sarcoma of soft tissue from malignant melanoma. *Mod Pathol* 18:1585-1590. PMID:16258500.

Peltomaki P [2003] Role of DNA mismatch repair defects in the pathogenesis of human cancer. *J Clin Oncol* 21:1174-9. PMID:12637487.

Pharoah PD, Guilford P, Caldas C [2001] Incidence of gastric cancer and breast cancer in CDH1 (E-cadherin) mutation carriers from hereditary diffuse gastric cancer families. *Gastroenterology* 121:1348-1353. PMID:11729114.

Phatak PD, Sham RL, Raubertas RF, et al [1998] Prevalence of hereditary hemochromatosis in 16031 primary care patients. *Ann Intern Med* 129:954-61. PMID:9867748.

Phillips AD, Schmitz J [1992] Familial villous atrophy: a clinico-pathological survey of 23 cases. *J Pediatr Gastroenterol Nutr* 14:380 PMID:1355534.

Pietrangelo A [2004] Hereditary hemochromatosis: a new look at an old disease. *N Engl J Med* 350(23):2383-2397. PMID:15175440.

Piippo K, Swan H, Pasternack M, et al [2001] A founder mutation of the potassium channel KCNQ1 in long QT syndrome: implications for estimation of disease prevalence and molecular diagnostics. *J Am Coll Cardiol* 37:562-8. PMID:11216980.

Pino MS, Chung DC [2010] Application of molecular diagnostics for the detection of Lynch syndrome. *Expert Rev Mol Diagn* 10(5):651-65. PMID:20629513.

Plante-Bordeneuve V, Said G [2000] Transthyretin related familial amyloid polyneuropathy. *Curr Opin Neurol* 13:569-73. PMID:11073365.

Poki HO, Holland AJ, Pitkin J [2005] Double bubble, double trouble. *Pediatr Surg Int* 21:428-31. PMID:15912365.

Press RD [1999] Hereditary hemochromatosis: impact of molecular and iron-based testing on the diagnosis, treatment, and prevention of a common, chronic disease. *Arch Pathol Lab Med* 123:1053-1059. PMID:10539907.

Prior TW, Bridgeman SJ [2005] Duchenne muscular dystrophy. *J Mol Diagn* 7(3):317-326. PMID:16049303.

Priori SG, Napolitano C, Giordano U, Collisani G, Memmi M [2000] Brugada syndrome and sudden cardiac death in children. *Lancet* 355:808-9. PMID:10711933.

Priori SG, Napolitano C, Tiso N, et al [2002] Mutations in the cardiac ryanodine receptor gene (hRyR2) underlie catecholaminergic polymorphic ventricular tachycardia. *Circulation* 102:r49-r53 PMID:11208676.

Pritchard KI, Shepherd LE, O'Malley FP, Andrulis IL, Tu D, Bramwell VH, Levine MN [2006] HER2 and responsiveness of breast cancer to adjuvant chemotherapy. *N Engl J Med* 354:2103-11. PMID:16707747.

Protonotarios N, Tsatsopoulou A, Anastasakis A, et al [2001] Genotype-phenotype assessment in autosomal recessive arrhythmogenic right ventricular cardiomyopathy (Naxos disease) caused by a deletion in plakoglobin. *J Am Coll Cardiol* 38:1477-84. PMID:11691526.

Pugliese A [2004] Genetics of type 1 diabetes. *Endocrinol Metab Clin N Am* 33:1-16. PMID:15053891.

Pyatt RE, Pilarski R, Prior TW [2006] Mutation screening in juvenile polyposis syndrome. *J Mol Diagn* 8(1) PMID:16436638.

Pyeritz RE [2005] Genetics and cardiovascular disease. In: *Braunwald's Heart Disease: A Textbook of Cardiovascular Medicine*, 7th ed. Philadelphia: Elsevier Saunders.

Qian Q, Li A, King BF, et al [2003] Clinical profile of autosomal dominant polycystic liver disease. *Hepatology* 37:164-71. PMID:12500201.

Ramasamy R, Haviland M, Woodard JR, Barone JG [2005] Patterns of inheritance in familial prune belly syndrome. *Urology* 65:1227. e26-1227.e27 PMID:15922438.

Ramirez-Seijas F, Granado-Villar D, Cepero-Akselrad A, et al [2000] Congenital nephrotic syndrome. *Int Pediatr* 15(2):121-122.

Rampazzo A, Nava A, Malacrida S, et al [2002] Mutation in human desmoplakin domain binding to plakoglobin causes a dominant form of arrhythmogenic right ventricular cardiomyopathy. *Am J Hum Genet* 71:1200-6. PMID:12373648.

Rapaport R [2004] Disorders of the gonads. In: *Nelson Textbook of Pediatrics*, 17th ed. Saunders, Philadelphia: Elsevier Science.

Raue F, Frank-Raue K, Grauer A [1994] Multiple endocrine neoplasia type 2. Clinical features and screening. *Endocrinol Metab Clin North Am* 23:137-56. PMID:7913021.

Ravine D, Gibson RN, Walker RG, et al [1994] Evaluation of ultrasonographic diagnostic criteria for autosomal dominant polycystic kidney disease 1. *Lancet* 343:824-7. PMID:7908078.

Redman JB, Fenwick RG Jr, Fu YH, Pizzuti A, Caskey CT [1993] Relationship between parental trinucleotide GCT repeat length and severity of myotonic dystrophy in offspring. *JAMA* 269:1960-5. PMID:8464127.

Reed MJ, Purohit A, Woo LWL, Newman SP, Potter BVL [2005] Steroid sulfatase: molecular biology, regulation, and inhibition. *Endocr Rev* 26(2):171-202. PMID:15561802.

Reid R, de Silva M, Paterson L, Ryan E, Fisher C [2003] Low grade fibromyxoid sarcoma and hyalinizing spindle cell tumor with giant rosettes share a common t(7;16)(q34;p11) translocation. *Am J Surg Pathol* 27:1229-1236. PMID:12960807.

Reynolds DM, Falk CT, Li A, et al [2000] Identification of a locus for autosomal dominant polycystic liver disease, on chromosome 19p13.2-13.1. *Am J Hum Genet* 67:1598-604. PMID:11047756.

Ribic CM, Sargent DJ, Moore MJ, et al [2003] Tumor microsatellite-instability status as a predictor of benefit from fluorouracil-based adjuvant chemotherapy for colon cancer. *N Engl J Med* 349:247-57. PMID:12867608.

Ridolfi RL, Jamehdor MR, Arber JM [2000] HER-2/neu testing in breast carcinoma: a combined immunohistochemical and fluorescence in situ hybridization approach. *Mod Pathol* 13(8):866-873. PMID:10955453.

Rijcken FEM, Hollema H, Kleibeuker JH [2002] Proximal adenomas in hereditary non-polyposis colorectal cancer are prone to rapid malignant transformation. *Gut* 50:382-386. PMID:11839719.

Rinaldo P, Yoon HR, Yu C, et al [1999] Sudden and unexpected neonatal death: a protocol for the postmortem diagnosis of fatty acid oxidation disorders. *Semin Perinatol* 23:204-10. PMID:10331471.

Rinaldo P, Matern D, Bennett MJ [2002] Fatty acid oxidation disorders. *Annu Rev Physiol* 64:477-502. PMID:11826276.

Rizzu P, Van Swieten JC, Joosse M, et al [1999] High prevalence of mutations in the microtubule-associated protein tau in a population study of frontotemporal dementia in the Netherlands. *Am J Hum Genet* 64:414-21. PMID:9973279.

Romeo G, Ceccherini I, Celli J, et al [1998] Association of multiple endocrine neoplasia type 2 and Hirschsprung disease. *J Intern Med* 243:515-20. PMID:9681852.

Rosenberg RN [2000] The molecular and genetic basis of AD: the end of the beginning. *Neurology* 54:2045-54. PMID:10851361.

Rosenblatt A, Brinkman RR, Liang KY, et al [2001] Familial influence on age of onset among siblings with Huntington disease. *Am J Med Genet* 105:399-403. PMID:11449389.

Rosenblatt A, Liang KY, Zhou H, et al [2006] The association of CAG repeat length with clinical progression in Huntington disease. *Neurology* 66:1016-1020. PMID:16606912.

Rossetti S, Strmecki L, Gamble V, et al [2001] Mutation analysis of the entire PKD1 gene: Genetic and diagnostic implications. *Am J Hum Genet* 68:46-63. PMID:11115377.

Rossetti S, Chauveau D, Walker D, et al [2002] A complete mutation screen of the ADPKD genes by DHPLC. *Kidney Int* 61:1588-99. PMID:11967008.

Rossetti S, Torra R, Coto E, et al [2003a] A complete mutation screen of PKHD1 in autosomal-recessive polycystic kidney disease (ARPKD) pedigrees. *Kidney Int* 64:391-403. PMID:12846734.

Rossetti S, Chauveau D, Kubly V, et al [2003b] Association of mutation position in polycystic kidney disease 1 (PKD1) gene and development of a vascular phenotype. *Lancet* 361:2196-201. PMID:12842373.

Rossi E, Olynyk JK, Cullen DJ, et al [2000] Compound heterozygous hemochromatosis: genotype predicts increased iron and erythrocyte indices in women. *Clin Chem* 46(2):162-166. PMID:10657371.

Rosso SM, Kamphorst W, de Graaf B, et al [2001] Familial frontotemporal dementia with ubiquitin-positive inclusions is linked to chromosome 17q21-22. *Brain* 124:1948-57. PMID:11571213.

Rowe SM, Miller S, Sorscher EJ [2005] Cystic fibrosis. *New Engl J Med* 352:1992-2001. PMID:15888700.

Rowley PT [2005] Inherited susceptibility to colorectal cancer. *Annu Rev Med* 56:539-54. PMID:15660526.

Ruijter E, Van De Kaa C, Miller G, Ruiter D, Debruyne F, Schalken J [1999] Molecular genetics and epidemiology of prostate carcinoma. *Endocr Rev* 20(1):22-45. PMID:10047972.

Rüschoff J, Dietel M, Baretton G, et al [2010] HER2 diagnostics in gastric cancer—guideline validation and development of standardized immunohistochemical testing. *Virchows Arch* 457(3):299-307. PMID:20665045.

Rustgi AK [1994] Hereditary gastrointestinal polyposis and nonpolyposis syndromes. *N Engl J Med* 331:1694-702. PMID:7969362.

Ryan MM, Schnell C, Strickland CD, et al [2001] Nemaline myopathy: a clinical study of 143 cases. *Ann Neurol* 50:312-20. PMID:11558787.

Saito M, Kawai H, Akaike M, et al [1996] Cardiac dysfunction with Becker muscular dystrophy. *Am Heart J* 132:642-7. PMID:8800037.

Sampson JR, Maheshwar MM, Aspinwall R, et al [1997] Renal cystic disease in tuberous sclerosis: role of the polycystic kidney disease 1 gene. *Am J Hum Genet* 61:843-51. PMID:9382094.

Sancandi M, Griseri P, Pesce B, et al [2003] Single nucleotide polymorphic alleles in the 5' region of the RET protooncogene define a risk haplotype in Hirschsprung's disease. *J Med Genet* 40:714-8. PMID:12960220.

Sandler A, Gray R, Perry MC, et al [2006] Paclitaxel-carboplatin alone or with bevacizumab for non-small-cell lung cancer. *N Engl J Med* 355(24):2542-2550. PMID:17167137.

Santoro M, Melillo RM, Carlomagno F, Vecchio G, Fusco A [2004] RET: normal and abnormal functions. *Endocrinology* 145:5448-51. PMID:15331579.

Santos GC, Zielenska M, Prasad M, Squire JA [2007] Chromosome 6p amplification and cancer progression. *J Clin Pathol* 60:1-7. PMID:16790693.

Saunders AM, Hulette O, Welsh-Bohmer KA, et al [1996] Specificity, sensitivity, and predictive value of apolipoprotein-E genotyping for sporadic Alzheimer's disease. *Lancet* 348:90-3. PMID:8676723.

Schmidt H, Bartel F, Kappler M, Wurl P, Lange H, Bache M, Holzhausen H, Taubert H [2005] Gains of 13q are correlated with a poor prognosis in liposarcoma. *Mod Pathol* 18:638-644. PMID:15540119.

Schrager CA, Schneider D, Gruener AC, Tsou HC, Peacocke M [1998] Clinical and pathological features of breast disease in Cowden's syndrome: An underrecognized syndrome with an increased risk of breast cancer. *Hum Pathol* 29:47-53. PMID:9445133.

Schuetz AN, Yin-Goen Q, Amin MB, et al [2005] Molecular classification of renal tumors by gene expression profiling. *J Mol Diagn* 7(2) PMID:15858144.

Schuppan D [2000] Current concepts of celiac disease pathogenesis. *Gastroenterology* 119:234-42. PMID:10889174.

Schwab M, Schaeffeler E, Marx C, et al [2003] Association between the C3435T MDR1 gene polymorphism and susceptibility for ulcerative colitis. *Gastroenterology* 124(1):26-33. PMID:12512026.

Schwartz PJ, Priori SG, Spazzolini C, et al [2001] Genotype-phenotype correlation in the long-QT syndrome: gene-specific triggers for life threatening arrhythmias. *Circulation* 103:89-95. PMID:11136691.

Sethi KD, Adams RJ, Loring DW, el Gammal T [1988] Hallervorden-Spatz syndrome: clinical and magnetic resonance imaging correlations. *Ann Neurol* 24:692-4. PMID:3202617.

Sharer N, Schwarz M, Malone G, Howarth A, Painter J, Super M, Braganza J [1998] Mutations of the cystic fibrosis gene in patients with chronic pancreatitis. *N Engl J Med* 339:645-52. PMID:9725921.

Shevell M [1992] Racial hygiene, active euthanasia, and Julius Hallervorden. *Neurology* 42:2214-9. PMID:1436542.

Shevell M [2003] Hallervorden and history. *N Engl J Med* 348(1):3-4. PMID:12510036.

Shia J, Tang LH, Vakiani E, Guillem JG, et al [2009] Immunohistochemistry as first-line screening for detecting colorectal cancer patients at risk for hereditary nonpolyposis colorectal cancer syndrome: a 2-antibody panel may be as predictive as a 4-antibody panel. *Am J Surg Pathol*. 33(11):1639-45. PMID:19701074.

Sholl LM, Lindeman NI [2010] Molecular diagnostics testing for lung adenocarcinoma—state of the art in 2010. *Pathol Case Rev* 15:103-110.

Sieber OM, Lipton L, Crabtree M, et al [2003] Multiple colorectal adenomas, classic adenomatous polyposis, and germline mutations in MYH. *N Engl J Med* 348:791-9. PMID:12606733.

Sipple JH [1961] The association of pheochromocytoma with carcinoma of the thyroid gland. *Am J Med* 31:163-166.

Sjögren H, Meis-Kindblom JM, Orndal C, et al [2003] Studies on the molecular pathogenesis of extraskeletal myxoid chondrosarcoma—cytogenetic, molecular genetic, and cDNA microarray analyses. *Am J Pathol* 162(3):781-792. PMID:12598313.

Skandalakis JE, Ellis H [2000] Embryologic and anatomic basis of esophageal surgery. *Surg Clin North Am* 80:85 PMID:10685146.

Smith VV, Eng C, Milla PJ [1999] Intestinal ganglioneuromatosis and multiple endocrine neoplasia type 2B: implications for treatment. *Gut* 45:143-6. PMID:10369718.

Smith JM, Kirk EP, Theodosopoulos G, et al [2002] Germline mutations of the tumour suppressor PTEN in Proteus syndrome. *J Med Genet* 39:937-40. PMID:12471211.

Smith RJH, Hone S [2003] Genetic screening for deafness. *Pediatr Clin N Am* 50:315-329. PMID:12809325.

Snover DC, Jass JR, Fenoglio-Preiser C, Batts KP [2005] Serrated polyps of the large intestine: a morphologic and molecular review of an evolving concept. *Am J Clin Pathol* 124:380-391. PMID:16191506.

Speiser PW, White PC [2003] Congenital adrenal hyperplasia. *N Engl J Med* 349:776-88. PMID:12930931.

Spiegel AM, Weinstein LS [2004] Inherited diseases involving G proteins and G protein-coupled receptors. *Annu Rev Med* 55:27-39. PMID:14746508.

Spillantini MG, Crowther RA, Kamphorst W, Heutink P, van Swieten JC [1998] Tau pathology in 2 Dutch families with mutations in the microtubule binding region of tau. *Am J Pathol* 153:1359-63. PMID:9811325.

Spitz L, Kiely EM, Morecroft JA, Drake DP [1994] Oesophageal atresia: at-risk groups for the 1990s. *J Pediatr Surg* 29:723-5. PMID:8078005.

Splawski I, Shen J, Timothy KW, et al [2000] Spectrum of mutations in long-QT syndrome genes: KVLQT1, HERG, SCN5A, KCNE1, and KCNE2. *Circulation* 102:1178-85. PMID:10973849.

Squitieri F, Gellera C, Cannella M, et al [2003] Homozygosity for CAG mutation in Huntington disease is associated with a more severe clinical course. *Brain* 126:946-55. PMID:12615650.

Stevens M, van Duijn CM, Kamphorst W, et al [1998] Familial aggregation in frontotemporal dementia. *Neurology* 50:1541-5. PMID:9633692.

Stewart DR, Von Allmen D [2003] The genetics of Hirschsprung disease. *Gastroenterol Clin N Am* 32:819-837. PMID:14562576.

Tabernero MD, Espinosa AB, Maíllo A, et al [2005] Characterization of chromosome 14 abnormalities by interphase in situ hybridization and comparative genomic hybridization in 124 meningiomas: correlation with clinical, histopathologic, and prognostic features. *Am J Clin Pathol* 123:744-751. PMID:15981814.

Tabib A, Loire R, Chalabreysse L, et al [2002] Circumstances of death and gross and microscopic observations in a series of 200 cases of sudden death associated with arrhythmogenic right ventricular cardiomyopathy and/or dysplasia. *Circulation* 108:3000-5. PMID:14662701.

Takahashi M, Asai N, Iwashita T, Murakami H, Ito S [1998] Molecular mechanisms of development of multiple endocrine neoplasia 2 by RET mutations. *J Intern Med* 243:509-13. PMID:9681851.

Takazawa Y, Sakurai S, Sakuma Y, et al [2005] Gastrointestinal stromal tumors of neurofibromatosis Type I (von Recklinghausen's disease). *Am J Surg Pathol* 29:755-763. PMID:15897742.

Tammaro A, Bracco A, Cozzolino S, et al [2003] Scanning for mutations of the ryanodine receptor (*RYR1*) gene by denaturing HPLC: Detection of 3 novel malignant hyperthermia alleles. *Clin Chem* 49(5): 761-768. PMID:12709367.

Tanaka R, Koyanagi K, Narita N, Kuo C, Hoon DSB [2011] Prognostic molecular biomarkers for cutaneous malignant melanoma. *J Surg Oncol* 104:438-446. PMID:21557225.

Tavill AS [2001] Diagnosis and management of hemochromatosis. *Hepatology* 33:1321-8. PMID:11343262.

Teunissen LL, Notermans NC, Franssen H, Van Engelen BG, Baas F, Wokke JH [2003] Disease course of Charcot-Marie-Tooth disease type 2: a 5-year follow-up study. *Arch Neurol* 60:823-8. PMID:12810486.

Thorner PS, Ho M, Chilton-MacNeill S, Zielenska M [2006] Use of chromogenic in situ hybridization to identify MYCN gene copy number in neuroblastoma using routine tissue sections. *Am J Surg Pathol* 30:635-642. PMID:16699319.

Thull DL, Vogel VG [2000] Recognition and management of hereditary breast cancer syndromes. *Oncologist* 9:13-24. PMID:14755011.

Tiebosch AT, Frederik PM, van Breda Vriesman PJ, et al [1989] Thin-basement-membrane nephropathy in adults with persistent hematuria. *N Engl J Med* 320:14-18. PMID:2909874.

Tiso N, Stephan DA, Nava A, et al [2001] Identification of mutations in the cardiac ryanodine receptor gene in families affected with arrhythmogenic right ventricular cardiomyopathy type 2 (ARVD2). *Hum Mol Genet* 10:189-94. PMID:11159936.

Torlakovic E, Skovlund E, Snover DC, Torlakovic G, Nesland JM [2003] Morphologic reappraisal of serrated colorectal polyps. *Am J Surg Pathol* 27(1):65-81. PMID:12502929.

Torres VE, Wilson DM, Hattery RR, Segura JW [1993] Renal stone disease in autosomal dominant polycystic kidney disease. *Am J Kidney Dis* 22:513-9. PMID:8213789.

Tortorelli S, Tokunaga C, Strauss AW, Winters J, Hahn SH, Matern D, Rinaldo P [2004] Correlation of genotype and biochemical phenotype in 106 patients with MCAD deficiency. *J Inherit Metab Dis* 27Suppl1:102.

Towbin JA [2004] Molecular genetic basis of sudden cardiac death. *Pediatr Clin N Am* 2004;51:1229-1255. PMID:15331282.

Trajkovskia M, Mziauta H, Schwarz PE, Solimenaa M [2006] Genes of type 2 diabetes in β cells. *Endocrinol Metab Clin N Am* 35:357-369. PMID:16632098.

Trpkov K, Gao Y, Hay R, Yimaz A [2006] No residual cancer on radical prostatectomy after positive 10-core biopsy: incidence, biopsy findings, and DNA specimen identity analysis. *Arch Pathol Lab Med* 130:811-816. PMID:16740032.

Tryggvason K, Patrakka J, Wartiovaara J [2006] Hereditary proteinuria syndromes and mechanisms of proteinuria. *N Engl J Med* 354:1387-401. PMID:16571882.

Van De Voorde R, Witte D, Kogan J, Goebel J [2006] Pierson syndrome: a novel cause of congenital nephrotic syndrome. *Pediatrics* 118;e501-e505 PMID:16864643.

Van den Bos M, Van den Hoven M, Jongejan E, et al [2004] More differences between HNPCC-related and sporadic carcinomas from the endometrium as compared to the colon. *Am J Surg Pathol* 28:706-711. PMID:15166662.

Van der Kooi AJ, Barth PG, Busch HF, et al [1996] The clinical spectrum of limb girdle muscular dystrophy. A survey in The Netherlands. *Brain* 119(5):1471-80. PMID:8931572.

Van Kessel AG, Wijnhoven H, Bodmer D, et al [1999] Renal cell cancer: chromosome 3 translocations as risk factors. *J Natl Cancer Inst* 91:1159-60. PMID:10393725.

Varley JM, Evans DG, Birch JM [1997] Li-Fraumeni syndrome--a molecular and clinical review. *Br J Cancer* 76:1-14. PMID:9218725.

Vasen HF, Watson P, Mecklin JP, Lynch HT [1999] New clinical criteria for hereditary nonpolyposis colorectal cancer (HNPCC, Lynch syndrome) proposed by the International Collaborative group on HNPCC. *Gastroenterology* 1999;116:1453-6. PMID:10348829.

Vatta M, Dumaine R, Varghese G, et al [2002] Genetic and biophysical basis of sudden unexplained nocturnal death syndrome (SUNDS), a disease allelic to Brugada syndrome. *Hum Mol Genet* 11:337-45. PMID:11823453.

Vaxillaire M, Froguel P [2006] Genetic basis of maturity-onset diabetes of the young. *Endocrinol Metab Clin N Am* 35:371-384. PMID:16632099.

Veugelers M, Bressan M, McDermott DA, et al [2004] Mutation of perinatal myosin heavy chain associated with a Carney complex variant. *N Engl J Med* 351:460-9. PMID:15282353.

Viitasalo M, Oikarinen L, Vaananen H, et al [2002] Differentiation between LQT1 and LQT2 patients and unaffected subjects using 24-hour electrocardiographic recordings. *Am J Cardiol* 89:679-85. PMID:11897209.

Vlahovic G, Crawford J [2003] Activation of tyrosine kinases in cancer. *Oncologist* 8(6):531-538. PMID:14657531.

Von Mehren M, Watson JC [2005] Gastrointestinal stromal tumors. *Hematol Oncol Clin N Am* 19:547-564. PMID:15939196.

Wagner KR [2002] Genetic diseases of muscle. *Neurol Clin N Am* 20:645-678. PMID:12432825.

Wang Q, Curran ME, Splawski I, et al [1996] Positional cloning of a novel potassium channel gene: KVLQT1 mutations cause cardiac arrhythmias. *Nat Genet* 12:17-23. PMID:8528244.

Wang DW, Viswanathan PC, Balser JR, et al [2002] Clinical, genetic, and biophysical characterization of SCN5A mutations associated with atrioventricular conduction block. *Circulation* 105:341-6. PMID:11804990.

Watanabe T, Wu TT, Catalano PJ, et al [2001] Molecular predictors of survival after adjuvant chemotherapy for colon cancer. *N Engl J Med* 344:1196-206. PMID:11309634.

Watson JC, Stratakis CA, Bryant-Greenwood PK, et al [2000] Neurosurgical implications of Carney complex. *J Neurosurg* 92:413-8. PMID:10701527.

Weinstein LS, Shenker A, Gejman PV, et al [1991] Activating mutations of the stimulatory G protein in the McCune-Albright syndrome. *N Engl J Med* 325:1688-1695. PMID:1944469.

Weiss FU, Simon P, Mayerle J, Kraft M, Lerch MM [2006] Germline mutations and gene polymorphism associated with human pancreatitis *Endocrinol Metab Clin N Am* 35:289-302. PMID:16632093.

Weksberg R, Nishikawa J, Caluseriu O, et al [2001] Tumor development in the Beckwith-Wiedemann syndrome is associated with a variety of constitutional molecular 11p15 alterations including imprinting defects of KCNQ1OT1. *Hum Mol Genet* 10:2989-3000. PMID:11751681.

West H, Harpole D, Travis W [2009] Histologic considerations for individualized systemic therapy approaches for the management of non-small cell lung cancer. *Chest* 136(4):1112-1118. PMID:19809052.

White PC, Tusie-Luna MT, New MI, Speiser PW [1994] Mutations in steroid 21-hydroxylase (CYP21). *Hum Mutat* 3:373-8. PMID:8081391.

Wicklund CL, Pauli RM, Johnston D, Hecht JT [1995] Natural history study of hereditary multiple exostoses. *Am J Med Genet* 55:43-6. PMID:7702095.

Wijsman EM, Daw EW, Yu CE, et al [2004] Evidence for a novel late-onset Alzheimer disease locus on chromosome 19p13.2. *Am J Hum Genet* 75:398-409. PMID:15248153.

Wilde AA, Antzelevitch C, Borggrefe M, et al [2002] Proposed diagnostic criteria for the Brugada syndrome. *Circulation* 106:2514-9. PMID:12417552.

Wilson PD [2004] Mechanisms of disease: polycystic kidney disease. *N Engl J Med* 350:151-64. PMID:14711914.

Wolff AC, Hammond MEH, Schwartz JN, et al [2007] American Society of Clinical Oncology/College of American Pathologists guideline recommendations for human epidermal growth factor receptor 2 testing in breast cancer. *Arch Pathol Lab Med* 131:18-43. PMID:19548375.

Worsham MJ, Wolman SR, Zarbo RJ [2001] Molecular approaches to identification of tissue contamination in surgical pathology sections. *J Mol Diagn* 3:11-15. PMID:11227066.

Wright TC Jr, Cox JT, Massad LS, Twiggs LB, Wilkinson EJ [2002] 2001 Consensus guidelines for the management of women with cervical cytological abnormalities. *JAMA* 287:2120-9. PMID:11966387.

Wright CL, Stewart ID [2003] Histopathology and mismatch repair status of 458 consecutive colorectal carcinomas. *Am J Surg Pathol* 27:1393-1406. PMID:14576472.

Wuyts W, Van Hul W [2001] Molecular basis of multiple exostoses: Mutations in the EXT1 and EXT2 genes. *Hum Mutat* 15:220-7. PMID:10679937.

Yamamoto H, Oda Y, Kawaguchi K, et al [2004] C-kit and PDGFRA mutations in extragastrointestinal stromal tumor (gastrointestinal stromal tumor of the soft tissue). *Am J Surg Pathol* 28:479-488. PMID:15087667.

Yang S, Farraye FA, Mack C, Posnik O, O'Brien MJ [2004] BRAF and KRAS mutations in hyperplastic polyps and serrated adenomas of the colorectum relationship to histology and CpG island methylation status. *Am J Surg Pathol* 28:1452-1459. PMID:15489648.

Yatabe Y, Kosaka T, Takahashi T, Mitsudomi T [2005] EGFR mutation is specific for terminal respiratory unit type adenocarcinoma. *Am J Surg Pathol* 29:633-639. PMID:15832087.

Young S, Gooneratne S, Straus FH, Zeller WP, Bulun SE, Rosenthal IM [1995] Feminizing Sertoli cell tumors in boys with Peutz-Jeghers syndrome. *Am J Surg Pathol* 19:50-8. PMID:7802138.

Zareba W, Moss AJ, Schwartz PJ, et al [1998] Influence of genotype on the clinical course of the long-QT syndrome. *N Engl J Med* 339:960-5. PMID:9753711.

Zenker M, Mayerle J, Lerch MM, et al [2005] Deficiency of UBR1, a ubiquitin ligase of the N-end rule pathway, causes pancreatic dysfunction, malformations and mental retardation (Johanson-Blizzard syndrome). *Nat Genet* 37:1345-50. PMID:16311597.

Zenker M, Mayerle J, Reis A, Lerch MM [2006] Genetic basis and pancreatic biology of Johanson-Blizzard syndrome. *Endocrinol Metab Clin N Am* 35:243-253. PMID:16632090.

Zhou X, Hampel H, Thiele H, Gorlin RJ, Hennekam RC, Parisi M, Winter RM, Eng C [2001] Association of germline mutation in the PTEN tumour suppressor gene and Proteus and Proteus-like syndromes. *Lancet* 358:210-1. PMID:11476841.

Zielenski J, Corey M, Rozmahel R [1999] Detection of a cystic fibrosis modifier locus for meconium ileus on human chromosome 19q13. *Nat Genet* 22:128-9. PMID:10369249.

Zielenski J [2000] Genotype and phenotype in cystic fibrosis. *Respiration* 67:117-33. PMID:10773783.

Zschocke J, Schulze A, Lindner M, Fiesel S, Olgemoller K, Hoffmann GF, Penzien J, Ruiter JP, Wanders RJ, Mayatepek E [2001] Molecular and functional characterisation of mild MCAD deficiency. *Hum Genet* 108:404-8. PMID:11409868.

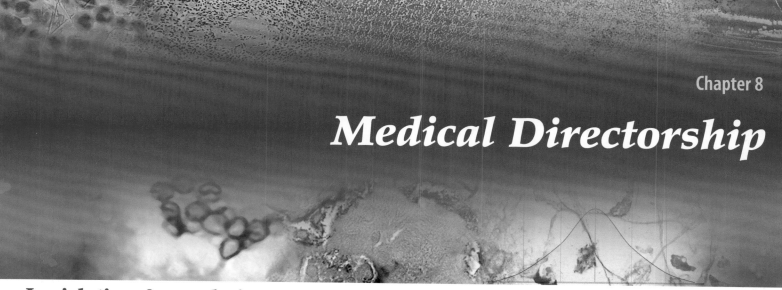

Chapter 8

Medical Directorship

Legislation & regulation, agencies & oversight

Legislation & regulations relating to laboratories

Clinical Laboratory Improvement Amendment of 1988 (CLIA '88)

CLIA was enacted in 1988 as an amendment to the Clinical Laboratory Act of 1967. It represents section 353 of chapter 42 of the Code of Federal Regulations. Its impetus was a series of stories in the lay press exposing Pap smear "mills" wherein laboratory testing was being performed for profit with inadequate regard for quality. CLIA was written to codify what are essentially good laboratory practices. The authority for executing the provisions of CLIA was given to the Centers for Medicare and Medicaid Services (CMS), a division of the Department of Health and Human Services (DHHS). Prior to CLIA, sporadic regulation existed at the state level, and the Clinical Laboratory Act of 1960 applied primarily to laboratories engaged in interstate commerce. CLIA applies to all laboratories that perform testing on "materials derived from the human body," including laboratories found in physician offices, whether or not they participate in Medicare or Medicaid. CLIA does not specifically regulate collection kits, workplace drug testing, testing for research purposes, or noninvasive testing (breath tests, transcutaneous bilirubin). About a decade passed before the final rules (regulations) for administration of CLIA were written; as part of the final rules, the CLIA Committee (CLIAC) was formed in order to arbitrate emerging issues.

According to CLIA, the Food and Drug Administration (FDA), also a division of DHHS, is responsible for classifying laboratory testing into 3 levels of test complexity t8.1, with stringency of requirements varying commensurately. Initially, test categories included waived, moderate complexity, and high complexity. Later, a category of provider-performed microscopy (PPM) was added, and moderate/high complexity tests were grouped into a single category of "nonwaived" tests. Subsequently, laboratories are classified according to the highest complexity of testing they perform.

When CLIA was first enacted, the waived test category included a list of 8 specifically named tests. Now there are many more on the list, and the waived category includes those specifically listed in addition to any test cleared by the FDA for home use. Each test submitted to the FDA is subjected to a scoring system based upon 7 criteria, worth up to 3 points each. A score of >12 makes a test nonwaived. There are no specific requirements for who may perform waived tests, but the performing laboratory must be in possession of at least a certificate of waiver. Note that waived tests are not synonymous with point of care (POC) tests. POC tests may be waived or nonwaived. POC testing is usually performed under the CLIA certificate of the hospital laboratory, whose responsibility it is to ensure that it is done properly.

t8.1 CLIA levels of test complexity

Test complexity	
Waived	If a lab performs only waived testing, then it must have certificate of waiver; waived tests are simple tests that have been cleared by FDA for home use, that are simple and accurate enough to be largely error-free, and that "pose no reasonable risk of harm to the patient if the test is performed incorrectly"
	Examples include the common urine dipstick tests, fecal occult blood testing, urine pregnancy tests, home glucose monitoring tests, spun hematocrit
	Requirements of those conducting waived testing are only that they follow manufacturer's instructions
Nonwaived (moderate & high complexity)	A scoring system is applied to nonwaived tests to determine whether they are of moderate or high complexity; in general, most automated tests are considered moderate, while those that have a significant manual component are high complexity (eg, parasite identification)
	If a test of moderate complexity is modified, it generally is then considered a high complexity test
	Requirements include qualified laboratory director & testing personnel, written procedures to assure proper specimen collection & procedure performance, the testing of positive & negative controls each day patient samples are tested, enrollment in proficiency testing, stipulations regarding record keeping & biennial (every other year) inspection
	Requirements of moderate & high complexity testing differs mainly in the personnel requirements
Provider-performed microscopy (PPM)	PPM is a subcategory of moderate complexity testing
	To be regarded as PPM, a procedure must be performed by a physician, dentist, or midlevel practitioner under physician supervision, and it must be performed during the patient visit during which the specimen is procured
	The primary instrument for performing the test must be a microscope, limited to bright field or phase contrast microscopy
	The specimen must be of the sort that a delay (in taking to a lab) would compromise it; control materials are not available for this type of test, and there is limited specimen processing required
	PPM examinations include, eg, direct wet mounts (eg, for fungi, parasites, bacteria), KOH preparations, pinworm examinations, ferning tests, examinations of urine sediment

CLIA requires federal certification for all laboratories. A CLIA certificate is required before a laboratory can perform testing on human samples, and certificates must be renewed every 2 years. The certificate holder is the laboratory medical director, and each medical director can hold no more than 5 certificates at any given time. There are several types of certification, including

1. certificate of registration

2. certificate of waiver

3. certificate for provider-performed microscopy (PPM)

4. certificate of compliance

5. certificate of accreditation

A laboratory that applies for certification will receive a certificate of registration, at which time testing can begin. If the laboratory chooses to be inspected by CLIA, then it will receive a certificate of compliance upon successful completion of its first CLIA inspection. A certificate of accreditation is awarded upon successful completion of inspection by an accrediting agency (eg, CAP).

Every certified lab must be externally inspected at least every 2 years, and must conduct an internal (interval) inspection during the intervening year. While CMS is the ultimate accrediting agency and reserves the right to perform its own inspections as needed, CMS extends "deemed" status to agencies such as the College of American Pathologists (CAP) who are normally entrusted with this activity. CAP inspections are "unannounced" inspections that take place within a known 3-month window that ends on the anniversary date of the last accreditation. CAP inspections are performed according to a checklist of items, and each checklist item is assigned a weight of either "phase I" or "phase II." Phase II citations are more severe and require documented corrective action within 30 days. Phase I citations must be corrected before the next internal inspection. "Phase 0" checklist items are not officially graded and usually represent items under development.

Laboratories may also be inspected as part of a hospitalwide inspection by The Joint Commission (TJC), and laboratories involved with blood products will be inspected by the FDA. Laboratories can be accredited by TJC, which like CAP has CLIA deemed status to accredit laboratories; in such instances, TJC laboratory inspection is usually distinct from the hospitalwide inspection. Laboratories that are CAP-accredited can choose to not be TJC-inspected; in this scenario, the hospitalwide TJC inspection may still involve the laboratory as part of TJC's tracer-style inspection. Lastly, laboratories that perform forensic drug testing (eg, drug testing for employers or government agencies) are certified under a separate DHHS registry.

CLIA requires that accredited laboratories participate in proficiency testing (PT), with criteria for acceptable performance defined by the regulations. PT vendors must be approved by CMS, and once a laboratory selects a vendor it must remain with the same vendor for 1 full year before switching to another. See p 449 for further discussion.

CLIA regulations articulate the minimum expectations for the preanalytic, analytic, and postanalytic management of patient testing. Preanalytic requirements include the use of written (or electronic) requisitions to document physician orders. The regulations further require the keeping of written procedure manuals and the keeping of maintenance records. Quality control practices are stipulated in the CLIA regulations, as are personnel requirements. Lastly, the regulations spell out the minimum requirements for result reporting (must be reported with a statement of the reference range on a form that properly identifies the patient) and result recordkeeping.

Medical devices & biologics

The FDA has 2 major roles in laboratory testing. It is tasked with regulating medical devices and biologics. Testing instruments and reagents are considered medical devices, and blood products are biologics.

Medical devices must be reviewed by the FDA before they are ready for market. A medical device is defined in the regulations as "any instrument, apparatus, or other article that is used to prevent, diagnose, mitigate, or treat a disease or to affect the structure or function of the body, with the exception of drugs." There are 2 echelons of review: clearance and approval. For FDA clearance, a premarket notification or 510(k) must be filed by the manufacturer to document that the device is substantially equivalent to another FDA approved device. For FDA approval, generally required of truly novel devices, a formal validation must be undertaken by the manufacturer and filed in the form of a premarket approval (PMA) application. The PMA process is much more rigorous than the 510(k) process.

There are some medical devices that do not require FDA review (510[k] exempt medical devices). Like FDA-cleared and approved devices, proper labeling, listing, reporting, and good manufacturing practices are still required. For these devices, part of proper labeling would include a statement that the device is not FDA-cleared or approved. The reporting requirement refers to the duty of users and/or manufacturers to report device malfunction; laboratories are subject to this mandate. Listing is primarily the responsibility of the manufacturer who must ensure that their device is FDA-listed. 510(k)-exempt devices are those that were marketed before enactment of the law on May 28, 1976 (preamendment or grandfathered devices) and newer devices that have been specifically exempted by regulation. Microscopes and microscope accessories, for example, are exempt.

Lastly, the FDA offers an exemption for Humanitarian Use Devices (HUDs). These are devices which are intended to be used in rare scenarios—for diagnosing or treating a condition that affects <4,000 individuals in the United States/year—such that the cost of research and development would exceed its market return. The premarket application in this case is meant to document safety rather than effectiveness. The institution in which an HUD is used must have an institutional review board (IRB) approval of the device.

The FDA classifies medical devices into one of 3 categories—class I, class II, and class III. The classification is largely based upon the risk associated with its use. Class I devices are deemed to be low risk and represent the vast majority of 510(k)-exempt devices. Dental floss is a class I medical device. Class II devices have higher risk associated with their use and are subject to tighter regulatory control. Class III devices include heart valves.

A particularly confusing topic in the medical device arena is that concerned with analyte specific reagents (ASRs) and laboratory-developed tests (LDTs). ASRs are defined as "antibodies, both polyclonal and monoclonal, specific receptor proteins, ligands, nucleic acid sequences, and similar reagents which, through specific binding or chemical reactions with substances in a specimen, are intended for use in a diagnostic application for identification and quantification of an individual chemical substance or ligand in biological specimens." This contrasts with general purpose reagents (GPRs) that are nonspecific. ASRs are the building blocks of LDTs. A reagent developed by a manufacturer for sole use in its test system (ie, reagent is not separately marketed by itself) is not an ASR. An antibody used in immunohistochemistry, for example, may be an ASR; the entire process that includes mounting the section, deparaffinizing it, incubation with antibody, peroxidase reaction, and interpretation comprises the LDT. Whether an antibody is or is not an ASR depends upon its labeling: those labeled as "for in vitro diagnostic use" (IVDs) are not ASRs. The FDA considers ASRs to be medical devices and therefore subject to its regulation. Under this authority, the FDA published "the ASR rule" in 1997. The FDA chose not to subject ASRs to the premarket process and instead to rely on the use of controls, good manufacturing practices, medical device reporting, and labeling. The ASR rule does 3 things:

1. classifies ASRs (class I, II or III)

2. imposes restrictions on the sale and use of ASRs

3. delineates labeling requirements

The labeling requirement is 2-fold.

1. Reports of test results must include the statement "this test was developed and its performance characteristics determined by (your laboratory). It has not been cleared or approved by the US Food and Drug Administration."

2. The ASR must be labeled with "Analyte Specific Reagent. Analytical and performance characteristics are not established." If a manufacturer wishes to make performance claims in its marketing, then the ASR must be submitted through the usual PMA process.

Given these requirements, the rule classifies most ASRs as class I devices. Some ASR are still categorized as class II and class III and therefore subject to FDA clearance or approval. Reagents used in blood bank testing, for example, are generally considered class II devices. Class III ASRs include those used independently to diagnose a condition that is likely to be fatal for which prompt and accurate diagnosis has public health impact (eg, TB), for donor screening of blood products, or for diagnosis or monitoring of HIV infection. In particular regard to immunohistochemistry (IHC), most antibodies are class I ASRs. For class I status, the IHC test must be adjunctive; that is, the primary diagnosis is made by conventional histopathology and IHC is used for further clarification or sub classification (eg, characterize tumor of unknown primary). Class II IHCs are generally those that are used to generate prognostic or predictive data that cannot be determined by routine histopathologic techniques and for which there is significant scientific validation (eg, hormone receptors in breast cancer). For these there are special requirements for control and guidance. Class III IHCs require PMA; these do not meet criteria for class I or II and generally imply a class II-like analyte for which there is not extensive scientific validation.

Blood falls under the FDA's Center for Biologics Evaluation and Research (CBER), which regulates blood and blood components, cell separation devices, blood collection containers and HIV screening tests that are used in the preparation of blood products. The FDA inspects all blood facilities at least annually, and participation is mandatory. One important peculiarity of FDA oversight is that, unlike CMS/CLIA in which the laboratory medical director is considered the ultimate leader, the FDA defines the "responsible head" as the facility owner; in most cases, the FDA defers to the hospital COO or CEO as the representative of the owner.

Agencies that set nonbinding standards

There are agencies that have no specific regulatory authority but offer useful standards for use by laboratories. These include the Clinical Laboratory Standards Institute (CLSI) and International Standardization Organization (ISO). CLSI initially went by the name of NCCLS (National Committee on Clinical Laboratory Standards). Its mission is to develop and publish best practices in laboratory testing through a consensus process that invites input from industry, government, and the health care professionals. For example, CLSI recently published a monograph on specimen labeling issuing a standard for font, font size, location, and orientation of labels. The standards are products that are available for purchase but are entirely voluntary. The American branch of the ISO is the American National Standards Institute (ANSI). ISO is primarily concerned with issuing standards concerned with quality management.

The Institute of Medicine (IOM) has emerged as an agency with significant weight in advising the federal government about the medical profession. The IOM is a division of the National Academy of Sciences (NAS); both the IOM and the NAS are private, nongovernmental organizations that utilize federal funds. The IOM has produced several reports, including the widely referenced *To Err is Human: Building A Safer Health System*.

Medicare, Medicaid & the Prospective Payment System

The Social Security Act of 1965 contained provisions for the establishment of Medicare and Medicaid. Medicare is a federal program administered by the Centers for Medicare and Medicaid Services (CMS), a division of DHHS. It extends benefits to 3 groups of people

1. age 65 and older

2. permanently disabled

3. end-stage renal disease

Care is reimbursed under parts A and B. Part A covers inpatient care (in addition to hospice care, skilled nursing facility care, and home health care), aside from physician services. Part B covers outpatient services and inpatient physician services according to a fee schedule (fee for service); importantly, private insurers refer to the Medicare part B fee schedule to benchmark their reimbursement rates. Unlike part A, though, beneficiaries must specifically enroll for and pay a premium, deductible, and co-payment for part B benefits (co-payment does not apply to the technical component [TC] of laboratory testing but does apply to the physician services or professional component [PC]). A current CLIA certificate is required for laboratories to be reimbursed by Medicare. There is a Medicare part C (Medicare+Choice) that is intended as an alternative to part B, in which beneficiaries may elect to be covered under a different model. Medicare claims are usually processed by nongovernmental contractors. These contractors are referred to as "fiscal intermediaries," who process part A claims, and "carriers," who process part B.

Medicare part A reimbursement operates under the Medicare Prospective Payment System, the "3-day rule," and the "14-day rule." Under this system, the inpatient care of Medicare beneficiaries is reimbursed to hospitals according to diagnosis related groups (DRGs). That is, hospitals get a single fixed sum for a patient's hospitalization, regardless of the costs incurred by the hospital. The important consequence is that, under these conditions, laboratory testing results in money lost for the hospital. Inpatient physician services are covered under part B; however, physician payment for most clinical pathology tests is included in a Medicare management fee, paid to the hospital. Contracted pathologists must negotiate with the hospital for a share of this fee. Tests with separate professional component billing codes, including anatomic pathology tests and a handful of clinical pathology tests, are paid directly from part B. The bill for part B professional services may be submitted by the hospital (eg, if the pathologist is a hospital employee) or by the pathologist (if an independent contractor). In addition, CMS wrote the "3-day rule" (sometimes incorrectly called the "72-hour rule") which affects prehospital testing. Under this rule outpatient diagnostic services furnished to a Medicare beneficiary by a hospital (or an entity wholly owned or operated by the hospital), on the date of admission or during the 3 calendar days immediately preceding admission, must be included on (bundled into) the Part A bill for the beneficiary's inpatient stay at the hospital. Physician professional services provided in the 3 days preceding admission, billed under part B, are not bundled in this way. The "14-day rule" pertains to testing performed after admission and concerns specimens obtained during the admission; as such, it primarily affects surgical pathology specimens. Under this rule, if a laboratory performs testing on such a specimen within 14 days following discharge, the date of service for payment purposes is the date on which the specimen was collected from the patient. This means that payment for the test must come from the hospital through its DRG payment and cannot be separately billed to Medicare.

Medicaid is a federal program that is administered by individual states, who are at liberty to set their own eligibility requirements and fee schedules. Medicaid is intended to extend benefits to low-income families.

Reimbursement

Billing for medical services is conducted in code. Both governmental and private payers recognize the International Coding of Disease (ICD) system, that describes the patient's medical problem, and the Health Care Procedural Coding System (HCPCS) system, that describes the services rendered. The ICD system was developed by the World Health Organization (WHO) for epidemiologic processes. A clinical modification of the ICD—the ICD-CM—was developed for the purposes of billing. The HCPCS codes are divided into levels I and II. Level I is described by Current Procedural Terminology

(CPT) codes (5-digit codes such as the 88305), which are published by the American Medical Association (AMA). Level II codes (a letter and 4 digits) are published annually by CMS. Level II codes essentially address services not covered by CPT (level I) codes. Both ICD codes and HCPCS codes must be provided in order to be paid.

One should use the most specific CPT code for the rendered service. If a specific CPT code cannot be found, then nonspecific methodology codes are used. This latter scenario applies most often to emerging technologies. CMS requires documentation of medical necessity in order to reimburse for pathology services rendered. Thus, an appropriate ICD code, provided by the clinician, must accompany claims.

For inpatient services, the typical scenario is that, after discharge, the patient's DRG and HCPCS codes are forwarded to CMS. CMS assigns each hospital a rate that is based upon its geographic location, setting (rural vs urban), and hospital type; it then multiplies the DRG reimbursement by the assigned hospital rate to calculate the actual reimbursement. Billing for professional services (professional component [PC] billing) are coded separately from the laboratory fee schedule. These codes are listed in the physician fee schedule and can be billed separately to Medicare (paid as Part B). TC work done in the clinical or anatomic pathology laboratory cannot be separately billed to Medicare—it is covered under the one-time DRG-related hospital payment. One notable exception is that independent anatomic pathology laboratories that process inpatient samples have traditionally been permitted to bill Medicare Part B for TC services rendered on hospital inpatients. Until recently, Medicare allowed this arrangement for enduring contractual arrangements between hospitals and independent labs that were in place before July 22, 1999 (the "grandfather clause"). The "grandfather clause" was permitted by congress to expire on July 1, 2012.

Medicare is obligated to pay only for laboratory services that it deems medically necessary. Furthermore, Medicare is reluctant to pay for laboratory tests that are not cleared by the FDA. Medicare does recognize that some tests without FDA clearance are medically necessary, and these may be covered as "investigational use." So-called "home brew" tests, better identified as laboratory-developed tests (LDTs), are most commonly encountered in the molecular arena; these are generally not covered. An exception is often made in the case of tests that utilize ASRs.

Invariably, Medicare will deny claims for some outpatient laboratory tests. If the patient is informed in advance that this may occur, then the patient may be billed for the services upon Medicare denial. Documentation of this is in the form of an advanced beneficiary notice (ABN); ABNs are mandatory at this time. Note that patients may not be billed for inpatient services that are not covered by Medicare.

Medicare Part B program covers payments for physician services (PC payments). Physician reimbursement is determined by the Physician Fee Schedule (PFS); the PFS, in turn, is based upon the Resource-Based Relative Value Scale (RBRVS). The RBRVS utilizes multiple variables to calculate a payment for each CPT code; the variables take into account physician work, practice expenses, and liability expenses and are generally referred to as "relative value units" (RVUs). The RBRVS variables are put into an equation and, finally, multiplied by a conversion factor (CF) to arrive at the final fee schedule amount. The CF is periodically adjusted, based upon economic conditions.

Laboratory test panels are a special case with regard to reimbursement. There are AMA-approved panels that, when performed, must be billed as a panel (not as individual tests). Billing separately in this scenario is referred to as "unbundling." The same is true for anatomic pathology codes (a uterus must be coded as a uterus and not be "unbundled" into its constituent parts for billing purposes). Furthermore, Medicare does not approve of laboratory-designed panels that are offered as a cohesive group for ordering purposes but billed separately.

Direct billing law, physician self-referral law (Stark law) & antikickback law

The direct billing law is contained in the Social Security Act and requires that Medicare be billed directly by the laboratory providing the service. This is intended to prevent ordering physicians from billing Medicare then paying a lower amount to the laboratory (providing an incentive for the ordering physician to order more tests).

The Stark law is intended to prevent physicians from working around the direct billing requirement by setting up "shell" labs, in which a "laboratory" that is owned by the physician does nothing other than refer testing out to actual laboratories and then bill Medicare directly. The Stark law that took effect in 1992 (Stark I) applied only to clinical laboratory services. The Stark law prohibited physicians from referring Medicare patients to laboratories in which they or an immediate family member has a financial relationship. In 1995, Stark was expanded by amendment to include additional "designated health services" (Stark II). These include physical therapy, radiology, dispensing of medications, and others. The Stark law does allow a number of exceptions, and it permits the Secretary to create additional exceptions.

In order for Stark to apply to an arrangement between a physician and an entity, Medicare/Medicaid patients must be involved, one of the designated health services must be involved, and there must be a financial relationship between the referring physician/family member and the entity. Even if these are all satisfied, Stark applies only if there are no relevant exceptions.

Note that the Stark law is distinct from the antikickback law, although both are titles of the Social Security Act. Kickbacks (inducements) are items of value provided to induce providers or patients to spend their Medicare benefits on your laboratory's services. As part of this prohibition, a laboratory that discounts the cost of lab testing for non-Medicare patients may not charge less than the cost of testing.

The Privacy Act & the Privacy Rule (HIPAA)

The Privacy Act (1974) protects records that can be retrieved by personal identifiers (eg, name, social security number) and prohibits disclosures without written consent unless a specified exception applies. Like the Freedom of Information Act (FOIA), the Privacy Act applied only to Federal agencies and records held by them.

The Privacy Rule (1996) is applicable to all health care entities. This rule (also known as Standards for Privacy of Individually Identifiable Health Information) is actually a set of rules issued by the DHHS for the implementation of the Health Insurance Portability and Accountability Act (HIPAA). The intent of the HIPAA law was 2-fold:

1. to ensure health insurance continuity when insured persons changed jobs

2. to create a simplified and efficient format for insurers and health care providers to share information

The privacy rules were meant to ensure that the free flow of health information did not get out of control. The Privacy Rule is enforced by the Office of Civil Rights (OCR) within the DHHS. The rules define several concepts, including a definition of "protected health information" and a definition of "covered entities." Protected health information refers to any individually identifiable health information; health information includes demographic data, health condition, or the fact that health care was provided. There is no restriction on the sharing of de-identified health information (not individually identifiable and provides no reasonable way to deduce the identity of an individual). Note that there are certain instances in which a covered entity is permitted to disclose protected health information (without patient permission) and additional instances in which it is required to do so. Sharing of information is permitted for the purposes of treatment, payment, or for laboratory operations (eg, quality control). Sharing of information is required when requested by DHHS as part of a legal investigation. Covered entities include health care providers, health plans, and health care clearinghouses.

The covered entities have a responsibility beyond limiting sharing of information. They are obligated to secure information to prevent unauthorized access. This requirement includes encryption of data, eg, password protection, the shredding of paper containing health information.

The Occupational Safety & Health Administration (OSHA)

OSHA is meant to protect workers in workplaces. It was created by the Occupational Safety and Health Act of 1970 as a division of the Department of Labor. Employers are required to be in compliance with OSHA regulations and with OSHA-approved state regulations (state regulations must meet or exceed federal OSHA standards for approval). OSHA regulations are concerned with a tremendous range of workplace hazards, from portable wooden ladders to bloodborne pathogens. Of particular interest to laboratories are the regulations concerning hazardous chemicals and bloodborne pathogens.

Hazardous chemicals

OSHA requires that laboratories create and execute a hazardous chemicals hygiene plan. The chemical hygiene plan specifies the use of personal protective equipment and procedures to ensure that protective equipment (eg, fume hoods) are functioning correctly. The plan describes the provisions for post-exposure evaluation and follow-up and procedures for investigating the circumstances surrounding an exposure. Furthermore, it specifies a Chemical Hygiene Officer and describes the record keeping requirements. Lastly, the hygiene plan includes employee training on such things as the OSHA occupational exposure standards, familiarity with the relevant hazardous chemicals and the associated hazards, permissible exposure limits (PELs) for the relevant hazardous chemicals, signs and symptoms associated with toxic exposures, methods of detecting hazardous chemicals, and procedures in case of a spill. Employees should be trained in the location and use of reference materials (usually in the form of Material Safety Data Sheets [MSDS]). Employers are required to ensure that employee exposures remain at or below PELs specified in OSHA standards. This means that exposures must be monitored if there is reason to suspect that exposures are regularly above a certain level (the "action level"). If measurements are found to be routinely above this level, then scheduled periodic monitoring of employees is required. The employer is responsible for applying the resources necessary to keep levels below PEL; if, despite process and physical interventions levels below PEL cannot be maintained, then respirators must be used. Employees must have the opportunity to receive medical attention, free of charge, if there is an exposure. Containers must be clearly labeled, and pertinent material safety data sheets (MSDS) readily available.

Bloodborne pathogens

Laboratories must create and execute an exposure control plan for employees. Components of an exposure control plan include the provision and required use of personal protective equipment (eg, gloves, face shields) and the use of universal precautions. It describes the provision of hepatitis B vaccination by the employer. The term "universal precautions" was adopted initially, to encourage the practice of treating every patient as potentially harboring a transmissible disease, and this was later replaced with the term "standard precautions." The exposure control plan should consider engineering and process controls to minimize risk of exposure and should specify the responsibility of housekeeping for minimization of contaminated material. It lists the procedures for identifying employee exposures, procedures for post-exposure evaluation and follow-up, and procedures for investigating the circumstances surrounding an exposure. Furthermore, it describes the record keeping requirements and the elements of employee training. In the plan, the person or department responsible for the plan is listed.

Financial considerations in the laboratory

Types of costs f8.1 & calculation of the breakeven point

Some costs are fixed (largely unaffected by the number of tests performed), and some are variable (change in proportion to the number of tests performed). Examples of fixed costs include instrument purchase, rent paid on laboratory space, and supervisor wages. If the number of tests performed grows beyond a certain threshold, however, you may need to acquire more instruments or pay for more laboratory space; thus, fixed costs may vary, but they do so in stepwise fashion. Nonetheless, it is simplest to think of laboratory costs in light of the fixed/variable dichotomy.

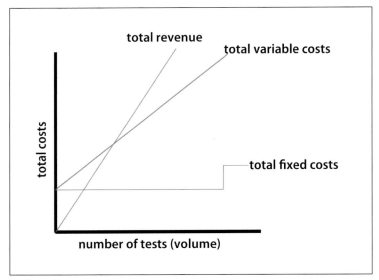

f8.1 Types of costs

Some costs are direct (incurred directly from the performance of tests), and some costs are indirect (overhead). Direct costs include instrument purchase, supervisor wages, technologist wages, and reagents. Indirect costs include rent paid on laboratory space, custodial services, and depreciation. In general, one can exercise the greatest control over direct costs and variable costs; the least over indirect costs and fixed costs.

Unit cost is the cost incurred in performing one test (cost/reportable). Generally, this is determined by adding the fixed and variable costs involved in performing the test. Note that variable costs/unit are the same regardless of the number of tests performed, whereas fixed costs/unit decrease as the number of tests performed increases t8.2.

t8.2 Relationship of total cost to unit cost

Assumptions: fixed cost is $500, variable cost is $5/test

Tests performed	100	200	300
Total cost	$500 + $500 = $1,000	$500 + $1,000 = $1,500	$500 + $1,500 = $2,000
Unit cost	$1,000 ÷ 100 tests = $10/test	$1,500 ÷ 200 tests = $7.50/test	$2,000 ÷ 300 = $6.66/test

The breakeven point is the number of tests you must perform to reach the point where total revenue equals total cost; ie, the point at which net income is zero. It is commonly necessary to determine the breakeven point when deciding whether to offer a test or send it out. What must be known, in addition to the costs, is what will be charged for the test (what revenue is expected).

In laboratory work, revenue can be tricky to predict, because we are rarely paid exactly what we charge (allowances) and in some instances we are not paid at all (bad debt). Revenue is then total charges minus allowances and bad debt. In this regard, it is common to estimate anticipated revenue based upon the known historical percentage of usual charges that the lab collects; with anticipated revenue calculated as this percentage times the total charges. In the example above, if 75% is the historical percentage that the lab collects, then we will not break even at 125 tests unless we charge more than $9 f8.2.

Net income = revenue (R) – fixed cost (FC) – variable cost (VC)

So, we seek the point at which net income is 0, or the point at which

$0 = R - FC - VC$

If Z is the number of tests performed, then the point we seek is

$0 = R \times Z - FC - VC \times Z$

This can be rearranged to

$FC = R \times Z - VC \times Z$ or

$FC = (R - VC) \times Z$

then rearranged to

$Z = FC \div (R - VC)$

So, if we repeat the assumptions of t8.2 and assume we will charge $9 per test, then

$Z = \$500 \div (\$9 - \$5) = 125$ tests

f8.2 Calculation of the break-even point

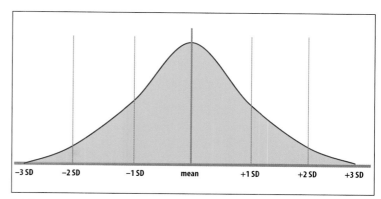

f8.3 Gaussian curve

Budgeting

Budgeting is the prospective process by which financial projections are made, generally encompassing a period of 1 year. The beginning date of the budgeting year varies from institution to institution, with many budgeting according to a fiscal year that begins on 1 October. Budgeting activities often begin ~6 months before the beginning of the budgeted year. Accurate budgeting is tricky and must take into account several factors. Usually one begins with assumptions that are based upon the performance of the past year; however, sometimes a clean slate is in order (so-called "zero-based" budgets). Wherever one begins, the budget for the next year must take into account projections of test volumes and case-mix, anticipated new testing and testing to be discontinued, anticipated changes in reimbursement and payer mix, and inflation.

In laboratories, there are generally ≥4 major parts of the budget: the capital budget, personnel budget, operating budget, and allocation budget. The capital budget is for "big ticket" items whose cost and return on investment may be mapped over several budget years (≥3 years, usually). One consideration, when capital is being restricted, is a lease (reagent-rental agreement). Under these circumstances, a new instrument can be accounted for in the operating budget instead of the capital budget, but reagents are usually more expensive under these arrangements. The personnel budget is the projection of personnel needs, generally expressed in full-time equivalents (FTEs). The personnel budget is built upon volume projections and productivity projections, with productivity generally taken to be the ratio of billable tests to FTEs. Thus, when personnel cannot be increased or is in fact being reduced, one must find ways to enhance productivity, such as through alternative methodologies that require less technologist time. The operating budget considers all the costs of day to day operations, including reagents and other consumables, the cost of reference lab tests, the costs of blood for the transfusion service, professional fees, depreciation, maintenance, and nonconsumable equipment ("small ticket" items such as computer monitors). Lastly, the allocation budget is the laboratory's allocated share of the hospital's fixed costs (eg, electricity, administration, marketing).

Statistical considerations in the laboratory
Definitions
Gaussian distribution, estimates of central tendency & estimates of variation

Gaussian refers to a distribution of data points that is arranged symmetrically around the mean with most values closest to the center. Since this distribution is describable by a mathematical equation, it is considered parametric. Random testing of a large population often results in a Gaussian normal distribution.

There are 3 estimates of central tendency: mean, median, and mode. In a perfect Gaussian distribution, mean, median, and mode are identical. Mean is the arithmetic average of a Gaussian set of data points. The mean is calculated as the sum of the individual values divided by the number of values. The median is the middle value of a range of values. The mode is the most frequently occurring value in a range of values. Some data sets are non-Gaussian—skewed positively or negatively—skews alter the mean and median but do not affect the mode. In a positively skewed set of data, mean > median > mode.

$$\text{Mean} = \Sigma x_i / n$$

The standard deviation (SD) is a reflection of variation (how wide is the Gaussian curve). Narrow curves have low SD and wide curves have high SD. The SD is also a calculation of an average: it is the average distance of an individual value from the mean.

$$SD = \sqrt{\Sigma(x_i - \text{mean})^2/(n - 1)}$$

In the ideal Gaussian distribution, 68.2% of the population falls within –1 SD and +1 SD, 95.5% falls within –2 SD and +2 SD, and 99.7% fall within –3 SD and +3 SD f8.3. Note that while reference intervals can be determined on this basis (ie, all values between –2 SD and +2 SD), it is recommended that a nonparametric analysis be used in most cases, because most data sets are not perfectly Gaussian.

Analytical accuracy & precision

Analytical accuracy is the extent to which a test result approximates the "true" value. Most often the "true" value is considered to be that obtained by the definitive method; ie, the method that uses the highest quality instrumentation available. A reference method is often used instead; it utilizes materials more widely available and has been validated by a definitive method. Accuracy has no numerical value. In the laboratory, accuracy is controlled through periodic calibration. Diagnostic accuracy (clinical accuracy) refers to the ability of a test to discriminate patient groups.

Precision refers to the reproducibility of a test result. It is affected by the random variability inherent in processes. Precision is assessed through daily testing of quality control (QC) reagents. The within-run precision is a function of analyte concentration: low concentrations usually have the least precision. Within-run precision for most analytes should run between 1-10%. Between-run precision (day to day precision) is affected by changing environmental conditions, and changing technologists (operator bias). Generally precision is expressed in terms of the coefficient of variation (CV). The CV describes the standard deviation as a percentage of the mean. Note that, since the CV is a function of the mean, it refers to the precision at a particular analyte concentration. Generally, CV increases as the analyte increases. Thus, one can assess test performance at critical cutoff values, if desired.

$$CV = SD/mean \times 100$$

Clinical sensitivity & specificity

Clinical sensitivity refers to the ability of the test to detect disease when present, or positivity in the presence of disease f8.4. Clinical sensitivity is distinct from analytical sensitivity (see below).

$$Sens = TP/(TP + FN)$$

Clinical specificity refers to the ability of the test to detect only the disease sought, or its negativity in the absence of disease f8.4.

$$Spec = TN/(TN + FP)$$

The clinical sensitivity and specificity should be distinguished from the analytical sensitivity and specificity which refer to the ability of the assay to detect small quantities of the analyte (analytical sensitivity) and its ability to accurately measure the analyte in the presence of multiple other substances (analytical specificity).

	disease	**no disease**
positive test	true positive (TP)	false positive (FP)
negative test	false negative (FN)	true negative (TN)

f8.4 Punnett square

Predictive value

Positive predictive value (PPV) is the percent of positive results that actually indicate disease f8.4. That is, if the test is positive, it is likely that the individual has the disease. The negative predictive value is the probability of no disease when the test is negative.

$$PPV = TP/(TP + FP)$$

$$NPV = TN/(TN + FN)$$

Disease prevalence affects the predictive value of a test. The pretest probability affects the performance of a test, and one of the most powerful estimates of pretest probability is the prevalence of the disease in the population. The practical consequence of this effect is that when disease prevalence is low, the PPV of a test declines (and the NPV increases). The converse is also true. Note that sensitivity and specificity are not mathematically influenced by prevalence, but positive and negative predictive values are.

Relative risk

Relative risk is the ratio of the risk in the presence of a risk factor to the baseline risk. It is the risk of an outcome "Y" in the presence of condition "X" as compared to the general population.

$$\text{Relative risk} = \frac{(\text{\# with X who develop Y/\# with X}}{(\text{\# in population who develop Y/\# in population})}$$

Types of variables

Tests may give results on scales that are nominal, interval, or ordinal. An interval scale is one that gives discrete numbers that have their usual mathematical meaning (eg, the sodium). An ordinal scale is one that gives a number with an assigned value (eg, the urine dipstick protein: 1+ to 4+). A nominal test is one that gives a category (positive, negative).

Diagnostic accuracy: receiver operating characteristic (ROC) curves

Diagnostic accuracy

Diagnostic accuracy refers to the ability of a test to distinguish between groups of patients (disease vs no disease). It is distinct from analytic accuracy which refers to the ability of a test to correctly measure analyte. The ROC f8.5 curve is a commonly used illustration of test accuracy. Another is the dot diagram.

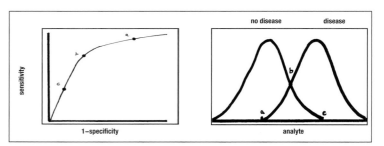

f8.5 ROC curve. On the left is a typical ROC curve with 3 arbitrarily selected points, a-c, labeled. On the right is a representation of two theoretical populations with the same points, a-c, labeled. It can be seen that if "a" is the selected cutoff, the test will have high sensitivity (all people with disease would be detected), but low specificity (a good number of people without disease test positive). If "c" were selected, the opposite would apply. Point "b" is an "ideal" cutoff, but, of course, this depends on what you want the test to accomplish.

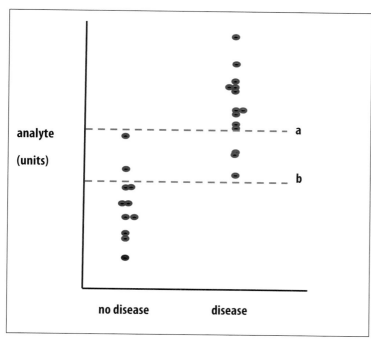

f8.6 Dot plot

The dot diagram **f8.6** allows one to quickly compare various test cutoffs and to see the degree of overlap in the results.

ROC curves

An ROC curve is used to assess the overall accuracy of a test; furthermore, it illustrates how a test performs, particularly at different cutoff values. An ROC curve is generated by plotting sensitivity (true positive rate) on the y axis and 1 − specificity (false positive rate) on the x axis for a range of different test cutoffs. Thus, the ROC curve displays a test's accuracy over a range of different cutoffs. One can also derive quantitative measures of accuracy, such as the area under the ROC curve (the c statistic). It is important to note that the ROC curve is independent of the prevalence of disease in the population (because the sensitivity is calculated entirely from data derived from the disease group and the specificity entirely from the nondisease group).

Despite the fact that it is stated as such throughout the literature, a diagnostic test does not have only one sensitivity or specificity, but many, depending upon the cutoff used. For any given test, one can always identify a cutoff (decision threshold, decision level) value and state a diagnostic sensitivity and specificity at that point. However, ROC plots provide a view of the whole spectrum of sensitivities and specificities, and this provides the most informative basis for comparisons between tests.

Each point on the ROC plot represents a sensitivity/specificity pair corresponding to a particular cutoff. A test with perfect discrimination would have an ROC plot that passes through the upper left corner, a point where sensitivity is 1.0 (100%, perfect sensitivity) and the false positive rate is 0 (specificity is 1.0). A test with no ability to discriminate would have an ROC plot that is a 45° diagonal line from the lower left corner to the upper right corner. A test with perfect discrimination has a c statistic of 1.0, and a test with no discrimination has a c statistic of 0.5. Most actual tests fall in between these 2 extremes, with tests having plots that most closely approach

the upper left corner deemed most accurate. In the ROC curve, an imaginary diagonal line with a slope of 1 beginning at the intercepts represents a test with no discrimination. Any curve above this line represents a test that performs better than chance. The greater the area under the curve, the better the test is performing.

Looking at the ROC curve, it should be clear that there are tradeoffs; that selecting a low cutoff results in high sensitivity but low specificity. A high cutoff will do the opposite. The cutoff selected depends on what you would like the test to do. For example, a screening test would require high sensitivity (with low specificity), while a confirmatory test would demand high specificity.

Reference intervals

Purpose of reference intervals

A test result must be interpreted in relation to what is normal. In laboratory medicine, normal is described as a reference interval. A reference interval is usually defined as the central 95% of measurements from a population of healthy individuals. Laboratories are required to report a reference interval with every test result. There are published and manufacturer recommended reference intervals for nearly every analyte; however, every laboratory is required by CLIA to "verify that the manufacturer's reference intervals…are appropriate for the laboratory's patient population." Generally this is taken to mean that the laboratory must either verify such reference intervals or establish their own. However, the universal need for this analysis is debatable, and many laboratories adopt manufacturer's reference intervals without further in-house testing, at the discretion of the medical director. In either case, the laboratory must document how their reference interval was established.

Establishing reference intervals

A reference population (a group of healthy individuals demographically comparable to the patient population) is tested for the analyte in question. CLSI recommends ≥120 such reference individuals (the minimum number required for 90% confidence at the 95th percentile reference limits [2.5% of individuals below the cutoff and 2.5% above]). The results are plotted; usually the plot recapitulates a Gaussian distribution but not exactly (a nonparametric distribution). It is for this reason that nonparametric calculations are advised (choosing the central 95th percentile rather than the central 2 SD). From this, reference limits are calculated; the reference interval is the values between the reference limits. For some analytes (eg, serum troponin), the 99th percentile is the chosen limit. Furthermore, some analytes (eg, serum troponin, serum prostate specific antigen) have no relevant lower limit.

A number of steps must be taken to ensure the validity of the foregoing analysis. First, a review of the literature is advised to look for factors that affect the assay (biologic variation and analytic interferences). Second, exclusion criteria must be articulated and potential members of the reference population screened by way of a questionnaire. Third, preanalytical and analytical conditions should be articulated and controlled. Lastly, the effect of partitioning factors should be analyzed in the data; ie, are separate intervals required based upon, eg, gender, race, age.

Laboratories usually adopt reference intervals rather than establish them anew. The source of the adopted reference interval may be literature, manufacturer, or the laboratory's own established reference interval (when a new instrument or method is being implemented). Before doing this, the adopted established reference interval is often verified (or validated) in the laboratory. This can be done in a number of ways. Most often, a set of 20 healthy individuals (the CLSI-recommended minimum) is tested. A more robust analysis can be gained with more subjects. In the 20 subject scenario, ≥18 should fall within the established reference range under consideration. The Student t test can be used to assess the laboratory's smaller population data set. Lastly, the laboratory-adopted reference interval should be compared to the manufacturer's reference interval; significant differences should be investigated, and one should hesitate to adopt a reference interval that differs significantly from the manufacturer. Such "outlier" reference intervals are often erroneous and reflective of either the inherent risk in testing small populations or a problem with in-house preanalytic or analytic methods. The medical director may simply review the manufacturer's reference interval and supporting literature and judge it essentially comparable to the laboratory's population.

Factors that confound reference intervals

Despite considerable international efforts to ensure method "harmonization," reference intervals remain largely method/instrument-dependent. One of the key requirements of an adopted reference interval is that it be derived from methodology/instrumentation identical to that employed in the adopting laboratory.

Despite large samples, the populations from which reference intervals are established are healthy and often younger than the population that submits for laboratory testing. The reference interval is deliberately chosen such that 5% of results from these healthy individuals are abnormal. Thus, a large number of "abnormal" laboratory tests are a consequence of statistical necessity.

Statistical population-based reference intervals cannot be applied to some laboratory tests, for which medical decision limits must be used instead. Examples include serum lipid levels, for which limits are established upon the basis of cardiac risk.

Lastly, some analytes differ so significantly between individuals that a population-based reference interval may be un-informative. For these analytes, individuals have unique "set points." An example is the mean corpuscular volume (MCV)—the population-based normal range for MCV spans 20 fL, but the intraindividual range is much tighter, perhaps 2-3 fL. Furthermore, separate individuals have widely disparate intraindividual ranges, though most individuals still fall within the population-based normal range. In such instances, intraindividual (subject-based) reference intervals may be more appropriate. In this context, an index of individuality has been determined for a large number of analytes. Low indices of individuality imply, somewhat counter-intuitively, that there is a high degree of individuality for that analyte; that is, the range within one person is likely to differ from the range within another, though both people are likely to fall within the population-based reference range. Conversely, a high index of individuality implies that there is little individuality.

$$\text{Index of individuality} = \frac{\text{within-subject variation}}{\text{between-subject variation}}$$

Implementation of new methods
Overview

When introducing new methods or instruments into the clinical laboratory, a process of evaluation must be undertaken. The extent of method evaluation depends upon the status of the method—whether FDA approved or not and, if approved, whether waived or not. Note that when moderate complexity laboratories perform "waived" tests, they do so under moderate complexity status; in such instances, the "waived" testing is held to the higher moderate-complexity standards. New assays that do not have FDA approval require formal validation; whereas FDA approved tests require only verification.

Method validation has all the ingredients of method verification plus assessment of sensitivity, specificity, and positive predictive value. Validation is required when implementing a laboratory-developed test or when using a modification of an FDA approved test. Validation is not required when FDA approved tests are used within the scope for which they were approved and without modification.

Method verification is the process by which a laboratory

1. verifies that it can reproduce manufacturer claims for

   - precision
   - accuracy
   - reportable range

2. verifies reference intervals

3. establishes the parameters for calibration and quality control

CLIA '03 specifically mandates verification of elements 1 and 2 (precision, accuracy, reportable range, and reference ranges). Furthermore, correlation studies with existing instrumentation or an outside "reference" laboratory may be undertaken as part of this process. Lastly, if more than one of any instrument is implemented, then correlations between them should be demonstrated. Reference ranges should be verified, and they may need to be altered as compared to prior laboratory reference ranges (this mandates communication with the medical staff, nursing, and often pharmacy). At the end of this process, it is the responsibility of the medical director to accept or reject the new method.

It is important to have a written validation plan that is approved by the medical director. A general validation plan checklist is helpful, and since most validations have the same elements, one can easily create a template or checklist for ease of production of future validation plans t8.3. The validation plan should list the validation elements, number of specimens to suffice for each element, and predetermined pass/fail points.

t8.3 Validation plan checklist

Calibration & calibration verification
Precision verification & establishment of quality control ranges
Establishment of reference intervals & critical values (if any)
Determination of analytic sensitivity
Determination of analytic specificity
Determination of accuracy/interferences
Method comparison (primary)
Method comparison (secondary), if any
Carryover tests
Establishment of analytical measurement range & clinical reportable range
Determination of specimen stability
Verification of interfaces & reports
Procedure written & approved by medical director
Application for proficiency testing
Training of laboratorians & competency assessment
Notification of clinicians

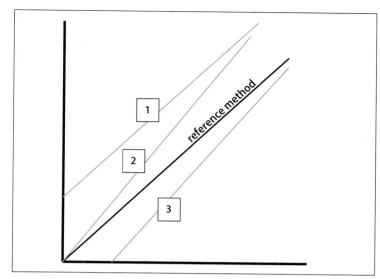

f8.7 Correlation study: 1 constant bias, 2 proportional bias, 3 mixed

Elements of method verification/ validation

Calibration & calibration verification

Calibration and calibration verification should be performed early in the process. The manufacturer's calibrators should be utilized, in accordance with the manufacturer's calibration instructions. Calibration is the process of adjusting the instrument to read out the known actual concentration of a calibrator. Calibration verification involves the use of several specimens with known concentrations (patient samples, commercial calibrators, proficiency testing survey material, controls) to ensure the validity of the calibrator over a wider range of results. Thus, calibration is analogous to "zeroing" a scale, and calibration verification is analogous to then testing the scale using a series of known weights. Calibration verification must be carried out at least once every 6 months and more frequently under some circumstances; eg, after major preventive maintenance.

Precision & establishment of quality control (QC) ranges

Precision refers to the reproducibility of a result. It is assessed by replicating measurements on same specimens. Usually QC reagents are assayed 20-40× over several days. The within-run and between-day standard deviations are calculated. Furthermore, the mean and standard deviation of these measurements are used to establish QC ranges for statistical quality control.

How many samples to test for this and other aspects of the verification procedure is a matter that must be considered on an individual basis. The "rule of thumb" dictates testing 20 samples, but there appears to be no statistical basis for this number.

Accuracy & inaccuracy (bias), method comparison, analytic specificity & interference

Accuracy refers to the correctness of a result, as compared to a known "true" value. Accuracy is verified by calibration, calibration verification, and method comparisons. A comparison is usually made with a previously validated method or with a reference method (method comparison). Results from testing on the new method are plotted on the y axis, and those from the reference method on the x axis f8.7. Linear regression analysis is a type of mathematical analysis that permits a straight line to be drawn that "best fits" a set of x and y data points. For the purposes of correlation studies, for example, where the x-axis data points are the reference test, least squares linear regression analysis is performed. In other instances, where neither is considered the reference, Deming regression analysis is performed. The correlation coefficient (r) is a number ranging from –1 to +1 that expresses the degree to which the "best fit" line actually fits the data points.

Method comparison should be carried out first with the previously validated assay, if any, or with a reference method (primary method comparison). Secondly, method comparison should be carried out between instruments, if more than one is in service (secondary method comparison).

A specific source of inaccuracy is interference. Analytical specificity (trueness) refers to the degree to which the analyte can be detected in the presence of interfering substances (bilirubinemia, lipemia, hemoglobinemia). Analytical specificity is tested in "recovery" experiments, in which quantities of interferents are added to known samples, and the amount of analyte measured ("recovered") is compared to the known amount.

Heterophile antibodies interference is a major problem in immunoassay-based testing. Human heterophile antibodies may interfere with immunoassays by binding to the animal antibodies used in the assay. Knowing how to detect heterophile antibody interference and how to avoid it are of paramount importance. Typically, the possibility of this sort of interference comes by way of a clinician phoning about an inexplicable laboratory result. Once there is suspicion of such interference, if the sample is still available, one can make serial dilutions of the sample. Heterophile antibody interference does not change linearly with dilution, whereas a true result will. Numerous strategies have been evaluated that are aimed at avoiding heterophile antibody interference. These include removal of immunoglobulins from a sample (eg, with PEG), modification of assay antibodies (in ways similar to those used in monoclonal antibody therapies) to make them less prone to react with heterophile antibodies, and the use of buffers to reduce interference.

Another sort of "interference" is the so-called solvent exclusion effect. This term refers to a falsely low analyte concentration that results from a higher than normal "solid phase." Each blood sample has a solid phase and an aqueous phase. An "indirect ISE" instrument measures, for example, a sodium concentration within the aqueous phase and calculates the sodium concentration for the entire volume of blood. When the solid phase is increased as, for example, in lipemia and high levels or paraprotein (myeloma effect), the apparent sodium concentration artifactually goes down.

Analytical sensitivity & functional sensitivity

Analytical sensitivity (limit of detection [LOD] or limit of blank) refers to the lowest analyte concentration detectable. Assays for which analytic sensitivity can be very important include the TSH, CRP, troponin, d-dimer, micro-albumin, and hCG. The analytical sensitivity can be determined by serially (20 times) measuring a zero standard, then calculating a mean and standard deviation. 2-3 SD above zero is taken as the analytical sensitivity (all within 2 SD of zero is considered "noise").

The concept of functional sensitivity was first introduced in relation to thyroid stimulating hormone (TSH) testing. Functional sensitivity (limit of quantitation [LOQ]) is the lowest analyte concentration reliably quantified. "Reliable" in this context is predetermined as some particular coefficient of variation (CV); often, the target is a CV of 20%. The LOQ may be equivalent to the LOD but is usually higher and, of course, cannot be lower. While the LOD is determined from the within-run precision of the zero calibrator, the LOQ is determined from between-run precision. Functional sensitivity is calculated from the 20% between-run coefficient of variation (CV) for the method and is meant to assess the minimum detection limit of the assay in clinical practice.

Carryover tests

Carryover can be a problem for analytes that, clinically, can have a wide range of concentration. For such analytes, carryover from one sample into another could have a major impact, such as β-hCG. Carryover studies are performed using a sample of known high analyte concentration and a sample of low concentration. The samples are loaded into the instrument in a way that will permit detection of significant carryover f8.8. The results from positions 1-3 are averaged, as are the results from 4 and 5. The percent carryover is calculated using the formula below. A percent carryover of <1.5% is desirable. High carryover suggests a problem in the dispensing/pipetting system which must be addressed.

$$\text{Percent carryover} = (\text{result of position 6}) - \frac{(\text{average 1-3})}{(\text{average 4-5})} \times 100$$

Clinical reportable range (CRR) & analytical measuring range (AMR)

The analytical measuring range (AMR), or linear range, is the range over which reliable measurements can be obtained. It is usually determined by serially diluting samples of known, usually high, concentration and plotting the results of ≥5 different concentrations. The plot may be examined visually, taking the

rack	sample
1	low
2	low
3	low
4	high
5	high
6	low

f8.8 Example of carryover test: rack loading order

limits of the AMR as the point of deflection in the line; alternatively, the data may be examined mathematically by

1. calculating the CV at various points
2. calculating the percent deviation from the expected value at various points

The clinical reportable range (CRR) refers to the highest and lowest values that can be reported accurately. The CRR is the range of quantitative results that may be reported, taking into account the ability to dilute samples that fall outside the upper limit of the AMR, if applicable. The low end of the CRR is typically identical to the low end of the AMR. The upper limit for the CRR may be the same as or higher than the upper limit of the AMR, depending upon the feasibility of specimen dilution. Some instruments are capable of automatically diluting samples that fall above the AMR; others require manual dilution. The laboratory may only report patient test results that fall within the CRR. The laboratory medical director must decide on limits of dilution and how the laboratory will report results that are outside of this range.

Reference intervals & critical values

Reference intervals are discussed on p 441. The laboratory must verify that the reference ranges provided by the manufacturer fit its patient population. Ultimately, the laboratory medical director may elect to use the manufacturer's suggested reference range, other published reference ranges, or a reference range validated by the laboratory. For many analytes, several reference ranges may be required (eg, age-based, gender-based). When known normal patients are tested, 95% of results should be within the reference range.

Specimen stability

Specimen stability refers to the length of time that a stored specimen will continue to produce reliable results. This may be assessed for specimens stored at room temperature, at refrigerator temperature, and/or for frozen specimens. Specimen stability must be verified for some analytes, depending upon whether robust published stabilities are available. To do this, patient samples are tested immediately and then at intervals under the defined storage conditions (room temperature, refrigerated, frozen). The maximum storage time is defined as the last time before significant, predefined, variation is noted. For example, one may choose to use 2 or 3 SD as defining significant variation.

Information systems

Manual entry of instrument results into the laboratory information system (LIS) is undesirable because it is error prone and raises labor costs. Instead, instruments should ideally be interfaced directly with the LIS. Often, there is need for software that intervenes between the 2 (generically, "middleware"), the purpose of which is to integrate logic that prevents reporting of suspicious results, ensures appropriate application of reflex testing, and insertion of predetermined interpretive comments. Often, there is then an interface between the LIS and the hospital information system (HIS) and possibly numerous additional proprietary information systems. At each of these interfaces, there is the potential for information to be mistranslated, garbled, or lost. Therefore, checking the integrity of these interfaces is a necessary component of any test validation.

One approach is to simply report a number of "test" patients across the various interfaces, originating with the instrument. A wide variety of possible results should be generated, eg, normal results, abnormal low, abnormal high, critical (if applicable). The report generated on the far side of the interface must then be checked to ensure that it faithfully reproduces the intended result, with no loss of interpretive comments, patient identification, units of measure, or reference ranges.

Written procedures

For each test there must be a written procedure. The procedure must address all aspects of the testing process, taking care not to contradict other laboratory procedures (eg, laboratory-wide quality control procedures, specimen collection procedures). A written procedure is a good one if an un-initiated but otherwise qualified technologist can reasonably perform the testing based upon what is written. Furthermore, a well written procedure is of immense value to the pathologist in dealing with questions that arise; when on call questions are raised by technologists, it is both informative and illustrious to respond with "what does the procedure manual say." Often the answer lies therein; if not, then the procedure probably needs work. In the words of Deming, a written procedure is the "liberator that relegates the problems that have already been solved to the field of routine, and leaves the creative faculties free for the problems that are still unsolved."

Written laboratory procedures should be crafted in a standard format, including the information listed in t8.4. Product inserts may form the basis for some of the information in the procedure, but do not suffice in their stead. Procedures must be reviewed by the medical director initially, each time a change is made, and annually.

t8.4 Elements of a laboratory procedure

Element	Notes
Test principle	An overview of the analyte, the methodology the test is based upon, and clinical utility of the test
Patient preparation	eg, fasting, nonfasting, preparation of venipuncture site
Specimen collection, labeling, handling & transport	What specimen is appropriate, how collected & into what container? Should the specimen be inverted several times immediately after collection? Can it be mailed, pneumatically tubed? Under what conditions & how quickly must it be transported to the laboratory?
Specimen storage, preservation & stability	Room temperature, refrigerator, or freezer storage, stability of analyte under various conditions, how quickly must it be centrifuged
Criteria for specimen acceptability	General "rejection criteria" are often discussed in a separate "lab-wide" procedure; herein list any criteria particular to this analyte or assay
Referral instructions	The laboratory must refer specimens for testing only to a CLIA-certified or CMS-approved laboratory. If the laboratory accepts referral specimens, written instructions must be available to clients, and must include the items listed above
Reagents	List of reagents, including proper storage (as applicable, temperature, humidity), concentrations, expiration dates
Procedures for microscopic examinations	If applicable, including the detection of inadequately prepared slides
Test procedure	Step by step
Reportable range	Determined at time of method verification/validation
Test calibration	How performed, how often
Quality control (QC) procedures	How performed, how often
Steps to be taken when calibration or QC fails	eg, retest the unacceptable control (one time only). If repeat acceptable, then no further action; if the repeat unacceptable, what actions are to be taken? This should include evaluating all patient test results obtained since the last acceptable QC to determine if the patient test results were adversely affected (before reporting the results and if necessary issuing corrected reports); at what point to notify clinicians of an anticipated delay?
Limitations of procedure	eg, interfering substances
Reference range	Determined at time of method verification/validation
Critical values	A lab-wide procedure should address the steps to be taken in reporting critical values; herein list the values considered critical, if any
Results reporting & calculations, if any	How results are entered into laboratory information system and any calculations that must be carried out
References	Sources of information for the procedure, including product insert, standard texts, published studies

Testing personnel must read and understand the procedures prior to testing and at regular intervals thereafter (annually, usually). Every change to the procedure must, likewise, be read and understood (the "read and sign" ceremony). Beyond this, it is important to write "competencies" or "quizzes" for testing personnel to ensure that the salient points are reinforced.

Ideally, written procedures should be maintained on a computerized document control program. Such procedures are usually accessible through an "intranet." A backup data source should be available for system down-times. If paper copies are maintained instead or in adjunct, diligence must be aimed at ensuring that all available copies represent the most recent iteration. In this regard, a document control flow sheet can be helpful. Any alterations to the written procedure must be made through a formal revision process; hand-written corrections should be strongly discouraged. All retired procedures must be archived for a set period of time.

By example and by fiat, zealous compliance with written procedures must be ingrained in the culture of your laboratory.

Education of laboratory staff & clinical staff

Before "going live" with the new assay, the relevant laboratory staff must review the new procedure and establish competency. A trainer is selected, usually the technologist who has performed the method verification/validation, who teaches each of the bench technologists who will be performing the new procedure. Competency is established and documented by having staff sign the procedure, to attest that they have read and understood it, and by written quiz of the salient points.

Before "going live," clinical staff must be notified of the new assay. The laboratory medical director should compose a communique (technical bulletin) and disseminate it by whatever routes are traditionally used by the hospital or independent laboratory. For changes that may create exceptional difficulty, confusion, or consternation among the medical staff, it is advisable to discuss these personally with key clinicians and/or clinical groups at their regularly scheduled departmental meetings. In such cases, it may be necessary to personally post notices in strategic locations, such as in physician lounges or on windshields in the physician parking lot. Such a communique should be brief, one side of one page is ideal t8.5.

t8.5 Suggested elements of test change communique (technical bulletin)

Element	Note	Examples
Headline	A one-line statement of what is about to happen	BHS Laboratory will discontinue the use of the X assay for measurement of Y and will be performing this measurement on the Z or BHS Laboratory will discontinue sending out testing for Y and will implement in-house testing on the Z instrument or BHS Laboratory introduces the Z assay for measurement of ___
Background	A brief paragraph about the reason for the change	The manufacturer no longer provides reagents for use on the X, and new instrumentation (Z) has been acquired or The performance of the Z assay for Y has been deemed superior to that of the X; for this reason, BHS laboratory has acquired the Z analyzer or BHS laboratory volume of testing for Y has been deemed sufficiently high to bring testing in-house; testing will be performed on the Z analyzer or Studies have determined that ___ can be accurately diagnosed/excluded by measurement of serum Y; BHS laboratory has acquired the Z analyzer for measurement of Y
Impact	What will this mean to the medical staff?	Turnaround time will be significantly improved or Test performance will be significantly improved or There will be a change in the reference range for Y from ___ (old reference range) to ___ (new reference range) or Specimen requirements differ significantly as follows: ___
Date of change	"Go live" date	
How ordered	The "test code"	The Z test may be ordered by the name ___

Quality management
Definitions
Quality

A suitable definition of quality in health care may be that offered by the Institute of Medicine: "…the degree to which health services for individuals and populations increase the likelihood of desired health outcomes and are consistent with current professional knowledge." The IOM publication *Crossing the Quality Chasm* offered the notion that all health care should be "safe, timely, effective, efficient, equitable, and patient centered." In recent years, the concept of patient safety has dominated health care quality discussions; patient safety can be thought of as the most fundamental element of overall health care quality—a modern embodiment of the Hippocratic edict "first, do no harm." From a practical standpoint, definitions of quality differ with the point of view of the stakeholder. Laboratorians tend to focus on accuracy and precision; clinicians often take these for granted and instead focus on timeliness and clarity. The global view, the perspective of the dutiful medical director, considers the net effect of all of these considerations upon patient care.

Quality management, quality improvement, quality control

The word "quality" is found in a variety of terms that at first seem synonymous. The dearth of inventive terminology may obscure the true insightfulness of their inventors. Quality and its manipulation at the organizational level was first considered in the early 20th century when the problem was unacceptable variability in the products of industrial manufacturing. Quality assurance of such products required a labor intensive inspection effort, wherein each product was inspected prior to distribution, the non-conforming ones discarded. The problem, of course, was that this wasted the effort of production, the raw materials, and the time of the inspectors.

A fresh point of view was offered by Walter Shewhart, a statistician. Perfection and exact reproducibility are impossible, he offered, and one should accept variability as inherent in all processes. The proper approach, therefore, is to define the limits of acceptability and adjust the process until the end products fall consistently within them. The aggregate data set generated from inspection of a representative sampling of the product could be analyzed to assess whether the products were largely within these limits; that is, whether the process was "in control." Out of control processes—those outside the bounds of random variation—must be inspected for "assignable causes." To analyze data, Shewhart plotted them on a control chart, a graph with lines demarcating the mean and several standard deviations. When Levey and Jennings proposed the use of Shewhart control charts in the clinical laboratory, the charts became known to laboratorians as "Levey-Jennings" charts. Shewhart analyses are now referred to as *statistical quality control (SQC)* or more simply as *quality control (QC)*. The practice of QC in the laboratory is discussed further below. 6 sigma is an extension of the SQC concept, the name referring to 6 standard deviations from the mean. The premise in 6 sigma is that a process design in which limits of acceptability are 6 standard deviations from the mean has a very low likelihood of failure; in fact, such a process should produce ~3.4 defects (errors)/

million (2 sigma produces 308,000/million, 3 sigma produces 66,800/million).

To examine processes that were out of control, Shewhart advocated the Plan-Do-Study-Act (PDSA) model. W Edwards Deming later expounded upon and promoted Shewhart PDSA methods and, finding no audience for them in the United States, exported them to Japan. There, he, Kaoru Ishikawa, and others revolutionized the quality movement with a great expansion in wealth to show for it. Japanese manufacturers not only embraced SQC but went beyond inspecting product to a vision of improving processes through the observations of the people involved in them; the sum of the Japanese approach that included SQC and internal process improvement was termed Total Quality Management (TQM). Lean is an example of TQM, in which a process is first mapped to illustrate the many steps within it. Each step is then examined with a view towards maximizing uniformity and efficiency.

Quality Assurance (QA) was a term promulgated by the Joint Commission on Accreditation of Healthcare Organizations (JCAHO, now TJC). QA is a retrospective approach to quality management, in which one responds to undesirable measures of predefined quality indicators. The laboratory selects its own quality indicators, monitors them, and, as needed, implements improvement efforts. In the 2003 amendment to CLIA, (CLIA '03), the term *quality assessment* was substituted for quality assurance.

Quality improvement (QI) is a broad term used to encompass efforts at improvement once suboptimal performance is identified. It is a prospective approach to quality management in which a process is examined and redesigned, as necessary, to improve future outcomes. Various models have been employed in the interest of QI; these include 6 sigma, continuous quality improvement (CQI), FADE (focus, analyze, develop, execute, evaluate), and PDSA (plan, do, study, act).

Quality & safety initiatives

It is the hope of every medical director to deliver the highest quality laboratory services. Doing so requires optimization of preanalytical, analytical, and postanalytical variables. Some types of optimization require 2 difficult factors: getting the support of the medical and nursing staff and getting money. For example, a reduction in blood utilization will require the support of the medical staff. An increase in the number of phlebotomists, improvements in software, and implementation of new instrumentation will require money from administration.

Winning the support of the medical staff is the trickier of the 2. No major change that affects them should be initiated until some support is garnered, and no needed change should be delayed until all are supportive. While some changes must be made quickly, most should be preceded by a campaign of one on one conversations with key "thought leaders" in the hospital—ideally, clinicians who are important to hospital revenue, respected by fellow clinicians, and vocal. The mere act of consulting people individually before the change is implemented will go a long way towards winning their support.

Getting money from administration is largely a matter of demonstrating that your proposed quality/safety initiative will save more money than it will cost. Proposing that something is simply "the right thing to do" will get you only moral

support and a mysterious failure of signatures to materialize. And while this at first seems daunting, it is in fact the case that most real improvements in quality and/or safety do save the hospital money. Cost offsets in other parts of the hospital budget, decreased lengths of stay, the ability to garner CMS quality bonuses, and enhanced physician or patient satisfaction are potential sources of such savings. Such proposals to administration customarily take the form of a *cost analysis*. Briefly, cost analyses take into account the cost of testing (labor plus consumables), anticipated reimbursement for testing, and projected cost savings within the laboratory and within other parts of the hospital budget. One component of this is establishing the breakeven point (see p 438).

Statistical quality control

Control specimens

Quality control specimens are most often samples provided by an outside source, usually the manufacturer of an instrument. They are designed to target values at or near the cutoff values. There are usually 2 or 3 controls for each test: a "low" QC reagent and a "high" QC reagent, sometimes a "midrange" QC reagent is added.

When a new control lot is received, it is reconstituted and run on the instrument in question several times (usually ≥20 times). The results from these several tests are used to calculate a mean and standard deviation (SD). Based on these, a Levey-Jennings (Shewhart) chart is created f8.9. Only one

Day	Interpretation	
2	Accept run	Control value is <2SD; run is in control
3	Accept run	Control value is <2SD; run is in control
4	Accept run	Control value is <2SD; run is in control
5	Accept run	Control value exceeds 2SD; No rules violated; run is in control
6	Reject run	Control value exceeds 2SD 2:2s rule violated
7	Accept run	Control value is <2SD; run is in control
8	Reject run	Control value exceeds 2SD 1:3s rule violated
9	Accept run	Control value is <2SD; run is in control
10	Accept run	Control value is <2SD; run is in control
11	Accept run	Control value is <2SD; run is in control
12	Accept run	Control value exceeds 2SD; no rules violated; run is in control
13	Reject run	Control value exceeds 2SD 2:2s (and 10:mean) rule violated
14	Accept run	Control value is <2SD; run is in control
15	Accept run	Control value is <2SD; run is in control
16	Accept run	Control value exceeds 2SD; no rules violated; run is in control
17	Accept run	Control value is <2SD; run is in control
18	Reject run	Control value exceeds 2SD; 4:1s rule violated

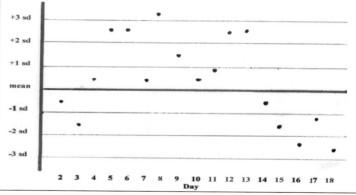

f8.9 Statistical quality control

Levey-Jennings chart is illustrated, but usually there is one for each level of control.

Among the most vexing issues with QC reagents is their stability. Most commercial QC reagents are stable, if appropriately stored, for the life of the lot. However, gradual deterioration of unopened reagents can be a cause of QC drift, and expedited deterioration of opened reagents may cause drifts and shifts in QC measurements. Furthermore, some reagents must be diluted, introducing the possibility of pipetting variation.

Commutable QC reagents are those that are biologically similar to patient samples; ie, the results obtained are directly commutable to a patient sample. Most QC reagents are non-commutable, because their matrix must be altered to achieve purity and stability.

Testing & evaluating controls

Controls samples are assayed at intervals (eg, with each run, once each day), depending on the type of test and its frequency. Frequency depends largely upon the stability of the test system—more stable systems require less frequent QC. At a minimum, CLIA '03 requires 2 levels of QC every 24 hours (if testing is performed during the 24-hour period) or as frequently as recommended by the manufacturer, whichever is more frequent.

The result obtained when the control is tested is plotted on the Levey-Jennings chart. If the control sample result falls within 2 SD of the mean, then the run is considered "in control," and the results of patient samples can be reported. If, however, the control sample result falls outside 2 SD of the mean, then the Levey-Jennings chart is interpreted in terms of Westgard rules. Based on this interpretation, the run is determined to be "in control" or "out of control." The results of "out of control" runs should not generally be reported.

The Westgard Rules, first published in 1981, provide a means of evaluating the results of QC reagent testing. There are a large number of rules, the most commonly employed of which are described in t8.6. Their purpose is to detect various kinds of error. As might be expected, application of a single rule would detect some kinds of error while missing others. For example the 1:3s rule is sensitive to marked imprecision but insensitive to systematic bias (a target of the 10:m rule). Therefore, multirule approaches are advised in most instances.

The Westgard website, www.westgard.com, is a rich source of guidance on the nuanced application of Westgard rules. No single set of rules is applicable to all tests, and the choice of rules should depend upon the known performance of individual assays. For example, methods with very good performance (low CV, low bias) may be amenable to single rule assessment. Very good performance is defined by Westgard according to the sigma metric, calculated as shown below. TEa is the CLIA-defined allowable error. Bias is defined during the validation of the test, as compared to a reference method, or from PT results. CV is also defined during the validation of the test or from QC assays. For example, if TEa is 10%, bias is 2%, and CV is 4%, then sigma is 2. The higher the sigma, the better the performance. When sigma is 6 or more, minimal QC is required. In such instances, single rule procedures and 2 QC measurements may suffice. When sigma is below 4, multirule QC with 4 QC measurements may be required.

$$Sigma = (TE_a - bias)/CV$$

The 1:3s, 2:2s, 4:s, and 10:mean rules are more sensitive to systematic error than random error. Systematic error may be caused by poor calibration, defective blanks, degraded reagents or instrument components, and poor temperature control.

The R:4s rule is most sensitive to random error. Random error may be caused by bubbles, underfilled tubes, technologist error, and autopipetting errors.

t8.6 Selected Westgard rules

Rule	Definition	Purpose
1:3s	1 value is found to be ± 3 SD from the mean	Detects imprecision
2:2s	2 consecutive values found to be >2 SD on the same side of the mean	Detects imprecision & systematic bias
R:4s	2 values within the same run are found to be >4 SD from each other	Detects random error
4:1s	4 consecutive values are found to be >1 SD on the same side of the mean	Detects systematic bias
10:mean	10 consecutive values are found to be on the same side of the mean	Detects systematic bias

Addressing "out of control" tests

When an adopted Westgard rule is violated, it is necessary to further evaluate the test system. The purpose of this evaluation is to determine the suitability of concomitant (and previous) patient results for reporting.

The first step is to check the reagents and the instrument. While it is tempting to hope that an "out of control" value will go away by repeating the assay of the control, this practice is not recommended. Instead, knowing that QC materials are subject to deterioration, it is acceptable after checking the system to repeat QC testing on a new aliquot of the QC reagent. Significant correction of the test suggests that the problem was caused by deterioration in the QC reagent; however, an acceptable repeat test that nearly approximates the previous out of control result suggests that a bias does indeed exist.

If repeat testing is not within acceptable limits, then a thorough check of the instrument and reagents must be undertaken. The suspected problems are corrected, and QC reagents are retested to ensure resolution. If this corrects the problem, then patient samples must be repeated before reporting.

The next step in the process is to repeat calibration and repeat testing upon the QC reagents, then repeat patient testing if appropriate. Persistence of an out of control assay at this point may require formal instrument maintenance. Testing should be shifted to the back-up instrument or sent to another laboratory in the meantime.

The type of error points towards the source of error. Out of control runs may be due to random or systematic errors, and different types of errors lead to violations of different Westgard rules. Rules that address widening distributions of results (13s and R:4s) are sensitive to random error or imprecision. Rules that address drifts and shifts (2:2s, 4:1s and 10:means) are sensitive to systematic error or bias. Systematic errors may be caused by, eg, improper preparation of reagent/calibrator reagents, deterioration of reagents over time, mechanical pipette problems, temperature changes, gradual deterioration of the light source. Random error may result from bubbles in reagents, bubbles in the lines, incomplete mixing of reagents, fluctuating temperature, fluctuating electrical supply, and intertechnologist variation.

Proficiency testing (external quality assessment)

Overview

CLIA requires each lab to enroll in a proficiency testing program for each area in which it performs testing. Proficiency testing must be administered by an agency approved by the CMS division of the Department of Health and Human Services. In proficiency testing programs, participants receive surveys 3×/year, each survey consisting of 5 "unknown" samples. The laboratory performs the indicated testing and reports results to the surveying agency.

To be in compliance, and to get the most information out of PT surveys, one must adhere to several principles. The laboratory must treat the survey sample as it would any other sample. The sample must not be sent out of the laboratory, even if under normal circumstances confirmatory testing is sought outside the laboratory. There must be no communication with other laboratories that do not share the same CLIA certificate. Testing of PT samples should be rotated amongst technologists.

Commutability is a term that refers to the degree to which a PT sample analytically resembles a patient sample. Noncommutable PT samples have a matrix related bias, such that results amongst labs using the same method are comparable, but results compared to patient samples are not. Thus, commutable samples could be used for method to method comparison, but noncommutable samples cannot.

Commutability impacts how target ranges are assigned. Commutable PT samples can be traced to a reference method, if available. In this circumstance, a "true" value can be assigned to the sample, with acceptability limits based upon the mean and standard deviation (SD) for the reference method (accuracy based evaluation). In the absence of commutability, or in the absence of a reference method, the mean and SD are most often determined from the peer group data. In this instance, the testing agency compiles the data and calculates the mean and SD from all the results generated by labs using the same methodology (the peer group). In compliance with CLIA, participants are graded as acceptable (<2 SD), needs improvement (2-3 SD) or unacceptable (>3 SD). For this determination, the proficiency testing agency calculates a standard deviation index (SDI) for each participant.

$$SDI = (\text{lab's result} - \text{mean for peer group}) \div \text{SD for peer group}$$

The lab must achieve acceptable results in ≥4 of 5 (80%) to be satisfactory. If an unsatisfactory result is obtained (3 or fewer correct out of 5), then the laboratory must exceed 80% on the next 2 surveys of that analyte. Failure to do so leads to additional scrutiny and the possible suspension of certification.

Unacceptable PT results must be investigated, and corrective action must be taken with appropriate documentation. It is wise to investigate even acceptable PT results that may indicate a trend towards unacceptability. The causes of PT failure are similar to those that cause QC failure, including reagent problems, instrument malfunction, calibration problems, and climate control problems. Investigation should include evaluation of QC data, maintenance data, and reagent logs around the time of PT performance. In general, a laboratory's likelihood of failing PT on a purely analytic basis is statistically unlikely if the laboratory's SD for the surveyed analyte is <33% of the SD allowed. Lastly, even successful PT performance can be a source of useful information. Is bias, drift or shift implied by the reported SDIs? Cembrowski and colleagues recommend a Westgard-like method of evaluating the data **t8.7**.

t8.7 Cembrowski rules for evaluation of PT data

Rule	Description	Implication
Screening rule	Do 2 or more of the 5 results exceed 1 SDI?	Proceed to evaluate data according to the following rules
Mean rule	Does the average of the 5 SDIs exceed ± 1.5?	Systematic error is significant
3 SDI rule	Any result beyond 3 SDI?	Random error is significant
4 SDI rule	Any 2 results >4 SDI apart?	Random error is significant

Prospectively, there are things you can do to ensure success in proficiency testing. In good laboratories that have well-trained staff and follow good laboratory practices, 1 of 5 incorrect responses on an occasional PT survey is a statistical likelihood (diligent investigation is still mandatory). In actual practice, PT failures often result from nonanalytic causes, including problems in reconstituting or mixing the PT samples, clerical errors in calculating conversions or in completion of PT documents, enrollment in the wrong peer group, and missed deadlines. This latter group of errors, while not necessarily identifying an analytic problem, is nevertheless cause for concern. This may point to a degree of carelessness that needs to be addressed. It may in fact reflect a greater problem with administration of the laboratory. Occasionally, a laboratory enrolls itself in the wrong peer group; ie, a peer group using a different instrument or different methodology. Because of matrix effects (that affect peer group members equally but may affect a laboratory in the wrong peer group disproportionately) this mistake will likely lead to PT failure. Past-due results will result in PT failure. A tracking system must exist in the laboratory, preferably overseen by the laboratory supervisor or designee, for ensuring that PT samples are received on schedule, expeditiously processed, and properly reported. Once the specimen is tested, one must verify correct transcription of the results onto the provided forms. Common errors in this step include, eg, wrong units, miscalculations, incorrect decimal point placement.

For some assays, PT is not available (unregulated analytes). This may be the result of the nature of the sample tested or the novelty of the assay. In such instances, the laboratory must engage in an alternative means of assuring proficiency. For example, one may split a patient sample and test it in duplicate with another laboratory (PT samples must never be split in this way).

Nonanalytic variables in laboratory medicine: preanalytic & postanalytic

Nonanalytic variables

It has always been indisputable that the surgeon is responsible for the preoperative preparation and postoperative care of the patient; attention is not confined solely to the surgical procedure. Likewise, while it is tempting to focus all resources upon the analytic phase of testing—ie, that which occurs in the laboratory and over which we can exercise somewhat direct control, attention to nonanalytic processes is mandatory for a number of reasons. First, errors in these processes, *particularly in the preanalytic phase*, account for the vast majority of errors in laboratory medicine. Second, the laboratory and therefore the medical director will in most instances be held liable, fairly or unfairly, for all errors arising in connection with laboratory testing, regardless of the root cause. Efforts to deflect blame are both unseemly and ineffectual. Third, as physicians we are duty-bound to prevent harm to patients. Lastly, it is not so daunting as it at first seems. It is important to initially attempt to map the hospital's administrative structure (chain of command) and the constitution of its committees. Over time, you will fill in these blanks with names and faces. But administrators come and go, are promoted and demoted. So take care to alienate no one. With each new issue encountered, knowledge of the hospital's anatomy improves. And while efforts to connect socially with key personnel—clinicians, nurses, administrators—are important, bonds are strongest when formed in adversity. So relish the opportunity.

Preanalytic variables

The preanalytic phase

The preanalytic phase encompasses all steps that precede the actual laboratory assay. Wresting control of the preanalytic phase represents one of the greatest challenges to quality in laboratory work. Many of the preanalytic variables are uncontrollable, such as patient age, but must be taken into account in the interpretation of laboratory tests. Some are controllable, and some are sources of error. Examples of preanalytic errors include inappropriate test selection, incorrect patient identification, inappropriate timing of specimen collection, and sample defects (hemolysis, aged samples, clotted samples, and low-quantity samples).

Patient identification

To fail in this is to render ineffective all our other efforts. Yet a disturbing number of "wrong blood in tube" errors occur, with an estimated frequency of 400/million (1 in 2,500) specimens. One sees mislabeling so frequently in practice that one soon learns to suspect it whenever laboratory results are questionable. In an effort to combat this, both the CAP and TJC require 2 patient identifiers on all samples (room number is not a patient identifier). Several technological solutions are commercially available, including "positive patient identification" systems that utilize bar codes and radiofrequency identification. Phlebotomists must be trained to properly identify patients by, when possible, asking the patient to state his or her name and date of birth, confirming with the wristband, and labeling at the bedside. Wristband errors occur frequently, however, with a rate of ~1%.

Age

Age has to be taken into account in the interpretation of many analytes. In particular, neonates can be expected to have noticeably different white cell differential than adults, with a relative increase in mononuclear cells. Adolescent children can have alarmingly high alkaline phosphatase, up to 5× the upper limit of normal for adults. In the elderly, a multitude of changes occur, including decreased creatinine clearance, decreased glucose tolerance, increased releasing hormones (TRH, ACTH), and increased lipids.

Gender

Among other differences, males can be expected to have an increased creatine kinase (CK) and LDL cholesterol.

Food intake

After meals, glucose concentration may be abnormally elevated or depressed, and it is never as reliable as in the fasting state. Triglycerides increase for 8-12 hours after a meal. Other analytes, such as gastrin and insulin, are also increased. Bilirubin is decreased following a meal. Fasting, so long as it is not prolonged, imparts a sort of steady state and is the best state in which to measure most analytes; however, it should be noted that prolonged fasting can alter several analytes as well, including elevated ketones, elevated bilirubin, decreased albumin, decreased potassium, and decreased magnesium.

Exercise

Recent exercise may increase the serum concentration of CK, lactase dehydrogenase (LD), and AST. In addition, rigorous exercise may induce neutrophil demargination, resulting in apparent neutrophilia.

Smoking

Cigarette smoking alters several analytes, including carbon monoxide, CEA, and serum catecholamines. Over the long term, the hematocrit may increase.

Posture

When a patient goes from the supine to the sitting or standing position, the increased hydrostatic pressure forces water out of the circulation and into the interstitial fluid. Small molecules such as electrolytes can easily follow the water, but larger molecules such as proteins, substances largely bound to proteins, and formed elements (blood cells) cannot. Thus, when sitting, the concentration of these 3 types of substances goes up relative to supine. The change is in the range of 5-15%. Though an electrolyte, calcium is largely protein bound and increases when the patient is upright, ~3-4%.

Time of day

Many analytes vary throughout the day. Most notably, serum cortisol has wide diurnal variation, peaking around 6-8 am, and should be measured at the same time every day.

Tourniquets

Tourniquets create an artificially hemoconcentrated and anaerobic region of the body after prolonged (>1-3 minutes) application. Such effects are made worse with fist clenching or if the tourniquet is released during blood collection. This is to be particularly avoided when drawing for lactate.

Order of draw

To maximize the integrity of samples obtained by venipuncture, it is important to draw tubes t8.8 in a particular order. Most laboratories have made the switch to plastic tubes instead of glass, and the appropriate order of draw is somewhat different t8.9.

t8.8 Selected blood collection tubes

Tube	Additive	Used for
Red	Glass—None Plastic—Silica clot activator	Serum chemistry & serology
Green	Heparin	Plasma chemistry
Blue	Citrate	Coagulation tests

Note: A 1:9 ratio of anticoagulant:blood is ideal; higher ratios lead to increased coagulation times, affecting the aPTT>PT; for polycythemic patients with Hct>60%, the PT and PTT can be prolonged due to decreased effective plasma

Tube	Additive	Used for
Black	Citrate (calcium chelation)	ESR
Lavender (purple)	EDTA (calcium chelation)	Cell counts
Yellow	Citrate & dextrose (ACD)	Blood bank tests, HLA typing
Gray	Sodium fluoride (inhibits glycolysis)	Glucose, lactate

t8.9 Order of draw

Priority	Glass	Plastic
First	Culture	Culture
	No additive tubes (red)	Coagulation test tubes
	Coagulation test tubes	No additive tubes (red)
	Serum separator tubes	Serum separator tubes
Last	Additive tubes (green then lavender then gray)	Additive tubes (green then lavender then gray)

Storage & transport conditions

During storage, blood cells continue to metabolize and slowly undergo lysis, serum proteins progressively degrade, and adsorption to tubes may occur. Some tests are performed on anticoagulated whole blood (eg, hematology), others on serum (clotted whole blood), and others on plasma (clot-inhibited centrifuged whole blood). For most purposes, serum and plasma give essentially similar results; serum must be used for SPEP and serologic assays, while plasma is required for coagulation tests. If not separated from blood cells, serum and plasma progressively change in several ways such that they no longer accurately reflect the in vivo state; for example, glucose progressively diminishes and lactate increases. Ideally, all tests should be run within 1-2 hours of blood collection, but this is not always practical. Blood not tested immediately should be stabilized. In the case of plasma tests, for example blood should be centrifuged within 1 hour and stored at 4-6 °C.

Serum vs plasma

For most measured analytes, serum and plasma are interchangeable. The clotting process in which plasma is converted to serum, however, results in the release of substances in which platelets are rich, including calcium, magnesium, LD, and potassium; thus, one should expect these analytes to be higher in serum than in plasma. Furthermore, the clotting process utilizes plasma proteins (notably fibrinogen), such that total protein is higher in plasma.

Underlying hematologic malignancy

Underlying conditions or the medications used to treat them can alter laboratory values. Many of these effects have not been well studied, with most attention having been focused on underlying hematologic disease. It is well known, for example, that paraproteinemia can drastically alter the measurement of a variety of analytes—either through direct interference with the assay or by altering the relative amount of the aqueous phase of plasma. High levels of paraprotein can lead to factitious hyperbilirubinemia, hyponatremia, hypouricemia, hypoalbuminemia, and hypercalcemia. With regard to hypercalcemia, a patient with paraproteinemia may

1. have factitious hypercalcemia caused by the turbidity of the paraprotein

2. have true total hypercalcemia, with normal ionized calcium, caused by increased calcium transport by paraprotein

3. have true total and ionized calcium caused by the myeloma itself

Patients with high leukemic cell counts (ALL, AML), and those with thrombocytosis (reactive and neoplastic), may have factitious hyperkalemia. Factitious hyperkalemia in this setting is significantly greater in serum than in plasma; whereas true hyperkalemia should be roughly equivalent in the 2 specimens. CML is notorious for spuriously high vitamin B_{12} levels.

Postanalytic variables

The postanalytic phase

This phase consists of the reporting and interpretation of test results. Errors in the postanalytic phase include errors in reports (transcription and proofreading errors), errors in reading reports (misreading or incorrectly hearing the result), errors in interpretation of the report, and incorrect responses to the information.

Result reporting

CLIA requires the following elements in laboratory reports: patient identification, date result is reported, specimen source, test(s) performed, result, units (if any), name and address of the laboratory. There is no industrywide standard on how laboratory reports should be formatted. Nonetheless, it is necessary to assess the format of the reports emanating from your laboratory for clarity and completeness. Furthermore, it is vital that both information and formatting be retained across all interfaces. It is sometimes necessary or desirable to report results verbally. Information is particularly vulnerable to corruption when transmitted verbally. Thus, it is important to insist upon read-back of such reports.

Critical values reporting

Critical values are test results that indicate the presence of a treatable condition that is immediately life threatening. It is important to have a procedure for notifying the treating health care provider of such results within a reasonable timeframe and for documenting notification. Some laboratories require that critical values be repeated before alerting the clinician, but universal adoption of this practice is of dubious value and should be adopted on an analyte by analyte basis, depending upon the reliability of the assay. What constitutes a critical value and what is a reasonable timeframe is a subject to discuss with your medical staff; the decision is usually made at the level of the medical executive committee.

Laboratory calculations

Reticulocyte proliferation index (RPI)

$$RPI = reticulocytes (\%) \times Hct/45 \times 1/MI$$

Hct = hematocrit, MI = maturation index t8.10
RPI >2 suggests an appropriate erythropoietic response; RPI <2 suggests ineffective erythropoiesis

t8.10 Maturation index

Maturation index	Hematocrit
1.0	36-45
1.5	26-35
2.0	16-25
2.5	≤15

International normalized ratio (INR)

$$INR = (PT_{patient}/PT_{normal})^{ISI}$$

$PT_{patient}$ = patient's measured PT
PT_{normal} = mean normal PT for the lab
ISI = international standardization index given in the package insert

Corrected (platelet) count increment (CCI)

CCI = observed increment × BSA ÷ number of platelets transfused

Observed increment = posttransfusion platelet count – pretransfusion platelet count

BSA = body surface area (in m²)
Number of platelets transfused = number of platelets in the product(s) if multiplied by 10^{11}; ie, 4 random donor platelet units contain ~2.0×10^{11} platelets, so in the formula you would plug in 2.0. 1 pheresis unit contains ~3.0×10^{11} platelets, so you would use 3.0.
Definitions vary, but CCI >10,000/µL is considered adequate response, while <5,000 is considered evidence of refractoriness

Anion gap

$$anion\ gap = [Na^+] - ([Cl^-] + [HCO_3^-])$$

Normal anion gap = 12 ± 4 (or 8-16)

Osmolal gap

$$osmolal\ gap = osmolarity\ measured - osmolarity\ calculated$$

$$osmolal\ gap = osmolarity\ measured - (2[Na] + [glucose]/18 + [BUN]/2.8)$$

Normal osmolal gap = <10 mOsm/kg

Friedewald equation

$$IDL = Total\ cholesterol - HDL - TG/5$$

Total cholesterol, high-density lipoprotein (HDL), and triglyceride (TG) are measured directly

Creatinine clearance (Cl_{Cr})

$$Cl_{Cr} = volume_{urine} \times urine_{creatinine}/plasma_{creatinine}$$

Cl_{Cr} is roughly = glomerular filtration rate (GFR)

Fractional excretion of sodium (FENa)

$$FENa = (urine_{Na} \times plasma_{creatinine})/(urine_{creatinine} \times plasma_{Na})$$

FENa <1% is indicative of primary glomerular disease and hepatorenal syndrome (HRS), while FENa >1% is found in acute tubular necrosis (ATN), prerenal azotemia, and postrenal azotemia.

Henderson-Hasselbalch equation

$$pH = pKa + log\ (base/acid)$$

Standard deviation (SD)

$$SD = \sqrt{\Sigma(x_i - mean)^2/(n - 1)}$$

Coefficient of variation (CV)

$$CV = SD/mean \times 100$$

Corrected serum sodium in hyperglycemia:

Na increases by 1.6 mmol/L/100 mg/dL of serum glucose

Corrected serum sodium in hyperlipidemia:

Na increases by 1.0 mmol/L for each 500 mg/dL of plasma lipid (triglyceride + cholesterol)

Corrected serum sodium in hyperproteinemia:

Na increases by 1.0 mmol/L for each 4.0 g/dL of plasma protein

Body surface area

$$BSA\ (m^2) = (height\ [cm] \times weight\ [kg] \div 3,600)^{1/2}$$

There are a number of similar formulae in use; there are also nomogram charts for quick reference

References

Armbruster DA, Pry T [2008] Limit of blank, limit of detection and limit of quantitation. *Clin Biochem Rev* 29(Supplement (i)):S49-S52 PMID:18852857.

Bjerner J, Børmer OP, Nustad K [2005] The war on heterophilic antibody interference. *Clin Chem* 51(1):9-11. PMID:15613705.

Bonini P, Plebani M, Ceriotti F, Rubboli F [2002] Errors in laboratory medicine. *Clin Chem* 48(5):691-698. PMID:11978595.

Boyanton L, Blick K [2002] Stability studies of twenty-four analytes in human plasma and serum. *Clin Chem* 48(12):2242-2247. PMID:12446483.

Boyd JC [1999] Laboratory statistics. In: *Professional Practice in Clinical Chemistry, A Companion Text.* Washington, DC: American Association for Clinical Chemistry. ISBN:978-1890883287.

Boyd JC [1999] Reference limits in the clinical laboratory. In: *Professional Practice in Clinical Chemistry, A Companion Text.* Washington, DC: American Association for Clinical Chemistry. ISBN:978-1890883287.

Boyd JC [1999] Statistical aids for test interpretation. In: *Professional Practice in Clinical Chemistry, A Companion Text.* Washington, DC: American Association for Clinical Chemistry. ISBN:978-1890883287.

Carraro P, Plebani M [1997] Errors in a stat laboratory: Types and frequency. *Clin Chem* 43(1):1348-1351. PMID:9267312.

Carraro P, Plebani M [2007] Errors in a Stat Laboratory: Types and Frequencies 10 years later. *Clin Chem* 53(7):1338-1342. PMID:17525103.

Cembrowski GS, Anderson PG, Crampton CA, et al [1996] Pump up your PT IQ. *MLO Med Lab Obs* Jan:46-51. PMID:10172547.

Cembrowski GS, Carey RN [2000] Adding value to proficiency testing programs. *Clin Chem.* 46:7-8. PMID:10620565.

Committee on the Quality of Health Care in America [2001] *Crossing the Quality Chasm: A New Health System for the 21st Century.* Washington, DC: National Academy Press. ISBN:978-0309072809.

Dalal BI, Brigden M [2009]. Factitious biochemical measurements resulting from hematologic conditions. *Am J Clin Pathol* 131:195-204. PMID:19141380.

Dufour DR [1999] Preanalytic variation, or what causes abnormal results (besides disease). In: *Professional Practice in Clinical Chemistry, A Companion Text.* Washington, DC: American Association for Clinical Chemistry. ISBN:978-1594250545

Edson DC, Russell D, Massey LD [2007] Proficiency testing: a guide to maintaining successful performance. *Lab Med* 38(3):184-186.

Friedberg RC, Souers R, Wagar EA, et al [2007] The origin of reference intervals: a College of American Pathologists Q-probes study of "normal ranges" used in 163 clinical laboratories. *Arch Pathol Lab Med* 131:348-357. PMID:17516737.

Howanitz PJ, Cembrowski GS [2000] Postanalytical quality improvement. *Arch Pathol Lab Med.* 124:504-510. PMID:10747304.

Howanitz PJ [2005] Errors in laboratory medicine: practical lessons to improve patient safety. *Arch Pathol Lab Med* 129:1252-1261. PMID:16196513.

Jhang JS, Chang CC, Fink DJ, Kroll MH [2004] Evaluation of linearity in the clinical laboratory. *Arch Pathol Lab* Med. 128:44-48. PMID:14692813.

Killeen AA [2009] Laboratory sanctions for proficiency testing sample referral and result communication: a review of actions from 1993-2006. *Arch Pathol Lab Med* 133:979-982. PMID:19492893.

Kroll MH, Præstgaard J, Michaliszyn E, Styer PE [2000] Evaluation of the extent of nonlinearity in reportable range studies. *Arch Pathol Lab Med.* 124:1331-1338. PMID:10975932.

Lahti A, Petersen PH, Boyd JC [2002a] Impact of subgroup prevalences on partitioning of Gaussian-distributed reference values. *Clin Chem* 48(11):1987-1999. PMID:12406985.

Lahti A, Petersen PH, Boyd JC, Fraser CG, Jørgensen N [2002b] Objective criteria for partitioning Gaussian distributed reference values into subgroups. *Clin Chem* 48(2):338-352. PMID:11805016.

Lohr K, Committee to Design a Strategy for Quality Review and Assurance in Medicare, eds [1990] *Medicare: A Strategy for Quality Assurance,* Vol. 1. Washington, DC: National Academy Press.

Miller WG [1999] Quality control. In: *Professional Practice in Clinical Chemistry, A Companion Text.* Washington, DC: American Association for Clinical Chemistry. ISBN:978-1890883287.

Miller WG, Jones GRD, Horowitz GL, Weykamp C [2011] Proficiency testing/external quality assessment: current challenges and future directions. *Clin Chem* 57:12 PMID:21965556.

Mosteller RD [1987] Simplified calculation of body surface area. *N Engl J Med* 317(17):1098 [letter] PMID:3657876.

Narayanan S [2000] The preanalytic phase: an important component of laboratory medicine. *Am J Clin Pathol* 113:429-452. PMID:10705825.

Obuchowski NA, Lieber ML, Wians FH Jr [2004] ROC curves in clinical chemistry: uses, misuses, and possible solutions. *Clin Chem* 50:1118-1125. PMID:15142978.

Pincus MR [1996] Interpreting laboratory results: reference values and decision making. In: *Clinical Diagnosis and Management by Laboratory Methods,* 19th ed. Philadelphia: WB Saunders Company. ISBN:978-0721660301.

Preissner CM, Dodge LA, O'Kane DJ, Singh RJ, Grebe SKG [2005] Prevalence of heterophilic antibody interference in 8 automated tumor marker immunoassays. *Clin Chem* 51(1):208-210. PMID:15613712.

Søreide K. [2009] Receiver-operating characteristic curve analysis in diagnostic, prognostic, and predictive biomarker research. *J Clin Pathol* 62:1-5. PMID:18818262.

Valenstein P [2005] *Quality Management in Clinical Laboratories: Promoting Patient Safety Through Risk Reduction and Continuous Improvement.* Northfield, IL: College of American Pathologists Press. ISBN:0930304888.

Weiss RL [2007] Coding, coverage, and compensation for pathology and laboratory medicine services. *Clin Lab Med* 27:875-891. PMID:17950903.

Westgard JO, Klee GG [1999] Chapter 17: Quality management. In: *Tietz Textbook of Clinical Chemistry,* 3rd ed. Philadelphia: WB Saunders Company. ISBN:978-0721656106.

Westgard JO, Barry PL, Hunt MR. [1981] A multirule Shewhart chart for quality control in clinical chemistry. *Clin Chem* 27:493-501. PMID:7471403.

Zweig MH, Campbell G [1993] Receiver-operating characteristic (ROC) plots: A fundamental evaluation tool in clinical medicine. *Clin Chem* 39(4):561-577. PMID:8472349.

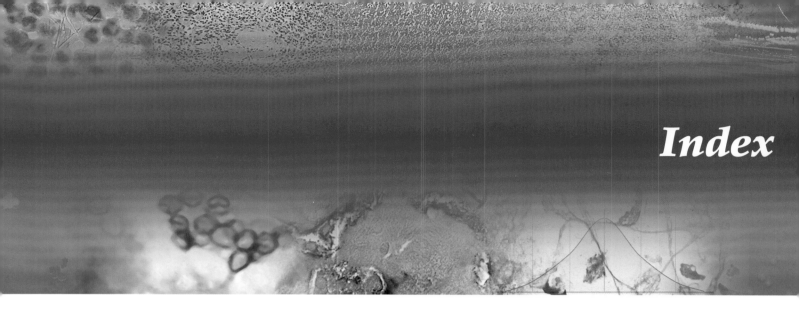

Index

Bold pages indicate figures. *Italic pages* indicate tables.

ISBN 978-089189-5985

Aspiration pneumonia, 115

Aspirin, 302

Astrocytoma, oligodendroglioma versus, **415**, *415*, 415-416

Astroviruses, 114

Ataxia-telangiectasia, 254, 340, 420

Attenuated familial adenomatous polyposis, 398

Atypical chronic myelogenous leukemia, 268

Atypical teratoid/rhabdoid tumor, 416

Austrian syndrome, 117, 118

Autoadsorption, 79

Autoantibodies, 82-84
methods for detection, 343-345, *345*

Autohemolysis test, 218

Autoimmune adrenalitis, 51

Autoimmune cholangitis, 351

Autoimmune diseases, 28, 342, 346-357

Autoimmune enteric disease, 387

Autoimmune hepatitis, 4, 350

Autoimmune hypoparathyroidism, 51

Autoimmune induction mechanism, 83

Autoimmune neutropenia, 233

Autoimmune pancreatitis, 349-350

Autologous blood, 95

Autologous donors, requirements of, 70

Autosomal dominant polycystic kidney disease, **378**, 378-379, 387

Autosomal inheritance, 303

Autosomal recessive polycystic kidney disease, 378, **378**

Avian influenza, 137

Azotemia, 22

B

Babesiosis, 106, **152**, 152-153

Bacillus anthracis, **192**, 192-193, **193**

Bacillus cereus, 193

Bacterial casts, 58

Bacteriology, 177-205

Bacteriuria, asymptomatic, 111

Bacteroides fragilis, 196

Bakers cyst, 347

Balamuthia mandrillaris, 143

Bannayan-Riley-Ruvalcaba syndrome

Barbiturates, 31

Barth syndrome, 233

Bartonella species, 205

Bartter syndrome, 18

Basal cell carcinoma, 414

Basophilic stippling, 34

Basophils, 331

B cell neoplasms, 241-255, 245-247, **249**, 251-254

B cells, *329*, 329-330, *330*

Becker muscular dystrophy, 381, 395, **395**

Beckwith-Wiedemann syndrome, 386, 420

Behçet disease, 354

Bence Jones protein, 13, 23

Benedict reaction, 55

Benign cold agglutinins, 82

Benign familial hematuria, 377

Benign familial hypercalcemia, 384

Benign familial neutropenias, 238

Benzodiazepine screening tests, 33

Bernard-Soulier syndrome, 91, 239, 302, 304

Bethesda assay, 300

Beuveria species, 168

Biclonal gammopathy, 13

Bilateral acoustic neuroma syndrome, 419-420

Bilateral adrenal hyperplasia, 51

Bilateral inferior petrosal sinus sampling, 51

Bile-esculin test, 181

Bilharziasis, 156, **156**

Biliary fibrocystic diseases, 387, **387**

Bilirubin, *3*, 3-4, *4*, 5, 56, *56*, 390

δ-Bilirubin, 3

Binet staging system, 243

Bioterrorism, CDC classification of agents of, 133, *133*

Bipolaris, 169

Birt-Hogg-Dubé syndrome, 407, **407**

Bisalbuminemia, 12

Biurate crystals, 58

Bivalirudin, 323

ISBN 978-089189-5985

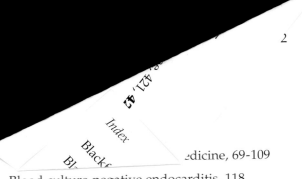

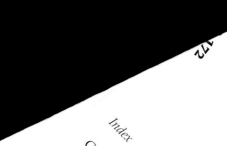

H

I

J

K

L

M

V

W